French's Index of
Differential Diagnosis

14TH EDITION

French's Index of Differential Diagnosis

An A–Z

Mark Kinirons BSc(Hons) MD FRCPI FRCP

Consultant Physician and Geriatrician, Department of Ageing & Health,
Guy's & St Thomas' Hospitals, London, UK

and

Harold Ellis CBE DM MCh FRCS

Professor and Clinical Anatomist in the Division of Anatomy, Cell and Human Biology,
Guy's, King's and St Thomas' School of Medicine, London, UK

Hodder Arnold

A MEMBER OF THE HODDER HEADLINE GROUP

LONDON

First published in Great Britain in 1912 by Butterworth Heinemann
Second edition 1917
Third edition 1917
Fourth edition 1928
Fifth edition 1936
Sixth edition 1945
Seventh edition 1954
Eighth edition 1960
Ninth edition 1967
Tenth edition 1973
Eleventh edition 1979
Twelfth edition 1985
Thirteenth edition 1996, reprinted 1997 (twice)
This fourteenth edition published in 2005 by Hodder Arnold, an imprint of Hodder Education,
a member of the Hodder Headline Group, 338 Euston Road, London NW1 3BH

http://www.hoddereducation.com

Distributed in the United States of America by
Oxford University Press Inc.,
198 Madison Avenue, New York, NY10016
Oxford is a registered trademark of Oxford University Press

© 2005 Hodder Arnold

Whilst the advice and information in this book are believed to be true and accurate at the date of going
to press, neither the author[s] nor the publisher can accept any legal responsibility or liability for any
errors or omissions that may be made. In particular, (but without limiting the generality of the preceding
disclaimer) every effort has been made to check drug dosages; however it is still possible that errors have
been missed. Furthermore, dosage schedules are constantly being revised and new side-effects recognized.
For these reasons the reader is strongly urged to consult the drug companies' printed instructions before
administering any of the drugs recommended in this book.

British Library Cataloguing in Publication Data
A catalogue record for this book is available from the British Library

Library of Congress Cataloging-in-Publication Data
A catalog record for this book is available from the Library of Congress

ISBN-10   0 340 810 475
ISBN-13   978 0 340 810 475

1 2 3 4 5 6 7 8 9 10

Commissioning Editor: Joanna Koster
Development Editor: Sarah Burrows
Project Editor: Heather Fyfe
Production Controller: Lindsay Smith
Cover Design: Sarah Rees

Typeset in 9/12 pts Minion by Charon Tec Pvt. Ltd, Chennai, India
www.charontec.com
Printed and bound in India

What do you think about this book? Or any other Hodder Arnold title?
Please visit our website at www.hoddereducation.com

A NOTE ON HERBERT FRENCH (1875–1951)

It might be of interest to readers to learn a little of the original editor of this volume. Herbert French was a scholar at Christ Church, Oxford and proceeded as a medical student to Guy's Hospital in 1898, with a University Scholarship. He was appointed Assistant Physician at Guy's in 1906 and Full Physician in 1917. He served in the first world war in the Royal Army Medical Corps with the rank of Lieutenant Colonel and was also for many years Physician to the Household of HM George V.

French was a prolific writer, and published *An Index of Differential Diagnosis of Main Symptoms* in 1912. His ambitious aim was to collect all the symptoms and signs that might arise in the course of disease. He was a man of wide erudition and wrote no less than half of the first edition himself, taking the whole of medicine as his province. The book was an immediate success and was reprinted in the same year and again in 1913 with a second edition appearing in 1917.

H.E.

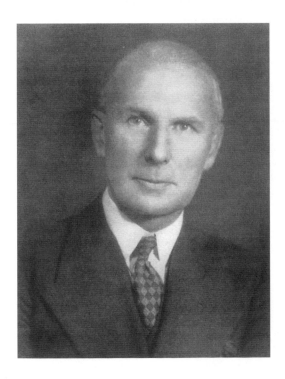

Contributors

Michael Baum MD(hc) ChM FRCS FRCR(hon)
Emeritus Professor of Surgery, University College London

Peter T. Blenkinsopp BDS LDS RCS MBBS FDS FRCS
Consultant Maxillofacial Surgeon, Kingston Hospital, Kingston, Surrey; and St George's Hospital, London

Duncan Churchill BA MBBS FRCP DTM&H
Consultant GU Physician, The Lawson Unit, Department of Genitourinary Medicine, Royal Sussex County Hospital, Brighton

Reginald Daniel MBBS DO FRCS FRCOphth
Emeritus Consultant Ophthalmic Surgeon, Guy's and St Thomas' Hospitals, London

Harold Ellis CBE DM MCh FRCS
Professor and Clinical Anatomist, Division of Anatomy, Cell and Human Biology, King's and St Thomas' School of Medicine, London

Michael Gleeson MD FRCS
Professor of Otolaryngology and Skull Base Surgery, Guy's Hospital; and The National Hospital for Neurology and Neurosurgery, London

Danielle Harari FRCP
Consultant Physician, Department of Ageing and Health, Guy's and St Thomas' Hospitals; and *Honorary Senior Lecturer*, King's College London

Fred Heatley MA MB BChir(Cantab) FRCS
Emeritus Professor of Orthopaedics, King's College London

Andrew D. Hodgkiss BA MBBS MD MRCPsych DCP
Consultant Liason Psychiatrist, South London and Maudsley NHS Trust; *Honorary Consultant Liason Psychiatrist*, Guy's and St Thomas' Hospitals, London; and *Honorary Senior Lecturer*, Guy's, King's and St Thomas' Medical and Dental School, London

Antony Hollingworth MB ChB FRCS(Ed) FRCOG DHMSA PhD MBA
Consultant in Obstetrics and Gynaecology, Whipps Cross University Hospital Trust; and *Honorary*

Senior Lecturer, Queen Mary and Westfield College, London

Dipak Kanabar MBBS MRCP FRCPCH
Consultant Paediatrician, Guy's Hospital, London

James Kelly
Stroke Fellow, Department of Ageing and Health, St Thomas' Hospital, London

Mark T. Kinirons BSc(Hons) MD FRCPI FRCP
Consultant Physician and Geriatrician, Department of Ageing and Health, Guy's and St Thomas' Hospitals, London

Boris Lams MBBChir MRCP MD
Consultant Respiratory Physician, St Thomas' Hospital, London

Melvin D. Lobo PhD MRCP
Lecturer in Clinical Pharmacology, Bart's and The London School of Medicine and Dentistry

John Meenan MD PhD FRCPI FRCP
Consultant, Department of Gastroenterology, St Thomas' Hospital, London

Barry E. Monk MA FRCP
Consultant Dermatologist, Bedford Hospital, Bedford

Sharon O'Byrne MD MSc MRCPI
Consultant Physician and Honorary Senior Lecturer, Department of Academic Medicine, Whittington Hospital, London

Julian Shah MB ChB LRCP FRCS
Senior Lecturer in Urology, Institute of Urology and Nephrology, University College London; and *Consultant Urologist*, St Peter's Hospital, Surrey, University College London and the Royal National Orthopaedic Hospital, Stanmore

David J. Werring BSc(Hons) MBBS MRCP PhD
Consultant Neurologist, National Hospital for Neurology and Neurosurgery, University College London Hospitals NHD Trust; and Watford General Hospital, Watford

Preface

French's '*Index*' was first published in 1912. The aim of this volume remains unchanged from the original statement by Herbert French in the first paragraph of his original preface; it is an alphabetic index to help in the differential diagnosis of any condition which may be seen in hospital or general practice. Essentially it is a book for the clinician. With modern transport, regional disease barriers have broken down. Moreover, the time it takes to get anywhere in the world is considerably less than the incubation period of almost all the infectious diseases. So, tropical illnesses are no longer confined to the tropics and one country's epidemic may appear anywhere else in the world in record time. This, together with the massive increase in iatrogenic diseases, makes the art and science of differential diagnosis more interesting than ever before – and vastly more complex too!

The first two editions of this book were edited by Herbert French. Subsequent editors, in turn, were Arthur Douthwaite, his colleague at Guy's Hospital, then Sir Adolphe Abrahams of Westminster Hospital, and then Frank Dudley Hart, also of Westminster. The thirteenth edition had as its editors Professor Ian Bouchier of Edinburgh, the late Peter Fleming of Westminster Hospital, and Harold Ellis. The current edition again has Harold Ellis, who is responsible for topics of a 'surgical' nature, and he is joined by Mark Kinirons, responsible for the sections on 'medical' subjects.

As for the contributors, we have retained a number of old friends and recruited new ones, all chosen carefully for their specialist knowledge and teaching skills. We thank them for their splendid work, although we take full responsibility for the contents of this book.

'French' has now been completely revised – many sections are largely rewritten, new ones added, diagnostic methods updated, many old illustrations replaced and others inserted. The emphasis, however, remains the same – the importance of a careful history, detailed clinical examination and the judicious use of laboratory and imaging investigations in the elucidation of the correct diagnosis.

We hope that this new edition of *French's Index* will continue to serve the medical profession, both in the United Kingdom and overseas, as it has done now for more than ninety years.

Mark Kinirons and Harold Ellis

Acknowledgements

Professor Heatley is particularly indebted to Mr R B Simons, curator of the Alan G Apley slide library held at St Peters Hospital, Chertsey, for providing over 60% of the illustrations in the orthopaedic sections.

Thanks are also due to the following colleagues from Guys and St Thomas Hospital, London: Dr J A Matthews for illustrations of the rheumatoid spine; Dr N Bateman for X-rays and CT scans of spinal tuberculosis; Mr J O'Dowd, Mr J D Lucas and Mr K S Lam for X-rays, CT and MRI scans of spinal deformity, disc disease, spinal stenosis and malignancy and Mr S A Corbett, for the CT scan of a rotator cuff tear.

In the upper limb section, Mr N J P Compson of King's College Hospital provided the illustrations of the rheumatoid hand, scapho-lunate disassociation and Dupuytrens contracture.

In the lower limb section, Dr J Healey, of Chelsea Westminster Hospital, provided MRI scans and Mr J Ritchie of King's College Hospital, the weight-bearing X-rays of knee osteoarthritis.

Springer-Verlag have kindly permitted reproduction of the radiology of hip osteoarthritis and the Maquet diagrams of forces across the knee.

Finally a special debt is owed to Mr S White, Robert James Orthopaedic hospital, Oswestry, for his concept of the classification of knee conditions which acted as a 'blueprint' for the differential diagnostic tables for the other peripheral joints.

The editors would also like to thank the following people for contributing images:

Elizabeth Graham FRCP DO FRCOphth
Consultant Medial Ophthalmologist, St Thomas' Hospital, London

Peter J A Moult MD FRCP
Consultant Physician and Endocrinologist (retired), Whittington Hospital, London

Sheila C Rankin FRCR
Consultant Radiologist, Guys and St Thomas' Foundation Trust, London

5-HIAA	5-hydroxy indole acetic acid	EPC	epilepsia partialis continua
5-HT	5-hydroxy-tryptamine	ERCP	endoscopic retrograde cholangiopancreatography
ABM	antibasement membrane		
ACTH	adrenocorticotrophic hormone	EUA	examination under anaesthetic
ADH	antidiuretic hormone	FEV$_1$	fixed expiratory volume in 1 second
ALS	acid-labile subunit	FSH	follicle-stimulating hormone
AME	apparent mineralocorticoid excess	FTA-ABS	fluorescent treponemal antibody absorption
ANCA	anti-neutrophil cytoplasmic antibodies		
ANDI	abnormalities of normal development and involution	FVC	forced vital capacity
		GHD	growth hormone deficiency
APTT	activated partial thromboplastin time	GIST	gastrointestinal stromal cell tumour
AZT	Zidovudine	GnRH	gonadotrophin-releasing hormone
BIPP	bismuth–iodoform paraffin paste	GORD	Gastro-oesophageal reflux disease
BMI	body mass index	GTN	glyceryl trinitrate
BPPV	benign positional paroxysmal vertigo	HAIR-AN	hyperandrogenism, insulin resistance, acanthosis nigricans (syndrome)
CADASIL	cerebral autosomal dominant arteriopathy with subcortical infarcts and leucoencephalopathy		
		hCG	human chorionic gonadotrophin
		HPO	hypothalamic–pituitary–ovarian axis
CDLE	chronic discoid lupus erythematosus	HPOA	hypertrophic pulmonary osteoarthropathy
CFS	chronic fatigue syndrome		
CIDP	chronic inflammatory demyelinating polyneuropathy	HRT	hormone replacement therapy
		HSG	hysterosalpingogram
CIN	cervical intra-epithelial neoplasia	HSMN	hereditary motor–sensory neuropathy
CMV	cytomegalovirus	HSV	herpes simplex virus
COPD	chronic obstructive pulmonary disease	HVS	hyperventilation syndrome
CPPD	calcium pyrophosphate dehydrate	IBS	irritable bowel syndrome
CRST	calcinosis, Raynaud's phenomenon, sclerodactyly, telangiectases (syndrome)	ICP	intracranial pressure
		IGF	insulin-like growth factor
		IGFBP	insulin-like growth factor binding protein
CSOM	chronic suppurative otitis media		
CT	computed tomography	IL-1	interleukin 1
CVA	cerebrovascular accident	IL-6	interleukin 6
DAT	direct antigen test	INR	International Normalized Ratio
DCIS	duct carcinoma-in-situ	ITP	idiopathic thrombocytopenic purpura
DHEA	dehydroepiandrosterone	IUCD	intra-uterine contraceptive device
DHEAS	dehydroepiandrosterone sulphate	JVP	jugular venous pressure
DIC	disseminated intravascular coagulation	LACI	lacunar infarction
DIDMOAD	diabetes insipidus, diabetes mellitus, optic atrophy, deafness (syndrome)	LDH	lactate dehydrogenase
		LH	luteinizing hormone
DISH	diffuse interstitial spinal hyperostosis	LHA	lateral hypothalamic nucleus
DRPLA	dentatorubropallidoluysian atrophy	LHRH	luteinizing hormone-releasing hormone
EAA	extrinsic allergic alveolitis	LSD	lysergic acid diethylamide
ECM	erythema chronicum migrans	MAOI	monoamine oxidase inhibitor
ECT	electroconvulsant therapy	MCV	mean corpuscular volume
ED	erectile dysfunction		

MD	muscular dystrophy	RAPD	relative afferent pupillary defect
MDM	mid-diastolic murmur	RAS	recurrent aphthous stomatitis
ME	myalgic encephalomyelitis	RAST	radioallergosorbent test
MEN	multiple endocrine neoplasia	REE	resting energy expenditure
MERRF	myoclonic epilepsy with ragged red fibers	REM	rapid eye movement
		RSI	Repetitive strain injury
MIBG	metaiodobenzguanidine	SHBG	sex hormone-binding globulin
MID	multi-infarct disease	SLE	systemic lupus erythematosus
MRI	magnetic resonance imaging	SSRI	selective serotonin re-uptake inhibitor
MSA-P	parkinsonian variant of multiple system atrophy	SUNCT	short-lasting unilateral neuralgiform headache attacks with conjunctival injection and tearing
MSH	melanocyte-stimulating hormone		
MTP	metatarsophalangeal	SVC	superior vena cava
NAFL	non-alcoholic fatty liver	T3	tri-iodothyronine
NASH	non-alcoholic steatohepatitis	T4	thyroxine
NIPTS	noise-induced permanent threshold shift	TACI	total anterior circulation infarction
		TAR	thrombocytopenia with absent radii
NITTS	noise-induced temporary threshold shift	TEN	toxic epidermal necrolysis
		TGA	transient global amnesia
NPY	neuropeptide Y	TIA	transient ischaemic attack
OCD	obsessive–compulsive disorder	TLC	total lung capacity
OCP	oral contraceptive pill	TNF	tumour necrosis factor
OSA	obstructive sleep apnoea	TPI	treponemal immobilization (test)
PACI	partial anterior circulation infarction	TRH	thyrotrophin-releasing hormone
PCOS	polycystic ovarian syndrome	TSH	thyroid-stimulating hormone
PEFR	peak expiratory flow rate	UMN	upper motor neurone
PID	pelvic inflammatory disease	UPPP	uvulopharyngopalatoplasty
PMD	post-micturition dribble	VMH	ventromedial hypothalamic nucleus
PMS	premenstrual syndrome	VOR	vestibulo-ocular reflex
POCI	posterior circulation infarction	VRDL	Venereal Disease Research Laboratory
PT	prothrombin time	vWF	von Willebrand factor
PTA	post-traumatic amnesia	XP	xeroderma pigmentosum
PUO	pyrexia of unknown origin		

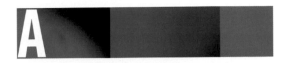

ABDOMINAL PAIN, ACUTE, LOCALIZED

A common and extremely important clinical problem is the patient who presents with acute abdominal pain. This may be referred all over the abdominal wall (see ABDOMINAL PAIN, general, p. 3), but here we shall consider those patients who present pain localized to a particular part of the abdominal cavity.

The causes are legion, and it is a useful exercise to summarize the organs that may be implicated together with the pathological processes pertaining to them so that the clinician can consider the possibilities in a logical manner:

1 Gastroduodenal
  - Perforated gastric or duodenal ulcer
  - Perforated gastric carcinoma
  - Acute gastritis (often alcoholic)
  - Irritant poisons

2 Intestinal
  - Small-bowel obstruction (adhesions, etc.)
  - Regional ileitis (Crohn's disease)
  - Intussusception
  - Sigmoid volvulus
  - Acute colonic diverticulitis
  - Large-bowel obstruction due to neoplasm
  - Strangulated external hernia (inguinal, femoral, umbilical)
  - Acute mesenteric occlusion due to arterial embolism or thrombosis or to venous thrombosis

3 Appendix
  - Acute appendicitis

4 Pancreas
  - Acute pancreatitis
  - Recurrent pancreatitis
  - Pancreatic trauma

5 Gallbladder and bile ducts
  - Calculus in the gallbladder or common bile ducts
  - Acute cholecystitis
  - Acute cholangitis

6 Liver
  - Trauma
  - Acute hepatitis
  - Malignant disease (primary or secondary)
  - Congestive cardiac failure

7 Spleen
  - Trauma
  - Spontaneous rupture (in malaria or infectious mononucleosis)
  - Infarction

8 Urinary tract
  - Renal, ureteric or vesical calculus
  - Renal trauma
  - Pyelonephritis
  - Pyonephrosis

9 Female genitalia
  - Salpingitis
  - Pyosalpinx
  - Ectopic pregnancy
  - Torsion of subserous fibroid
  - Red degeneration of fibroid
  - Twisted ovarian cyst
  - Ruptured ovarian cyst

10 Aorta
  - Ruptured aneurysm
  - Dissecting aneurysm

In addition to causes from intra-abdominal, retroperitoneal and pelvic organs, it is important to remember that acute localized pain may be referred to the abdomen from other structures:

11 Central nervous system
  - Herpes zoster affecting the lower thoracic segments. Posterior nerve root pain (e.g. from prolapsed intervertebral disc or collapsed vertebra from trauma or secondary deposits)

12 The heart and pericardium
  - Myocardial infarction
  - Acute pericarditis

13 Pleura
  - Acute diaphragmatic pleurisy

Occasionally, patients are seen who are often well known in the Accident and Emergency Department, presenting with simulated acute abdominal pain due to hysteria or malingering.

Patients with acute abdominal pain present one of the most testing trials to the clinician. In the first place, diagnosis is all important, since a decision has to be made whether or not the patient requires urgent laparotomy – for example, for a perforated peptic ulcer, acute appendicitis or acute intestinal obstruction. The history and examination are often difficult to elicit, particularly in a very ill patient who is in great pain and hardly wishes either to answer a lot of questions or to submit to prolonged examination. Finally, there are very few laboratory or radiological aids to diagnosis. Acute appendicitis, for example, has no specific tests. A raised white blood count suggests intraperitoneal infection, but something like one-quarter of the cases of acute appendicitis have a white blood cell count below 10 000 per mm[3]. Plain X-rays of the abdomen may indicate free gas when there is a perforated hollow viscus, but this is not invariably so. Intestinal obstruction may be revealed by distended loops of bowel on a plain X-ray of the abdomen, but in some 10 per cent of small-bowel obstructions the X-rays are entirely normal, since the distended loops of bowel are filled with fluid only so that the typical gas-distended loops of bowel are not present.

Ultrasonography of the abdomen may be used to demonstrate distended loops of bowel, fluid collections, gallbladder pathology, the presence of gall stones, a pathological appendix and intussusception. However, accurate diagnosis is heavily observer-dependent and requires the help of an expert ultrasonographer.

One of the few investigations that the surgeon relies upon heavily is a raised serum amylase activity. When this is above 1000 units per 100 ml serum it is almost pathognomic of acute pancreatitis, although every now and then a fulminating case of pancreatitis is seen in which the amylase is not elevated.

Every effort must therefore be made to establish the diagnosis on a careful history and examination.

One of the important aspects in the assessment of the acute abdomen in the establishment of a trend. Increasing pain, tenderness, guarding or rigidity indicates that there is some progressive intra-abdominal condition. This is also suggested by a rising pulse rate on hourly or half-hourly observations, and it is also suggested by progressive elevation of the temperature. In a doubtful case, repeated clinical examination – together with sequential recordings of the temperature and pulse – will enable the clinician to decide whether the intra-abdominal condition is either subsiding or progressing.

General features

General inspection of the patient is all important and must never be omitted. The flushed face and coated tongue of acute appendicitis, the agonized expression of the patient with a perforated ulcer, the writhing colic of a patient with ureteric stone, biliary colic or small-bowel obstruction are all most helpful. The skin is inspected for the pallor suggestive of haemorrhage, and for the jaundice which may be associated with biliary colic with a stone impacted at the lower end of the common bile duct. In such a case there will also be bile pigment which can be detected in the urine.

Abdominal examination

The patient must be placed in a good light, and the entire abdomen exposed from the nipples to the knees. The abdomen is inspected. Failure of movement with respiration may suggest an underlying peritoneal irritation. Abdominal distension is present in intestinal obstruction, and visible peristalsis may be seen from rhythmic contractions of the small bowel under these circumstances. Retraction of the abdomen may occur in acute peritonitis so that the abdomen assumes a scaphoid appearance, e.g. following perforation of a peptic ulcer.

Guarding – a voluntary contraction of the abdominal wall on palpation – denotes underlying inflammatory disease, and this is accompanied by localized tenderness. *Rigidity* is indicated by an involuntary tightness of the abdominal wall and may be generalized or localized. Localized rigidity over one particular organ suggests local peritoneal involvement, for example, in acute appendicitis or acute cholecystitis.

Percussion of the abdomen is useful. Dullness in the flanks suggests the presence of intraperitoneal fluid (e.g. blood in a patient with a ruptured spleen). A resonant distended abdomen is found in obstruction, and loss of liver dullness suggests free gas within the peritoneal cavity in a patient with a ruptured hollow viscus.

In intestinal obstruction the bowel sounds are increased and have a particular 'tinkling' quality. In some cases, borborygmi may be audible without using the stethoscope. A complete absence of bowel sounds suggests peritonitis.

Examination of the abdomen is not complete until the hernial orifices have been carefully inspected and palpated. It is easy enough to miss a small strangulated inguinal, femoral or umbilical hernia which, surprisingly enough, may have been completely overlooked by the patient.

A rectal examination is then performed. In intestinal obstruction the rectum has a characteristic 'ballooned' empty feel, although the exact mechanism of this is unknown. In pelvic peritonitis there will be tenderness anteriorly in the pouch of Douglas. A tender mass suggests an inflamed or twisted pelvic organ, and this can be confirmed by bimanual vaginal examination.

The urine and special investigations

The presence of blood, protein, pus or bile pigment in the urine may help to distinguish a renal or biliary colic from other causes of intra-abdominal pain. As well as routine testing of a urine specimen, a drop placed under the microscope and viewed with a 1/6th lens (staining is not required) constitutes a useful test. It is the work of a few minutes to see if pus cells or red cells are obvious. In obscure cases of abdominal pain, the urine should be examined for porphyrins to exclude porphyria, particularly when the attack appears to have been precipitated by barbiturates.

The clinical assessment of the patient with acute localized abdominal pain, based on a careful history and examination together with examination of the urine, may be supplemented by laboratory and radiological investigations. A full blood count, plain X-ray of the abdomen, and estimation of the serum amylase in suspected pancreatitis may all be helpful although, as mentioned above, the findings must be interpreted with caution. Ultrasound of the pelvis may be helpful if a twisted ovarian cyst or some other pelvic pathology is suspected. Ultrasonography is also valuable in demonstrating gall stones in acute cholecystitis. An emergency intravenous urogram is indicated when a ureteric stone or some other renal pathology is suspected. An electrocardiogram and appropriate cardiac enzyme estimations are performed if it is suspected that the upper abdominal pain is referred from a myocardial infarction, and a chest X-ray may demonstrate a basal pneumonia. It must be stressed, however, that the clinical features take precedence over all other diagnostic aids.

Nothing can be simpler, nor more difficult, than diagnosing a patient with the so-called 'acute abdomen'.

Particular difficulties will be encountered in infants (where history may be difficult, and examining a screaming child most demanding), and in the elderly, where again it is often difficult to obtain an accurate history and where physical signs are often atypical. The grossly obese patient and the pregnant patient are two other categories where particular difficulties may be encountered.

When faced with a patient with severe abdominal pain the main decision that must be taken, of course, is whether or not a laparotomy is indicated as a matter of urgency. If careful assessment still makes the decision difficult, then repeated observations must be carried out over the next few hours to observe the trend of the particular case. This will nearly always enable a definite decision to be made as to whether laparotomy or further conservative treatment is indicated.

Harold Ellis

ABDOMINAL PAIN (GENERAL)

(See also ABDOMINAL PAIN, acute, localized, p. 1) Most abdominal pain is localized, for example that due to a renal stone or biliary stone, acute appendicitis, peptic ulceration, and so on. There are, however, a number of causes of generalized abdominal pain, the commonest of which are peritonitis and intestinal obstructions.

A list of causes to be considered includes:

1 General peritonitis
2 Tuberculous peritonitis
3 Intestinal obstruction
4 Lead colic (rare)
5 Gastric crises (rare)
6 Functional abdominal pain
7 General medical diseases:
   ■ malaria
   ■ porphyria
   ■ diabetic ketosis
   ■ blood dyscrasias
   ■ Henoch's purpura
   ■ Sickle cell anaemia
   ■ Hypercalcaemia

Acute peritonitis

Peritonitis must be secondary to a lesion which enables some clue in the history to suggest the initiating disease. Thus, the patient with established peritonitis may give a history of onset which indicates acute appendicitis or salpingitis as the source of origin. Where the onset of peritonitis is sudden, one should suspect an acute perforation of a hollow viscus. The early features depend on the severity and the extent of the peritonitis. Pain is always severe, and typically the patient lies still on its account – in contrast with the restlessness of a patient with abdominal colic. An extensive peritonitis which involves the abdominal aspect of the diaphragm may be accompanied by shoulder-tip pain. Vomiting often occurs early in the course of the disease. The patient is obviously ill and the temperature frequently elevated. If initially the peritoneal exudate is not purulent, the temperature may be normal. It is a good aphorism concerning the two common causes of this condition that peritonitis due to appendicitis is usually accompanied by a temperature above 38°C (100°F), whereas the temperature in peritonitis due to a perforation of a peptic ulcer seldom reaches this level. The pulse is often raised and tends to increase from hour to hour.

Examination of the abdomen demonstrates tenderness, which may be localized to the affected area or is generalized if the peritoneal cavity is extensively involved. There is marked guarding, which again may be localized or generalized, and rebound tenderness is present. The abdomen is silent on auscultation, although sometimes the transmitted sounds of the heart beat and respiration may be detected. Rectally, there is tenderness of the pelvic peritoneum.

As the disease progresses, the abdomen becomes distended, signs of free fluid may be detected, and the pulse becomes more rapid and feeble. Vomiting is now effortless and faeculent, and the patient, though still conscious and mentally alert, demonstrates the Hippocratic facies with sunken eyes, pale, cold and sweating skin, and cyanosis of the extremities.

An X-ray of the abdomen in the erect position may reveal free subdiaphragmatic gas in peritonitis due to hollow viscus perforation (e.g. perforated peptic ulcer), but its absence by no means excludes the diagnosis.

The main differential diagnoses are the colics of intestinal obstruction or of ureteric or biliary stone. Intraperitoneal haemorrhage, acute pancreatitis, dissection or leakage of an aortic aneurysm, or a basal pneumonia are also important differential diagnoses.

Tuberculous peritonitis

In Great Britain this is now a rare disease. When it is encountered in this country, the patient is usually an immigrant from the Third World. Usually, there is a feeling of heaviness rather than acute pain. The onset of symptoms is gradual, with abdominal distension, the presence of fluid within the peritoneal cavity, and often the presence of a puckered, thickened omentum, which forms a tumour lying transversely across the middle of the abdomen.

Intestinal colic (see also ABDOMINAL PAIN, acute, localized)

Intestinal obstruction

This is a common cause of generalized abdominal pain. In peritonitis there is no periodic rhythm, whereas waves of pain interspersed with periods of complete relief or only a dull ache are typical of obstruction. In contrast to the patients with peritonitis who wish to remain completely still, the victim of intestinal obstruction is restless and rolls about with the spasms of colic. Usually, there are the accompaniments of progressive abdominal distension, absolute constipation, progressive vomiting (which becomes faeculent), and the presence of noisy bowel sounds on auscultation. An X-ray of the abdomen usually reveals multiple fluid levels on the erect film, together with distended loops of gas-filled bowel which are obvious on the supine radiograph.

The presence of a scar (or scars) of previous abdominal surgery, performed no matter how long previously, strongly suggests postoperative adhesions or bands as the cause of the obstruction. Careful examination of the hernial orifices – inguinal, femoral and umbilical – is mandatory to diagnose a strangulated external hernia. Surprisingly, the patient may be completely ignorant of its presence. The author has seen a distinguished anaesthetist who correctly diagnosed his own acute bowel obstruction, but had not noticed his strangulated inguinal hernia.

Lead colic

Lead colic may cause extremely severe attacks of general abdominal pain. There may be preceding anorexia, constipation and vague abdominal discomfort. The severe pain is usually situated in the lower abdomen and radiating to both groins; it may also sometimes be associated with wrist-drop (due to peripheral neuritis), and occasionally with lead encephalopathy. There may be a blue 'lead line' on the gums if oral sepsis is present, due to the precipitation of lead sulphide. Frequently there is a normocytic hypochromic anaemia with stippling of the red cells (punctuate basophilia). Inquiry about the patient's occupation may well be the first clue to the diagnosis. Other signs of lead poisoning are considered on p. 247.

Gastric crises

Gastric crises in neurosyphilis, although rare, may cause general abdominal pain. The patient has other evidence of tabes dorsalis, with Argyll Robertson pupils, optic atrophy and ptosis, loss of deep sensation (absence of pain on testicular compression or squeezing the tendo Achillis), and loss of ankle- and knee-jerks. The pain is severe and lasts for many hours or even days. There may be accompanying vomiting, and there may also be rigidity of the abdominal wall. The visceral crisis may be the sole manifestation of tabes. The mere fact that a patient has tabes dorsalis does not, of course, mean that their abdominal pain must necessarily be a gastric crisis. The author has repaired a perforated duodenal ulcer in a patient with all the classic features of well-documented tabes dorsalis.

Abdominal angina

Abdominal angina occurs in elderly patients as a result of progressive atheromatous narrowing of the superior mesenteric artery. Colicky attacks of central abdominal pain occur after meals, and this is followed by diarrhoea. Complete occlusion with infarction of the intestine is often preceded by attacks of this nature. Occlusion of vessels to small or large intestine – as is seen in a number of vasculopathies such as systemic lupus erythematosus or polyarteritis nodosa – may cause generalized abdominal pain and proceed to gangrene, perforation and general peritonitis.

Functional abdominal pain

One of the most difficult problems is the patient (female more often than male) who presents with severe chronic generalized abdominal pains and in whom all clinical, laboratory and radiological tests are negative. Inquiry will often reveal features of depression or the presence of some precipitating factor producing an anxiety state. In some cases the abdomen is covered with scars of previous laparotomies at which various organs have been reposited, non-essential viscera removed, and real or imaginary adhesions divided. Some of these patients prove to be drug addicts, others are frank hysterics, and others seek the security of the hospital environment, but in still others the aetiology remains mysterious. This forms one type of the so-called 'Munchausen syndrome', described by the late Dr Richard Asher.

Abdominal pains in general disease

Acute abdominal pain may occur in a number of medical conditions not already considered. These include sudden and severe pain complicating malignant malaria, familial Mediterranean fever, and cholera, or may accompany uncontrolled diabetes with ketosis, that rare condition known as porphyria (see p. 5), and any of the blood dyscrasias; the best examples are Henoch's purpura in children and the abdominal colic of acute sickle cell crisis (see p. 61). Bouts of abdominal pain may occur in the hypercalcaemia of hyperparathyroidism.

Harold Ellis

ABDOMINAL PULSATION

A pulsatile swelling in the abdomen may be due to:

- a prominent aorta – normal or arteriosclerotic;
- an abdominal aortic aneurysm;
- transmission of aortic pulsations through an abdominal mass; or
- a pulsatile, enlarged liver.

Prominent aorta

The pulsations of the normal aorta may be felt in perfectly normal but thin subjects along a line extending from the xiphoid to the bifurcation of the aorta at the level of the fourth lumbar vertebra. This is on a line joining the iliac crests, about 2 cm below and a little to the left of the umbilicus. In the arteriosclerotic and hypertensive subject, it may be difficult to decide whether or not the aorta is merely thickened and tortuous, or whether it is aneurysmal. If the two index fingers are placed parallel, one on either side of the aorta, the distance between the fingers can be measured. According to the size of the patient, a gap of 2–3 cm between the fingertips may be considered normal, but any measurement above this is suspicious of aneurysmal dilatation.

If in doubt, visualization of the aorta by means of ultrasound or computed tomography (CT) enables accurate measurement of the aorta to be made.

Abdominal aortic aneurysm

There is no doubt that arteriosclerotic abdominal aneurysms are becoming more frequently encountered, as is the serious emergency of leakage or rupture of such an aneurysm. The majority of patients are aged more than 60 years, and the great majority are men. The aneurysm may be entirely symptomless or the patient may complain of epigastric or central abdominal discomfort which frequently radiates into the lumbar region. The patient himself may actually detect the pulsating mass in the abdomen.

The pulsation may be visible in the upper abdomen, above the umbilicus, and – if large enough – may actually appear as a pulsating mass. On palpation, the aneurysm is a midline swelling which bulges over to the left side, away from the adjacent inferior vena cava. If the mass extends below the level of the umbilicus it suggests implication of the iliac arteries. The characteristic physical sign is that the mass has an expansile pulsation. The index fingers are placed one either side of the mass, which enables the diameter to be assessed. If the diameter is more than 3 cm, this certainly suggests aneurysmal dilatation of the aorta; if the diameter is above 5 cm, the clinical diagnosis is all but certain. Typically, the fingers are pushed apart with each pulse, and not up and down. The latter sign suggests *transmission* of the pulsation (see section below).

Usually the aneurysm is resonant to percussion due to overlying loops of intestine. However, an extremely large aneurysm will displace the bowel laterally to reach the anterior abdominal wall and will then give a dull percussion note. Auscultation may reveal bruits over the lower extremity of the aneurysm. This suggests turbulent flow of blood caused by relative stenosis at the aorto-iliac junctions.

Rectal examination may reveal a pulsatile mass when one or both of the internal iliac arteries are involved in the aneurysmal process.

Leakage or rupture of the aneurysm is an acute abdominal emergency. The patient presents with the features of massive blood loss (pale, sweating, clammy skin, a rapid pulse and low blood pressure) together with severe abdominal pain, lumbar pain and marked abdominal tenderness and guarding. Because of the low blood pressure and the associated peri-aneurysmal haematoma, as well as the overlying guarding, the aneurysm may be quite difficult to palpate and, unless sought carefully, is easy enough to miss.

The diagnosis of aortic aneurysm is often readily confirmed by means of a plain abdominal X-ray (Fig. A.1) which frequently delineates the aneurysm because of the associated calcification in its wall. Typically, the aneurysm is seen to bulge over to the left side of the abdomen. More accurately, an ultrasound or computed tomogram of the abdomen visualizes the aneurysm and enables its length and diameter to be measured accurately.

Transmission of aortic pulsations through an abdominal mass

A large intra-abdominal or retroperitoneal solid mass, pressing against the aorta, may exhibit transmitted aortic pulsation. Typical examples are a large carcinoma of the body of the stomach, a carcinoma or cyst of the pancreas, and a large ovarian cyst. Indeed, when the whole abdomen is filled by a cystic mass it may be quite difficult to distinguish between such a mass and extensive ascites. Percussion, of course, is helpful since ascites gives dullness in the flanks as compared with the central dullness of a large intra-abdominal mass. The two index fingers, when placed on the mass, will perceive that the pulsation is transmitted *directly forwards* from the aorta and is not expansile, as would be found in an aneurysm.

Pulsatile liver

It is unlikely that an enlarged pulsatile liver will be mistaken for any other kind of pulsatile tumour. It occurs in cases of chronic failure of cardiac compensation, generally from mitral stenosis or tricuspid stenosis. There is associated cyanosis, oedema of the legs and ascites. It is not, however, every liver which seems to pulsate that really presents expansile pulsation. An impression of pulsation may be given

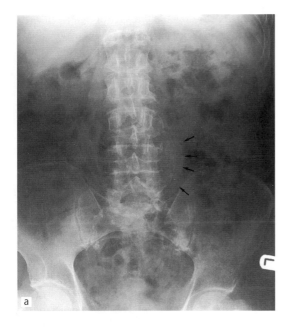

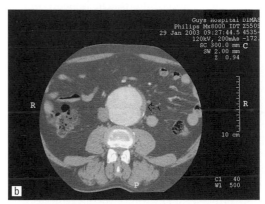

Figure A.1 (a) Plain X-ray of the abdomen, showing large calcified aortic aneurysm (arrowed). (b) Aortic aneurysm on CT scan (arrow). [Dr Sheila Rankin, Guy's Hospital.]

by the movements transmitted directly to the liver by the hypertrophied right heart.

Harold Ellis

ABDOMINAL RIGIDITY

Rigidity of the abdomen is a sign of utmost importance, since in most cases it indicates serious intra-abdominal mischief requiring immediate operation. It is the expression of a state of tonic contraction in the muscles of the abdominal wall. The responsible stimulus may be in the brain or basal ganglia, or in the territory of the six lower dorsal nerves that supply the abdominal wall. The extent of the rigidity will depend on the number of nerves involved, and its degree on the nature and duration of the stimulus. The analysis in Table A.1 may be considered.

The patient should be examined lying on the back with the whole abdomen and lower thorax exposed, but with the shoulders and legs well covered. The room must be warm. The examiner, seated on a level with the patient, should first watch the abdomen to

Table A.1 The extent of abdominal rigidity

Site of stimulus	Causative agent	Characters of rigidity
Cerebral cortex or basal ganglia	Nervousness, anticipation of pain, cold	Affects the whole abdominal wall; varies in intensity, can be abolished by appropriate means
Dorsal nerve-trunks	Pleurisy; infections of the chest wall	Limited to one side of the abdomen; varies in extent and degree
Nerve-endings in abdominal wall	Injury or infection of muscles	Limited to injured or infected segment
Nerve-endings in peritoneum	Irritation by any intraperitoneal foreign substance: infection, chemical irritant, or blood	Degree varies with nature of irritant and suddenness with which stimulus has arrived. Extent corresponds to area of peritoneum involved. Both degree and extent remain approximately constant during the period of examination

see whether it moves with respiration or not, and whether one part moves more than another; at the same time he or she may observe other things which will help in the diagnosis, such as asymmetry of the two sides, local swelling, or the movement of coils of bowel. While watching – and later when examining – he/she should engage the patient in conversation, encouraging him to talk in order to allay nervousness and to remove any part of the rigidity which is due to a voluntary contraction. Some nervous patients – especially if the room is cold – hold their abdomens intensely rigid, and can be induced to relax only after gentle persuasion; a request to take a few deep breaths, or to draw the knees up and keep the mouth open, will often help. During this preliminary examination, one (well-warmed) hand may be laid gently on the abdomen and passed over its surface with a light touch that cannot possibly hurt; this manoeuvre will help to allay the patient's anxiety still further and give the examiner an idea of the extent, intensity and constancy of the rigidity which he or she must later investigate in more detail.

For a more exact examination, the observer should sit at the patient's side facing their head, and place both hands on the abdomen, examining comparable areas of both sides, simultaneously, and taking in turn the epigastrium, right and left hypochondria, umbilical region, both flanks as far back as the erector spinae (for the rigidity of a retrocaecal appendix may only affect the posterior part of the abdominal wall), the hypogastrium, and both iliac fossae. First, the whole hand should be applied with light pressure; next, the fingers held flat should be pressed more firmly to estimate the extent of the rigidity and to discover deep tenderness; lastly, a detailed examination may be made in suspected areas with the firm pressure of one or two fingers. Evidence is not complete without percussion and auscultation. A rectal examination is indispensable.

After a leisurely examination with warm hands in a warm room, during which the physician has also been able to sum up the patient, his temperament, and whether he is really ill or not, the rigidity of anxiety or cold will have been dispelled or recognized. The abdominal rigidity due to a lesion in the chest or chest wall usually involves a wide area limited to one side – a distribution most unusual with intra-abdominal mischief, which, if it has spread widely but not everywhere, tends to be limited to the upper or lower half. The extent and degree of rigidity in chest affections also vary widely during examination. Other things such as a flushed face, rapid respiration, movement of the alae nasi, or a temperature of more than 39°C (102°F), may suggest that the lesion is not abdominal, and a friction rub may be felt or heard in the chest.

Auscultation and rectal examination dispel any remaining doubts, for in chest conditions peristaltic sounds remain normal, and there is no tenderness in Douglas's pouch.

Examination of the blood may show a high leucocytosis (up to 30 000 or 40 000 per mm^3), whereas in peritonitis the count is seldom over 12 000 per mm^3. Chest X-rays (including a lateral film) will demonstrate the intrathoracic lesion.

Injuries of the abdominal wall, and particularly those caused by run-over accidents, lead to very marked rigidity of the injured segment. Here, the rigidity is not necessary to establish a diagnosis, for the injury is already known, but its degree and extent should be carefully noted. There must always be a doubt as to whether the abdominal viscera are damaged as well as the walls, and this point can only be settled by careful observation. The patient is put to bed and kept warm, the pulse is charted every 15 minutes, and the abdomen is re-examined from time to time. In the case of a mere contusion, the collapse will soon disappear, the abdomen will become less rigid, and the pulse rate will fall. If the contents of a hollow viscus have escaped, rigidity will extend beyond the area of the damaged muscles, and the signs of peritonitis will develop rapidly.

An X-ray of the abdomen, in the erect position, will demonstrate free gas beneath the diaphragm. If there is internal bleeding (e.g. from a ruptured spleen or liver) there is pallor and progressive elevation of the pulse, together with a falling blood pressure. Dullness in the flanks (especially on the left side, in rupture of the spleen) is often detected, as blood collects in the paracolic gutters.

Peritonitis

The commonest and the most important cause of general abdominal rigidity is peritonitis, and it is a safe rule when meeting true rigidity to diagnose peritonitis until it can be excluded. Actually, rigidity means no more than that the parietal peritoneum lining the abdominal cavity is in contact with something differing from the smooth surfaces which are its normal environment. The *presence of rigidity* therefore announces a change in the coelomic cavity that is probably infective in origin. When gallstone colic is followed by rigidity of the right rectus, it means not only that a stone is blocking the cystic duct but also that the wall of the gallbladder is inflamed. Intestinal obstruction of mechanical origin (such as that due to a band or adhesion) gives colic referred to the umbilicus, but no guarding of the muscles; local rigidity accompanying the clinical picture of intestinal obstruction indicates that there is also a local inflammatory focus such as a strangulated loop of bowel, while a more diffuse rigidity suggests changes such as thrombosis of the superior mesenteric artery, affecting a large segment of bowel. In appendicitis, rigidity denotes that infection has spread beyond the coats of the appendix.

The *degree of rigidity* varies with the nature of the irritant, the rapidity with which the peritoneum is attacked, and the area involved. At one extreme is the rigidity of a gastric or duodenal perforation, where the abdomen is suddenly flooded with gastric contents. Here, the whole abdominal wall is fixed in a contraction that can best be described as board-like: there is no respiratory movement, and no yielding to the firmest pressure. At the other extreme is the relatively minor degree of rigidity which accompanies the presence of small amounts of blood or urine in the peritoneal cavity; there is perhaps only a slightly increased resistance when the hands are pressed on the abdomen. Perforation of a gastric or duodenal ulcer produces the most intense rigidity; the escape of amylase in acute pancreatitis leads to less rigidity, and the escape of other sterile fluids, urine for instance, or blood, still less. Bacterial invasion of the peritoneum produces marked rigidity. The degree of muscle contraction also alters during the development of a case. The board-like abdominal wall of a perforation is considerably softer after 3–4 hours when the peritoneum has recovered from the shock of the first insult. The slight resistance apparent when sterile urine escapes from a ruptured bladder rapidly increases as infection supervenes.

The *extent of the rigidity* usually corresponds to the area of peritoneum affected. The whole abdomen may be rigid, the upper or lower part only, one side, or a restricted part. Total rigidity should mean a total

peritonitis, but because the peritoneum reacts immediately to invasion by forming adhesions which localize the mischief, a general peritonitis is only seen when an irritant or infected fluid is suddenly discharged in large quantities – as in duodenal perforation, pancreatitis, or the bursting of a large abscess or distended viscus – or when the infection is brought by the bloodstream and reaches all parts simultaneously. Occasionally, and particularly in children, the reaction to a sudden infection may be excessive and the muscles contract over a wide area in response to a purely local infection, for instance of the appendix, though this exaggerated response rapidly disappears. Conversely, the aged patient – with atrophic abdominal muscles – may exhibit only slight rigidity, even in generalized peritonitis. Local peritonitis starts around some site of infection, and as it spreads it is guided by certain peritoneal watersheds, of which the most important is the attachment of the great omentum to the transverse colon, dividing the abdomen into supra- and infra-colic compartments. Rigidity accompanies the infection. Thus, localized rigidity is found over any inflamed organ, and as the infection and the guarding spread, they tend to involve the upper or the lower half of the abdomen as a whole. When we have mapped out the extent of the rigidity, we should – from a knowledge of the organs at that site and of the watersheds that guide the spread of infection – be able, in conjunction with the history, to make a diagnosis.

The influence of natural subdivisions in guiding intraperitoneal extension must always be taken into account. Infections in the right supracolic compartment tend to pass down between the ascending colon and the right abdominal wall, while one in the pelvis is guided by the pelvic mesocolon to the left side of the abdomen as it ascends. Thus, rigidity in the right iliac fossa may indicate a leaking duodenal ulcer, and in the left may be due to a pelvic appendix.

Since the diagnosis of peritonitis in most cases means immediate operation, every endeavour must be made to confirm the diagnosis, particularly by the simple tests of percussion, auscultation and rectal examination. Percussion may reveal the outline of some dilated hollow organ, such as the caecum; it may disclose free gas which has escaped from a perforation as a shifting circle of resonance or a tympanitic note where liver dullness should be; it may map out an abnormal area of dullness where there is an abscess or a collection of blood; or it may indicate free fluid in the peritoneum. Auscultation is even more important, for with peritonitis peristalsis ceases: in a normal abdomen peristaltic sounds can be heard every 4–10 seconds; in obstruction they are increased in loudness, pitch and frequency; in peritonitis there is complete silence. Rectal examination nearly always reveals tenderness when there is intra-abdominal infection, even if it is distant and localized.

Other signs must be mentioned: the patient lies still, sometimes with the knees drawn up, and resists interference. The abdomen gradually becomes distended, tense and tympanitic. The tongue is brown and dry. Vomiting is to be expected at the onset of any abdominal catastrophe, but except in intestinal obstruction it usually ceases; with advancing peritonitis it reappears, and the vomit becomes first bile-stained, later brownish and faecal-smelling, and is allowed to dribble from the corner of the mouth in contrast to the projectile vomiting of obstruction. There may be diarrhoea at first, but absolute constipation soon succeeds it. The temperature tends to fall; the pulse is small and rapid, rising progressively. In late stages the sunken cheeks, wide eyes and anxious expression of the patient form a characteristic feature – the Hippocratic facies.

These signs are indications of a peritonitis discovered too late, and are the heralds of approaching death. Abdominal rigidity, abdominal silence, rectal tenderness and a rising pulse are a tetrad that calls for immediate definitive treatment.

A more detailed diagnosis is usually possible when the history and other signs are taken together, but a consideration of all the alternatives is out of the question in this section. Abdominal paracentesis with a fine needle may clinch the presence of pus, blood or urine in the peritoneal cavity, but a false negative tap may delay rather than aid diagnosis. A list of the more common conditions associated with rigidity may, however, help the inquiry:

- Stomach or duodenum
  - ◆ Perforation of peptic ulcer
- Gallbladder
  - ◆ Acute cholecystitis
  - ◆ Rupture of gallbladder
- Pancreas
  - ◆ Acute pancreatitis
- Small intestine
  - ◆ Strangulation of a loop
  - ◆ Traumatic perforation

- ◆ Mesenteric vascular thrombosis or embolism
- ◆ Meckel's diverticulitis
- ◆ Acute ileitis
- Large intestine
  - ◆ Appendicitis
  - ◆ Volvulus
  - ◆ Diverticulitis with perforation
- Peritoneum
  - ◆ Acute blood-borne peritonitis:
    - Streptococcal
    - Pneumococcal
    - Gonococcal
- Female generative organs
  - ◆ Twisted ovarian cyst
  - ◆ Ruptured ectopic pregnancy
  - ◆ Acute salpingitis
  - ◆ Torsion or red degeneration of fibroid
  - ◆ Perforation of uterus or posterior fornix of vagina in attempted abortion
- Spleen and/or liver
  - ◆ Traumatic rupture
- Aorta
  - ◆ Ruptured aneurysm

Perforation of a peptic ulcer is characterized by the most sudden onset, the worst agony, and the most extreme abdominal rigidity that the physician is ever likely to see. Radiation of pain to the right shoulder tip (referred pain from diaphragmatic irritation) may be experienced. Immediately afterwards, the patient is motionless and speechless, in a state of obvious collapse. A few hours later pain, rigidity and shock have all diminished and only the traumatic history and persistent abdominal and rectal tenderness may remain to indicate the seriousness of the condition.

Acute pancreatitis is seldom accompanied by the severe pain described in textbooks, or indeed by pain as bad as that of gallstone colic. The abdominal rigidity is more marked in the upper abdomen but is not profound. On the other hand, the patient shows a degree of toxaemia out of all proportion to the physical signs in the abdomen. The diagnosis is confirmed by a considerable rise in the serum amylase.

A *ruptured ectopic pregnancy* may simulate a lower abdominal peritonitis, but the signs of bleeding predominate and rigidity is not well marked. If the patient is a woman of child-bearing age who is known to have missed a period, the onset of abdominal pain and pallor suggest the diagnosis. Extravasated blood will be felt in the pelvis, together with acute tenderness on vaginal and rectal examinations.

Blue discoloration of the skin around the umbilicus – Cullen's sign – may be associated with rigidity. This discoloration is due to extravasated blood coming forwards from the retroperitoneal space. The sign is seen in ruptured kidney, leaking abdominal aneurysm and acute pancreatitis. Occasionally, it is seen in ruptured ectopic pregnancy, when the blood gains entry to the subperitoneal space through the broad ligament. Although pancreatitis may produce this sign, it is more common to see a green discoloration in the loins (Grey Turner's sign).

Harold Ellis

ABDOMINAL SWELLINGS

(See also VARICOSE VEINS, ABDOMINAL, p. 772) This may be acute or chronic, general or local, and caused by abdominal accumulations that are gaseous, liquid or solid. They may arise in the abdominal cavity itself or in the abdominal wall.

Swellings in the abdominal wall

Swellings situated in the abdominal wall itself can be recognized by their superficial position, by their adherence to the skin, subcutaneous fascia or muscles, or by their failure to follow the movements of the viscera immediately underlying the abdominal wall (Fig. A.2). It may be impossible to differentiate, for

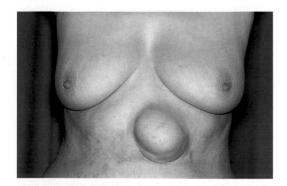

Figure A.2 A large, subcutaneous lipoma in the epigastrum. This moved freely on the anterior abdominal wall, even when the underlying muscles were tightly contracted, thus excluding the diagnosis of an epigastric hernia.

obvious reasons, an intra-abdominal mass that has become attached to the abdominal parietes, either as an inflammatory or malignant process. A simple test which should be applied to all abdominal masses is to ask the patient to raise either their legs or shoulders from the couch. This procedure tightens the abdominal muscles; if the lump is intraperitoneal it disappears, but if it is situated in the abdominal wall itself it persists.

Inflammatory swelling of the abdominal wall most commonly complicates a laparotomy incision, and the diagnosis is obvious. A superficial cellulitis may complicate infection of a small abrasion or hair follicle infection. Inflammation of the abdominal wall may be secondary to an extension of an intraperitoneal abscess, particularly an appendix abscess in the right iliac fossa, or, on the left side, a paracolic abscess in relation to diverticular disease of the sigmoid colon or to perforation of a carcinoma of the large bowel.

Inflammatory swelling of the umbilicus in newborn infants is rare, except in primitive communities where the cord is not divided with the niceties of modern aseptic practice. Suppuration at the umbilicus in adults is not uncommon if the navel is deep and narrow.

A tender haematoma in the lower abdomen may result from rupture of the rectus abdominis muscle, or tearing of the inferior epigastric artery which may occur as the result of a violent cough.

Tumours of the abdominal wall are usually subcutaneous lipomas. These may be multiple, and may be a feature of Dercum's disease (adiposa dolorosa). Lipomas should be carefully differentiated from irreducible umbilical or epigastric hernias containing omentum.

A desmoid tumour may arise in the lower part of the abdominal wall, and malignant fibrosarcomas or melanomas may also occasionally be encountered. A neoplastic deposit may sometimes be palpated at the umbilicus, and represents a transcoelomic seeding, usually from a carcinoma of the stomach or large bowel.

General abdominal swellings

Every medical student knows the mnemonic of the five causes of gross generalized swelling of the abdomen: Fat, Fluid, Flatus, Faeces and Fetus.

In *obesity* the abdomen may swell either in consequence of the deposit of fat in the abdominal wall itself, or as the result of adipose tissue in the mesentery, the omentum, and in the extraperitoneal layer. In very obese persons it is rarely possible to diagnose the exact nature of an intra-abdominal mass by the usual clinical methods. Indeed, tumours of quite remarkable size – including the full-term fetus – may remain occult to even the most careful examiner.

Distension of the intestines with gas occurs in *intestinal obstruction*, and is particularly marked in cases of volvulus of the sigmoid colon, chronic large-bowel obstruction and megacolon. It also occurs in adynamic ileus. The whole of the abdomen, or, in special cases some part of it, is distended and gives on percussion a highly resonant or tympanitic note. The outlines of the gas-distended viscera are often visible; loops of dilated small bowel, one above the other, may produce a characteristic 'ladder pattern'. The increased size of the inflated intestine may produce displacement of the other viscera; the dome of the diaphragm is pushed up into the chest, shifting the apex beat of the heart upwards. The liver is similarly displaced. The distended *stomach* may occasionally be gross enough all but to fill the abdomen in very advanced cases of pyloric stenosis and in acute gastric dilatation.

The causes producing an accumulation of liquid in the peritoneal cavity can be listed as:

- congestive cardiac failure;
- cirrhosis;
- the nephrotic syndrome;
- carcinomatosis peritonei; and
- tuberculous peritonitis.

In severe cases of *chronic constipation*, abdominal distension may result from the accumulation of faeces in the large intestine, particularly where megacolon exists. The scybala may be felt, usually soft and plastic in the region of the ascending colon, and hard and nodular in the descending and sigmoid colon. Rectal examination often reveals an enormous accumulation of faeces. In some cases of tuberculous peritonitis semi-solid inflammatory masses may bring about a general swelling of the abdomen. General swelling of the abdomen may occur in *malignant disease involving the peritoneum* due to the growth of numerous secondary nodules in addition to a concomitant ascites. *Pseudomyxoma peritonei* may follow rupture of a pseudomucinous cystadenoma of the ovary or of a mucocele of the appendix. The whole abdominal cavity becomes distended with gelatinous material.

Local intra-abdominal swellings

These may be due to some general cause, or to a mass arising in a specific viscus.

Swellings due to general causes

Causes which ordinarily produce general swelling of the abdomen may sometimes give rise to only a local swelling. Thus, with encysted ascites left after an acute diffuse peritonitis or accompanying tuberculous peritonitis, an accumulation of fluid bounded by adhesions between the adjacent viscera may be found in any part of the peritoneal cavity, most often in the flanks or pelvis. A reliable history may be a clue to the nature of such a mass, although its cause may not be revealed until a laparotomy has been performed.

Abdominal swellings may occur in *tuberculous peritonitis* resulting from the rolled-up, matted and infiltrated omentum, doughy masses of adherent intestine, or enlarged tuberculous mesenteric lymph nodes. The amount of ascites in such cases varies considerably from a gross degree to almost complete absence (the obliterative form). Discovery of a tuberculous focus elsewhere in the body is support for the diagnosis.

Hydatid cysts may occur in any part of the abdominal cavity. They are usually single. The liver – particularly the right lobe – is the most common situation, and more rarely the spleen, omentum, mesentery or peritoneum. The cyst grows slowly and is spherical except in so far as it is moulded by the pressure of adjacent structures. It contains a clear fluid in which may be found hooklets, scolices and secondary or daughter cysts detached from the walls of the parent cyst. Unless large enough to cause mechanical pressure, the single hydatid cyst gives rise to little pain, or indeed to any complaint of any kind. It may produce a smooth, rounded, tense bulging of the overlying abdominal wall. It is dull on percussion, and it may yield a 'hydatid thrill' as may any other cyst; this thrill is the vibratory sensation experienced by the rest of the hand when, with the whole hand laid flat over the tumour, a central finger is percussed. Occasionally, there may be pain and fever due to inflammation within these cysts, and rupture into the peritoneal cavity may cause a severe anaphylactic reaction. Rupture of a hydatid cyst of the liver into a bile duct may cause jaundice due to biliary obstruction by daughter cysts. Hydatid disease is rare except in countries where the inhabitants live in close association with dogs that are the hosts of *Taenia echinococcus* (Australasia, South America, Greece, Cyprus, and, in the British Isles, North Wales). About one-quarter of patients demonstrate eosinophilia. A complement fixation test gives a high degree of accuracy. X-rays of the abdomen may reveal calcification of the cyst wall in long-standing cases.

Any part of the abdomen may swell from the formation of an abscess. A subphrenic abscess following a general peritonitis is occasionally large enough to produce an upper abdominal swelling. The patient is usually seriously ill with a swinging fever, rapid pulse, leucocytosis and all the general manifestations of toxaemia. However, in this antibiotic era, an increasing number of examples are being seen of a more insidious and chronic progress of the disease, with onset delayed weeks or even many months after the initial peritoneal infection. X-ray examination, together with screening of the diaphragm, is extremely useful, and at least 90 per cent of patients with subphrenic infection have some abnormality on this investigation. On the affected side the diaphragm is raised and its sharp definition is lost. Its mobility on screening is diminished or absent. There is frequently a pleural effusion, collapse of the lung base or evidence of pneumonitis. About 25 per cent of patients have gas below the diaphragm, frequently associated with a fluid level. This gas is usually derived from a perforated abdominal viscus, but occasionally is formed by gas-producing organisms. On the left side, gas under the diaphragm may be confused with the gastric bubble. An important differential feature is that the gas shadow of the stomach rarely reaches the lateral abdominal wall; however, if there is doubt a mouthful of barium is given in order to demarcate the stomach. Ultrasonography and computed tomography usually clinch the diagnosis.

Pus may localize in either the right or left paracolic gutter or iliac fossa. On the right side this commonly follows a ruptured appendix, or occasionally a perforated duodenal ulcer. On the left, a perforation of an inflamed diverticulum or carcinoma of the sigmoid colon is the usual cause. A large pelvic abscess frequently extends above the pubis or into one or other iliac fossa from the pelvis and can be palpated abdominally as well as on pelvic or rectal examination. About 75 per cent result from gangrenous appendicitis, and the remainder follow gynaecological infections, pelvic surgery, or any general peritonitis.

Regional diagnosis of local abdominal swellings

For clinical purposes, the abdomen may be subdivided into nine regions by two vertical lines drawn upwards from the mid-inguinal point midway between the anterior superior iliac spine and the symphysis pubis, and by two horizontal lines, the upper one passing through the lowest points of the 10th ribs (the subcostal line), the other drawn at the highest points of the iliac crests – the supracristal plane (Fig. A.3).

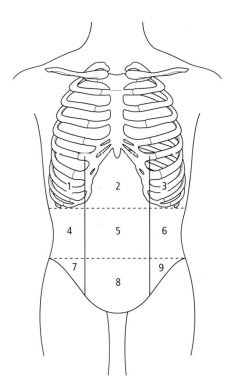

Figure A.3 The regions of the abdomen. Identification numerals are listed in Table A.2.

The three median areas thus mapped out are named, from above downwards, the epigastric, umbilical and hypogastric (or suprapubic) regions; the six lateral areas are, from above downwards, the right and left hypochondriac, lumbar and iliac regions.

The viscera, or portions of viscera, commonly situated in the areas thus demarcated are listed in Table A.2.

The abdominal swellings that may be felt in and about these nine regions, excluding the tumours

Table A.2 The normal contents of the abdominal regions

1 Right hypochondriac region Liver Gallbladder Hepatic flexure of colon Right kidney Right suprarenal gland **2 Epigastric region** Liver Stomach and pylorus Transverse colon Omentum Pancreas Duodenum Kidneys Suprarenal glands Aorta Lymph nodes **3 Left hypochondriac region** Liver Stomach	Splenic flexure of colon Spleen Tail of pancreas Left kidney Left suprarenal gland **4 Right lumbar region** Riedel's lobe of the liver Ascending colon Small intestine Right kidney **5 Umbilical region** Stomach Duodenum Transverse colon Omentum Urachus Small intestine Aorta Lymph nodes	**6 Left lumbar region** Descending colon Small intestine Left kidney **7 Right iliac fossa** Caecum Vermiform appendix Lymph nodes **8 Hypogastric region** Small intestine Sigmoid flexure Distended bladder Urachus Enlarged uterus and adnexa **9 Left iliac fossa** Sigmoid flexure Lymph nodes

situated in the abdominal wall itself that have already been described, are as follows:

Right hypochondriac region

Most tumours in this area are connected with the liver or gallbladder, and their differential diagnosis is discussed under LIVER, ENLARGEMENT OF (p. 375) and GALLBLADDER, PALPABLE (p. 232).

An easily made mistake is to regard the firm and rounded swelling produced by the upper segment of the right rectus abdominis muscle, especially in a well-developed subject, as a tumour of the liver or gallbladder. In such cases the characteristic dull note of the liver on percussion over the lower right chest ceases at the costal margin.

Tumours in connection with the hepatic flexure of the colon, scybalous collections in the hepatic flexure region, or the head of an intussusception may present as masses in this area.

Epigastric region

Enlargement of the *liver* may be felt in this area, and indeed it is common to feel the normal liver in this region, especially in infants and in adults with an acute costal angle. The dilated stomach produced by pyloric stenosis in either children or adults may present as a visible swelling demonstrating waves of peristalsis travelling from left to right. A succussion splash is usually elicited. Tumours of the stomach, apart from malignant growth, are rare. A hundred years ago a hair ball or trichobezoar was frequently encountered as an epigastric mass in hysterical girls who chewed and swallowed their hair, which then formed an exact mould of the stomach. Hairballs are only rarely encountered these days, and modern textbooks hardly mention them; however, as fashions and hair styles change they may reappear on the clinical scene (Fig. A.4). Other foreign bodies are sometimes ingested by mental defectives and form a palpable mass. In congenital pyloric stenosis a tumour the size of a small marble is palpable at the right border of the right rectus.

The *transverse colon* usually passes across the upper part of the umbilical area, and may be palpated when it is the site of a carcinoma, when it is impacted with faeces, or when it is distended by a large-bowel obstruction placed distal to it.

Swellings in connection with the *omentum* may be due to tuberculous peritonitis or, more commonly, due to infiltration with secondary malignant deposits.

Swellings arising from the *pancreas* push forward from the depths of the abdominal cavity towards the epigastric and the upper part of the umbilical areas, and present themselves as vaguely palpable deeply seated masses. They have the stomach, or the stomach and colon, in front of them and are fixed to the posterior abdominal wall, thus moving but little on respiration.

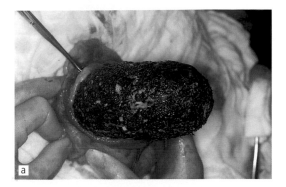 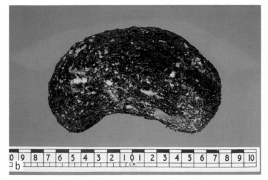

Figure A.4 Gastric hairball (trichobezoar). This formed a large, mobile epigastric mass in a young woman with long hair. (a) The mass being removed at gastrotomy. (b) The removed specimen.

They may transmit a non-expansile pulsation from the subjacent aorta. Unless extremely large, such swellings are resonant on percussion, due to the overlying air-filled gut. A pancreatic swelling may be carcinomatous, in which case wasting, anaemia and jaundice are likely to be observed. There may be clay-coloured stools and dark urine, and it is important to note that frequently the onset of jaundice is preceded by deeply placed abdominal pain, or pain in the back. Glycosuria of recent origin in an elderly patient also raises suspicion of a pancreatic carcinoma. In about half the patients with jaundice due to carcinomatous obstruction the gallbladder is palpably distended (Courvoisier's law). Occasionally, the mass may result from chronic pancreatitis; the swollen pancreas of acute pancreatitis has only exceptionally been palpated before laparotomy.

Pancreatic cysts are the pancreatic swellings which are most commonly palpable. Only 20 per cent are true cysts; these are either single or multiple retention cysts which usually result from chronic pancreatitis, neoplastic cysts (cystadenoma and cystadenocarcinoma) and the rare congenital polycystic disease of the pancreas and hydatid cyst of the pancreas. Far more often the cysts are not in the pancreas itself but comprise a collection of fluid sealed off in the lesser sac due to closure of the foramen of Winslow (pseudocyst of the pancreas). This may occur after trauma to the pancreas, following acute pancreatitis or, much less commonly, resulting from perforation of a posterior gastric ulcer. They may reach an enormous size and fill the whole upper part of the abdomen.

Retroperitoneal cysts are rare. The majority arise from remnants of the mesonephric (Wolffian) duct and occur in adult women. Others are teratomatous, lymphangiomatous or dermoid.

Retroperitoneal tumours (apart from those arising in the pancreas, suprarenal gland or kidney) originate in the mesenchymal tissues, the sympathetic chain and the para-aortic lymph nodes.

Swellings in connection with the *duodenum* are exceedingly rare. They may result from an inflammatory mass developing around a penetrating duodenal ulcer, or be due to a duodenal malignant tumour, but the latter is a pathological curiosity. Those in connection with the *kidneys* and *suprarenal glands* are found in the epigastrium only if very large. Their diagnosis is considered below.

Enlargement of the *spleen* may bring its anterior edge into the epigastric area; a splenic swelling always lies in contact with the anterior wall of the abdomen (see SPLENOMEGALY, p. 667).

Lymph nodes, which are numerous in the para-aortic retroperitoneal tissues and in the mesentery, may become palpable in reticuloses, tuberculous peritonitis, or malignant disease as nodulated chains or masses.

Left hypochondriac region

An abnormal lobe or a tumour in the left lobe of the *liver* may appear as a superficial tumour in this area. Much of the *stomach* normally lies in the left hypochondrium; the diagnosis of gastric swelling has been considered above, and a gastric tumour is commonly felt in this region. On physical signs alone it must be differentiated from a swelling of the adjoining *spleen*. A barium-meal X-ray examination, ultrasound or CT scan help considerably in differentiating between a gastric and a splenic swelling.

The diagnosis of a tumour of the splenic flexure of the *colon*, whether scybalous or malignant, is arrived at in the same way as a case of a tumour of the hepatic flexure or transverse colon (see 'Right hypochondriac region' and 'Epigastric region').

The diagnosis of various causes of enlargement of the *spleen* is discussed under SPLENOMEGALY (p. 667). The distinguishing features are that the spleen comes down from under the left costal margin in direct contact with the anterior abdominal wall (and is therefore dull on percussion), descends on inspiration, has a smooth surface, and a notch may be palpable on its inner margin. A splenic swelling may be identified on a plain X-ray of the abdomen and differentiated from a renal mass by means of pyelography. A barium-meal examination may show displacement and indentation of the adjacent stomach. Ultrasound or CT scan will clinch the diagnosis.

Tumours of the *pancreas* may project into the left hypochondrium, as may retroperitoneal tumours and cysts (see 'Epigastric region').

Tumours of the left *kidney* and *suprarenal gland* have the stomach and colon in front of them and therefore, unless extremely large, are resonant on percussion. Since they arise in the loin, these masses can usually be balloted by bimanual palpation.

Right lumbar region

Occasionally, a congenital projection of the liver, known as Riedel's lobe, may appear as a superficial tumour continuous with the liver above it in this zone. It may be mistaken for a dilated gallbladder.

The *ascending colon* may be palpable due to contained faecal masses, owing to thickening as a result of long-standing colitis, Crohn's disease or hyperplastic tuberculosis, or due to malignant disease.

The ascending colon can be felt in acute or chronic *ileocaecal and ileocolic intussusception* as a sausage-shaped tumour, at first situated in the right flank, then moving across the abdomen above the umbilicus and finally down the left flank into the pelvis. The vast majority of these cases occur in infants or young children, commonly aged between 3 and 12 months. Boys are affected twice as often as girls. The history is of paroxysms of abdominal colic typified by screaming and pallor. There is vomiting and usually the passage of blood and mucus per rectum, giving the characteristic 'red-currant jelly stool'. A rectal examination nearly always reveals this typical feature, and rarely the tip of the intussusception can be felt. In infants there is usually no obvious cause, but the mesenteric lymph nodes in these cases are invariably enlarged. In adults a polyp, carcinoma or an inverted Meckel's diverticulum may form the apex of the intussusception.

Tumours in connection with the *right kidney* and *suprarenal gland* usually appear deep down in this region, having the ascending colon and small intestine in front of them. They can be lifted forwards en masse from behind by a hand placed at the back of the loin and thus palpated bimanually. For their diagnosis, see KIDNEY, PALPABLE (p. 360). The lower pole of the right kidney can be felt in some normal persons on deep abdominal palpation, especially in thin females. When abnormally low and mobile, the whole of the otherwise normal kidney may be palpable. Its shape and consistency are characteristic. Renal swellings move on respiration and, unless very large, are resonant on percussion due to the anteriorly related gut. However, Riedel's lobe of the liver, an enlarged gallbladder, masses in the ascending colon and secondary deposits in the omentum have all been mistaken for it, although they are more superficially placed and lie in contact with the anterior abdominal wall. Other wandering masses, for example those arising from the ovary, Fallopian tube and mesentery, as well as hydatid cysts, are all liable to the same error of identification.

Imaging by means of ultrasound or CT scanning is invaluable in assistance with the differential diagnosis.

Umbilical region

The grossly dilated *stomach* resulting from long-standing pyloric obstruction may occupy the umbilical region; indeed it may descend below it down into the pelvis.

Tumours in connection with the *transverse colon* have been considered in 'Epigastric region' and 'Right lumbar region' above.

Tumours in connection with the *omentum* are common in this region; those arising from the small intestine are much rarer, although the thickened small bowel in Crohn's disease may form a palpable mass.

Swellings arising from the *kidneys, suprarenal glands, pancreas, retroperitoneal tissues, para-aortic nodes* and *mesentery* may all present themselves in the deeper parts of the umbilical region, usually as more or less fixed masses arising from or connected with the posterior wall of the abdomen.

The aorta bifurcates 1 cm below and to the left of the umbilicus in the supracristal plane, as shown in Fig. A.3 (at the level of the 4th lumbar vertebra). In thin patients, pulsation of the normal aorta can often be felt and indeed seen in this region, and may lead to the incorrect diagnosis of an abdominal aneurysm. Careful examination, however, will show that this pulsation is no more than a throbbing, an up-and-down movement, and is not laterally expansile. Aneurysm of the abdominal aorta forms an expansile mass situated above the umbilicus itself, and may be accompanied by pain in the back from erosion of the bodies of the lumbar vertebrae. Often, X-rays of the abdomen in such cases will reveal calcification in the aneurysmal wall. Ultrasound and CT enable accurate delineation of the size and extent of the aneurysm. These methods are also valuable in the visualization of the other retroperitoneal masses enumerated above.

Left lumbar region

An enlarged *spleen* (see 'Left hypochondriac region') may protrude into this area. It forms a firm mass which is in contact with the abdominal wall, and its dullness to percussion continues with its thoracic dullness, which extends back up into the axilla along the line of the 9th or 10th ribs. Tumours in connection with the *right kidney*, the *right suprarenal gland* and the *descending colon* give similar features to those considered in 'Left hypochondriac region' above.

Right iliac fossa

An inflammatory mass in this region is most commonly associated with an *appendix abscess*. Less commonly, there may be a *paracaecal abscess* in relation to a perforated carcinoma of the caecum, or a solitary caecal benign ulcer. A *pyosalpinx* may result from salpingitis and, rarely, inflammatory swellings may arise in connection with suppurating *iliac lymph nodes* or a *psoas abscess*.

An important differential diagnosis is between an appendix mass and a carcinoma of the caecum. Usually, in the former there is a preceding episode of an acute abdominal pain, typical of appendicitis, with fever and leucocytosis. The inflammatory mass subsides progressively over 2–3 weeks, and the occult blood test in the stools is negative. A carcinoma of the caecum may be suspected if there is a preceding history

of bowel disturbance in a middle-aged or elderly patient, if the mass fails to resolve rapidly, and if the occult blood test in the stools is repeatedly positive. If there is any clinical doubt, a barium-enema X-ray examination should be carried out and, if necessary, resort made to laparotomy.

It is not at all rare for a soft 'squelchy' caecum to be palpable in a perfectly normal thin female subject.

Occasionally, a grossly distended *gallbladder* may project down as far as the right iliac fossa and a low-lying *kidney* may form a palpable mass in this region. An *ovarian tumour* or cyst or a pedunculated *fibroid* of the uterus may project into this area.

Hypogastric region

The commonest mass to be felt in this region, after the pregnant uterus, is the distended *bladder*. This may reach as high as, or slightly above, the umbilicus. Not uncommonly this midline structure tilts over to one or the other side. A distended bladder has been tapped as ascites, operated upon as an ovarian cyst or fibroid, or mistaken for the pregnant uterus. No diagnostic opinion should be advanced, and no operative procedure undertaken respecting a tumour in this situation, until the bladder has been emptied, either by voluntary micturition or by the passing of a catheter.

Abdominal swellings arising from the *uterus*, *ovaries*, *Fallopian tubes* and *uterine ligaments* may all rise up out of the pelvis and present themselves as swellings in this region; as they grow larger they may be spread into any part of the abdomen. While they remain comparatively small and are manifestedly connected with some intrapelvic organ, their origin is not difficult to determine (see PELVIS, SWELLING IN, p. 523). However, when they have extended into the abdomen or have acquired a long pedicle, or have become fixed by adhesions to some distant part of the abdominal wall or to some other viscus, these pelvic tumours may give rise to signs and symptoms which bear no relation to pelvic disease. In such cases they may only be correctly diagnosed at laparotomy. The discerning clinician will always remember the possibility of pregnancy in every female patient between the menarche and menopause.

Tumours of ileal Crohn's disease arising in the *small intestine* may be felt in the hypogastric area.

The *urachus* is a fibrous cord running in the middle line in front of the peritoneum from the fundus of the bladder to the umbilicus. Occasionally, it becomes the seat of cyst formation, more often in women than in men. The urachal cyst is a rounded tumour lying between the umbilicus and the pubic symphysis, which occasionally becomes infected.

Left iliac fossa

The *pelvic colon* can often be felt in normal subjects as a tube-like cord, either when empty and in spasm, or else when distended with faecal masses. The region is a common site for carcinoma of the colon, and there are usually symptoms of chronic intestinal obstruction, or bowel disturbance with the passage of blood and mucus in the stools. It is clinically impossible to differentiate between such a mass and that associated with diverticular disease of the sigmoid colon. Similarly, a paracolic abscess in this region may equally well be associated with suppuration of an inflamed colonic diverticulum or a perforating carcinoma. Rarely, such an abscess may be due to perforation of the tip of a long *appendix* passing over the left iliac fossa, or as an extreme rarity due to local perforation of a left-sided appendix in transposition of the viscera. The diagnosis of this would be suggested by finding the cardiac apex beat to lie on the *right* side.

Harold Ellis

ALCOHOL

While some patients readily declare alcohol misuse, many do not. There are a number of common presentations that oblige the doctor to enquire carefully about the possibility of alcohol misuse. These are most readily grouped into *medical* (e.g. falls, fits, head injuries, haematemesis, jaundice), *psychiatric* (e.g. panic attacks, amnesic blackouts, confusional states, deliberate self-harm) and *social* (e.g. road traffic accidents, victim or perpetrator of violent crime, domestic violence, rough sleeping). These may be the current presenting complaint or prominent in the past history. It is estimated that up to 20 per cent of UK medical admissions are for conditions caused by alcohol misuse, yet too few medical admissions have their drinking habits adequately assessed.

The assessment of alcohol misuse has three aims: (i) to quantify use; (ii) to catalogue any alcohol-related problems the patient has; and (iii) to detect alcohol dependence syndrome if present.

Quantifying use by direct questioning is not always doomed to fail. The aim is to establish how many units the individual consumes in a typical week (or on a 'heavy session' if the pattern is binge drinking rather than regular drinking). One unit of alcohol is a small glass of 13 per cent wine or a half-pint (270 ml) of 3 per cent lager. Consumption exceeding 21 units per week for a woman, or 28 units per week for a man, will inevitably prove harmful to health in the long term. A high percentage of the UK population, including many teenagers, currently exceed these recommended limits.

The distinction between alcohol-related problems and alcohol dependence (addiction) is very useful. Alcohol dependence syndrome consists of:

- withdrawal symptoms (i.e. tremor, sweating, retching, anxiety);
- relief drinking (i.e. drinking alcohol specifically to avoid or reduce withdrawal symptoms, perhaps in the morning);
- tolerance (i.e. requiring ever-increasing quantities of alcohol to achieve the same effect);
- a stereotyped pattern of drinking taking precedence over other activities;
- craving; and
- rapid reinstatement after abstinence (i.e. immediately resuming heavy drinking after a period of abstinence).

Alcohol-related problems should be systematically sought and catalogued in the past medical history, past psychiatric history and social history.

Medical problems

These include: gastrointestinal irritation and bleeding, cirrhosis, epileptic fits, head injuries, accidents, fractures, osteoporosis, gynaecomastia, testicular atrophy, neuropathy, pancreatitis and diabetes mellitus.

Psychiatric problems

These include: anxiety, panic attacks, agoraphobia, dysphoria, deliberate self-harm, delirium tremens, amnesic blackouts, alcoholic hallucinosis, morbid jealousy, Wernicke's encephalopathy, amnesic syndrome and dementia.

Social problems

These include: debt, dismissal from accommodation, work and relationships, drink-driving offences, shoplifting and domestic violence.

The features of alcohol dependence can develop insidiously in the absence of any alcohol-related problems in some people, classically in the wealthy professional who comfortably affords the alcohol, and is generally well nourished and well supported. Conversely, it is possible to accrue several alcohol-related problems in a single evening of heavy drinking with no alcohol dependency at all.

Andrew Hodgkiss

ALOPECIA

Hair loss has a psychological impact which is out of all proportion to its physical significance, although disorders causing hair fall may also sometimes be a marker for systemic disorders. Convenient clinical division of the possible causes of alopecia can be made by considering: (i) whether obvious scalp skin abnormality is present or not (Table A.3); or (ii) the distribution of hair loss, e.g. localized, generalized or male-patterned.

Patchy hair, thinning/balding with obvious scalp skin disease

Hair loss is surprisingly uncommon in eczema and psoriasis of the scalp, even when these conditions are

severe. Allergic contact sensitivity to hair dye is a common cause of a severe eczematous eruption of the scalp, face and neck, but hair loss is rarely a major feature. Small infants with a severe generalized atopic eczema may produce a patch of alopecia at the occiput through habitual rubbing of the head on the pillow.

One or more localized bald areas on the scalp associated with broken stubbly hairs, and scaling of the affected area of the scalp, is always suggestive of tinea capitis (scalp ringworm) (see SCALP AND BEARD, FUNGUS AFFECTIONS OF, p. 628). The degree of surrounding inflammation and scaling is very variable, and depends on the fungus responsible, and the host response. Cattle ringworm (*Trichophyton verrucosum*) may produce a particularly violent reaction, with swelling, discharge, and local lymphadenopathy. Microscopical examination and subsequent cultural identification confirms the diagnosis. *Bacterial folliculitis*, if extensive enough, sometimes perpetuated by infestation with head lice, can cause patchy hairfall. Pustules should be easily found, and there will be draining lymphadenopathy A sterile inflammatory folliculitis (folliculitis decalvans) is a rare cause of patchy balding in middle-aged scalps.

Scarring alopecia

Should the scalp skin be obviously tethered and scarred around the balding area, a search should be

Table A.3 Characteristics of alopecia

Characteristic	Scalp skin abnormal	Scalp skin normal

Patches of hair thinning/balding	Dermatitis
	  Seborrhoeic
	  Contact allergic
	Tinea capitis
	Folliculitis
	  Bacterial
	  Decalvans
	Lupus erythematosus
	Lichen planus
	Morphoea
	Hot-combing
	Radiotherapy
	Lupus vulgaris
	Pseudo-pelade
		Alopecia areata
		Secondary syphilis
		
		Trichotillomania
		Traction alopecia

Diffuse hair thinning/balding		Alopecia totalis Telogen effluvium: 3/12 post-trigger event Anagen effluvium: drugs and poisons Endocrinopathy
Male-patterned hair thinning/balding		Androgenic alopecia

made for signs of lupus erythematosus (fixed, sharply demarcated patches of erythema, scaling with follicular plugging and telangiectasia, often with marginal activity and central depigmentation), or lichen planus (Fig. A.5) (flat-topped papules on the wrists, lace-like white areas on the buccal mucosae). More esoteric causes of scarring alopecia include radiotherapy, lupus vulgaris (Figs A.6 and A.7), hotcombing in Negroes and pseudo-pelade of Brocq. If scarring is linear, and especially if it extends to the forehead and has a violaceous edge, then localized scleroderma (morphoea) may be the cause. The whole lesion has the appearance of an exaggerated scar – en coup de sabre.

Patchy hair, thinning/balding with normal underlying scalp

Alopecia areata (Fig. A.8) is the commonest cause of patchy baldness. The patches are asymptomatic, and are often discovered by relatives or hairdressers. Patients of any age are affected, especially those in late childhood or early teens. The hallmark of this disease is a neat, sharply localized patch of billiard-ball baldness with no obvious inflammation or scaling at the edge of lesions, where the diagnostic exclamation-mark hairs should be searched for. There are usually two or three patches, and sometimes these coalesce at an alarming rate and may even cause *alopecia totalis* of the scalp, or *alopecia universalis* (Fig. A.9) where beard and all body hairs are lost. The course and prognosis are highly variable, but generally good. On average, two or three patches appear, remain stable

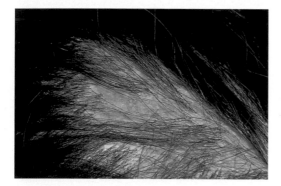

Figure A.5 Lichen planus with scarring alopecia (Graham – Little syndrome).

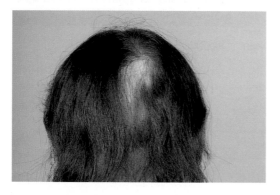

Figure A.6 Alopecia secondary to sarcoidosis.

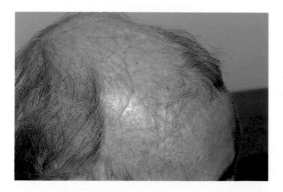

Figure A.7 Alopecia secondary to radiation.

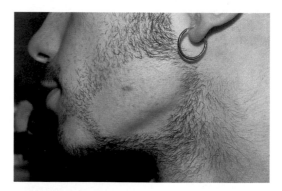

Figure A.8 Alopecia areata.

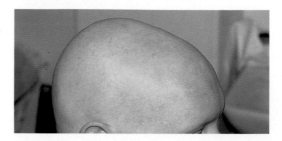

Figure A.9 Alopecia universalis.

for anything up to 6 months, and then regrow without trace within 12 months. Initially regrowth is often white. The cause is unknown. There is a family history in 30 per cent of cases, and it is occasionally associated with autoimmune diseases such as vitiligo, thyroid disease, pernicious anaemia or Addison's disease. A convincing preceding history of emotional shock is given by a proportion of patients, and may be a trigger factor.

Syphilis is uncommon nowadays, but is a diagnosis that must not be overlooked. Patchy alopecia may be a feature of the secondary phase. The appearance is of an asymptomatic patchy 'moth-eaten' baldness. On examination there is no scaling or obvious scalp disease and, in contrast to alopecia areata, the baldness is partial rather than complete. Exclamation-mark hairs are not seen, and the patches are more numerous and accompanied by fever, sore throat and lymphadenopathy. The serology is positive, and the hair regrows after antibiotic treatment.

Trichotillomania is the rather cumbersome title given to what often amounts to only a 'habit tic'. If hair is twirled between the fingers it eventually breaks, leaving patches of shortened hairs. Microscopic examination reveals obvious fractured ends to affected hairs. Some psychiatrically disturbed individuals pursue hair pulling and produce bald patches. The fractures may be seen at the scalp surface, or even at the roots.

Traction alopecia is seen at the hair margins and is due to regular hair-dressing techniques pulling on the hairs; examples include rollers, braiding, ethnic plaiting (Fig. A.10) and tight pony tails.

Diffuse alopecia without scalp disease

Telogen effluvium

A growing (anagen) hair has a large bulb which is easily seen with a hand lens on plucking. When growth ceases, the bulb shrinks and the hair enters a resting (telogen) phase for 3 months before falling (catagen). In healthy adults some 50–100 hairs enter telogen daily and thus fall some 3 months later. Not surprisingly, certain events upset the hair cycle, whereupon a larger number of hairs cease growing and enter telogen. Three months later they will fall as a so-called 'telogen effluvium'.

Triggering events include childbirth, stopping the contraceptive pill, a febrile illness, blood loss, an

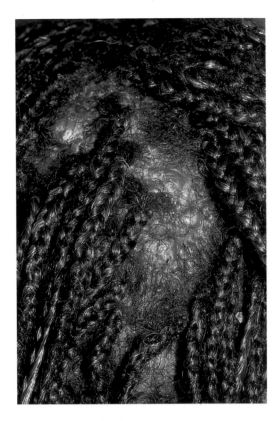

Figure A.10 Traction alopecia.

operation, myocardial infarction, stroke, rapid weight loss, bereavement or other psychological stress. The patient often complains of a worrying increase in hairfall, but on examining the scalp no obvious abnormality is seen, although if the hair is gently grasped between thumb and finger many telogen hairs may be detached. Further evidence can be obtained by asking patients to collect their daily hairfall from hair brushes and pillows. Normally, between 50 and 100 hairs can be collected, and 300–400 can fall daily in telogen effluvium. The prognosis is excellent.

Anagen effluvium

Fall of growing hairs also causes diffuse hair shedding, and may occur after exposure to certain drugs or poisons, for example cytotoxics, isotretinoin, thiouracil, anticoagulants, excess vitamin A and thallium poisoning.

Diffuse hairfall occurs in endocrinopathy, for example myxoedema, hypopituitarism and hypoparathyroidism (Fig. A.11). Myxoedema is regularly

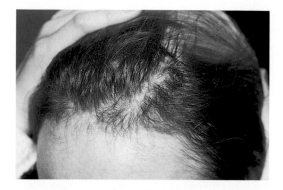

Figure A.11 Diffuse hair thinning with myxoedema.

accompanied by hair thinning. The mechanism is unknown, and may not be directly related to serum thyroxine level as adequate replacement therapy may fail to reverse the process. Hair loss may be a feature of systemic lupus erythematosus, and may even be the presenting symptom.

Male-pattern baldness without obvious scalp disease

Male-pattern baldness is not a disease, but rather an accelerated physiological process, being especially pronounced in those with a genetic predisposition. Males and females progressively lose androgen-dependent scalp hairs with increasing age – in males with successive thinning of bitemporal, occipital and pate areas, and in females with a more diffuse patterned thinning over most of the vertex. Some individuals have increased sensitivity of their hair follicles to normal levels of circulating androgens and lose their androgen-dependent hair earlier. Such hairfall does not occur in castrates and oestrogens, and anti-androgenic drugs appear to have a protective effect. The prognosis for regrowth is poor, although it may be retarded by therapy with finasteride or minoxidil.

Barry Monk

AMENORRHOEA

Amenorrhoea can be defined as the absence of menstruation, which can be either temporary or permanent. It may occur as a normal physiological event

before puberty, as a result of pregnancy and subsequent lactation or the onset of the menopause. It may be a symptom of a non-physiological problem which may be systemic or gynaecological in origin.

Primary amenorrhoea is the failure to menstruate by the age of 16 years when the girl has developed normal secondary sexual characteristics **OR** failure to menstruate at the age of 14 years in the absence of any secondary sexual characteristics. This definition aids the diagnostic differentiation of causes which include reproductive tract anomalies, gonadal quiescence or gonadal failure. Primary amenorrhoea may result from congenital abnormalities in the development of the ovaries, genital tract (Figs A.13 and O.1, p. 497) or external genitalia or disturbance of the normal

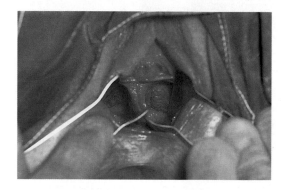

Figure A.12 Double vagina.

endocrinological events at the time of puberty. Some of these structural abnormalities may lead to cryptomenorrhoea, where menstruation is taking place but the menstrual flow is unable to escape due to some closure of part of the genital tract.

Most of the non-genital tract causes of secondary amenorrhoea (see below) can also cause primary amenorrhoea if these conditions occur before puberty. Delay in the onset of puberty is often constitutional. It is important to exclude the possibility of primary ovarian failure or dysfunction of the hypothalamic–pituitary axis. As a general rule, 40 per cent of cases of primary amenorrhoea are due to endocrine disorders and the remainder (60%) are due to developmental abnormalities.

The definition of *secondary amenorrhoea* has usually been taken to be the cessation of menstruation for six consecutive months in a woman who has had regular periods, though recently it has been suggested

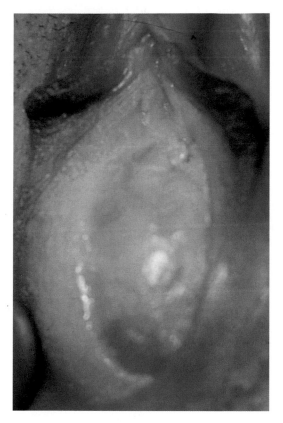

Figure A.13 Imperforate hymen with bluish tinge of blood distending the hymen.

important to exclude pregnancy. Serum investigations should include prolactin, gonadotrophins [follicle-stimulating hormone (FSH) and luteinizing hormone (LH)] and the thyroid function tests.

Raised serum prolactin levels >1500 iu/l may indicate the need for a CT or MRI scan of the pituitary fossa to exclude a hypothalamic tumour. Serum FSH levels >40 iu/l usually suggest irreversible ovarian failure. Raised serum FSH and LH levels usually suggest ovarian failure, but raised LH levels alone may indicate polycystic ovarian syndrome (PCOS) which can be confirmed by ultrasound scan of the ovaries. PCOS amenorrhoea is secondary to acylical ovarian activity and continuous oestrogen production. Abnormally low serum levels of FSH and LH suggests failure at the level of the hypothalamus and pituitary, giving hypogonadotrophic hypogonadism. Kallman's syndrome is associated with hypogonadotrophic hypogonadism, and these patients have hyposmia and/or colour blindness.

Chromosomal abnormalities (e.g. Turner's syndrome 45XO) can be diagnosed by karyotyping. Auto-antibody screens should be undertaken in women with a premature menopause. Premature menopause can be associated with an increased risk of heart disease, and consequently it may be useful to check serum cholesterol levels in these patients. Women with PCOS and prolonged amenorrhoea have an increased risk of endometrial hyperplasia and carcinoma, and endometrial sampling may be useful if any abnormal bleeding occurs.

Primary amenorrhoea

Chromosomal

In *Turner's syndrome* (gonadal dysgenesis) there is also dwarfism, web-neck, cubitus valgus, and an XO sex-chromosome pattern. This is the commonest form of gonadal dysgenesis, and these women may develop spontaneous menstruation, though premature ovarian failure is common. The gonadotrophin levels may be raised, and these individuals may require hormone replacement therapy (HRT). Spontaneous conceptions have been reported, but many would require some form of assisted conception in order to have an intrauterine pregnancy.

In *testicular feminization* (which is in reality androgen insensitivity), the form is female with well-developed breasts but absent or sparse pubic and

that cessation of periods for 3–4 months may be considered pathological and warrant investigation.

Regardless of the type of amenorrhoea, a thorough history and examination should be undertaken. Examination needs to include the stature and body form of the individual, and the height and weight should be measured and converted into a body mass index [BMI = weight in kg/(height in metres)^2]. Inspection should concentrate on the presence or absence of secondary sexual characteristics and the appearance of the external genitalia. It is essential that this be undertaken before requesting any investigations. Most cases of secondary amenorrhoea, by definition, would exclude congenital anomalies unless the individual had been using the oral contraceptive pill which would induce a withdrawal bleed each month. Vaginal examination may be inappropriate in someone under the age of 16 years or who had not been sexually active. Abdominal ultrasound scanning is very useful to define the anatomy. It is ALWAYS axillary hair, while the gonad – which may be found in the groin or in the abdomen – is a testicle. The gonadal tissue should be removed because of the increased risk of malignancy. In ovarian dysgenesis, there are streak ovaries, an infantile uterus and absent secondary sexual characteristics (Fig. A.14). In these cases, a buccal smear for sex chromatin and a chromosome analysis on a sample of peripheral blood are indicated. In ovarian dysgenesis there is a chromatin negative smear, but only 45 chromosomes; a single X chromosome (XO); in testicular feminization the smear is also chromatin-negative but there are 46 chromosomes, XY. Gonadal biopsy is also helpful in diagnosis.

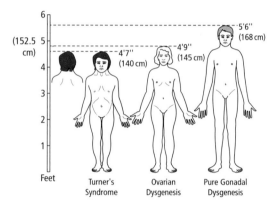

Figure A.14 Characteristics of ovarian dysgenesis. [Prof. Paul Polani.]

Müllerian duct abnormalities

The Wolffian (mesonephric) ducts regress in the embryo after the sixth week if there is no Y chromosome present. The Müllerian (paramesonephric) ducts will develop into the tubes and uterus, and fuse caudally with the urogenital sinus to produce the vagina. Abnormalities may occur in the process of fusion, and these may be medial or vertical and give rise to primary amenorrhoea. Complete or partial Müllerian agenesis may occur. In these cases, the genotype is 46XX with normal secondary sexual characteristics and normal ovarian tissue, but the vagina is short and may require surgery. There may also be associated urinary tract abnormalities.

The commonest form of abnormality is that of an imperforate hymen, and this leads to primary amenorrhoea or cryptomenorrhoea (hidden menses). The secondary sexual characteristics are normal. The individual may complain of cyclical pain and abdominal distension. It is not unusual for these cases to present with retention of urine and on inspection have a bulging hymen. A cruciate incision releases the menses, and that is all that is necessary.

Secondary amenorrhoea

Genital tract abnormalities

There is potential for scarring anywhere within the genital outflow tract. Ashermann's syndrome is a condition where intrauterine adhesions develop which prevent normal endometrial growth. This is an uncommon condition, but it may occur following vigorous curettage at the time of an evacuation of the uterus or suction termination of pregnancy.

Cervical stenosis can cause cryptomenorrhoea with development of a haematometra, and may occur due to repeated treatment of the cervix for precancerous lesions. Radiotherapy may have an effect on the cervix and uterus if used for advanced cancer of the cervix, and may possibly cause vaginal stenosis. In these cases the amenorrhoea is more likely be related to the radiotherapy effect on the ovaries than to outflow obstruction.

Systemic disorders

Chronic disease may cause menstrual disorders as a consequence of the general disease state, weight loss or effects on the hypothalamic–pituitary axis. Certain disorders will affect gonadal function directly. Chronic renal disease will act by increasing the serum LH level and also prolactin levels, possibly due to reduced clearance.

Weight-related amenorrhoea

Body weight/BMI can have a significant effect on the regulation and release of serum gonadotrophins. Menstruation will not occur regularly if the BMI falls below 18–19 kg/m^2, and it is estimated that 22 per cent of female body weight should be fat to ensure ovulatory cycles. Fat in the form of adipose tissue is a source of oestrogen by the aromatization of androgens to oestrogen. This ensures the appropriate feedback mechanism of the hypothalamic–pituitary–ovarian (HPO) axis. The weight loss may be due to illness, exercise or dieting. Potential sequelae of the condition may be long-term effects on the bone.

Stress in itself is unlikely to give amenorrhoea lasting longer than 2 months, unless it is associated with debilitation. Exercise – particularly in endurance events – is a common cause of amenorrhoea, and this is usually related to the BMI and body fat content as described above.

Hypothalamic causes

These are uncommon and include craniopharyngioma, gliomas and dermoid cysts. The mechanism of action may be to destroy local tissue or disrupt dopamine production, resulting in hyperprolactinaemia. Treatment is usually surgical and possibly radiotherapy; HRT may be necessary, together with other hormonal supplementation.

Other causes would include systemic conditions in the form of tuberculosis or sarcoid. Head injury or irradiation may have a similar effect. Profound hypotension following delivery can cause Sheehan's syndrome, which affects the pituitary to cause necrosis, as it is an end artery with no collateral supply to protect it in this situation. Appropriate agents may induce ovulation.

Table A.4 Classification of amenorrhoea

- **Physiological**
  - Before puberty
  - After the menopause
  - During pregnancy
  - During lactation
- **Hypothalamic**
  - Primary hypothalamic–pituitary failure
  - Following oral contraceptive use
  - Anterior pituitary failure (Sheehan's disease)
- **Pituitary**
- **Ovarian**
  - Congenital absence of ovaries (rare)
  - Ovarian agenesis
  - Gonadal dysgenesis (Turner's syndrome)
  - Destruction of both ovaries by double ovarian growths
  - Polycystic ovary disease
  - Resistant ovarian syndrome
  - Certain rate-functioning tumours of the ovary: arrhenoblastoma; granulosa-cell tumour
- **Genital outflow (uterine, cervix, vagina and vulva)**
  - Imperforate vagina
  - Imperforate hymen
  - Absence of the vagina
  - Imperforate cervix
  - Double uterus with retention
  - Congenital absence of uterus
  - Uterine hypoplasia of infantile type
  - Uterine hypoplasia of adult type
  - Haematocolpos
  - Haematometra
  - Haematosalpinx
- **Acquired**
  - Ashermann's syndrome
  - Pelvic inflammation
  - Closure of the vagina
    - Due to radiotherapy
    - Due to injury
  - Closure of the cervix
    - Due to injury
    - Following operations (e.g. loop cone biopsy)
- **Endocrine**
  - Myxoedema
  - Addison's disease
  - Thyrotoxicosis
  - Adrenal hyperplasia
  - Adrenal cortical tumours
  - Acromegaly
- **Iatrogenic**
  - Pelvic irradiation
  - Hysterectomy
  - Depo-Provera
  - Progesterone-only contraception
  - Mirena coil
- **General**
  - Anaemia
  - Leukaemia
  - Hodgkin's disease
  - Malignant growths
  - Tuberculosis
  - Prolonged suppuration
  - Diabetes
  - Late stages of nephritis
  - Late stage of some forms of heart disease
  - Late stage of cirrhosis of the liver
  - Dietetic deficiencies, the result of attempts to slim
  - Toxic
  - During and after specific fevers
  - Chronic poisoning by lead, mercury, morphine, alcohol
  - Anorexia nervosa or loss of weight
  - Obesity
  - Dystrophia adipose-genitalis (Frohlich's syndrome)
  - Cretinism
  - Stress

Pituitary causes

The commonest pituitary cause of amenorrhoea is hyperprolactinaemia; this may be physiological due to lactation, or it may be iatrogenic or pathological. A non-functioning tumour or pituitary adenoma may affect dopamine secretion levels, as may prothiazines and metoclopramide. The consequence is a rise in prolactin level. Galactorrhoea may occur in up to one-third of patients, and very occasionally there may be visual field impairment.

Unless the serum prolactin level is markedly raised, it is unlikely to show any effect on the sella turcica on a lateral skull X-ray. CT or MRI scanning may be a more appropriate investigation. Treatment involves the use of a dopamine antagonist – usually bromo-criptine or a related drug. This treatment may be discontinued if the patient becomes pregnant. There may be an increase in the size of the adenomas caus-ing hyperprolactinaemia in a quarter of the women who subsequently become pregnant.

Treatment must be given to correct the amenorrhoea and oestrogen deficiency, improve libido and effect tumour shrinkage in cases with hyperprolactinaemia. It is safe to use the combined oral contraceptive pill in these women if they require contraception.

Ovarian causes

Premature ovarian failure may occur and is defined as the cessation of periods before the age of 40 years. This may be due to chromosomal abnormalities, which have already been discussed. The most common causes include autoimmune disease, as well as infec-tion, previous surgery, chemotherapy or radiotherapy.

Tumours are unusual causes of amenorrhoea, but arrhenoblastomas can cause virilism as well as amen-orrhoea, atrophy of the breasts and hirsutism.

Iatrogenic causes

The obvious causes include radiotherapy and chemo-therapy for malignant disease. Others that may need to be considered are forms of contraception including Depo-Provera, the progesterone-only pill, the mirena coil, 'post-pill' amenorrhoea as well as gonadotrophin-releasing hormone (GnRH) analogues.

Classification of amenorrhoea

The classification of amenorrhoea is listed in Table A.4.

Antony Hollingworth

AMNESIA (MEMORY DYSFUNCTION)

Memory is the ability to store and subsequently retrieve past experience, and is fundamental to many cognitive functions. Amnesia can be defined as a loss of previous memories and an inability to form new ones. Altered alertness, attention, language and motiv-ation may all confound the clinical assessment of memory function, and must be absent for the term amnesia to have clinical usefulness. Memory is con-ventionally divided into: registration (which includes perception in all modalities); encoding and storage; and retrieval. Learning includes encoding and initial storage of information.

Classification and nomenclature

Memory is not a unitary function, and can be divided up in many different ways. One classification is presented in Table A.5. It is conventional to divide memory into short-term (also called primary, imme-diate or working) memory and long-term (also called secondary) memory. *Long-term memory* may be fur-ther subdivided into recent (from initial learning to hours) and remote (extending back to childhood). *Short-term memory* is tested at the bedside by digit span testing, although poor attention can confound this test. A normal person's digit span is seven or eight digits, which are forgotten over about 30 seconds unless rehearsed. Long-term memory has been

Table A.5 Memory nomenclature

Suggested name	Immediate memory	Recent memory	Remote memory
Alternatives	Primary, short-term, working memory	Secondary memory	Semantic memory (not absolutely synonymous but conceptually similar)
Method of bedside assessment	Digit span test up to seven digits (repeating after no delay)	Recall for three to five items after 5 min	Personal history, vocabulary, beliefs

traditionally regarded as a consolidated form of short-term information, but this concept does not explain patients with impaired digit span but normal learning and long-term memory. Ribot's law states that there is an inverse relationship between memory strength and recency (i.e. older memories are better preserved), and is a useful guiding principle often seen clinically. *Semantic memory* refers to an individual's store of previously acquired facts, concepts, words and beliefs, and is conceptually rather similar to long-term memory. *Procedural memory* is outside conscious awareness, and allows the patient remember how to perform tasks, for example driving or cycling. It may be relatively resistant to disease processes that profoundly affect the recent memory system, such as Korsakoff's syndrome or Alzheimer's disease.

Functional anatomy of memory

Functional imaging of cerebral blood flow suggests that the prefrontal cortex is important for tasks involving working memory. Recent memory function involves a pathway that includes the hippocampus and the adjacent entorhinal cortex, which are richly connected to multimodal neocortical association areas. The hippocampus is thought to form new associations between ordinarily unrelated events, and damage therefore impairs learning. Midline structures, such as the medial and anterior thalamic nuclei and mamillary bodies, are also critical for recent memory. Functional imaging studies show that the hippocampus is activated during encoding; furthermore, material that evokes the most parahippocampal gyral activation is most likely to be remembered. There are anatomical links between the hippocampal formation and the midline structures, but the interaction between these structures is not well understood. The bilateral representation of the midline structures critical for memory means that bilateral cerebral damage is usually necessary to produce a severe amnesic syndrome.

Functional links between the working memory system (involving prefrontal cortex) and recent memory system (involving hippocampus, parahippocampal gyri, and midline structures) must be important in creating long-term memories, which are likely to be stored in the neocortex.

The cholinergic neurotransmitter system plays a key role in recent memory, as shown by the damage to forebrain cholinergic projections in Alzheimer's disease.

Furthermore, cholinergic antagonist drugs (e.g. scopolamine) markedly impair recent memory and learning.

The synaptic basis for encoding and storage of memories is an area of active research. The process of long-term potentiation (the modification of a synapse's strength by the neural traffic across it) has been the most widely cited mechanism by which neural networks 'learn'.

Memory disorders

Memory disorders are common, and when making a diagnosis in a clinical setting it is useful to divide them according to whether the onset is rapid or gradually progressive, and whether they are of short duration or persistent. These types of memory loss are now considered.

Recent memory loss of rapid onset and short duration

Transient global amnesia (TGA)

This is the prototype syndrome of recent memory loss with preserved attention. It occurs in middle-aged and elderly patients who develop sudden amnesia and bewilderment lasting for several hours. There is amnesia for the recent past, as well as anterograde amnesia. They typically ask questions about their circumstances over and over again: 'Where am I?', 'How did I get here?', and 'What time is it?' There is no impairment of consciousness and the ability to do even complex tasks (procedural memory) is preserved. Patients remain capable of high-level intellectual performance throughout. Normal memory function will return within minutes to hours, and the patient has no subsequent recall for the period of amnesia and a brief spell before the attack. Most patients suffer only a single attack, but there is an annual risk of recurrence of about 5 per cent. The cause of this syndrome is uncertain, but antecedent events are commonly identified, including emotion or stress, cold-water exposure, sexual intercourse and mild head trauma. It has been suggested that TGA is due to an unusual form of complex partial seizure activity or cerebral ischaemia. Recent data from diffusion-weighted magnetic resonance imaging showed restricted diffusion in the left mesial temporal lobe in seven of 10 patients during an attack, suggesting that TGA may have similarities with the cortical spreading depression thought to underlie migrainous aura propagation. A history of migraine is often found in patients with TGA.

In clinical practice, the important conditions to be considered in the differential diagnosis of TGA are complex partial seizures (which are shorter and involve altered awareness and other characteristic features; see FITS AND CONVULSIONS, p. 222), and posterior circulation ischaemia (which will usually cause add-itional brainstem symptoms and signs). Transient ischaemic attacks involving isolated ischaemia of the thalamus or hippocampi may produce selectively impaired recent memory and a TGA-like syndrome. Once the diagnosis of TGA is secure, the patient can be reassured that the condition is notably benign, with no increased risk of ischaemic stroke.

Ictal amnesia

Amnesia for the duration of the seizure is usual in tonic–clonic seizures, complex partial and absence seizures, due to disrupted electrical activity in com-ponents of brain memory systems. There may be brief retrograde amnesia prior to attacks as well as a period of post-ictal amnesia. Memory loss may occa-sionally be the only symptom of an epileptic seizure involving temporal lobe structures, though observers usually describe speech or motor disturbance, or auto-matic behaviours. The brief episodes of memory dis-turbance seen in childhood 'petit mal' absence may cause problems with learning and behaviour. Rarely, complex partial seizures in adults may result in pro-longed non-convulsive status epilepticus, which may last for days or weeks for which the patient is sub-sequently amnesic.

Electroconvulsive therapy

Temporary impairment of memory is almost invari-able following electroconvulsive therapy (ECT). It may be retrograde as well as anterograde. Unilateral ECT has much less effect on memory than has bilateral ECT.

Persistent recent memory loss

The disorders in which recent memory is persistently impaired are listed in Table A.6, and will now be briefly outlined.

Korsakoff's syndrome

Korrsakoff's syndrome – which was first described between 1887 and 1891 – is a dramatic example of the amnesic syndrome. It is related to thiamine deficiency and commonly associated with long-term alcohol

Table A.6 Causes of persistent recent memory loss

Korsakoff's syndrome
Head injury
Hypoxia post cardiac arrest
Anterior cerebral artery aneurysm rupture
Cerebral infarction
- Hippocampi
- Medial thalamic nuclei
Herpes simplex encephalitis
Limbic encephalitis
Structural lesions of hypothalamic–mammillary body region
- Tumours
- Granulomatous disease, e.g. sarcoidosis
Dementias
- Vascular dementia
- Alzheimer's disease
- Dementia with Lewy bodies
Frontotemporal dementias
Huntington's disease

abuse, though it can also result from other causes of thiamine deficiency such as persistent vomiting (including hyperemesis gravidarum), intestinal obstruction, malabsorption, puerperal sepsis and metastatic carcinoma. It usually follows or accompa-nies Wernicke's encephalopathy, which is character-ized by confusion, ophthalmoplegia and ataxia. The definition of a pure Korsakoff's syndrome requires that the patient be awake and attentive, responsive, and capable of understanding language, making appropriate deductions and solving problems. Newly presented information is correctly registered but can-not be retained for more than a few minutes (antero-grade amnesia or learning failure). There may be an associated variable dysfunction of recall of older memories – days, weeks or even years – that is, retro-grade amnesia. Confabulation, or falsification of memory, is commonly (but not invariably) seen. If recovery occurs, the period of retrograde amnesia shrinks but leaves the gap in memory for the period of anterograde amnesia following the illness onset. Neuropathological studies have shown degeneration of neurons and loss of myelin in the mamillary bod-ies, the anteroventral and pulvinar nuclei of the thal-amus and the fornix.

Head injury

A severe head injury, sufficient to impair conscious-ness, invariably results in amnesia for the period of unconsciousness. It is also apt to cause retrograde amnesia, which extends for seconds, minutes or sometimes hours prior to the injury, and post-traumatic amnesia (PTA), which extends for days, weeks or, rarely, months after the injury. PTA is associated with reduced orientation and difficulty in learning, and therefore has major impact on rehabilitation. The duration of the retrograde amnesia will tend to shrink with time, whereas the anterograde amnesia is more persistent. The duration of PTA is of considerable value in assessing the severity of injury and prognosis: the longer the PTA the more severe the head injury and the poorer the prognosis. As a guide, in patients with PTA duration of less than an hour, 95 per cent can be expected to return to work within 2 months; however, if the amnesia lasts over 24 hours, then only 80 per cent will return to work at 6 months. The most severely injured may remain permanently disabled. Patients who have recovered consciousness may appear capable of conversing and carrying out normal activities, yet are unable to recall these activities later when recovery is complete because they are still in a state of PTA. This can impair their rehabilitation and must be taken into account. Following recovery from PTA, patients may be forgetful and complain of problems with memory for two or three years. A residual defect remaining this long is likely to be permanent. Assessment of memory loss after head injury is difficult, and is sometimes influenced by litigation. Formal psychometric assessment of memory function should always be undertaken, though this may be difficult or impossible in the context of profound PTA.

Head injuries that do not cause loss of consciousness are unlikely to result in severe amnesia. Penetrating wounds of the head, unless they specifically injure the medial temporal lobes, are also unlikely to cause problems with memory. Permanent memory defects may follow single severe acute head injuries or repeated minor traumas, as in the case of boxers (dementia pugilistica). The pathology of memory loss after closed head injury varies. Trauma can result in cerebral oedema followed by infarction of the hippocampus and cingulate gyri. Memory loss may be due to diffuse microscopic injuries causing diffuse axonal injury. Figure A.15 demonstrates burr holes to treat extensive extradural haemorrhage in a young footballer following a clash of heads.

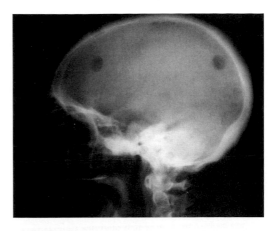

Figure A.15 Bilateral burr holes in young man.

Vascular disease

Bilateral limbic structure infarction (including hippocampi and medial thalamic nuclei) may cause persistent amnesia. There are often associated neurological signs to indicate posterior cerebral artery territory infarction, including visual disturbances, cortical blindness, aphasia or alexia. Unilateral infarction in the same areas may rarely cause problems with memory. Isolated frontal infarcts have also been reported to cause memory impairment. Patients who suffer rupture of an anterior communicating artery aneurysm, or who undergo surgical treatment for such a lesion, may suffer ischaemia (due to vasospasm) and consequent infarction in the distribution of the small penetrating branches of the anterior communicating artery. This results in damage to posterior inferior medial frontal areas and to the anterior portion of the fornix and corpus callosum. These patients may present with acute amnesia, which may recover in those in whom the ischaemia is temporary and related to vasospasm.

An acute hypoxic cerebral insult, such as that resulting from cardiac or respiratory arrest, or after carbon monoxide poisoning, may produce an irreversible amnesic syndrome because of involvement of the medial temporal lobes and thalamus.

Encephalitis and other inflammatory conditions

Herpes simplex encephalitis is a striking cause of an acute persistent amnesic syndrome. Patients with this severe illness typically present with seizures, behavioural change, encephalopathy, dysphasia and hemiparesis; because of the predilection of the virus to cause haemorrhagic infarction in the temporal lobes, there may be a specific amnesic syndrome. If memory deficits persist for one month or more, the prognosis for recovery is likely to be poor. In addition to herpes simplex infection, any pathological process involving the functional networks underlying memory systems, particularly limbic structures, can cause amnesia. Subtle cognitive decline frequently occurs in multiple sclerosis, and in rare cases there may be specific and severe memory impairment. Neurosarcoidosis, cerebral lupus and neurological Behçet's disease may also cause memory impairment. In patients with small cell lung carcinoma there is an associated form of 'limbic encephalitis' in which memory defects occur as a non-metastatic distant manifestation of the cancer. Specific antibodies to neuronal components (most commonly anti-Hu antibodies) may be identified in serum or cerebrospinal fluid. More rarely this syndrome can be associated with other tumours, including testis or breast carcinoma.

Cerebral tumour

Amnesic syndromes are rare as the presentation of cerebral tumours. They do nevertheless occur with masses arising in the diencephalic–mamillary body region in the midline. Causes include corpus callosum tumours (e.g. astrocytoma) arising in the region of the fornix. The fornix may be damaged after removal of a colloid cyst of the third ventricle, causing postoperative amnesia.

Memory loss associated with dementias

Insidious recent memory loss is the most common presenting symptom in Alzheimer's disease, and it becomes increasingly severe as the condition progresses. Other neurodegenerative conditions including the frontotemporal dementias may also involve memory function, though recent memory is typically preserved for longer into these illnesses than in Alzheimer's disease. Dementia with Lewy bodies, progressive supranuclear palsy and corticobasal degeneration may all involve progressive recent memory impairment, but should have other neurological features to suggest the correct diagnosis. Vascular dementia is another common cause of progressive (classically 'step-wise') memory impairment, and infarctions in the thalamus, hippocampi, or in white matter pathways connecting these regions to the neocortex are the probable cause. In all of these conditions the progression of memory loss is usually associated with intellectual, perceptual, linguistic, praxic, attentional, personality and mood disturbances indicating the diffuse evolving nature of the underlying pathology.

Other types of memory loss

Drug-induced

Many drugs impair memory as part of a central nervous depressant effect, but others have a more specific amnesic effect. The latter include cannabis, organic solvents, heavy metals (e.g. lead and mercury), anticonvulsants, anticholinergics and benzodiazepines. Older anticonvulsant drugs – particularly phenytoin and the barbiturates – have marked effects on memory in normal volunteers and in patients with epilepsy. The new anticonvulsant topiramate may also cause mental slowness and verbal learning disturbance. Other new anticonvulsant drugs including gabapentin and lamotrigine appear to have fewer cognitive side effects than older medications.

'Psychogenic amnesia'

Complaints of memory impairment are common in depression and anxiety, but formal assessment with psychometry will usually reveal that reduced attention motivation or low mood is the cause for the symptom. More florid psychogenic amnesic states do occur, but differ from organic amnesia in the pattern of the memory defect and in the time-course of onset and recovery. Loss of personal identity is common in psychogenic amnesia, but extremely rare in organic amnesia. The common setting of the 'psychogenic fugue', in which the patient is discovered wandering, often a long distance from home, is associated with loss of personal identity and amnesia. There may be a triggering event such as financial or marital problems. Recovery of normal learning and alertness is often sudden, but loss of personal identity and profound retrograde amnesia may persist, unlike the usual temporal memory gradient and gradual recovery seen in organic amnesias. Inability to recognize their spouse or partner is also typical. The retrospective forgetting of circumscribed periods from the past is often found after distressing events, as in wartime, but may include periods of alleged criminal activity in malingerers. Feigned amnesia may be detected by the 'two-choice' recognition test of memory, in which malingerers will score significantly worse than they would by chance.

David Werring

ANGIOMATA AND TELANGIECTASIA

An angioma is a proliferation of blood vessels and occurs as a developmental or an acquired vascular abnormality. Telangectasia (Fig. A.16) is the term applied to skin lesions composed of a network of fine visible blood vessels in the skin: it may arise in a number of congenital and acquired disorders.

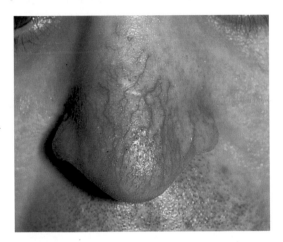

Figure A.16 Telangiectasia.

Developmental vascular abnormalities

Vascular birthmarks

Transient small salmon-pink macular birthmarks – naevus flammeus – are remarkably common, and are thought to occur in over 50 per cent of live births, affecting the sexes equally. They are most commonly on the nape of the neck, forehead or eyelids. Those on the face usually resolve within months, but the flame naevus on the nape of the neck more often persists into adult life.

The most important distinction which must be made in children is between a *vascular naevus* and a *haemangioma*. Vascular naevi, most commonly arising from a developmental anomaly of the dermal capillaries, are known as *port wine stains* (Fig. A.17).

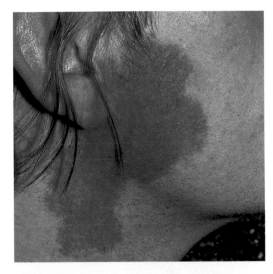

Figure A.17 Port wine stain.

They are present from birth, and persist throughout life, growing in proportion as the child grows and tending to darken in adult life. Not infrequently they have a dermatomal distribution, and when arising in relation to the trigeminal nerve may be associated with ipsilateral vascular anomalies of the brain (*Sturge–Weber syndrome*), which may manifest itself with fits, mental retardation or spasticity. Ateriovenous malformation (Fig. A.18) presents with pulsatile lesions, which may bleed torrentially following injury. By contrast, the *strawberry naevus* is a haemangioma, absent at birth, and appearing in the early weeks of

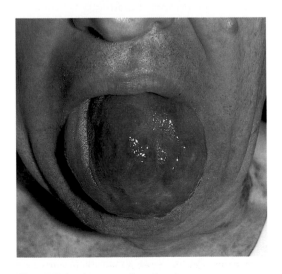

Figure A.18 Arteriovenous malformation.

life. Its alarming rate of growth may be disconcerting to the parents, but spontaneous regression will follow by the age of 8 years, and active intervention is only required if the lesion interferes with the visual axis or with feeding. Rapidly growing strawberry naevi may ulcerate, and this may be associated with haemorrhage (Fig. A.19). Rarely, a massive cavernous haemangioma may sequestrate platelets and lead to a bleeding tendency (Kasabach–Merritt syndrome).

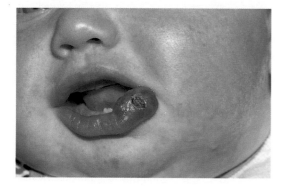

Figure A.19 Ulcerating strawberry haemangioma.

Hereditary haemorrhagic telangiectasia (Osler–Weber–Rendu syndrome) is a common genetic condition manifested by multiple small vascular lesions in the skin, associated with mucosal lesions. Cases commonly present with recurrent epistaxis, or with bleeding from the gastrointestinal tract, and female patients may suffer from menorrhagia. Occasionally, there are associated vascular anomalies in the lungs. *Generalized essential telangiectasia* may be distinguished by sparing of the mucosae, but the body is more widely affected with telangiectases, which are arborizing rather than spider. *Ataxia–telangiectasia* (Louis–Bar syndrome) is a recessively inherited immunodeficiency syndrome. Affected children are small of stature, and develop progressive cerebellar ataxia from the age of 2 years; telangiectases appear on bulbar conjunctivae, ears and cheeks from the age of 3 years.

Acquired vascular abnormalities

Cherry angiomata (Campbell de Morgan spots) develop on the trunks of almost all persons past middle age. They are usually small, from 1–3 mm in

diameter, bright red, globular and soft. They are of no systemic significance, but are said to involute spontaneously should the 8th decade of life be reached. Larger cavernous lesions, especially on the lower lips, are common in old age (*venous lakes*). Small angiomas surmounted by a variable amount of hyperkeratosis (angiokeratoma) (Fig. A.20) are common on the scrotum (angiokeratomas of Fordyce), but also occur scattered in the bathing trunk area in the extremely rare *Anderson–Fabry disease* (alpha-galactosidase deficiency) (Fig. A.21). This X-linked recessive disorder is a condition in which the diagnosis is often delayed due to the inconspicuous nature of the angiokeratomas, but it is important to recognize because renal and vascular involvement can lead to early death.

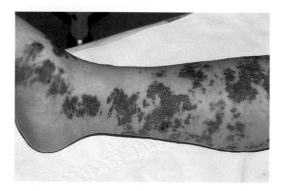

Figure A.20 Angiokeratoma.

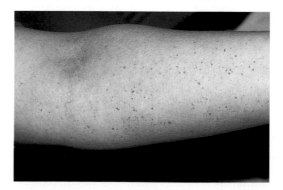

Figure A.21 Anderson–Fabry disease (alpha-galactosidase deficiency).

Pyogenic granuloma has a characteristic morphology, growing on a stalk surrounded by a collarette of normal skin. These rapidly growing angiomas are seen on the chest and extremities of young people, and because of their tendency to bleed they are often the cause of alarm. A *glomus tumour* (glomangioma) also occurs on the extremities, often beneath a nail, and is composed of a bluish-red, rounded firm papule a few millimetres in diameter. Lesions can be excruciatingly painful on pressure.

Kaposi's sarcoma is a form of angiosarcoma which, in its classical form, grows indolently on the extremities of elderly Jewish or Southern Italian persons. An endemic form, more aggressive and metastasizing, was described in younger people in subequatorial East and Central Africa in the 1950s. The *epidemic* of aggressive Kaposi's sarcoma seen in the last 20 years is largely associated with HIV infection.

Acquired telangiectases are common. Isolated spider naevi (Fig. A.22) appear on children's faces, and during late pregnancy over half of the mothers develop several scattered over the face, upper chest,

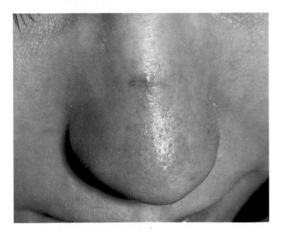

Figure A.22 Spider naevus.

arms and hands. These usually disappear within 6 weeks of delivery. Similar lesions appear in *thyrotoxicosis* and *liver disease*, and also in two conditions where vasodilatory agents are released into the circulation intermittently – the *carcinoid syndrome* and *systemic mastocytosis*. Other cutaneous manifestations of chronic liver disease include palmar erythema, leukonychia and clubbing. Telangiectasia on exposed skin is related to the gradual disappearance of support tissue that occurs with age, and more particularly with cumulative sun exposure. This is extremely rare in older Negroes. Similar mechanisms cause telangiectasia after X-radiation, and following the abuse of *topical corticosteroids*. They are also seen

in localized skin disorders such as *rosacea* and *poikiloderma*, as well as in collagen–vascular disorders such as *scleroderma* (matt-telangiectases), *dermatomyositis* and *lupus erythematosus*.

Barry Monk

ANORECTAL PAIN

Where there is an evident cause, the history of anorectal pain is usually of relatively short duration, and treatment is frequently successful in relieving symptoms. A small subgroup exists, however, in which symptoms are longstanding and no organic cause is found; these patients present a major therapeutic challenge to the clinician.

Classification of major causes

Acute causes

- Anal fissure
- Perianal haematoma
- Herpes simplex infection
- Perianal abscess
- Intersphincteric abscess

Chronic causes

- Proctalgia fugax
- Coccydynia
- Idiopathic
- Sometimes associated with descending perineum syndrome
- Gynaecological disorders
- Anorectal malignancy
- Presacral tumours or cysts
- Cauda equina lesions
- Tumours
- Trauma
- Anal fistula
- Chronic perianal sepsis
- Crohn's disease
- Anorectal tuberculosis

Short history of pain

Acute disorders in the perianal region usually give rise to severe pain because of the profusion of sensory nerve endings prevalent in the squamous epithelium at and below the level of the dentate line. A sudden onset of pain in association with a dark blue oedematous perianal swelling are the characteristic features of a *perianal haematoma*, which is thrombosis of a large venous dilatation in the external venous plexus (Fig. A.23). A history of anal pain initiated by defaecation and lasting for a variable period up to an hour

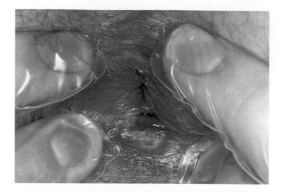

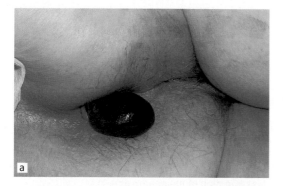

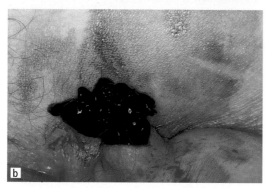

Figure A.23 (a) Perianal haematoma, a particularly large example. (b) The clot evacuated under local anaesthetic, with immediate relief of pain.

afterwards is usually diagnostic of an *acute anal fissure*. The lesion is observed on inspection of the anus usually in either the anterior or posterior midline positions, and may be associated with an oedematous 'sentinel' skin tag at its more caudal margin (Fig. A.24). Digital examination or instrumentation of the anal canal causes severe pain and tenderness associated with marked spasm of the internal anal sphincter. Chronicity or multiplicity of a fissure observed in unusual sites around the circumference of the anal canal should arouse suspicions of underlying *Crohn's disease*. Infection with *herpes simplex virus* is extremely common and may present with pain due to anal lesions. Lesions are typically shallow ulcers that crust

Figure A.24 Acute anal fissure. The edges of the anal verge are gently retracted by the examiner's fingers to reveal the fissure in the 6-o'clock position. The skin tag ('sentinel pile') is seen at its inferior position.

over and heal within days to weeks; tender enlargement of the inguinal lymph nodes during an attack is typical. The frequency of recurrent attacks is very variable; they affect the same anatomical site. The diagnosis of herpes simplex should be confirmed by a swab for viral culture.

The association of a short history of pain with fever and purulent anal discharge usually signifies *perianal sepsis*. The primary source is usually an infected anal gland, and if the sepsis remains localized an intersphincteric abscess is the result. The diagnosis can be notoriously difficult because there may be no overt signs of infection; exquisite tenderness on digital examination of the anal canal may be the only physical finding. Usually, pus in the infected anal gland extends to the surface (i.e. to the perineum or buttock), in which case a fistula opening will be clearly visible and an area of induration corresponding to the fistula track will be palpable.

Pain of chronic duration

Patients with chronic perineal pain may be found to have organic disease, although in many, after exhaustive investigation, no cause is apparent. *Proctalgia fugax* is a common source of perineal pain in which no structural abnormality is apparent. The pain is spasmodic, with episodes lasting up to 30 minutes, and is probably the consequence of paroxysmal contraction of the levator ani musculature. *Coccydynia* is a rather loose term applied to a history of vague tenderness and ache in the region of the sacrum and coccyx. Sometimes the pain radiates to the back of the thighs or buttocks and is usually provoked by sitting. Symptoms, without any convincing evidence, have been considered to arise from the coccyx. Idiopathic perineal pain is sometimes associated with the *descending perineum syndrome*, a disorder of the pelvic floor in which the pelvic floor becomes denervated, and on examination the perineum is seen to 'balloon' well below the bony pelvis as represented by the level of the ischial tuberosities. The pain, in these patients, may arise from stretching of the pudendal nerves, or alternatively from the mucosal prolapse which occurs secondarily to loss of muscle tone. Characteristically the pain is provoked by prolonged standing or walking and is relieved by lying flat.

Of the treatable underlying disorders, malignancy in the rectum or anus must be excluded early on by digital examination and sigmoidoscopy. Gynaecological and presacral pathology should be excluded by pelvic examination, ultrasound and CT scanning of the pelvis. If the history of pain accompanies motor disorder of the anorectum and bladder, a cauda equina lesion should be suspected and excluded by MRI examination. Finally, chronic perianal sepsis should always suggest a possible inflammatory disorder such as Crohn's disease or anorectal tuberculosis.

Harold Ellis

ANXIETY

Anxiety is a universally experienced emotion, the presentations of which require an understanding of both its adaptive role and the relationship between personality and coping.

Anxiety is the emotional component of the 'fight or flight' reaction – the physiological response to threat. In 'fight or flight', the individual has both a choice to make and to prepare for taking either option. Once fight or flight are enacted, anxiety subsides, its job done; thus, anxiety is the emotion of indecision or conflict and of preparation for action. Anxiety contrasts with fear, which is the emotion of a non-conflictual, known, threat and it precedes depression, the emotion of loss, which develops when the consequences of the threat become evident. In daily living anxiety enhances both physical performance

(e.g. in sport) and mental performance (e.g. in examinations). Being anxious occasionally makes the difference between surviving or not, but often facilitates action to ward off potential threats such as illness, pain, helplessness, punishment, separation, or to one's status or social functioning.

How the anxiety that is generated to deal with a potential menace – whether internal or external, real or imaginary – is disposed of depends upon the individual's personality attributes, and especially the array and efficiency of mental defence mechanisms that have been developed. To simplify, the 'normal', mature, balanced personality deals with anxiety effectively, either through initiating appropriate actions or through the utilization of various defence mechanisms that produce an adaptive response. An example would be a student who feels anxious about a romance and settles their uncertainty or sublimates this emotion by intensifying their study. The immature or disordered personality cannot handle anxiety – either because the correct, relieving actions are not undertaken, or because a dearth, imbalance or inadequacy of defence mechanisms lead to a maladaptive response. In such a case the student who feels anxious about a romance may take an overdose or dissociate from this emotion by becoming severely depersonalized and so be unable to work.

Defence mechanisms therefore are unconsciously operated mental tricks for disposing of anxiety that might otherwise overwhelm the individual. At least 30 mechanisms have been described, and both heredity and upbringing are involved in determining their presence and application. Common examples are regression, repression, denial, rationalization, projection and introjection. It follows that many types of psychological problem can develop from the failure to manage anxiety – from the interaction of personality and stress, and from the combination of coping strategies and defence mechanisms that are employed.

It should be evident that excessive amounts of anxiety may be generated in spite of a sound personality if the stress is great enough. This is the origin of neurotic reactions named by their association with major life-threatening events like accidents and shell-shock, battle neurosis, post-traumatic stress disorder – how the ordinary individual copes with the extraordinary event.

Excessive stress is also the basis of the adjustment reaction, a common phenomenon in medical practice when patients face the threats and uncertainty of illness – cancer or not, transplant or not, survival or not. These reactions tend to follow the pattern of the illness, being florid and severe in acute, life-threatening illness and persistent and less severe in chronic disabling disorders. In adjustment reactions anxiety figures predominantly in the early stages, and depression latterly, as the uncertainty becomes certainty and the loss apparent. Sometimes there is an unwelcome tendency for any overt emotional response to be interpreted as pathological and so to be treated with drugs: in adjustment reaction the best approach is inquiry and explanation, exploring the patient's concerns, reassuring when appropriate, expediting investigations and treatment when appropriate, being a good listener. Indeed, this is an excellent opportunity to forge a therapeutic alliance with the patient that facilitates not only in the recognition and prevention of further emotional distress but also in coping with developments, setbacks and even mistakes as the illness unfolds.

It is when anxiety is inappropriate in degree or duration that the basis for diagnosing generalized/chronic anxiety disorder is established. Maladaptive responses to anxiety are topics of other sections.

The diagnosis of generalized anxiety disorder rests upon: (i) excessive anxiety and worry; (ii) other clinical features (Table A.7); and (iii) the exclusion of underlying physical or mental disorders.

In addition to the emotion being excessive for the circumstances, anxiety states are characterized by generalization of worries – the patient may or may not be concerned about everything, but their anxieties will certainly extend beyond the single-issue worry which is more typical of phobias, obsessive–compulsive disorder, anorexia nervosa, panic disorder and hypochondriasis.

The features of anxiety are direct consequences of increased activity of the autonomic nervous system. The symptom pattern varies considerably from patient to patient, but physical symptoms are frequently presented as the primary complaint with anxiety and other psychological concomitants interpreted as a secondary response.

Somatization, the presentation of psychological distress with physical symptoms which are attributed to organic disease, takes this process further with the emotional origins of the presentation denied, or further still when all emotional aspects are denied – even

Table A.7 Clinical features of anxiety

Somatic
- Breathlessness
- Palpitations
- Accelerated heart rate
- Sweating but cold and clammy
- Dry mouth
- Lump in throat
- Nausea
- Butterflies in the stomach
- Diarrhoea
- Urinary frequency, hesitancy, urgency
- Dizziness
- Faintness
- Lightheadedness
- Tension headache
- Musculoskeletal aches
- Restlessness
- Coarse tremor
- Trembling, shaking

Hyperalertness
- Feeling keyed-up, on edge
- Feelings of dread or threat
- Irritability
- Increased sensitivity to stimuli
- Poorly sustained concentration
- Inability to relax
- Initial insomnia

overt depression and anxiety. Somatization arises partly from the misinterpretation of altered or amplified physiological functions, but there are other important elements: the stigma of mental illness, the belief that doctors are more interested in and sympathetic towards physical disorders, the inability to express emotions either because of lack of awareness of emotional responses or inarticulateness (alexithymia), and sociocultural factors such as older age, lower social class and previous physical illnesses. Doctors also play their part in promoting somatization through neglecting to consider and pursue the emotional dimension and by overzealous physical investigations.

Any feature in Table A.7 may be the presenting complaint, but particularly common are headaches, dizziness, chest pain, palpitations, gastrointestinal symptoms, tremor, fatigue and emotional upset. Of course likely physical illnesses must be excluded, even in the overtly anxious patient, and the very act of treating the symptom seriously can be therapeutic, for anxious people usually respond to reassurance.

Table A.8 Causes of anxiety

Commonest
- Normal/stress related
- Adjustment reaction
- Generalized or chronic anxiety state

Less common
- Drugs
  - Stimulants: cocaine, amphetamines, caffeine
  - Sympathomimetics
  - Hallucinogens
- Drug withdrawal
- Physical disorders
  - Thyroid dysfunction
  - Hypoglycaemia
  - Hyperventilation
  - Migraine
  - Temporal lobe epilepsy
  - Brain tumour
  - Head injury
- Psychiatric disorders
  - Depression
  - Mania
  - Schizophrenia
  - Phobias
  - Hysteria
  - Malingering
  - Obsessive–compulsive disorder
  - Post-traumatic stress disorder
  - Panic
  - Depersonalization
  - Hypochondriasis

Rare
- Drugs
  - Antihypertensives
  - Penicillin
  - Sulphonamides
  - Cannabis
  - Nicotine
  - Inhalers
  - Anticholinergics
- Endocrine disorders
  - Pituitary dysfunction
  - Parathyroid dysfunction
  - Adrenal dysfunction
- Neurological disorders
  - Cerebrovascular disease
  - Subarachnoid haemorrhage
  - Encephalitis
  - Neurosyphillis
  - Multiple sclerosis
  - Wilson's disease
  - Huntington's chorea
- Gastrointestinal disorders
  - Hiatus hernia
  - Peptic ulcer disease
  - Ulcerative colitis
  - Crohn's disease
- Cardiorespiratory disorders
  - Congestive cardiac failure
  - Chronic respiratory failure
  - Cardiac arrhythmias
  - Myocardial infarction

- Hypertension
- Anaemia
- Emphysema
- Asthma
- Auto-immune disorders
  - SLE
  - Rheumatoid arthritis
  - Polyarteritis nodosa
  - Temporal arteritis
- Toxicological disorders
  - Benzene and derivatives
  - Carbon disulphide
  - Mercury
  - Arsenic
  - Lead
  - Organophosphates
- Other causes
  - Vitamin B_{12} deficiency
  - Pellagra
  - Aspirin intolerance
  - Brucellosis
  - Infectious mononucleosis
  - Carcinoid syndrome
  - Systemic malignancy
  - Porphyria
  - Uraemia
  - Electrolytes disturbances
  - Anaphylaxis
  - Premenstrual tension syndrome

The differential diagnosis of anxiety is lengthy and complicated by the fact that anxiety frequently overlaps other disorders. This is particularly true when considering the psychiatric differential diagnoses, with *panic* and *hyperventilation* both being cause and effect. The most important practical distinction is from *depression*, although once again anxiety and depression frequently co-exist – particularly in the less severe forms of emotional disorder typically met in general practice. The crux is to identify major depressive states in which agitation is marked. Usually, patients with agitated depression have developed typical biological and cognitive depressive changes; however, if there is doubt then it is preferable to err on the side of misdiagnosing an anxiety state as an agitated depression than vice versa.

Medical disorders that may cause or present with physical or psychological manifestations of anxiety are numerous (see Table A.8). Within this list there are several conditions which merit further discussion. Hyperthyroidism is justifiably the best-known differential diagnosis, first because the state of metabolic overactivity induced by thyroxine is similar in many respects to primary anxiety, and second because anxiety is a common emotional presentation of the disorder. Symptoms that point towards hyperthyroidism are increased cold tolerance, increased appetite and significant weight loss, while distinguishing signs (in addition to the classical findings in the eye and neck) are warm extremities and fine (versus coarse) finger tremor. Excluding thyroid disorder is also desirable when no obvious stressor can be established and there is no evident predisposition to anxiety.

Drugs – both stimulants (especially caffeine) and abstinence from alcohol or benzodiazepines – are another common factor: a detailed inquiry into drug-taking habits and recent changes is essential, and this should include coffee and tobacco consumption.

In general, an anxiety state arising without adequate explanation in a middle-aged or elderly person is highly suspicious of either an underlying physical disorder or depressive illness.

Finally – and central to the whole issue of diagnosing anxiety disorders – it is usually not the illness that is masked but the doctor who is blind. By confining enquiries to physical systems, the correct questions are not asked and consequently the correct diagnosis is missed. Perhaps the doctor may justifiably feel sometimes that a psychological line of inquiry could upset the patient and might damage their relationship, but there are usually ways round this – either by exercising tact and judgement as to how far and fast to make the approach, or by speaking to and involving relatives. Undue delay or inappropriate referrals, investigations and treatments aggravate rather than ameliorate anxiety states, and hence make the task of helping the patient more difficult.

Andrew Hodgkiss

APPETITE, DISORDERS OF

Loss of appetite

Loss of appetite is so common and non-specific that its presence is rarely of assistance in making a diagnosis. It can be a feature of many physical or psychological disorders, as well as a transient phenomenon in stress or even ordinary living. When a patient complains of diminished appetite, a useful pointer to the importance and clinical significance is the presence and amount of accompanying weight loss. Without confirmed weight loss or other evidence of illness it is inappropriate to pursue investigations of loss of appetite.

Gastrointestinal disorders which are characteristically associated with loss of appetite include the *prodromal stage of viral hepatitis, gastric carcinoma, gastric ulcer* and *coeliac disease*. In coeliac disease, however, the patient may occasionally compensate for the malabsorption with an increase in appetite, and under these circumstances a loss of weight is not a problem. Patients with *roundworm* infestation may also have a loss of appetite but, uncommonly, the patient may have an increase in appetite.

Anorexia may be a prominent feature of chronic diseases such as *advanced malignant disease, chronic*

alcoholism, uraemia, severe congestive heart failure, chronic pulmonary disease and *cirrhosis of the liver.* Adrenal insufficiency is constantly associated with anorexia and loss of weight. On the other hand, both *thyrotoxicosis* and *diabetes mellitus* may lead to a marked loss of body weight in the absence of any impairment of appetite.

Anorexia may feature prominently in patients with psychiatric illness, including *anxiety, stress* and *depression.* However, there are two psychiatric illnesses in which a disorder of eating features prominently, namely *anorexia nervosa* and *bulimia,* which may affect 5–10 per cent of adolescent girls and young women, with a significant morbidity and mortality. It is rare for these syndromes to occur in males. Anorexia nervosa usually begins in a teenage girl who is either overweight or believes herself to be so. There is a refusal to maintain normal body weight, a loss of more than 25 per cent of original body weight, a disturbance of body image, an intense fear of becoming fat, and there is no associated medical illness leading to weight loss. There are many accompanying physical abnormalities in the patient with established anorexia nervosa. These include amenorrhoea, osteoporosis, abnormal temperature regulation, bradycardia and hypotension, decreased glomerular filtration rate, renal calculi, oedema, constipation, and abnormality of liver biochemistry. The patient will become anaemic with leucopenia and thrombocytopenia.

Increased appetite

An increase in appetite will occur normally in individuals exercising strenuously, and transiently in those recovering from an illness. An increased appetite can occur in *mania* and *hyperthyroidism. Hypoglycaemia –* such as occurs with an insulinoma – may be associated with an increased appetite, but this is an uncommon manifestation of the disease. Occasionally the *depressed* or *hysterical* patient may eat to excess.

Bulimia is characterized by recurrent episodes of binge eating. There is consumption of high-calorie, easily ingested foods taken in a binge and terminated by abdominal pain, sleep or vomiting. In between binges, there are repeated attempts to lose weight, and the body weight can fluctuate rapidly over short periods of time by more than 5 kg. The patient usually is aware that there is an abnormal eating pattern, but she fears that she will not be able to stop voluntarily.

After the eating binge the patient becomes depressed. Physical features in bulimia include menstrual abnormalities, hypokalaemia, acute gastric dilatation, parotid gland enlargement, dental-enamel erosion, the risk of Mallory–Weiss tears and aspiration pneumonia.

Perverted appetite (pica)

A perverted appetite may be a striking manifestation of iron-deficiency anaemia. Affected individuals may crave earth or clay (geophagia), starch (amylophagia) or ice (pagophagia). Perversion of the appetite is also seen in other psychiatric disorders. Pica may also occur during the course of pregnancy, and is of no special significance.

John Meenan

APRAXIA

Apraxia is an impairment in the execution of learned (or skilled) movements not caused by weakness, paralysis, incoordination, extrapyramidal disorders or sensory loss. It is thought that the (dominant) left temporoparietal cortex is where visual, auditory and somatosensory information is integrated to form the motor programmes (engrams) for skilled movement of both hands. These engrams then pass to the left premotor cortex before being transferred to the right hemisphere premotor cortex via the anterior corpus callosum. Thus, lesions in the dominant temporoparietal cortex, the anterior corpus callosum or in either premotor cortex can cause apraxia, and the deficits can be predicted from the above model. Apraxia can be divided into three main types (affecting progressively 'higher' elements of the motor system) – kinetic (limb), ideomotor and ideational – as well as a number of other specific disorders of praxis.

Classification

Limb kinetic apraxia

This is a loss of the components of motor engrams, resulting in coarse or unrefined movements that no longer have the expected appearance of being practised over time. These apraxias are usually contralateral to a hemisphere lesion.

Ideomotor (ideokinetic) apraxia

This is the most common type of apraxia. It involves a loss of the volitional ability to perform learned movements. A lesion in the dominant hemisphere, in the premotor area, anterior corpus callosum or inferior parietal lobe, can cause ideomotor apraxia.

Ideational apraxia

Ideational apraxia is an impairment of ideational (conceptual) knowledge resulting in a loss of the links between tools and their actions, as well as the ability to sequence movements correctly. Movements may be left out, produced in the wrong order, or attempted with incorrect tools. This condition may result from diffuse brain disease or dominant parietal lobe lesions.

Apraxia of speech

Some patients who have disturbances of motor speech are considered to show an apraxia of buccolingual movements, though this may co-exist with – and be difficult to distinguish from – aphasia. The region of damage involves the insula in the dominant frontal lobe.

Dressing and constructional apraxia

In patients with lesions of the non-dominant parietal lobe there may be an inability to put on clothes in the correct order, or to identify items that have been turned inside out. Such patients will also show constructional apraxia (i.e. they will have difficulty in copying a diagram, drawing a clock or constructing a figure from matchsticks). This disorder is best considered as a type of visuospatial dysfunction rather than a true apraxia.

Oro-facial apraxia

Oro-facial apraxia may be seen with lesions that affect the dominant supramarginal gyrus or motor association cortex. Patients will be unable to lick the lips or pretend to blow out a match, though they will be able to perform these tasks if there is jam on the lips or if a lighted match is held in front of them.

Conduction apraxia

Conduction apraxia causes selective difficulty in copying movements, so that patients can pantomime a sequence on command better than they can imitate it. This is similar in concept to conduction aphasia (see SPEECH, ABNORMALITIES OF, p. 657). The location of the lesion is not known.

Apraxias are unusual in that the problems are often not evident to the patient, and are easily overlooked by the examining doctor. The special types of testing required to fully appreciate apraxias may be extremely difficult because of co-existing neurology, such as aphasia or agnosia.

Clinical assessment of praxis

Apraxia should be considered when the patient has functional disability that seems out of keeping with the degree of motor impairment shown on neurological testing. Ideational apraxia may be suggested when components of a complex task can be performed individually, but not integrated together as a whole. Some simple suggestions for bedside testing are summarized in Table A.9.

Table A.9 Bedside testing of praxis

Limbs
Ask the patient to:
- Mime use of common tools, e.g. comb, toothbrush, pen
- Imitate use of comb, toothbrush, pen
- Use comb, toothbrush, pen

Orofacial
Ask the patient to:
- Whistle
- Stick out tongue
- Blow cheeks out
- Cough

Serial actions
Ask patient to mime serial task, e.g. '… mime each step, from the beginning, of how you clean your teeth.' The patient should then be observed to mime the following:
- Open tube of toothpaste
- Put toothpaste on brush
- Brush teeth
- Rinse mouth with water
- Spit out water and rinse toothbrush

Differential diagnosis

Comprehension disorders, movement disorders and language disorders (aphasias) must be carefully evaluated before a diagnosis of apraxia is made. Impaired object recognition (visual agnosia) must be ruled out if patients select the wrong tool for a task. The patient must be able to name the tool or describe its function and purpose in order to establish that they have apraxia and not visual agnosia.

The main causes of apraxia are listed in Table A.10.

Table A.10 Differential diagnosis of apraxia

- Stroke
- Traumatic brain injury
- Cerebral tumour
- Neurodegenerative conditions
  - Cortico-basal-ganglionic degeneration
  - Progressive supranuclear palsy
  - Alzheimer's disease
  - Frontotemporal dementias
  - Multiple system atrophy

The history of onset and associated physical signs should point towards the correct diagnosis. For example, stroke is usually of sudden onset without progression, in contrast to the subacute onset of deficits due to a mass lesion and the slower progression of symptoms due to a degenerative condition. In clinical practice it is unusual to see apraxia in isolation. Thus, in corticobasal ganglionic degeneration, progressive supranuclear palsy, fronto-temporal dementias and Alzheimer's disease there will be associated neurological features: these may include bradykinesia and rigidity, supranuclear gaze palsy, altered behaviour or memory loss, respectively.

David Werring

ARCUS CORNEALIS (ARCUS SENILIS)

Arcus cornealis is an extremely common and asymptomatic bilateral peripheral corneal condition associated with hypercholesterolaemia and/or ageing. It is a type of degeneration which is found in 60 per cent of people between the age of 40 and 60 years. It is more common in blacks than other races, and increases in frequency with age.

The opacity (Fig. A.25) is due to deposition of lipid droplets in the superficial and deep layers of the cornea forming a yellowish-white ring about 2 mm in width, with a clear space between it and the junction

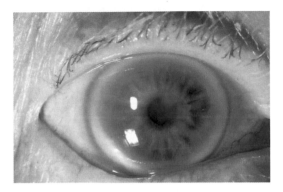

Figure A.25 Opacity seen in arcus cornealis.

of the cornea and the sclera (the limbus). It may also arise from hyaline degeneration of the lamellae and cells of the cornea. Some individuals with corneal arcus due to hypercholesterolaemia may merit lipid-lowering treatment according to their absolute levels of cardiovascular risk.

Melvin Lobo

ARM, PAIN IN

This section deals primarily with pain referred into the arm from the neck and thorax. In addition, pain arising in the brachial plexus and peripheral nerves is included, as also are lesions at the shoulder, elbow, wrist and hand which specifically or characteristically affect the upper limb. The causes of such pain are summarized in Table A.11. Lesions which may arise at any site such as arthritis, bone tumours, injuries and skin disease are excluded.

Pain referred into the arm falls into two major categories:

1 Sharp, well-localized neuralgia often associated with paraesthesiae is usually attributed to nerve root or trunk compression.

2 Dull, diffuse discomfort in the limb, which is often difficult for the patient to describe and which may be accompanied by changes in skin temperature, vascularity and sweating and is often ascribed to involvement of autonomic pathways. In the case of this 'cylindrical' limb pain an origin within the thorax or the thoracic spine should be considered.

Table A.11 Causes of pain specific to the arm

Lesions in the neck
- Disc prolapse
- Spondylosis
- Syringomyelia
- Fracture dislocations
- Post-herpetic neuralgia
- Radiculitis – paralytic/viral (neuralgic amyotrophy)
- Spinal abscess
  - tuberculous
  - *Brucella*
  - pyogenic
- Epidural abscess
- Pachymeningitis cervicalis
- Tumours
  - spinal cord
  - meninges
  - nerve roots
  - vertebrae
    - primary
    - secondary

Lesions of the brachial plexus
- Cervical rib
- Malignant infiltration
- Costoclavicular compression
- Subclavian aneurysm
- Scalenus anterior syndrome

Lesions of the thorax and thoracic spine
- Cardiac ischaemia
- Syphilitic aortitis
- Thoracic disc
- Oesophagitis

Lesions at the shoulder
- Periarthritis/capsulitis
- Subacromial bursitis
- Calcific tendonitis
- Bicipital tendonitis
- Shoulder–hand syndrome

Lesions at the elbow
- Epicondylitis
- Olecranon bursitis

Lesions of the forearm, wrist and hand
- Carpal tunnel syndrome
- Tenosynovitis
- Ulnar neuritis
- Trigger finger
- Algodystrophy
- Hypertrophic osteoarthropathy
- Pachydermoperiostitis
- Repetitive strain injury (RSI) (e.g. writer's cramp)

Lesions in the neck

X-ray changes of cervical spondylosis are a normal finding after the age of 40 years. Over the age of 60, neurological symptoms and signs referred from the cervical roots are common. Great care must be taken, therefore, before ascribing a patient's symptoms to spondylosis.

Cervical spondylosis can produce three clinical syndromes which may occur alone or in combination. Pain and stiffness of the neck is often recurrent and may be aggravated by tension, anxiety and posture. Radicular pain radiating down one or both arms may or may not be associated with muscle wasting, weakness and reflex changes referred to as brachial neuralgia. Finally, compression of the cervical cord may produce three sets of symptoms and signs:

- Weakness, wasting and fibrillation in the upper limbs with reduction or loss of the tendon reflexes at the level of the compression.
- Paraesthesiae in the arms and legs with or without impaired sensation in the hands and feet.
- Pyramidal involvement with weakness, spasticity, hyper-reflexia and extensor plantar responses in the legs.

The combination of weakness and wasting in the arms and spastic weakness in the legs resembles *amyotrophic lateral sclerosis*; spondylosis may usually be distinguished from this by the history of paraesthesiae, evidence of sensory impairment and radiographic or MRI evidence of cord compression. *L'Hermitte's sign* may be demonstrable.

Disc herniation at the C5/6 and C6/7 intervertebral spaces is a common cause of pain in the upper limb. Onset may be acute, with well-localized pain radiating from the back of the neck across the back of the shoulder down the arm and forearm to the wrist or fingers; more commonly, onset is less dramatic, often after a period of recurrent aching and stiffness in the neck. Pain may be aggravated by movements of the neck, by downward pressure on the head and by changing the position of the arm. Pain may radiate downwards into the scapular region and to the upper chest. *Sensory disturbances* are uncommon, but may be detected in a dermatomal distribution (Fig. A.26) and muscle weakness may be detected in the appropriate muscles. The clinical signs associated with the most common root lesions are indicated in Table A.12. Depression of the biceps jerk may indicate a lesion of

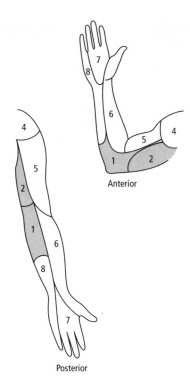

Figure A.26 Dermatomal distribution of pain referred to the arms. [Redrawn with permission from Doherty, MacFarlane and Maddison (1985), *Rheumatological Medicine*, Churchill Livingstone, Edinburgh.]

the C5 root, paraesthesiae in the thumb and index finger with depression of the supinator jerk indicate a lesion at the C6 root, and paraesthesiae in the index and middle fingers with loss of the triceps jerk are associated with a lesion of the C7 root. *Paraesthesiae in the feet* with spasticity in the legs and extensor plantar responses indicate pyramidal damage associated with cord compression. X-rays of the cervical spine may show disc space narrowing especially at the C5/6 or C6/7 levels with lipping of the adjacent margins of the vertebral bodies. In the acute stage, X-rays may not reveal a relevant abnormality. Protrusion of a disc may be demonstrated by contrast myelography or MRI. A spinal fluid examination is usually required to make a diagnosis.

Other causes of *brachial neuralgia* are uncommon. Viral, bacterial and fungal infections should be considered. Herpes zoster may give rise to persistent pain in the arm, especially in the elderly. The history of a vesicular rash and residual pigmented scars in dermatomal distribution is usually diagnostic; weakness

Table A.12 Signs and symptoms associated with common nerve root lesions affecting the arms

Root	Paraesthesiae/Numbness	Muscle weakness	Reflex change
C5	Radial aspect of forearm	Shoulder abduction Elbow flexion	Biceps jerk diminished
C6	Thumb and index finger	Wrist extension and pronation	Supinator jerk diminished
C7	Middle finger, back of hand	Elbow extension and finger extension	Triceps jerk diminished
C8	Little finger, ulnar border of hand	Finger and wrist flexion	
T1	Ulnar border of forearm (see Fig. A.26)	Intrinsic muscles of hand	

of one or more muscles in the limb with cutaneous hyperalgesia or hypoaesthesia may also be present in a minority of cases.

Vertebral and *paravertebral abscesses* may result from tuberculosis or brucellosis, or be caused by more common pyogenic organisms such as *Staphylococcus aureus*. In drug addicts and immunocompromised individuals (including those with AIDS), fungal or parasitic lesions may occasionally develop. Such lesions may or may not be accompanied by fever, and the initial symptoms may closely resemble cervical disc prolapse. Occasionally, there are no other pointers to a septic lesion so that severe root symptoms in the arms in the absence of clear radiographic abnormalities should prompt CT or MRI examination of the neck. *Pachymeningitis cervicalis hypertrophica* is a rare condition, sometimes syphilitic in origin, which causes diffuse pain in both arms together with paraesthesiae, widespread atrophy, loss of reflexes and variable sensory loss; more than one root is implicated. Positive syphilitic serology should not be taken to indicate this rare condition in the absence of other diagnostic features. *Primary or secondary neoplasms* of the vertebral bodies may give rise to root pain with or without motor, sensory and reflex changes. X-ray examination may be diagnostic with destructive damage, though isotope bone scanning is more helpful. Spurious hot spots may be seen in the presence of marked degenerative disease of the spine, while plasmacytomas and myeloma produce a normal bone scan. CT and MRI scanning may be helpful in early lesions. Tumours of the meninges and roots usually cause symptoms in the legs, from compression of the pyramidal and sensory tracts, as well as pain in the arm. Root lesions in the presence of multiple cutaneous neurofibromata (*von Recklinghausen's disease*) should raise the possibility of the development of a neurofibrosarcoma. Specialized spinal imaging is necessary for diagnosis. Where a neural tumour is

suspected, MRI scanning will provide the most sensitive diagnostic information. *Syringomyelia* occasionally causes pain in the arm, but only as a late feature. By this stage the classical features of dissociated sensory loss, muscle wasting and hyporeflexia in the arms with pyramidal signs below the level of the lesion are likely to be apparent. Fracture dislocations of the cervical spine are especially likely in the presence of rheumatoid arthritis or ankylosing spondylitis. In the former, atlantoaxial and/or subaxial subluxation of the spine may lead to upper- and lower limb symptoms, and fused segments of spondylitic spine are particularly at risk of fracture with or without displacement. Fractures of cervical vertebrae due to osteoporosis are unusual.

Lesions of the brachial plexus

Compression of the neurovascular bundle (including the brachial plexus) may occur at several sites, giving rise to characteristic features classified as *thoracic outlet syndromes*. Symptoms include paraesthesiae of the fingertips, especially in the night or early morning; the ulnar border of the hand is typically affected (in contrast to carpal tunnel syndrome, which affects the radial border), but numbness on waking may extend to the distal forearm. Symptoms may be aggravated by carrying heavy weights, though this is not diagnostic. Typically, pain is felt behind the clavicle and down the inner aspect of the arm, and there may be atrophy of the hypothenar eminence and interossei. Paraesthesiae and hypoaesthesia in the C8 and T1 dermatomes with associated vasospastic features are common findings. The diagnosis is usually based on induction of paraesthesiae and numbness by abduction of the arm to 90° with external rotation, detection of an arterial bruit in the supraclavicular fossa during this manoeuvre, and disappearance of symptoms and bruit with return of the arm to the neutral position. Finding a position of the arm in which the radial pulse is obliterated has been considered a key diagnostic finding. However, this may be demonstrated in normal subjects and symptoms may be due to compression of the brachial plexus, without involvement of the subclavian artery. The diagnosis is not, therefore, dependent on demonstration of arterial compression. When chronic or recurrent subclavian artery compression is present this may lead rarely to the development of aneurysmal dilatation of the subclavian artery. Causes include the position of the scalenus anterior muscle, the presence of a cervical rib, and stretching of the plexus over a normal first rib by drooping of the shoulder, which may occur in middle life. In a few patients the accessory rib may be palpable and visible on X-ray; not infrequently the rib is vestigial, occurring as a fibrous band which cannot be detected. In the majority of instances in which the diagnosis of thoracic outlet syndrome is considered an alternative cause, such as cervical spondylosis, cervical disc lesion or peripheral nerve lesion will be detected.

Pain in the arm is occasionally due to pressure on, or infiltration of, the brachial plexus by malignant tumours. *Lymphadenopathy* associated with lymphomas or carcinoma will usually be detectable by palpation of the axilla and of the posterior triangle of the neck, though infiltration of the plexus by metastatic carcinoma (especially from the breast) may take a long time to become detectable. Involvement of the plexus by upward spread of an apical bronchial carcinoma (Pancoast tumour), or more rarely by apical inflammatory lung disease, may produce unilateral Horner's syndrome in addition to arm pain. Such lesions can usually be detected on a chest X-ray. In each of these conditions the pain may be very severe without any accompanying signs in the early stages. Further infiltration usually leads to paralysis, with relative sparing of sensation.

Lesions of the thorax and thoracic spine

In contrast to the characteristically searing localized pain of nerve root involvement, pain in the arm originating in the chest has a dull, poorly localized quality, sometimes described as cylindrical. Such pain may also be associated with alterations in autonomic functions, including temperature of the limb and sweating.

Pain associated with *myocardial infarction* or pain of *angina pectoris* is usually readily recognized and confirmed by ECG or exercise testing. Syphilitic aortitis may induce similar referred pain. Oesophagitis may also produce cylindrical arm pain with or without more classical 'heartburn'. Such pain may also be accompanied by ECG abnormalities, so that accurate distinction from myocardial ischaemia may rest upon cardiac enzyme analysis (troponin T and creatinine kinase), exercise testing, and visualization of the upper gastrointestinal tract. Referral from the thoracic spine is a major (but little recognized) cause of aching in the arm or 'fibrositis'. *Thoracic disc prolapse* usually leads to benign thoracic pain, though it may also cause referral to the upper limb. Onset is usually insidious, and back pain may not be present. However, physical examination of the spine usually reveals local thoracic spine tenderness, often with rib and sternal tenderness and pain on thoracic rotation. Other causes of stiffness of the thoracic spine, including spondylosis, may lead to similar symptoms. Infections of the discs also produce radicular pain. *Discitis* due mainly to blood-borne infection is increasingly recognized as MRI has become the investigation of choice in back imaging.

In a minority of instances myocardial infarction leads to the development of pain and stiffness at one shoulder with varying degrees of pain, swelling, osteoporosis and vasomotor disturbance more distally in the limb. This 'shoulder–hand syndrome' is discussed further below.

Lesions around the shoulder, elbow and wrist

In the absence of swelling, many painful lesions in the arm are referred from the spine, even in the presence of local tenderness. Thus, even apparently discrete lesions of the shoulder and elbow may originate from spinal lesions.

Degenerative arthritis at the shoulder joint is unusual. Pain around the shoulder radiating to the outer aspect of the upper arm with pain and reduction of glenohumeral movement in all planes is referred to as *capsulitis* or *peri-arthritis*. A painful arc on abduction of the shoulder, especially with tenderness at the shoulder tip, is typical of supraspinatus tendonitis or subacromial bursitis. Transient calcification around the supraspinatus tendon may be seen on X-ray. Similarly, tenderness of the long head of biceps (bicipital tendonitis) may be noted, usually in association with capsulitis of the shoulder. The pain of tendonitis at the shoulder is usually exacerbated by resisted movement of the appropriate muscles: (a) supraspinatus – abduction; (b) infraspinatus – external rotation; (c) subscapularis – internal rotation; and (d) biceps – supination and flexion of elbow.

Swelling of the olecranon bursa, due to trauma, gout or infection, may produce pain over the extensor aspect of the elbow with limitation of movement.

Nerve palsies can all cause arm pain. Inflammatory or traumatic lesions at the medial aspect of the elbow may lead to *ulnar neuritis* with characteristic pain, tingling and numbness radiating down the ulnar border of the forearm and hand with impaired intrinsic muscle function. This is especially common after prolonged bed rest where prolonged pressure is applied to the elbows. Radial nerve injury, producing wrist drop with pain, numbness or tingling over the back of the hand is more likely to result from pressure or trauma above the elbow, where the nerve runs around the posterior aspect of the humerus in the radial groove. Median nerve dysfunction produces characteristic pain, numbness and tingling in the thumb, index and middle fingers. Symptoms are often worse at night and first thing in the morning. This is most commonly caused by *carpal tunnel syndrome*, especially in the presence of hypothyroidism, pregnancy or inflammatory arthritis at the wrist. Pressure may also be exerted on the median nerve where it passes between the two heads of pronator teres in the forearm. A positive Tinel's sign with wasting and weakness of abductor pollicis brevis and slowed median nerve conduction on electromyography confirm the diagnosis.

A variety of *repetitive strain syndromes* are now described. These soft tissue syndromes relate to repeated or sustained actions of the upper limb, and produce local pain, fatigue and a decline in performance. Symptoms are commonest in young adults, especially keyboard workers, and a variety of factors including poor posture, stress, inadequate rest periods, poor training and worker's compensation may contribute to their development. Both work and recreational activities may be implicated. *Writer's cramp*, with pain in the wrist and shoulder associated with an excessively tight grip of the pen and a tense posture whilst writing, may be a related condition. *Acute viral radiculitis* (paralytic brachial radiculitis, neuralgic amyotrophy) produces severe pain in the shoulder and upper arm, often with rapid onset of muscle wasting and weakness. Symptoms usually subside after a few days, though there may be some persisting weakness and ache. Tenderness over the lateral epicondyle sometimes extending to involve the superior radioulnar joint is referred to as 'tennis elbow', and over the medial epicondyle as 'golfer's elbow'.

Miscellaneous conditions

Reflex sympathetic dystrophies may affect the upper limb, being usually referred to as *shoulder–hand syndrome*, *causalgia* or *algodystrophy*. This condition is characterized by pain, swelling, vasomotor disturbances and trophic skin changes usually affecting the distal part of the limb. This may follow peripheral nerve injury or myocardial infarction, though in at least 50 per cent of cases no cause is demonstrable. In the later stages, contractures may also develop.

Hypertrophic (pulmonary) osteoarthropathy (HPOA) may affect many sites, but in particular the elbows, wrists and fingers. Onset of joint pain is often acute with stiffness and weakness, and there may be marked tenderness of distal long bones associated with radiographic appearances of periostitis. Clubbing of the fingers is also present. HPOA is usually associated with malignancy of the lung, pleura or diaphragm, though it may occasionally be benign or hereditary; it is usually bilateral and symmetrical. Only the upper limbs are affected in association with Pancoast's syndrome and aortic aneurysms. Similar changes of periostitis and clubbing associated with thickening of the skin, especially in the scalp, may develop soon after puberty in the syndrome of pachydermoperiostitis. The condition is benign, and gradually becomes inactive after a few years.

Fibromyalgia

Fibromyalgia is a syndrome of unknown cause that manifests as episodic pain and tender muscles of the upper body, including the arms. It is made worse by stress. Its pattern of symptoms are not consistent with a specific musculoskeletal abnormality.

Mark Kinirons

ATAXIA

Ataxia is defined as uncoordinated movements which are not caused by weakness, altered tone or involuntary movements and results either from damage to afferent sensory inputs (sensory ataxia) or to the cerebellum and its connections (cerebellar ataxia).

Cerebellar ataxias

The cerebellum is involved in the regulation of muscle tone, the coordination of movement, and the control of posture and gait. Cerebellar dysfunction will arise with lesions of the cerebellum itself or its connections in the cerebellar peduncles, midbrain, pons or medulla (Fig. A.27). The cerebellar hemispheres relate ipsilaterally to the limbs, and therefore unilateral lesions of the cerebellar hemisphere will result in ataxia which is most marked on the same side of the body. Midline cerebellar lesions tend to manifest with severe gait ataxia. As well as ataxia, lesions of the cerebellum and its connections may give rise to additional signs such as hypotonia, pendular reflexes, dysarthria (due to incoordination of the muscles of voice production, leading to 'scanning' or 'staccato' speech) and nystagmus.

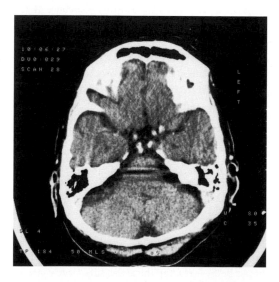

Figure A.27 Computed tomogram of the head, demonstrating cerebellar atrophy in a man with a long history of alcohol abuse.

Limb ataxia is demonstrated using the finger–nose and heel–shin tests. An intention tremor may be present in the upper limbs, together with evidence of dysdiadochokinesis on rapid alternating movements of the upper and lower limbs. Patients with *gait ataxia* tend to walk with a broad-based gait and persistently grab for support. If mild, this becomes most evident on heel–toe walking. *Truncal ataxia* is a feature of midline cerebellar lesions and manifests as an inability to sit or stand without assistance, and to fall backwards. Many different pathologies may result in cerebellar ataxia.

Cerebellar ataxia of abrupt onset

The sudden onset of cerebellar ataxia implies an aetiology which is vascular, demyelinating or inflammatory, most commonly due to posterior circulation stroke or multiple sclerosis (Fig. A.28).

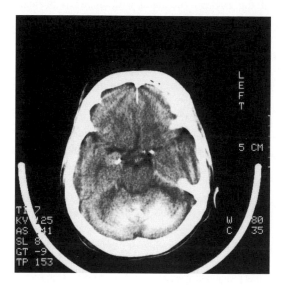

Figure A.28 Computed tomogram of the head, demonstrating extensive cerebellar haemorrhage.

Subacute evolution of cerebellar ataxia

The subacute evolution of an ataxic syndrome should raise the possibility of a mass lesion within the posterior fossa, most commonly secondaries. *Haemangioblastomas* and *medulloblastomas* also occur. *Cerebellar abscesses* are relatively rare, except in patients with evident infection in the middle ear; encephalitides are extremely uncommon. In some patients with lung cancer there is a form of paraneoplastic cerebellar ataxia which develops subacutely and which affects particularly the limbs.

Chronic cerebellar ataxia

Chronic alcoholism, severe hypothyroidism, vitamin B_{12} deficiency, phenytoin toxicity, anoxic injury including carbon monoxide poisoning and head trauma can all cause chronic cerebellar ataxia.

The slow development of a cerebellar ataxia may also occur in the context of the hereditary ataxias, the best known of which is the autosomal recessive *Freidrich's ataxia*. The cardinal features include gait and limb ataxia, dysarthria, areflexia, sensory loss and corticospinal tract signs. Skeletal abnormalities, diabetes and cardiomyopathy may also occur.

Sensory ataxia

The term 'sensory ataxia' is used to describe the incoordination that is seen in patients who have lost proprioception in a limb or limbs. Afferent proprioceptive impulses travel from the muscles and joints, providing information to the cerebellum and cerebrum about the movements of muscles. In the absence of this sensory information, or if it is distorted, the corticospinal system is unable to coordinate normal movements. Such proprioceptive sensory loss may be seen in patients with peripheral neuropathies, spinal cord disease affecting the posterior columns (e.g. subacute combined degeneration of the cord due to vitamin B_{12} deficiency, multiple sclerosis) and in lesions of the thalamus and sensory cortex. The resulting ataxia is most apparent when visual guidance is removed. Associated signs include loss of touch and joint position sense and pseudo-athetosis of the fingers (the patient is unable to keep the fingers still in the outstretched position).

The gait is typically wide-based, and the feet may strike the ground with extreme force, causing a stamping gait. When asked to stand with the feet together and the eyes closed, the patient will sway (Rombergism). In the upper limbs the phenomenon may be demonstrated by asking the patient to hold the arms outstretched and to close the eyes. The patient is likely to have great difficulty in undertaking fine movements which are outside the normal range of vision, such as fastening the top button of a shirt, or tying a tie.

James Kelly

ATHETOSIS

The word 'athetosis' derives from the Greek for 'unfixed' or 'changeable'. The condition is characterized by slow, writhing, continuous movements often affecting the limbs, but also the axial muscles including the neck, face and tongue. They are often confined to the upper limbs, and are most pronounced in the digits and hands. When absent at rest, the movements in one region can be brought out by asking the patient voluntarily to move other parts of the body; for example, speaking may induce athetosis in the limbs, neck, face or tongue. This phenomenon is called 'overflow'.

Within the patterns of movement it is possible to identify extension, pronation and flexion–supination of the forearm, and flexion–extension of the fingers with the thumb often being trapped by the flexed fingers as the hand closes. In the lower limbs there is typically eversion–inversion of the foot; in the face, there is retraction and pursing of the lips and alternate constriction and relaxation of the forehead with opening and closing of the eyes. The neck and torso are prone to rotatory twisting movements.

In general, the movements of athetosis are slower and less jerky than those described in chorea, but gradations between the two forms of involuntary movement are seen; in some cases the distinction is impossible and the term 'choreoathetosis' is used. The commonest cause of athetosis is damage to the basal ganglia in early life (neonatal or infancy).

In children – particularly in association with hemiplegia due to cerebral palsy – athetosis can be unilateral, though bilateral ('double') athetosis may also occur. Both the arms and face are involved; speech and swallowing are also affected. Such children are usually slow in gaining their motor milestones and have learning difficulty. Athetosis in infants usually involves slow twisting movements, and is most appropriately considered as a form of dystonia.

In adults, athetosis may occur as an episodic or permanent abnormality in hepatic encephalopathy, as a manifestation of chronic intoxication with phenothiazines or haloperidol and, most commonly, as an effect of chronic administration of L-dopa in patients with Parkinson's disease. Athetosis is part of the involuntary movement seen in patients with Huntington's chorea and may also be seen in patients with Wilson's disease, Hallervorden–Spatz disease and Leigh's disease. The movements of adult athetosis may be almost as fast and jerky as those of chorea, and so are often termed choreoathetosis.

Athetosis, like most forms of involuntary movement, ceases during sleep, and may be brought out at the bedside by distraction, for example by asking the patient to close both eyes and recite sequential numbers or days of the week.

David Werring

AURA

An aura may be defined as a premonitory symptom, which is commonly related to an epileptic attack. The term may also be used to describe the focal cerebral symptoms occurring before the development of headache in migraine.

One of the main differentiating features between the aura of an epileptic seizure and the aura of migraine is duration. The aura in migraine may last from a few minutes to an hour or more, though a good rule of thumb is that if the symptoms last for over 30 minutes then another cause, such as a cerebrovascular event, should be considered. In epilepsy the aura is usually shorter, lasting from seconds to minutes.

Seizure aura

A seizure aura has been defined as that part which occurs before consciousness is lost (or automatisms begin), and which can be remembered subsequently. The typical characteristics of an epileptic aura are: it is spontaneous, normally in the context of otherwise good health, begins abruptly, and lasts for seconds only. Auras are most commonly seen in patients who have complex partial seizures arising in a focal brain area, and reflect where the seizure starts. Thus, a motor aura may include involuntary movement of a limb, or occasionally a more coordinated movement such as running. A sensory aura is more common, and may be described as discomfort, tingling or occasionally a more complex sensation moving along a limb. A visual aura may be simple, consisting of shimmering lights or colours within the field of vision, implying an origin in the occipital lobes; or it may be a complex hallucination, such as flowers or a brightly-coloured pattern, which suggests an origin in the lateral temporal neocortex.

Seizures arising in the medial temporal lobes are likely to be associated with a psychical aura, involving feelings of apprehension, a sense of unreality or a 'dreamy state', consisting of vivid memory-like hallucinations, or the sense of having previously lived through exactly the same situation before (déjà vu). There are often associated epigastric phenomena (e.g. an abnormal sensation beginning in the stomach and welling up into the throat) and fear. These symptoms may progress to a loss of contact with the environment, oro-alimentary automatisms (e.g. chewing, lip-smacking, sucking or blowing movements), and then simple gestural automatisms. With involvement of the temporal lobe uncus there may also be an olfactory or gustatory aura in which patients may describe disturbances of smell or taste, which are usually unpleasant.

The most important aspect of the aura in epilepsy is in helping to classify the seizure type, which can guide investigation and treatment. A *focal aura* indicates that the epilepsy is arising at a focus within the brain and is therefore a form of partial seizure. Thus, a patient who describes an aura consisting of a sensory disturbance in the left hand will be likely to have a lesion in the contralateral parietal lobe; one who describes an aura beginning in the right visual field will be likely to have a lesion in the left occipital lobe. An aura of movement beginning in the right thumb and spreading in Jacksonian fashion up the arm implies a lesion in the left motor strip (precentral gyrus of the left frontal lobe). All patients with focal aura must be investigated with cerebral imaging using CT or MRI if these are available. Traditionally, carbamazepine has been the first-line treatment for partial seizures.

The second importance of an aura in epilepsy is that it provides evidence of continuing seizure activity. Patients with seizures may be able to describe minor episodes in which their usual aura does not proceed to a full attack, thus indicating to the physician that, although control is partially achieved in reducing the severity of the attacks, the epileptogenic focus continues and the patient requires an increase in anticonvulsant therapy.

Migraine aura

Migraine affects about 10 per cent of the population. Most suffer from common migraine (migraine without aura) in which headache, usually unilateral, is associated with nausea, photophobia, phonophobia and nausea or vomiting. One in ten migraineurs have classical migraine (migraine with aura), in which some or all of the attacks are preceded by symptoms that are typically positive (i.e. an excess of normal perceptions or other neurological phenomena) attributable to focal alterations in brain activity. The commonest is a *visual aura*, classically a black-and-white zigzag (fortification) in part of the field of vision. Other auras include complex disturbances of function such as shimmering loss of vision ('scintillating scotomas'), aphasia, or sensory-motor dysfunction of part of the body. Zigzag visual forms are generally considered pathognomonic of migraine. The aura may evolve over a few minutes and continue (generally up to about 30 minutes, to a maximum of about 1 hour). If the symptoms are negative (i.e. a loss of function such as numbness or paralysis) or prolonged, then the possibility of a vascular event including migrainous infarction must be considered. Other pathologies that can cause migraine-like symptoms include cerebral arteriovenous malformations, syndromes associated with anticardiolipin antibodies (including Hughes' syndrome) or the rare familial disorder of cerebral autosomal dominant arteriopathy with subcortical infarcts and leukoencephalopathy (CADASIL), in which a progressive dementia and family history should suggest the diagnosis.

Migraine auras are usually – but not always – followed by a typical lateralized, throbbing headache. Aura without headache is termed *acephalgic migraine*, and quite commonly develops in middle to late adult life, especially in women. The diagnosis of transient ischaemic attack (TIA) may be considered with recurrent episodes of aura without headache, but TIAs may be distinguished by an abrupt, non-evolving onset, and must mimic a known vascular territory syndrome. Migrainous aura is commoner than TIA at all ages. It should also be noted that the character of a migranous aura may change in an individual at different stages of their life; sometimes in women aura changes are clearly related to hormonal changes.

The most commonly accepted explanation of pathophysiology for migraine aura is spreading cortical depression that moves across cerebral areas at the same rate as symptoms evolve clinically, and has recently been demonstrated on functional brain imaging. Similar studies indicate that the 'neuronal generator' for migraine is in the midline brainstem structures including the periaqueductal grey matter, dorsal raphe nuclei and locus coeruleus, with subsequent activation of the trigeminovascular system (see HEADACHE, p. 278).

David Werring

AXILLARY SWELLING

Classification

The differential diagnosis of axillary swelling is best carried out by considering the individual anatomical structures present in the axilla and the lesions that can arise therefrom:

Skin and subcutaneous tissue

- Abscess
  - Acute
  - Chronic
- Accessory breast
- Lipoma

Lymph nodes

- Acute adenitis
- Chronic adenitis (tuberculosis)
- Lymphomas
- Secondary malignant deposits

Chest wall

- Cold abscess
- Tumours
  - Benign
  - Malignant

Axillary blood vessels

- Axillary aneurysm
  - Traumatic
  - Subacute bacterial endarteritis

A swelling in the axilla in the majority of cases is due to enlargement of the lymph nodes. An *acute lymphadenitis* will be secondary to infection in the cutaneous area drained by the axillary nodes, that is to say, the whole of the upper limb, the breast and the skin and subcutaneous tissues of the trunk, front and back, down to the level of the umbilicus. The whole of this area must be carefully searched in an effort to find a primary focus. Any form of tumour other than involvement of the axillary nodes by secondary deposits is distinctly rare, but unfortunately it is common to find the axillary nodes to be the site of metastases from carcinoma of the breast. Skin tumours, especially melanoma, in the cutaneous area already defined are a not uncommon source of axillary node deposits. The differential diagnosis is considered in more detail in the following sections.

Acute abscess

An acute axillary abscess may be recognized by the well-marked signs of local inflammation, usually accompanied by the general features of pyrexia and malaise. The patient resists movement of the arm on account of the pain, and there is usually some cause, such as a paronychia, to account for the source of infection.

Although most examples of axillary abscess are due to *Staphylococcus aureus*, the remainder are caused by mixed anaerobes, often complicating hydradenitis suppurativa of the axillary skin. This is a chronic infection of the axillary apocrine sweat glands, with sinuses, scarring and a history of intermittent purulent discharge.

Rarely, an empyema points in the axilla (empyema necessitans). There are generally, but not always, abnormal lung signs to suggest the diagnosis, but the underlying lesion will be revealed on chest X-ray.

Tuberculous abscess

A tuberculous abscess forms a single fluctuating non-tender swelling in the axilla. It may result from breaking down of the tuberculous axillary lymph nodes, or from a cold abscess originating in one of the upper thoracic vertebrae which tracks round the intercostal bundle and results in a fluctuant swelling at any point along the chest wall, commonly in the mid-axillary line.

Occasionally, a cold abscess will result from a BCG injection administered in the deltoid region.

Axillary lymphadenopathy

If the examination proves that the swelling is not an abscess, the next most likely diagnosis is lymphadenopathy. This may present as a single enlarged node, a number of discrete individual nodes or a mass of matter glands.

For a detailed differential diagnosis, see LYMPHADENOPATHY (p. 423). It is sufficient here to enumerate the principal causes. These are acute infection and metastatic deposits. Much less often encountered are chronic infection with tuberculosis, or one of the lyphomas.

An acute lymphadenopathy is suggested by the presence of septic focus in the drainage area of the axillary nodes, although not infrequently the primary focus (e.g. a splinter in the finger) has disappeared and can only be ascertained from the history. The story of a scratch on the hand from a cat, which again by now might have completely healed, suggests the possibility of cat scratch disease.

The most likely primary tumours to give rise to axillary deposits are carcinoma of the breast and a malignant melanoma of skin (Fig. A.29). Occasionally, a node or group of nodes in the axilla appears malignant and, upon being removed for histological examination, are found to be infiltrated with metastatic carcinoma, yet no source of the primary lesion can be found. The most likely site for such a hidden primary is undoubtedly an occult tumour in the breast, and this will be identified on mammography. Occasionally, a primary tumour will be discovered in the lung on chest X-ray.

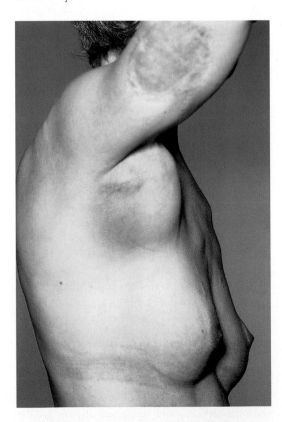

Figure A.29 A huge mass of melanotic deposits in the axillary nodes following previous resection of malignant melanoma of the posterior of the upper arm. Note the skin graft at this site.

Accessory breast

Occasionally, a woman will present with a soft, subcutaneous axillary mass, resembling a lipoma which is, in fact, an accessory breast. The history of the swelling will go back to puberty, and careful examination will usually reveal an overlying nipple, which will clinch the diagnosis.

Primary tumours of the axilla

The only common tumour of the axilla is a lipoma (Fig. A.30) which may attain a large size and extend up under the pectoral muscles. The mass slowly grows over a period of years, is subcutaneous, has a definite outline, is freely mobile, lobulated and gives the sign of fluctuation. This is not, of course, because fat is liquid at body temperature, but rather that each fat cell acts as a micro cyst.

This condition may be confused with a *cystic hygroma* of the axilla. It usually arises in infancy or is even present at birth, and is associated with the more common cystic hygroma of the cervical region, and which is brilliantly transilluminable.

Unusually, a mass on the medial wall of the axilla proves to have its origin from the underlying ribs, chondroma or bony secondary deposit.

Axillary aneurysm

An axillary aneurysm is rare, but the diagnosis should be obvious as it presents with an expansile pulsating mass along the line of the axillary artery. A bruit may be elicited on auscultation.

There is usually a preceding history of trauma, such as a stab wound which has a produced a true or a false aneurysm.

In the absence of any history of local injury, or in cases of an apparently spontaneous aneurysm, there may be the symptoms and signs of bacterial endocarditis.

Harold Ellis

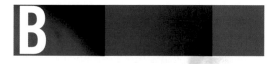

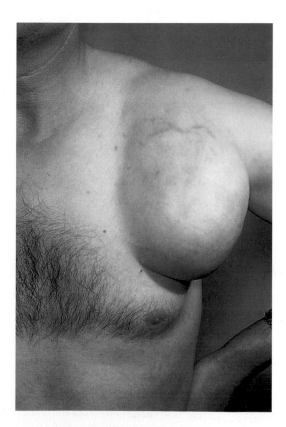

Figure A.30 A massive, but benign, lipoma of the axilla.

BACK, PAIN IN

(See also SPINE, TENDERNESS OF, p. 664)
Pain in the back is one of the most common complaints in general and specialist practice. No speciality is immune from it, and the differential diagnosis therefore covers most of medicine. The classical approach with a long list of differential diagnoses separated out into the standard categories – traumatic, degenerative, inflammatory, infective, etc. – is indeed formidable, as illustrated in the Table B.1. A close inspection will rapidly reveal that even this is abbreviated, and probably incomplete. Furthermore, few of us will retain this whole list in our brain each time we see a patient with backache, and if we did we would probably never finish our day's work!

Mechanical backache – that is, musculoskeletal causes – accounts for the overwhelming majority of patients presenting with backache, no matter whether it be acute or chronic. The skill in dealing with this

Table B.1 Causes of backache

1 Mechanical: traumatic and degenerative
- low back pain; postural – fatigue – obesity; pregnancy
- fractures and fracture dislocations
- ligament sprains and facet joint injuries (while these are probably a common source of acute backache, they are unfortunately impossible to confirm, even with modern imaging techniques such as MRI. This group falls into the category of acute self-limiting back pain)
- intervertebral disc lesions
- osteoarthritis of the facet joints, ankylosing hyperostosis with bony spondylophytes extending from vertebral bodies around the discs
- spinal stenosis and nerve root impingement at exit foramina
- lumbar instability syndromes – spondylosis, spondylolisthesis including the degenerative type, i.e. secondary to facet joint osteoarthritis (see SPINE, DEFORMITY OF, p. 661)
- spinal deformity – scoliosis postural, structural. Scheuermann's disease (see SPINE, DEFORMITY OF, p. 660)

2 Metabolic
- Osteoporosis
- Osteomalacia
- Paget's disease of bone
- Hyper- and hypoparathyroidism
- Ochronosis; fluorosis
- Hypophosphataemic rickets

3 Inflammatory
- Ankylosing spondylitis
- Spondylitis associated with Reiter's syndrome, psoriasis, ulcerative colitis, Whipple's and Crohn's diseases
- Polymyositis and polymyalgia rheumatica
- Arachnoiditis (this low-grade inflammatory condition was a complication caused by the contrast medium used for myelography. Fortunately, this investigation has now been superseded by MRI and CT scanning)

4 Infective
- Osteomyelitis
  - acute – pyogenic (see SPINE, TENDERNESS OF; Figs S.49, S.50 and S.51)
  - subacute – *Salmonella* (typhoid and paratyphoid fever)
  - chronic – tuberculosis, brucellosis (undulant fever – *Brucella abortus* and *melitensis*), syphilis, yaws, Weil's disease (*Leptospirosis icterohaemorrhagica*).
- Intervertebral disc – pyogenic discitis, iatrogenic discitis (secondary to surgical exploration or investigations)
- Spinal 'space' infection, acute and chronic meningitis, subarachnoid abscess, epidural abscess.

5 Neoplastic
- Metastatic (by far the most common malignant tumour found in bone): carcinoma of the breast, prostate, bronchus, kidney, thyroid and colon are the most common primary sites. Direct invasion can occur from carcinoma of the oesophagus
- Myeloma, leukaemia, lymphoma
- Primary tumours of spinal canal and nerve roots: neurofibroma, lipoma, ependymoma, glioma, angioma, meningioma, chordoma
- Primary bone tumours and tumour-like conditions, osteoblastoma, osteoid osteoma, aneurysmal bone cyst (see LOWER LIMB, PAIN IN and around the knee, p. 403), haemangioma

6 Haemorrhagic/blood disorders
- Sickle cell crisis
- Acute haemolytic state
- Haematomas following surgery or anaesthesia, for example epidural haematoma

7 Referred pain
- Vascular/cardiac. Thoracic or abdominal aneurysm. Grossly enlarged left atrium in mitral valve disease. Myocardial infarction only very rarely presents as backache
- Gastrointestinal conditions. Perforating posterior gastric or duodenal ulcer. Pancreatitis, acute or chronic. Referred pain from biliary calculi. Retroperitoneal neoplasms (particularly pancreatic carcinoma). Retroperitoneal fibrosis
- Renal and genitourinary causes. Carcinoma of kidney. Calculus. Hydronephrosis. Polycystic kidney. Necrotizing papillitis. Pyelitis and pyelonephritis. Perinephric abscess. Prostatic carcinoma
- Gynaecological conditions (backache is often attributed to this group, but this is in fact uncommon and is usually an error!). Chronic salpingitis, pelvic abscess, chronic cervicitis, tuberculous disease. Uterine prolapse or retroversion (very rare cause of backache)

8 Drug-related
- Complications of drug therapy:
  - Corticosteroids – a potent cause of increased osteoporosis and vertebral fractures
  - Methysergide (taken over long periods to prevent migraine may be complicated by retroperitoneal fibrosis)

9 Psychogenic and hysterical (see SPINE, TENDERNESS OF, p. 665) condition is to be able to recognize the small percentage of cases who present with non-mechanical backache and have a serious underlying disease. To avoid mistakes the following 'rules' are helpful.

History

In taking the history, note the following:

- The patient is well and fit, has not lost weight, does not have night sweats, etc.
- The pattern of pain. Mechanical backache is nearly always episodic. Beware the patient who has severe constant pain localized to a particular site in the spine. This suggests underlying bone pathology, for example infection (tuberculosis is on a rapid increase throughout the world due to its association with AIDS), or malignancy.
- Always enquire about urinary symptoms. Central compression of the cauda equina is rare, often rather atypical in presentation, and may not have associated abnormal peripheral neurology. However, if it is missed, and hence allowed to progress to bladder paralysis, it is devastating to the patient's quality of life.
- Pay attention to the age of the patient. Men of 55 and upwards presenting with their first episode of backache that has persisted for more than 2–3 weeks should be presumed to have carcinoma of the prostate with spinal secondaries, until proven otherwise. Classical disc disease often starts in the late teens or early twenties with acute backache that only later progresses to episodes of sciatica. The main differential diagnoses in this younger age group are: (a) spondylolisthesis, i.e. a stress fracture of the pars interarticularis; (b) an inflammatory discitis; and (c) ankylosing spondylitis. Females aged over 60 presenting with acute onset of severe backache have a stress fracture of a vertebra, until proven otherwise. Do not presume that these are all osteoporotic, for they may be metastatic. Osteomalacia is another diagnostic 'blind spot'.

Examination

On examination:

- Look for fixed deformities, especially a kyphos.
- Check the spinal movements. Mechanical disease nearly always has a full or almost full range of movement in at least one direction. For example, a patient presenting with an acute disc and a lumbar tilt/scoliosis will usually have very reasonable range of movement to the side in

the direction of the tilt. A totally rigid spine with loss of movement in all directions should be presumed to have underlying serious disease until proven otherwise.
- Examine the peripheral neurology. If this is abnormal, check carefully that it fits with the diagnosis in the back. If a nerve is already 'irritable' due to an underlying neurological disease, it will be at risk of paralysis from much less compression than a normal nerve. For example, a patient with motor neurone disease or a peripheral neuropathy may present with a profound foot drop in association with a recurrent episode of acute backache from a 'minor' disc protrusion. Also beware a patient who has a definite loss of a knee jerk since this has a dual root innervation. (In theory, this is supplied by L2, 3 and 4, but is predominantly L3 and 4.) While a disc protrusion taking out both these nerve roots can occur, it is very uncommon. Note that in clinical practice there is no reflex for L5, and you need to test the power of big toe extension for the L5 root (extensor hallucis longus and brevis).
- Always do the Babinski (plantar) response. On the sensory side, the most important of all signs is loss of sensation in the saddle area – S3, 4 and 5, which control the bladder via the parasympathetics (S2, 3 and 4).

Investigations

In considering plain X-rays it is 'normal' for the spine to show degenerative changes in patients aged over 60; indeed, these will be present in many patients aged over 50. It is all too easy to miss the absence of a pedicle which is frequently the earliest X-ray change in metastatic disease. At least 50 per cent of metastatic deposits will probably not be visible on routine X-rays. In particular, the spinal X-ray may be 'normal' in early cases of multiple myeloma. Involvement of two bodies and the intervening disc is the characteristic feature of infection. Finally, destructive lesions in the sacrum and sacroiliac joints are difficult to spot on plain films due to presence of overlying bowel shadows.

Do not neglect simple blood investigations such as haemoglobin, white count, acid phosphatase and erythrocyte sedimentation rate (ESR). In particular, if the ESR is normal one is unlikely to have missed either the inflammatory or infective group of diseases.

In summary, to diagnose mechanical disease with confidence it is necessary to have a fit patient; a past history in which the backache and/or radicular pain has been episodic; a pattern of spinal movements in which a range of movement in at least one direction is largely preserved; neurological signs – if present – must fit to the mechanical signs; an X-ray that is 'normal' for the patient's age group; and normal routine blood tests. Having diagnosed a mechanical problem, beware of the patient who may have cauda equina compression. Fortunately this is rare but, when present, symptoms can be surprisingly vague and easily overlooked by the unwary.

Mechanical causes

This group accounts for the vast majority of backache. The principles of diagnosis and the pitfalls to be avoided before concluding that backache is indeed mechanical have already been set out in the preceding paragraphs.

Disc degeneration

The intervertebral disc is an ingenious structure. The central nucleus is highly hydrophilic and exerts high osmostic pressure. It is contained by the endplates above and below, and the annulus circumferentially. It acts rather like an elastic ball, the range of movement between the endplates being constrained by the annulus, the ligaments and the shape of the facet joints. With increasing age the nucleus desiccates, losing its ability to maintain the osmotic pressure, the annulus develops fissures and nuclear material herniates in all directions including superiorly and inferiorly into the adjacent vertebral bodies, which is manifest on X-ray as a Schmorl's node. Marginal osteophytes form around the endplates and the bulging annulus to complete the picture of spondylosis seen on a routine X-ray. Posteriorly, the facet joints lose their congruity and, since they are synovial joints, they develop osteoarthritis. The nerve root exit canals narrow due to osteophyte intrusion and a change in shape secondary to the loss of disc space height. These pathological changes set the scene in which a nerve root entrapment in the younger patient is caused predominantly by disc protrusion, while in the older patient it is secondary to entrapment at the exit foramen. These changes are most marked in the distal lumbar segments (i.e. L4/5 and L5/S1). The common disc protrusion is posterolateral, and will therefore catch the nerve root exiting under the pedicle of the vertebra below – that is, L5/S1 disc will most commonly compress the S1 nerve.

Classically, *disc prolapse* (Fig. B.1) first occurs in young adults – the 20- to 30-year age group. Initially there is an episode of acute backache following lifting or bending. Spinal movements are restricted and there is often a tilt. Frequently, this initial episode settles and only with subsequent episodes does it become clear that there is nerve root compression. Pain in the lower back is poorly localized and is referred over a wide area, particularly to the region of the posterior superior iliac spine and into the buttock. Clinically, to diagnose sciatica one requires the pain to radiate down below the knee into the calf, preferably to the ankle. The straight leg raise will be limited. The presence of abnormal neurological signs is clearly helpful in localizing the nerve root under compression.

Plain X-rays are not particularly helpful in disc disease since in younger patients they are usually normal, whilst in the older patient one can expect to see signs of degeneration. MRI is the investigation of choice. The main indication for surgical decompression is the persistence of severe leg pain, not necessarily the presence of abnormal neurology. Finally, beware of the patient who has had sciatica first down one leg then down the other, since this may represent a central disc prolapse. Always enquire about micturition, and test for perineal 'saddle' anaesthesia.

The bony spinal canal is, like the cranial cavity, a 'closed box', and nerve compression therefore can result from any space-occupying lesion. The situation in the spinal column is complicated by the fact that the shape and size of the bony canal is different at different levels in the spine. Furthermore, the spinal cord, which ends opposite L1, is more at risk of compression than the cauda equina. It is fortunate that thoracic disc herniation is rare in clinical practice, even though small prolapses are quite frequently seen on MRI imaging, since thoracic discs have a much greater incidence of neurological complications (e.g. lower-extremity weakness, bowel and bladder symptoms), and there may be a sensory level, while upper motor neurone signs may be present in the lower limbs.

Spinal stenosis (Fig. B.2) is seen in patients, predominantly men, over the age of 50 years (see also LOWER LIMB, PAIN IN, Diagnosis of neurogenic claudication, p. 380). Classically, it presents with neurogenic claudication. While this is a well-recognized syndrome, the precise source of pain is poorly understood. It is easily confused with arterial claudication. Patients normally give a long history of low lumbar backache.

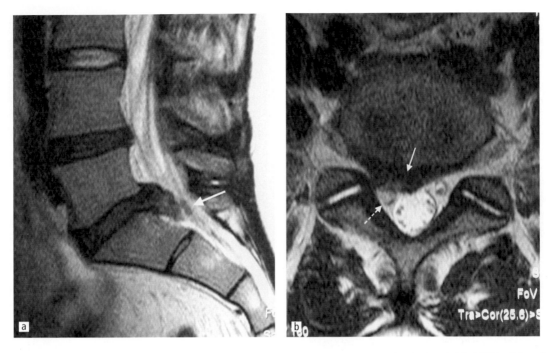

Figure B.1 A prolapsed L5/S1 disc (MRI scanning). (a) Sagittal scan; note the large disc protrusion into the spinal canal at the L5/S1 level. A small part of the disc has actually sequestered (separated and lying loose) (arrowed). (b) Axial view across the L5/S1 level. The prolapsed disc (solid arrow) is impinging not only into the spinal canal, but also into the exit foramen. Note the displacement of the S1 nerve root (dotted arrow). The patient had severe right-sided sciatica with pain radiating down the back of the thigh, the back of the calf and into the foot. The ankle jerk was diminished.

The symptoms in the legs are varied – pain, weakness and tiredness – and these characteristically worsen on walking until they cause the patient to stop. Classically, this is aggravated by walking down a slope when the spine is extended, and eased by going up a slope when the spine is flexed. The symptoms disappear after resting. The lumbar spine is particularly affected (achondroplastics are particularly at risk due to their short pedicles). Within the normal population there is a natural variation in the cross-sectioned shape of the bony canal, but the trefoil pattern – in which the lateral recesses are narrow – has an increased incidence. Old disc disease, facet joint osteoarthritis and bony encroachment spondylosis will clearly reduce the space even further. Specific causes of narrowing include spondylolisthesis (especially the degenerative type), Paget's disease of bone and, rarely, post-traumatic fracture dislocations. Compression at two levels has a much greater risk of precipitating neurogenic claudication than stenosis at one level. It is postulated that this is due to venous congestion and reduced blood flow in the intervening segment of the nerve root. (See further discussion under LEG PAIN OF RADICULAR OR VASCULAR ORIGIN, p. 378.)

Nerve root entrapment at the exit foramen may often be aggravated by walking, and is easy to confuse with spinal stenosis. However, with entrapment, the pain tends to be constant and is often present even at rest. Root tension signs, for example a limited straight leg raise, are usually found.

Spinal deformity

A *structural scoliosis* is rarely painful except when degenerative disease has superimposed later in life. *Scheuerman's disease* – an increased thoracic kyphosis in adolescence – is usually painless, but can sometimes produce aching discomfort. Like scoliosis, it can cause backache in later life (see SPINE, DEFORMITY OF, p. 658).

Metabolic causes

Osteoporosis is of increasing concern in many populations as the percentage of the elderly rises. There are

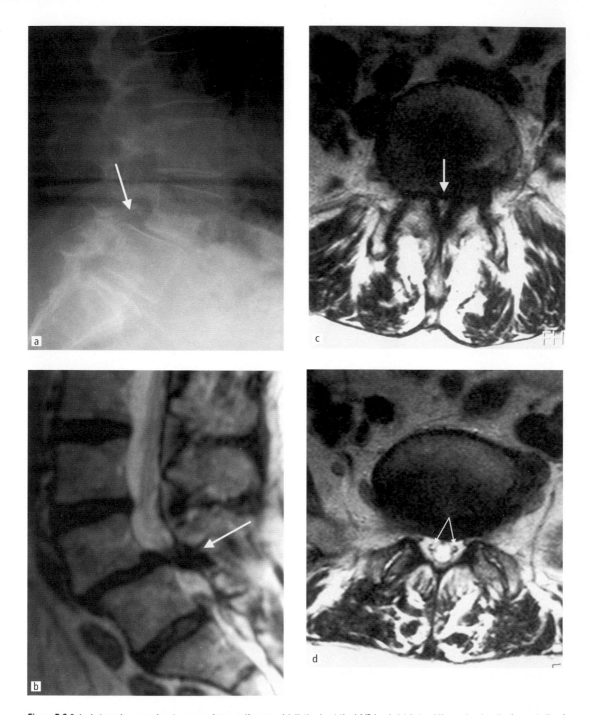

Figure B.2 Spinal stenosis, secondary to severe degenerative spondylolisthesis at the L4/5 level. (a) Lateral X-ray showing the forward slip of L4 on L5 (arrow). (b) MRI sagittal cut. Note the sharp cut-off at the L4/5 level. (c) MRI axial scan at the L4/5 level. Note the severe diminution of the spinal canal; compare this to (d). (d) MRI axial scan across the body of L5, where the spinal canal is again patent. The dural sac is clearly outlined, as are both S1 nerve roots, which are just exiting in their dural sheaths (arrowed). The epidural fat is clearly displayed (white).

three well-recognized orthopaedic entities: wrist fractures; hip fractures; and vertebral fractures, all of which cause much morbidity and much expense for healthcare systems. The surprising feature about vertebral osteoporosis is that it is so often relatively symptom-free. The patient loses height and becomes round-shouldered as the vertebral bodies, especially the thoracic spine, collapse and wedge anteriorly. The posterior elements remain intact. For most patients there is a slow subsidence rather than an acute collapse. When the latter occurs there is a sudden onset of pain, often following a minor fall. This pain usually settles over a few weeks, but occasionally it may be associated with intercostal nerve root entrapment. This is easily overlooked and results in unnecessary suffering since this condition often responds well to injections of long-lasting local anaesthetic, which also of course confirms the diagnosis. Many patients suffer from multiple vertebral body fractures, and in severe cases the rib cage comes to rest on the iliac crest and can be a source of considerable discomfort. Fortunately, neurological problems secondary to spinal cord compression are very rare, even with multiple fractures. Patients may however have difficulty walking if the thoracic and lumbar deformities are so severe that they struggle to get their centre of gravity in line with their feet and consequently topple forwards.

It is important to realize that when radiologists refer to a bone being osteoporotic they are using this purely as a descriptive term – 'the bones appear osteoporotic'. This merely means that there is less calcium present to absorb the X-rays and therefore the radiograph appears darker. Several important and serious conditions can produce 'radiological osteoporosis'. These include multiple myeloma, metastases and osteomalacia. Osteoporosis is best defined as 'reduced mass of bone per unit volume of bone'. On densitometry measurements, osteoporosis is two standard deviations below the sex age-related mean, while osteopenia is one standard deviation below. In osteoporosis, routine blood investigations, including the ESR, are normal. The ESR is usually raised in metastatic disease and often reaches high levels of 80–100 mm/hour (Westergren) in myeloma. Marrow studies and electrophoresis will clinch the diagnosis in myelomatosis, but if there is any doubt as to the aetiology of a crush fracture then a biopsy under X-ray control should be carried out. Radiologically, beware of the crush fracture which involves both endplates, as there is a greater incidence of malignancy or osteomalacia. In osteoporotic fractures it is usually the superior endplate which collapses down.

In *osteomalacia*, as in rickets, there is inadequate mineralization of bone, and unmineralized osteoid seams accumulate on the surfaces of new bone. There is often a history of dietetic and/or intestinal insufficiency, chronic disease or a previous gastrectomy – that is, the inadequacy of calcification may be due to calcium deficiency or to a defect anywhere along the metabolic pathway of vitamin D. The serum alkaline phosphatase is often elevated, serum calcium and plasma phosphate are normal or decreased, whilst urinary 24-hour calcium output is low. Clinically, these patients present with diffuse backache, in contradistinction to the localized severe pain of a crush fracture from osteoporosis. The backache is usually eased by rest and aggravated by activity. Classically, X-rays of the spine show a biconcave appearance to the vertebral bodies – the 'cod fish vertebrae' – while X-rays of the pelvis may show Looser's zones and, in some instances, protrusio acetabuli.

Hyperparathyroidism may present with generalized backache and tenderness. Radiographs show 'osteoporosis', the serum calcium is raised (one may need repeated estimations to confirm this), plasma phosphorus may be low (though it rises with renal failure), and the alkaline phosphatase is usually, but not invariably, raised. There may be other features of hypercalcaemia such as nausea, vomiting, muscle weakness or a true myopathy, corneal calcification (band keratitis), nephrocalcinosis and renal tract calculi. Peptic ulceration and pancreatitis may occur. The syndrome is usually due to primary hyperparathyroidism, secondary to hyperplasia or an adenoma of the parathyroid gland, but may occur secondary to renal or other diseases in which the serum calcium can be normal. The finding of plasma chloride levels consistently less than 100 mmol/l in the presence of hypercalcaemia virtually excludes the diagnosis of primary hyperparathyroidism. Finally, there may be other bone changes, including bone cysts (secondary to brown tumours of von Reckinghausen); subperiosteal reabsorption of the phalanges and distal end of the clavicles is also characteristic.

Paget's disease, in which there is increased bone turnover involving both deposition and resorption, can be a cause of severe backache, though it is often an incidental finding. The characteristic X-ray feature is of an enlarged vertebral body with coarse trabeculation. Severe pain of a radicular origin is caused by a nerve root entrapment at the exit foramen. Paget's disease can occur in a single bone or in many bones. An onset of pain or an exacerbation of pain in an old Paget's bone may signify malignant change to an osteosarcoma, which carries a very poor prognosis. Skeletal pain secondary to Paget's usually responds to calcitonin. However, the pain is often difficult to distinguish from that of osteoarthritis, which is common if the Paget's disease involves a joint. Osteoarthritic pain will, however, not respond to calcitonin.

Inflammatory conditions (spondyloarthropathy)

The best example is idiopathic *ankylosing spondylitis*. Here, the patient is usually a male aged between 16 and 36, and in 90 per cent of cases the histocompatability antigen HLA-B27 is found. The spine is stiffened and restricted in movement *in all planes*. Neck movements are often restricted (see NECK, PAIN AND/OR STIFFNESS, p. 475, Fig. N.19) and intercostal expansion at nipple level reduced from the normal 5–7.5 cm to 2–5 cm or less. This intercostal restriction occurs early in the course of the disease, and is not a late complication but an essential and early part of the clinical picture. Diaphragmatic movement is normal. Evidence of active or old iridocyclitis is present in over 20 per cent of the patients, in most cases seen as iritic adhesions or dark spots on the posterior surface of the cornea. Tender heels or tender areas over the pelvic brim, ischial tuberosities, or greater trochanters are not uncommon. Peripheral arthritis occurs in some 24 per cent of cases initially and hydrarthrosis of knees in about 7 per cent. Occasionally, the disease presents as an inflammatory arthropathy of one of the large joints, for example the hip. It is easy to overlook fixed flexion deformity of the hip and erroneously to attribute the inability of the patient to stand upright solely to the spinal disease (Figs B.3 and B.4). The ESR is elevated in almost all cases, but sheep-cell agglutination and latex tests are negative. Nodules do not occur, nor does lymphadenopathy or splenomegaly.

The most common initial symptom is aching in the buttocks, the patient drawing his/her hand down the back of the buttocks and thighs at the site of discomfort, but lumbar backache and stiffness soon occur and may be the initial symptoms. Two radiographs help in early diagnosis: a posteroanterior view of the sacroiliac

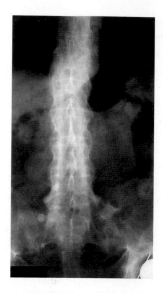

Figure B.3 Ankylosing spondylitis. Anteroposterior X-ray of the thoracolumbar spine showing extensive spondylophytic fusion to form a 'bamboo spine'. The sacro-iliac joints are also fused.

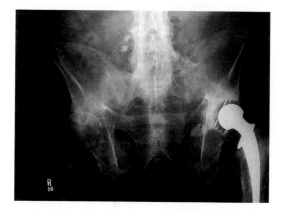

Figure B.4 Ankylosing spondylitis. Associated inflammatory arthropathy of the hips. Note the ovoid shape of the obturator foramina due to the fixed flexion deformity to which hip disease is a potent additional contributor. This patient's ability to stand upright and see ahead improved when the second hip was replaced. Ankylosing spondylitis was one of the original indications when hip replacement was being developed; hence the old-fashioned design shown here, a McKee–Arden prosthesis.

joint; and an anteroposterior film of the dorsolumbar spine D8–L3, but X-ray changes may not be present until symptoms have been present for 2–3 years or more. The earliest radiological sacroiliac changes are blurring of the joint outlines with para-articular ilial sclerosis, erosions and apparent widening of the joint space, gradually giving way over the years to narrowing and obliteration of the joint. Small syndesmophytes, resembling bony 'stalagmites and stalactites', are usually seen, first along the edges of the intervertebral discs between the vertebral bodies of D10 and L2; this is where the 'bamboo spine' usually first becomes evident. Lytic lesions with periosteal elevation and 'whiskering' may be seen in the pelvis or in the spine primarily, girdle joints (hips and shoulders) secondarily, and peripheral joints least often, in contrast to the distribution of joint involvement seen in rheumatoid arthritis, where initial involvement is usually feet, hands and wrists. The spondylitic pattern of disease may also be seen occasionally in Whipple's disease and Behçet's disease and, very rarely, in polymyalgia rheumatica. Some male cases of juvenile chronic polyarthritis progress to the spondylitic picture. In the diagnosis of ankylosing spondylitis these variants should always be considered.

Infective conditions

A spinal infection is easy to overlook, and as a consequence there is often a considerable delay in diagnosis. For example, with tuberculosis it is uncommon to make the diagnosis within six months from the onset of backache, and a delay of a year is frequent. *Pyogenic osteomyelitis* can also be deceptive, especially when it occurs in patients who are ill, for example, in intensive care units or those who are immunocompromised, have AIDS, or are drugs addicts. A wide variety of organisms can be encountered, and a bacteriological diagnosis is mandatory.

The cardinal features are backache and a fever. Spinal infection is, surprisingly, a diagnostic blind spot in considering a pyrexia of unknown origin (PUO). In the early stages, the backache is often mild, though persistent. It is present at rest, although since it is aggravated by activity, it is all to easy to attribute pain to a mechanical cause. In the established disease, night sweats and weight loss become prominent. Spinal infection is even harder to diagnose when there is no fever, as can happen with a low-grade infection in susceptible ill patients. The author has known cases in which a technetium bone scan, performed in desperation on account of continuing unexplained weight loss, showed a hot spot in a vertebral body. Whole-body MRI scans also occasionally discover 'hidden infection'.

The hallmarks as regards the clinical signs are local tenderness, presence of a kyphos, muscle spasm and restricted movements in all directions. These signs are also easy to miss. Look for localized tenderness and a kyphos by examining the patient prone. The sharp angle of the kyphos is best felt by running a finger down the whole length of the spinous processes. Tenderness is best elicited by 'springing' of the spine (see SPINE, TENDERNESS OF, p. 652). In comparing the thoracic and lumbar spines, a kyphos is more prominent in the thoracic spine, whereas in the lumbar spine the natural lordosis merely flattens; however, muscle spasm and loss of mobility is more obvious in the lumbar spine since the thoracic spine is splinted by the ribs.

The classic radiological picture is the involvement of two bodies and the intervening disc reflecting the embryological segmental pattern. However, there is considerable variation and the infection may involve purely the body, the posterior elements or the disc (see SPINE, TENDERNESS OF, Figs S.49–S.50). The extent of bone destruction is usually much more marked than is expected on the basis of the symptoms and signs. Inflammatory markers, the ESR and C-reactive protein, are raised. A technetium bone scan can be helpful in localizing the site of the bony infection in patients presenting with a PUO. CT and MRI scans clearly delineate the extent of the bony and soft tissue involvement. The longer the delay in making the diagnosis, the greater the risk of: (i) bony destruction causing significant deformity; (ii) the formation of abscesses; and (iii) neurological complications secondary to either compression of the cauda equina dependent on the level of the lesion, or the entrapment of nerve roots secondary to compression/deformation at the exit foramina. In all cases of spinal infection it is essential not only to examine the distal peripheral neurology but also to check perineal sensation and enquire about bladder control. A neurological deficit secondary to a compression by 'soft tissue' (i.e. abscess and inflammatory oedema) has a much better prognosis than when it is caused by angulation of the cord over a sharp bony prominence.

It is mandatory to establish the precise bacteriological diagnosis. This is best done by aspiration and biopsy under radiological or CT-guided control (see Fig. S.50). A bony specimen should be sent for histology as well as bacteriology. *Staphylococcus aureus* is the most common pyogenic infection, but a wide variety of other organisms can be found, for example a

Pseudomonas infection in drug addicts. The differential diagnosis for the more chronic tubercular infection is from typhoid, both *Salmonella typhi* and *S. paratyphi*; *Brucella abortus* from cattle, *B. melitensis* from goats, and *B. suis* in pigs. Weil's disease (caused by *Leptospirosis icterohaemorrhagica*), which is characterized by fever, high white blood cell count, jaundice and haemorrhagic manifestations, can also cause acute backache at the time of the infection and may lead on to subsequently marked degenerative change and chronic backache.

Primary disc space infection occurs in children and adolescence prior to the closure of the endplates. In adults, it is nearly always iatrogenic – that is, secondary to a procedure involving the disc (e.g. a discogram). Backache, which is often severe, is usually localized to the affected area – particularly so when a lumbar disc is involved – and there may be referred pain to the buttocks or thighs. The tenderness is localized, but the muscle spasm is usually widespread. The white cell count is often within normal, but the C-reactive protein and ESR are usually raised. In children, the condition was well recognized in pre-antibiotic days and was termed 'benign osteomyelitis', as it was self-resolving. Initially the X-rays are normal, but after 2–3 weeks disc space narrowing becomes apparent and this eventually progresses to bone fusion. Primary extradural abscesses are uncommon, but when they occur they most frequently affect the thoracic spine. They cause severe pain which radiates along the relevant thoracic nerve root. Epidural infection is fortunately rare since it spreads rapidly throughout the spine, precipitating paraplegia and death.

Neoplastic conditions

Metastatic disease is by far the most common malignant tumour found in bones. However, by comparison with the very high incidence of mechanical backache, metastatic spinal disease is an uncommon entity and it is all too easy to fail to diagnose malignancy when backache is the presenting symptom and the primary is unknown. Only a good thorough history will prevent the clinician from making this mistake, since in the early stages, the physical signs are subtle – localized tenderness and muscle spasm. The cardinal features are: (i) backache that is persistent, unremitting, not relieved by rest, and indeed is often worse at night; (ii) weight loss; and (iii) no past history of mechanical

backache. A useful rule states that a man presenting in his mid-fifties with his first ever episode of *significant backache* should be presumed to have prostatic cancer until proven otherwise.

On X-ray there is considerable variation. Metastatic tumours may be sclerotic (prostate, sometimes breast) or lytic, solitary or multiple. Any part of the vertebra can be involved, and one of the classic radiological patterns is loss of a pedicle on the AP X-ray. Unfortunately, this is all too easy to overlook (see Figs S.52 and S.53). A technetium bone scan can be very helpful in defining the extent and number of metastases, and hence in defining which part of the skeleton should be closely studied by CT and MRI scanning. If the primary lesion is unknown, it is often easier for the patient, as well as for the doctor, to establish diagnosis by performing a CT-guided biopsy rather than carry out extensive medical investigations. The diagnosis can be particularly difficult when the presenting feature is as a solitary metastasis, as the differential diagnosis then includes the whole range of malignant bone tumours in addition to the search for a primary. Renal carcinoma (hypernephroma) is often silent, and quite commonly presents with a destructive expansile lytic bone secondary. These are highly vascular. Indeed, if the metastasis is in a superficial bone (e.g. the skull) a defect will not only be palpable but also pulsatile.

Metastatic disease in the spine can also present with acute severe pain secondary to collapse on the vertebral body. This can be accompanied by acute-onset distal paralysis. This is a surgical emergency as the cord or cauda equina will need to be decompressed and the spine stabilized if the patient is to have any relief from their severe pain and to regain any quality of life.

Multiple myeloma nearly always involves the spine (see NECK, PAIN AND/OR STIFFNESS, p. 473, Fig. N.16). The skull, ribs, sternum and pelvis are other common sites. The patient is usually aged over 50 years, and men are affected twice as often as women. The ESR is usually raised and a monoclonal protein is found on serum electrophoresis. Radiologically, there are round, punched-out lytic areas with no surrounding sclerotic margin. However, there is occasionally an altogether different picture of diffuse osteoporosis. This pattern can be easily overlooked – especially on poor-quality X-rays – and even when it is recognized it is all too easy to dismiss it as osteoporosis. A *plasmacytoma* is a solitary form of myeloma; the majority of which (70%) will progress to multiple myeloma. This solitary type carries a very good prognosis in the other 30 per cent of lesions if adequately treated.

Malignant lymphoma involves the skeleton in 20 per cent of cases, the bony lesions being distributed, one-third to the lower limb, one-third to the spine and pelvis, and one-third to the rest of the skeleton. Primary bone lymphomas without general involvement are uncommon, but they do carry the best prognosis. Normally they present with local pain, and as the patient is usually in good general health, the diagnosis can be difficult in the early stages. Skeletal pain is the presenting symptom in 25 per cent of children and 5 per cent of adults with *acute leukaemia*. Eventually, X-ray changes will be found in as many as 70–90 per cent of patients, but there is a very wide variation pattern which varies from transverse lucent metaphyseal lines in children to generalized osteopenia and osteolyitic destruction.

Spinal tumours

Tumours of the central nervous system are an important group, particularly in children. Most are intracranial, but 15 per cent are intraspinal, of which 33 per cent are intramedullary, 22 per cent intradural and 45 per cent extradural. Symptoms are often rather vague, and localizing signs may take a long time to develop. Plain X-rays may show widening of the canal, scalloping of the vertebral bodies or enlargement of an intervertebral foramen. The most common intramedullary tumours are ependymomas and astrocytomas. In children, astrocytomas predominate and tend to involve the cervical and thoracic regions, while in adults the majority are ependymomas and involve the lumbosacral region.

Meningiomas, neurofibromas and *haemangioblastomas* are the most common extramedullary intradural spinal tumours seen in adults. The classic dumbbell neurofibromas cause intra- and extradural expansion and usually arise from the spinal roots, the posterior more often than the anterior. These may be either single or multiple, and may or may not be part of the generalized neurofibromatosis. Extradural tumours, of course, include the whole range of bone tumours as well as tumours which can arise from the neural crest, of which ganglioneuromas are usually benign and neuroblastomas usually malignant. These usually present as large paraspinal masses which are visible on abdominal or chest X-rays. Among this large group of benign bone tumours and tumour-like conditions

the most common to be encountered in the spine are haemangiomas, aneurysmal bone cysts, osteoblastomas and osteoid osteomas. Even these are rare. *Osteoid osteomas* classically produce a painful scoliosis in a teenager or young adult. Characteristically the pain is well relieved by analgesics (see Figs S.45–S.47). Haemangiomas can lead to extensive bone destruction, although the common X-ray pattern is for the vertebral body to show vertical sclerotic striations.

Backache can be a prominent feature in some patients during a sickle cell crisis. Localized bleeding in the form of an epidural haematoma is a complication of spinal anaesthetics. In the early stages, the fluid content gives a high signal on the T2 image, which later changes to a low T2 signal as fluid is absorbed and haemosiderin deposited.

Referred pain

Backache may be caused by cardiovascular and intrathoracic disorders, of which a good example is the intense, demoralizing, boring pain of an aneurysm invading the spine. Features of syphylitic aneurysm of the arch and upper descending aorta will probably be present with signs of an aortic reflux, collapsing arterial pulses, and possibly signs of neurosyphilis. Dissecting aneurysms of the descending aorta below the arch are less apparent; unequal or delayed pulses in the arms and legs should be noted. An arteriosclerotic aneurysm of the abdominal aorta often causes pain in the lower part of the back as well as in the upper abdomen, the groin and occasionally in the testicles; a pulsating mass can be felt in the abdomen. A carcinoma of the bronchus or oesophagus may cause backache.

A rare cause is an enormous enlargement of the left atrium with mitral disease. The pain in such cases is usually relieved by leaning forwards and to the left. The pain from myocardial infarction only rarely radiates to the back.

Chronic pancreatitis and carcinoma of the pancreas may cause a dull, persistent, upper lumbar ache which is usually (but not always) associated with upper abdominal pain and discomfort. The pain is eased by leaning forwards. A penetrating ulcer on the posterior wall of the stomach or first part of the duodenum quite characteristically gives a boring pain in the upper lumbar region; the pain is related to meals and may be relieved by antacid therapy. Enlargement of the liver from any cause may give a dull ache felt to the right of the lower thoracic spine, in addition to aching discomfort in the abdomen and lower chest. The pain of cholecystitis and cholelithiasis is felt over the liver, or a little higher, in addition to the upper abdomen.

Backache is commonly found in association with renal and genitourinary disease. Pyelitis and pyelonephritis can cause lower thoracic and lumbar backache. Renal tumours (in particular carcinoma; see above) often remain silent as haematuria and the findings of a palpable mass in the flank only tend to occur late in the onset of the disease. Backache in association with prostatic metastases is all too easy to confuse with mechanical backache (see above).

Gynaecological conditions are a rare cause of low lumbar and sacral backache. It is common for all varieties of pain (including backache) to be worse during menses, but this does not equate to having a gynaecological cause. Thus, whilst backache may occasional occur in association with diseases of the ovaries or fallopian tubes, this diagnosis should only be made by excluding other causes. Backache due to retroversion of the uterus is a diagnosis of despair and should be discarded as a mistake.

Psychogenic factors

Psychogenic factors are important to assess, especially in patients complaining of chronic backache. It is however important to remember that pain by itself is rarely a hysterical symptom, for these are much more dramatic as well as visibly obvious (e.g. blindness, paralysis, etc.). The problem with pain is assessing the severity. Pain, out of proportion to the underlying pathology, is a common diagnostic problem. 'Inappropriate signs' are a helpful indicator, for example excessive spinal tenderness, a false straight leg raise, etc. Characteristically, with the former even the lightest touch to the skin of the back causes severe pain and often the patient may wobble and lose balance. In a false-positive straight leg raise, the leg can hardly be lifted off the couch with the patient lying supine, but the patient can be deceived into sitting up to 90° with the legs fully extended. Before attributing a stocking glove sensory loss to being psychogenic, a peripheral neuropathy must be excluded. Benign intraspinal tumours; cauda equina compression from spinal stenosis or from a central prolapsed lumbar disc; a prolapsed thoracic disc; and myelopathy due to compression in the cervical spine for example in rheumatoid disease, are all entities which can be associated with long, rather vague symptoms and subtle signs. It is all too easy to label such patients as 'hysterical'.

Fred Heatley

BEHAVIOUR, ANTISOCIAL

All societies generate long lists of behaviours that are considered antisocial. These vary over time and from place to place, and reflect the values and prejudices of the whole community. It is a matter of great current debate how wise doctors are to have involved themselves in this domain at all. Accusations of medicalizing wrongdoing, being agents of social control or being apologists for criminals all haunt psychiatrists in particular. Yet the fact remains that a proportion of those who behave antisocially do so because of a definite psychiatric or medical disorder, and we would wish to avoid punishment of those not responsible for their acts.

The most contentious areas are the concepts of conduct disorder in children and antisocial personality disorder in adults (discussed in the past as juvenile delinquency and psychopathy, respectively). These are syndromes which are defined to a large extent by the antisocial behaviour of the individual, yet are offered by psychiatrists to explain this behaviour! Professional regret about suggesting medical science has something useful to offer in this instance is at something of a peak in the UK at present. This is because the government is asking psychiatrists to identify dangerous individuals with severe personality disorder so they can be incarcerated in psychiatric settings, sometimes prior to committing serious offences. Estimates vary about the number of people who will fall into this category, but the demand from government has sharpened minds.

Conduct disorder is one of the most common diagnoses made by child psychiatrists. It refers to behaviours ranging from truancy, lying, drug misuse and defiance to firesetting, stealing, serious assaults and deliberate self-harm. While testing of boundaries and challenging authority are part of the normal psychological work of adolescence, there is a growing number of young people in the UK whose antisocial behaviour is seriously damaging themselves and others (Table B.2). One fashionable theory is that the absence of

Table B.2 Causes of delinquency

Most common
- Normal
- Socially determined

Less common
- Neurotic
- Stress reaction
- Conduct disorder (antisocial personality)

Rare
- Organic, especially epilepsy
- Psychotic, especially schizophrenia
- Mental impairment

Table B.3 Differential diagnosis of antisocial behaviour in adults

Commonest
- No medical or psychiatric component

Less common
- Stress reaction
- Adjustment reaction
- Neurological disorders
  - Cerebrovascular accident
  - Encephalitis
  - Neurosyphillis
  - AIDS
  - Multiple sclerosis
  - Subdural haematoma
  - Head injury
  - Epilepsy
  - Dementia
  - Delirium
- Alcohol
- Illicit drugs
  - Stimulants
  - Opiates
  - Hallucinogens
- Prescribed drugs
  - Benzodiazepines
- Drug withdrawal
- Learning disability
- Major psychiatric disorder

- Schizophrenia
- Delusional disorder
- Schizoaffective disorder
- Mania
- Major psychotic depression
- Antisocial personality disorder

Rare
- Prescribed drugs
  - Tricyclic antidepressants
  - Monoamine oxidase inhibitors
  - Anticholinergics
  - L-tryptophan
  - Dopaminergics
  - H_2 receptor blockers
  - Corticosteroids
  - Narcotic analgesics
- Psychiatric disorders
  - Hysteria
  - Malingering
  - Post-traumatic stress disorder
- Other conditions
  - Premenstrual tension syndrome
  - Diogenes syndrome
  - Hypoglycaemia

adequate fathering or male role models is compensated for by extreme herd behaviour, in which groups of adolescent males form gangs and set their own norms of behaviour (which may include extreme risk taking and offending). The child psychiatrist must exclude causes of antisocial behaviour such as emotional disorder, early-onset psychosis, learning disability and epilepsy. After that, there is a lack of consensus as to how best to intervene through the criminal justice system or mental health services.

Adult antisocial behaviour

Antisocial behaviour in adults tends to decrease with age. A medical or psychiatric basis should be suspected when the behaviour occurs acutely, unexpectedly, or after a recent stressful life event. Apparently motiveless behaviours occurring in bursts are suspect. Perpetrators who are female, older and without a criminal record merit close attention. Assessment should include consideration of a detailed and accurate account of the behaviour itself from a reliable impartial informant and a description of the premorbid personality and past mental health of the perpetrator. Planning before, and actions and attitudes after, the event should be elicited. The mental state examination (MSE) should exclude disinhibition, mood disturbance, impaired judgment, delusions, hallucinations and cognitive impairment (Table B.3).

There are recognized associations between certain offences and particular psychiatric disorders: murder followed by suicide in psychotic depression, infanticide in severe post-natal depression, shoplifting and depression, morbid jealousy and wife murder, schizophrenia and matricide, psychoses and attacks on the famous. Diagnosing a major psychiatric disorder in

an offender should be the beginning rather than the end of considering their responsibility for their behaviour. As a professor once remarked, 'there is nothing about hearing voices that obliges you to hit someone' (irresistible command hallucinations are indeed a rarity). There is considerable attention now being paid to the personality of psychotic patients who offend.

The offences related to alcohol and drug misuse have a sad familiarity and predictability, but the individual is generally held legally responsible for these. Persistent antisocial behaviour beginning in adolescence and continuing into adulthood points to *antisocial personality*. To make a convincing diagnosis (if diagnosis is the right word) of *antisocial personality disorder* the doctor needs to demonstrate a lack of remorse, lack of empathy, a failure to learn from punishment and poor impulse control in the patient. There is usually a pattern of fractured relationships and work record along with polysubstance misuse.

There is little optimism about the treatment of this disorder outside forensic psychiatry services.

Andrew Hodgkiss

BLEEDING

(See also BRUISES, PURPURA, p. 84)

Within the context of a normal haemostatic system, excessive haemorrhage tends to occur secondary to a structural lesion, such as a peptic ulcer. Recurrent bleeding mainly from one site may point to the location of a pathological lesion. More generalized bleeding is seen with abnormal haemostasis, examples of which are isolated coagulation defects (e.g. haemophilia), platelet disorders (e.g. thrombocytopenia) and drug effects (e.g. aspirin). Certain medical disorders, such as liver and renal disease, are associated with a haemorrhagic state of multifactorial origin. The severity of the haemorrhagic diathesis is in general proportional to the severity of the underlying disorder. The maintenance of blood within the vascular system depends upon the integrity of the coagulation mechanism, the presence of a reasonable number of functional platelets as well as endothelial-lined vessels capable of constriction when severed.

Platelets are responsible for controlling the initial onset of haemorrhage by adhering to subendothelial components (e.g. collagen and microfibrils) and forming a plug in the severed vessel. Platelets circulate for 7–10 days after being released from bone marrow megakaryocytes. They have a complex structure suitable for responding rapidly to breaches in vascular integrity. Platelets have cell surface receptors for various activated components of the coagulation cascade (such as thrombin), and possess delta granules containing vasoactive amines (e.g. ATP and 5-hydroxy-tryptamine, 5-HT) and alpha granules containing protein components of the haemostatic system (e.g. von Willebrand factor [vWF] and factor V). Inadequate platelet function or a low platelet count typically results in mucosal bleeding, such as purpura, easy bruising, epistaxis, gastrointestinal haemorrhage or menorrhagia.

The *von Willebrand factor* is a plasma protein, secreted by endothelial cells, that promotes adhesion of platelets to damaged vessel walls. It also acts as a

carrier protein for factor VIII; hence in von Willebrand's disease the plasma level of factor VIII is often reduced because without its carrier it is unstable and has a reduced plasma half-life. As the vWF is essential for platelet adhesion to traumatized vessels, patients with von Willebrand's disease present with similar bleeding patterns as individuals with platelet functional disorders (i.e. mucosal haemorrhage).

The *coagulation cascade* consists of a series of proenzymes. Initially, each acts as an enzyme substrate; after activation they act as enzymes activating the subsequent proenzyme in the cascade (Fig. B.5). The rate of many of the steps in the coagulation cascade are enhanced if they occur on the platelet surface, although these reactions can also occur in plasma. This procoagulant property is due to specific platelet receptors for components of the coagulation cascade.

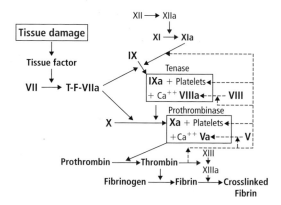

Figure B.5 The coagulation cascade.

Conventionally, the coagulation system is considered to be composed of two parts – the intrinsic and extrinsic components – although recent research has revealed that the system is considerably more complicated. Deficiencies in the coagulation system may be either single (e.g. haemophilia) or multiple (e.g. warfarin therapy). Bleeding can occur due to the presence of an inhibitor (usually an IgG antibody) against one or more of the coagulation factors or platelets (e.g. idiopathic thrombocytopenic purpura, ITP). Single coagulation deficiencies tend to cause haemarthrosis or muscle haematoma, while multiple abnormalities may cause almost any bleeding manifestation. In haemophilia, the primary haemostatic mechanism involving platelets is normal so the

Table B.4 Haematological changes in bleeding-related conditions

Condition	Platelet count	Bleeding time	APTT	Prothrombin ratio	Fibrinogen	D-dimer
Thrombocytopenia	↓	↑	N	N	N	N
von Willebrand's disease	N	↑	N or ↑	N	N	N
Haemophilia A or B	N	N	↑	N	N	N
Warfarin/liver disease	N	N	N	↑	N	N
Disseminated intravascular coagulation	↓	↑	↑	↑	↓	↑

bleeding often stops immediately after trauma. However, haemorrhage will then start several hours later because the platelet plug is not consolidated by the deposition of fibrin.

History-taking of a patient presenting with possible excessive bleeding should focus on the following important aspects:

- The duration of symptomatology indicates whether the possible haemorrhagic predisposition is congenital or acquired.
- The bleeding pattern indicates which component of the haemostatic system may be deficient; thrombocytopenia and platelet disorders give rise to purpura and bleeding into mucosal surfaces, while a coagulation defect usually results in muscle and joint haemorrhage.
- Bleeding timing is also relevant. Bleeding starting at the time of trauma (e.g. dental extraction) indicates failure of platelet plug formation and therefore a platelet disorder, or von Willebrand's disease.
- Spontaneous haemorrhage indicates a more severe bleeding disorder than that associated with provocation by trauma.
- Dental extractions, tonsillectomy and circumcision are all potent stresses of the haemostatic mechanism. If a patient has undergone any two of these procedures without excessive blood loss, they are unlikely to have a clinically significant bleeding problem.
- Family history is important, as many congenital conditions have a familial predisposition.
- The drug history is essential because almost all medicines can, by one mechanism or another, predispose towards bleeding. Ingestion of warfarin or aspirin has to be identified. Exposure to toxins or solvents at work or with hobbies may result in hypoplastic anaemia.
- The general medical history is essential to identify the many disorders that may result in thrombocytopenia or coagulation disturbances, such as liver disease, renal failure and connective tissue diseases.

Clinical examination should identify all the sites of haemorrhage. The buccal cavity and optic fundi should therefore always be looked at, as superficial bleeding at these sites indicates severe platelet dysfunction. It may be necessary to use imaging procedures (e.g. CT scanning or ultrasound) to fully document the extent of internal haematoma formation. Initial screening tests include a complete blood count, examination of a blood film, bleeding time, activated partial thromboplastin time (APTT; intrinsic system), prothrombin time (PT; extrinsic system), fibrinogen and D-dimers (measure of fibrinolysis) (see Table B.4).

If either the APTT or PT is found to be prolonged, the tests must be repeated after addition of normal plasma, when the test time should become normal. Failure to normalize the clotting time raises the suspicion of the presence of an inhibitor.

Table B.5 Causes of bleeding

Cause	Example
Structural lesion	Peptic ulcer, aortic aneurysm, arteriovenous malformation, subarachnoid haemorrhage, angiodysplasia (colonic bleeding), endometriosis, Osler–Weber–Rendu syndrome (hereditary haemorrhagic telangectasia – epistaxis or gastrointestinal bleeding)
Coagulation defect	Haemophilia, von Willebrand's, disseminated intravascular coagulation, thrombocytopenia (autoimmune, marrow failure)
Medication	Warfarin (especially with drug interactions), heparin (can also cause thrombocytopenia), aspirin
Systemic illness	Liver disease, renal failure, malabsorption (vitamin K deficiency)
Infection	Schistosomiasis (haematuria), tuberculosis (haematemesis), Ebola virus
Other	Snake bite venom, scurvy (vitamin C deficiency)

Any patient with thrombocytopenia for which the cause is not immediately and unequivocally apparent should have a bone marrow aspirate and/or trephine performed. This will allow assessment of megakaryocyte numbers. These are reduced in conditions of under-production of platelets (e.g. hypoplastic anaemia), but increased when there is increased destruction and/or pooling of circulating platelets (e.g. splenomegaly). A trephine biopsy is particularly useful for assessing whether the bone marrow is infiltrated with carcinoma cells (Table B.5).

Danielle Harari

BLOOD PRESSURE, HIGH

An isolated (casual) elevated blood pressure reading can have three possible explanations:

1 An error due to either faulty or inappropriate apparatus or faulty technique (observer error).

2 Temporary elevation of blood pressure at the time of measurement (elevation due to biological variability).

3 Sustained blood pressure elevation in the subject not attributable to environmental stimuli (elevated basal pressure).

Observer error

This may be due to instrument design and maintenance, inadequate cuff size, technique of measurement and criteria used for determining systolic and diastolic pressures.

Faulty or inappropriate apparatus

Aneroid sphygmomanometers lose accuracy with time and require regular calibration. Dirt in the escape valve may cause irregular deflation and add to inaccuracy of reading. Incorrect readings may be obtained if, in the case of a mercury sphygmomanometer, the mercury column does not read zero before inflation. If the mercury column is not vertical, the readings will overestimate the blood pressure.

If the rubber bladder contained within the sphygmomanometer cuff is too short, the blood pressure will be over-estimated as pressure is not fully transmitted to the artery. The bladder should therefore cover at least 80 per cent of the circumference of the arm. A 35-cm bladder is recommended for normal or lean arms, while longer bladders (up to 42 cm) are necessary for heavily muscled or obese arms. Too narrow a bladder also leads to over-estimation of blood pressure, although this causes fewer problems than too short a bladder. The width of the bladder should be at least 40 per cent of the circumference of the arm.

Faulty technique

The cuff should be inflated to at least 30 mmHg above the point at which the radial pulse disappears. The cuff should then be deflated at a rate of 2–3 mmHg per second over the critical points. When using mercury sphygmomanometers, the eye should be level with the meniscus; otherwise parallax will give rise to erroneous readings. Rapid re-inflation of the cuff or failure to deflate properly before repeating blood pressure measurement may increase the level at which the Korotkoff sounds appear, and so over-estimate systolic blood pressure level. Rounding up or down to the nearest figure ending in a zero or five (digit preference) may make a small contribution to erroneous readings. Normally, readings can be rounded to the nearest even number. A pre-determined threshold for the diagnosis of hypertension or for treatment may also unconsciously influence the observer's record (observer bias). In clinical trial work, observer bias is eliminated by the use of special sphygmomanometers (e.g. the Hawkesley random zero sphygmomanometer or the London School of Hygiene and Tropical Medicine sphygmomanometer). In both cases, the blood pressure is measured without the observer being aware of the true final value.

The arm should be supported at the mid-sternal level. If the arm is held in a dependent position, the diastolic and systolic blood pressures can be over-estimated by up to 10 mmHg.

Where the phase of muffling (phase IV Korotkoff sounds) is used for estimating diastolic blood pressure levels, values 5–10 mmHg higher are obtained than when the point of disappearance of the Korotkoff sounds is used (phase V Korotkoff). Generally, phase V values correlate better with intra-arterial pressures, and reproducibility between observers is superior.

Subject (biological) variability

Anxiety, recent physical activity, recent cigarette smoking, cold temperature and physical pain all cause elevation of blood pressure through activation of the autonomic nervous system. The first reading obtained by a doctor is usually higher than subsequent readings, either on the same occasion or on later occasions. Thus, significant blood pressure falls have been recorded with the passage of time in placebo-treated patients in clinical trials. These important pressor effects can be minimized by careful explanation of the procedure to the patient beforehand, a comfortable environment, and allowing a 2- to 3-minute period of rest before the blood pressure is measured. The final decision about the presence or absence of hypertension should not normally be made before blood pressure has been measured on three or more occasions, unless other evidence such as the presence of significant target organ damage is found or unless very high blood pressure levels are observed. Some patients show a consistent pressor response to the presence of a doctor or to blood pressure recording ('white coat' hypertension). This should be suspected where high blood pressure levels are repeatedly recorded in the absence of any fundal, electrocardiographic or echocardiographic evidence of hypertensive organ damage. It should also be suspected in patients who appear consistently tense or anxious during the measurement procedure. Under these circumstances, ambulatory monitoring of blood pressure or self-monitoring at home using an electronic digital device should be used.

Blood pressures should, on the first occasion, always be measured in both arms since minor degrees of inequality are quite common. If there is a reproducible difference of 20 mmHg for systolic blood pressure and 10 mmHg for diastolic blood pressure, simultaneous measurements should be carried out: the higher values should be taken as more representative for clinical management of the patient. The time at which antihypertensive drugs are taken may also influence blood pressure. For patients receiving once-daily treatment it is probably best to measure blood pressure just before the patient takes their daily dose.

Raised blood pressure: assessment

In unselected populations, blood pressure is distributed as a smooth, unimodal curve. There is therefore no natural line of demarcation between normal and abnormal blood pressures in unselected subjects. The incidence of cardiovascular disease (i.e. stroke, ischaemic heart disease and peripheral vascular disease) is related to blood pressure level in a curvilinear fashion, with no evidence

for a threshold. It is impossible therefore to define hypertension by reference to a value above which a patient is at risk. The level of blood pressure at which drug treatment is indicated also provides uncertain guidance, since practice in this respect varies considerably not only from one country to another but also between different clinicians in the same country.

There are nevertheless great clinical advantages in selecting an arbitrary criterion. The most commonly used criteria are those of the World Health Organization (5th Korotkoff phase). These are:

- *Normal range:* equal to or below 140/90 mmHg.
- *Hypertensive range:* 160/95 mmHg and above.
- *Borderline or intermittent:* 140–159/90–94 mmHg.

The presence of either systodiastolic hypertension, diastolic hypertension or (isolated) systolic hypertension are all associated with increased cardiovascular risk in individuals, and the decision to treat is nowadays made with reference to national guidelines based upon assessment of absolute cardiovascular risk.

Since both systolic and diastolic blood pressures rise with age (Fig. B.6), the apparent prevalence of hypertension will also rise with age. Furthermore, where a single reading is used rather than average reading over several measurements, the apparent prevalence of hypertension will be much higher since blood pressure tends to fall with repeated measurements (see above). Thus, approximately 40 per cent of untreated middle-aged and elderly men will have a diastolic blood pressure of 90 mmHg or over on single readings, but this figure will fall by 15–20 per cent on repeated measurement.

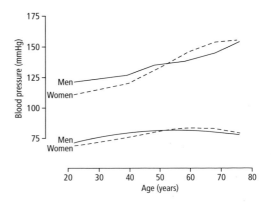

Figure B.6 Blood pressure levels (systolic and diastolic) at different ages in American men and women.

There is little justification in taking age into account in defining hypertension in the adult population since the risks of high blood pressure at least up to extreme old age (i.e. 80 years and above) are related to absolute blood pressure level. In children, however, the same criteria used to define hypertension in adults clearly cannot be applied. Blood pressure rises rapidly in the first few days of life, slightly more slowly over the next few weeks, and then shows little change between 6 weeks and 6 years of age when blood pressure begins to rise again slowly. Thus, in infancy blood pressures of 80–90/50–60 mmHg are observed, whilst in children aged 10 years the blood pressures are 90–100/60–70 mmHg. Blood pressure levels which would be acceptable in adults are poorly tolerated by children, and the arbitrary values used in adults therefore have to be adjusted and related to age. The American Task Force on Blood Pressure Control in Children has recommended that sustained blood pressure levels (obtained on at least three separate occasions) above the 95th centile for age should be considered abnormal in this context.

The malignant or accelerated phase may occur in hypertension from any cause. Whilst the term *malignant hypertension* was previously reserved for patients with papilloedema, it is now recognized that, when untreated, the prognosis is just as bad in patients who show hypertensive haemorrhages or exudates (Grade III retinopathy), and it is now customary to term hypertension associated with Grade III or IV retinopathy as malignant. Malignant hypertension is more common in males. It is usually associated with a diastolic blood pressure of 130 mmHg or more and, compared with other hypertensive patients, these patients are relatively young (most often 40–50 years of age). The clinical picture of malignant hypertension reflects the pathological process – that is, acute severe vascular damage. Symptoms are much more frequent than with 'benign' essential hypertension. They include blurring of vision, mental impairment, haematuria or haematospermia and clinical features of target organ damage.

Hypertensive haemorrhages in malignant hypertension are of two sorts. *Flame-shaped haemorrhages* are more superficial and owe their character to constraints imposed by nerve fibres. *Dot and blot haemorrhages* are deep to the nerve fibres and so are not limited in the same way. Haemorrhages are a sign of recent severe vascular damage and usually disappear after a few weeks of effective blood pressure control. Exudates are of two types:

- Hard or waxy exudates represent the end result of fluid leakage into the fibre layers of the retina from damaged vessels often with associated nerve fibre damage. Fluid is reabsorbed, leaving a protein lipid residue which is slowly removed by macrophages, and finally leaving a hyaline deposit which may sometimes persist. Like retinal haemorrhages, hard exudates are forced into a radial spoke-like distribution by the nerve fibres around the macula ('macular star').
- Soft exudates or cotton wool patches are quite different, both aetiologically and ophthalmoscopically. They are usually larger than hard exudates and have a woolly ill-defined edge. They are not true exudates but nerve fibre infarcts caused by hypertensive vascular occlusion. Unlike hard exudates, these lesions disappear within a few weeks of establishing adequate hypertensive therapy.

Papilloedema is associated with increased pressure within the optic disc secondary to severe vascular damage. Venous distension is followed by increased vascularity of the optic disc which has a pink appearance with blurring of the disc margins and loss of the optic cup. Raising of the optic disc with anterior displacement of the vessels occurs later. Often, the surrounding retina shows oedema, small radial haemorrhages and cotton-wool exudates.

Raised blood pressure: causes

Essential hypertension

No identifiable cause can be found in the vast majority of patients who present with sustained blood pressure elevation (essential hypertension). High blood pressure in such individuals is believed to be multifactorial, with a substantial contribution from both genetic and environmental factors. Studies of hypertension prevalence in families and in monozygotic and dizygotic twins have confirmed the importance of the genetic factor. The advent of the 'molecular medicine' era has heralded the development of newer techniques to study mechanisms and genes determining blood pressure control. As yet, genome-wide screening has not identified any novel genes implicated in blood pressure control, although a few promising chromosomal regions have been identified.

Epidemiological studies have also emphasized the importance of other factors which are associated with blood pressure elevation. These include obesity and heavy alcohol intake. In addition, higher blood pressure levels are noted in American (although probably not British) blacks. Extensive investigation of patients with essential hypertension may show a variety of minor changes – for example, slight elevation in haematocrit, increase in renal vascular resistance, decreased renal plasma flow and increased filtration fraction. All of these changes are, however, probably secondary to structural changes induced in the blood vessels by hypertension. One possible clue to the aetiology is provided by evidence for sympathetic nervous systemic activation in young hypertensives, who often have a cardiac output in the upper part of the normal range, increased heart rate and slightly elevated circulating noradrenaline levels. Later in the course of hypertension this evidence for increased nervous system activity disappears, and blood pressure is maintained by elevated peripheral resistance alone. There is no evidence that other powerful pressor systems (e.g. the renin–angiotensin system or sodium retention) are responsible for blood pressure elevation in essential hypertension.

The vast majority of patients with essential hypertension are diagnosed either at routine examination or incidentally when attending a doctor for other medical problems. The early stages of hypertension are, in most cases, asymptomatic. Occipital headaches which are throbbing in nature and worse in the morning are described as classical, but are only seen in a small minority of patients. In most cases headaches are probably unrelated to hypertension, although the frequency of headaches in a hypertension clinic decreases with effective blood pressure control. Epistaxes are more frequent in hypertensive patients but are an unusual manifestation. The other manifestations of hypertension are due to target organ damage. Dyspnoea due to left ventricular failure is a very late manifestation. Besides reflecting increased load against which the left ventricle works, it may also be due to associated ischaemic heart disease which is of course more common in hypertension. Visual disturbances are only seen with advanced (Grade III or Grade IV) retinopathy, although, occasionally, arteriovenous nipping – seen in less severe retinopathy – can cause a branch retinal vein occlusion. Renal impairment is extremely rare in patients who have only Grades I or II retinopathy (so-called benign essential hypertension). Nocturia is, however, frequently seen in hypertension of all grades, reflecting a disturbance in the normal circadian rhythm of urine formation. Focal neurological signs may reflect either a cerebrovascular accident (cerebral haemorrhage or thrombosis) or be due to focal oedema (hypertensive encephalopathy). This disorder is characterized by transient focal neurological signs associated with very high blood pressure levels. It is due to systemic blood pressure exceeding the upper autoregulatory range of cerebral blood flow control so that focal hyperaemia and oedema occur. Peripheral vascular disease is due to hypertension-induced atheroma in the large arteries and aorta.

Secondary hypertension

High blood pressure can be attributed to a specific disorder or drug only in a minority of patients. The quoted incidence of secondary hypertension has been as high as 20–30 per cent. However, such figures come from specialist clinics where patients are referred because of the high suspicion of secondary hypertension. The true incidence of secondary hypertension in unselected populations is much lower. Where such populations have been screened intensively for renal or adrenal hypertension, the observed prevalence in patients with elevated blood pressure has been less than 1 per cent. The incidence of iatrogenic hypertension is more difficult to assess, since drugs may contribute to hypertension in individuals already predisposed to essential hypertension. It seems likely however that oral contraceptive pill hypertension is more frequent than either renal or adrenal hypertension. Other causes of hypertension are rarer still. A list of the causes of secondary hypertension (excluding renal causes) is given in Table B.6.

Renal hypertension

There are three different groups of disorders which cause renal hypertension. These are diseases of the renal artery or its smaller branches (renovascular hypertension), diseases of the renal parenchyma, and renin-secreting tumours which are derived from the cells of the juxtaglomerular apparatus. The last-named is an extremely rare cause of hypertension occurring in children or young adults. There are also case reports of hypersecretion of renin by Wilms' tumour, renal carcinoma, bronchial carcinoma and pancreatic adenocarcinoma. Hypertension is caused by the high renin levels, with associated secondary aldosteronism, although structural changes in the

Table B.6 Causes of secondary hypertension other than renal causes

Endocrine and metabolic
- Mineralocorticoid:
  - ◆ primary hyperaldosteronism
  - ◆ isolated secretion of corticosterone/deoxycorticosterone/18-hydroxy-deoxycorticosterone
  - ◆ ovarian dysgenesis and mineralocorticoid excess
  - ◆ heritable disorders (17α-hydroxylase and 11β-hydroxylase deficiency, syndrome of apparent mineralocorticoid excess, glucocorticoid-remediable aldosteronism)
- Glucocorticoid: Cushing's syndrome
- Phaeochromocytoma
- Acromegaly
- Myxoedema
- Other heritable disorders: Liddle's syndrome, Gordon's syndrome

Other causes
- Coarctation of the aorta
- Hypertensive disorders of pregnancy: chronic hypertension, gestational hypertension, pre-eclampsia
- Neurological: bulbar, raised intracranial pressure, spinal

Drug-related causes of hypertension
- Corticosteroids, oestrogens (contraceptive pill)
- Alcohol, amphetamines, ecstasy (MDMA and derivatives) and cocaine
- Migraine medications ($5HT_1$ agonists)
- Ciclosporin, erythropoietin
- Nasal decongestants
- Monoamine oxidase inhibitors
- Anti-hypertensive medications (e.g. clonidine) on sudden discontinuation – rebound hypertension

resistance vessels help to maintain blood pressure when hypertension has been maintained for prolonged periods. Renovascular and renoparenchymal hypertension are not entirely discrete categories. Thus, renal parenchymal disease such as pyelonephritis or glomerulonephritis gives rise to renal ischaemia and frequently hypersecretion of renin can be demonstrated. The other known factor which plays a role in some patients with bilateral renovascular or renoparenchymal disease (or disease in a single kidney) is *sodium retention*. This is particularly notable in acute glomerulonephritis and in advanced renal failure where oedema is often associated with hypertension. Unfortunately, from the diagnostic point of view, in many patients with renovascular or renoparenchymal disease there are neither high renin levels nor evidence of sodium retention. In some cases it seems likely that chronic hypertension has given rise to structural changes in the resistance vessels which then maintain blood pressure, even after the precipitating factor is no longer in evidence. It also seems likely, however, that the kidney regulates blood pressure in other less well-understood ways. For instance, the renal medulla secretes vasodepressor material, and this mechanism may be impaired in some forms of renal hypertension.

Because of the multiplicity of renal mechanisms and because secondary changes may maintain blood pressure even after the initial mechanism has ceased to act, the diagnosis of renal hypertension is frequently extremely difficult. Clinical and biochemical features are often conspicuous by their absence. Certain clues may however be suggestive. Thus, severe hypertension presenting in a young patient (e.g. below the age of 30 years) in the absence of a family history of hypertension makes a renal cause more likely. A renal cause is more likely to be found in patients with malignant hypertension and in those in whom the blood pressure rises rapidly. A renal bruit – particularly when it occurs both in diastolic and systolic phases – is more suggestive of a renovascular cause, although such bruits are frequently heard in the absence of any lesions of the renal arteries. Generalized oedema suggests acute glomerulonephritis. This may be post-streptococcal, or it may be a manifestation of systemic disease such as Henoch–Schönlein purpura, Goodpasture's syndrome, polyarteritis nodosa or Wegener's granulomatosis. Clinical evidence of uraemia – perhaps associated with dependent oedema – suggests advanced renal disease, most probably due to end-stage chronic glomerulonephritis or chronic pyelonephritis. It must be borne in mind, however, that severe hypertension can give rise to hypertensive nephropathy and renal failure, so that uraemia can be an effect rather than a cause of hypertension. This is more likely in patients with Grade III or IV retinopathy. Whilst a history of urinary tract infections (UTI), perhaps in childhood or many years previously, may suggest chronic pyelonephritis, in the majority of cases of chronic pyelonephritis and hypertension there is no previous history of UTI. In some patients, there may be a history of previous reflux uropathy in childhood. A history of renal disease in the family suggests polycystic kidneys or, less commonly, hereditary nephritis. Relevant features in the history may less commonly indicate such causes as gouty nephropathy, diabetes, irradiation nephritis, amyloidosis, renal tuberculosis or heavy-metal poisoning.

In only a minority of cases with renal hypertension will the history and examination yield the diagnosis. Urine dipstick testing and microscopy are simple, useful and inexpensive investigations which may provide evidence of renal pathology. Measurement of serum electrolytes, urea and creatinine may indicate the presence of renal disease in a few patients. Plasma renin and aldosterone are often normal, and may indeed be subnormal where renin secretion has been suppressed by sodium retention. In addition, severe and malignant hypertension often is associated with elevated plasma renin levels, even where there is no primary renal disease. Further investigation of renal hypertension requires renal imaging with ultrasonography in the first instance. Screening for renovascular hypertension involves duplex ultrasound/nuclear renal imaging/ magnetic resonance angiography/CT angiography depending upon which centre the patient is in. Definitive diagnosis of the lesion in renovascular hypertension demands renal angiography.

There is considerable debate amongst medical professionals as to how best to manage renovascular hypertension, although it seems likely that advances in the field of renal artery stenting will profoundly influence the landscape.

Hypertension in pregnant women

Hypertensive disorders are the most common medical complications of pregnancy and are, broadly speaking, classified into three varieties: chronic hypertension; gestational hypertension; and pre-eclampsia. *Pre-eclampsia* is unique in being a self-limiting form of hypertension. Classical pre-eclampsia occurs for the first time during the third trimester of pregnancy, and blood pressure falls immediately after delivery. Blood pressure elevation is associated with significant proteinuria and oedema. Classically, pre-eclampsia is observed during the first pregnancy only, and is more common in older women, diabetic patients, multiple pregnancies and hydatidiform mole. It must be differentiated from essential hypertension which has been exacerbated by pregnancy (chronic hypertension). In this case, hypertension occurs during the first trimester and becomes progressively worse with successive pregnancies. The difference between the two conditions is often not clear-cut, and the diagnosis may have to be delayed until the course of blood pressure after gestation can be observed. *Gestational*

hypertension is defined as the development of hypertension without features of pre-eclampsia after 20 weeks' gestation in a previously normotensive woman. This form of hypertension tends to be associated with a good prognosis, and may not even require blood pressure-lowering therapy in many instances.

Endocrine and metabolic hypertension

Primary aldosteronism is associated with either a single adenoma or bilateral hyperplasia of the adrenal cortical zona glomerulosa. The latter may take the form of diffuse hypertrophy, or there may be multiple small adenomata (micronodular hyperplasia). It is important to distinguish between a single adenoma and hyperplasia, as the treatment of the first condition is surgical, and the second medical. Very rarely, the lesion may be carcinomatous, and occasional cases have been described with no histological lesion. Primary aldosteronism probably accounts for less than 0.1 per cent of cases of hypertension. The clinical picture may be indistinguishable from that of essential hypertension. The most characteristic symptom is generalized muscle weakness, although cramps, tetany and polyuria occasionally occur. Malignant hypertension is comparatively rare in primary aldosteronism, perhaps because the rise in blood pressure is gradual rather than rapid. The biochemical features which suggest primary aldosteronism are a low serum potassium associated with serum sodium which is in the upper part of, or just above, the normal range. Further investigations will demonstrate suppression of plasma renin and elevation of blood and urinary aldosterone. It is important to differentiate between primary and secondary aldosteronism (which is frequently seen in severe hypertension or in diuretic-treated patients). In *secondary aldosteronism*, the serum sodium is low and plasma renin elevated. Tumours may be visualized by contrast-enhanced CT scanning, although in some centres external isotope scanning of the adrenal glands after administration of technetium or iodine-labelled cholesterol is the imaging method of choice. If uncertainty still exists, differential adrenal venous sampling should be carried out.

Very rarely, cases have been described with isolated secretion of other mineralocorticoids such as deoxycorticosterone. 11β-Hydroxylase deficiency occurs in children, and is associated with virilization (adrenogenital syndrome). 17α-Hydroxylase deficiency is associated with sexual immaturity as the production of sex hormones is impaired. In all of these conditions, mineralocorticoid-induced sodium retention and hypokalaemia occur with suppression of plasma renin. *Liddle's syndrome* is an autosomal dominant condition characterized by early-onset hypertension with hypokalaemic alkalosis. It is caused by activating mutations in the renal collecting tubular epithelial sodium channel, leading to increased sodium-retaining and potassium-secreting activity. Thus, although the biochemical features of primary aldosteronism are present with a low potassium and renin level, aldosterone is also very low. *Glucocorticoid-remediable aldosteronism* (also called dexamethasone-suppressible hyperaldosteronism) is another autosomal dominant trait in which early-onset hypertension is associated with haemorrhagic stroke. It has the biochemical features of primary aldosteronism, but the biochemistry is corrected by suppressing adrenocorticotrophic hormone (ACTH) with dexamethasone. This is due to a mutation producing a chimeric gene encoding a protein with aldosterone synthase enzymatic activity, the expression of which is regulated by ACTH. Other rare causes of heritable hypertension include the syndrome of apparent mineralocorticoid excess (AME, autosomal recessive) and pseudohypoaldosteronism type II (Gordon's syndrome, autosomal dominant).

The *hypertension of Cushing's syndrome* is usually associated with hypersecretion of glucocorticoids, although mineralocorticoids such as deoxycorticosterone may also occasionally be elevated. The hypertension arises due to cortisol-mediated activation of the mineralocorticoid receptor secondary to supersaturation of the enzyme 11β-hydroxysteroid dehydrogenase type 2, which would normally inactivate cortisol by metabolizing it to cortisone.

Phaeochromocytomas are tumours of sympathetic tissue which produce hypertension by the secretion of catecholamines (adrenaline, noradrenaline and, occasionally, dopamine). They are probably responsible for hypertension in less than 0.1 per cent of hypertensive patients. Although the tumours usually originate in the adrenal medulla (when adrenaline secretion tends to predominate), they may also arise from sympathetic ganglia associated with the abdominal, and rarely thoracic, aorta and the bladder wall. Tumours are frequently multiple and occasionally malignant. Classically, suspicion of phaeochromocytoma is raised on clinical grounds. The patient has short periods of high blood pressure associated with

other features of sympathetic activity. These include sweating, flushing and throbbing headache, abdominal or chest pain and weight loss. The anxiety usually associated with such attacks is presumably a manifestation of visceral feedback. Examination during attacks usually shows either tachycardia or bradycardia and severe hypertension. Attacks may be provoked by specific movement, exercise, micturition or by abdominal palpation or at surgery (Fig. B.7): indeed, occasional fatalities have been described during clinical examination. In addition, some patients have a low standing blood pressure, and this may cause symptoms of *postural hypotension*. Occasionally, very high circulating catecholamine levels have been associated with a condition which resembles cardiogenic shock, and post-mortem focal myocardial lesions have been observed. Glucose tolerance is frequently impaired, the basal metabolic rate elevated, and free fatty acid levels are raised. In some cases the tumour is associated with neurofibromatosis (von Recklinghausen's disease). A rare combination of endocrine disorders is inherited as autosomal dominant: this comprises multiple phaeochromocytomas, medullary carcinoma of the thyroid and hyperparathyroidism (Sipple's syndrome or multiple endocrine adenomatosis Type II). Other associations are tuberose sclerosis and the Sturge–Weber syndrome. Diagnosis is made by finding either unchanged catecholamines or catecholamine metabolites (such as vanillyl mandelic acid or normetadrenaline and metadrenaline) in the urine. Significant numbers of false negatives occur, particularly if the urine collection does not

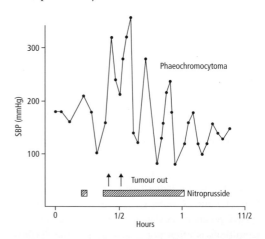

Figure B.7 Systolic blood pressure fluctuation during manipulation of the tumour at operation in a patient with phaeochromocytoma.

coincide with a pressor attack. For this reason, if the diagnosis is seriously being considered, multiple urine collections are necessary. Additionally, plasma catecholamines can be measured while the patient is under observation. Elevated levels associated with tachycardia and raised blood pressure are suggestive. The main differential diagnosis here is anxiety. Administration of clonidine results in a lowering of plasma catecholamine levels in patients with anxiety, but has no effect upon the high catecholamine levels observed in phaeochromocytoma. Tumours can be imaged either by CT scanning or by isotope studies using metaiodobenzguanidine (MIBG). If no adrenal tumour is seen, venous sampling for catecholamines at different levels in the inferior and superior vena cava may help to locate an ectopic tumour.

Blood pressure is elevated in about 30 per cent of patients with *acromegaly*, although different clinical series quote wide-ranging prevalence of 20 to 60 per cent. The exact mechanisms underlying the development of hypertension in acromegaly remain unclear, although it is recognized that growth hormone induces sodium retention. Consistent with this finding is the observation that plasma renin is often suppressed in acromegalic patients. There is also an association between adrenal adenomata and acromegaly which may be relevant in some patients.

High blood pressure is approximately twice as common in *hypothyroid patients* as in the general population. In most cases, blood pressure falls when thyroid deficiency is corrected. Hypertension cannot be clearly related either to increased renin secretion or to sodium and water retention. It has been suggested that there may be an abnormality in vascular smooth muscle produced by thyroid hormone deficiency.

Other causes of hypertension

Coarctation of the aorta is the most common cardiovascular cause of hypertension. In this condition there is narrowing usually situated distal to the origin of the left subclavian artery at or near the insertion of the ligamentum arteriosum. The so-called infantile type of coarctation in which the ductus is patent is irrelevant to hypertension. Uncomplicated coarctation may present as mild blood pressure elevation in childhood, and occasionally hypertension becomes suddenly more severe. Infants with other cardiac lesions present with congestive failure. The young adult usually presents

with asymptomatic hypertension or with the complications of hypertension. Unless there is an associated cardiac lesion, the clinical symptoms are usually indistinguishable from those of essential hypertension beginning at an unusual age, although diminished circulation through the legs may cause cramps. Physical signs which suggest the diagnosis are: raised blood pressure in the arms associated with normal or low blood pressure in the legs (a wide-leg cuff has to be used to determine this); delayed, weak or absent femoral pulses; an ejection systolic murmur heard best posteriorly between the left scapula and the spine; and pulsatile collateral vessels situated around the scapulae and in the posterior intercostal spaces: these are more noticeable on sitting the patient forward. There are usually associated bruits. There may also be an aortic systolic ejection murmur due to a biscuspid aortic valve which is present in 50 per cent of cases. A firm diagnosis can often be made from the chest X-ray. The characteristic double aortic knuckle is made up of the dilated left subclavian artery and post stenotic dilatation of the descending aorta. Another, almost pathognomonic, sign is notching of the lower borders of the ribs. These are not to be confused with defects of an erosive nature in the superior margins of the ribs seen rarely in poliomyelitis, hyperparathyroidism, rheumatoid arthritis and scleroderma. The diagnosis can finally be confirmed and the extent of the coarctation delineated by aortography.

Neurological disease causes hypertension only very rarely. Raised intracranial pressure probably causes hypertension through brainstem compression and ischaemia activating sympathetic efferent outflow from the vasomotor centre. Transient blood pressure elevation may be seen after head injury, presumably for the same reason. Vascular disease, brainstem encephalitis and poliomyelitis also occasionally produce hypertension through involvement of the brainstem centre. Lesions of the upper part of the spinal cord may cause severe hypertension through interference with cardiovascular reflexes. Such hypertension may be paroxysmal, as a result of an acute pressor response to stimulation of viscera such as the bladder or rectum.

In addition to the *contraceptive pill* and *corticosteroid therapy*, many drugs can either cause hypertension or exacerbate pre-existing hypertension. Hypertension and tachycardia are common findings in patients attending accident and emergency departments who have abused recreational drugs such as ecstasy and cocaine. Non-steroidal anti-inflammatory drugs (NSAIDs) raise blood pressure probably through inhibition of renal prostaglandin synthesis, which plays a role in the regulation of sodium and water output. Usually, the degree of blood pressure elevation is mild, but administration of NSAIDs may cause loss of blood pressure control in patients on antihypertensive therapy. Anti-migraine preparations of the serotonergic variety ($5HT_1$ agonists or 'triptans') can produce a transient increase in blood pressure.

Nowadays, rarely used *monoamine-oxidase inhibitors* (e.g. phenelzine and tranylcypromine) can produce severe paroxysmal hypertension. This is particularly likely to occur when used in combination with tyramine-containing foods (of which mature cheese is the most important) and amphetamines. Clinically, the resulting syndrome resembles that observed in phaeochromocytoma. Sympathomimetic amines (e.g. amphetamine, ephedrine, metaraminol and other synthetic agents) are often used as nasal decongestants, and may cause significant hypertension. Liquorice and carbenoxolone raise blood pressure through inducing a syndrome which resembles primary aldosteronism with a hypokalaemic alkalosis; in addition the patients may be oedematous. This is due to direct inhibition of 11β-hydroxysteroid dehydrogenase Type II which normally metabolizes cortisol to cortisone and thereby allows the mineralocorticoid effects of cortisol (which has equal affinity to aldosterone for the mineralocorticoid receptor) to predominate.

Ciclosporin and *erythropoietin* cause high blood pressure by mechanisms which have not been elucidated. Withdrawal of the centrally acting antihypertensive agent clonidine causes paroxysmal hypertension due to increased efferent sympathetic nerve activity. Certain medical preparations contain large amounts of sodium; these include resonium A, paraminosalicylate, sodium carbenicillin and some antacid mixtures. Whilst these have no effect on blood pressure in healthy individuals, hypertension may be caused in patients with renal failure.

Melvin Lobo

BLOOD PRESSURE, LOW

The lower half of the blood pressure distribution curve in healthy unselected populations is just as smooth as the upper half, with no evidence for a discrete group of hypotensive subjects (see BLOOD PRESSURE, HIGH, p. 66). The diagnosis of low blood pressure is therefore just as arbitrary as the diagnosis of high blood pressure. The clinical significance of the diagnosis is, however, quite different. Both high and low blood pressure are most commonly multifactorial – that is, the result of the interaction of genetic and environmental factors (biological variability). High blood pressure carries an increased cardiovascular risk, although it is only infrequently due to a specific disease. However, low blood pressure – when it is attributable only to biological variability – carries a lower risk of cardiovascular disease than the population average. Its only clinical significance therefore is when it causes symptoms (see FAINTS, p. 212), or when it is a manifestation of disease. In epidemiological studies it has been associated with increased prevalence of psychoneurotic symptoms. Additionally, in some studies a low diastolic blood pressure in treated hypertensive patients has been associated with an increased risk of cardiac death. Whether this is a result of treatment or not is controversial. The causes of low blood pressure are listed in Table B.7.

Low blood pressure can result from underactivity of any of the systems which maintain blood pressure. Since these systems assume particular importance when the subject stands, *postural hypotension* may be the only manifestation of low blood pressure. It is seen commonly, therefore, when fluid is lost from the gastrointestinal tract as a result of vomiting or diarrhoea, when renal fluid losses occur as in the excessive use of diuretics, in Addison's disease or in some patients with chronic pyelonephritis and a sodium-losing tendency. It is also observed when fluid is lost as a result of bleeding or burns. In wasting conditions, or after prolonged bed-rest, venous return to the heart and cardiac output may be reduced as a result of loss of skeletal muscle bulk; a low blood pressure is therefore frequently seen in this situation. Hypotension may result less commonly when cardiac output is reduced as a result of primary cardiac disease or cardiac tamponade, or as a result of obstruction to outflow of blood from the right or left side of the heart from, for example, valvular lesions.

Impairment of autonomic circulatory reflexes is often observed in diabetics and elderly patients with postural hypotension. In the latter case, this is probably due to rigidity of the carotid artery and aorta in

Table B.7 Causes of low blood pressure

Cardiac
- Disturbances of rate and rhythm
  - Heart block
  - Dysrhythmias
- Obstruction to flow
  - Aortic or pulmonary valvular stenosis
  - Hypertrophic obstructive cardiomyopathy
  - Atrial myxoma
  - Primary pulmonary hypertension
  - Pulmonary embolism
  - Cardiac tamponade
  - Mitral and tricuspid stenosis
  - Cor triatriatum
  - Tetralogy of Fallot
  - Eisenmenger's syndrome
- Impaired ventricular function
  - Myocardial infarction
  - Bilateral cardiomyopathy

Impaired vasomotor control
- Vasovagal syncope
- Glossopharyngeal neuralgia
- Micturition, deglutition or post-tussive syncope
- Baroceptor dysfunction in the elderly
- Autonomic degeneration (diabetes and Shy–Drager syndrome)
- Carotid sinus hypersensitivity

Impaired venous return
- Haemorrhage and dehydration
- Muscle wasting and prolonged bed-rest

Metabolic and endocrine
- Phaeochromocytoma
- Serotonin-secreting tumours
- Hyporeninaemic hypoaldosteronism
- Addison's disease
- Monogenic diseases: aldosterone synthase deficiency, 21-hydroxylase deficiency, pseudohypoaldosteronism type I, Gitelman's syndrome, Barter's syndrome

Drugs
- Antihypertensives (particularly centrally acting agents, ganglion-blockers, post-adrenergic ganglion blockers, alpha-receptor-blockers and diuretics)
- CNS depressants
- Anti-arrhythmic drugs (e.g. flecainide, disopyramide, propafenone)
- Anti-anginal drugs (nitrates, nicorandil)
- Thrombolytic agents

the region of the baroreceptors. Lesions of central pathways less commonly cause hypotension. Efferent pathways are interfered with particularly by ganglion-blocking drugs and alpha-receptor-blocking agents such as prazosin or terozsin. However, antihypertensive drugs of any class may lead to hypotension. Degeneration of sympathetic pathways occurs in the rare Shy–Drager syndrome. The renin–angiotensin system does not assume great importance in blood pressure control unless patients are fluid-depleted, so inhibition of this system does not normally cause a low blood pressure. However, a syndrome of hyporeninaemic, hypoaldosteronism has been described in elderly subjects with postural hypotension.

Melvin Lobo

BODY IMAGE, DISORDERS OF

Broadly, disorders of body image can be divided into two categories differentiated by whether or not the problem is the presenting complaint for which the patient seeks correction (Table B.8).

Table B.8 Causes of disorders of body image

Not the presenting complaint
- Commonest
  - Anorexia nervosa
  - Bulimia nervosa
  - Parietal lobe lesions
  - Temporal lobe epilepsy
- Rare
  - Migraine
  - Depersonalization
  - Schizophrenia
- Drug-related
  - LSD
  - Mescaline

The presenting complaint
- Common
  - Dysmorphophobia
  - Personality disorder (body dysmorphic disorder)
  - Stress reaction
- Rare
  - Transsexualism
  - Schizophrenia
  - Monosymptomatic hypochondriacal psychosis
  - Major depression

Not the presenting complaint

The classical organic presentation is *hemiasomatognosia*, the unilateral misperception of one's own body which is associated with parietal lobe lesions. There is a conscious form of hemiasomatognosia occasionally found in epilepsy or migraine when the disturbance is transient and may be related to lesions in either cerebral lobe. Much more common and spectacular is *unconscious hemiasomatognosia*, when the patient believes and behaves as if half the body no longer exists. This can be subdivided into three forms:

- Anosognosia for left hemiplegia, the denial of the existence of paralysis which is usually confined to the first 2 weeks after onset (right parietal lobe).
- Neglect syndromes, hemi-inattention and spatial neglect which is permanent (either parietal lobe).
- Gerstmann's syndrome, which consists of finger agnosia, acalculia, agraphia and right/left disorientation, and is associated with autopagnosia – the failure to localize, recognize or name parts of the body (left parietal lobe).

Macrosomatognosia or *microsomatognosia*, the experience that parts (or the whole) of the body have enlarged or shrunk, is associated most notably with temporal lobe epilepsy, but may also occur in depersonalization, migraine, schizophrenia and LSD or mescaline abuse. Similarly, changes in body shape, weight, colour or familiarity may occur in any of these conditions.

Over-estimation of body width is a recognized feature of both anorexia nervosa and bulimia nervosa. The patient's over-estimation of size does not involve their height or other people's body width. It is an inconsistent finding among patients, although characteristic of the group, while its clinical significance lies in the observations that it is a useful indicator of treatment response and the likelihood of relapse. This phenomenon has been reported to a lesser extent in young women without eating disorders, and it is postulated that over-estimation of body width reflects the degree of personal value attached to body shape and size.

The presenting complaint

In *gender dysphoria* (or *transsexualism*), the individual's dissatisfaction with their body stems from a deeply held belief that they belong to the opposite gender from their physical sexual characteristics. Sex reassignment surgery is sought so that the external sexual characteristics of the desired sex may be acquired. These patients usually live, dress and act as if they belong to their chosen gender, and may 'shop around' for hormonal and surgical correction. Prolonged specialist assessment is always required before proceeding to definitive surgery.

A commoner presenting complaint of body image disorder is *body dysmorphic disorder* (or *dysmorphophobia*), when the patient asserts to being physically misshapen or defective in some way which cannot be substantiated, or is grossly exaggerated upon objective examination, such that they seek cosmetic surgery. An important aspect of this condition is the concern – and sometimes the certainty – that the defect is noticed by others. The most frequent sites for complaint are the nose or breasts, but the ears, chin, other facial features and genitals are not uncommon. While recognizing a dysmorphophobic presentation is usually straightforward it can be difficult – and sometimes impossible – to determine whether the belief is held with delusional conviction or is an over-valued idea. Generally, the more unusual the site and the more bizarre the belief, the more likely the presentation is a delusion, occasionally in the setting of major depression but more often as a feature of schizophrenia or monosymptomatic hypochondriacal delusional state. When doubt exists about whether the presentation is delusional, a treatment trial with a neuroleptic has been advocated and reported to be effective, although many patients will baulk at the prospect of this management approach.

The second problem is to determine whether cosmetic surgery will help the patient whose dysmorphophobia is neurotically or personality-based. It used to be considered that surgical correction in dysmorphophobic patients was inappropriate as it would neither affect their beliefs nor prevent the psychological problems that many of them subsequently suffered. However, it has become apparent that following corrective surgery for minor deficits the level of psychological disturbance falls and the change in appearance is frequently regarded as satisfactory by the patient. This has led to an important distinction developing between patients who have trivial deformities and those who have none, notwithstanding such a delineation can prove difficult to define.

In patients who have minor defects the key is to understand the significance of the problem from the patient's perspective. A middle-aged male doctor is likely to view a small bump on the nose quite differently from a teenage girl, and it is important to acknowledge it is her viewpoint that should be the more relevant. Sometimes, minor physical defects can have major cultural, social or financial implications for the patient.

Patients who should not be operated upon are first, of course, those in whom corrective surgery is technically inappropriate either because there is no defect, or the likelihood is that surgery will make matters worse or unchanged, or there is no corrective procedure for the patient's complaint. Second, patients who have vague complaints and no specific treatment in mind, yet expect surgery both to be performed and to create perfection, should not be operated upon; most of these individuals suffer fundamentally from personality disorders – over-sensitive, insecure, schizoid, narcissistic and obsessional traits are all described. Third, seeking corrective surgery following a major life event is likely to be a method of coping maladaptively with adjustment and loss; a characteristic presentation is the middle-aged woman wanting mammoplasty after her successful husband has left her for a younger women. For this group of patients, psychiatric intervention can prove particularly helpful, but although psychiatric treatment has been advocated generally for dysmorphophobic patients in whom surgery is considered inappropriate, in practice this is rarely acceptable to the patient, and even when it is, successful interventions are the exception rather than the rule.

Andrew Hodgkiss

BORBORYGMI

'Borborygmi' is the term applied to rumbling noises of varying quality and intensity produced by peristaltic movements of the bowel propelling mixed gaseous and liquid contents.

These sounds, although normally inaudible to the patient or to other persons, and detected only by auscultation by means of a stethoscope, may occasionally be annoyingly obtrusive. They may occur in perfectly normal people, especially when the alimentary canal is relatively empty, for instance when a meal is overdue, and they may occur as a result of nervous air-swallowing. They may be due to the powerful peristaltic waves of a bowel that is hypertrophied and dilated above a slowly developing obstruction of the large bowel; here there will usually be accompanying progressive constipation, colicky abdominal pains and distension. Some people are able to produce a loud sound by forcibly

contracting the muscles of the anterior abdominal wall and splashing the fluid content of the stomach.

The carcinoid syndrome may feature loud borborygmi as well as flushing of the face, trunk and limbs, pulmonary stenosis, cramping abdominal pains and diarrhoea.

In contrast, the absence of borborygmi, resulting in complete silence in the abdomen on auscultation for several minutes, is seen in adynamic ileus and peritonitis.

Harold Ellis

BREAST LUMPS

(See also NIPPLE, ABNORMALITIES OF, p. 483)

Method of examination

The patient should sit stripped to the waist, so that a clear view of both breasts, the thorax, axillae and supraclavicular fossae may be obtained. The surgeon should sit with his or her eyes level with the patient's nipples. Both breasts should first be looked at as a whole, to see whether they are symmetrical in size, contour and level, and whether the two nipples are in the same site and of the same circumference, prominence and inclination. One breast may always have been smaller or one nipple inverted, but any recent change is highly significant. The patient should then sit on a couch, and the breasts studied in detail for any evidence of local enlargement or shrinking, and for abnormalities such as redness of the skin, dilatation of veins, tumour or ulcer. If no difference is at first noticed, the patient should be asked to raise both arms slowly above the head and bring them down again to the side, since differences which were previously invisible – particularly dimpling of the skin from attachment of a lump – may come into view as the breast glides over the chest wall. Next, the breasts are felt, using first the flat of the hand, passing systematically over all parts, examining comparable sectors on the two sides simultaneously; afterwards, the fingers are used for more detailed examination of any irregularity that may have been discovered or suspected. The axillae should also be palpated carefully for enlarged nodes, with particular attention being paid to the inner wall, along the pectoralis minor and to the apex. In cases of suspected cancer the supraclavicular and infraclavicular fossae should also be examined for fullness or enlarged nodes, and the chest and liver should be investigated for signs of secondary growth. An examination from behind, with the patient sitting, may be used to check any abnormalities seen, felt or suspected whilst in the lying position.

Alternative posture for 'difficult' or pendulous breasts

When dealing with a woman with large, obese or pendulous breasts, the conventional posture for examination is often unsatisfactory. An alternative posture is to arrange the woman in a semi-recumbent position, rotated obliquely with a pillow behind the scapula of the side under examination and the shoulder fully abducted, with the hand tucked behind the head. This fixes the pectoralis major and allows the breast disc to 'float' over a rigid base.

Classification

Swellings of the whole breast

- Bilateral
  - ◆ Pregnancy
  - ◆ Lactation
  - ◆ ANDI (abnormalities of normal development and involution)
  - ◆ Hypertrophy
  - ◆ In males from stilboestrol administration
  - ◆ Acute mastitis
- Unilateral
  - ◆ Hypertrophy of the newborn
  - ◆ Puberty
  - ◆ Unilateral hypertrophy

Discrete lumps in breast

- Benign
  - ◆ Fibroadenoma
  - ◆ Simple cyst
  - ◆ Galactocele
  - ◆ Lipoma
  - ◆ Plasma cell mastitis (peri-ductal mastitis) (Rare: fat necrosis; tuberculous abscess)
  - ◆ Phylloides tumour
- Malignant
  - ◆ Carcinoma (Rare: sarcoma; lymphoma)

Multiple swellings, usually involving both breasts

- ◆ ANDI
- ◆ Multiple cysts

Swellings that are not of the breast

- ◆ Retromammary abscess:
  - From disease of rib
  - Chronic empyema
- ◆ Chondroma of chest wall
- ◆ Deformities of the ribs
- ◆ Mondor's disease

Swelling in pregnancy and lactation

Swelling in these cases is normal, and only liable to cause confusion when the patient is unaware of her condition. Both breasts are enlarged equally, and feel tense and nodular. The superficial veins are usually prominent, and on gentle squeezing a few drops of milk are discharged from the nipple. Montgomery's tubercles will be evident.

Unilateral enlargements

These are usually found in the undeveloped breast. In the *newborn*, one breast is often enlarged to the limits of its infantile size, and may discharge a little serous fluid from the nipple. The enlargement used to be attributed to the manipulation of midwives, but it is more probably due to an endocrine imbalance consequent on the withdrawal of the maternal hormones in the fetal circulation, and subsides rapidly. In girls at *puberty* one breast may enlarge several months before the other, and may distress a solicitous mother; however, unless there are obvious signs of an inflammatory change, no notice need be taken of unilateral enlargement of the breast in girls between the ages of 10 and 13 years. Uniform enlargement of one breast also occurs in *men*, usually after the age of 40, and nodular plaques may appear in both sexes at puberty as a result of endocrine disturbance.

On no account should the breast disc of an adolescent girl be biopsied, as this may cause failure of either a quadrant or the whole breast to develop, and would be a legitimate reason for litigation.

Acute mastitis

Acute mastitis usually occurs during lactation, occasionally during pregnancy, and is most often due to infection with pyogenic organisms which have gained entrance through cracks in the nipple. At the beginning of the illness there is shivering, followed by fever and a feeling of weight and pain in the breast; the pain soon becomes very acute. In the early stages the swelling is limited to one part of the breast, which feels more resistant than normal; the skin is not reddened at first, nor are the lymphatic nodes enlarged. Pressure over the swelling may cause extrusion of a drop of pus from the nipple, and this is distinguished from milk by its viscidity and yellow colour. Later, fluctuation may become evident and, as the inflammation approaches the skin, this becomes red and oedematous, and ultimately an abscess may point and burst through it. At the same time, other foci of suppuration form, until the breast may be a bag of pus. The presence of fever and the intense tenderness of one portion of the breast are sufficient to distinguish acute mastitis from physiological engorgement.

It is not uncommon to find a small *areolar abscess,* which represents an infected gland of Montgomery.

Duct ectasia/plasma cell mastitis (periductal mastitis)

There is a common group of diseases which are generally poorly recognized, that cluster together under this heading. Their aetiology is unknown. For example, it is even uncertain whether the inflammatory process comes first, followed by ectasia of the duct, or whether ectatic ducts are the primary phenomenon with sloughing duct epithelium responsible for initiating the process of periductal mastitis. Assuming the latter sequence of events, then the cycle of clinical features may develop in the following way. The terminal lactiferous ducts dilate and often become hugely ectatic. As a consequence of this, the epithelial lining loosens and liquefies, causing plugs of cellular debris to fill up the ectatic ducts. The first clinical symptom of this condition is the extrusion of viscous, multi-coloured discharge from multiple duct orifices on the nipple surface. The milk ducts then become permeable to cellular and lipid contents normally contained within the lumina, and these then excite a chemical periductal inflammatory process, which is characterized by infiltration with plasma cells and foreign body giant cells. At this stage, a hard indurated mass with overlying inflammation may appear at the areolar margin. Commonly, this condition resolves spontaneously within a week or two. Less often, the inflammatory mass becomes secondarily infected with anaerobic organisms liquefying to produce a periareolar abscess. This may point at the areolar margin and spontaneously discharge. If the condition is not recognized and treated appropriately, then a pathological communication between the ducts of the nipple and the skin develops, forming a so-called mammillary duct fistula. In the acute phase, antibiotics covering both aerobic and anaerobic organisms may abort the process. Over the years, a series of clinical or subclinical episodes of periductal mastitis produces fibrosis along the ducts, causing them to shrink and pull in the nipple, producing a typical slit-like indrawing at the centre. Ultimately, the condition burns itself out with age. This complex of conditions is most common postmenopausally, but if it occurs in premenopausal women it tends to be more florid and often bilateral, leading to multiple abscesses and fistulae.

The mammillary duct fistula should be treated by laying open the fistula track and excising the chronic inflammatory tissue. Recurrent episodes of periductal mastitis and troublesome nipple discharge should be treated by removing surgically the whole of the subareolar system.

Tuberculous abscess

Tuberculous abscess is rare, but a certain number of cases of chronic mastitis and chronic abscess are really tuberculous, particularly in developing countries. The disease is insidious, starting as a painless irregular swelling, the periphery of which is hard and the centre soft. Later, the skin becomes reddened, and an abscess forms which may burst and leave a sinus. It differs from an acute abscess in that the duration is much longer, there is little or no pain or fever, and the pus, if examined, reveals no organisms on culture unless there has been secondary infection. Direct examination of stained films of the pus may show tubercle bacilli. The facts that the history is a long one, that the swelling or the edges of the abscess are hard, and that the axillary nodes may be enlarged, render this condition liable to be confounded with carcinoma.

Local fat necrosis

If this follows a blow on the breast it may give rise to a tumour that is almost indistinguishable from cancer. It is hard, irregular in outline, and fixed to the skin. Points of distinction are the previous history of severe injury at the exact spot where the swelling lies, the impression given on palpation that the lump is on rather than of the breast, and the absence of hard nodes in the axilla. Sometimes, a period of 2–3 weeks' observation is justifiable, during which time a traumatic swelling should decrease in size. However, if there is any real doubt about its nature, the lesion should be excised and submitted to section.

Contrary to popular myth, this is a rare condition of the breast. It is usually wise to ignore a history of trauma to the breast and to investigate the lump fully with mammography and biopsy.

Galactocele

A cyst containing milk, this is formed by dilatation of one of the larger ducts owing to obstruction. Galactoceles occur only during lactation and very rarely during the later months of pregnancy. They form oval, fluctuating swellings lying in the central zone of the breast just outside the areola, and on pressure milk can sometimes be squeezed out of the nipple. Aspiration both confirms the diagnosis and cures the condition.

Simple cysts

Simple cysts are common in the 30- to 60-year age group. They present as well-defined mobile lumps with a texture like an inflatable rubber ring. However, some are so tense as to be confused with a solid lump. Diagnosis is easy with a characteristic ultrasound image of a black, well-defined ovoid with a strong posterior acoustic enhancement. The diagnosis is confirmed and the condition treated by cyst aspiration. The cyst fluid should not be sent for cytological examination.

Benign tumours

A fibroadenoma is the only common innocent tumour of the breast. It is an encapsulated tumour, generally single, but sometimes multiple, and varying in size. It is more common (and often multiple) in Afro-Caribbean women. It is firm, with the consistency of hard rubber, rounded, or with irregular rounded projections, and clearly outlined. Most characteristic is the ease with which it can be moved under the skin and in the substance of the breast, to neither of which does it appear to have any attachment; hence, the

term 'breast mouse' which is applied to this lesion. These tumours generally occur between the ages of 18 and 30 years, and although they are quite painless they are so firm that they are usually discovered by the patient. Although a carcinoma of the breast is rare in this age group, it is wise to complete the 'triple assessment' with an ultrasound scan and fine-needle aspiration cytology. If the diagnosis is confirmed by imaging and pathology, it is safe to reassure the young woman and to discharge her from the clinic.

A lipoma may occur in the breast as elsewhere, and has the same characteristics.

However, always beware the 'pseudolipoma' which may be the earliest sign of a small invasive duct cancer which, by infiltrating Cooper's ligaments, may extrude fatty lobules forming a mushroom-like umbrella over the primary focus.

Malignant tumours

Malignant tumours of the breast are nearly always primary. Sarcoma is very rare, but carcinoma is common and the most important tumour that affects the breast. It is essentially a disease of the female breast, with only about 1 per cent of cases occurring in males. It is common in both married and unmarried women, and may occur at any age after puberty, though the majority are in women aged between 35 and 60. In advanced cases the disease is obvious (Fig. B.8), with the tumour being large and hard. It is attached to and ultimately, if not removed, will fungate through the skin and become fixed to the chest wall; the axillary nodes are enlarged and hard. Such cases are beyond

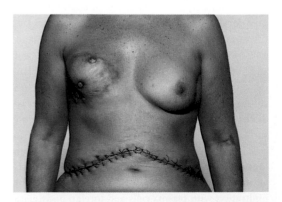

Figure B.8 Massive carcinoma of the right breast. Note the incipient skin ulceration and elevation and retraction of the nipple. The abdominal scar is from a recent bilateral adrenalectomy.

any but palliative treatment, and the importance of diagnosis lies in recognition of the early case, where the only sign is a small lump which the patient has probably discovered accidentally. Usually, there is no pain and the patient looks and feels perfectly well. The lump may lie in any part of the breast, but typically it is intermediate between the nipple and the periphery, and is more commonly in the upper and outer quadrant than in the other three. It can usually be felt with the flat of the hand. These lumps may be stony hard, but any consistency may be met with. Its outline is usually not sharply defined. In the early stage it is freely movable over the pectoral muscles and under the skin, but it is less movable in the breast substance than a fibroadenoma. Very soon, bands of fibrous tissue that connect the breast with the skin become involved, and by their contraction prevent free movement of the skin over the swelling. This first causes dimpling when the tumour is displaced, and later on puckering is visible all the time. If the tumour is anywhere near the centre of the breast, the nipple becomes retracted (Fig. B.9); a nipple may have been always inverted, but if one which was previously well

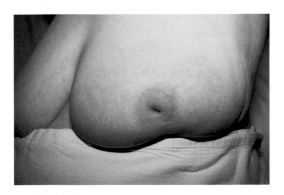

Figure B.9 Recent nipple inversion in carcinoma of the breast.

formed becomes retracted then the sign is of serious importance. Fixation to the deep fascia, which usually comes later, can be demonstrated by making the patient press her hands on the iliac crests to fix the pectoralis major, at which point the involved breast will be found to move less on the muscle than the normal breast. Many cancerous tumours – even when extensive infiltration has occurred – cause shrinkage, so that the affected breast may appear smaller than the healthy one, and in the atrophic form it may almost disappear. In the ordinary form it will be rare

to find any discharge from the nipple. After a while, the axillary nodes become enlarged and hard. Too much attention should not be given to the absence of palpable nodes; in a fat patient these may be enlarged but impalpable, and in any case it is hoped to recognize cancer before the nodes are involved.

Duct carcinoma-in-situ

The earliest premalignant condition affecting the breast ducts is referred to as duct carcinoma-in-situ (DCIS). Rarely, the condition starts within the lobules, where it is referred to as lobular carcinoma-in-situ. In most cases the condition is impalpable, and may only be discovered at a chance biopsy of a coincidental benign lump. More commonly these days DCIS may be discovered as a result of a breast screening programme, where the condition shows itself as a cluster of microcalcifications on mammography, accounting for 20 per cent of screen-detected 'cancers'. Rarely, a large mass of DCIS of the comedo variety may present as a clinical mass or, if the in-situ disease is close to the nipple, may present as a bloody nipple discharge or Paget's disease (see NIPPLE, ABNORMALITIES OF, p. 484).

Phylloides tumour

A phylloides tumour is a rare clinical and pathological entity which presents with all the features of a giant fibroadenoma. In the past, this condition was referred to as a cystosarcoma phylloides. However, the majority of these lesions are completely benign. The term phylloides means 'leaf-like'; this refers to the slit-like clefts arranged in a 'botanical' manner when viewed on a cut section. Rarely, the stromal elements of these tumours become hyperplastic and atypical, adopting some of the features of a sarcoma. This tumour is then referred to as a malignant phylloides tumour. These lesions have a tendency to recur locally if not widely excised at the first attempt and, with each recurrence, their malignant potential is more pronounced.

Sarcoma of the breast

Sarcoma of the breast is rare. It generally occurs in women under the age of 40 years. In the early stages it is not easily distinguishable from a fibroadenoma, particularly one which is enlarging rapidly on account of a cyst or intracycstic growth. The lesion is soft and vascular, and grows quickly, at first seeming to push the breast aside, but later infiltrating its tissues and eventually fungating through the skin.

Abnormalities of normal development and involution (ANDI) (Extremes of physiological variability)

When a woman presents at the clinic complaining of a lump in the breast, the first step on clinical examination is to distinguish between a discrete lump and an area of lumpiness or nodularity. Although these lumpy areas in the breast of a young woman are extremely common (perhaps affecting 30% of the female population), there is enormous confusion among the medical profession as to the correct terminology. In the past, these lumpy areas have been referred to by a series of terms, such as fibrocystic disease, fibroadenosis, mammary dysplasia, cystic hyperplasia, Schimmelbusch's disease, chronic cystic mastitis, cystic mastopathy, Koenig's disease and mastoplasia. Whatever name is given to these lumpy breasts, there are no consistent pathological features which explain the varying textures palpable in different quadrants of the breast. For that reason, a group of clinicians in the University Hospital of Wales headed by Professor Hughes has devised a rational description of these conditions, which can be grouped together under the catchy acronym ANDI, standing for abnormalities of normal development and involution.

These abnormalities vary in extreme from normal physiological processes, which may be considered as benign disorders of little significance, to the other extreme where the pathology can produce particular problems of discomfort or anxiety to the young woman. For example, during the developmental phase of the breast architecture, duct lobular overgrowth can lead to a fibroadenoma, which may cease growing at 2 cm or continue to grow to the extreme of a giant fibroadenoma, reaching sizes of 4–5 cm. Normal cyclical changes can produce premenstrual swelling and epithelial hyperplasia. Physiological abnormalities in the sensitivity of the duct epithelium to cyclical hormone changes can lead to cyclical mastalgia, nodularity and intraduct papilloma. Taken to its extreme, the intraduct epithelial hyperplasia can progress to atypia, which is known as a risk factor predicting the development of breast cancer. Finally, normal lobular involution may progress to the formation of cysts, sclerosing adenosis and duct ectasia. If a lumpy area of breast tissue is biopsied, almost all these features can be seen under the microscope to one extent or another.

Since these conditions are aberrations of normal physiological development or involution, it can be accepted that in most cases the woman with a lumpy breast or a painful lumpy breast can be reassured. However, if the condition extends beyond the menopause into the cancer age group, clinical diagnosis can be extremely difficult and it is in this area that ultrasound scanning and X-ray mammography is of great value. In addition it should be remembered that invasive lobular cancer, which accounts for about 5 per cent of all malignant disease of the breast, may present as diffuse nodularity and atypical mammographic appearances. When in doubt, a core-cut biopsy is mandatory.

Multiple cystic disease

Multiple cystic disease of the breast is usually regarded as a variety of ANDI. One breast (but sometimes both) becomes filled with cysts (some microscopic, others as large as walnuts, but with all intermediate sizes) so that the organ has a 'bossy' appearance. The diagnosis is usually simple, but it can be confirmed by aspiration of the cysts. This is a simple outpatient procedure, which is also curative, although several aspirations may sometimes be necessary.

Diagnosis of solitary lump in breast

The diagnosis of a single lump in the breast, where cancer must be taken into consideration, may cause considerably difficulty. A lump which is definite enough to be felt with the flat of the hand and hard enough to resemble cancer is a fibroadenoma or a tense cyst or a carcinoma. A fibroadenoma is usually found in women aged under 30, is less hard than a carcinoma, and is of rounded outline, but its contour may be obscured by surrounding fibroadenosis. A cyst is usually round and elastic, but if it is deep its outline is obscured, and if it is tense it may feel hard. A carcinoma is undoubtedly solid, and has an ill-defined outline; where these characters are present, or where there is the slightest suggestion of skin dimpling, local flattening of the breast or alteration in the nipple, then cancer must be diagnosed.

The diagnosis of cancer at this early stage is intensely important, for only then is the prospect of cure high. If there is the possibility that the lump is a cyst, this can easily be confirmed by ultrasound scanning, after which aspiration is attempted under local anaesthetic.

If clear fluid is obtained and the lump disappears, then you can be certain that the diagnosis is one of simple cyst. If no fluid is obtained, or only a few drops of blood, smears should be made for cytological examination, a core-cut biopsy taken, or arrangements must be made for urgent excision and microscopic examination of the specimen. Local resection of a doubtful lump is imperative.

Swellings pushing the breast forwards

These are often mistaken by the patient for breast tumours. A *retromammary abscess* is most commonly tuberculous, arising in an underlying rib or in a mediastinal abscess that has tracked along a branch of the internal thoracic artery. Sometimes, an empyema points beneath the breast, usually in the 5th or 6th intercostal space in the midclavicular line. A *chondroma* is a hard nodular swelling springing from one of the ribs and tilting the breast, or pushing it aside. More common is a swelling of one or more of the costal cartilages, especially the 2nd and 3rd, which may be bilateral and tender. This condition, termed costochondritis or *Tietze's syndrome*, is entirely benign and requires no treatment.

Deformities of the ribs may also cause confusion; the commonest is a prominence of the costochondral junction of the 3rd rib, which may be forked and join two cartilages. The condition is often bilateral, and may be associated with other abnormalities of the ribs or vertebrae.

Role of X-ray mammography and ultrasound scanning

It is now well established that routine X-ray mammography for women over the age of 50 who are otherwise asymptomatic may be of value in preventing premature death from breast cancer by the detection of subclinical cancers (Fig. B.10). In addition, no patient with breast cancer should be managed without mammography, as this will describe the extent of the disease within the ipsilateral breast and exclude the presence of synchronous contralateral cancers. Ultrasound scanning may help distinguish a solid from a cystic lump, and may also help to define a discrete lump within an area of diffuse nodularity (see ANDI, above).

Mondor's disease

Although strictly speaking not a lump in the breast, it is difficult to know how to classify this condition. If a

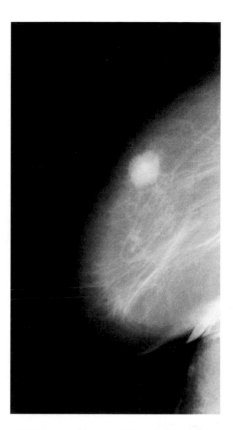

Figure B.10 Mammogram demonstrating a dense shadow of a carcinoma in the upper outer quadrant of the breast.

woman presents with characteristic guttering over the surface of the breast, this a pathognomonic sign of Mondor's disease, which is due to spontaneous thrombophlebitis of a superficial vein coursing over the thorax and breast. It has an indurated feel, and can be mistaken for the dimpling of an underlying cancer, except for its linearity. The author has reported a case where Mondor's disease was the only presenting sign of a cancer, which was detected on mammography. Other such cases have been reported, but it is uncertain whether this may be coincidental or casual.

Michael Baum

BREAST, PAIN IN

Pain in the breast (mastalgia) is a common symptom encountered in general surgical practice.

When pain in one breast is the chief symptom, the first step is to palpate both breasts with a view to detecting any abnormality which might suggest an early carcinoma. The methods of such examination are described on p. 77. Unfortunately, pain does not occur as an early symptom in carcinoma of the breast, and by the time it is pronounced there may be an obvious stony-hard tumour.

Other causes of pain in the breast are:

- Pregnancy
- Menstruation (cyclical mastalgia)
- The onset of puberty
- Lactation
- Cracked nipple
- Inflammation of the nipple
- Cyst of the breast
- Galactocele
- Breast abscess
- Submammary abscess
- Mastitis, acute mastitis, periductal
- Tuberculous disease of the breast
- The after-effects of a blow or injury
- Anxiety state
- Angina
- Cervical spondylosis
- Herpes zoster

The differential diagnosis of most of these conditions is discussed under the heading of BREAST LUMPS (p. 77). Pain in the breast due to intrauterine or to ectopic pregnancy will generally be bilateral and will be associated with the other signs of pregnancy. Suggestive indications are the dark brown colour of the nipples, and the broad secondary areola and swollen Montgomery's glands.

The pains in the breast which precede menstruation are also bilateral, and their relationship may be indicated by their development synchronously with the fast menstruation or their periodic recurrence before each menstrual period. This common condition is best described as pronounced cyclical mastalgia.

Pronounced cyclical mastalgia

Most young women notice some soreness and discomfort in the outer quadrants of their breasts during the week preceding a period, and this is a normal consequence of cyclical changes in their hormonal environment. In about one in 10 women, this condition is sufficiently pronounced to cause anxiety, distress and insomnia. Characteristically, the pain is felt in the upper outer quadrants of both breasts, reaching a crescendo 2 or 3 days before the menses. Immediately after this, 2 weeks of comfort are experienced and then the pain starts building up during the luteal phase of the cycle. The cyclical mastalgia may or may not be associated with lumpiness, and the two conditions should be considered separately. In the majority of such cases simple reassurance with advice on mild analgesia is all that is needed. However, in severe cases, it is worth asking the woman to keep a diary, and if the pattern is clearly cyclical, then a 6-month course of prolactin inhibitors can be prescribed (bromocriptine, danazol). In addition, there is some circumstantial evidence that oil of evening primrose and the withdrawal of caffeine may benefit the condition, although it is notorious for this self-limiting disease to respond remarkably well to suggestion or placebo. By common consent, cyclical mastalgia has nothing to do with water retention, and therefore diuretics are not indicated. The underlying pathology is thought to relate to a hypersensitivity of the duct epithelium to biologically active prolactin.

Mammography is only indicated in women over the age of 35, or if pain is non-cyclical and localized to one area of the breast.

Michael Baum

BRUISES

Subcutaneous bleeding may present as bruises (ecchymoses) which will vary in colour from dusky red to green, yellow, purple or black depending on the duration of the bruise and the various haemoglobin breakdown products. Superficial crops of small capillary haemorrhages are called *petechiae*, and are best seen in the skin, mucous membranes and retina, although they also occur on the internal organs. Ecchymoses result from the confluence of petechiae or from haemorrhages from vessels larger than capillaries. Multiple bruises characterize bleeding disorders (q.v.), whereas petechiae suggest an abnormality of either the platelets or the vessel wall. Multiple skin petechiae and ecchymoses are collectively referred to as *purpura* (q.v.). Bruising frequently occurs after trauma which may be minimal (or unobserved) in elderly persons, and isolated ecchymoses are normal in women and young children.

There are several acquired vascular defects which promote skin bruising. Senile purpura affects older people, usually on sun-exposed areas such as the hands and forearms, and takes several weeks to resolve, leaving brownish discoloration (hemosiderin deposit). Corticosteroid use causes easy bruising and characteristic purple striae, particularly on the abdomen. Other vascular causes are vasculitis, connective tissue diseases, and scurvy (highly characteristic perifollicular haemorrhage, though gum bruising is also seen). Painful bruising syndrome occurs in women, and is associated with tingling sensation followed by bruising over the trunk and limbs, with spontaneous resolution.

Danielle Harari

BULLAE AND VESICLES (BLISTERS)

A *blister* is a circumscribed elevation of the skin containing free fluid. Blisters less than 5 mm in diameter are termed vesicles, while larger blisters are termed *bullae*. However, blisters of differing sizes may co-exist in some disorders, so the two presentations are best considered together. Blisters can be a feature of a number of important skin disorders (see Table B.9).

Traumatic disorders

Normal skin is a cohesive, multilayered tissue which is remarkably resistant to friction, and only neonatal skin blisters easily. In adults, localized blistering of the skin occurs following thermal or chemical burns and sometimes frostbite. Friction due to ill-fitting footwear may cause blistering of the feet, whilst palmar blisters follow unaccustomed manual toil. Spontaneous blistering always has a pathological cause (Fig. B.11).

Genetic disorders

Rather rarely, a child is born with an inherited defect in the cohesion between the layers of the skin; electron microscopy and genetic studies have now identified several forms of *epidermolysis bullosa*. The severest forms may be associated with mucosal (including laryngeal) involvement and severe blistering from birth, whilst

Table B.9 Bullae and vesicles (blisters)

Traumatic
- Friction, thermal, caustic
- Dermatitis artefacta

Genetic
- Epidermolysis bullosa
- Incontinentia pigmenti
- Porphyria cutanea tarda

Infective
- Insect bites
- Jelly-fish
- Scabies
- Bullous impetigo
- Staphylococcal scalded skin syndrome
- Herpes simplex
- Eczema herpeticum
- Herpes zoster
- Varicella
- Variola
- Hand, foot and mouth disease

Inflammatory
- Eczema: contact dermatitis, pompholyx
- Fixed drug eruption
- Erythema multiforme
- Toxic epidermal necrolysis
- Mastocytosis (urticaria pigmentosa)
- Vasculitis

Immunobullous
- Pemphigus
- Pemphigoid
- Dermatitis herpetiformis
- Linear IgA disease
- Epidermolysis bullosa acquisita
- Herpes gestationis

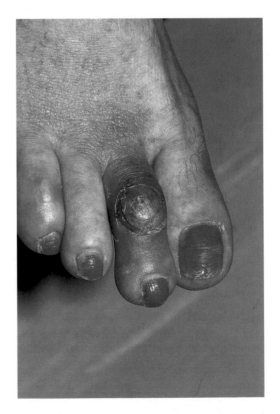

Figure B.11 Orf.

other forms are associated with a rather milder degree of blistering, only occurring with friction. Another uncommon, but important genetic cause of blistering in infants is *incontinentia pigmenti*, in which the linear pattern of blistering may lead the unwary to make the incorrect diagnosis of herpes zoster. This is an X-linked disorder, is generally fatal in the affected male, and is associated with a number of ocular and neurological disorders in affected females.

Infectious disorders

A number of infections can cause blistering eruptions in infants and young children. *Bullous impetigo* (Fig. B.12) is caused predominantly by superficial infection with *Staphylococcus*. Sometimes, the predominant lesion is the honey-coloured oozing crust, but quite marked blistering may occur. The roof of the blisters is fragile and easily ruptured, leading to an appearance which has been likened to a cigarette burn, and which may lead to false accusation of child abuse or neglect. Microbiology swabs will demonstrate the causative organism, and there is a rapid response to topical antibiotics. Some strains of *Staphylococcus* produce an exotoxin which causes a dramatic superficial exfoliation of the skin resembling that caused by a burn (staphylococcal scalded skin syndrome); this must be distinguished from *toxic epidermal necrolysis* (TEN), a condition which may arise at any age, usually as a result of an idiosyncratic reaction to a drug, in which extensive areas of skin apparently dissolve leaving raw weeping areas; the mortality is high.

Another cause of blistering in young children that may cause diagnostic confusion is *scabies*; this is an infection of the skin with the mite *Sarcoptes scabiei*, which is passed from person to person by direct physical contact. The classic lesion of scabies is the burrow; this is an irregular serpiginous track which is most commonly found around the wrists or finger webs, and from which the live mite may be extracted on the end of a needle and demonstrated under the microscope. In babies, blistering on the soles of the feet may be found, and should prompt examination of other family members (especially the mother).

The sudden onset of a widespread vesicular rash, associated with mild fever and constitutional upset, may suggest chickenpox (*varicella*) (Fig. B.13). Blisters appear in crops, so will be at different stages of evolution, and mucosal blistering may be evident in the mouth. In patients with any form of immunodeficiency, or who are receiving immunosuppressive drugs, chickenpox may present with a violent haemorrhagic blistered eruption; pulmonary involvement may occur, and there is a significant mortality.

The cropped eruption of chickenpox is one of the features which may distinguish it from smallpox

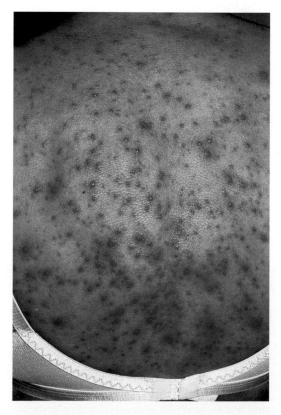

Figure B.13 Chickenpox in an immunosuppressed patient.

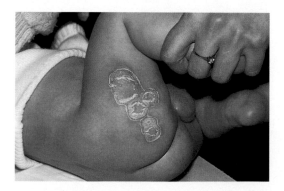

Figure B.12 Impetigo.

(*variola*), in which the lesions erupt together and are thus much more monomorphic. A generalized vesicular or pustular eruption is a rather uncommon sequel to smallpox vaccination.

Perhaps the commonest of all infections to cause blistering is *herpes simplex* (Fig. B.14). The typical lesion of herpetic infection is a cluster of small vesicles, arising on an erythematous background, which crust and heal over a period of 7–10 days, only to recur repeatedly on the same site. When herpetic vesicles occur on mucosal surfaces, the appearance may be somewhat modified; vesicles become macerated and the roofs rub off, leaving painful round erosions or shallow ulcers. The commonest sites affected are the lips, the face, the buttocks and the genitalia. Although genital herpes simplex (Type II herpes) typically occurs on the genitalia, Type I infections may also arise on this site. The first episode of herpes simplex is usually more severe, and associated with more pain and constitutional upset than subsequent episodes.

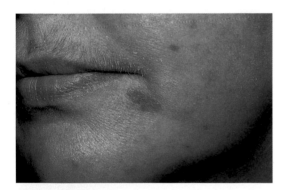

Figure B.14 Herpes simplex.

The history of recurrent blistered lesions at the same site is characteristic of herpes, but is also the hallmark of another blistering disorder, *fixed drug eruption*; in this dramatic and intriguing condition a blister on an erythematous base recurs in exactly the same location (commonly including the orogenital mucosae) each time affected individuals are exposed to certain medicaments (e.g. phenolphthalein laxatives, codeine, tetracyclines and sulphonamides). The blister resolves, leaving a round patch of post-inflammatory pigmentation, which will then be the site of the next episode. It is remarkable how rarely patients associate the recurrent painful blistering with taking the offending medication.

Herpes simplex, whilst usually causing a localized blistering, may be responsible for a widespread eruption in patients with atopic eczema, who appear to be incapable of mounting an appropriate immune response to the virus, *eczema herpeticum* (*Kaposi's varicelliform eruption*). Typically, the subject has quite active eczema, and presents with a sudden onset of a diffuse or generalized eruption composed of umbilicated vesicles or crusted erosions. The lesions are often painful, and there may be a severe fever and constitutional disturbance. The condition may be fatal, especially if unrecognized and appropriate treatment not instituted.

Herpes zoster (shingles) causes a band of vesicles along a dermatome. It is caused by a secondary activation of *varicella* virus lying dormant in nervous tissue following primary (chickenpox) infection, sometimes as long as 60 years previously. The condition is uncommon in childhood (except, curiously, in blacks) and more common with increasing age. It also occurs in those immunosuppressed by drugs or HIV disease, systemic illness or malignancy, where it may be accompanied by toxicity and disseminated chickenpox lesions.

Pain usually precedes obvious skin changes by up to 48 hours. The first sign in the skin is erythema on which grouped clear vesicles appear, which later become umbilicated and haemorrhagic. Smears from the base of vesicles show multinucleated giant cells. The limitation to one side of the body, the distribution in one or more dermatomes and the pain usually suffice to distinguish herpes zoster from erythema multiforme and dermatitis herpetiformis. When the trunk is affected the preceding pain may be mistaken for pleurisy or some intra-abdominal condition. The pain may also simulate myocardial infarction, slipped disc, orchitis or venous thrombosis depending on the site affected. When the second division of the trigeminal nerve is affected, involvement of the tip of the nose with vesicles indicates infection of the nasociliary branch of the ophthalmic nerve and hence is a sign that keratitis may occur.

Sometimes, the bites and stings of insects cause bullous reactions and present as discrete large blisters on the lower legs, especially in children (Fig. B.15). The sting of jellyfish produces a bullous reaction. In *dermatitis artefacta*, bullae may be artificially induced by patients themselves (e.g. with acids, alkalis and phenolics). Blisters can be a feature of acute severe eczema of

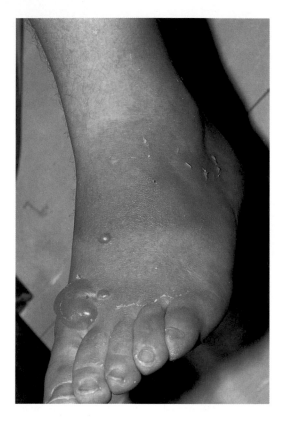

Figure B.15 Insect bite reaction.

any cause (Fig. B.16). This is seen on the palms, sides of fingers and soles in *pompholyx* and in acute contact dermatitis. Some plants, especially of the umbelliferae family, produce a toxin that is activated by ultraviolet light. Typically, it presents in gardeners who have been clearing a patch of overgrown land on a sunny day, and wearing short sleeves or short trousers.

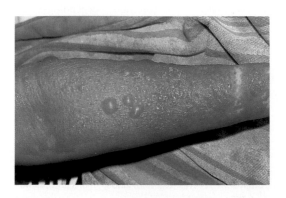

Figure B.16 Phototoxic reaction to a sunscreen cream.

Inflammatory disorders

Another condition characterized by blisters provoked by sun exposure is *porphyria cutanea tarda;* small vesicles occur on the backs of the hands and are associated with an acquired fragility of the skin. The urine will fluoresce when examined under ultraviolet light. Blistering on the legs may occur in patients with renal failure on haemodialysis; its cause is unknown.

Erythema multiforme (Fig. B.17) is an acute eruption which may be triggered by a large number of provoking factors, including viral infections, drugs and radiotherapy. Recurrent episodes occur if the provoking cause recurs (e.g. herpes simplex infection). The characteristic 'target' lesions on the dorsa of hands and feet, over knees and elbows, and sometimes more widely, owe their pattern to two erythematous rings of different shade, surrounding a central blister. In severe cases blistering may be extensive and associated with fever, prostration and occasionally pneumonitis. Involvement of the mucous membranes may be a prominent feature (Stevens–Johnson syndrome) (Fig. B.18).

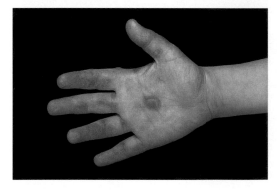

Figure B.17 Bullous erythema multiforme.

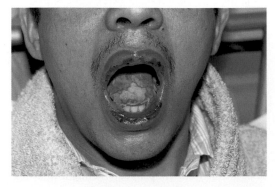

Figure B.18 Stevens–Johnson syndrome.

Immunobullous disorders

Three uncommon conditions – pemphigus, pemphigoid and dermatitis herpetiformis – share the features of being chronic blistering eruptions, in which characteristic patterns of deposition of antibodies in the skin can be demonstrated.

Pemphigus comprises a group of disorders, possibly arising in those with a genetic predisposition, in which there is formation of blisters *within* the epidermis. Both the skin and mucous membranes are affected. *Pemphigus vulgaris* begins in the third and fourth decades of life, with equal gender-related incidence. The mucosa of the mouth is often affected before the skin. Fragile intra-epidermal cutaneous blisters occur at any site and quickly become erosions. These are often extensive, slow to heal, and become secondarily infected. The uncomfortable oral lesions are the most constant, persisting even when blistering elsewhere is controlled, and making eating difficult. The blistering is thought to be due to a circulating auto-antibody directed against the intercellular substance. This is detectable in the blood by an indirect immunofluorescence technique on a suitable substrate tissue (e.g. primate oesophagus), and the titre of this antibody is related to the severity and progress of blistering. Fluorescence may also be demonstrated in unfixed skin biopsy specimens. Affected patients also have a higher incidence of organ-specific autoimmune diseases, and thymoma. A milder form of pemphigus with positive immunofluorescence may arise in patients under treatment with penicillamine.

Chronic familial benign pemphigus (Halley–Hailey disease) is unrelated, but has histological similarities. Affected family members show a vulnerability of flexural skin to friction, producing characteristic fissured erosions on the sides of neck, axillae, perineum and oral and vulval lips. Circulating auto-antibodies have not been detected.

Bullous pemphigoid (Fig. B.19) is usually a disease of the over-sixties. Bullae of 2–5 cm diameter arise on an erythematous, urticated background on the limbs, and this later becomes generalized: indeed, 200–300 blisters can appear within a few days. The blisters are thick-roofed and can last for many days; initially, their constituent fluid is clear, but it soon becomes cloudy or haemorrhagic. Scratching may lead to extensive erosions which, unlike pemphigus, heal fairly rapidly. Once the multiple large blisters occur the diagnosis can be easily made. However, widespread pruritus, erythema

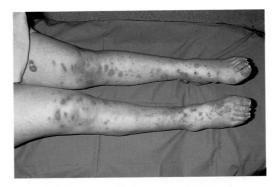

Figure B.19 Bullous pemphigoid.

and urticaria may precede the blistering by several weeks or months, and at this stage diagnosis is difficult. There is also a circulating auto-antibody, but in this case directed at the dermo-epidermal junction. The mucosae can be affected with similar tense bullae, but this is a much less constant feature than in pemphigus.

Cicatricial pemphigoid (benign mucous membrane pemphigoid) (Fig. B.20) is a variant where the blister forms just below the dermo-epidermal junction, so that healing takes place with scarring. Blisters appear on mucosae rather than skin, particularly the eyes, frequently causing blindness.

In *dermatitis herpetiformis* blisters are subepidermal and tend to be short-lived, as, being intensely

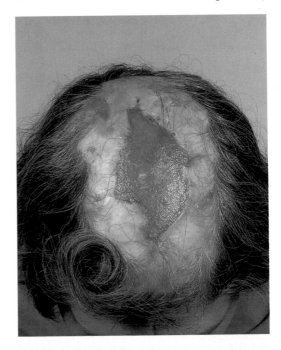

Figure B.20 Cicatricial pemphigoid.

pruritic, they are quickly excoriated. The condition chiefly affects the extensor surfaces of shoulders, buttocks, knees, forehead and scalp, sparing the mucosae. There appears to be a related gastrointestinal gluten hypersensitivity, and direct immunofluorescence of frozen skin reveals diagnostic deposits of IgA in the dermis. The condition responds dramatically to the antileprosy drug dapsone, its action being anti-inflammatory rather than antimicrobial.

Barry Monk

BUTTOCK, PAIN IN

See LOWER LIMB, PAIN IN (p. 381).

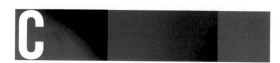

CALF AND SHIN, PAIN IN

See LOWER LIMB, PAIN IN (p. 409).

CATARACT

A cataract is an opacity within the lens of the eye; the opacity may be located in the centre of the lens (nuclear), in the cortical region, or in the posterior subcapsular area. It has little clinical significance unless interference with vision results. Cataracts are frequently bilateral, but the severity and rate of progression in each eye usually varies. Most cataracts are associated with ageing, but they can result from a wide variety of causes. Cataracts may have a congenital or acquired aetiology, and sometimes occur secondary to other eye diseases such as iritis, glaucoma and retinitis pigmentosa. Cataracts can result from trauma, and are often associated with some systemic disorders (e.g. diabetes mellitus) and certain drugs used topically or systemically (e.g. corticosteroids) (Table C.1).

Most cataracts are not visible to the casual observer until they are advanced and causing profound visual loss (Fig. C.1). In the early stages, cataracts are best diagnosed by examining the red reflex of the fundus

Table C.1 Causes of cataract

1 Age-related (senile) cataract
2 Cataract associated with ocular disease
  - Congenital disorders
  - Acquired disorders
    - Uveitis
    - Glaucoma
    - Neoplasia
    - Topical drug therapy – steroids and miotics
    - Trauma – mechanical, chemical or radiation
3 Cataract associated with systemic disease
  - Maternal infection
    - Rubella
    - Cytomegalovirus
  - Hereditary disorders, e.g. Down's syndrome, dystrophia myotonica, Alport's syndrome, Fabry's disease, Lowe's syndrome
  - Metabolic disorders, e.g. diabetes mellitus, galactosaemia, mannosidosis, hypoparathyroidism, hypothyroidism
  - Systemic drugs, e.g. corticosteroids, antimitotics, phenothiazines, and anticholinesterases
  - Dermatological disorders, e.g. atopic dermatitis, and ichthyosis

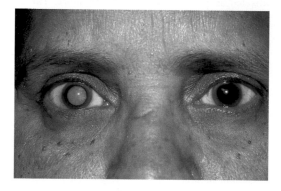

Figure C.1 Presence of cataract in the eye. [Moorfields Eye Hospital.]

with an ophthalmoscope through a well-dilated pupil, or by slit-lamp examination. The most common symptom caused by cataract is decreased visual acuity. Other symptoms include increasing myopia, monocular diplopia, and glare where vision is much worse in conditions of bright illumination.

The rate of progression of cataract is very variable, and when the visual loss is interfering significantly with the patient's daily living, surgery is indicated. Lens extraction with the insertion into the lens capsular sac of an intraocular lens implant manufactured from polymethylmethacrylate, silicone or acrylic material restores vision very successfully. On rare occasions it may not be possible to implant an artificial lens, and in these cases either contact lenses or cataract spectacles are necessary to attain a satisfactory result. Intraocular lens implants have become extremely refined, and usually achieve excellent postoperative vision with a very low complication rate. Implants have considerable optical advantages over cataract glasses, which are associated with disturbing problems of image magnification, lens aberrations and limited visual field. Contact lenses overcome these optical problems, but many elderly or handicapped patients experience management and handling problems.

Reginald Daniel

CHEST DEFORMITY

The chest wall is an integral part of the 'pump' that ventilates the lungs. Minor chest wall deformities with no significant effect on respiration may cause concern and are relatively common. These are described together with the infrequent but more serious conditions which adversely affect cardiorespiratory function.

Normal configuration of the chest is influenced by age, sex and physical build of the individual. It is determined by the condition of the spine, ribs and sternum, the overlying muscles and soft tissues, and the underlying lung and pleura. In infants, the chest wall is almost circular in cross-section, the ribs lie horizontally, and the anteroposterior and transverse thoracic diameters are similar. With growth the chest becomes flattened anteroposteriorly, wider transversely and the ribs adopt an oblique, downward-sloping position.

The shape of the adult chest is dependent upon body build. In stocky mesomorphic individuals the chest wall tends to be circular with relatively deep posteroanterior and wide transverse diameters. The heart may lie horizontally. The vertical height from sternal notch to the diaphragm is proportionally reduced. In contrast, the chest in ectomorphic individuals is long in proportion to the overall width, shallow anteroposteriorly, and the heart adopts a more vertical position (Fig. C.2). Variation in normal body build is not associated with predisposition to respiratory disease, although morbid obesity may cause respiratory failure either directly by influencing chest wall function or indirectly by provoking obstructive sleep apnoea.

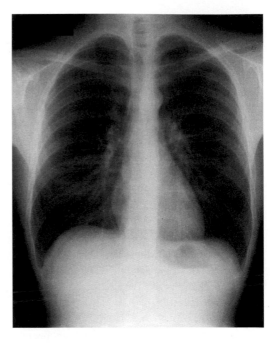

Figure C.2 Radiograph of a normal chest. Patient of tall thin build with vertically disposed heart.

Congenital defects

Rib abnormality

- Bifid ribs are common, particularly in the upper six ribs, and may cause confusion if the abnormality is not appreciated on the chest radiograph.
- Cervical ribs, usually arising from the seventh cervical vertebra, occur in 0.5 per cent of the population, in 80 per cent are bilateral, and vary greatly in size and shape. They are seldom a cause of symptoms and often are a chance discovery on either routine chest radiography or at physical examination when a deep bony mass is discovered in the supraclavicular fossa. Symptoms due to compression are more prevalent in females, and commoner on the left side. Neurological symptoms include pain and weakness in the arm with paraesthesiae of the fingers and wasting of the intrinsic muscles of the hand. Vascular symptoms may mimic Raynaud's phenomenon and subclavian artery obstruction, or thrombosis may cause distal gangrene.

Pectus carinatum or pigeon-chest deformity

The sternum is prominent, forming an anterior ridge and the ribs inclined forwards causing a greatly increased anteroposterior diameter. The condition can be acquired (asthma), but if congenital is due to premature obliteration of the sternal sutures during growth or to malattachment of the anterior portion of the diaphragm to the posterior portion of the rectus sheath rather than, as normally, to the xiphoid process, with consequent distorting mechanical effects.

Pectus excavatum or funnel-chest deformity

The costal cartilages are prominent, curve inwards, and the body of the sternum is depressed backwards towards the spine from the manubrio-sternal joint downwards with maximum recession at the xiphoid.

In severe cases the lower sternum forms a deep concavity, and may almost touch the spine. The heart is displaced to the left side of the chest. Radiographic displacement of the heart to the left and rotational changes of the electrocardiogram may be wrongly interpreted as evidence of heart disease. The electrocardiogram may show persistence of the juvenile pattern with T-wave inversion in the right precordial leads, incomplete right bundle branch block and right axis deviation. Because of cardiac rotation there may be P-wave inversion and a QR pattern in lead VI. Minor lung function abnormalities occur with reduced total lung, maximum breathing and vital capacities. The condition does not predispose to cardiac or respiratory disease in later life. Surgery is rarely required because of symptoms, but is occasionally sought for cosmetic reasons.

Incomplete fusion of the sternum

An unusual abnormality, apparent at birth, produces the appearance of a split sternum with indrawing of the soft tissue over the central fissure during inspiration and bulging on expiration. This paradoxical respiratory movement is much increased when coughing or in the presence of respiratory obstruction.

Partial or complete absence of the pectoral muscle

This is a rare congenital abnormality, usually unilateral and mostly involving the lower portion of the pectoralis major. The condition produces no symptoms, but if it is of a severe degree the rib cage is deformed and the anterior chest wall on the affected side is under-developed and shrunken because it is not subject to the lateral pull of the pectoral muscle. The chest radiograph may show abnormal transradiancy of the affected side, which may give rise to an erroneous impression of pulmonary disease.

The straight back syndrome

This is an absence of the normal physiological dorsal kyphosis of the spine associated with a reduced anterioposterior diameter of the chest. A mild insignificant restrictive defect of lung function may be present, but cardiac complications are more likely to occur. Examination may reveal a palpable left parasternal systolic impulse and exaggerated splitting of the second heart sound on auscultation, presumably caused by compression of the pulmonary outflow tract and great vessels between the spine and sternum. The ECG may show an RSR pattern in lead VI.

Acquired skeletal deformities of the chest

Scoliosis

Acquired abnormalities of the vertebral column may directly impair respiration should they interfere with the mechanical action of the ribs and diaphragm, or prevent full expansion of the lungs.

Scoliosis is a lateral curvature of the vertebral column, sometimes accompanied by abnormal flexion (kyphoscoliosis) or by rotation of the spine and adjacent viscera. In about 80 per cent of cases the cause is obscure – idiopathic scoliosis. In the remainder it is secondary to a variety of conditions (see Table C.2).

Scoliosis may be either functional (non-structural or postural) or structural. Functional scoliosis is reversible, the curvature being abolished by forward flexion of the spine, whereas in structural scoliosis the deformity persists on forward flexion. Idiopathic scoliosis may be seen at any age during growth and at all spinal levels. It occurs most frequently in girls from 10–15 years of age who most commonly present with midthoracic scoliosis to the right. The sideways curvature is usually accompanied by some spinal rotation. The vertebral bodies of the most prominent part of the curve rotate to a greater extent than is indicated by external inspection of the line of spinous processes, and this rotation is the cause of the significant rib displacement that so often accompanies apparently moderate spinal scoliosis.

The ribs are prominent posteriorly on the convex side of the curvature, and bulge anteriorly on the concave side. The shoulder tends to droop on the concave side. If there is a double thoracic spine curve the chest wall deformities are more complex.

The higher the structural curve in the spine the worse the outcome, for the prognosis depends upon

Table C.2 Causes of scoliosis

Idiopathic: 80%
Secondary scoliosis: 20%
■ Non-structural (postural)
  ◆ Compensatory (short leg)
  ◆ Sciatica
  ◆ Hysterical
  ◆ Postural
■ Structural
  ◆ Idiopathic
  ◆ Bone disorders
    ■ Congenital
      hemivertebra
    ■ Osteogenesis
      imperfecta
    ■ Osteoporosis
    ■ Bone lysis
    ■ Tuberculosis
    ■ Malignancy
    ■ Spondylolistheses
■ Neurological disorders
  ◆ Syringomyelia
  ◆ Friedreich's ataxia
  ◆ Neurofibromatosis
  ◆ Poliomyelitis
■ Muscular disorders
  ◆ Duchenne's muscular
    dystrophy
  ◆ Faciohumeroscapular
    dystrophy
■ Connective tissue disease
  ◆ Marfan's syndrome   } Dominant
  ◆ Ehlers–Danlos syndrome } inheritance
  ◆ Homocystinuria   } Recessive
  ◆ Morquio's syndrome   } inheritance
■ Thoracic disorders
  ◆ Thoracoplasty
  ◆ Fibrothorax (secondary
    to empyema)
  ◆ Lung fibrosis
  ◆ Pneumonectomy
  ◆ Thoracic burns
  ◆ Chest irradiation

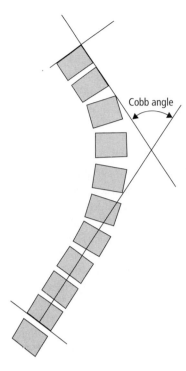

Figure C.3 The measurement of a thoracic scoliosis by Cobb's angle.

failure in those with high curves greater than 100 degrees, leading to chronic hypercapnia, pulmonary hypertension, right heart failure and death.

Neuropathic (poliomyelitis) and myopathic conditions are usually associated with a worse prognosis for a given degree of curvature, owing to associated muscle weakness causing ventilatory problems.

Ankylosing spondylitis

This is an inflammatory arthritis, affecting the axial skeleton of young men, the great majority of whom are HLA-B27-positive. The condition results in the fusion of costotransverse and vertebral joints with relative fixation of the rib cage in an inspiratory position. Sternomanubrial and sternoclavicular joints may also be affected. Clinical examination of the chest may reveal a dorsal kyphosis and diminished chest expansion with corresponding increase in abdominal expansion. Changes in the relative proportion of diaphragmatic and chest wall movement alter the normal relationship of ventilation to perfusion in the upper lobes. Most of the ventilatory movement is performed by the diaphragm and abdomen. With advanced disease, signs of apical fibrosis, consolidation

the angle of the curvature. This is measured as shown in Figure C.3; lines are drawn parallel to the upper and lower vertebral bodies lying beyond the structural curvature, and the angle of curvature is measured where the perpendicular lines intersect.

In scoliosis, the total lung volume is reduced and, if the deformity has been present since infancy, the alveolar growth may also be deficient. The spectrum of symptoms varies from none in young mild scoliotics to severe disability and chronic respiratory or cavitation may be present. The posteroanterior chest radiograph may demonstrate the characteristic bilateral apical cavitating lesions, and the lateral radiograph the classical 'bamboo' calcification of the anterior spinal ligaments. The clinical picture is completed if there is an aortic diastolic murmur and cardiac failure due to aortic valve disease.

Rickets (osteomalacia)

Rickets – either nutritional, due to renal disease or to inherited enzyme defects (1-alpha-hydrolase) – may cause important skeletal deformity, with disorganization of the bone growth plate and faulty replacement of calcified cartilage. In active childhood rickets, the costochondral junctions enlarge producing the so-called 'rickety rosary'. The soft plastic ribs are readily moulded. The upper ribs tend to be indrawn by inspiratory forces, while the lower chest is supported at the costal margins by the underlying abdominal viscera. A depression is produced above the costal margins with a flaring outwards of the costal margin itself. This deformity may remain and is known as Harrison's sulcus.

Pigeon chest

This condition may be congenital (rare), due to rickets, or most commonly accompanies chronic bronchopulmonary disease in childhood. This is most frequently seen as a skeletal manifestation of severe uncontrolled asthma. It is, to a considerable extent, reversible if the asthma is treated adequately and sufficiently early. It should be a rarity. Pigeon-chest deformity may also occur in bronchiectasis.

Barrel chest

Barrel chest is the name given to the deep chest, in which the anteroposterior diameter is increased often to equal the transverse diameter, the subcostal angle is abnormally wide, and the horizontal position of the ribs is accentuated. This appearance is most constantly related to over-inflation of the lungs, and may be observed in acute attacks of asthma and in chronic obstructive pulmonary disease, usually associated with irreversible structural emphysema, especially when associated with alpha-1 protease deficiency. Radiologically, the lungs are hyperinflated and hypertransradiant, the heart is narrow and lies vertically, and the diaphragm adopts a low position.

General expansion of one side of the chest

General expansion of one side of the chest is unusual. It may occur in children and young adults, but is unlikely in older subjects with more rigid chest walls. Clinically detectable expansion of one hemithorax may accompany large rapidly accumulating pleural effusions, large tension pneumothoraces, especially in patients undergoing assisted ventilation; or unilateral obstructive emphysema associated with partial bronchial obstruction causing a check valve effect allowing air to enter the lung segment and preventing its escape, and to over-expansion of giant air-containing cysts in the lung.

General contraction of one side of the chest

General contraction of one side of the chest is due to loss of volume of the underlying lung. This may follow lung collapse, lung fibrosis, surgical resection of the lung tissue, or pleural thickening preventing inflation of the underlying lung. Pleural thickening may result from chronic empyema (Fig. C.4) (bacterial and tuberculous) and malignant infiltration from adenocarcinoma or mesothelioma. Unilateral pulmonary fibrosis may result from lung inflammation due to pulmonary tuberculosis, chronic lung abscess or organizing pneumonia. The whole hemithorax may appear shrunken, with abnormalities most apparent in the upper anterior chest showing obvious

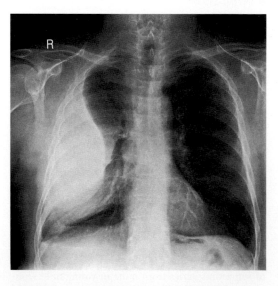

Figure C.4 Empyema due to HIV-related recurrent chest infections.

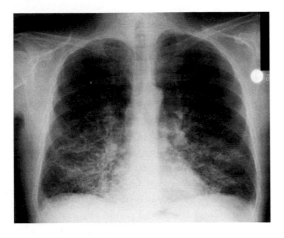

Figure C.5 Extensive basal fibrosis of lung in man exposed to coal dust.

flattening and reduced respiratory excursion (remember the adage, 'flattening equals fibrosis'). The contracted fibrotic lung due to chronic pulmonary suppuration is frequently the site of bronchiectasis (Fig. C.5).

When unilateral contraction of the chest with gross pleural thickening arises from any cause during childhood or adolescence, the resulting scoliosis may become extreme as growth proceeds.

Localized chest wall disease

Disorders of the chest wall which may present as localized swellings are listed in Table C.3.

Table C.3 Causes of localized swelling of the chest wall

Infectious inflammations	
Tuberculosis of the chest wall	See text
Osteomyelitis	— in children — staphylococcal infection involving the ribs
	— in adults — usually staphylococcal in drug addicts following a blow
Osteochondritis of costochondral junction	— Tietze's syndrome (uncommon); see text
	— typhoid fever (very rare); see text
Syphilitic gumma	Starts in anterior mediastinum and presents at the front of an intercostal space. Now very rare
Actinomycosis	See text
Fungal infections	Blastomycosis, coccidiodomycosis and cryptococcosis can cause osteolytic rib lesions
Benign soft tissue tumours	
Lipoma	Commonest benign tumour of the chest wall. CT scan confirms the presence of fat
Haemangioma	Mass may pulsate. Bruit heard. Phleboliths in the tumour on chest radiograph diagnostic
Cystic hygroma	A rare hamartomatous lymphatic malformation producing a thin-walled cystic tumour lined with endothelium
Neurofibromatosis	Multiple fibromas present in one or more intercostal spaces. Café au lait patches, etc.
Malignant soft tissue tumours	
Fibrosarcoma	Commonest malignant soft tissue primary tumour of the chest wall; can arise in soft tissues in older women many years after radiotherapy to the breast
Benign bony tissue tumours	
Osteochondroma (exostosis)	Small hard tumour fixed to a rib or the sternum in children and young adults. May cause severe pain
Chondroma	Tends to become carcinomatous; see Chondrosarcoma
Diaphysical aclasias	Generalized disorder of skeleton. The rib excrescences resemble chondromas
Osteoclastoma	Rarely affects ribs. About 10% can become malignant
Malignant bony tissue tumours	
Metastases	Primary is usually in lung, breast, prostate, thyroid or kidney in adults and is usually a neuroblastoma in children
Multiple and solitary myeloma	Monoclonal hypergammaglobulinaemia
Chondrosarcoma	Initial silent painless growth — may stop growing for a time only to become painful and invasive
Ewing's sarcoma	Aggressive, commonest in those under 30 years of age. Involves the ribs and rarely scapula or sternum
Osteogenic sarcoma	May occur in rib of patient with Paget's disease or in a woman many years after radiation therapy to the breast

Tuberculosis of the chest wall

Tuberculosis of the chest wall usually arises from the breakdown of intercostal lymph nodes, and presents as a painless fluctuating cold abscess that may be mistaken for a lipoma. Diagnosis is made by aspiration of caseous pus or during histological examination. There are two main groups of intercostal lymph nodes. The first group lies at the angle of the ribs, while the second group lies along the internal thoracic (internal mammary) vessels, a finger's breadth from the edge of the sternum. From here, pus may track backwards with the posterior primary division of the intercostal nerves to present near the erector spinae muscles or forwards with the anterior division of the intercostal nerve to present in the lateral chest wall. Abscesses may arise from nodes in the region of the internal mammary artery, from which pus may present near the costochondral junction.

Tuberculosis of the sternum can cause a cold abscess over the anterior chest wall. Rib tuberculosis is rare, but may give rise to local pain, swelling and sinus formation. Radiologically, there is an initial small area of bone destruction which progresses to periosteal elevation and soft tissue swelling. Multiple cold abscesses of the ribs may accompany spinal tuberculosis (Pott's disease) with paravertebral abscess formation pointing over the back and lower ribs.

Tietze's syndrome (costochondritis)

This condition of obscure aetiology results in pain, swelling and tenderness of one or more of the upper six costal cartilages. The second costal cartilage is most often affected. This syndrome may present at any age, but is most common in young adults. The onset may be insidious or abrupt, the pain variously described as aching, gripping, sharp or dull, and the condition – which is self-limiting – can persist for weeks, months or rarely years. It has been suggested that asymmetrical rib growth, prolonged coughing or hyperventilation may be the cause, but it is often idiopathic.

Osteomyelitis of the ribs, spine or sternum

Osteomyelitis is a well-known, albeit rare, consequence of bacteraemia. Classically difficult to diagnose, patients present with chronic symptoms of pain, fever, thoracic cage swelling and radiographic evidence of erosion and bony sclerosis. *Staphylococcus aureus* is the most common agent. *Staphylococcus epidermidis* has emerged in recent years as a frequent cause from infected intravenous lines and prosthetic implant material. Gram-negative organisms are often responsible for haematogenous vertebral osteomyelitis, especially in patients with sickle cell anaemia. Intravenous drug abusers are especially susceptible to a wide range of bacterial and fungal causes of osteomyelitis.

Actinomycosis

Thoracic actinomycosis may spread from the lungs to cause a diffuse indurated swelling of the chest wall; if the condition is undiagnosed and untreated it progresses to destructive rib lesions associated with periostitis and multiple sinuses discharging 'sulphur granule pus'.

Empyema necessitatis

A localized swelling of the chest wall may be caused by a neglected empyema pointing externally to produce a soft diffuse fluctuant swelling which sometimes gives an impulse on respiration or coughing.

Tumours

Tumours may originate or metastasize to the chest wall (see Table C.3).

Aortic aneurysms

Aortic aneurysms involving the ascending part of the aorta may cause pulsating swellings over the upper anterior chest; they should be easily recognizable by the characteristic expansile pulsation and by other signs and symptoms of aneurysm. The commonest situation for such a swelling is to the right of the sternum at the first, second and third intercostal spaces. In the presence of a grossly enlarged heart the precordium may become prominent, a condition most often seen in children suffering from severe rheumatic or congenital heart disease.

Boris Lams

CHEST PAIN

Pain in the chest is one of the commonest of all complaints. However slight it may be, it only too often conjures up in the mind of the sufferer a vision of serious organic disease of the lungs or, more often, of the heart. Accurate diagnosis depends, to a considerable extent, on physical examination and special investigations but, most of all, on a detailed and precise history of the site and radiation of the pain, of its character and duration, and of factors by which it is aggravated or relieved. A useful clinical classification of pain in the chest is into pain felt mainly in the centre of the chest or in its lateral aspects; each of these categories can be further subdivided into: (i) pain of sudden onset, often presenting as an emergency; and (ii) pain which, on presentation to the physician, has been present for several days or weeks. The common, and some of the less common, causes of chest pain are listed in this way in Table C.4. Pain in the precordium will be included in the discussion of central chest pain. The adjectives 'central' and 'precordial' are not of course synonymous – the precordium being that area of the anterior chest wall

Table C.4 Causes of chest pain

Acute	Chronic
Central or precordial	
Common	*Common*
Myocardial infarction	Angina of effort
Unstable angina	Oesophageal spasm or reflux
Pericarditis	Cervical spondylosis
Dissecting aortic aneurysm	Prolapsed mitral cusp
Massive pulmonary embolism	Da Costa's syndrome
Less common	*Less common*
Upper abdominal catastrophe	Pulmonary hypertension
Precordial catch	Peptic ulcer
Acute anxiety	Gallbladder disease
Tracheitis	Chronic pancreatitis
Mycoplasma pneumonia	Ankylosing spondylitis
Pericardial fat necrosis	Tietze's disease
	Lesions of sternum
	Mediastinal tumour
Lateral	
Common	*Common*
Pleurisy: infective, infarction, connective tissue disease	Spinal disease: infection, tumours, spondylosis
Trauma, e.g. fractured rib	Chronic trauma
	Bronchial carcinoma
Less common	*Less common*
Superficial lesions, e.g. herpes zoster	Rib metastases
Bornholm disease	Aortic aneurysm
Trichinosis	

circumscribed by the surface markings of the heart – but the two sites are naturally associated in the diagnosis of pain which arises, or is thought to arise, from the heart. Before proceeding to the main discussion, a brief account will be given, for the sake of completeness, of several causes of chest pain which are immediately obvious on superficial examination.

Pain due to superficial lesions

Pain due to inflammation of the superficial tissues of the chest wall poses no great diagnostic problem. It is important to remember, however, that the inflammation may have spread from a deeper lesion such as an empyema. Herpes zoster, which involves thoracic nerve roots in at least 50 per cent of cases, is also obvious once the eruption has appeared, but pain and paraesthesiae may be present for a few days before this and cause temporary diagnostic confusion. The vesicles are implanted on an erythematous base and may be discrete or confluent; they are strictly unilateral, and occupy the area of one or more dermatomes. Fever and malaise occur in a few patients, and the axillary lymph nodes may be enlarged. Scabs form and the lesions heal in a week or two, without scarring unless they have become secondarily infected. Post-herpetic neuralgia may, occasionally, cause severe pain for a long period after the eruption has disappeared, especially in the elderly. Very rarely, *Mondor's disease*, which is phlebitis of the subcutaneous anterior thoracic veins, produces pain which is either pleuritic in type or is provoked by raising the arms. The inflamed vein may be palpable as a tender cord. Resolution occurs in a few weeks or a month or two.

Central chest pain

Much the most important cause of central chest pain is myocardial ischaemia. Three separate clinical syndromes are recognized – angina of effort, unstable angina, and myocardial infarction – although there is some overlap, at least between the first two.

The diagnosis of *angina* turns, in the great majority of cases, on an accurate history. The pain is typically symmetrical in the chest, or nearly so, being felt in the region of the sternum, or slightly to the left, and radiating laterally towards the axillae and down the inner sides of the arms. The left is involved a little more often than the right, but this is of no diagnostic importance as bilateral radiation is the rule.

Radiation to the epigastrium, the side of the neck, jaw and tongue also occurs. Very occasionally the pain is felt in the midline of the back or in one or other scapular region. The pain is described as 'tight', 'gripping' or 'like indigestion', or the patient may deny actual pain and describe only a feeling of pressure or of tightness. A particularly revealing gesture is the clenched fist placed on the sternum to indicate both the site and, presumably, the character of the sensation. A pain described as 'stabbing' is probably not angina, but patients do not always choose their words with care, and each statement must be carefully analysed to ascertain the patient's meaning exactly. Certainly a pain which comes in sharp jabs, lasting a second only, is unlikely to be angina, and adjectives such as 'shooting' and 'stabbing' are suspect on this account. The typical duration of an attack is a few minutes only, and a pain lasting for a much longer or shorter time than this is unlikely to be angina; there are exceptions, however, which will be discussed.

Perhaps the most important aspect is the relationship to exertion. A pain in the anterior part of the chest which is consistently provoked by effort and relieved by rest must be presumed to be angina, unless there is overwhelming evidence to the contrary. The pain may be provoked more easily after meals or in cold weather, but it is the relationship to effort which is of paramount importance provided that the pain develops *during* the exercise; a pain starting *after* exercise is not angina. The effect of sublingual glyceryl trinitrate (GTN) may be of diagnostic importance but, again, the time relationship is important. If the pain is relieved within a minute by GTN, angina is probable; patients are, however, unfamiliar with such a rapid effect from oral medication and may claim that GTN relieves their pain, omitting the essential fact that the pain does not cease until, perhaps, half an hour after the tablet was taken. Occasionally, variants of angina are seen such as pain felt only in one of the distal sites of radiation; even 'tennis elbow' and 'toothache' may prove to be angina if the constant relationship to exertion can be elicited.

Apart from exercise, angina may be precipitated by sympathetic over-activity. This is the mechanism of angina provoked by emotion, as in the case of John Hunter who said, some time before he died after an acrimonious Board Meeting, 'My life is in the hands of any rascal who chooses to annoy and tease me.' Nocturnal angina is also related to sympathetic over-activity, as it has been shown to occur after a period of REM (rapid eye movement) sleep which is associated with dreaming. Angina decubitus, provoked by lying down, is probably due to the increase in cardiac output in this posture; it is rather characteristic of syphilitic aortic valve disease. In general, angina which is easily provoked or occurs, apparently spontaneously, at rest is associated with severe disease involving all three coronary arteries (right, left circumflex and anterior descending).

In the majority of cases of angina no abnormal physical signs are found, but two important signs should be specifically sought. A left atrial impulse may be palpable at the apex and an atrial gallop rhythm heard, particularly during an actual attack of pain. Paradoxical splitting of the second heart sound is less common and is difficult to elicit but, if present, implies prolongation of left ventricular systole and a serious disturbance of left ventricular function. The electrocardiogram is usually normal at rest, but the typical depression of the RS-T segment may be present to confirm the diagnosis of ischaemia; evidence of previous infarction may also be present or non-specific changes such as bundle-branch block. Recording the electrocardiogram during exercise to demonstrate RS-T depression and, sometimes, other changes is a reliable method of confirming the diagnosis of myocardial ischaemia. Radio-isotope scanning of the myocardium using, for example, thallium-201 is also helpful in delineating areas of ischaemia which develop during exercise. In the majority of patients with angina and a positive exercise test, coronary angiography will show occlusive lesions of one or, usually, several coronary arteries. In a few, however, the arteries are normal or nearly so, and in such cases the most likely cause of the ischaemia is coronary artery spasm. This concept is an old one, but was convincingly revived by Maseri et al. It can occur in otherwise normal arteries or in association with occlusive disease of any degree of severity.

In a large majority of cases of angina the underlying lesion is coronary atherosclerosis. In addition, other forms of arterial disease can, occasionally, cause ischaemia. Angina is a well-recognized, though rare, symptom of polyarteritis nodosa and giant-cell arteritis; smaller vessels may be involved in rheumatoid arteritis and in association with livedo reticularis. Another inflammatory cause of angina is involvement of the coronary ostia in syphilitic aortitis;

the attacks of pain tend to last longer and to occur rather characteristically at night, although the relationship to effort is as in other varieties of angina. Ischaemic pain is aggravated by left ventricular hypertrophy due to hypertension and, particularly, aortic valve disease. In these conditions, and in hypertrophic obstructive cardiomyopathy, the disease of the coronary arteries themselves may be trivial and the pain due to relative ischaemia of the hypertrophied muscle. Severe anaemia (e.g. pernicious anaemia or following gastrointestinal haemorrhage), thyrotoxicosis and tachycardia can also cause angina in patients with minor coronary disease only. All of these factors must be borne in mind, particularly when dealing with a case of angina in a premenopausal woman. Coronary atherosclerosis is rare in such patients, and angina is likely to be due to one of the precipitating factors mentioned or to premature atherosclerosis resulting from hyperlipidaemia, as in diabetes, myxoedema or hereditary hypercholesterolaemic xanthomatosis (Type II hyperlipidaemia in Fredrickson's classification).

Unstable angina is one of a number of terms used to describe cases in which prolonged cardiac pain occurs at rest without evidence of myocardial necrosis. Other terms used include 'acute coronary insufficiency', 'preinfarction angina' and 'crescendo angina' which carry the (often correct) implication that myocardial infarction is imminent. A variant of this condition is the so-called 'angina inversa', described by Prinzmetal, in which RS-T *elevation* occurs briefly in association with ischaemic pain at rest or on exercise; this is believed to be due to severe ischaemia of a rather localized area of myocardium due to severe arterial disease or, sometimes, spasm. RS-T depression can also occur in similar circumstances, and it is probable that the elevation of 'angina inversa' is produced merely by the relationship of the site of ischaemia to the electrode position.

Myocardial infarction is nearly always due to occlusion of a coronary artery by atherosclerosis, with or without superadded thrombosis; a much rarer cause is coronary embolus in association with, for example, atrial fibrillation or infective endocarditis. The pain of myocardial infarction has exactly the same character and areas of radiation as angina. It is not, however, related to exercise and typically lasts for several hours, if untreated, rather than the few minutes of an anginal attack. Myocardial infarction can, rarely, be painless, especially in the elderly in whom it may manifest itself as syncope or an arrhythmia or as otherwise unexplained left ventricular failure. In contrast to the paucity of physical signs in angina, it is unusual to find no abnormal physical signs in a case of myocardial infarction, provided that frequent examination is carried out as many of the signs may be very transient. Some fall in blood pressure is common but may not be detected if the previous level is unknown. Slight elevation of the jugular venous pressure is seen in many cases and an audible or palpable atrial gallop is found even more frequently. Paradoxical splitting of the second sound may occasionally be detected and, after a day or two, a pericardial rub may be heard.

The three most common complications are arrhythmias, cardiac failure and shock, in that order. Continuous monitoring has demonstrated that over 90 per cent of cases of myocardial infarction have some form of arrhythmia, of which ventricular extrasystoles are the most common and may presage ventricular tachycardia and fibrillation. Supraventricular arrhythmias also occur, often in association with cardiac failure. Atrioventricular block is an ominous complication, especially if it develops in a case of anterior infarction. Congestive heart failure or frank pulmonary oedema occur from time to time, but lesser degrees of left ventricular failure are common. As a result of the consequent pulmonary venous congestion, with the probable addition of multiple alveolar collapse, mild arterial hypoxaemia is seen very frequently, the arterial PO_2 being around 9 kPa; this often causes sufficient hyperventilation to reduce the arterial PCO_2 to about 5 kPa. The term 'cardiogenic shock' should be reserved for cases with severe hypotension, cold, clammy skin, oliguria and clouding of consciousness.

Less common complications include rupture of the infarct, which will usually cause rapidly fatal haemopericardium or, if a papillary muscle is involved, acute mitral regurgitation with pulmonary oedema; rupture of the interventricular septum causes acute right ventricular failure. Systemic embolism from a mural thrombus is not uncommon; pulmonary embolism arises most often from thrombosis of the leg veins secondary to enforced recumbency. Later sequelae are ventricular aneurysm, which may rarely calcify, Dressler's syndrome of recurrent pericarditis and pleurisy and the shoulder–hand syndrome, which consists of 'frozen shoulder' and Raynaud's phenomenon, usually on the left.

Electrocardiography remains the most commonly used method of confirming a diagnosis of myocardial infarction, but estimation of various serum enzymes is also valuable particularly in the (not infrequent) cases in which the electrocardiographic signs are equivocal. There are three cardinal electrocardiographic signs of myocardial infarction: a pathological Q wave, at least a third the amplitude of the R wave in the same lead and at least 0.04 seconds in duration; RS-T segment elevation with an upward convexity; and T-wave inversion which may not be seen until the RS-T segment is returning to the iso-electric line, as it does during the first few weeks after the episode. The T wave may also return to, or towards, normal after some months, but the Q wave – the sign of irreversible muscle necrosis – virtually always remains indefinitely. These changes are seen in leads of which the positive terminals face the infarcted area of myocardium; in leads 'facing' the diametrically opposite part of the heart reciprocal changes are seen which may, occasionally, be of diagnostic significance. For descriptive purposes, infarcts are subdivided into anterior, inferior (or diaphragmatic) and 'true' posterior. Originally, the term 'posterior' was applied to the diaphragmatic surface of the heart, but now that it is possible to diagnose infarction of the small part of the left ventricle which lies posteriorly, the anatomically more correct term 'inferior' is preferred. To avoid confusion with the older nomenclature, infarcts at the back of the left ventricle are designated true posterior (Figs C.6–C.9).

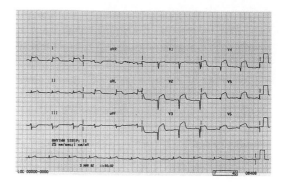

Figure C.7 Acute anterior myocardial infarction.

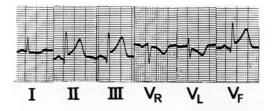

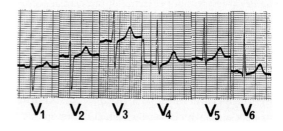

Figure C.8 Acute inferior myocardial infarction.

ST SEGMENT ABNORMALITIES

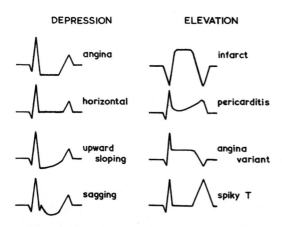

Figure C.6 Diagrammatic representation of common abnormal ECG changes.

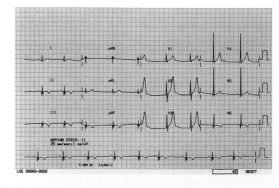

Figure C.9 Acute posterior myocardial infarction.

Many intracellular enzymes are released into the circulation from the infarcted myocardium, and the rise and fall of their serum levels can be of great diagnostic value. Those most commonly estimated clinically are aspartate amino-transferase (previously known as 'glutamic-oxaloacetic transaminase'), creatine phosphokinase and lactate dehydrogenase (LDH). The first two remain elevated for 3–4 days only, but elevation of the serum LDH persists for up to 2 weeks. Greater specificity for myocardial damage can be achieved by estimating the iso-enzymes of LDH separately; the iso-enzyme released in largest amounts from the myocardium also acts upon hydroxybutyrate, and can be conveniently estimated as hydroxybutyrate dehydrogenase. Apart from the changes in the serum enzymes, non-specific evidence of tissue necrosis is also present following myocardial infarction; such evidence includes pyrexia, leucocytosis and raised erythrocyte sedimentation rate. Such changes, although characteristic, are of little or no diagnostic value.

The pain of *pericarditis* is, in some respects, similar to that of myocardial infarction and, as localized pericarditis is common in the latter, the differentiation may present some difficulty. Pericardial pain is felt in the sternal region and towards the left, and may radiate to the epigastrium, neck, back, shoulders and, occasionally, to the arms. The severity varies markedly, from a mild discomfort to extreme agony, and the pain is described either as 'stabbing' or 'like a knife', or in terms very reminiscent of those used to describe the pain of myocardial ischaemia. It is aggravated by deep breathing, coughing and by twisting movements involving the muscles of the chest wall. There is therefore some relationship with exertion, on account of the associated hyperventilation, but the aggravation by specific movements such as turning over in bed serves to distinguish it from angina. The pain is also worse in the recumbent position and is relieved by sitting up; it may also be aggravated by swallowing. The characteristic physical sign is the friction rub, heard over all or part of the precordium (see RUB, PERICARDIAL, p. 624). The third cardinal feature of pericarditis is the electrocardiogram. RS-T elevation is seen in all epicardial leads, that is in all the leads of a conventional 12-lead record except a VR (Fig. C.10). The RS-T elevation is concave upwards, unlike that of myocardial infarction; pathological Q waves are, of course, absent. Later in the course of the disease, T-wave inversion appears and, at this stage, the

differentiation from myocardial ischaemia may be difficult. The diagnosis of pericarditis is incomplete unless the aetiology is determined. Common causes include virus infection (often Coxsackie B), connective-tissue disorders such as systemic lupus erythematosus (SLE), rheumatic fever, rheumatoid arthritis, bacterial infections and Dressler's and other similar syndromes. Chronic renal failure is a well-known cause, but the commonest cause of all is myocardial infarction; in that condition the pericarditis probably contributes little to the pain.

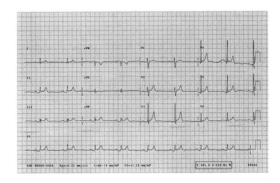

Figure C.10 Acute pericarditis.

Pericardial fat necrosis is a rare cause of pain simulating that of pericarditis. No friction rub can be heard, and the electrocardiogram is normal. A paracardiac mass may be visible in the chest radiograph.

Dissecting aneurysm causes very severe anterior chest pain which radiates to the neck, back and, later, to the abdomen; it rarely spreads to the arms. With dissection of the descending thoracic aorta the pain may begin in the back. The resemblance to myocardial infarction is close and, indeed, if the dissection involves a coronary artery, infarction may, in fact, occur and confuse the diagnostic issue further. Important differentiating features include the absence of one or more peripheral pulses, particularly if a pulse disappears while the patient is under observation, or other evidence of arterial occlusion such as hemiparesis, blindness in one eye, or haematuria. The development of aortic regurgitation, due to involvement of the aortic valve ring by the dissection, is a valuable diagnostic feature. The blood pressure is little changed compared with the fall commonly seen in myocardial infarction. The severity of the pain is of some diagnostic significance; chest pain which is hardly influenced by morphine or diamorphine may well be due to a dissecting aneurysm. The electrocardiogram is normal unless a coronary artery is involved or pre-existing hypertensive changes are present. Much reliance is placed on radiography in diagnosis: gross dilatation of the thoracic aorta may be seen, but this is not always easy to distinguish from unfolding unless a previous film is available. Also the dilatation may not be very marked in the early stages. In practice, a firm diagnosis is rarely possible from the plain radiograph. If available, contrast CT is the investigation of choice; otherwise the definitive diagnosis can only be made by aortography, though even this can be misleading at times.

Another important cause of sudden anterior chest pain is massive *pulmonary embolism*. Smaller pulmonary emboli cause pulmonary infarction (this is discussed below, among the causes of lateral, pleuritic chest pain). Pulmonary embolism occurs commonly in the postoperative period or during a period of enforced recumbency associated with a low cardiac output, as after myocardial infarction or in cardiac failure. In young women, oral contraceptive agents have been incriminated as the cause of the initiating venous thrombosis. The same complication may, of course, occur in pregnancy. The source of the embolism is commonly thrombosis in the veins of the leg or pelvis, but this may not have been clinically manifest except, perhaps, as a small 'spike' of temperature. The patient rapidly becomes severely ill with central chest pain which is almost identical to that of myocardial infarction, breathlessness and, often, faintness or even loss of consciousness. Peripheral cyanosis is present, the pulse is rapid, and the blood pressure very low. Elevation of the jugular venous pressure is nearly always present; it is usually a good deal higher than in myocardial infarction causing a comparable degree of hypotension. Gallop rhythm may be heard over the right ventricle. The electrocardiogram may show classic changes of a deep S wave in lead I, in addition to a Q wave and inverted T wave in lead III – the S1Q3T3 pattern. Other patterns include T-wave inversion in V1–V4 and right axis deviation. In some cases the electrocardiogram may be normal or reveal only a tachycardia. The chest radiograph may show dilatation of one or both main branches of the pulmonary artery, and one lung (or part thereof) may appear unusually translucent (Westermark's

sign). The chest X-ray may however be normal or reveal only a pleural effusion. Ventilation perfusion scanning may reveal multiple areas of mismatch. Doppler ultrasound of the legs may reveal a source for the emboli from the deep venous system. CT pulmonary angiography may demonstrate central pulmonary emboli. Pulmonary angiography, which is less hazardous than might have been expected in this situation, may show occlusion of the pulmonary artery.

Chronic *pulmonary hypertension*, as in mitral stenosis or the Eisenmenger syndrome, can produce a pain which is indistinguishable from angina. The cause, indeed, is almost certainly myocardial ischaemia as a result of the severely limited cardiac output. Severe *pulmonary stenosis* can cause a similar pain.

The anterior chest pain associated with *prolapse of a mitral valve cusp* is not usually ischaemic in origin. This lesion is not uncommon, with a prevalence of between 4–5% in otherwise healthy individuals and is often associated with a mid-systolic click and late systolic murmur. The diagnosis can be confirmed by echocardiography or angiocardiography. The pain is very variable in site, duration and severity, and has no clear-cut diagnostic features.

Pain arising from the oesophagus is felt in the midline of the chest, with radiation to the jaw, back, shoulders and, to a small extent, down the inner sides of the arms. The resemblance to angina is close, and oesophageal pain may even have some relationship to exertion, although this is never constant. The pain may be due to *oesophageal spasm* without any other lesion, it may occur early in the evolution of *achalasia of the cardia*, or it may be due to *hiatus hernia* with oesophageal reflux and oesophagitis. Heartburn, with radiation of sternal pain upwards from the xiphoid, is very characteristic of the last condition. Helpful diagnostic features include the association of the pain with taking food and relief with belching; the pain of oesophageal reflux is commonly worse in the recumbent position or in other postures favouring regurgitation, such as bending forward or the cramped position of the driver of a small car, especially if wearing a tight safety belt. If the pain can be reproduced by the instillation of 0.1 N hydrochloric acid into the lower oesophagus, this is good evidence that it is due to reflux. The demonstration of a hiatus hernia by a barium swallow is only too easy. Most hiatus hernias produce no symptoms at all, and chest pain in a patient in whom such a lesion has been demonstrated is as likely to be due to myocardial ischaemia or other conditions as to the hernia. There is no substitute for a detailed analysis of the symptoms.

Other upper abdominal lesions can cause pain felt in the midline of the front of the chest. The frequency with which angina is regarded as 'indigestion' – even by experienced physicians suffering from this condition – bears witness to this. Catastrophes such as perforated peptic ulcer and acute pancreatitis must be remembered in the differential diagnosis of myocardial infarction. Gastric distension due to aerophagy or other causes can cause substernal discomfort, but peptic ulcer and chronic relapsing pancreatitis are less common causes of confusion; in the former, the relationship of the pain to meals is obviously important.

Finally, there is the (almost mystical) association of gallbladder disease with ischaemic heart disease. Both conditions are common, and can certainly coexist. Much debate has centred around whether this co-existence occurs more commonly than would have been expected by chance; many experienced clinicians have a strong impression that this is so, but none of the theories to account for it is very convincing. Suffice it to say that gallbladder pain can certainly radiate into the front of the chest and simulate angina; also, central chest pain with a constant relationship to exertion must be regarded as angina, even if gallbladder disease is present in addition.

There are numerous musculoskeletal causes of anterior chest pain. Local *trauma is* usually obvious, but recurrent mild trauma – for example in some particular occupation – may not be mentioned by the patient as a possible cause for his/her pain. The pain may be a dull ache on one or other side of the chest, rarely exactly in the midline, or it may be possible to relate it to particular movements if anterior thoracic muscles are the site of origin. Pain from *spondylosis* or spondylitis of the thoracic (or even the cervical) spine can be referred to the front of the chest. The distribution can occasionally simulate that of angina, and radiological proof of the spondylosis is of little diagnostic significance. Relief of the pain from wearing a cervical collar is, however, good evidence of a skeletal origin. Less obvious spinal disease may also be a cause of pain felt diffusely over the precordium or in the corresponding area on the right. Experimentally, the injection of hypertonic saline into an interspinous ligament produces pain referred to the anterior part of the corresponding dermatome with some radiation

upwards and downwards. It is difficult to prove this aetiology in any particular patient, but it has been suggested that chronic mild trauma to interspinous ligaments, for example due to scoliosis, may be a cause of otherwise unexplained precordial pain.

Less common musculoskeletal lesions include *Tietze's disease.* This causes pain of sudden or gradual onset in one or more upper costal cartilages. The pain is worse on coughing or deep breathing, and the affected cartilage is swollen and tender. *Xiphoidalgia* is a similar condition involving the xiphisternum which is possibly a variant of Tietze's disease or, more likely, due to recurrent mild trauma. Ankylosing spondylitis can cause a diffuse pain in the anterior chest wall often associated with local tenderness over the sternum and costal cartilages. Pain arising in the sternum itself may be due to *myelomatosis*, *metastases*, *ankylosing spondylitis*, *osteomyelitis* or *fracture*. The sudden, sharp pain at or near the cardiac apex (known as *precordial catch*) is probably quite common, although rare as a spontaneous complaint. There is rarely any diagnostic confusion with other causes of chest pain as the history is quite characteristic. The pain occurs most often when the subject is seated and lasts for a few minutes only. It can be relieved by a single, painful, deep inspiration.

Respiratory disease most often causes pain, if at all, in one or other side of the chest, but *tracheitis* should be mentioned as a cause of upper sternal pain. It is aggravated by the hyperventilation of exercise and may thus, very occasionally, have to be distinguished from angina. *Mycoplasma pneumonia*, unlike other varieties of pneumonia, is never associated with pleurisy, but may cause a substernal pain aggravated by coughing. *Dyspnoea* itself – especially if it is associated with obstruction of airways – may be described as 'tightness in the chest', and an injudicious series of leading questions may persuade the patient that he or she has a 'tight pain' across their chest and lead to an erroneous diagnosis of angina.

Two psychological conditions are important in the differential diagnosis of anterior chest pain. The terrifying panic of an attack of *acute anxiety* can be confused with a myocardial infarction or other intrathoracic vascular catastrophe. The patient, very often a woman, complains of dizziness, palpitations, dyspnoea and precordial oppression or pain. Angor animi – the fear of impending death – is a prominent feature, much more so than in genuine myocardial ischaemia, and further exacerbates the anxiety. The circumstances in which the attack occurs – and the complete absence of objective evidence of organic disease – are important distinguishing features, and doubt about the nature of the condition should rarely persist for long. Chronic anxiety is the commonest underlying disorder in *Da Costa's syndrome*; the non-committal eponymous title is preferred to the numerous other terms, such as 'effort syndrome', 'cardiac neurosis' and 'disordered action of the heart', which have been used (with no great semantic accuracy) to describe this condition. Apart from the pain, the features of the syndrome are dyspnoea, palpitation, fatigue and dizziness. The pain is most commonly felt in the left submammary region, although it may be nearer the midline or, indeed, anywhere on the left side of the chest, even radiating into the left arm. In character it is sharp and stabbing, with occasional momentary twinges superimposed on a dull ache which persists for many hours at a time. It often occurs *after* – but rarely during – exertion; this important point may be elicited only after careful questioning. In summary, it differs from angina in almost all respects except in the rare, difficult case in which it has a more constricting quality and is felt near the left border of the sternum. The mechanism of the pain is unknown, but it seems likely that, in some cases at least, the original cause was a minor musculoskeletal abnormality. The pain convinces the patient that their heart is diseased and is perpetuated by the anxiety engendered by this conviction.

Lateral chest pain

Almost all tissues of the lateral chest wall, the pleura, muscles, ribs and intercostal nerves, can be the site of painful lesions. Frequently, the pain is closely related to respiration, as exemplified most clearly in *pleurisy*. The visceral pleura is insensitive, but the parietal pleura is plentifully supplied with pain fibres from the intercostal nerves. The pain is felt, therefore, in the cutaneous areas supplied by these nerves which, it is important to remember, include a large area of the anterior abdominal wall. Apart from inflammation of the pleura itself, there is some evidence that spasm of the intercostal muscles may be a factor in producing the pain. The pain is characteristically sharp, superficial, of any degree of severity, and is aggravated by deep breathing and by coughing. Inspiration is abruptly halted by the pain so that respiration is often

very shallow. Holding the breath in expiration will usually relieve the pain completely, and a change in the patient's posture in bed can produce considerable relief or exacerbation. The only physical sign of pleurisy, in the absence of effusion, is the pleural friction rub – a characteristic creaking sound present during inspiration and expiration. The sound is difficult to describe, but easy to recognize with a little experience. The pain is not at all closely related to the rub as one may be present without the other; neither alone is essential for the diagnosis of pleurisy. The pain of diaphragmatic pleurisy is typically referred to the shoulder; this is a common feature of pleurisy due to subdiaphragmatic lesions such as liver abscess or subphrenic abscess.

Pleurisy may be due to pulmonary infections such as lobar pneumonia or tuberculosis, to vascular lesions such as pulmonary infarction, or to connective-tissue disorders such as SLE. In many of these conditions, the clinical picture is modified by the development of an effusion which usually results in the disappearance of the pain and the rub.

A pain identical to that of pleurisy is felt in epidemic pleurodynia or *Bornholm disease*, due to Group B Coxsackie viruses. The pain is the presenting symptom and may be extremely severe; fever quickly develops and headache and malaise are common. Recovery is usually rapid, but relapses are frequent and may continue for several weeks. *Trichinosis*, involving the intercostal muscles, can also produce pleuritic pain; the diagnosis would be supported by finding periorbital or generalized oedema, and by eosinophilia in the peripheral blood. Pain arising from the capsule of the spleen is also related to respiration; it is commonly due to *splenic infarction*, and may be accompanied by a friction rub so that the resemblance to pleurisy is very close. Splenic pain is not uncommon in Hodgkin's disease and in other similar conditions.

The pain of *spontaneous pneumothorax* is usually abrupt in onset, and pleuritic in type (Fig. C.11). Some patients however complain only of a dull ache or a sense of tightness, and a few have no pain at all. The typical physical signs are a diminution in movement and in breath-sounds on the affected side, often with a hyperresonant percussion note and – especially if the pneumothorax is under tension – deviation of the trachea towards the normal side. Dissection of the air into the mediastinum may cause central chest pain and the patient may notice a 'crunching' sound over

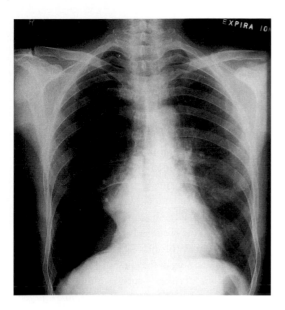

Figure C.11 Complete right pneumothorax.

the heart which is also audible on auscultation. The diagnosis of spontaneous pneumothorax can be confirmed by radiography, but careful study may be needed if the pneumothorax is shallow; a film taken in expiration will show the lesion more clearly.

Involvement of the intercostal nerves in many pathological processes can cause pain in the corresponding areas of the chest wall. *Spinal disease* has already been mentioned as a cause of referred pain in the anterolateral regions of the chest. Direct pressure on nerves may occur in fracture of the thoracic spine, from malignant metastases in that region, or in tuberculosis of the spine. Spondylosis with disc protrusion is not common as a cause of nerve-root compression in the thoracic spine. Neurofibromatosis may affect the thoracic nerve roots, but does not often cause pain.

Aortic aneurysm is not a common lesion, although in former years it was an important cause of chest pain. Aneurysm of the ascending aorta may cause chest pain by eroding the sternum, but much more often causes no symptoms at all. Aneurysm of the arch and descending thoracic aorta can cause very severe radiating pain by vertebral erosion and pressure on nerve roots. Other symptoms and signs result from pressure on mediastinal structures. Thus, pressure on the left recurrent laryngeal nerve will cause paralysis of the left vocal cord, whilst cough and stridor may follow pressure on the trachea, and dysphagia results from pressure on the

oesophagus. Pressure on the left main bronchus may cause collapse of the left lung with subsequent infection; a tracheal tug is a well-known physical sign of aneurysm depressing the left main bronchus.

Primary or secondary intrathoracic *malignant disease* may cause pain in various ways. Direct invasion of the pleura by a bronchial carcinoma can cause pleurisy, often with effusion; more often, pleural pain occurs as a result of infection in the lung distal to a blocked bronchus. Primary tumours of the pleura (e.g. mesothelioma) cause pleuritic pain directly. Apart from the pleura, the ribs and intercostal nerves may be involved by tumour with the production of severe pain. Metastases in the thoracic spine have been mentioned as a cause of intercostal pain; secondary deposits in the ribs can also be extremely painful. Rarely, tumours in the mediastinum can apparently cause a poorly localized central chest pain without other pressure symptoms; the mechanism is not known.

Boris Lams

CHEST, TENDERNESS IN

Chest pain is one of the most common symptoms given for seeking medical advice. Because there is no clear relationship between the intensity of discomfort and aetiology, all complaints of chest pain must be considered carefully. (See also CHEST PAIN, p. 96). This section deals exclusively with tenderness which is, in fact, rarely complained of in the absence of pain.

Tenderness in the chest, an ache or discomfort, perhaps with increased sensitivity and often accompanied with pain, can be difficult for the patient to describe. It is best classified according to the situation or character of the responsible lesion. Pains referred from visceral lesions may sometimes be associated with local tenderness in the chest wall. The parietal pleura is exquisitely sensitive to painful stimuli and unpleasant sensations may also arise from lesions in the tracheobronchial tree.

Classification

Lesions of the chest wall

■ Inflammation of the skin and underlying tissues, including the breasts

- Intercostal myositis
- Myalgia
- Inflammation of the ribs and sternum
- Blood diseases
- Intercostal neuritis and neuralgia
- Injury of the intercostal nerves
- Ankylosing spondylitis
- Herpes zoster
- Tietze's syndrome

Lesions of the thoracic and abdominal viscera

- Lungs
- Heart and aorta
- Diaphragm
- Stomach and oesophagus
- Liver/gallbladder

Lesions of the chest wall

Discomfort in the chest wall can result from respiratory diseases as well as from primary musculoskeletal lesions. Patients with chronic cough, dyspnoea or asthmatics subject to chest tightness often complain of anterolateral chest wall tenderness.

Tenderness is always present in *superficial inflammatory lesions* of the chest wall, such as bruises, burns, cuts, mastitis and superficial infections, the diagnosis of which will usually be evident on examination.

Pain will be the chief complaint in the so-called *intercostal myositis* that occurs after injury or strain of an intercostal muscle, the affected muscle being tender to deep pressure. The condition is also known as *intercostal myalgia* or *pleurodynia*. It is distinguished from pleurisy by the absence of a pleural friction rub. Similar, but more transient, pain with a variable degree of tenderness may accompany the *stitch* to which some athletes are prone.

The acute pain of Bornholm disease, epidemic myalgia due to Coxsackie virus B infection, may be accompanied by hyperaesthesia of skin, but less often by muscle tenderness. The myalgia of *Phlebotomus* (Sandfly) fever and dengue may also be accompanied by tenderness, which is often mild.

Tenderness of the *breasts* in the absence of mastitis is a common occurrence at or just before the menstrual periods and with high-dosage oestrogen therapy. Gynaecomastia in males, whatever the cause, is accompanied by tenderness of the breasts. It is not uncommon in chronic male alcoholics with cirrhosis of the liver.

Tenderness in the chest may result from *disease or injury of a rib or the sternum* when it will be localized to the injured spot; fracture, inflammation, tuberculosis or new growth may be the immediate cause. If *fracture is* present, X-radiography may show the lesion or crepitus between the fragments on movement may be obtainable. *Sternal* or *costal osteitis* or *periostitis* may follow injury and may also occur in such diseases as typhoid or paratyphoid fever, or tuberculosis. The local signs of inflammation (pain, redness, heat, swelling) will usually – but not invariably – be present. The chest wall may be invaded by local extension of a peripheral primary bronchial carcinoma or secondary tumour. Tenderness in the chest due to *malignancy* in a rib or in the sternum – such as multiple myeloma, sarcoma, secondary deposit from carcinoma – is generally a late occurrence, the existence of malignant disease elsewhere having usually been established. Tenderness of the ribs and sternum occurs in certain *blood diseases* such as leukaemia. Diagnosis depends on examination of the blood and marrow biopsy. Tenderness over the sternum and ribs also occurs as part of the clinical picture of ankylosing spondylitis. In this disease the sternomanubrial and sternoclavicular joints may become acutely swollen and tender, causing considerable discomfort.

The particularly tender spots in the course of an *intercostal nerve* are three in number, corresponding to the points at which the posterior, the lateral cutaneous and the anterior cutaneous branches are given off, near the spinal column, in the mid-axillary line and at the sternal margin, respectively. Such tenderness may be marked in so-called *intercostal neuritis*, when some intrathoracic disorder such as pneumonia or pleurisy is present and in cases of pressure on an intercostal nerve, as for example by *abscess* about the spinal column, *aneurysm* of the descending aorta or *malignancy* invading the spinal canal. Local tenderness may more commonly result from external pressure by, for instance, the buckle of the braces or some tool carried in a breast pocket – a simple detail, but one not infrequently overlooked.

Pain and tenderness along an intercostal nerve are common in *herpes zoster*, and may be present before, during and after the appearance of the characteristic rash. Tenderness can often be elicited at the three spots mentioned above; in particular, when herpes occurs past middle age it may be followed by a long period of pain and tenderness along the course of the affected nerve. The rash, once seen, can hardly be mistaken; to anticipate it on the type and site of the pain is a diagnostic *tour de force*. Similar pain and tenderness may follow thoracotomy, and occasional patients experience intractable postoperative discomfort.

Tietze's syndrome is an unexplained disorder in which pain and swelling are found in the upper costochondral junctions of the anterior chest wall. Biopsies of costal cartridges show nothing characteristically abnormal. One or more costal cartilages, usually on one side only, the second and third most often, may be affected. Spontaneous remission occurs in weeks, months or occasionally years.

Lesions of the underlying viscera

Tenderness in the chest may sometimes be a symptom of disease in the thoracic or abdominal viscera. The tenderness is as a rule superficial, confined to the skin and subjacent areolar and fatty tissues. Tactile hyperaesthesia or the production of unpleasant sensations or pain by the lightest touch may occur in neuralgia, neuroses, following thoracotomy or in cases of referred pain. A similar hyperaesthesia for cold (or less often for heat) sometimes occurs in the chest of tabetic patients. Hyperalgesia, where a normally painless stimulus becomes transformed into an acutely painful sensation, may be regarded as a form of 'tenderness' in the chest. This occurs in patients suffering from anxiety states, often with added depression. Further, perversions of sensation sometimes occur in organic nervous diseases, such as syringomyelia or tabes.

Tenderness of the chest may occur in *pleurisy*. The tenderness is as a rule deeply seated, and not in the skin and subcutaneous tissues. However, chest wall pain can mimic pleurisy and conditions in the chest wall can cause confusion. Tenderness due to the straining or tearing of thoracic muscles can be severe and painful, and may be exacerbated by coughing and confused with pleurisy.

The sternum may be tender as the result of *mediastinal inflammation, tumour* or *aneurysm*. The diagnosis in these cases is made by physical and X-ray examination. Tenderness with pain over the precordium may occur in *pericarditis*, accompanied usually by a pericardial rub. It may be so severe as to preclude percussion or even the application of a stethoscope. Similar pain and

tenderness may also be found in the epigastrium and upper costal angles.

Chest tenderness is sometimes found in cases of *acute* or *chronic disease of the lungs*, particularly *tuberculosis*. The tenderness may be either superficial or deep. It is generally felt most about the region of the apices of the lungs, the curve of the shoulder or the scapula. Similar tenderness is experienced occasionally *in acute bronchitis* or in *chronic bronchitis* and *emphysema*. Tenderness along the lower chest wall anteriorly may be found after vigorous coughing, probably from trauma in the soft tissues, the muscles particularly. A rib may be fractured by vigorous coughing.

Direct tenderness about the precordium is almost never due to *heart disease*. It is more generally associated with cardiac neurosis than with organic heart disease. Tenderness at the area of the apex beat is common in the Da Costa syndrome ('soldiers heart' or 'neurocirculatory asthenia'), a nervous condition in which there is no cardiac abnormality. The tenderness (which may be extreme) that is felt by some patients with heart disease, such as mitral stenosis, at the cardiac apex is due to anxiety rather than to an organic lesion.

Tenderness in the right side of the chest near the costal margin is not rare in *diseases of the liver* and *gallbladder* corresponding to the cutaneous distribution of the D7, D8 and D9 nerves; for the most part, however, the pain and tenderness are in the epigastrium and the right hypochondrium. The right phrenic nerve (C3–C5) sends branches to the liver and gallbladder, so that tenderness and pain may also be felt in the right shoulder, as in the case of disorders of the diaphragm. It is particularly in cases of gallstone or biliary colic that these areas of tenderness are likely to be found. In patients with hepatic abscess the spread of inflammation to the chest wall may give rise directly to pain and tenderness.

Boris Lams

CHEYNE–STOKES RESPIRATION

This well-known abnormality of respiration, described independently by John Cheyne in 1818 and William Stokes in 1846, is probably referred to in the Hippocratic writings in an account of a patient whose breathing was '… like that of a man recollecting himself, and rare and large'.

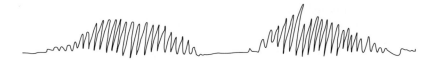

Figure C.12 Spirogram from a patient with severe cerebral vascular disease. Two cycles of Cheyne–Stokes breathing are shown over a period of 143 seconds.

Cheyne–Stokes respiration – the commonest form of periodic breathing – consists of alternating periods of apnoea and hyperventilation, beginning with hardly perceptible movements, gradually increasing until the tidal volume is much above normal, and then dying away to end in apnoea (Fig. C.12). The apnoeic period lasts for 10–30 seconds or more, and the hyperpnoeic phase comprises 30 or more breaths and usually lasts between 1 and 3 minutes. The condition is obvious to the experienced observer, but an untrained person will often describe the hyperpnoeic phase as 'breathlessness'. The patient may be unaware of the breathing abnormality. As Cheyne–Stokes breathing is accentuated during sleep, the hyperpnoea may disturb the patient's sleep and the symptoms may be confused with those of paroxysmal nocturnal dyspnoea due to cardiac failure.

The mechanism responsible for Cheyne–Stokes breathing is complex. In health, there is an oscillating balance between changes in arterial blood gas tensions and respiratory drive. The system is controlled by peripheral and central chemoreceptors, the rate of response of which is dependent upon the time it takes the circulation to carry arterial blood from the lungs to the carotid bodies and to the brain. The effect of these functional changes is most apparent when the predominant regulator for breathing is by the chemical control system that occurs in non-REM sleep. Thus, in stages 1 and 2 of non-REM sleep, periodic breathing is normal and is initiated by a change in the homoeostatic set point for ventilation induced by the onset of sleep. Physiological periodic breathing is accentuated at altitude.

Pathologically, Cheyne–Stokes respiration – which is an extreme form of periodic breathing – occurs almost exclusively during non-REM sleep and typically ceases during REM sleep. Periodic breathing commonly signifies cerebral or cardiac disease, and is most common following a stroke or in cases of left ventricular failure. At least three mechanisms have been postulated. First, in patients with an increased respiratory drive due to chronic hypoxaemia, a further fall in arterial oxygen gas tension (PaO_2) at the onset of sleep may result in periodic breathing by a mechanism analogous to that occurring in healthy subjects at altitude. Second, there is an inevitable circulatory delay in $PaCO_2$ changes produced by altered ventilation and the detection of blood gas changes by the central chemoreceptors. The lung to brain circulation time may be prolonged in certain cardiac or cerebrovascular diseases. Third, the chemoceptors may be over-responsive to changes in PaO_2 due to loss of normal inhibitory influences on the metabolic control system, such as may occur in bilateral pyramidal tract destruction.

Thus, in normal subjects, voluntary hyperventilation with air will lead to a short period of apnoea followed by a few cycles of Cheyne–Stokes breathing. It is therefore possible to reduce the $PaCO_2$ to such a level that even a healthy respiratory centre fails to discharge normally; this does not occur after hyperventilation with 5 per cent CO_2. The slow decline in arterial oxygen saturation and rise in carbon dioxide during the apnoea begins to stimulate the respiratory centre, and respiration is resumed either normally or leading to a second fall in $PaCO_2$ with repetition of the cycle. The changes in the blood gases during the cycle are shown in Figure C.13.

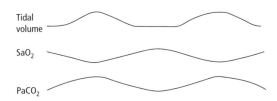

Tidal volume

SaO_2

$PaCO_2$

Figure C.13 Diagram of changes in tidal volume, arterial oxygen saturation (SaO_2) and partial pressure of carbon dioxide in arterial blood ($PaCO_2$) over two cycles of Cheyne–Stokes breathing.

Cheyne–Stokes respiration occurs in normal subjects not only after hyperventilation but also at high altitude, where the hypoxic stimulus to respiration reduces the $PaCO_2$. It may also be seen in apparently healthy elderly subjects during sleep; it is difficult however to exclude minor degrees of cardiac or cerebrovascular disease causing depression of the respiratory centre in such cases. In clinical practice the commonest cause is left ventricular failure. Periodic breathing occurs especially in patients with degenerative arterial disease in whom the blood supply to the brainstem may be reduced as a result of the low cardiac output and local arterial disease. Cheyne–Stokes respiration is commonly regarded as indicating a poor prognosis in left ventricular failure, but it may disappear with treatment for the failure and, rarely, may persist for many months in patients in whom the other symptoms and signs of failure are unimpressive.

Bronchopneumonia or other *respiratory infections* may also precipitate Cheyne–Stokes breathing in the elderly. However, it must be realized that in chronic respiratory failure in which a raised rather than a lowered $PaCO_2$ is the rule, Cheyne–Stokes respiration does not occur. Occasionally, there may be a few cycles in the recovery period following a Stokes–Adams attack. Respiration continues during the period of circulatory arrest, and the first blood which enters the cerebral circulation after cardiac action is resumed contains very little carbon dioxide. The sensitivity of the respiratory centre is reduced by hypoxia during the circulatory arrest, and this combines with the hypocapnia to cause Cheyne–Stokes breathing. Rarely, Cheyne–Stokes breathing is complicated by cardiac arrhythmias, including junctional rhythm and atrioventricular block, which occur intermittently in phase with the respiratory arrhythmia; the mechanism of this is unknown.

Primary depression of the respiratory centre in the absence of much change in the $PaCO_2$ can also cause Cheyne–Stokes respiration. Thus, it occurs in many diseases of the central nervous system. These include cerebral vascular disease with or without haemorrhage or thrombosis, cerebral tumours (especially those involving the brainstem), and severe head injuries. Cheyne–Stokes respiration is always more prominent during sleep, and can be precipitated by the administration of narcotic hypnotic drugs such as morphine, or occasionally benzodiazepines. It is also seen quite often in uraemia, but is probably not due to the renal failure *per se*. Hyperventilation in renal failure is caused by acidosis, the effect of which persists despite the fall in $PaCO_2$. Left ventricular failure resulting from renal hypertension may be responsible for Cheyne–Stokes breathing in this situation, although it may occur in patients whose blood pressure is normal.

Cheyne–Stokes respiration may be confused with other periodic breathing patterns which typically show a shorter, less symmetrical, and regular contour. In pontine brainstem lesions or if the intracranial pressure is raised abruptly, short clusters of hyperpnoeic breathing may be interrupted by abrupt spasms of apnoea (Biot's breathing). Ataxic respiration may be seen with medullary lesions which can provoke a grossly irregular breathing pattern. Respiratory apraxis is recognized by a monotonously regular pattern of breathing which cannot be modified, and is seen in the 'locked in' syndrome when subjects suffer bilateral pyramidal lesions. Central neurogenic hyperventilation is seen occasionally in midbrain lesions.

Boris Lams

CHOREA

Chorea is derived from the Greek word for 'dance', and refers to involuntary, irregular, purposeless, nonrhythmic movements of a rapid and jerky type that flow from one part of the body to another. This is in contrast to the slow writhing movements of athetosis. Choreiform movements may be either simple or elaborate, and typically flit from one region to another unpredictably. They are purposeless, but attempts may be made to incorporate them into functional movements by the patient. The movements may affect the face, causing grimacing; there may be movements of the tongue and also peculiar grunting sounds on respiration. The involuntary movements, which may affect any of the muscles of the body, are made worse by attempted voluntary movement, excitement and by the maintenance of posture. Normal volitional movements are possible but frequently are interrupted by the chorea. If the patient is asked to grip the examiner's hand, the force will be felt to vary; this physical sign is termed motor impersistence or 'milk-maid's grip'.

It is frequently difficult to dissociate chorea from the slower, writhing movements of athetosis, and the term 'choreoathetosis' is sometimes used to describe involuntary movements that have characteristics of both. It is also important to differentiate chorea from myoclonus, the main distinguishing features being that myoclonus is much more rapid, and does not flow from one muscle to another like chorea. There are many causes of chorea, some of which are listed in Table C.5. A few of the more important causes are discussed further below.

Table C.5 Selected causes of chorea

- Cerebral palsy (anoxia, kernicterus)
- Senile chorea
- Hereditary: Huntington's, neuroacanthocytosis, olivopontocerebellar atrophy, Hallevorden–Spatz disease, Friedreich's ataxia, Wilson's disease, lysosomal storage disorders, mitochondrial disorders
- Drug-induced: neuroleptics, levodopa, amphetamine, cocaine, tricyclics, oral contraceptives
- Toxins: carbon monoxide, manganese, mercury
- Metabolic: hyperthyroidism, hypoparathyroidism, pregnancy, electrolytes (hyponatraemia, hypomagnesaemia, hypocalcaemia, hypo- or hyperglycaemia)
- Nutritional (pellagra, beri-beri, vitamin B_{12} in infants)
- Infectious: Sydenham's, encephalitis lethargica, Creutzfeldt–Jakob disease
- Immunological: SLE, anticardiolipin, multiple sclerosis, Neuro-Behçet's, polyarteritis
- Vascular: subcortical infarction or haemorrhage

Sydenham's chorea is a disease that follows rheumatic fever due to group A beta-haemolytic *Streptococcus*. The mechanism has recently been postulated to involve antibodies, generated as part of the response to infection, which cross-react to basal ganglia structures. *Chorea gravidarum* occurs during pregnancy and in patients taking oral contraceptives, and may follow an earlier episode of rheumatic fever.

Huntington's chorea is an inherited autosomal dominant disorder with onset usually in middle age or later, in which patients develop dementia and involuntary movements. The latter tend to be a mixture of chorea and choreoathetotic posturing. Long-term treatment with neuroleptic drugs or levodopa can also cause chorea or choreoathetosis.

Senile chorea is sometimes used to describe the development of involuntary movements in the sixth and seventh decades of life. Patients do not show any evidence of dementing illness, and although it is possible that this represents a *forme fruste* of Huntington's chorea, it carries a more benign prognosis. Some cases previously ascribed to this category may in fact have been due to cerebral small vessel disease affecting the basal ganglia.

Congenital chorea is sometimes seen in association with congenital hemiplegia and diplegia, but is less common than congenital athetosis. Choreoathetosis in the young may be seen in a number of rare inherited degenerative metabolic disorders (see Table C.5).

Hemichorea is often due to a structural lesion (vascular damage or neoplasm). A strikingly violent movement disorder related to, but distinct from, chorea is *hemiballismus*. This is seen most often in elderly patients with diabetes and hypertension due to small vascular lesions (lacunar infarction), classically within the contralateral subthalamic nucleus. The syndrome begins abruptly, but the movements tend to decrease in magnitude and the patient may be left only with minor irregular flexion or extension movements of the wrists and fingers.

David Werring

CLONUS

Clonus refers to a series of rhythmic, monophasic (i.e. unidirectional) contractions and relaxations of a group of muscles. This is in contrast to tremors, which are always bidirectional. Myoclonus refers to shock-like contractions of a group of muscles, which are irregular in rhythm and amplitude and usually asynchronous and asymmetrical. If such contractions occur singly, or only a few times, in a restricted group of muscles, they are referred to as *segmental myoclonus* or *myoclonus simplex*; however, if they are widespread and repetitive they are termed *polymyoclonus* or *myoclonus multiplex*. If myoclonus affects the whole body at once, it can be termed 'generalized'. The classification of clonus and myoclonus is important, as each subtype has different diagnostic implications. Myoclonus is often stimulus- or activity-sensitive, in which case it can be termed 'reflex myoclonus' or 'action myoclonus', respectively. Myoclonus may be generated by disease in the cerebral cortex, brainstem, cerebellum or spinal cord. The causes of clonus and myoclonus are summarized in Table C.6.

Clonus in upper motor neurone lesions

Clonus is one of the positive (excess) motor phenomena that characterize the upper motor neurone (UMN) syndrome. The UMN syndrome results from damage

Table C.6 Causes of clonus and myoclonus

Clonus
- Upper motor neurone pathway damage (hemisphere or descending pathways), e.g. stroke, tumour or trauma
- Epilepsia partialis continua
- Palatal myoclonus

Myoclonus simplex
- Juvenile myoclonic epilepsy
- Benign Rolandic epilepsy
- West syndrome

Myoclonus multiplex
- Paramyoclonus multiplex (essential and progressive forms)
- Myoclonus with ataxia
- Opsoclonus-myoclonus
- Post-anoxic (Lance–Adams)
- Ramsay Hunt dyssynergia cerebellaris myoclonica
- Progressive myoclonic epilepsies: Unverricht–Lundborg disease, Lafora body disease, Baltic myoclonus, mitochondrial myoclonic epilepsy, neuronal ceroid lipofuscinosis (Kuf disease), Tay–Sachs disease
- Myoclonus with dementia: prion diseases (e.g. Creutzfeld–Jacob disease), subacute sclerosing panencephalitis, Alzheimer's, Lewy body dementias, Whipple's disease, corticobasal degeneration, dentatorubropallidoluysian atrophy (DRPLA), AIDS dementia
- Metabolic and toxic myoclonus: hypoxia, uraemia, Hashimoto encephalitis
- Drug-induced: lithium, haloperidol, phenothiazines, cyclosporin
- Hepatic encephalopathy (negative myoclonus of outstretched arms)
- Tetanus

Spinal myoclonus
- Myelitides: herpes zoster, demyelination (multiple sclerosis), trauma, spinal arteriovenous malformation
- Spinal interneuronitis

to descending pathways to the lower motor neurones (anterior horn cells) in the spinal cord, especially the corticospinal tract. Damage to these pathways – which can be at a spinal or cerebral level – interrupts the supraspinal control of spinal reflexes, causing the positive phenomena of clonus, spasticity, hyperreflexia and reflex spread. These features often, but not always, occur together. Clonus is a series of rhythmic involuntary muscle contractions occurring at a frequency of 5–7 Hz in response to an abruptly applied and sustained stretch stimulus; it is frequently seen at the ankle, but may also be elicited at the patella. It depends upon voluntary relaxation of the muscles, the integrity of the spinal stretch reflex mechanisms, sustained hyperexcitability of the alpha and gamma motor neurones, and synchronization of the contraction–relaxation cycle of the muscle spindles.

Several beats of clonus (less than five or six) may be elicited normally at the ankle by abrupt dorsiflexion of the foot. More numerous beats – or sustained clonus – imply an upper motor neurone lesion above the level of the first sacral segment, and will usually occur in association with an extensor plantar reflex. When the upper motor neurone lesion is above the third and fourth lumbar segments, patellar clonus may also be elicited.

Palatal myoclonus

This rhythmic form of clonus is sometimes classified as a tremor because it is continuous. There is an essential form, where there is rhythmic contraction of the tensor veli palatini muscles (up to about 7 Hz) causing a repetitive auditory click. There is no known pathological cause. The second, and more common (symptomatic), form involves the levator palatini muscles (up to about 3 Hz), with rapid elevation of the uvula and palate. There may be oscillopsia and cerebellar signs, and it persists in sleep. The condition is seen when lesions interrupt the tegmental tracts that connect the midbrain nuclei to the inferior olivary complex (Mollaret's triangle). The cause may be vascular, demyelinating, neoplastic or traumatic.

Epilepsia partialis continua

Epilepsia partialis continua (EPC) is a type of focal motor epilepsy characterized by persistent, rhythmic monophasic clonus in a group of muscles, often in the face, arm or leg. Typical muscles affected include the distal arm or leg muscles, especially the flexors of the hand or fingers; the corner of the mouth; or the eyelids. The movements may continue for weeks, months or years, are reduced but not abolished in sleep, and do not generalize. The disorder is best considered as a very focal form of status epilepticus, of cerebral origin and associated with focal electroencephalographic (EEG) abnormalities. The cause may be a range of acute or chronic cerebral lesions, commonly ischaemic stroke, or focal encephalitis (especially Rasmussen's encephalitis). Because it does not generalize, there is not the same urgency to control this seizure activity as there is in generalized status epilepticus. Indeed, EPC is often very resistant to therapy. Clobazam is a helpful treatment in some cases, but tolerance may develop.

Myoclonus simplex

This is either a single contraction or several rapid contractions of muscles in a part of or throughout the body. It may be seen in patients with idiopathic epilepsies, but there is usually no progressive mental or physical deterioration (in contrast to the progressive myoclonic epilepsies; see below). In benign epilepsy with Rolandic spikes, myoclonic jerks occur unilaterally. Myoclonus may also be seen with petit mal, and in akinetic seizures in the childhood Lennox–Gastaut syndrome, causing sudden loss of postural tone and collapse. Diffuse myoclonus is typical of juvenile myoclonic epilepsy, a common disorder in children where myoclonus is classically worse after awakening in the morning, and the EEG shows 3-Hz spike-and-wave discharges. West syndrome is a seizure disorder of infancy characterized by sudden extension or flexion of the arms and trunk ('salaam' attacks). Small-amplitude, brief myoclonic jerks may also be a feature of typical absence seizures in adolescence.

Myoclonus multiplex (diffuse myoclonus or polymyoclonus)

Paramyoclonus multiplex

This condition, first described by Friedreich in 1881 and perhaps the first use of the term myoclonus, is a sporadic form of widespread muscle jerking in adult life. The jerks may be symmetrical, may vary in site, and commonly occur when the patient is at rest in bed, though they disappear during sleep. They are usually prevented by voluntary movement, and may vary from being almost unnoticed to being severe enough to throw the patient to the floor. The condition may be familial (autosomal dominant). In the 'essential' form the myoclonus continues without other features for many years, but there sometimes there are associated neurological dysfunction and progression to severe disability. The status of paramyoclonus multiplex as a nosological entity remains insecure and its continued usefulness as a diagnostic label is not clear.

Myoclonic epilepsies

Myoclonus associated with epilepsy has many causes. The more benign forms associated with myoclonus simplex, including juvenile myoclonic epilepsy, have already been discussed. More severe forms with polymyoclonus and other neurological features with onset in childhood or adolescence are conventionally considered separately as the progressive myoclonic epilepsies (see Table C.6). The typical features are severe and progressive myoclonus, generalized tonic–clonic seizures, dementia and ataxia. In young patients with this syndrome the following conditions must be considered in the differential diagnosis. *Lafora body disease* is familial (autosomal recessive), has onset in late childhood or adolescence, and is characterized by polyglucosan-Schiff-positive inclusion bodies in the brain, liver, muscle or skin (eccrine sweat glands). *Unverricht–Lundborg disease* is also familial, and is characterized by stimulus-sensitive myoclonus, tonic–clonic seizures, EEG abnormalities (paroxysmal generalized spike and wave activity and photosensitivity), *ataxia* and mild dementia with an onset at 5 to 15 years. *Baltic myoclonus* is another familial form with loss of Purkinje cells, but no inclusion bodies. It has a relatively favourable prognosis, and often responds well to treatment with sodium valproate. Disorders of lysosomal storage can also cause progressive myoclonic epilepsy. In these conditions there is a deficiency of one or other enzymes responsible for the breakdown of intracellular lipids (sphingolipids) or other complex molecules such as mucolipids or glycoproteins. These molecules thus accumulate in neurones, causing progressive and widespread neurological dysfunction. Neuronal ceroid lipofuscinosis (*Batten disease*) presents with seizures, myoclonus, dementia and visual loss (in the childhood forms), and is characterized by curvilinear inclusion bodies (lipofuscin) in the brain, eccrine glands, muscle and gut. *Sialidosis* is a storage disorder associated with a 'cherry-red spot' on fundoscopy and dysmorphic facial features. *Tay–Sachs disease* is a disorder of sphingolipid storage with an infantile onset, marked startle response, profound motor and cognitive delay, spasticity, visual loss, a cherry-red spot, seizures and death age 3–5 years. The late childhood-onset form of *Gaucher disease* is associated with supranuclear gaze palsies, ataxia and splenomegaly; characteristic abnormal histiocytes (Gaucher cells) are seen on marrow, liver or spleen biopsy. *Myoclonic epilepsy with ragged red fibres* (MERRF) is maternally inherited (transmitted by mitochondrial DNA), and may be diagnosed by increased serum and CSF lactate and 'ragged-red' fibres on muscle biopsy. In the adult-onset patient with progressive myoclonic epilepsy, *dentatorubropallidoluysian atrophy* (DRPLA) should be considered, especially (but not exclusively) in Japanese patients. This disorder has a wide phenotype, which may include dystonia or a bradykinetic–rigid syndrome.

Myoclonus with dementia

In middle and later life, polymyoclonus with dementia must raise the suspicion of *Creutzfeldt–Jakob disease* or *Alzheimer's disease*. Much rarer causes include *Whipple's disease* of the central nervous system (which causes the rare but pathognomonic movement disorder of oculomasticatory myoarrhythmia), corticobasal degeneration (in which an asymmetric bradykinetic–rigid syndrome with alien limb are typically seen), dentatopallidoluysian atrophy and AIDS dementia. In children with prolonged polymyoclonus and encephalopathy, subacute sclerosing panencephalitis – a rare entity related to measles virus infection – should be considered.

Myoclonic ataxia

Progressive myoclonic ataxia (*Ramsay Hunt syndrome*) is a syndrome distinguished from progressive myoclonic epilepsy by the relative lack of dementia and prominent ataxia, and has a number of causes. These include mitochondrial encephalomyopathy, coeliac disease, late-onset neuronal ceroid lipofuscinosis, biotin-responsive encephalopathy, adult Gaucher disease, action myoclonus–renal failure syndrome, neurodegenerative diseases including spinocerebellar degenerations, olivopontocerebellar atrophy, and DRPLA. Hypoxic damage to the brain causes polymyoclonus in the acute phase, but as recovery occurs a striking form of intention or action myoclonus becomes apparent, which is always associated with cerebellar ataxia. This is termed post-anoxic or *Lance–Adams myoclonus*. When an attempt is made to move a limb, large-amplitude myoclonic jerks occur that are distinct from classical intention tremor. This disabling syndrome may improve with clonazepam or valproate treatment.

Opsoclonus–myoclonus is a condition that consists of dramatic, chaotic eye movements due to ocular clonus (or marked ocular dysmetria) associated with polymyoclonus and ataxia. It is a non-metastatic, immunologically mediated manifestation of cancer (i.e. a paraneoplastic syndrome). In children, it is usually associated with medulloblastoma, but in adults it is mainly associated with breast and small cell lung cancer. Rarer associations are with melanoma and lymphoma. The relevant antineuronal antibodies can be detected in specialized laboratories to confirm the diagnosis.

The causes of *metabolic and toxic myoclonus* are listed in Table C.6, and it may present at any age.

Spinal myoclonus

Myoclonus may arise from pathology in the spinal cord rather than the cortex, cerebellum or brainstem. Important causes are herpes zoster myelopathy, spinal trauma, and the myelopathy associated with spinal cord demyelination in multiple sclerosis.

David Werring

CONFUSION

Confusion is the term used to indicate that a subject is temporarily unable to think in a clear and logical fashion. The value of the term in diagnosis is, however, much diminished by imprecise definition. In a confusional state, some or all of the following features are found: an impairment of concentration and attention span with an inability to shift attention to new external stimuli; memory impairments; disorientation in time, space or person; speech which is rambling, irrelevant or incoherent; an impaired ability to properly grasp the meaning or significance of surrounding events. These features are extremely common and are found in a wide range of disorders which fall into the following main categories: *acute confusional states* or *delirium*; *chronic confusional states* (chronic organic reactions or the dementias); *the functional psychoses*; *dissociative states* and other neurotic conditions. The term should be considered as a convenient clinical description of a certain qualitative change in consciousness.

Acute confusional states

The term acute confusional state and acute brain syndrome should be considered synonymous with delirium. The speech is incoherent and rambling, indicating disordered thinking. Questions have to be repeated because the subject's attention is poor. There is altered level of consciousness; this may be reduced in approximately 30 per cent of patients, but is increased in 70 per cent. The onset is usually rapid, and the course often fluctuating. There is a disturbance of the sleep–wake cycle. Fearfulness is common, and many patients experience visual hallucinations.

The range of possible causes of delirium is large. These causes frequently lie outside the nervous system, and include infectious, metabolic and toxic states due to alcohol and drugs (pharmaceutical and recreational). A careful history, complete physical examination and laboratory investigations suggested by the features of the case will generally be sufficient to identify the cause (Table C.7).

Chronic confusional states (chronic organic reactions)

(See also MEMORY, DISORDERS OF, p. 429)
These are sometimes broadly defined as 'the dementias'. Dementia is defined as impairment in two or more areas of higher cortical function with consequent social impact. Examples include forgetting money, misplacing items and getting lost on the way home. Alzheimer's disease accounts for approximately 60 per cent of all cases of dementia; the remainder are due to multi-infarct dementia (30%) and miscellaneous causes (5–10%) (see Table C.8) (Fig. C.14).

The commonest presenting feature is impairment in short- and long-term memory, often accompanied by other features of higher cortical dysfunction such as impairment of abstract thinking and judgement. Relatives may notice a gradual personality change and a depressive, irritable, disinhibited or euphoric mood disturbance. The memory loss initially may be mild and most marked for recent events. The person forgets names, loses objects round the house, or experiences distressing confusion in unfamiliar surroundings due to loss of spatial memory. As the condition progresses new information is not retained, and the person may become forgetful enough to become a danger to themselves by leaving tasks undone and taps and switches left on. Impairment in abstract thinking is suggested when the patient cannot cope with new tasks, thinking becomes more literal and concrete and the repertoire of conversation is narrowed. There may be impaired judgement, the person becoming disinhibited with inappropriate behaviour in social situations. Marked disinhibition can be a feature of

Table C.7 Causes of acute states of confusion (delirium)

Common	
Hypoxia (due to cardiac and respiratory disorders)	*Thiamine deficiency (Wernicke's encephalopathy)*
Metabolic disorders	*Vitamin B$_{12}$ deficiency*
▪ Electrolyte imbalances	*Substance intoxication and*
▪ Hypoglycaemia	*withdrawal*
▪ Uraemia	▪ Alcohol (delirium tremens)
▪ Hepatic failure	▪ Barbiturates
Systemic infections	▪ Heroin
▪ Septicaemia	▪ Opiates
▪ Bronchopneumonia	▪ Stimulants (amphetamine,
▪ Urinary tract infections	cocaine)
▪ Malaria	▪ Digoxin
Cerebral infections	▪ Lithium
▪ Meningitis	▪ Steroids
▪ Encephalitis	▪ L-dopa
▪ Brain abscess	*Post-ictal state*
Non-infective cerebral causes	
▪ Head injury	**Less common**
▪ Raised intracranial pressure	Focal lesions of right parietal lobe
▪ Hypertensive encephalopathy	Porphyria
▪ Tumours	Hyperparathyroidism
▪ Cerebral haemorrhage	Hypoparathyroidism
▪ Cerebral embolism	Hypopituitarism
Endocrine disorders	Cushing's disease
▪ Diabetic keto-acidosis	
▪ Myxoedema	

frontal lobe impairment. Other neurological deficits including aphasias and apraxias are common, as are changes in mood, usually to depression and irritability.

Alzheimer's-type dementia is diagnosed by the clinical findings and the exclusion of other causes of a progressive dementia. In multi-infarct dementia there may be hypertension and a stepwise progression of impairment with a history of transient ischaemic episodes. Computed tomography (CT) scanning may show old infarcts, whereas in Alzheimer's dementia the CT scan may be either normal or show selective cerebral atrophy of the temporal lobes and ventricular enlargement.

Metabolic disorders giving rise to chronic confusional states include vitamin B$_{12}$, folate and thiamine deficiencies. The latter (Wernicke–Korsakoff syndrome) is commonly associated with chronic alcoholism, but may be due to gastric carcinoma or malabsorption. Cerebral anoxia due to anaemia, respiratory or cardiovascular disease also causes symptoms of confusion, although these latter causes are more likely to present with acute confusion.

Table C.8 Causes of chronic states of confusion

Common

Vascular brain disease
■ Subarachnoid haemorrhage
■ Subdural haematoma
■ Infarct (multi-infarct dementia)
Head injury
Intercranial space-occupying lesion
Brain degenerative diseases
■ Alzheimer's type dementia
■ Huntington's disease
Infections
■ Viral encephalitis (including HIV encephalopathy)
Systemic
■ Myxoedema
■ Anoxia (anaemia, cardiac and respiratory failure)
■ Vitamin deficiency (B_{12}, folate, thiamine)

Less common

Parkinson's disease
Multiple sclerosis
Pick's disease
Normotensive hydrocephalus
Depressive pseudodementia

Uncommon

Binswanger's leucoencephalopathy
Tertiary syphilis

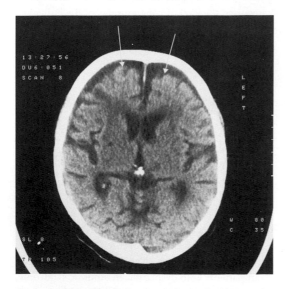

Figure C.14 Computed tomogram of the head, demonstrating bilateral chronic subdural haematoma (arrows).

Brain degenerative conditions giving rise to dementia include Huntington's chorea, which is an autosomal dominant condition usually presenting in the age range of 35–45 years, with involuntary movements and cognitive changes. A proportion of patients with *multiple sclerosis* develop a steadily progressive illness with severe impairment of higher cortical function. There are usually other signs and symptoms disseminated in time and place. In *normal-pressure hydrocephalus* a dementia is typically accompanied by apraxic gait and urinary incontinence which occurs early in the dementing illness, in contrast to Alzheimer's disease, when it is late. *Pick's disease,* which is the most common of a family of frontotemporal dementing syndromes, is a rare condition that develops usually in older patients, typically with a marked personality change consistent with frontal lobe impairment and a speech disorder which progresses to mutism. This is due to selective loss of nerve tracts to the frontal cortex. Recent advances have identified gene defects leading to frontotemporal dementia in certain families. Signs of cognitive impairment are found in *Parkinson's disease,* especially in older patients who have had the condition for a long time. *Binswanger's leucoencephalopathy* is a very rare progressive degenerative disease with signs on CT scan of focal areothosis.

Central nervous system infections which give rise to features of dementia include viral encephalitis. The human immunodeficiency virus is neurotropic as well as lymphotropic, and people with AIDS may develop a confusional state with fever leading to a state of lethargy, apathy and ataxia due to a subacute encephalopathy. *Tertiary syphilis is* now rare in the West, but is still an important, treatable, cause of dementia worldwide. *Creutzfeldt–Jakob spongiform encephalopathy* caused by a prion protein is also quite rare, and has features including limb weakness with spasticity, myoclonus cerebellar degeneration and other movement disturbances. EEG changes are common. Variant Creutzfeldt–Jakob disease is also very rare, being due to the ingestion of prion protein particles in the diet or through surgery. There have been cases reported worldwide.

Psychiatric illness can present as confusion. *Schizophrenia,* which may remain undiagnosed until relatively late in life, can present with a degree of intellectual deterioration, impaired volition, disordered thinking and confused speech. A detailed history may reveal a family history or earlier episodes of psychotic illness, but memory loss is not a feature. *Pseudodementia* is a condition of patients with major depressive illness which presents a dementing-like picture of poor memory, impoverished thinking and reduced intellectual abilities, and may mimic an organic dementia. This condition is diagnosed by careful history-taking from the patient and relatives, and it should be borne in mind that in every case of 'dementia' the depression can be cured by treatment. Very rarely, a *factitious disorder* may mimic acute or chronic confusional states, but careful assessment will usually reveal inconsistencies in the patient's account of symptoms and their performance in tests of higher cerebral function. Epileptic *twilight states* and automatisms are characterized by an abrupt onset and ending, a duration of hours or rarely days, and the occurrence of apparently purposeless acts. The subject has impaired consciousness. A history of seizures and EEG evidence of epileptic activity should be sought, and would be essential evidence for a patient facing prosecution for offences claimed to have been perpetrated during a state of epileptic automatism.

Mark Kinirons

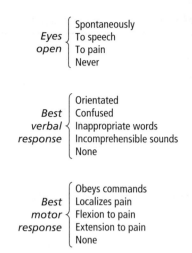

Figure C.15 The Glasgow Coma Scale.

CONSCIOUSNESS, DISORDERS OF

Consciousness is the state of awareness of the self and the environment when provided with adequate stimuli. Patients who are in normal wakefulness will be fully responsive to stimuli, and will display correct behaviour and speech in response to these stimuli. Physiological changes in consciousness occur during sleep when the patient may be easily aroused by external stimuli. Pathological impairment of consciousness occurs in states of injury, disease or intoxication.

The *Glasgow Coma Scale* provides a useful measure to assess the level of consciousness (Fig. C.15). It is based on the observation of levels of response to graded stimuli in three modes: eye opening; motor function; and verbal utterance. In the first mode, spontaneous eye opening and blinking score the highest grade, eye opening in response to voice the next highest, eye opening in response to painful stimuli the next, and finally no response of eye opening to stimuli the lowest. The highest motor response is voluntary movement to command, followed by localizing response to painful stimuli, withdrawal from painful stimuli, a pathological flexor response (sometimes called decorticate), a pathological extensor response (sometimes called decerebrate), and finally no response at all to pain. In terms of verbal response, the highest level is orientated conversation, the next disorientated conversation, followed by the use of occasional recognizable words, no recognizable words but groaning in response to pain, and finally no response of a verbal nature. By allocating a point in each of these categories, the level of consciousness of the individual patient may be recorded and monitored in order to measure progress. The maximum score is 14.

Several terms are used to define altered states of consciousness, as follows.

Confusion (see also CONFUSION, p. 113)

Confusion, or clouding of consciousness, is characterized by an impaired capacity to think clearly and to perceive, respond to and remember current stimuli. There is usually disorientation. There may be a gradation between an initial clouding of consciousness and a more profound confusional state in which the main elements are reduced attention, an inability to express thoughts clearly, together with a defect in memory and drowsiness. The differential diagnosis is from patients with dysphasia, an amnesic syndrome, an acute psychosis or severe retarded depression. Patients with confusion frequently have a generalized disturbance of cerebral function which may be associated with widespread EEG changes. A reduction in cerebral oxygen consumption has been demonstrated in such patients. Confusion is most commonly the result of toxic or metabolic abnormalities, and it occurs particularly in the elderly.

Delirium

This is a state of severely disturbed consciousness with motor restlessness, disorientation and delusions. Patients are out of touch with reality, frightened, irritable, and frequently have visual hallucinations. Delirium is associated with a diffusely abnormal EEG, and is commonly seen with toxic and metabolic disorders. Delirium may be mimicked by degenerative brain disease, acute psychosis or hypomania, but patients with these conditions do not usually show the depressed alertness which is a cardinal feature of delirium. Both confusion and delirium are more common in the elderly. They are more likely to occur when there is underlying degenerative disease, and may be the precursor of coma.

Stupor

The patient, though not unconscious and still rousable, exhibits little or no spontaneous activity. The patient may seem to be asleep but will not respond to vigorous stimulation and will show relatively limited motor abilities, tending to lapse back into sleep when the stimulus ceases. The differential diagnosis is from catatonic schizophrenia and severe depression; the finding of catatonia, posturing of the limbs or flexibilitas cerea is more common with psychiatric disturbances. In organic stupor the EEG is invariably diffusely abnormal, whereas in psychiatric disease it will usually be normal. The exception to this is Gjessing's syndrome, in which periodic stupor may occur with minor EEG abnormalities.

Coma

This is a condition of absolute unconsciousness judged by the absence of any psychologically understandable response to external stimulus or internal need. It may more simply be defined as a state of 'unrousable unconsciousness'. The patient will appear to be asleep, but is incapable of sensing or responding normally to external stimuli. The condition may vary in depth from the deepest levels in which there will be no eye opening, motor or verbal response, to a level in which there may be eye opening to pain, a weak flexor response of the limbs to pain and groaning, without recognizable words, in response to pain.

States of altered consciousness will be seen in patients who have suffered from *head injury, intoxication* with drugs or alcohol, *metabolic* disturbances, *infections* or *vascular* disturbances, and as the result of *hypoxic* or *ischaemic injuries.*

Rarely, patients without evident organic illness may appear to have disturbances of consciousness, or pseudocoma. The distinction between pseudocoma and organic disease may be established by testing the oculo-vestibular reflex in response to the instillation of ice water into the external auditory meatus. In patients in organic coma, the normal reaction of nystagmus will not been seen, but in patients with pseudocoma nystagmus will occur and the patients will usually reveal their responsiveness.

Mark Kinirons

CONSTIPATION

Acute constipation

Acute constipation may be:

- due to acute intestinal obstruction;
- a symptom of some general disease or of some other acute abdominal disease; or
- due to a sudden alteration in daily habits, e.g. admission to hospital.

Acute intestinal obstruction

The following points help in the distinction between acute intestinal obstruction and severe cases of acute constipation of other origin:

- In other conditions the constipation is incomplete, in that flatus – and even a small quantity of faeces – may be passed spontaneously. A rectal examination should always be made. In organic intestinal obstruction the rectum is usually empty. If it contains faeces these may be present below an obstruction or, if impacted, may themselves be responsible for the occlusion, but it is exceedingly rare for faecal impaction to produce symptoms quite comparable in severity with those due to acute obstruction. In doubtful cases, it used to be the custom to carry out the two-enema test; the first enema generally brought away a certain amount of faeces, even if obstruction was complete; the second enema, given at an interval of 30 minutes to 1 hour, resulted in the passage of faeces or flatus if obstruction was incomplete, whereas in complete obstruction the second enema was either retained or expelled unaltered. This test should never be employed; it is exhausting to the patient, time wasting, and the information obtained is often equivocal. Diagnosis can usually be made on clinical grounds supplemented by abdominal radiographs.

■ Vomiting is rarely a feature of constipation, whereas it is frequently present in small-bowel obstruction, and in late cases becomes faeculent.

■ Visible peristalsis, accompanied by noisy borborygmi, is never present except in obstruction.

■ Obstruction is accompanied by progressive distension of the abdomen.

■ Pain is usually the first symptom of intestinal obstruction and is colicky in nature; its severity is out of all proportion to the mild abdominal discomfort that may accompany simple constipation.

Plain radiographs of the abdomen are essential in the diagnosis of intestinal obstruction and in attempting to localize its site. A loop or loops of distended bowel are usually seen, together with multiple fluid levels. Small bowel is suggested by a ladder pattern of distended loops, by their central position, and by striations which pass completely across the width of the distended loop and which are produced by its circular mucosal folds (Fig. C.16). Distended large bowel tends to lie peripherally and to show the corrugations produced by the taenia coli (Fig. C.17). A small percentage – perhaps 5 per cent of intestinal obstructions – shows no abnormality on plain radiographs. This is due to the small bowel being completely distended with fluid in a closed loop and thus without the fluid levels which are produced by coexistent gas.

Aetiology of acute intestinal obstruction

The causes of intestinal obstruction may be classified as:

■ In the lumen:
  ◆ faecal impaction;
  ◆ food bolus;
  ◆ gallstone ileus;
  ◆ meconium ileus in the neonate.

■ In the wall:
  ◆ Congenital atresia of the small intestine
  ◆ Crohn's disease
  ◆ tuberculous stricture
  ◆ diverticular disease of the colon
  ◆ tumours – especially carcinoma of the colon.
■ Outside the wall:
  ◆ adhesions and bands (post abdominal surgery or intra-abdominal sepsis)
  ◆ strangulated hernia (external or internal)
  ◆ intussusception
  ◆ volvulus (of small bowel, caecal or sigmoid colon).

Before considering any other possibility, all the hernial apertures should be examined, even in the absence of local pain, as a small strangulated femoral hernia in an obese woman, for example, may easily be overlooked.

The following points should be considered in determining the cause of the acute intestinal obstruction:

Age Intestinal obstruction in the newborn should always be suspected in the presence of bile-vomiting: the rectum should be examined first for the presence of an imperforate anus. Other possibilities are congenital atresia or stenosis of the intestine, volvulus neonatorum, meconium ileus and Hirschsprung's disease. In infants, the commonest cause of intestinal obstruction is intussusception, but Hirschsprung's disease, strangulated inguinal hernia and obstruction due to a band from the tip of a Meckel's diverticulum should also be considered. In young adults and patients of middle age, adhesions and bands from previous surgery or intraperitoneal inflammation are common, but strangulated hernia and Crohn's disease are also encountered. In older patients, strangulated hernias, carcinoma of the bowel and diverticular disease, as well as postoperative adhesions, are all common conditions.

History The history of a previous abdominal operation, or of inflammatory pelvic disease in females, strongly suggests the possibility of bands or adhesions. A history of biliary colic or of the symptoms, which may result in cholecystitis, may suggest that obstruction might be due to impaction of a gallstone in the ileum. Obstruction following a period of increasing constipation, perhaps with blood or slime in the stools or spurious diarrhoea, in a middle-aged or elderly

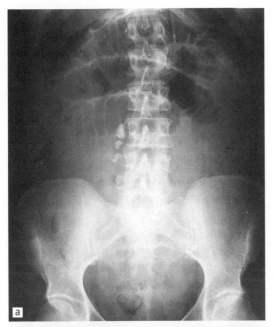

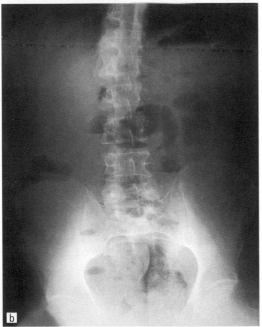

Figure C.16 Small-bowel obstruction. (a) Plain X-ray of the abdomen, supine film. (b) Plain X-ray of the abdomen, erect film. Note the fluid levels.

patient, suggests cancer or diverticular disease of the colon. The history in an infant or child that blood or mucus have been passed per rectum is suggestive of an intussusception.

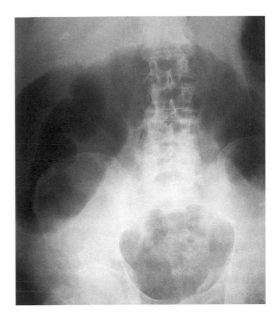

Figure C.17 Large-bowel obstruction due to carcinoma of the sigmoid colon; supine plain X-ray.

Abdominal examination The importance of searching specifically for a strangulated hernia has already been mentioned. The presence of a recent or old laparotomy immediately suggests the diagnosis of postoperative adhesions. Gross distension generally means that the obstruction is in the colon; if occurring very soon after the onset of symptoms, it suggests volvulus of the sigmoid or, less commonly, the caecum. If distension has been present to a less extent for some time before the onset of acute symptoms, a growth is likely. In infants and small children great distension suggests Hirschsprung's disease. Slight distension occurs when the obstruction is in the duodenum or high in the jejunum.

The diagnosis of intussusception can be made with certainty only when the characteristic sausage-shaped tumour situated somewhere in the course of the colon is felt. In acute obstruction due to cancer, the tumour is often not palpable as it may be disguised by the dilated intestine; however, large masses are sometimes felt, especially when present in the right or left iliac fossa. On the right side, they are generally due to cancer of the caecum, on the left to cancer of the sigmoid colon or diverticular disease.

Rectal examination A growth of the rectum should be recognized easily, although this is rather unusual as a cause of obstruction. Sometimes, a growth of the pelvic colon can be felt through the front wall of the rectum. In infants, the tip of an intussusception may be felt in the lumen of the rectum, and the typical red-currant jelly stool (a mixture of blood and mucus) will be seen on the examining finger. Occasionally, the mother will report that a sausage-like structure actually prolapses from the child's anal verge during the attacks of colic accompanying the intussusception. The present author has only seen this on one occasion. A much-ballooned rectum suggests obstruction in the colon; this is an undoubted fact, but its cause is obscure.

Vomiting The more frequent the vomiting and the earlier the onset of faeculent vomiting, the higher in the intestine is the obstruction likely to be. Its onset is later and its occurrence less frequent in cases of colonic obstruction.

Symptomatic

In acute general diseases

Constipation beginning acutely is a frequent symptom of a large variety of acute infective and other diseases. It is never so severe as to become a presenting symptom, and the other features in the majority of cases are so much more striking that the presence of constipation has little influence on making a diagnosis.

In acute abdominal conditions

Constipation is a conspicuous symptom in most acute abdominal conditions. However, once again, other symptoms are often so well marked that the question of intestinal obstruction hardly arises. Thus, it frequently accompanies acute appendicitis, salpingitis, perforation of a peptic ulcer, and biliary and renal colic. In lead colic, the constipation is not absolute and the occupation of the patient, the blue line on the gums and the presence of punctate basophilia point to the diagnosis.

Changes in daily routine

These may precipitate constipation, as in patients admitted to hospital, children going to boarding school, or patients suddenly being confined to bed from illness.

Chronic constipation

Constipation can be defined as delay in the passage of faeces through the large bowel, and is frequently associated with difficulty in defecation. Most people empty the bowel once in every 24 hours, but there is a considerable range of variation in perfectly normal individuals. In one study of a large working population this varied from three bowel actions daily to one act every three days.

The abnormal action of the bowel in constipation may manifest itself in three different ways:

1 Defecation may occur with insufficient frequency.

2 The stools may be insufficient in quantity and a certain amount of faeces is retained, although the bowels may be opened once daily or more often (cumulative constipation).

3 The bowels may be open daily, yet the faeces are hard and dry owing to prolonged retention in the bowel, dehydration, or insufficient residue in the food consumed.

The commoner causes of chronic constipation are as follows:

1 Organic obstructions, for example carcinoma of the colon or diverticular disease.

2 Painful anal conditions, e.g. fissure *in ano* or prolapsed piles.

3 Adynamic bowel, as may occur in Hirschsprung's disease, senility, spinal cord injuries and diseases, Parkinson's disease and myxoedema.

4 Drugs which decrease the peristaltic activity of the bowel – including codeine, probanthine and other ganglion-blocking agents, and morphine.

5 Habit and diet, for example dehydration, starvation, lack of suitable bulk in the diet, and dyschezia.

It is comparatively rare for a patient to consult a doctor on account of constipation without having already attempted to cure themselves with aperients. The symptoms generally ascribed to 'auto-intoxication' caused by intestinal stasis are usually really caused by the purgatives themselves, which may produce depletion of sodium and potassium in the resultant watery stools, or from the abdominal colic and flatulence produced by powerful aperients.

In spite of probable protests, the patient is instructed to see what happens if no drugs are taken for a few days, an attempt being made to open the bowels each morning on a normal diet containing plenty of fruit and vegetables. In most cases, he/she loses the abdominal pains and so-called 'toxic' symptoms. During this test, the bowels are often opened daily, in which case a diagnosis of functional pseudoconstipation can be made, the patient having come to believe, as a result of faulty education combined with advice of friends and with the reading of pernicious advertisements, that he or she was constipated and required aperients to keep well. Frequently, a little psychotherapy in the form of an explanation of the physiology of the bowels and the origin of the symptoms, and persuading the patient to try to open the bowels each morning without artificial help, results in a cure.

The investigation of constipation entails a careful and accurate history and full examination, including an examination of the rectum and sigmoidoscopy, followed, in some cases, by special laboratory tests, a barium-enema X-ray examination and colonoscopy.

Organic obstructions

The two common causes of narrowing of the lumen of the large bowel are diverticular disease and carcinoma of the colon. Other non-malignant strictures are rare, but they include Crohn's disease of the large bowel, stricture complicating ulcerative colitis and tuberculous stricture.

Organic stricture of the colon is most commonly due to carcinoma. The possibility of cancer should always be considered when an individual above the age of 40, whose bowels have been regular previously, without change of diet or habit develops constipation of increasing severity, or when a patient who is habitually constipated becomes more so without obvious reason. The constipation is at first intermittent, and may alternate with diarrhoea, or rather with a frequent desire to go to stool without effective evacuation. Aperients become steadily less helpful. There may be colicky pain and episodes of distension and the patient may notice blood, pus and mucus in the faeces. An examination of the abdomen may reveal a palpable mass due to the presence of the tumour itself, or to inspissated faeces which have become impacted above a cancerous stricture which is itself impalpable. Progressive loss of weight and strength, anorexia and anaemia are rather late features of the disease. A rectal examination reveals usually an empty rectum, but not infrequently a carcinoma in the sigmoid colon can be felt through the rectal wall as the mass in this loop of bowel prolapses into the pelvis.

An occult blood test on any faecal material is often positive. Sigmoidoscopy or colonoscopy may visualize the tumour and biopsy and histological examination can confirm its nature. A barium enema examination is invaluable (Fig. C.18).

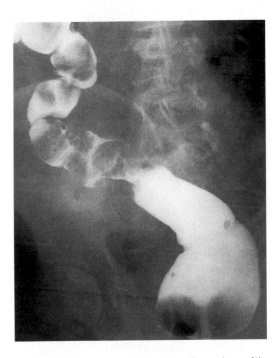

Figure C.18 Barium enema showing an obstructing carcinoma of the sigmoid colon.

Diverticular disease of the sigmoid colon can mimic carcinoma exactly, and indeed the surgeon – even at laparotomy – may not be able to differentiate between the two conditions. The barium enema examination (Fig. C.19) is often helpful, but the radiologist may have difficulty in distinguishing a stricture due to one or other cause; indeed, not infrequently these two common diseases may co-exist. Again, colonoscopy will often be useful in making the differential diagnosis.

Occasionally, extracolonic masses may press upon the rectum or sigmoid colon with resultant constipation; for example, the pregnant uterus, a mass of fibroids, a large ovarian cyst or other pelvic tumours.

Painful anal conditions

When defecation is painful, reflex spasm of the anal sphincter may be produced with resultant constipation.

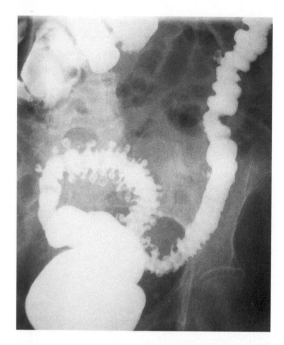

Figure C.19 Barium enema showing extensive diverticulosis of the sigmoid colon.

A local cause of the pain such as a fissure-in-ano, strangulated haemorrhoids or a perianal abscess is obvious on careful local examination of the anal verge and surrounds.

Adynamic bowel

In Hirschsprung's disease (aganglionic congenital megacolon) there is always a history of constipation dating from the first few months of life. The abdomen becomes greatly enlarged soon after birth, and the outline of distended colon can be seen, often with visible peristalsis. The abdomen finally becomes enormous and it is then tense and tympanitic. There may be eversion of the umbilicus and marked widening of the subcostal angle.

A rectal examination reveals a narrow empty rectum above which faecal impaction may be felt; this examination is usually followed by a gush of flatus and faeces.

The condition is due to the absence of ganglion cells in the wall of the rectosigmoid region of the large bowel, although in some cases a more extensive part of the colon may be involved. Some 80 per cent of the patients are males.

A barium enema examination reveals gross dilatation of the colon leading down to a narrow funnel in the aganglionic rectum (Fig. C.20). Rectal wall biopsy shows complete absence of ganglion cells.

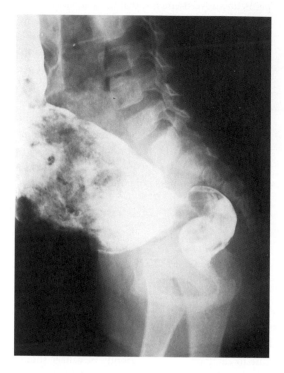

Figure C.20 Barium enema in a child with Hirschsprung's disease.

The differential diagnosis is *acquired megacolon*, a condition of severe chronic constipation, commencing usually at the age of 1 or 2 years, often in a mentally retarded child. Rectal examination in such cases is typical, impacted faeces being present right up to the anal verge. If necessary, a rectal biopsy may be indicated and will show the presence of normal ganglion cells.

Deficient motor activity of the bowel may be due to senile changes in the elderly, and may be a prominent feature of myxoedemic patients. Constipation may occur in the course of organic nervous diseases, including Parkinson's disease, tabes dorsalis, spinal compression from tumour, transverse myelitis and disseminated sclerosis, as well as cord transection in trauma. This is due to disturbance of the motor and sensory pathways responsible for defecation.

Drugs

Many commonly employed drugs have a constipating effect on the bowel; these include codeine, morphine and the ganglion-blocking agents. Constipation accompanied by abdominal pain may be a feature of lead poisoning.

Habit and diet

By far the greatest number of patients complaining of constipation falls into this group. When the faeces are abnormally hard as a result of dehydration, inadequate liquid intake or inadequate cellulosic material in the diet, rectal examination will reveal impacted faeces of rock-like consistency. This may occur as an acute phenomenon following a barium meal examination, when masses of inspissated barium may lodge in the rectum.

Dyschezia

Dyschezia is the term applied to difficulty in defecation due to faulty bowel habit. The patient ignores the normal call to stool, the rectum distends with faeces with eventual loss of the defecation reflex. The very same patient who gets into this habit is probably one who lives on the modern synthetic diet which is grossly deficient in roughage. As mentioned above, the so-called symptoms of constipation usually result from the purgatives that the patient ingests after becoming anxious about the scarcity of bowel actions. A rectal examination in such individuals often reveals large amounts of faeces in the rectum, and more scybala may be palpated in the sigmoid colon. Dyschezia is, of course, present in those patients who have to remove faeces from the rectum digitally.

Harold Ellis

CORNEAL DISEASE

The main symptoms of corneal disease are pain, reduced vision, photophobia, lacrimation and haloes seen around light sources. The cornea – the principal refracting surface of the eye – has a rich sensory nerve supply from the ophthalmic division of the trigeminal nerve, stimulation of which can result in severe pain with secondary excess lacrimation. Reduced vision is due to loss of corneal transparency which may be secondary to corneal oedema, cellular infiltration, or scarring. Haloes are due to epithelial oedema producing diffraction of light.

The cornea is examined by ophthalmologists using the slit-lamp (biomicroscope), but may be examined with the naked eye by the non-ophthalmologist, using focal illumination and magnification (pentorch and magnifier). Corneal epithelial defects (such as ulcers or abrasions) can be most easily detected by instilling sodium fluorescein, which will stain any epithelial defects. Corneal disease can conveniently be classified into ulcers which may be infective or immune, nutritional and metabolic disorders and corneal degenerations.

Corneal degeneration

The most common degenerative condition of the cornea is arcus senilis, a concentric grey opaque crescent of lipid deposition in the peripheral cornea which, with time, completely encircles the cornea. The ring is about 1–1.5 mm wide, and follows the contour of the limbus but is separated from it by a clear zone. The outer edge of the ring is a sharp line, but the inner edge shades off gradually. Arcus senilis has no clinical significance except, perhaps, in younger patients in whom it may be associated with serum lipid abnormalities. *Band keratopathy* (Fig. C.21) is the name given to characteristic hyaline degenerative changes with calcareous deposits which appear across the interpalpebral area of the cornea in certain eyes. It is rarely found in otherwise healthy

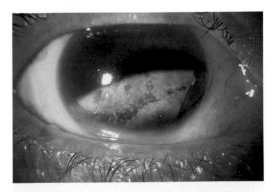

Figure C.21 Band-shaped degeneration of the cornea. [Moorfields Eye Hospital.]

eyes, but occurs frequently in blind, shrunken eyes and following prolonged uveitis. *Keratoconus* (Fig. C.22) or conical cornea is due to an abnormal thinning of the central cornea, and results in a cone-shaped cornea. This condition usually commences around puberty and progresses slowly, although sometimes it develops an acute progressive phase causing sudden visual deterioration and eye discomfort.

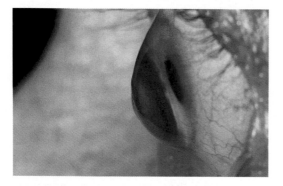

Figure C.22 Keratoconus. [Moorfields Eye Hospital.]

Corneal ulcer

The cornea can be infected by viruses, bacteria or fungi. The herpes simplex virus is a common pathogen, producing the typical dendritic ulcer (Fig. C.23). Early lesions comprise opaque epithelial cells which later desquamate to form the branching pattern of the dendritic ulcer that can be demonstrated by fluorescein staining. It is a very painful condition, with much lacrimation and photophobia, and in the absence of proper treatment tends to last for weeks or even months. It can produce dense stromal scarring which, if centrally situated, leads to visual impairment. The virus can remain dormant but may easily be reactivated in the future by a variety of trigger factors such as poor general health or exposure to excessive sunlight or topical steroids. Hence, herpes simplex keratitis is frequently a recurrent condition.

The herpes zoster virus, when involving the ophthalmic nerve, can also produce corneal lesions in the form of microdendritic ulcers and corneal opacities. Both herpes simplex and herpes zoster infection can reduce corneal sensation permanently. Corneal sensation can be assessed by touching the cornea with a wisp of cotton-wool and comparing the blink reflex of the two eyes. Damage to the corneal sensory nerves can result in ulceration of neurotrophic keratitis. The corneal epithelium requires an intact sensory nerve supply to permit normal healing, and neurotrophic ulcers show little tendency to heal, often requiring a tarsorrhaphy.

Bacterial ulcers or abscesses often follow minor trauma to the cornea. The most common pathogens are *Streptococcus pneumoniae* and *Staphylococcus aureus*, but β-haemolytic *Streptococcus*, *Pseudomonas*, *Proteus*, *Klebsiella*, *Escherichia coli* and *Neisseria* can also be causative. Clinically, the ulcer appears as a yellowish irregular opacity associated with corneal stromal necrosis. It is usually associated with reactive iritis with outpouring of white blood cells into the anterior chamber; these cells settle inferiorly to form a pus level or hypopyon (Fig. C.24). The causative organism is identified and the appropriate antibiotics given. The ulcer may heal without perforating, but if the resulting scar is both large and centrally placed, ultimately the vision is often much impaired. If perforation does occur, the underlying iris may adhere to the site of

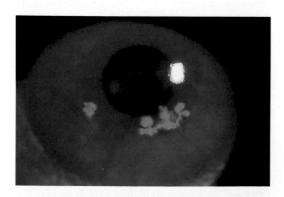

Figure C.23 Herpes simplex dendritic ulcer. [Moorfields Eye Hospital.]

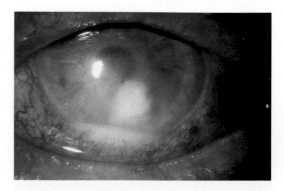

Figure C.24 Hypopyon ulcer. [Moorfields Eye Hospital.]

perforation with subsequent dense corneal scar formation, which may then distend to form a bulging anterior staphyloma.

Marginal ulcers situated around the periphery of the cornea, with a clear zone between the ulcer and the limbus, tend to remain superficial. They most commonly follow *Staphylococcus aureus* conjunctivitis or blepharitis, and are produced as an immunological reaction against staphylococcal exotoxins.

Interstitial keratitis is a late manifestation of congenital syphilis that produces stromal corneal opacities with the associated stigmata.

Keratomalacia due to vitamin A deficiency is characterized by desiccation and subsequent necrosis of the cornea and conjunctiva. It affects undernourished infants, and is extremely rare in the UK. Urgent administration of vitamin A is required, together with attention to the corneal hydration.

Reginald Daniel

COUGH

Healthy persons seldom cough; their scant bronchial secretions result in a thin sheet of mucus which is constantly carried up the tracheobronchial tree towards the larynx by the action of cilia. On reaching the pharynx, the secretions raised in this way are disposed of into the alimentary tract by unconscious acts of swallowing.

Coughing is an essential defence mechanism that protects the airways from the adverse effects of inhaled noxious substances, and also serves to clear them of retained secretions. Patients recognize that coughing indicates an abnormality, and this symptom is one of the most frequent reasons given for seeking medical advice.

Coughing may be produced voluntarily, but more often it results from reflex stimulation. To a lesser extent it can be suppressed voluntarily. The involuntary initiation of a cough takes place in a reflex arc. Extrathoracic cough receptors are present in the nose, oropharynx, larynx and upper trachea. Intrathoracic irritant receptors are located in the epithelium of the lower trachea and large central bronchi, which are the air passages from which coughing effectively expels retained secretions or foreign material. Efferent pathways include the recurrent laryngeal nerves to cause

closure of the glottis, and the corticospinal tract and peripheral nerves to cause contraction of the thoracic and abdominal musculature. The cough receptors may accommodate to repeated stimuli – as they often do in cigarette smokers who may only cough after the first cigarette of the day. The cough reflex becomes less sensitive in the elderly, and is lost in anaesthesia and unconsciousness, leading to an increased danger of aspiration pneumonia.

The act of coughing occurs in three phases. The first phase is a preliminary deep inspiration, and the second is closure of the glottis, relaxation of the diaphragm and contraction of the thoracic and abdominal expiratory muscles generating a positive pressure of 100–300 mmHg within the thorax. Because the positive pressure in the pleural space is higher than the luminal pressure in the trachea and central bronchi, a pressure difference is created that causes the posterior membranous portion of the airway walls to fold inwards and partially obliterate the lumen. When the third phase occurs – namely sudden relaxation of the glottis – the linear velocity of airflow through the narrow channels is markedly increased, thus creating forces that dislodge secretions and particles from the mucosal surface. During cough, the volume rate of flow out of the lungs (litres/s) is very similar to that obtained during a forced expiratory manoeuvre – a fact that is not always appreciated. In patients with severe airflow obstruction, high rates of flow cannot be generated because the airways are already narrowed; such patients may have prolonged wheezy coughs which sometimes cause the involuntary effects of a Valsalva manoeuvre and resultant cough syncope which occasionally is accompanied by convulsions mimicking epilepsy.

In general, the diagnosis of the cause of cough depends not only on an analysis of the cough itself but also on the other symptoms and physical signs and, above all, the chest radiograph. When the chest radiograph shows a significant abnormality such as lobar collapse (Figs C.25–C.27), carcinoma (Fig. C.28), bronchopneumonia (Fig. C.29) or pulmonary tuberculosis (Figs C.30 and C.31), the reason for the cough is established and the next step is to initiate appropriate treatment. Diagnostic problems arise in those patients in whom the chest radiograph appears normal. The disorders that need to be considered are listed in Table C.9 on page 128. Some helpful diagnostic clinical clues and signs and further investigations are listed in the same

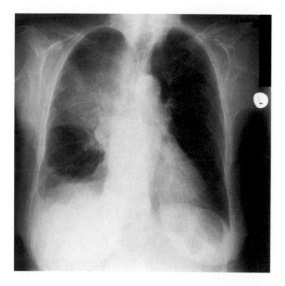

Figure C.25 Collapse of the right upper lobe due to lung carcinoma.

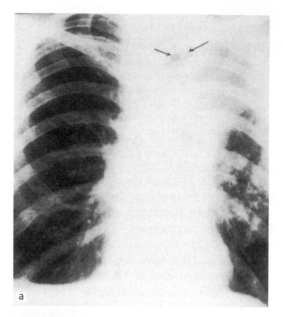

a

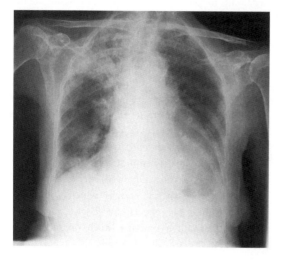

Figure C.26 Right upper lobe pneumonia.

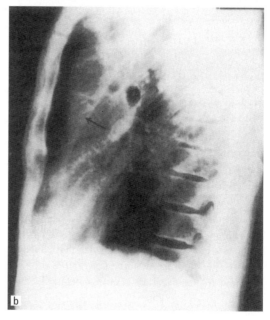

b

Figure C.27 (a,b) Left upper lobe collapse in a man with cancer metastases to the liver and suprarenal glands.

table. Enquiry about the presence or absence of sputum, whether the cough is occasional or persistent, provoked by any activity or situation, and especially where there is disturbed sleep, will provide helpful pointers to diagnosis. When the causes of the chronic cough are analysed, asthma frequently heads the list, and indeed chronic non-productive cough – especially at night – may be the sole presenting complaint of patients subsequently proven to have bronchial asthma.

Dry cough is also a feature of lung fibrosis from any cause. Typically, the chest radiograph will be

abnormal but, if equivocal, thoracic high-resolution CT scanning is helpful in confirming or refuting the presence of structural lung disease. An intractable dry cough is now recognized as an important side effect of angiotension-converting enzyme inhibitors.

In *pertussis*, the characteristic cough is paroxysmal and occurs in bouts which may last for a minute or two

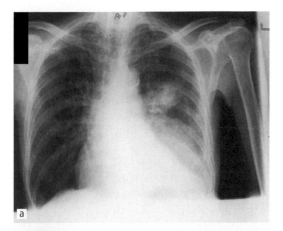

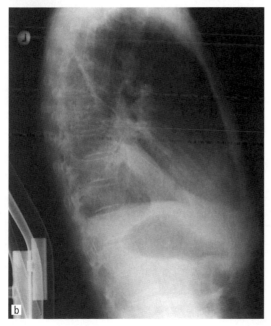

Figure C.28 (a,b) Frontal and lateral chest X-ray demonstrating left lung neoplasm.

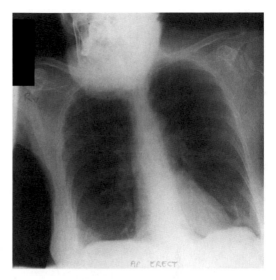

Figure C.29 Patient with bilateral basal consolidation.

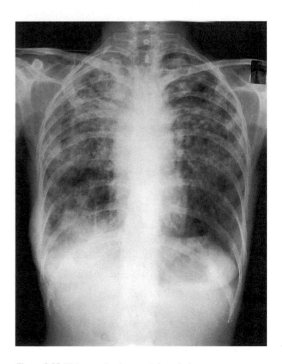

Figure C.30 Widespread pulmonary tuberculosis.

and culminate in vomiting, in addition to a characteristic terminal inspiratory whoop. In severe paroxysms the child may become cyanosed. On examination, the most striking finding in the chest is a negative one, the rhonchi characteristic of ordinary acute bronchitis being generally absent. A sublingual ulcer on the fraenum linguae due to the friction of the protruding tongue on the lower front teeth during long paroxysms of coughing is a helpful finding, as is a history of exposure to infection.

A cough which an adult patient has had intermittently since childhood is more likely to be associated with bronchiectasis than one for which the onset can be dated more recently.

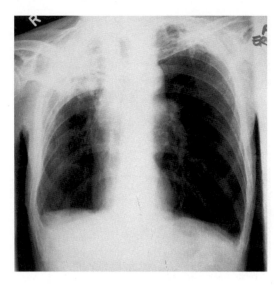

Figure C.31 Right upper lobe tuberculous infection.

In children and even young adults with a persistent or recurrent cough, the possibility of cystic fibrosis must be borne in mind; the presence of associated bowel symptoms should lead to an estimate of sweat sodium levels.

A cough appearing and persisting for the first time in a young adult – especially if an Asian – must give rise to suspicion of pulmonary tuberculosis, and calls for complete investigation including a chest radiograph and sputum examination. Similarly, a cough appearing for the first time in middle age – especially in a man – must raise suspicion of bronchial carcinoma which should only be dismissed after a complete investigation.

The characteristic morning cough of the cigarette smoker is due to a chronic pharyngotracheobronchitis; many cigarette smokers regard it as a normal part of their lives, and refer to it as 'clearing the throat'. It is in fact the first symptom of chronic bronchitis. The frequency with which chronic bronchitis and bronchogenic carcinoma co-exist – both being directly associated with tobacco consumption – has led to the important axiom that any change in the character or pattern of a chronic cough warrants investigation for carcinoma of the lung. Chronic nasal sinusitis may produce or contribute to this symptom, secretions which have trickled down into the trachea during sleep being expelled when the patient wakes. A cough which appears on first lying down at night or on some other changes of posture is suggestive of localized

Table C.9 Causes of cough to be considered when the chest radiograph does not show any gross abnormality

Acute conditions	**Helpful diagnostic clinical clues**
Acute specific fever, e.g. measles, typhoid or paratyphoid	Other features, e.g. Koplik's spots and rash of measles
Pneumocystis pneumonia	Features of HIV disease (oral thrush, weight loss, skin disease, etc.)
Whooping cough (pertussis)	Characteristic cough and whoop (see text)
Acute laryngitis	Associated with hoarseness
Acute tracheobronchitis	Painful cough with retrosternal soreness
Exposure to noxious gases	Obvious history
Inhaled foreign body	Usually a young child, usually no history
Chronic or recurrent conditions	**Diagnostic investigations**
Chronic sinusitis	Sinus radiographs
Chronic laryngitis	
Laryngeal papilloma, carcinoma, }	Laryngoscopy
tuberculosis, syphilis	
Cystic fibrosis	Chest radiograph may be characteristic
	Sweat test
Chronic bronchitis }	
Bronchial asthma }	PEFR or FEV measurement
Bronchiectasis	Bronchoscopy, CT scan of lungs
Carcinoma or adenoma or foreign body only partly	Flow volume loop may be characteristic
obstructing the trachea or main bronchus	Bronchoscopy
Mediastinal lymphadenopathy or tumour pressing on a bronchus	Tomography and/or mediastinoscopy
Diaphragmatic irritation due to subphrenic abscess or hepatic abscess	Ultrasound and fluoroscopy

bronchiectasis or chronic pulmonary suppuration. In older people, recurrent aspiration is a not uncommon cause that is often overlooked. It may be related to oesophageal regurgitation, stricture or neurological disease affecting swallowing. Asthma and cardiac failure also commonly cause cough in the elderly, but this may be especially prominent at night. Asthmatic patients sometimes complain of cough as a predominant feature of their attacks, and wheezing and dyspnoea may be relatively trivial. In typical asthma, cough may also occur on exercise or nocturnally, waking patients from sleep. A cough with dyspnoea or orthopnoea waking the patient from sleep may also be due to pulmonary congestion or oedema due to left ventricular failure in hypertension, aortic valvular disease or disorders of the myocardium. Because such nocturnal attacks of paroxysmal dyspnoea in these conditions may be accompanied by wheeziness, they are sometimes referred to as 'cardiac asthma'. The important findings that might help to differentiate bronchial and cardiac asthma are listed in Table C.10.

Table C.10 Differentiation of bronchial and cardiac asthma

Bronchial asthma	Cardiac asthma
History of previous bronchial asthma	History of hypertension, valvular or ischaemic heart disease
Often young – sometimes old	Rarely young – usually old
Expiratory wheezing	Sometimes also expiratory wheezing
No crackles	Many basal crackles
	Gallop rhythm/cardiac failure
	Evidence of pre-existing cardiac disorder
ECG normal	ECG often abnormal
Chest radiograph shows hyperinflation of lungs	Chest radiograph shows enlargement of left ventricle
	Kerley's septal lines and other evidence of pulmonary venous congestion and/or pulmonary oedema
Bronchial hyperactivity (PEFR measurements)	No evidence of bronchial hyperactivity
Methacholine or histamine challenge	

The presence or absence of expectoration and the quality of expectoration are important diagnostic features of any cough. It should be remembered that many patients find it difficult to expectorate, and habitually expel small amounts of secretion through the larynx by cough and then swallow it. This is the rule in children. A dry cough, or one producing only scant mucoid sputum, may be due to inflammation or tumour of the larynx when there will be associated hoarseness. Laryngeal involvement in syphilis is a very unusual cause of a dry cough with hoarse voice. Another cause of cough associated with a weak voice often described as 'hoarseness' is carcinoma of the bronchus with recurrent laryngeal nerve involvement. A dry cough may be a manifestation of nervousness, but should not be accepted as such without proper investigations. A dry cough may also be due to external pressure on a bronchus by a mediastinal mass such as benign or malignant tumour, or by enlarged mediastinal lymph nodes due to reticulosis or tuberculosis; the latter should be particularly considered in Asians. Cough due to external pressure on the trachea is usually described as 'brassy' or 'bovine'.

If a cough is productive, the quality and mode of production of the sputum should be noted. Frankly purulent sputum suggests bronchiectasis, lung abscess, primary or secondary to bronchial obstruction by new growth, foreign body, or cavitating pulmonary tuberculosis. The odour of the sputum is important: a malodorous sputum almost invariably indicates infection with anaerobic organisms and suggests bronchiectasis, inhalation pneumonia, lung abscess or bronchopleural fistula with expectoration of a putrid empyema. (See also SPUTUM, p. 668.) Cough due to a bronchopleural fistula is characteristically dependent on position; the cough is worse when the patient lies on their good side, and is relieved by lying on the side of the lesion.

Coughing seems to provoke more coughing. Paroxysms of coughing as in pertussis may terminate in vomiting which seems to break the cycle. Paroxysmal attacks may also terminate in syncope. At times, severe coughing attacks have continued to the point of utter exhaustion. The muscular force developed during coughing may be sufficient to cause occasional fractures of ribs (cough fractures) and even compression fractures of vertebral bodies. In some cases, no physical cause for the cough may be detected, and in some of these patients psychogenic factors are important.

Boris Lams

CRAMPS

Cramps are involuntary, painful, sudden spasms of voluntary muscles which become hard and 'knotted'. Cramps may be initiated by a sudden voluntary contraction, but they usually occur at rest. They may persist for seconds or minutes, and can generally be relieved by a slow passive extension of the affected muscle. Electromyography of a muscle in cramp shows fluctuating high-frequency bursts of motor unit activity.

Cramps are a common symptom, and only infrequently indicate disease, particularly if they occur in the legs. Underlying medical causes however include salt depletion, hypocalcaemia, muscle ischaemia, myopathy and neurological disease.

Cramps may occur in normal people under certain physiological (rather than disease) conditions. They often occur during *pregnancy*. Excessive *unaccustomed exercise* can cause cramps; thus, athletes and swimmers commencing training are often affected, the cramps disappearing with increasing fitness. Cramp of the intercostal muscles (stitch) may occur during and after exercise in untrained individuals. Excessive use of combinations of small muscle groups can cause cramps (e.g. writer's or musician's cramp). These are *focal dystonias* (without generalized neurological disease) which make it hard to perform that particular motor task. Medications and psychotherapy are generally unhelpful, but botulinum toxin has been shown to be effective (its use should however be justified by the severity of the condition). *Night cramps* typically occur in older people, and may be painful enough to wake patients from sleep. The foot and calf muscles are most commonly affected, the thighs less often. Quinine is moderately effective at preventing nocturnal leg cramps.

Chronic muscle ischaemia due to atherosclerosis causes *intermittent claudication*, most commonly in the calves, where walking a certain distance (often consistent in any one individual) causes a cramping pain forcing the person to stop. Rest will tend to relieve the pain, and patients with claudication are advised to increase their daily exercise to walking at least four half-hour walks each week. Signs of disease are absent lower-limb pulses, duskiness of feet on hanging the legs down, atrophic skin, and if severe, cold white leg and punched-out ulcers.

Hypocalcaemia causes cramp, most strikingly seen in the forearm and hand muscles as carpopedal spasm (tetany). Hypoparathyroidism, malabsorption and inadequate dietary calcium intake can cause hypocalcaemia. Acute alkalosis from hysterical hyperventilation can also lower ionized calcium in plasma and cause carpopedal spasm. *Chronic renal failure* may also result in hypocalcaemia and, with hypomagnesaemia, be a cause of cramp. In these patients cramps may be particularly troublesome during dialysis. Salt depletion as a result of hard physical work in a hot environment, profuse sweating, and hypotonic fluid replacement (i.e. water) causes *heat cramps*, typically presenting as severe spasms of the extremities. Rectal temperature is usually normal, and treatment consists of rest and salt replacement (preferably by food and fluids containing sodium chloride, rather than by salt tablets). Cramps may also occur from *salt and water imbalance* due to diarrhoea and vomiting, burns, diuretic use, fistula, and small-bowel obstruction.

Neurological diseases affecting the spinal cord or peripheral nerves can cause cramps. Flexor spasms of the legs may be seen in patients with *spinal cord injury* and myelitis due to *multiple sclerosis*. Diseases of the peripheral nerves such as *alcoholic or diabetic neuropathy* tend to cause cramps of the legs and feet, whereas forearm cramps raise the possible diagnosis of *motor neurone disease*.

In addition to diuretics, *drugs* associated with cramps are beta-adrenoreceptor stimulants (e.g. terbutaline), steroids, calcium-channel antagonists (e.g. nifedipine), statins (myopathy) and phenothiazine-type neuroleptics. The latter cause a particular form of cramp and spasm of the facial and neck muscles (orofacial and nuchal dyskinesia).

Very rarely, cramps may be due to *enzyme disorders of muscles*; for example, phosphoglycerate mutase, phosphoglycerate kinase and adenylate deaminase deficiency. *Tetanus* is a form of cramp due to infection by *Clostridium tetani*. The spasm appears first in the facial muscles and then spreads over the body. Cramps due to *lead poisoning* or *strychnine* are rarely seen, and are only of historical interest.

Danielle Harari

CREPITUS

Crepitus is a term which is generally used to denote the grating or crackling sensation and noise produced when two rough substances rub together, as for instance the grating that can be felt and heard between the fractured ends of a bone. Crepitus from within a joint should be distinguished from sharp cracking sounds occurring in normal or abnormal joints after temporary immobility, and from the slipping of tendons and ligaments over bone surfaces on movement.

Articular crepitus arises most commonly from osteoarthrotic degenerative changes in joints, most commonly the knee, where subpatellar fine friction can be felt with the hands in many cases, often early in the degenerative process. The patient should be reassured that it is not a serious finding and is felt by most middle-aged or elderly persons at some time in their lives.

A common and unimportant observation after middle age is the awareness of a grating sensation in the neck, apparent to both patient and clinician. In acromegaly, gross crepitus throughout the full range of articular movement is often found in large peripheral joints as it may in other syndromes be associated with hypermobile joints, such as Marfan's and Ehlers–Danlos syndromes. A coarser crepitation may be felt after trauma and in chondromalacia patellae. Coarse crepitation or 'crackling' may be felt with the hands or heard with the ear wherever degenerative changes occur, for instance in the neck or shoulder, but is more common in the more mobile weight-bearing joints, where cartilage has become worn and degenerated, as in, most commonly, the knee.

In rheumatoid arthritis a fine 'rubbing' crepitus occurs which can be felt over the joints in relatively early cases; this may become coarser as the disease advances. At the shoulder, inflammatory or degenerative processes may produce crepitus at scapulohumeral or acrominclavicular joints, and a peculiar sensation may be experienced with the hand over the scapular border as though the bone were moving over soft marbles; this, again, is not a sign of serious disease and the patient can in most cases be fully reassured.

On palpation of a joint with hydrarthrosis, the so-called 'silken crepitus' can occasionally be felt, as if two silken surfaces were being rubbed together by the examiner's hands. *Tenosynovitis*, especially around the flexor tendons at the wrist, can also produce a feeling of crepitus, to both the patient and examiner.

When there is an enlargement of a bone without fracture, and when on palpation a feeling of crepitus or eggshell crackling is obtained, it indicates that some tumour is eroding the overlying cortex. Radiography will be necessary to establish the diagnosis. Rarefraction of the bones of the skull, either as the result of syphilitic lesions in adults, or of *hydrocephalus* or *craniotabes*, especially in the occipital region of congenitally syphilitic and rickety infants, may make the skull bones so thin that they bend readily on pressure, and sometimes the result is a sensation of crepitus. The diagnosis is generally obvious. The condition is very rare.

Apart from bony, arthritic or synovial changes, a characteristic feeling of crepitus may be felt beneath the skin when gas or air has accumulated in the subcutaneous tissues as the result of surgical emphysema.

Mark Kinirons

CRUSTS

Crusts or scabs are secondary skin lesions formed when serum, blood, sebum, purulent exudate or a *mixture* of these dries on the surface of the skin (Fig. C.32). In addition, they may contain dirt and the remains of local applications (e.g. calamine lotion). It is important to distinguish crusts from scales (see SCALY ERUPTIONS, p. 630), the causes being quite distinct. In addition to arising in a variety of dermatoses, crusts may result from scratching, or the application of irritant or caustic chemicals. They vary considerably in thickness, from the light crust of dermatitis to the thick barnacle-like scabs seen in keratoderma blennorrhagica. It may sometimes be necessary to remove crusts by prolonged soaking in order to make a diagnosis of the underlying lesion. This is particularly important when a crust overlies a neoplasm (e.g. rodent ulcer on the scalp) (see Table C.11). *Impetigo is* the classic cause of

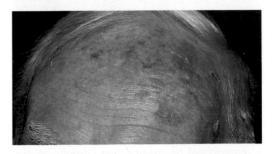

Figure C.32 Actinic keratoses.

Table C.11 Crusts

Impetigo
Eczema
Trauma – thermal, chemical, factitial
Herpes simplex, eczema herpeticum
Herpes zoster
Pemphigus
Stasis ulcers
Pyoderma gangrenosum
Keratoderma blennorrhagica (Reiter's syndrome)
Syphilis – rupiod
Yaws

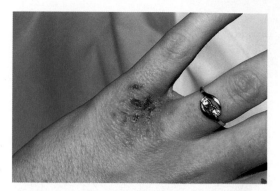

Figure C.34 Eczema with secondary infection.

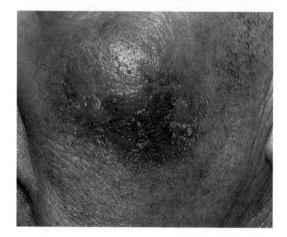

Figure C.35 Pemphigus.

golden-coloured crusts on the skin (Fig. C.33). These are commonest around the mouth and face of children, but can be very widespread or affect any age group. Acute vesicular 'wet' *eczema* results in crust formation, usually with a brownish colour; if this becomes golden-coloured, secondary impetiginization due to infection with *Staphylococcus aureus* should be suspected (Fig. C.34). Crusting rapidly follows secondary degree *burns*, or chemical burns, which may on occasion be factitial. *Herpes simplex* sores become crusted on the fourth or fifth day, and crusting is prolonged if there is a secondary impetigo. The same may occur in *herpes zoster*, but here crusts are often haemorrhagic. In *eczema herpeticum* (Kaposi's varicelliform eruption), crusting can be very extensive and pose a difficult nursing problem.

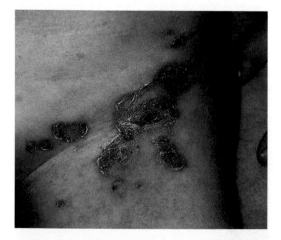

Figure C.33 Impetigo.

Pemphigus (Fig. C.35) is the bullous disorder that is characterized by crusting, and erosions because the blisters are superficial and therefore very fragile.

A search should be made for the characteristic mucosal erosions. These crusts are notoriously slow to heal, and are probably the only situation where the application of a potent topical corticosteroid can speed re-epithelialization.

Scabbing can be profuse around stasis ulcers, particularly if a *dermatitis medicamentosa* (e.g. to lanolin or topical antibiotic) has developed. The crusting over *pyoderma gangrenosum* overlies the characteristic cribriform fibrous scarring.

In *keratoderma blennorrhagica*, the skin eruption of Reiter's syndrome, crusty rupioid nodules may be seen on the limbs accompanying the pustular crusted lesions of palms and soles. In the rupial form of secondary syphilis the crusts are greenish or blackish, and consist of several layers, each smaller than the one immediately below it, so that a pyramidal structure is formed resembling a barnacle. Removal of these crusts exposes a foul-smelling ulcer. One of the features of yaws (framboesia) is heavily encrusted flexural granulations.

It should not be forgotten that scabbing ulcers and erosions which fail to heal with appropriate anti-infective treatment may be self-inflicted (dermatitis artefacta).

Barry Monk

CYANOSIS

Cyanosis is an abnormal blue discoloration of the skin and mucous membranes which is seen whenever the cutaneous and subcutaneous vessels contain an excess of reduced haemoglobin. There is wide inter-observer variation in the detection of mild cyanosis. The long-held belief that cyanosis was detectable when 5 g/dl or more of reduced haemoglobin was present is not consistently true. Cyanosis can either be central or peripheral.

Central cyanosis is due either to arterial hypox aemia or to the presence of the abnormal pigments methaemoglobin or sulphaemoglobin. Central cyanosis is seen in the mucous membranes, particularly the lips and tongue, as well as on the skin, and in good lighting can be identified by most observers when the arterial oxygen saturation falls below about 87 per cent. In anaemia, greater desaturation will occur before cyanosis is apparent as less reduced haemoglobin will be present at a given saturation.

Peripheral cyanosis is due to reduced blood flow in the skin, allowing more oxygen to be extracted than normal. Peripheral cyanosis may result from local vasoconstriction, from a low cardiac output, or from a combination of both. It is apparent in exposed areas such as fingers, ears, nose and cheeks, but not in mucous membranes or the warmer parts of the skin.

Central cyanosis

Respiratory disease

The commonest mechanism for arterial hypoxaemia due to respiratory disease is the impairment of matching of ventilation to perfusion. Poorly ventilated but well-perfused alveoli will have a low oxygen tension, and will contribute poorly oxygenated blood to the systemic arterial circulation. Alveolar hypoventilation will also result in arterial hypoxaemia, usually in association with hypercapnia.

Virtually any diffuse lung disease, if sufficiently severe, will result in central cyanosis. The commonest respiratory cause of central cyanosis is chronic obstructive pulmonary disease (COPD, previously termed chronic bronchitis and emphysema). Central cyanosis is the hallmark of the 'blue and bloated' form of COPD, and is then due to a combination of ventilation/perfusion mismatching and hypoventilation. Patients with the 'pink and puffing' form of COPD have impaired ventilation/perfusion matching, but avoid marked arterial hypoxaemia by maintaining adequate ventilation at the cost of developing dyspnoea. Central cyanosis is a feature of advanced pulmonary fibrosis from whatever cause, when it results from ventilation/perfusion mismatching. Ventilation/perfusion mismatching is also the cause of cyanosis in pulmonary embolism, pulmonary oedema and pneumonia.

Alveolar hypoventilation is the cause of central hypoxaemia following excess sedation and in patients with ventilatory failure due to impaired chest wall movement. Impaired chest movement may result from kyphoscoliosis or from paresis of the respiratory muscles. Alveolar hypoventilation may also cause cyanosis in patients with sleep apnoea/hypopnoea (a condition characterized by daytime sleepiness and loud snoring), or the obesity hypoventilation syndrome (a condition characterized by obesity and episodes of hypoventilation occurring principally at night and leading to type II respiratory failure and consequent hypoxia, the 'Pickwickian syndrome') (see SLEEP, DISORDERS OF, p. 653). Alveolar hypoventilation also occasionally occurs following obstruction to a major airway. For example, the larynx may be obstructed by aspiration of a foreign body, by laryngeal oedema (usually due to angioneurotic oedema), or bilateral abductor, or paralysis following thyroidectomy. Tracheal obstruction from thyroid carcinoma, haemorrhage into a thyroid cyst, malignant lymph nodes, primary tracheal tumours or benign tracheal stenosis following tracheostomy or intubation are all rare causes of cyanosis due to alveolar hypoventilation.

Cardiovascular disease

Although the commonest cardiac cause of mild hypoxaemia is left heart failure – usually on the basis of ischaemic heart disease – this is rarely severe enough to cause cyanosis, except during acute attacks of pulmonary oedema. Although cyanotic congenital heart disease is a less common cause of hypoxaemia, it is a much more common and more dramatic cause of cyanosis. An important point which differentiates cyanosis due to a central veno-arterial shunt from that due to lung disease is the response to breathing oxygen. In lung disease, cyanosis will disappear and arterial hypoxaemia greatly improve as a result of breathing 100 per cent oxygen, unless many perfused alveoli are completely unventilated. In cyanotic congenital heart disease, oxygen produces little change in arterial oxygen saturation as the blood in the shunt does not participate in gas exchange. Other features common to all types of cyanotic congenital heart disease are clubbing of the fingers and toes and polycythaemia. In severe cases, the haemoglobin concentration may be well over 20 g/dl.

Fallot's tetralogy is by far the most common congenital cardiac lesion to cause cyanosis. The four classic features are pulmonary stenosis, ventricular septal defect, overriding aorta, and right ventricular hypertrophy. Of these features, the last is the direct haemodynamic consequence of the pulmonary stenosis; the overriding aorta, although characteristic, is not a major factor in determining the presence or severity of cyanosis. An associated anomaly in several cases is a right-sided aortic arch; this must not be confused with dextro-position of the aorta – a synonym for overriding. Cyanosis is not often present at birth, but develops (with clubbing) during the first year or two of life. The symptoms include dyspnoea (which is relieved by squatting) and syncope associated with deepening of the cyanosis (see DYSPNOEA, p. 159 and FAINTS, p. 211). The arterial and venous pulses are unremarkable except for, occasionally, a dominant 'a' wave in the jugular venous pulse. The apex beat is little displaced, and there may be a slight or moderate right ventricular impulse at the left sternal border. The systolic murmur is rather short and often loud enough to be accompanied by a thrill; the second sound is single. The definitive diagnosis can be made by echocardiography or angiocardiography.

Pulmonary atresia is embryologically related to Fallot's tetralogy, and usually produces very severe cyanosis. The differentiation is easily made by the absence of the systolic murmur of pulmonary stenosis in atresia and its replacement by a subclavicular continuous murmur, usually bilateral, due to large anastomoses between the bronchial and pulmonary arteries. Other conditions which may be more difficult to distinguish clinically from Fallot's tetralogy are: (i) pulmonary stenosis with reversed interatrial shunt; and (ii) Eisenmenger's complex, properly so-called, that is pulmonary hypertension with reversed interventricular shunt. Tricuspid atresia is another cause of cyanosis, characterized by an unusual ECG pattern suggesting right atrial and left ventricular hypertrophy.

Transposition of the great arteries is a relatively common form of cyanotic congenital heart disease in infancy, although few untreated patients survive. The aorta arises from the right ventricle and the pulmonary artery from the left. Clearly, communications between the two circulations – at either the atrial or ventricular level – must also be present if life is to be maintained. Pulmonary stenosis or pulmonary hypertension may also be present to complicate the haemodynamic situation. The physical signs vary with the associated abnormalities, but the X-ray may be of diagnostic value. The vascular pedicle of the heart is rather narrow in the posteroanterior view, and pulmonary plethora is nearly always present. As oligaemia of the lung fields is the rule in most types of cyanotic congenital heart disease, the association of cyanosis with plethora is very suggestive of transposition. Angiocardiography is diagnostic, showing, in the lateral view, the aorta arising anteriorly from the right ventricle and the pulmonary artery posteriorly from the left. Very rare types of cyanotic congenital heart disease include drainage of the superior or inferior vena cava into the left atrium, and some cases of Ebstein's anomaly of the tricuspid valve with reversed interatrial shunt.

Pulmonary arteriovenous malformations may cause central cyanosis if the shunt is large enough. They are frequently associated with cutaneous telangiectases, especially on the lips, and may occur in the familial condition, hereditary haemorrhagic telangiectasia. Continuous murmurs may be heard over the aneurysms, which may be multiple. In the radiograph, one or more round opacities are visible, and a CT scan will often reveal the feeding artery and draining vein.

Pigmentary cyanosis

Cyanosis is a major feature of a group of conditions in which ferric (Fe^{3+}) rather than ferrous (Fe^{2+}) iron is present in haemoglobin, producing methaemoglobin. Sulphaemoglobin is a poorly characterized substance which can be produced by the action of hydrogen sulphide on haemoglobin. Small amounts of these pigments, for example, 1.5 g methaemoglobin or 0.5 g sulphaemoglobin, are said to produce as marked cyanosis as 5 g of deoxygenated haemoglobin.

Methaemoglobinaemia may be either congenital or acquired. *Congenital methaemoglobinaemias* due to a deficiency of NADH-methaemoglobin reductase have a recessive inheritance. Methaemoglobinaemia may also result from congenital abnormalities of the alpha or beta globin chain of haemoglobin, rendering the molecule unresponsive to methaemoglobin reductase, and these varieties may be inherited as autosomal dominant characteristics. Acquired methaemoglobinaemia can result from the ingestion of a large group of chemicals, including oxidizing agents such as nitrites and chlorates. Nitrates can be converted to nitrites in the bowel, and cyanosis has been reported in infants in association with a high nitrate content of drinking water. Poisoning with potassium chlorate can also produce methaemoglobinaemia, apart from its more serious effects. Aniline dyes have also been incriminated: these compounds can be absorbed through the intact skin. Phenacetin can also cause methaemoglobinaemia and cyanosis, though due to its declining use this is now rare. The symptoms of methaemoglobinaemia are those of severe anaemia (to which the condition is closely analogous), namely dyspnoea on exertion and dizziness. The diagnosis can be confirmed by spectroscopic analysis which will detect a band at 630 pm that disappears with the addition of a reducing agent.

Sulphaemoglobinaemia is a poorly defined condition which may occur in conjunction with methaemoglobinaemia following the ingestion of nitrates, nitrites, aniline dyes and phenacetin. It has also been reported in conjunction with chronic constipation and with malabsorption. There is no congenital form of this condition. Sulphaemoglobinaemia is usually asymptomatic.

Peripheral cyanosis

When red cell transit through cutaneous vessels is delayed, continued oxygen extraction will decrease the oxygen saturation of the haemoglobin, and cyanosis will appear. This may result either from increased resistance to blood flow, from decreased cardiac output, or from increased blood viscosity.

Increased resistance in blood flow

The commonest cause of peripheral cyanosis is the transient and appropriate vasoconstriction in response to cold. The best-known medical conditions associated with peripheral cyanosis are *Raynaud's disease* and *Raynaud's phenomenon* (see FINGERS, DEAD, p. 218).

Acrocyanosis is a relatively benign condition caused by spasm of smaller cutaneous arteries and arterioles. The hands and fingers are cold and mottled red and blue, but pain is not a feature. Arteriolar spasm is also the mechanism of *erythrocyanosis*, a disease that is almost confined to young women in which cyanotic blotches are seen in the lower parts of the legs. Cyanosis of the affected leg or legs occurs occasionally following deep venous thrombosis, particularly if collateral drainage is poor. This condition has been termed 'phlegmasia caerulea dolens'. Similarly, cyanosis of the face may occur, together with gross venous engorgement and oedema, as a feature of *superior vena caval obstruction* from whatever cause. This mechanism may contribute to the so-called *traumatic cyanosis* following crush injury to the chest, although hypoxaemia due to lung trauma may contribute.

Decreased cardiac output

The ashen grey appearance of patients with severe shock is a typical example of peripheral cyanosis due to a marked fall in cardiac output, and it occurs irrespective of the cause of the shock. The low cardiac output and vasoconstriction which occur with left ventricular failure can also cause peripheral cyanosis, although central cyanosis will usually co-exist. Similarly, cyanosis in massive *pulmonary embolism* is usually both central and peripheral. The classical malar flush in mitral stenosis is an example of local peripheral cyanosis, but why this should be so sited is unknown.

Increased blood viscosity

Cyanosis may occur in *polycythaemia rubra vera*, despite a normal arterial oxygen saturation. This is presumed to result from decreased cutaneous blood flow due to increased viscosity.

Boris Lams

D

DEAFNESS

Deafness is rarely total or complete. The term 'hearing loss' is a better term to use as it implies that there may be degrees of deafness. Hearing loss is an extremely common problem, and constitutes one of the major handicaps affecting mankind. Most of us will have experienced a temporary hearing loss in one or other ear at some time, perhaps when flying or associated with a cold, and should be able to appreciate how incapacitating permanent and more severe loss of hearing must be. In fact, almost 60 per cent of the population will have acquired a significant degree of hearing loss by the time they retire from full-time employment.

From a clinical standpoint, three types of hearing loss are recognized, namely conductive, sensorineural, and mixed.

- **Conductive hearing loss**: this is caused by lesions in the external and/or middle ear that attenuate or prevent sound reaching the cochlea.
- **Sensorineural hearing loss**: this is caused by lesions within the cochlea or affecting the auditory nerve and/or higher pathways.
- **Mixed hearing loss**: this is caused by a combination of conductive and sensorineural elements.

Hearing tests

These tests are undertaken to determine the nature and severity of hearing loss. Both psycho-acoustic and objective tests have been devised and are employed in clinical practice.

Voice tests

An initial assessment of hearing loss can be gained by occlusion of the contralateral ear while speaking or whispering into the ipsilateral ear. The patient should be told to repeat exactly what the examiner says, and be positioned so that they cannot see the examiner's lips. Anyone with normal hearing will be able to hear a whispered voice at a distance of 60 cm (2 feet).

Hearing in the contralateral ear is usually masked by gentle pressure on the tragus, or by holding paper over the ear and scratching it when speaking. An alternative and better method of masking the non-test ear is by use of a Barany box; this is a sound-generating device that is inserted into the contralateral ear canal and emits a loud noise while testing the other ear. More accurate measures of the spoken voice can be obtained with sound pressure meters.

Tuning-fork tests

With these simple, chair-side tests it is possible to distinguish between conductive and sensorineural hearing losses. Only 256 cps or 512 cps tuning forks should be used. Lower-frequency tuning forks are appropriate for vibration sense tests only.

The Rinne test

The tuning fork is struck and its base held firmly on the patient's mastoid process until they no longer hear the tone. The fork is then rapidly transferred so that the vibrating forks are close to the external auditory meatus. If the patient continues to hear the sound it is considered that they hear better by air conduction than by bone conduction – a positive test result. In fact, in patients with normal middle-ear function the sound is usually perceived as being much louder. Patients with either normal hearing acuity or with a sensorineural hearing loss perceive the tuning fork better by air conduction than by bone conduction. Conversely, patients with conductive losses hear the tuning fork better by bone conduction than air conduction – a negative test result.

The Weber test

In this test, the tuning fork is placed in the middle of the forehead or on the vertex, and the patient is asked to signify in which ear they hear the sound louder. In the Weber test, the sound is either heard better by one ear (in other words, it lateralizes), or it is heard equally by both ears. The sound lateralizes to the ear with the better hearing in sensorineural hearing loss, or to the ear with the greater conductive hearing loss in patients with conductive hearing losses. The normal response is to hear the sound equally in both ears, but this result can also be obtained in patients with equal sensorineural or conductive hearing loss.

The absolute bone-conduction test

In this test an assessment is made of the patient's ability to hear by bone conduction. This is a measure of sensorineural deafness, and the patient's response is compared to the examiner's perception of the tone. If the examiner has roughly normal hearing, then the patient ought to hear a tuning fork placed on their mastoid as long as the examiner does. If they hear it for less time, then it is considered that their bone conduction is diminished and they have worse hearing than the examiner, probably a sensorineural hearing loss.

Audiometry

Pure-tone audiometry

A pure-tone audiometer produces tones of varying intensity (0 to 120 dB) and frequency (125 Hz to 8000 Hz). The test is performed with the patient wearing earphones, usually but always in a sound-proofed environment. Test sounds at different intensities and frequencies are introduced via the earphones, and the patient is asked to indicate when they hear the sound. Threshold values at each frequency are determined and plotted on a graph – an audiogram (Fig. D.1). Normal thresholds have been established by the National Physics Laboratory, and young adults should have threshold values across the test range of 0 to 10 dB, with 0 dB being the sound pressure level considered to be threshold for 18-year-olds.

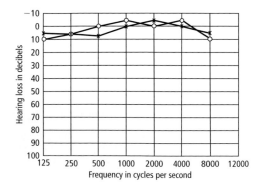

Figure D.1 Audiogram showing hearing that is within 'normal limits'. It is conventional to represent hearing by air conduction in the right ear by 0–0, and in the left ear by X–X.

Bone conduction is considered to be equivalent to cochlear function as it bypasses the middle-ear conduction mechanism. To obtain bone conduction, a vibrating disk is applied to the patient's mastoid process. The test is then carried out in the same manner as for air conduction, and the auditory thresholds are obtained and plotted on the audiogram. In this way it can be seen if bone conduction is better than air conduction (conductive deafness), or if bone conduction and air conduction are roughly equal (normal or sensorineural deafness).

Speech audiometry

It is possible for a patient to produce a normal pure-tone audiogram yet be unable to interpret or discriminate speech. A more discriminatory test of hearing is a speech audiogram, where the patient has to respond to a list of test words played at threshold levels through earphones. Either a graph can be made of the patient's speech responses at each test level, or a simple raw speech discrimination score can be recorded. The threshold level at which approximately 50 per cent of the words are interpreted correctly (the half-peak level) is about equivalent to the pure-tone average. A difference between the half-peak level of a speech audiogram and the pure-tone average audiogram is indicative of malingering. Patients with pure conductive losses achieve 100 per cent discrimination at an elevated sound presentation level, and sustain this increased sound pressure level. Conversely, patients with sensorineural hearing losses rarely achieve 100 per cent discrimination, and with increased sound pressure levels the scores deteriorate – a phenomenon known as 'roll over'.

Tympanometry

Tympanometers measure middle-ear compliance. Sound is injected into the ear canal, and the reflected sound level is measured while the atmospheric pressure of the ear canal is varied. The reciprocal value of the reflected sound – the compliance – is plotted against the atmospheric pressure. The compliance of the middle ear is greatest when the external ear canal pressure is the same as that in the middle ear. This test can diagnose middle-ear effusions, ossicular disruptions or discontinuity and Eustachian tube dysfunction. Low compliance levels are seen in severe otosclerotic fixation of the stapes footplate. Changes in middle-ear compliance produced by stapedius muscle contraction can also be measured by injecting high-intensity sound (threshold +80 dB) to elicit the stapedial reflex. An absence of the reflex or abnormal decay of reflex activity is of diagnostic importance in otosclerosis, ossicular discontinuity and retrocochlear hearing loss.

Evoked response audiometry

Sound transduction into the neural activity can be detected throughout the auditory pathway. In the cochlea, contraction of the outer hair cells produces echoes that can be heard by sensitive microphones; depolarization of the first-order neurones can be recorded by electrocochleography and the passage of neural flux in the auditory pathways documented by brainstem and cortical techniques. All of these techniques have specific indications, but find universal use for screening neonates for hearing loss, detecting non-organic hearing loss in medicolegal problems, and investigating patients with endolymphatic hydrops.

Hearing tests in children

Deafness should be diagnosed in infants as early as possible. The earlier that deafness is diagnosed, the more chance there is of the child developing normal language skills and not falling behind their peer group from an educational standpoint. Every child born in the UK has a hearing test by specially trained nurses at 6 weeks and at the end of the first year of life. Children at particular risk of hearing loss (e.g. those born to deaf parents), premature births requiring intensive care, and infants with abnormal facies, etc. are tested within days of birth or discharge from hospital. Where the nurse does not receive an unambiguous response indicating normal hearing from her/his simple clinical tests, the child is referred to a special children's speech and hearing clinic. There, further clinical tests are undertaken which may include evoked response audiometry.

If a child is found to be deaf, then special education is set in hand at a very early age and amplification devices are fitted to the child, depending on the severity of the deafness. Those found to be profoundly deaf are considered for cochlear implantation.

Conductive deafness

The common causes of conductive deafness are listed in Table D.1.

Conductive deafness is often less severe than sensorineural deafness. Complete disruption of the

Table D.1 The causes of conductive deafness

Congenital lesions
1 Atresia of the external meatus and middle ear usually with microtia (see Fig. D.2)
2 Atresia associated with other facial defects
3 Middle-ear deformities
- Some syndromes (frequently associated with sensorineural loss in addition to the conductive loss)
  - Mandibulofacial dysostosis (Treacher–Collins syndrome)
  - Crouzon deformity
  - Marfan's syndrome
  - Klippel–Feil syndrome
  - Trisomy D and E
  - Cretinism
  - Cleft palate
  - Submucous cleft palate
  - Osteogenesis imperfecta (van der Hoeve–de Kleyn triad)
  - Thalidomide
  - Rubella

External auditory meatus
- Wax
- Foreign bodies
- Otitis externa
- Exostoses (diver's ear; wet ear)

Middle-ear lesions
- Trauma
- Blood
- Ossicular disruption
- Perforated tympanic membrane
- Acute otitis media
- Eustachian malfunction
  - Atelectasis of middle ear
  - Serous otitis ('glue ear')
- Otitic barotrauma
- Chronic otitis media
- Haemotympanum
- Malignant disease
- Glomus tumour
- Otosclerosis

sound-transmitting mechanism imparts a 60 dB hearing loss, while a simple perforation inflicts a hearing loss of 25–30 dB. Many of these conductive hearing losses are amenable to surgical correction (e.g. otosclerosis, middle-ear effusions or perforations), and some can be cured by medication (e.g. acute otitis media). Others can be overcome by hearing aids.

Congenital syndromes

There are a number of congenital syndromes associated with deafness, and most are sensorineural in nature. Where there is a conductive element to the hearing loss, it is often associated with a cochlear abnormality as well as resulting in a mixed hearing loss. It is quite impossible to list all the possible combinations of congenital abnormalities, but the golden rule is that if one abnormality is observed, a careful search for others must be made and that, during this search, deafness must never be forgotten. Some of the more common congenital syndromes associated with hearing loss are listed.

Goldenhar's syndrome

The anomalies characteristically present in this maldevelopment of the 1st and 2nd branchial arches are microtia, total atresia of the external auditory canal, ossicular abnormalities, absent middle-ear muscles and anomalous facial nerve pathway. Abnormalities of the inner ear may be present as well as hemifacial microsmia (Fig. D.2).

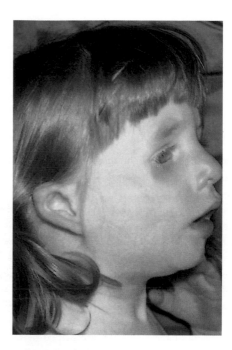

Figure D.3 Treacher–Collins syndrome, showing typical appearance of the eye, micrognathia, depressed malar bone and ptosis of the ear.

Crouzon deformity

Crouzon's syndrome is a craniofacial dysostosis characterized by exophthalmos, a divergent squint, hypoplastic maxillae, a short upper lip, hyperteliorism, beak-shaped nose and deafness caused by atresia and middle-ear abnormalities.

Marfan's syndrome

This comprises an inherited collagen disorder, abnormally long extremities, subluxation of the lens, cardiovascular abnormalities and deafness. The auricles are very large in this condition, and the cartilaginous canals tend to collapse.

Klippel–Feil syndrome

This is a syndrome in which there are malformed cervical vertebrae and a webbed neck in association with hearing loss caused by ankylosis of the ossicles. Some patients also have rudimentary inner ears.

Trisomy D and E

Patients with this condition have low-set ears, preauricular tags, atresia of the external auditory canals and an absence of the middle-ear cleft.

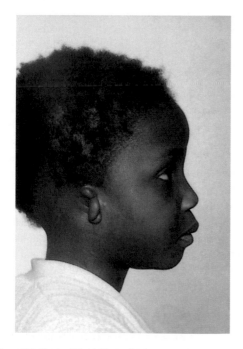

Figure D.2 Atresia of the right ear, showing absent external auditory meatus and deformed auricle.

Treacher–Collins syndrome

This comprises micrognathia, depressed malar bones, eyes sloping downwards and outwards with notched lower lids, ptosis of the auricles and middle-ear abnormalities with deformed ossicles (Fig. D.3).

Osteogenesis imperfecta

Sometimes known as the van der Hoeve's syndrome, the classical triad is deafness caused by stapedial fixation and incudo-stapedial fragility, blue sclera and fragile bones. It is fortunately an uncommon condition, with a frequency of 2–3 per 100 000 population.

Cleft-palate

Cleft palate is one of the most common congenital deformities, with a frequency of about 1 in 1000. It is also a cause of deafness. The palatal muscles (tensor palati and levator palati) play an important part in Eustachian tube opening and closure. Nearly every cleft-palate child has a middle-ear effusion, and some go on to develop atectasis of the middle-ear cleft. Closure of the palatal defect does not influence Eustachian tube function. Submucous clefts of the palate in which there is a deficiency of the muscular layer are equally disruptive to Eustachian tube function. Some of these children are helped by reconstructive surgery. This can be a difficult condition to recognize but, in a few, a bifid uvula may be present and draw attention to the abnormality (Fig. D.4).

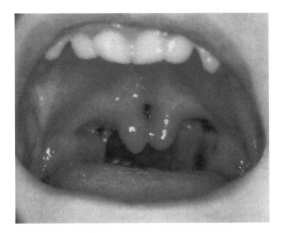

Figure D.4 Submucous cleft palate with deeply bifid uvula typical of this rare condition.

Other syndromes associated with hearing loss

The hearing losses found in these syndromes are often predominantly sensorineural, with relatively minor conductive elements. Examples are Pendred's syndrome in which hearing loss is associated with thyroid deficiency, rubella infection and thalidomide toxicity.

Abnormalities of the external auditory canal

Diseases of the external auditory meatus rarely cause deafness, as hearing is retained while there is still the smallest airway past the obstruction to the tympanic membrane. However, sudden deafness can develop when wax becomes impacted or wet when it expands and closes the canal. Similarly, the oedema associated with *otitis externa* can also cause occlusion of the ear canal and a conductive hearing loss.

Middle-ear causes of hearing loss

Most of these are easily identified by a thorough and careful otoscopic examination.

Otitis media with effusion (syn., secretory otitis media, 'glue ear')

This is an extremely common condition and is present in 4 per cent of all children aged between 5 and 15 years. This means that almost every classroom in the country will contain one child with a temporary hearing loss caused by 'glue ear'. The resulting hearing loss is variable, but may be sufficient to impair education. Fairly typical changes occur in the eardrum, which becomes retracted and develops a yellowish glaze. Occasionally, fluid levels and bubbles can be seen through the eardrum, but in other instances there may be no observable clinical signs. The diagnosis is made by tympanometry where a flat compliance curve is recorded. In adults, otitis media with effusion may be the first sign of Eustachian tube obstruction by a nasopharyngeal carcinoma. Although less common among Europeans, this condition is of very definite clinical significance in the Chinese, where nasopharyngeal carcinoma is the most common head and neck tumour. Drainage of the effusions and the insertion of grommets (ventilation tubes) restores hearing.

Acute otitis media

This is a common viral or bacterial infective disorder of childhood caused by *Streptococcus pneumoniae*, *Haemophilus influenzae*, *Moraxella catarrhalis* and, less frequently, *Streptococcus pyogenes* or *Staphylococcus aureus*. Acute otitis media often accompanies or complicates upper respiratory tract infections. The child becomes unwell and pyrexial, and complains of a hearing loss in the affected ear and increasing earache. Occasionally, instead of complaining of earache, a child may complain of abdominal pain. Eventually, the eardrum ruptures to release pus that has accumulated in the middle-ear cleft. Pain diminishes rapidly once the pus has drained, as do any toxic symptoms and signs. Over the course of the next few days, the infection resolves and the ruptured eardrum seals spontaneously in most cases. There is a considerable dichotomy of opinion about the value of antibiotics in the management of this condition. One body of opinion suggests that it can be managed just as successfully by symptomatic treatment with analgesics, while others feel that antibiotics should always be prescribed.

Chronic otitis media

Two types of chronic otitis media are recognized, *tubo-tympanic* and *attico-antral* disease. Tubo-tympanic disease is characterized by a persistent central perforation, while attico-antral disease is associated with ingrowth of skin from the attic or posteromarginal region of the tympanic membrane into the mastoid antrum, mastoid and middle ear – cholesteatoma. Both groups of patients develop hearing loss in the affected ear and are subject to chronic discharge. In the case of tubo-tympanic disease, this discharge is mucoid and not particularly offensive. By contrast, patients with attico-antral disease have a watery and offensive discharge.

Both conditions are potentially dangerous, as uncontrolled infection may spread to cause meningitis, brain abscess and facial palsy. Persistent perforations can often be repaired surgically, but those that cannot should be kept dry and free from water contamination. Episodes of infection are treated with topical antibiotics. Attico-antral disease almost always requires surgical treatment in the form of a mastoid exploration. Some small cholesteatomas can be managed by suction clearance on an intermittent basis, but these cases are relatively rare.

Otosclerosis

This is a form of deafness caused by fixation of the stapes by the development of new bone around its footplate. It tends to affect young adults, and is a progressive form of deafness that increases as the footplate becomes more and more fixed. In females, the deafness is often made worse by pregnancy. Pure-tone audiometry demonstrates a conductive loss often with an increased loss at 2 kHz, the so-called 'Carhart's notch'. Treatment of this condition is determined by the degree of hearing loss it inflicts, the likely benefit derivable from surgical intervention, and the patient's wishes. Oral fluoride therapy can retard progression. Those with significant hearing loss will certainly benefit from a hearing aid, and some by removal of the stapes and replacement by a prosthesis (stapedectomy).

Sensorineural deafness

Although there may be some overlap, it is probably better to separate those conditions that generally arise in childhood (see Table D.2) from those that develop in adult life. The importance of early diagnosis of hearing deficit in childhood has already been mentioned. The normal development of an infant is greatly dependent upon hearing, the understanding of speech being the one function of human behaviour that sets man apart from animals. Failure to hear speech not only prevents the development of language but also inhibits the formation of personal and social relationships. Much can be achieved nowadays to minimize the handicap of hearing loss by cochlear implantation or provision of suitable hearing aids and peripatetic care.

Infants who have a family history of deafness, maternal infection during pregnancy or perinatal problems, who are late to talk or who have other congenital defects, must be considered as being 'at risk' of a significant hearing deficit, and should be carefully tested. The frequency of sporadic cases of deafness makes testing of all babies important. In this respect, the mother's views should never be ignored; if she thinks her child is deaf, the diagnosis should be presumed correct until demonstrated to be otherwise. It must be remembered also that mild or moderate conductive deafness may be an additional handicap in this age group. This added handicap may be the decisive factor that prevents a child from hearing at all without amplification.

Genetically determined syndromes

There are a very large number of genetically determined syndromes that include sensorineural hearing loss. The most common have been listed together here with a brief description of their main characteristics.

Table D.2 Causes of deafness in children

1 Pre-natal
a. Genetic
- Scheibe type
- Bing–Siebenmann type
- Waardenburg's syndrome
- Pendred's syndrome
- Mondini–Alexander type
- Michel type
- Usher's syndrome
- Endemic cretinism
- Klippel–Feil syndrome

b. Non-genetic
- Diseases occurring in pregnancy
  - Rubella and other viral illnesses
  - Toxaemia
  - Diabetes
  - Syphilis
  - Nephritis
- Drugs taken in pregnancy
  - Streptomycin
  - Quinine
  - Salicylates
  - Thalidomide

2 Peri-natal
- Prematurity
- Jaundice-haemolytic disease and kernicterus
- Anoxia due to birth trauma

3 Post-natal
a. Genetic
- Familial degenerative deafness
- Otosclerosis
- Alport's syndrome

b. Non-genetic infectious diseases
- Measles
- Mumps
- Meningitis
  - Meningococcal
  - Pneumococcal
  - Viral
  - Tuberculous
- Trauma
- Otitis media
- Ototoxic antibiotics
  - Streptomycin
  - Neomycin
  - Gentamicin

Four main types of *structural abnormality* associated with severe hearing loss have been described:

1 The *Scheibe* structural abnormality is characterized by failure of sacculo-cochlear development.

2 The *Mondini* type of dysplasia in which both vestibular and cochlear structures are deformed.

3 The *Bing* abnormality, in which there is a normal bony labyrinth but the membranous labyrinth is malformed or degenerate in both the cochlea and vestibule. In children with this malformation other central nervous system abnormalities may be present.

4 The *Michel* group of abnormalities mainly affect the otic capsule with almost complete lack of development of the inner ear. This particular type of abnormality is often associated with mental retardation.

Non-genetically determined syndromes

These include the following:

- Waardenburg's syndrome: this is an example of the group of integumentary system disease and deafness. A white forelock and heterochromia of the iris are combined with familial genetic deafness.
- Pendred's syndrome: this is a syndrome which comprises congenital goitre and hypothyroidism with severe abnormalities of the labyrinth in both the vestibular and cochlear parts.

A large group of abnormalities is described where hearing loss is associated with eye disease, retinal abnormalities, myopia, optic atrophy and corneal degeneration. For example, *Usher's syndrome* is deafness combined with retinitis pigmentosa.

Late-onset genetic deafness is now considered to be an important cause of deafness in childhood and later life than had been previously thought. *Alport's syndrome* is an example of this, and is also representative of a group of syndromes where genetic hearing loss is associated with nephritis and lenticonus.

Non-genetic prenatal influences are also well recognized as causes of significant hearing loss. Rubella is the most widely known example, and one that is potentially preventable by the use of vaccination programmes. Other peri-natal causes of hearing loss are also potentially preventable, for example peri-natal anoxia or jaundice.

Post-natal causes of profound sensorineural hearing loss include *mumps* and *meningitis*. Curiously, the hearing loss acquired with mumps is nearly always unilateral, and this serves to identify it on occasion.

The proportion of the various groups of conditions causing congenital deafness has been estimated as one-quarter each of genetic, maternal rubella, perinatal causes and unknown. Genetic causes – either alone or as a contributory factor by increasing the liability to other influences – are being increasingly implicated. In areas of the world where consanguineous marriages are common, genetic sensorineural deafness is reported to comprise 70–80 per cent of cases. A careful family history is most important in making a probable diagnosis.

A different scheme of classification is appropriate for adults (Table D.3).

More common causes of sensorineural deafness

Many of these conditions in adults have been considered above. Some, however, require further attention.

Refsum's disease is yet another syndrome combining eye disease (retinitis pigmentosa), polyneuritis, cerebellar ataxia and a genetic late-onset deafness. The inheritance is autosomal recessive.

Acoustic trauma from noise is wholly preventable, and entirely untreatable. It may be diagnosed from the history and the audiogram that shows a typical curve, sharply falling in the higher frequencies with a characteristic dip at 4 kHz (Fig. D.5). Noise-induced hearing loss may be demonstrated audiometrically as either temporary (noise-induced temporary threshold shift, NITTS) or permanent (noise-induced permanent threshold shift, NIPTS) and may be caused by sudden loud sounds such as gunfire or by continuous trauma such as traffic noise, industrial noise,

Table D.3 Causes of deafness in older children and in adults

1 Cochlear lesions
- Late-onset genetic deafness
  - Familial degenerative
  - Alport's syndrome
  - Refsum's syndrome
  - Otosclerosis (later cochlear effects)
- Inflammatory (labyrinthitis)
  - Bacterial
  - Late-onset rubella
  - Syphilis
  - Mumps
  - Herpes
  - Measles
- Trauma
  - Fracture of temporal bone
  - Acoustic trauma
    - Temporary
    - Permanent
- Vascular lesions
  - Atherosclerosis
  - Hypertension
  - Vascular accident of end-artery
  - Ménière's disease (labyrinthine hydrops)
  - Lermoyez's syndrome
  - Leukaemia
  - Malaria
- Degenerative (partly vascular)
  - Presbyacusis
- Vitamin deficiency
  - Vitamin B deficiency
- Dietary
  - Tropical ataxic neuropathy
- Hormonal
  - Myxoedema
  - Pregnancy

- Drug-induced deafness
  - Antibiotics
    - Aminoglycosides
      - Streptomycin
      - Neomycin
      - Gentamicin
    - Others in large doses
  - Aspirin (reversible deafness)
  - Quinine
  - Chloroquine
  - Chemotherapeutic agents for malignant disease
- Unknown

2 Retrocochlear lesions
a. Neural
  - Acoustic neuroma (VIIIth nerve neurilemmoma)
  - Meningitis
    - Leptomeningitis
    - Syphilitic
    - Tuberculous
  - Cerebello-pontine angle tumour
  - Trauma
  - Carcinomatous neuropathy
  - Vogt–Koyanagi syndrome
  - Harada's disease
  - Unknown
b. Central
  - Multiple sclerosis
  - Encephalitis
  - Meningomyelitis
  - Pontine glioma
  - Concussion
  - Vascular accidents
  - Brainstem damage from head injury
  - Psychogenic–hysterical
  - Unknown

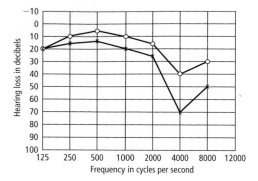

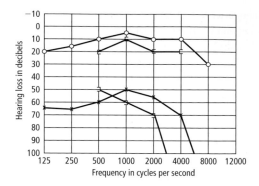

Figure D.5 Audiogram showing the typical findings in noise-induced hearing loss. In this case the patient had been shooting for some years with a 12-bore gun; the left ear, being nearer the muzzle, has sustained greater damage than the right.

Figure D.6 Audiogram in a case of Menière's disease affecting the left labyrinth. Careful investigations are required to exclude acoustic neuroma if unilateral sensorineural deafness such as this is found.

agricultural noise or even 'pop' music. Compensation is awarded on a very large scale to workers exposed to noise in industry who have not been provided with and made to use noise protection. This affects mainly ship-yard and railway workers, motor car industry workers and miners. Unfortunately, no amount of compensation can make up for the hearing loss or impaired quality of life. Tinnitus is very frequently present in noise-induced hearing loss and contributes to the misery experienced by those deafened by this means.

Vascular lesions of the inner ear are the cause (or part cause) of many cases of deafness. Sudden, small vascular accidents in the end-arterioles may cause deafness by damaging part or the whole of the organ of Corti.

The cause of *Menière's disease* (Fig. D.6) is not fully known and is probably multi-factorial, but the end result is an increase in endolymphatic pressure. Episodes of increased pressure give rise to a sensation of fullness in the affected ear that is followed by intense rotatory vertigo and impaired hearing. After a period of hours, the vertigo subsides and hearing improves. With repeated attacks, permanent damage is sustained by both the organ of Corti and the vestibular sensory epithelium. The effect of repeated attacks is cumulative. The diagnosis of Menière's disease is made from the typical history. The disease shows periods of remission between paroxysms of attacks. *Lermoyez's syndrome* is a variant of Menière's disease where the hearing improves very suddenly after an attack of vertigo and tinnitus. It is thought that the membranous labyrinth ruptures, releasing the endolymphatic pressure and restoring cochlear function. Other conditions can

also cause endolymphatic hydrops, for example, myx-oedema, post-meningitic and head-injury syndromes.

Leukaemia causes haemorrhage in the inner ear, whilst in *malaria* destruction of the blood cells results in pigment being left in the cells. Deafness in this disease may also be caused by antimalarial drugs.

Presbyacusis (senile deafness) is common to mankind, and loss of hearing in the higher frequencies is almost invariable with age, though the rate is dependent upon genetic background, exposure to noise (city dwellers lose their hearing more rapidly than country dwellers) and vascular changes associated with atherosclerosis. The audiogram in Fig. D.7 shows an increasing depression in the high frequencies. Failure to discriminate speech ('I can hear you talking, but I cannot hear what you say'), particularly in background noise, is characteristic of this high tone hearing loss as the consonant sounds that give speech its intelligibility are carried in this part of the frequency spectrum.

Drug-induced deafness, *ototoxicity*, results not only from systemic treatment but can also develop following excessive use of topical eardrops. Amino-glycoside antibiotics, loop diuretics, cytotoxic agents, quinine and aspirin are the most commonly implicated substances. Among the neural and central lesions *vestibular schwannomas* (*acoustic neuromas*) are important because they are silent, slow-growing, difficult to diagnose and potentially lethal if not found when reasonably small. They are usually solitary, but in patients with neurofibromatosis type 2 (NF2) are characteristically bilateral and associated with other intracranial tumours. The presentation of these tumours is usually with a progressive unilateral sensorineural deafness

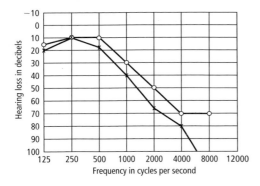

Figure D.7 Audiogram showing the fairly symmetrical hearing loss for high tones in presbyacusis.

often accompanied by tinnitus. Vertigo or unsteadiness is also not uncommon, and is frequently misdiagnosed as Ménière's disease. As the tumour becomes larger, trigeminal symptoms arise that include progressive sensory deficits or even trigeminal neuralgia. Diagnosis of acoustic neuroma, after clinical, audiometric and vestibular tests is made by MRI (Fig. D.8).

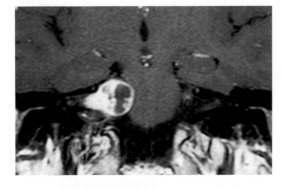

Figure D.8 A magnetic resonance scan showing an acoustic neuroma compressing the brainstem.

The *Vogt–Koyanagi syndrome*, from which it is thought that the artist Goya suffered, is a sudden and rare illness with severe headache and malaise which goes on to uveitis, alopecia, vitiligo and deafness. *Harada's disease* is very similar, but with retinal detachment instead of uveitis. The deafness is usually permanent but the uveitis recovers. The depressing effects of sudden complete deafness on a sensitive artist such as Goya explains his change of style from brightly coloured, happy pictures of handsome men and pretty girls to those of his later 'Black

Period' and the 'Disasters of War'. This is an indication of the severe psychological effects that deafness may bring.

Michael Gleeson

DELUSIONS

A delusion has been defined as a false unshakeable conviction which is out of keeping with the patient's educational, cultural and social background. It is a belief which is held with great certainty, and patients themselves may not complain of this symptom but will come to medical attention because they have acted on a delusional belief or relatives have become aware of their unusual or bizarre content. A delusion should be distinguished from an *over-valued idea*, which is a comprehendible conviction held beyond the bounds of reason. For example, morbid jealousy is an over-valued idea when a spouse who is unduly preoccupied by thoughts of their partner's suspected infidelity can be reassured after lengthy persuasion that their belief is irrational. In delusional jealousy on the other hand, such reassurance would not be possible because the spouse would be convinced of infidelity in the face of all evidence to the contrary. Delusions are also to be distinguished from obsessional ideas which may be bizarre but trouble the patient and are seen by them as intrusive, unwanted and requiring some response (see OBSESSION, p. 494). Similarly, religious and political non-conformity – however extreme – does not represent delusional belief when it is in keeping with the culture to which the person belongs.

Delusions may be caused by organic disease, by drug or substance abuse, or they may be signs of a functional psychotic illness (Table D.4).

Organic delusional state

Delusions may be a prominent feature of a number of quite diverse conditions, and organic causes should be considered in any patient, particularly if delusions arise for the first time in someone over the age of 35 years. Substances such as amphetamines, cocaine and phencyclidine – if taken intravenously – cause an initial feeling of well-being and confidence. Intoxication with high doses may however lead to an episode of paranoid delusions with visual, auditory and tactile

Table D.4 Delusions

Common causes	
Schizophrenia	■ Bromocriptine
Depression	■ L-dopa
Mania	■ Corticosteroids
Delusional disorders	Alzheimer's-type dementia
Substance abuse	Multi-infarct dementia
■ Alcohol	Temporal lobe epilepsy
■ Amphetamines	Hyperthyroidism
■ Methylphenidate	Encephalopathies including HIV
■ Cocaine	Head injury
■ Cannabis	
■ Hallucinogens (e.g. LSD)	**Rarer causes**
■ Phencyclidine	Neurosyphilis
Delirium	Cerebral abscess
Drugs	Multiple sclerosis

hallucinations, incoherent speech and anxious mood. Associated with these mental phenomena are tachycardia, pupillary dilatation, elevated blood pressure, sweating and sometimes nausea. Full recovery is usual within 48 hours, but cessation of regular heavy use may lead to a withdrawal state which again may be associated with paranoid delusions and suicidal ideation, fatigue, depression and agitation persisting for several days. Cocaine, shortly after intake, leads in some users to the rapid onset of a delusional disorder which can persist for over a week and occasionally for several months. Delusions are usually persecutory, and other features are body image distortion, the feeling of insects on the skin (cocaine bug) and sometimes aggression directed against imagined persecutors. Cannabis and hallucinogens such as LSD may also cause paranoid delusions in some users.

An organic delusional state may develop in some subjects with temporal lobe epilepsy who show interictal features similar to schizophrenia.

Delusions in functional psychoses

In the absence of organic causes, delusional thinking is commonly a symptom of *schizophrenia*, the *delusional disorders*, *mania* or *depression*. To distinguish these possibilities, considerable stress is placed on whether or not the contents of the delusions are congruent or incongruent with the prevailing mood of the patient. For example, when a depressed patient expresses the delusion that there is a plot to kill him, this is in keeping with the depressed mood – as is the case with a manic patient who believes he has been invested with special powers and has a mission to save the world. These delusions are said to be secondary because an understandable connection can be made between the patient's mood and the content of the delusion. Moreover, these beliefs will disappear when the mania and depression have responded to treatment. In schizophrenia, by contrast, the content of delusional thinking is often bizarre and out of keeping with the patient's mood state, and the beliefs often persist. *Primary delusions* describe those beliefs which take the form of sudden convictions that come into the patient's mind in response to what the ordinary observer would consider a totally unrelated experience. For example, a patient when reading the number plate of a passing car suddenly became convinced that the driver was accusing him of being a homosexual. Primary delusions of this sort are observed more often in schizophrenia than affective illness. Schizophrenic patients may also experience *delusional mood* when they are perplexed, unsettled and convinced that something self-referential is occurring but are unable to understand what it is. There is no hard and fast distinction between the types of delusions found in schizophrenia, mania and depression, but clinical observation suggests that certain types of delusion are more commonly associated with schizophrenia. These include the delusion that the body is being influenced by outside forces and the subject is being 'made' to perform certain acts, think certain thoughts or, rarely, to feel certain emotions. The patient may complain that alien thoughts have been inserted into their head, or that their own thoughts have been removed. Some commonly encountered delusions which may occur just as frequently in schizophrenia as affective illness include persecutory beliefs, grandiose delusions and delusions of guilt, poverty, worthlessness and hypochondriacal beliefs. Both *grandiose* and *depressive delusions* are often set in a religious context, although beliefs in influence by radio, radar and other real or imagined physical forces are also common.

Monosymptomatic delusions sometimes occur in a patient whose thinking, mood and behaviour show none of the disturbances normally associated with schizophrenia or affective psychosis. Morbid jealously, the total conviction of the spouse's infidelity – although sometimes associated with the psychoses, alcohol abuse or psychopathic personality – may also occur as the only symptom when it must nevertheless be taken seriously by the clinician as a significant cause of domestic violence and even homicide. Other delusions which occur in isolation as well as in the context of major psychotic illness include delusions of love (*de Clerambault's syndrome*) in which the patient believes that some person, usually an authority figure, is in love with them, and delusions of misidentification (*Capgras syndrome*) in which the patient believes that someone close to them, for example a wife, has been replaced by an impostor pretending to be that person. *Somatic* (*hypochondriacal*) delusions take several forms. The person may be convinced that certain parts of the body (brain, intestine, stomach) are not functioning, or in extreme cases are not there at all. There may be conviction of an internal parasite or infestation on or in the skin. The body may be held to be misshapen or ugly, or there may be a belief that a foul smell is emanating from it. Hypochondriacal delusions are frequently found in depression, and may include the belief that the patient is dying from an incurable disease such as cancer. However, such beliefs may also occur in the absence of other overt psychiatric abnormality. Delusions concerning the face, mouth, teeth and gums may be accompanied by frequent and persistent demands for medical and dental investigations, and be the basis for litigation. Some patients with monosymptomatic delusions are considered depressed or schizophrenic, but in others the condition is not well understood and difficult to treat.

Delusions on their own have little diagnostic significance, and their assessment must take account of all aspects of the patient's physical and mental state as well as their cultural background. Brief delusional ideas may develop in normal people following severe sleep deprivation, and delusions – often of a persecutory nature – will develop in a person in strange or unusual surroundings, especially when under stress. In delirium, delusions develop when consciousness is clouded and the cause of the condition may be apparent. Delusions in the delirious (acutely confused) patient tend to be fleeting, poorly formed and drawn from the immediate environment (e.g. '… the nurses are trying to poison me'). Similarly, in chronic organic states delusions will rarely be the only presenting feature, and the diagnosis will be suggested by the memory disturbance and cognitive and other deficits. The differential diagnosis of substance abuse, schizophrenia and mania gives most difficulty particularly

because drug abuse is common in patients with functional psychosis, and may be the precipitant as much as the cause of the delusional state (see also HALLUCINATIONS, p. 273). A careful history and urine drug screen should elucidate the role of stimulants and hallucinogens in a psychotic episode.

Andrew Hodgkiss

DEPERSONALIZATION

Depersonalization is the experience of losing the accustomed sense of one's own reality, and should be distinguished from the very much rarer delusion of not being real occasionally elicited in schizophrenia. A variety of unusual phenomena can accompany depersonalization:

- derealization (a sensation that the outer world is not real)
- emotional numbing
- bodily change (particularly enlargement of head or limbs, lifelessness, unfamiliarity)
- autoscopy
- doubling (perceptions linked to an independently existing double)
- automaton experience with self or others appearing to act or think in a contrived, forced fashion
- disturbance of time sense
- dizziness (a particularly common associated symptom).

Typically, depersonalization is alarming and distressing, which contrasts sharply with the subjective inability to feel emotions: insight is invariably retained (Table D.5).

Depersonalization can be a *normal experience*, occurring in 30–70 per cent of the population. It is commonest in late adolescence and early adulthood, when it is usually mild, transient, associated with fatigue, and of no clinical significance. Depersonalization also occurs physiologically in the rare states of sleep deprivation, sensory deprivation and the near-death experience.

Depersonalization can be generated by the mental mechanism of dissociation as an anxiety-reducing response in stress; hence, *dissociative depersonalization* tends to be less unpleasant or alarming, and not a focus for complaint. This process permits a temporary emotional respite and better coping in circumstances such as battle, accident, admission to hospital

Table D.5 Causes of depersonalization

Commonest	Psychiatric disorders
Normal	■ Phobia
Stress reaction (dissociative	■ Panic
depersonalization)	■ Depression
Anxiety	■ Obsessive–compulsive disorder
	■ Schizophrenia
Less common	■ Post-traumatic stress disorder
Drugs	Insomnia
■ Alcohol	Primary depersonalization
■ Hallucinogens	syndrome
■ Stimulants	
■ Cannabis	**Rare**
■ Anticholinergics	Psychiatric disorders
■ Benzodiazepines	■ Hysteria
Drug withdrawal	■ Malingering
Fever	Sleep deprivation
Neurological disorders	Sensory deprivation
■ Head injury	Near-death experience
■ Brain tumour	Brain-washing
■ Encephalitis	
■ Multiple sclerosis	
■ Epilepsy	

or appearance in court, and during the early stages of grief. It can also precede anticipated trauma, and indeed in deliberate self-injury (especially multiple cutting) it may even facilitate the act through diminution of pain. If the stress is prolonged, then dissociative depersonalization can persist equally long, for months or even years, as recounted in the experiences of concentration camp survivors.

Depersonalization in the setting of *psychological disorders is* also common, but it is unusual for this feature to persist or to be the main complaint. The commonest primary conditions are *anxiety, agoraphobia* and *depression*. In anxiety, agoraphobia, panic disorder and chronic hyperventilation syndrome depersonalization is rarely intense or is accompanied by associated experiences apart from derealization, while the amount of anguish and self-concern is substantial, with the fear of going mad frequently expressed. In depression and post-traumatic stress disorder, emotional numbing characteristically accompanies depersonalization, and can even be the predominant feature – bodily change (especially physical lifelessness) may be reported in severe depression. In schizophrenia, depersonalization is usually an early, transient phenomenon with more typical disturbances of identity either present or emergent soon afterwards;

autoscopy, often with emotional detachment, tends to occur when the illness is acute and established.

Drug intoxication or withdrawal can precipitate depersonalization, the commonest associations being reported with *LSD, mescaline, cannabis* and *anticholinergics. Brain disease* or *brain damage* may precipitate or even present with depersonalization. Post-concussional syndrome is usually apparent from the history and accompanying features. However, in temporal lobe disease and/or epilepsy depersonalization may not only be the prime symptom but can also precede positive findings upon neurological examination and investigation. This possibility ought to remain under consideration when the state of depersonalization is severe and persistent, autoscopy or perceptual distortions are present, and there are no apparent stressors or evidence of a primary emotional illness.

Primary depersonalization syndrome is an uncommon condition which presents abruptly in early adulthood with recurrent bouts of severe depersonalization, usually with many of the concomitant features. There are characteristic personality traits associated with this condition, the typical sufferer being described as intelligent, obsessional, introspective, sensitive and hypochondriacal. These patients often have particular difficulty in establishing personal relationships and coping with the general upheaval of adolescence. Their disorder tends to be chronic, readily precipitated by stress and anxiety, but with minimal impairment in social functioning – they are prone to hypochondriasis in later life.

Andrew Hodgkiss

DEPRESSION

Depressed mood is one of the commonest conditions for which patients seek help. Unhappiness is an understandable response to loss of any sort. Depression refers to a more severe and qualitatively different mood change when the patient may describe feelings of hopelessness, misery, tiredness and fatigue and the mood state is communicated by facial expression, gesture, posture, tone of voice and general demeanour. However, not infrequently one has to rely on a history from the patient, their friends and employers to recognize severe depressive illness in some people who do not themselves acknowledge mood change (smiling or masked depression). For cultural and other reasons, some patients have no words for moods and may communicate their distress by hypochondriacal complaints or by seeking advice for marital, employment or a variety of other difficulties.

In uncomplicated bereavement a patient responds to loss by an initial experience of shock, numbness and feelings of emptiness. There is an initial tendency to deny that the loss has occurred, but this gives way to a depressed mood, often with symptoms of anxiety and panic. There may be poor appetite with weight loss, insomnia, impaired concentration and feelings of guilt surrounding the death. Auditory and visual hallucinations of the deceased are commonly reported. The state of grief is resolved as the person accepts the loss and begins to redirect their life and activities. Many cases of depression follow a real or imagined loss or threatening situation, and symptoms are not dissimilar to those of bereavement. However, *major depressive illness* may develop without any clear-cut relation to loss or helplessness, and classification may be based on symptoms, severity and outcome without making any aetiological assumptions. In *major depression* there is a distinct quality of depressive mood which is perceived by the patient as being distinctly different from the feelings of loss experienced in bereavement. These patients describe a loss of pleasure in all their activities (*anhedonia*), and they cannot be even temporarily cheered out of their depression by something good happening in their life. This type of depressive illness is often associated with diurnal variation of mood, the depression being worse in the morning; early morning wakening; psychomotor retardation or agitation; significant appetite impairment; and excessive guilt. In the most severe forms the patient may express delusions of poverty, ill health and persecution congruent with depressed mood and hallucinations which are often voices critical of the patient. There is a high risk of suicide, and suicidal ideation must always be specifically asked about. There is frequently a family history of depression, and although the illness may develop suddenly without a recognizable precipitant, adverse stressful life events will often have occurred during the weeks preceding the onset of the illness. Major depressive illness can be usefully subdivided into *bipolar depression* (patients have at some stage in their lives experienced an episode of mania) and *unipolar depression* (patients have bouts of depression without mania). Recurrent mild unipolar depression, sometimes described as dysthymia, is a chronic depressed mood persisting for most of the time for 2 years or more. Such patients may present with inability to cope with everyday life, low self-esteem, tiredness, sleep disturbance, somatic complaints and frequently symptoms of anxiety.

Difficulties may arise in the diagnosis of depression, especially when a patient presents with physical symptoms such as headache, low back pain, weight loss, constipation, loss of libido, loss of energy or anorexia. Some patients are worried that they may have cancer, venereal disease, angina or memory loss, and the physician's attention is directed towards an investigation of these physical conditions. In the elderly, depression may present as a *pseudodementia* which may be initially difficult to distinguish from dementia but which should respond well to standard anti-depressant measures.

Anxiety may be a principal feature of depressive illness, and such cases may be termed *agitated depression*. The patient may be restless and unable to relax during the interview, wringing hands, pulling hair, shifting legs, or pacing around the room. *Obsessional symptoms* can develop during a depressive illness, and these will generally improve when the depression is treated. However, patients with obsessive personality or obsessive–compulsive disorder are also very prone to develop depressive episodes.

Depression in other psychiatric illnesses

Depression is a common accompaniment of almost all other psychiatric disorders. An episode of depression may herald the onset of a schizophrenic illness, and patients with schizophrenia are more prone to suffer from depression – perhaps because of the nature of their symptoms, the social and other handicaps of the illness, or perhaps because mood change is an integral part of the disease itself. Depression is particularly common and difficult to treat immediately following the resolution of an acute exacerbation of schizophrenia.

Physical disease and depression

A number of possible mechanisms account for the very high instance of depression in almost all types of

Table D.6 Physical causes of depression

1 Physical diseases which may cause depression
Infections
- Influenza
- Hepatitis
- Infectious mononucleosis
- Brucellosis
- Toxoplasmosis

Endocrine disorders
- Hypothyroidism
- Hyperadrenocorticalism
- Hypoadrenocorticalism
- Hypoparathyroidism
- Hypopituitarism
- Pancreatic, pulmonary, thyroid carcinomas
- Acute intermittent porphyria
- Disseminated lupus erythematosus
- Folate, vitamin B_{12} deficiency

Neurological diseases
- Multi-infarct dementia
- Alzheimer's dementia
- Pick's disease
- Huntington's chorea
- Multiple sclerosis
- Parkinson's disease
- Temporal lobe epilepsy
- Head injury
- Cerebrovascular disease and stroke
- Subdural haematoma
- Subarachnoid haemorrhage
- Cerebral tumour
- Encephalitis
- Neurosyphilis
- AIDS

2 Drugs which can cause depression
- Reserpine
- Alpha-methyldopa
- Beta-blockers
- Corticosteroids
- Oral contraceptives
- L-dopa
- Indomethacin
- Isoniazid
- Cycloserine
- Withdrawal from alcohol
- Withdrawal from amphetamine and related drugs (fenfluramine, diethylproprion)
- Withdrawal from cocaine and phencyclidine
- Use of hallucinogens
- Opioid intoxication

physical disease (Table D.6). Pain, incapacity and loss of health, independence and social status are entirely understandable causes of depression during and following illness. Some illnesses, however, are more specifically linked with depression. Several endocrine disorders may present as depression, including *hypothyroidism, hypo-* and *hyperadrenocorticolism, hypoparathyroidism* and *hypopituitaryism.* Certain forms of *carcinoma,* particularly those of the pancreas, thyroid and lung, may cause depression months before other symptoms of the tumour are manifest, possibly due to brain-active peptides being synthesized and released from the tumour. With most central nervous system diseases depression is a common accompaniment. In multi-infarct and Alzheimer's-type dementia, depressive symptoms may arise because the patient is aware of their failing powers, but direct cerebral damage may also be implicated. An interaction between a normal response to incapacitating illness and the direct effects of brain damage probably account for mood disturbances found in Huntington's chorea, multiple sclerosis, Parkinson's disease, temporal lobe epilepsy, certain types of head injury and cerebral vascular disease.

Drugs which can cause depression

These include both therapeutic agents and drugs of abuse. The former include antihypertensive agents, steroids and antibiotics. Withdrawal from alcohol is a very common cause of depression; withdrawal from amphetamines, the appetite-suppressants fenfluramine and diethlypropion, cocaine and phencyclidine may precipitate mood change, particularly in chronic users. Intoxication with opioids and the use of hallucinogens may trigger severe mood disturbance.

Depression may present at any age, and the diagnosis in children is more difficult. In prepubertal children there may be somatic complaints, agitation, anxiety disorders, avoidance behaviour and phobias. In adolescents, a mood disturbance may be accompanied by negativistic or antisocial behaviour, abuse of alcohol and illicit drugs and feelings of restlessness, aggression, withdrawal from social activities, poor school performance and complaints of not being understood.

Andrew Hodgkiss

DIARRHOEA

This term is taken to imply the passage of frequent, poorly formed stools. It is important to ensure that both patient and healthcare worker alike are talking about the same thing when this symptom is being discussed. It should be borne in mind that the patient's and the physician's ideas of normality with respect to bowel function may be quite different.

The terms osmotic (impaired fluid absorption) and secretory (excessive fluid excretion) have been used to classify diarrhoea with respect to underlying physiology; examples include malabsorptive states and certain bacterial infections, respectively. The nature of the diarrhoea gives some indication as to the potential site of pathology; frequent, small-volume stools suggest a large-bowel origin, whereas less frequent but large-volume, often watery stools indicate a possible small-bowel cause. The association of other symptoms such as passage of blood per rectum or abdominal pain yields information as to specific underlying pathology:

- Frequent small, usually formed, stools: colorectal cancer, diverticular disease, adenomatous polyps, solitary rectal ulcer or normal bowel.
- Frequent, poorly formed stools: colorectal cancer, diverticular disease, adenomatous polyps, infection (*Salmonella*, *Campylobacter*, *E. coli*, *Staphylococcus*, *Bacillus cereus*, *Yersinia*, *Clostridium difficile*, tuberculosis, schistosomiasis, cytomegalovirus, small-bowel bacterial overgrowth, worms), inflammatory bowel disease (Crohn's disease and ulcerative colitis), gluten enteropathy, tropical sprue, small-bowel lymphoma, medications (laxatives, non-steroidal anti-inflammatory drugs, proton-pump inhibitors, fluoxitine), exocrine pancreatic insufficiency (cancer, chronic pancreatitis, cystic fibrosis), infiltrative disorders (scleroderma, amyloid), hyperthyroidism, Whipple's disease.
- Frequent, watery bowel motions: collagenous/lymphocytic colitis; bile salt malabsorption (secondary to terminal ileal resection, Crohn's disease), infection (giardiasis, cryptosporidiosis) surgery (vagotomy, cholecystectomy, gastrectomy, small-bowel resection), enteric fistula, rapid transport (osmotic effect due to food), Crohn's disease, arthropathy-associated terminal ileitis (ankylosing spondylitis), diet (fruit), disaccharidase deficiency, post-infectious irritable bowel syndrome, terminal ileal Crohn's disease.
- Frequent large volume, watery bowel motions: neuroendocrine tumours (vipoma, gastrinoma), enteric fistula, infection (Norwalk/Rotavirus, cryptosporidiosis, blastocystis hominis, cholera), drugs, surgery.

As there are myriad causes for diarrhoea, it is important to relate this symptom to the patient's history:

- elderly (cancer, polyps, diverticular disease, ischaemic colitis)
- female (collagenous/lymphocytic colitis)
- young/thin female (laxative abuse)
- predominant constipation (spurious diarrhoea)
- travel/local conditions (infection, post-infectious irritable bowel syndrome)
- previous episodes (inflammatory bowel disease, irritable bowel syndrome)
- medications (recent broad-spectrum antibiotics, NSAIDs, proton-pump inhibitors, fluoxitine, immunosuppressants, etc.)
- other conditions (cystic fibrosis, scleroderma)
- recent-onset diabetes mellitus (pancreatic cancer with insufficiency)
- systemic features (inflammatory bowel disease, ankylosing spondylitis)
- previous surgery (vagotomy, Polya gastrectomy, cholecystectomy, terminal ileal resection, blind loop, recent coeliac axis neurolysis, transplant)
- family history (inflammatory bowel disease, gluten enteropathy, colorectal cancer/polyposis, multiple endocrine neoplasia)
- gluten enteropathy with recent deterioration (lymphoma).

The presence of blood in the stool suggests a large-bowel cause: cancer, adenomatous polyps, ischaemic colitis, infection (*Shigella*), inflammatory bowel disease (ulcerative colitis and Crohn's colitis), solitary rectal ulcer, neutropenic colitis, Loeffler's syndrome (Fig. D.9). Bleeding due to diverticular disease is generally of large volume, although a mild non-specific colitis often associated with this condition may give rise to passage of lesser amounts. Tumours of the proximal colon are increasingly common, and may present with melaena.

Colicky abdominal pain – particularly with associated bloating – might be suggestive of irritable bowel syndrome or of a small-bowel cause. Crohn's disease and ileocaecal tuberculosis may present with the paradoxical combination of subacute obstructive-like symptoms and diarrhoea. Protracted lower abdominal pain, particularly after defaecation, can be associated with distal ulcerative/Crohn's colitis. A sensation of incomplete evacuation can accompany the presence of a rectal tumour.

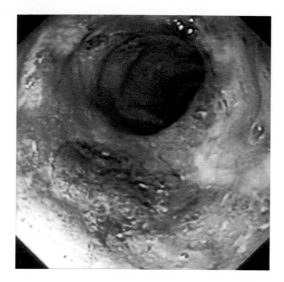

Figure D.9 Sigmoid colon with characteristic oedematous, haemorrhagic mucosa suggestive of acute ulcerative colitis.

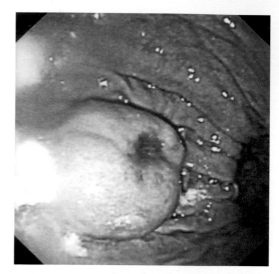

Figure D.10 Submucosal gastric polypoid lesion with apical ulceration suggestive of gastrointestinal stromal cell tumour (GIST) or leiomyoma. Endoscopic ultrasound guided Tru-cut biopsy demonstrated CD117-positive cells characteristic for a GIST.

History and physical examination can only narrow the range of likely conditions present, and specific tests are always required in order to make a firm diagnosis. It is of paramount importance that cancer be excluded in patients over the age of 50 years (or younger in those with a family history), even if the symptoms appear trivial.

The single most important test is colonoscopy, to the terminal ileum where possible, with serial biopsies. Barium enema, CT enema, virtual colonoscopy, flexible sigmoidoscopy and rigid sigmoidoscopy are helpful procedures, but their use involves some degree of compromise. A small-bowel barium meal or enteroclysis (jejunal intubation with instillation of barium) may identify malabsorptive states and conditions such as Crohn's disease and lymphoma. Capsule wireless videoendoscopy is rarely helpful for investigating diarrhoea, and is not indicated for identifying colonic pathology (Figs D.10 and D.11).

Gastroscopy with distal duodenal biopsy will identify some enteropathies (particularly coeliac disease), but this latter condition may be more easily screened for by serology (anti-endomysial or tissue transglutaminase antibodies). False-negative serology may occur in patients with low levels of IgA, so serum protein electrophoresis can be a helpful adjunctive test.

Absorptive tests (pancreolauryl test), stool testing for fat and trypsinogen levels and MRI with secretin

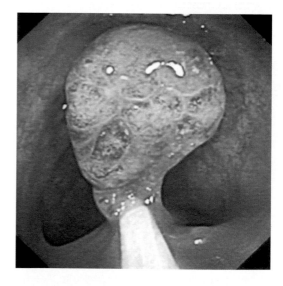

Figure D.11 Snare polypectomy of a pedunculated sigmoid adenoma.

provocation or endoscopic ultrasound yield information on pancreatic function and structure. Today, endoscopic retrograde cholangiopancreatography (ERCP) is less commonly used for diagnostic studies on account of the risk of inducing acute pancreatitis (about 5%).

Stool cultures for culture and ova/parasites is always important, even in known cases of inflammatory bowel disease. A specific request must be made for *Clostridium difficile* Toxin A if pseudomembranous colitis is suspected. Peri-anal sampling with adhesive tape may identify pin worms. Stool levels of calprotectin in association with small-bowel sugar permeability testing can be used to triage young patients with suspected irritable bowel syndrome for colonoscopy; low levels are rarely seen with mucosal pathology of the colon or terminal ileum such as Crohn's disease.

John Meenan

DIPLOPIA

Diplopia, or double vision, is the earliest symptom apparent to the patient with dysconjugate gaze of the two eyes. It is seen with ocular paresis or following loss of normal binocular control. It is usually binocular in nature, and is rarely described in monocular form. Usually, an object is seen singly with each eye separately but appears double when both eyes are open.

Binocular diplopia

Physiological diplopia

This is a normal phenomenon in all binocular vision. Since the two eyes observe an object from different directions, the retinal images differ, but the double vision is not apparent since the dissimilar images are combined by the visual centres in the brain to form a single solid conception of the object viewed. This physiological appearance of the two retinal images is called 'disparateness'. Such physiological diplopia is sometimes noticed by an individual who realizes that, when fixing on a particular object, other objects which are closer or further away than the object of fixation may be seen double. Patients who are anxious or unduly introspective may need reassurance about this normal phenomenon. If the centre in the brain which controls the fusion of the two images is disturbed, as after the excessive consumption of alcohol, the normal balance of the muscular mechanisms of the eyes may be lost and diplopia experienced.

Pathological diplopia

In normal binocular vision both eyes are aligned so that the image of the object fixated falls upon the central and most sensitive part of the retina. Other objects form images upon more peripheral areas of the retina, and are less well observed. When an individual is looking at a particular point ahead, the image of any object lying to the right of the eyes will fall upon the nasal side of the right retina and the temporal side of the left retina, and these different areas of the retinas will always correspond and, in normal circumstances, will always be stimulated simultaneously. If the relative position of the two eyes is upset, the image of an object no longer falls upon the two corresponding areas of the retina, erroneous forms of projection occur, and there is consequent diplopia. An examination of this diplopia leads to the ascertainment of the type of displacement of the eye.

In a paralytic strabismus where one of the eyes is not able to move normally in one direction, the image seen by the affected eye, lying away from the macula of the retina, is usually less distinct. A more reliable way of distinguishing which image is the false one is by finding the direction of gaze in which the images are most displaced, and then performing a 'cover test' in which each eye is alternately covered; the eye which subtends the more distal image is the one which has the paralysed muscle. Alternatively, the use of a red glass test or a Maddox rod test – the former to create red and white images with white light, and the latter to create a white pin-point image and a red line image – may be used to identify the images arising from the different eyes. For example, if the greatest horizontal separation of images is on looking to the right, either the right lateral rectus or the left medial rectus is weak. The image which is projected farther from the centre is that arising in the paretic eye and by covering one eye after the other this may be determined.

Binocular diplopia may be caused by paralysis of any extraocular muscle, and it will also be seen when there is displacement of one of the globes, as with an intraorbital tumour, abscess, haemorrhage or cavernous sinus thrombosis. It may also be seen following an operation on the extraocular muscles if the excursion of one eye is limited by scarring. Binocular diplopia arising from disease within the orbit will frequently be associated with pain or discomfort, and often with proptosis. The investigation of such syndromes is optimally undertaken with CT or MRI scanning of the orbits.

Double vision may be seen in the elderly after local cerebral ischaemic events; it is usually thought to be of intrinsic-brainstem origin, and is often temporary.

Patients with true paralytic strabismus will be identified as having lesions affecting the IIIrd, IVth or VIth cranial nerves, either singly or in combination, and investigations of the relevant areas may then be undertaken with CT or MRI imaging, cerebrospinal fluid (CSF) examination and possibly angiography. Rarely, orbital myositis will cause problems in eye movement and result in diplopia. Occasionally, neuromuscular junction disorders will affect the eye as in ocular myasthenia. The diagnosis may be confirmed by the use of intravenous edrophonium and by single-fibre electromyography (EMG) studies (Table D.7).

Diplopia may occasionally be seen in patients with pituitary exophthalmos or with thyroid disturbances resulting in dysthyroid eye disease.

Table D.7 Differential diagnosis of binocular diplopia

True ocular palsy: due to lesion of IIIrd, IVth or VIth cranial nerve, or of extraocular muscles

1 Lesion of IIIrd, IVth or VIth nerve
- Congenital, e.g. agenesis, malformation
- Inflammation, e.g. encephalitis, neurosyphilis, disseminated sclerosis, herpes zoster, Tolosa–Hunt syndrome, pseudotumour of orbit
- Neoplasms, e.g. primary or secondary intracranial, meningeal tumour
- Toxic, e.g. alcohol, carbon monoxide, lead
- Vascular, e.g. thrombosis, haemorrhage, embolism, aneurysm (intracavernous), cavernous sinus thrombosis, giant cell arteritis, diabetes, hypertension, ophthalmoplegic migraine
- Traumatic
- Raised intracranial pressure
2 Lesion of extraocular muscle
- Congenital, e.g. agenesis, malformation, Möbius' syndrome
- Traumatic, including postoperative scarring or surgical overcorrection
- Myopathy, e.g. endocrine, ocular myopathy, carcinomatous, iatrogenic
- Inflammation, e.g. ocular myositis
- Disorder of neuromuscular transmission, e.g. myasthenia gravis

Relative ocular palsy: due to lesion in orbit resulting in deviation of visual axis
- Traumatic, e.g. damage to supports of eyeball, fracture of orbital floor
- Space-occupying lesion of orbit causing exophthalmos, e.g. tumour, haemorrhage, inflammatory lesion, mucocele, endocrine conditions

Ocular palsies may be central, that is due to a lesion of the nucleus or of the parenchymal portion of the cranial nerve. Alternatively, they may be peripheral, arising along the tract of the cranial nerve within the posterior or middle fossa or in the orbit itself. Lesions which can damage individual cranial nerves subserving eye movement include posterior communicating artery aneurysm, classically causing IIIrd nerve palsy, aneurysms within the cavernous sinus, raised intracranial pressure, resulting in VIth nerve palsy, and vascular lesions of the trunk of the nerve; these are the commonest cause of IVth nerve palsy. The VIth nerve may also be affected near the apex of the petrous bone when involvement with a local infective process or a nasopharyngeal tumour have to be included in the differential diagnosis.

The rare occurrence in children of episodes of ocular palsy in conjunction with unilateral headache may be recognized as ophthalmoplegic migraine. There is a rare condition in which an inflammatory or granulomatous process in the anterior portion of the cavernous sinus or superior orbital fissure may involve any one of the nerves responsible for eye movement (Tolosa–Hunt syndrome).

The acute development of a bilateral ophthalmoplegia is most commonly seen in brainstem lesions or in post-infective cranial neuropathies (Guillain–Barré syndrome), whereas the chronic development of a bilateral ophthalmoplegia is most often seen with ocular myopathy, as in one of the mitochondrial cytopathies.

There are rare examples of pseudoparalysis of ocular muscles. In dysthyroid eye disease a tight inferior or superior rectus muscle may limit upward and downward gaze respectively, and occasionally muscle enlargement may be demonstrated by CT scanning. The Duane syndrome, due to congenital fibrosis of the lateral rectus, causes retraction of the globe on adduction, giving rise to diplopia. However, since it is life-long it is rarely a symptom to the patient, and is more likely to be discovered by the unsuspecting examiner.

Monocular diplopia

This is infrequently found, and may be due to early cataract, or irregularity of the corneal surface, for example following inflammation.

Reginald Daniel

DROP ATTACKS

The term 'drop attack' is applied to a fall occurring without warning and without loss of consciousness or post-ictal confusion. The patients are usually elderly. They suddenly drop to the floor whilst walking or standing; the knees buckle, there is no dizziness or other preceding symptoms, and they usually fall forwards, striking the knees and sometimes the nose upon the ground. Some patients will describe loss of power in the legs, and they are unable to raise their hands to stop the face hitting the ground, implying that normal tonus may be lost in both the lower and the upper limbs. After the episode the patient is able to rise and move immediately. Not infrequently, the falls result in lacerations to the knees and abrasions to the face. Attacks without apparent cause may occur for a few weeks and then stop. They have a benign prognosis, and there is no effective therapy.

It is probable that most 'drop attacks' occur as a result of *brainstem ischaemia*, though a relationship to cardiovascular or cerebrovascular disease is not striking. The fact that some patients describe episodes of double vision, and that some identify weakness and inability to move the arm in association with attacks, suggests involvement of the brainstem, and a form of vertebrobasilar insufficiency is an attractive (though unproven) theory of causation.

'Drop attacks' can occur rarely in the presence of *hydrocephalus* or a *third ventricular tumour*. Although these are important in the differential diagnosis, they are uncommon in the elderly group who are the most liable to 'drop attacks'.

Mark Kinirons

DYSMENORRHOEA

This term comes from the Greek meaning difficult monthly flow; however, it is taken to mean painful menstruation. It is a symptom complex, which includes cramping lower abdominal pain radiating to the back and legs, associated with some gastrointestinal upset, malaise and headaches. The problem can be divided into:

■ *Primary dysmenorrhoea*, when the periods are painful and no organic or psychological cause can be found. It

usually occurs at the beginning of reproductive life when the girl starts ovulating. The pain starts with the onset of menstruation, and is generally associated with ovulatory cycles. There is an abnormally high production of endometrial prostaglandins, which causes excessive uterine contractions. Examination findings are usually normal and further investigation may only be necessary if treatment fails to alleviate the symptoms. The options for treatment include the combined oral contraceptive pill to inhibit ovulation, or non-steroidal anti-inflammatory agents, which act as prostaglandin synthetase inhibitors to decrease the concentration of local prostaglandins and thereby reduce pain and also menstrual loss.

■ *Secondary dysmenorrhoea* occurs when the woman experiences painful periods where an organic or psychosexual cause can be found. The differential diagnosis includes:
  ◆ Pelvic inflammatory disease
  ◆ Endometriosis (Fig. D.12) or adenomyosis
  ◆ Fibroids
  ◆ Intrauterine contraceptive device
  ◆ Cervical stenosis following treatment for precancer
  ◆ Ovarian tumour
  ◆ Previous pelvic or abdominal surgery
  ◆ Previous history of sexual abuse or other psychological problems.

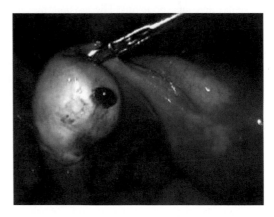

Figure D.12 Endometriosis on an ovary; laparoscopic appearance.

Detailed history is important, and may take time if there is a psychosexual element. A pelvic examination should be performed, and swabs taken if indicated. A tender uterus will usually indicate the possibility of adenomyosis; restricted mobility or a fixed retroverted uterus may suggest the presence of adhesions secondary to endometriosis, pelvic inflammatory disease or previous surgery. A previous history of cone biopsy or other excision procedures for cervical intra-epithelial neoplasia (CIN) might suggest the possibility of cervical stenosis and may require dilatation of the cervix.

Investigations will depend on the history, and in many cases laparoscopy may be indicated to exclude a particular pathology. If the findings are normal, then often reassurance in itself may be sufficient.

Antony Hollingworth

DYSPAREUNIA

Dyspareunia is defined as pain on intercourse, and is probably the most common sexual difficulty which presents to the gynaecologist. This pain may be classified as:

- Superficial, when the pain arises at the vaginal introitus or
- Deep when the pain is felt within the pelvis.

The pain may be either continuous or intermittent in nature, and continue after intercourse is finished. The main question that needs to be asked is whether it prevents intercourse occurring. These symptoms can be further divided into:

- Primary dyspareunia, when intercourse has always been painful; this condition often has a psychological background and may need expert counselling.
- Secondary dyspareunia, when the symptoms have been acquired; this is usually to an organic problem.

Dyspareunia may lead to vaginismus, which is involuntary spasm of the pubococcygeus muscle such that penetration is difficult, or impossible. It may occur after one episode of pain, but may become regular in an attempt to prevent subsequent episodes of pain.

Superficial dyspareunia can be classified according to the local anatomical factors.

Vulval causes of dyspareunia

- Infective vulvitis can occur with herpes or candidal infections. Relevant swabs and antibiotics or antiviral agents are needed.
- Atrophic changes, particularly in post-menopausal women, respond to HRT or topical oestrogens. If oestrogen is

contraindicated, then lubrication with KY jelly may be of value, as may local moisturising preparations (Replens).
- Bartholinitis may be due to local infection of the Bartholin's gland, but can be a site for gonorrhoea. Marsupialization is the standard treatment to drain the cyst and create a new duct for the gland.
- Skin conditions affecting the vulva, including lichen sclerosus (pruritus vulvae), may cause pain as a result of the development of cracks and fissures in the skin.
- Neoplasms – either malignant or premalignant – may cause these symptoms, and would require appropriate diagnosis and treatment.

Urethral causes of dyspareunia

These are very much anatomical problems and are not seen very often in a general gynaecological clinic.

- Urethritis and cystitis may require local swabs or a midstream urine specimen for culture and sensitivity.
- Caruncle should be clearly seen on inspection; this usually occurs in post-menopausal women, and may become inflamed and tender.
- Diverticulum of the urethra is an uncommon condition to present to the gynaecologist.

Vaginal causes of dyspareunia

- Vaginismus, as previously described.
- Atrophic vaginitis; treatment is as above for the atrophic vulva.
- Infective vaginitis with *Candida*, *Trichomonas*, herpes and gonorrhoea. Routine local swabs need to be undertaken, and appropriate treatment instituted.
- Anatomical problems may come to light in the form of vaginal atresia or imperforate hymen. These may require scanning to see if there are further anatomical problems within the pelvis, and an examination to determine the extent of the problem.
- Contractures post surgery – especially for episiotomy or perineal tear repair – which can lead to narrowing of the entrance to the vagina. The introitus may be very tight and require further surgery to relieve the local tightness from the original repair.
- Post radiotherapy; this can be prevented to a great extent by the use of vaginal dilators around the time of initial treatment.

Disproportion in size is rarely in itself of importance, as the vagina is very distensile, but if in addition there is any local lesion the pain will be accentuated. Anal fissure and thrombosed and inflamed piles are recognized by careful examination of the anus and rectum by the finger or speculum. Arthritis of the hips or lumbar spine may cause dyspareunia, though it may not be so well localized.

Deep dyspareunia is due to deep stretching at the time of coitus of the involved pelvic tissues, which include a fixed retroverted uterus, the uterosacral ligaments or rectovaginal septum, or pressure on enlarged ovaries. There may be no pain on penetration and no difficulty, but coitus with deep penetration gives acute pain at the time or leads to dull aching in the pelvis after intercourse. Clinically, the symptoms can be mimicked with vaginal examination. The following are usual causes:

- Pelvic inflammatory disease, where the pelvic organs may be inflamed and adhesions may fix the tissues in place. If this is an acute episode, then antibiotics can be used and it is important to ensure that the partner is also treated. If this is a chronic picture, then pelvic clearance of the genital organs may be a final stage option.
- Endometriosis is a common cause of deep dyspareunia, especially when the uterosacral ligaments are involved (Fig. D.13). The degree of endometriosis does not always mirror the symptoms, the diagnosis being confirmed by diagnostic laparoscopy. Treatment options will depend on the degree of endometriosis, and may involve surgery.
- Ectopic pregnancy may cause peritoneal irritation, which in turn causes dyspareunia. It is not a common presentation for ectopic pregnancy.
- Chronic pelvic pain syndrome with prominent vasculature of the pelvis may be diagnosed at laparoscopy, and can be treated with progestogens.
- Ovarian neoplasm is an unusual cause of dyspareunia.
- Any pelvic pathology that will affect the peritoneum.

Severe constipation can cause dyspareunia in a number of women, and this may be noted at the time of vaginal examination. Diagnostic laparoscopy is used to determine an obvious gynaecological cause, but if the laparoscopy is negative it can serve to reassure the woman that there is no pathology and break the cycle of expecting, and experiencing, pain.

Antony Hollingworth

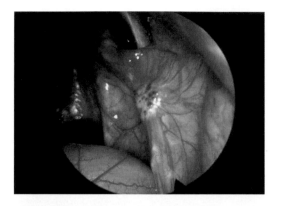

Figure D.13 Endometriosis of the uterosacral ligament; laparoscopic appearance.

DYSPHAGIA

Dysphagia describes the sensation of difficulty in swallowing; the term odynophgia is used to describe painful swallowing. Luminal, mural and extraluminal pathologies may give rise to dysphagia *cancer*, but is the single most important differential diagnosis.

The luminal causes of dysphagia include: adenocarcinoma (usually distal); squamous cell carcinoma (usually proximal, but may be distal); invasive lung or mediastinal tumours (primary and metastatic);

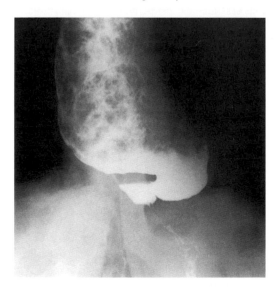

Figure D.14 Achalasia showing gross oesophageal dilatation. The filling defects in the column of barium are due to retained masses of food.

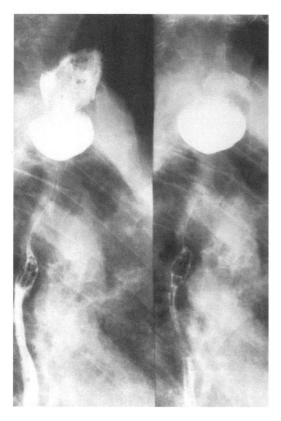

Figure D.15 Diverticulum of the pharynx (pharyngeal pouch), demonstrated on barium swallow.

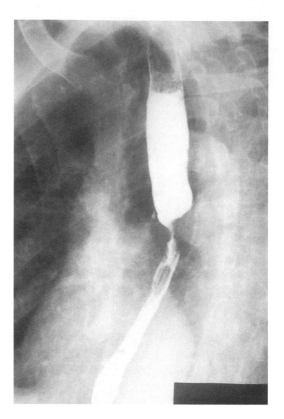

Figure D.16 Carcinoma of the oesophagus, the typical 'rat tail' deformity on barium swallow.

Kaposi's sarcoma; hiatus hernia (especially rolling type); reflux oesophagitis; peptic or lye stricture; epidermolysis bullosa (usually proximal strictures); Crohn's disease; pemphigus; infection (viral: cytomegalovirus, herpes simplex; fungal/yeast: *Candida*; bacterial: tuberculosis); web formation (Plummer–Vinson syndrome associated with iron deficiency); Zenker's diverticulum (pharyngeal pouch); pulsion/traction diverticulum; and foreign bodies.

Diffuse infiltrating conditions such as scleroderma and amyloid, neuropathic states including Chagas' disease (trypanosomiasis, South America) and achalasia (myenteric plexus denervation), as well as bulbar/pseudobulbar palsies may all give rise to dysphagia. Large bronchogenic/re-duplication cysts and massive varices may cause luminal obstruction. When diagnosing achalasia, it is important to be wary of the potential for pseudo-achalasia due to submucosal malignancy of the gastro-oesophageal junction.

A broad range of extraluminal pathologies such as enlargement of the thyroid (carcinoma, cyst, adenoma), thymus (carcinoma) and mediastinal lymph glands (lymphoma, metastatic cancer, tuberculosis, sarcoid) may give rise to dysphagia (Figs D.14–D.17). Primary (sclerosing mediastinitis) or secondary (post-radiotherapy) mediastinal fibrosis may cause dysphagia, even in the absence of obvious luminal compression at endoscopy or on barium studies. This may be due to oesophageal tethering causing dysmotility. The term 'dysphagia lusoria' is used to describe difficulty with swallowing, particularly in children, that results from an aberrant right subclavian artery compressing the oesophagus.

The investigation of dysphagia is a matter of urgency on account of the potential presence of an underlying cancer. The main tool for this investigation is gastroscopy. Evidence of luminal pathology or dysmotility may be garnered from a barium swallow, particularly if swallowing is induced by combining the barium with soft foods such as bread or marshmallows. Oesophageal manometry is combined with subsequent ambulatory 24-hour pH measurement to identify acid

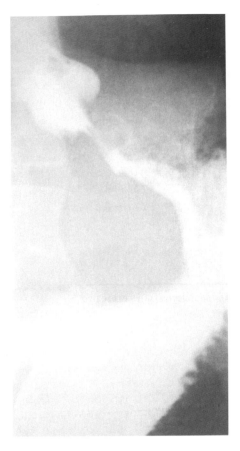

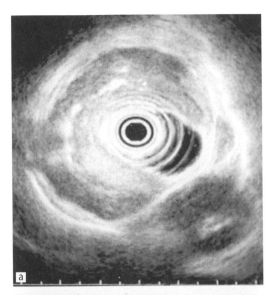

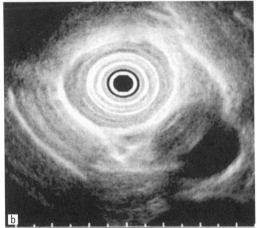

Figure D.17 Barium meal of a patient with severe dysphagia due to an extensive carcinoma of the cardia.

reflux or dysmotility states such as achalasia. Infusion of dilute acid in a blinded fashion (Bernstein test) identifies an 'acid-sensitive' oesophagus. Both CT scanning and endoscopic ultrasound (Fig. D.18) permit the identification of mediastinal pathology, the latter technique allowing tissue sampling. Endoscopy in cases of achalasia is always completely normal, with absolutely no inhibition to scope the passage.

John Meenan

Figure D.18 Endoscopic ultrasound appearances of a distal oesophageal adenocarcinoma (a) before and (b) after neoadjuvant chemotherapy.

DYSPNOEA

Dyspnoea is the clinical word for breathlessness. Although it is the ordinary Greek word for breathlessness, it is not an everyday term for English-speaking people. Thus, the word breathlessness, rather than dyspnoea, will be used throughout this section to emphasize that we are dealing with a sensation or symptom, not a physical sign. Most people intuitively know what is meant by breathlessness, but would find it hard to describe in words. A useful definition is that offered by Comroe in 1966: '... difficult, laboured, uncomfortable breathing; it is an unpleasant type of breathing, though it is not painful in the usual sense of the word'. Most definitions of the term involve concepts of effort and awareness of a need to breathe.

Breathlessness may be a single sensation or, like pain, several related sensations. It is not clear to what extent the breathless sensation is the same in physiological circumstances (e.g. on vigorous exercise in normal subjects) and pathological circumstances, such as in respiratory disease; it is also not clear whether the breathlessness of different disease states is qualitatively the same. These issues, although intriguing, are rarely of practical importance in the clinical situation.

Conditions associated with breathlessness can be grouped into three main categories, which are not mutually exclusive. Breathlessness occurs in conditions where there is: an increased chemical or neurological drive to breathe; an increased work of breathing; or a decreased neuromuscular power. In all these situations, there is likely to be an increased drive to breathe, whether primary or secondary, and whether or not accompanied by an actual increase in ventilation. Recent experimental work on breathlessness, in both normal subjects and patients with respiratory disease, has led to a general hypothesis for the genesis of the sensation. This suggests that breathlessness occurs when a drive to breathe exists that is abnormal, either qualitatively or quantitatively, and is translated in the medulla into a descending motor command to the respiratory muscles.

The important causes of breathlessness, in terms of the three categories described above, are listed in Table D.8. In practice, many of these conditions have their effects via more than one mechanism. There are some conditions associated with increased ventilation that are only rarely associated with breathlessness.

Table D.8 Causes of breathlessness

Conditions associated with an increased chemical or neurological drive to breathe

Common causes	*Uncommon causes*
Pulmonary oedema	Acidosis
Pulmonary embolus	Pregnancy
Pneumothorax	Cyanotic congenital heart disease
Pneumonia	High altitude
Lobar collapse	Arteriovenous fistula
Pulmonary fibrosis	
Anaemia	

Conditions associated with an increased work of breathing
Obstructive ventilatory defects

Common causes	*Uncommon causes*
Chronic obstructive airways disease	Upper airways obstruction
Emphysema	
Asthma	
Bronchiectasis	
Cystic fibrosis	
Byssinosis	

Restrictive ventilatory defects

Common causes	*Uncommon causes*
Sarcoidosis	Large tumours
Fibrosing alveolitis	Large hiatus hernia
Extrinsic allergic alveolitis	Lymphangitis carcinomatosa
Pneumoconioses	Connective tissue diseases
Large pleural effusion	Aspiration pneumonitis
Extensive lung resection	Infections
Chest wall deformity	
Pulmonary oedema	
Left ventricular dysfunction	

Conditions associated with decreased neuromuscular power

Common causes	*Uncommon causes*
Myasthenia gravis	Poliomyelitis
Polyneuritis	Motor neurone disease
	Muscular dystrophies

Conditions associated with decreased neuromuscular power are all relatively rare causes of breathlessness.

When increased ventilation is voluntary, the descending path from the cortex to the respiratory anterior horn cells bypasses the medullary respiratory centre, and breathlessness is much reduced or absent. This is evidence for the origin of the sensation in the region of the respiratory centre. In many forms of acidosis, if the respiratory apparatus is normal, breathlessness is rare despite the increased ventilation.

Respiratory function tests

In most respiratory conditions severe enough to cause breathlessness, sophisticated tests of function are not necessary as the problem is obvious. However, respiratory function tests can be of use in determining patterns of impairment that can help in diagnosing the cause of the problem, and are particularly useful for monitoring changes in function over time or in response to treatment. Most respiratory function testing is done at rest, but important information about the cardiorespiratory system can also be obtained from measurements made during exercise.

The basic and most useful indices of lung function can be measured using a spirometer to record expired volume over time. Many machines are now available, with results produced either as flow-volume curves (Fig. D.19) or as volume–time curves (Fig. D.20). The major variables obtained from spirometry during forced expiration are the forced expiratory volume in 1 second (FEV_1), the forced vital capacity (FVC) and the peak expiratory flow rate (PEFR). Other variables that can be obtained from the same manoeuvre include flows at different points in the expiration such as at 50 per cent and 75 per cent of the vital capacity (VC). The relaxed VC can be measured using the same equipment, but with a slow expiration. The PEFR can also be measured by simpler, cheaper peak flow meters; these are convenient when repeated estimates of PEFR are required, for example to diagnose variable airflow limitation in asthma.

To estimate other lung volumes it is necessary to use helium dilution to give an estimate of residual volume (RV, the volume remaining in the lungs at the end of a full expiration). Total lung capacity (TLC) is the sum of the RV and the VC. Another aspect of lung function is gas exchange between the alveoli and the blood. This can be assessed by measuring the transfer factor for carbon monoxide. Of course, arterial oxygen tension is also a good indication of gas exchange,

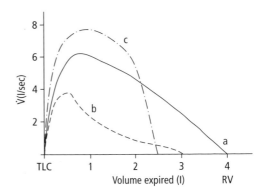

Figure D.19 Superimposed expiratory flow–volume curves. (a) Normal; (b) obstructive airways disease; (c) restrictive lung disease.

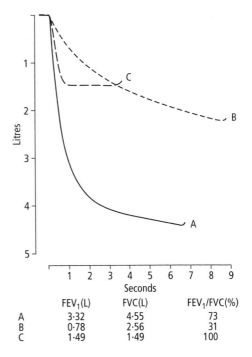

	FEV_1(L)	FVC(L)	FEV_1/FVC(%)
A	3·32	4·55	73
B	0·78	2·56	31
C	1·49	1·49	100

Figure D.20 Superimposed tracings of expiratory spirograms in normals (A), obstructive airways disease (B) and restrictive lung disease (C). The measurements derived from these records are given below the graph.

and a fall during exercise is a sensitive means of detecting interstitial lung disease affecting gas exchange. Measurement of arterial blood gas tensions requires arterial puncture, which can be uncomfortable and even hazardous and, in the absence of an indwelling arterial line, difficult to repeat frequently.

It is also possible to measure arterial oxygen saturation non-invasively using oximeters. These function by shining different wavelengths of light through the tissue (usually the ear lobe or fingertip); they can be left in place for several hours, for example during exercise testing or during sleep. Similarly, it is now possible to measure arterial blood CO_2 tension (PCO_2) non-invasively, using a sensor strapped to the skin.

Exercise tests can assess the functioning of the cardiorespiratory system under stress. Commonly, exercise of progressively greater severity is performed on the treadmill or bicycle ergometer. Variables such as ventilation, heart rate, O_2 consumption and CO_2 production can be measured; it is also possible to obtain the subject's assessments of degree of breathlessness during the test. Such testing is mainly of research interest, but can sometimes elucidate the cause of breathlessness on exercise in someone with relatively normal results at rest (for example, an exercise-induced cardiac arrhythmia or a profound fall in arterial PO_2 due to a reversal of an arteriovenous shunt).

The pattern of lung function abnormality is particularly useful in deciding what type of disease is present. In airways obstruction, such as is found in chronic obstructive pulmonary disease (COPD) or asthma, spirometry typically shows a reduction in FEV, and in the FEV_1/FVC ratio. If a flow–volume curve is examined, the descending part of the curve tends to be concave due to reductions in flow at low lung volumes (Fig. D.19). In some cases, there is quite a marked reduction in FVC, due to air-trapping during the forced expiration. This is especially likely in COPD. Spirometry alone in such cases cannot distinguish between obstruction with air-trapping and a mixed obstructive/restrictive defect. Restrictive lung conditions, such as diffuse pulmonary fibrosis, typically produce a reduction in FVC but have less effect on the FEV, so that the FEV_1/FVC ratio tends to be high. A typical flow–volume curve in restrictive lung disease is shown in Figure D.19.

Additional tests are not always necessary to distinguish between obstructive and restrictive conditions. Static lung volumes are uniformly reduced in restrictive conditions, with a normal RV/TLC ratio, and there is frequently a reduction in gas transfer factor. In obstructive conditions, it is common to find that the relaxed VC is greater than the FVC, and that the RV/TLC ratio is increased, both due to air trapping. If emphysema is present, destruction of lung tissue often results in a reduction in gas transfer factor.

Blood gases can become abnormal in any severe lung disease. In respiratory failure secondary to chronic obstructive airways disease, the PO_2 is reduced and there is a tendency for the PCO_2 to increase due to alveolar hypoventilation. In asthma, a reduction in PO_2 is the main feature, and the PCO_2 tends to be low due to hyperventilation in response to the hypoxaemia, only rising as a late event in life-threatening asthma. In restrictive lung conditions, a low PO_2 with a low PCO_2 is the usual pattern. In all these situations, including restrictive lung conditions, the hypoxaemia is mainly secondary to a mismatch between ventilation and perfusion of alveoli rather than to an actual diffusion defect.

The various conditions associated with breathlessness will be discussed under the headings used in Table D.8. Many of these produce breathlessness by several different mechanisms, but are classified according to the primary mechanism operating in most cases.

Conditions associated with an increased chemical or neurological drive to breathe

A characteristic of increased ventilation due to chemical or neurological stimulation is a high respiratory frequency and a low arterial PCO_2. Hypoxia and acidosis are the important chemical drives to breathe. Potential sources of neurological drives to breathe include pulmonary receptors, chest wall receptors and other skeletal muscle receptors. Neurological drives to breathe are probably important in parenchymal lung conditions associated with breathlessness, such as *pulmonary oedema* and *pulmonary infarction secondary to pulmonary embolus*. There may also be a mechanism for the breathlessness associated with *pneumonia* and *lobar collapse* (e.g. secondary to bronchial obstruction produced by *bronchogenic carcinoma*). It has been demonstrated that the increased ventilation associated with lobar collapse occurs even when the collapsed segment is small and there is little or no hypoxia. Breathlessness, due perhaps to stimulation of lung receptors, is a prominent early symptom of *Pneumocystis jiroveci* (formerly known as *Pneumocystis carinii*) pneumonia associated with HIV infection (Fig. D.21). This condition typically has an insidious onset and a long history stretching back weeks or months with a dry cough a prominent feature; the

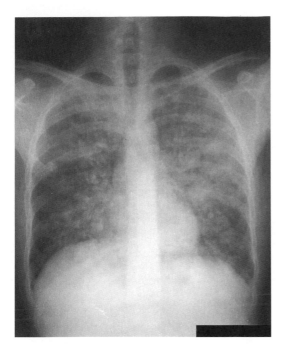

Figure D.21 Extensive bilateral shadowing due to *Pneumocystis jiroveci* infection.

chest radiograph may be normal, but arterial oxygen desaturation on exercise is usual. The breathlessness that accompanies a relatively small *spontaneous pneumothorax* is often quite marked, especially in the early stages, and cannot be explained by mechanical difficulties with ventilation. Again, it is possible that stimulation of lung receptors plays a part.

Hypoxia from any cause can lead to breathlessness via stimulation of ventilation, for example in *cyanotic congenital heart disease*, *high altitude* (mountaineers) and *parenchymal lung disease* such as the various types of *pulmonary fibrosis*. It is not clear whether hypoxia can act as a direct stimulus to breathlessness, independent of its effects on ventilation; experiments have produced conflicting results.

In *cyanotic congenital heart disease*, such as Fallot's tetralogy, the mixed venous oxygen saturation falls on exercise due to increased extraction by the exercising muscles (this is a normal phenomenon); some of this venous blood passes into the aorta via the ventricular septal defect, causing a steep fall in arterial oxygen saturation. This stimulates ventilation and leads to severe breathlessness on exercise. Children with Fallot's tetralogy are often observed to squat. This produces some obstruction of venous return from the exercising

muscles of the legs, reducing the fall in arterial oxygen saturation and the resultant increased ventilation and breathlessness.

Severe arterial hypoxaemia occurs in *respiratory distress syndrome of the newborn*. Due to a lack of pulmonary surfactant, parts of the lung fail to expand and there is marked mismatching of ventilation and perfusion in the lungs. Perfusion of unventilated segments contributes to the arterial hypoxia. There is profound stimulation of ventilation, with respiratory rates of up to 100 per minute. It is, of course, only speculation to suggest that this is accompanied by breathlessness in these infants.

Hypoxia is a common feature of many types of *parenchymal lung disease*; it is more often due to mismatching of ventilation and perfusion than to an actual block to diffusion (see above). A more important cause of breathlessness in many of these conditions is the increased work of breathing, due to decreased compliance of the lung tissue, and these points are discussed more fully below.

Anaemia is frequently accompanied by a complaint of breathlessness. The mechanism is probably inefficient oxygen delivery to exercising muscles, with a resultant increase in anaerobic metabolism and lactate production which drives ventilation. The breathlessness that sometimes accompanies *pregnancy* and *arteriovenous fistula* may in part be due to a similar mechanism, with changes in distribution of the cardiac output leaving some muscle groups relatively hypoxic. In late pregnancy, mechanical difficulties with ventilation are likely to be more important. Other causes of acidosis also produce an increase in ventilation, such as *renal failure* and *diabetic keto-acidosis*. In practice, these conditions are rarely accompanied by breathlessness unless there is concomitant lung disease. In the case of keto-acidosis this may be because consciousness is obtunded, but it remains unclear why there is relatively little breathlessness associated with other causes of acidosis.

Isocapnic *voluntary hyperventilation* is not accompanied by breathlessness in the experimental situation, as discussed above. Similarly, breathlessness is a relatively rare complaint in the *hyperventilation syndrome*; symptoms such as nausea, light-headedness and paraesthesiae are much more common. Although it has been suggested that some people with lung disease have *disproportionate dyspnoea*, associated with various psychiatric symptoms, true *psychogenic dyspnoea* is a very rare phenomenon and should never be diagnosed without very thorough investigation, including exercise testing. It should be noted, however, that the sighing respiration of *cardiac neurosis* may be referred to by the patient as 'breathlessness'.

Conditions associated with an increased work of breathing

Obstructive ventilatory defects

The term *chronic obstructive pulmonary disease* (*COPD*) refers to the situation where there is chronic, more or less irreversible, obstruction of the airways, especially the smaller airways. It is sometimes referred to by other names, such as *chronic airflow limitation*, *chronic obstructive airways disease*, *chronic bronchitis and emphysema* or *chronic obstructive lung disease*. The most important association is with cigarette smoking, but general atmospheric pollution also plays a part, and it is common in some dusty occupations. The old term 'chronic bronchitis' should probably no longer be used, as it is unclear whether it refers to chronic mucus hypersecretion (it was often diagnosed on the basis of this) or to airways obstruction. There is now convincing epidemiological evidence that the two conditions are distinct, connected through cigarette smoking, and that it is only the airways obstruction that is related to increased mortality.

COPD remains a very common condition and an important cause of breathlessness due to the increased drive to breathe required to overcome the increased resistance to airflow. It is diagnosed by the finding of airflow limitation, not reversible by bronchodilators, usually with a history of cigarette smoking and productive cough. The main differential diagnosis is asthma (see below).

In advanced COPD, the chest becomes chronically over-inflated with an increased anteroposterior diameter – the so-called 'barrel chest'. The chest radiograph shows a loss of normal lung markings, flattened domes of the diaphragm, and sometimes the presence of bullae. The lung function defect is obstructive, with collapse of the airways during expiration partly due to lack of support from the surrounding lung tissue. Other common lung function findings are an increased RV, an increased TLC, an increased RV/TLC ratio, and a decreased transfer factor. Occasionally, large bullae may act as space-occupying lesions and

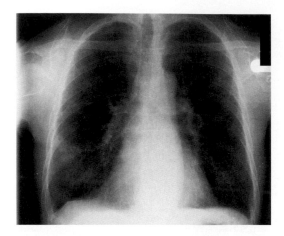

Figure D.22 Advanced emphysema.

add a restrictive component to the picture. There is debate about whether resection of the bullae relieves breathlessness in these cases. *Emphysema* is defined as an increase in size, due to destruction of the alveolar walls, of the air spaces distal to the terminal bronchioles (Fig. D.22). It is a pathological diagnosis, and is part of the pathology of COPD. A particular type of emphysema is that related to inherited deficiency of alpha-l-proteinase inhibitor; the emphysema is panacinar rather than centrilobular, and tends to affect the upper, rather than the lower, lobes.

Breathlessness due to chronic irreversible obstructive airways disease presents as a major feature in a well-known clinical picture. Expiratory wheezes at the mouth and on auscultation are common, but not invariable. Respiratory failure, with hypoxia and often hypercapnia, develops. Cor pulmonale, with peripheral oedema, develops in some cases. Two extremes have been described, depending on the degree to which the respiratory centre retains its sensitivity to carbon dioxide. Where sensitivity is lost, the PCO_2 rises, oedema is present, and there is cyanosis due to hypoxia and sometimes secondary polycythaemia; this is the so-called 'blue bloater'. Where CO_2 sensitivity is retained, there tends to be a greater drive to breathe, with correspondingly more severe breathlessness, but relatively normal blood gases until a late stage of disease; this is described as the 'pink puffer'. In practice, there is considerable overlap between these two extremes.

Bronchiectasis is associated with breathlessness if there is appreciable airways obstruction present and if the lung destruction is extensive. The diagnosis is suggested by a history of production of copious purulent sputum, often with haemoptysis. Clubbing may be present with extensive disease. A bronchogram is the traditional way to confirm the diagnosis, but a more recent, non-invasive, alternative is computed tomography. The lung disease of *cystic fibrosis* in children is similar to bronchiectasis of adults, with destruction of lung tissue and airways obstruction.

One common cause of breathlessness in all age groups is the episodic airways obstruction of *asthma*. The cardinal feature of asthma is the variable nature of the airways obstruction, with partial or complete reversal after bronchodilator treatment. The typical history is of episodes of breathlessness, accompanied by wheezing, coughing or chest tightness, occurring especially at night and *after* exercise. During an attack, there is over-inflation of the chest, wheezing and rapid ventilation. The breathlessness is made worse by the ventilatory stimulation from the accompanying hypoxia. A palpable 'paradox' of the arterial pulse is often present during a severe episode due to the large intrathoracic pressure swings. There are some particular causes of asthma that merit mention. *Bronchopulmonary aspergillosis* may provoke episodes of asthma or worsen pre-existing asthma. The chest radiograph may show transient pulmonary infiltrations, and there is often an eosinophilia in the peripheral blood. A rare cause of asthma is *polyarteritis nodosa*, where it may be an early manifestation of this more general condition. Recently, *occupational asthma* has been recognized with increasing frequency, and should always be considered, especially when asthma fails to respond to usual treatments. A careful occupational history should be taken in all cases of asthma.

Airways obstruction is the main feature of *byssinosis*, a lung condition caused by the inhalation of cotton and other vegetable dusts. The typical history is of breathlessness and chest tightness occurring on the first day back at work after a break, then gradually progressing so that it is constantly present. The late stages of byssinosis are indistinguishable from other causes of chronic obstructive airways disease.

Upper airways obstruction is an uncommon cause of breathlessness, but it is important to recognize because it can be rapidly fatal, but can be quickly relieved by intubation or tracheostomy. Obstruction at the level of the larynx may be due to severe *laryngitis*, which may still be secondary to *diphtheria*, or to *laryngeal oedema* as part of an allergic reaction. Severe *laryngotracheobronchitis*, as occurs in croup, can rapidly produce life-threatening respiratory obstruction and breathlessness, and respiratory embarrassment can occur with severe *tonsillitis*. Obstruction can also be due to an impacted *foreign body* or to problems with the vocal cords themselves, as in *bilateral abductor paralysis*. Obstruction at the level of the trachea can be produced by intrinsic *carcinoma of the trachea* or by external compression from *carcinoma of the thyroid, haemorrhage into a thyroid cyst, neoplastic glands* in the neck or mediastinum, *aortic aneurysm* or *dermoid tumour* of the mediastinum. Obstruction of the upper airways may be accompanied by inspiratory stridor, and the flow–volume loop shows a characteristic truncation of the inspiratory part of the loop.

Restrictive ventilatory defects

The most obvious form of restrictive ventilatory defect is when there has been actual loss of lung tissue, following *surgical resection* of a lung or lobe. Breathlessness following pneumonectomy is more likely when there is disease of the remaining lung, such as obstructive lung disease in a smoker who has had a pneumonectomy for lung cancer. Space-occupying lesions can produce a similar effect. Examples are a large *pleural effusion* or *spontaneous pneumothorax*. Part of the breathlessness associated with these conditions is probably due to a neurological drive to breathe, but the effusions also produce a restriction of lung tissue when large. A pleural effusion must be very large before it produces noticeable breathlessness in young, healthy adults, but even a small effusion can lead to a worsening of breathlessness when it occurs in association with left ventricular failure, when there may already be pulmonary hypertension and oedema. Common features of a spontaneous pneumothorax are chest pain, often pleuritic in nature, and moderate breathlessness. A tension pneumothorax, actively increasing in size and compressing lung tissue, produces extreme breathlessness and often cardiovascular collapse and requires urgent relief through insertion of a cannula. Physical signs of a large pneumothorax are reduced movement and reduced (or absent) breath sounds on the affected side. Large *tumours* can behave as space-occupying lesions, a particularly unpleasant example being a *mesothelioma* secondary to asbestos exposure. At post-mortem examination, the tumour is often seen to have replaced most of the original lung volume. A large *hiatus hernia* can occasionally cause breathlessness by acting as a space-occupying lesion within the chest.

Lung restriction can result from conditions of the chest wall. Deformity of the thoracic cage, such as occurs in severe *kyphoscoliosis, ankylosing spondylitis* or after a *thoracoplasty*, reduces the inspiratory volume that can be achieved, and may be associated with breathlessness as a result. Extensive pleural fibrosis or calcification can similarly produce a restrictive ventilatory defect; this may be found following *tuberculosis* or secondary to *asbestos exposure*. In severe cases, the lungs become encased in a rigid shell of pleura, sometimes called a 'cuirass'. Restrictive ventilatory defects due to conditions outside the lung itself are characterized by reduced lung volumes, but a normal or even increased transfer factor for carbon monoxide. This is because the lung tissue itself is normal, though compressed, and there may be a higher blood flow in the smaller volume of tissue causing the increase in transfer factor.

The largest group of conditions producing restrictive ventilatory defects are those involving the lung parenchyma itself. *Fibrosing alveolitis* is a generalized condition of the lung parenchyma which begins as an inflammatory process and frequently progresses to established fibrosis. There are a number of variants of this condition, differing in their rate of progression and response to treatment with corticosteroids or immunosuppressants. The most acute form, sometimes known as the Hamman–Rich syndrome, progresses to severe disability and death within weeks or months. Other forms can be present for years before causing severe symptoms. Common features are breathlessness on exertion, dry cough, clubbing of the fingers (and toes) and inspiratory crackles, especially at the lung bases. The chest radiograph shows reticulonodular shadowing, usually more marked in the lower zones.

In most cases of fibrosing alveolitis the cause is unknown. A somewhat similar clinical picture can develop in some cases of extrinsic allergic alveolitis which develops in response to inhaled organic dusts. The major mechanism is a type III allergy, with IgG antibodies against the allergen present in the blood.

The best-known example of typical extrinsic allergic alveolitis (EAA) is farmer's lung. Acute episodes follow heavy exposure to the allergen, in this case spores of fungi such as *Micropolyspora faeni* contaminating damp hay. There is fever, breathlessness, cough, sometimes cyanosis, and crackles are audible in the chest. Hypoxia and a restrictive ventilatory defect are present, and there are scattered small, nodular shadows on the chest radiograph. Such acute episodes are often difficult to distinguish from atypical pneumonia, although the presence of precipitating antibodies can help. If exposure to the responsible agent continues, chronic disease develops. This is characterized by persistent breathlessness and dry cough, sometimes with clubbing and cyanosis. Airways obstruction can develop in addition to the restrictive defect, and there may be emphysema as well as fibrosis in the lungs. The diagnosis is helped if there is a history of preceding acute episodes. In some types of EAA these are rare; for example, in budgerigar fancier's lung an insidious development of fibrosis is common, probably because of the continuous low level exposure in this case. There are numerous other causes of EAA, including: fungal spores, involved in bagassosis of sugar-cane workers, in suberosis of cork workers, in sequoiosis of redwood sawyers, and in lung disease of mushroom workers, malt workers, maple-bark strippers and cheese makers; animal proteins in pigeon fancier's lung; and bacterial or amoebal proteins in humidifier fever (as distinct from legionnaires' disease, where lung infection is involved).

Extrinsic allergic alveolitis has some clinical and pathological features in common with sarcoidosis, although in the latter no causative agent has been identified. Acute, subacute and chronic forms of *sarcoidosis* are described. The acute form may have little in the way of respiratory symptoms, and is characterized by bilateral hilar lymphadenopathy, often with fever, erythema nodosum and arthralgia. In the subacute and chronic forms there is a granulomatous infiltration in the lungs with increasing breathlessness. The chest radiograph shows pulmonary infiltration, said to be characteristically peri-hilar but often more generalized (Fig. D.23). Sarcoidosis is a systemic condition, and many organs apart from the lungs can be affected, including the eyes (iridocychtis), the lacrimal and salivary glands, the lymph nodes, the liver, the skin and the central and peripheral nervous

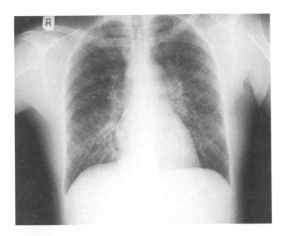

Figure D.23 Pulmonary sarcoidosis in a man complaining of breathlessness.

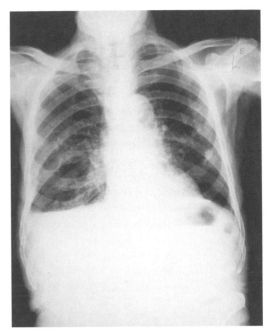

Figure D.25 Man with pleural plaques from previous asbestos exposure and emphysema.

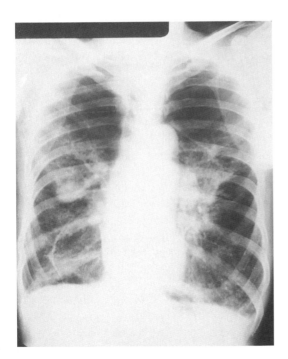

Figure D.24 Coalminer's pneumoconiosis.

systems. The Kveim test is positive in acute disease, but may be negative in the chronic form. A useful diagnostic feature of sarcoidosis, and EAA, is the presence of a large number of lymphocytes in the bronchoalveolar lavage fluid. In idiopathic fibrosing alveolitis, on the other hand, the fluid contains increased numbers of neutrophils.

Pneumoconiosis is a general term for lung disease due to dust inhalation, but it is used mainly to describe the conditions associated with inhaling inorganic dusts where allergy is not an important mechanism. *Silicosis* is still an important disease world-wide. Breathlessness develops gradually, and the restrictive pattern of deficit is frequently complicated by airways obstruction due to airways disease and lung distortion by fibrotic masses. The fibrosis of silicosis is nodular rather than diffuse, and the chest radiograph shows distinct nodules which tend to coalesce to form large masses. In *coalworker's pneumoconiosis*, the chest radiograph shows a background of small nodular opacities, with large masses as the disease progresses (Fig. D.24). Disability is due mainly to the associated emphysema, which may be severe. *Asbestosis* is a very common cause of restrictive lung disease in the industrialized world (Fig. D.25). Symptoms and signs of lung disease tend to develop after exposure over many months or years. The lung fibrosis associated with asbestos exposure is diffuse and affects especially the lower lobes. It is frequently accompanied by pleural thickening or plaques, which may calcify. An important complication is lung cancer, or more rarely mesothelioma. The restrictive lung function deficit and breathlessness of asbestosis is only poorly related to the severity of the radiographic changes. A number of other dusts can produce forms of pneumoconiosis. *Berylliosis*, caused by exposure to beryllium, has many features in common with sarcoidosis, and sometimes responds to treatment with corticosteroids.

Carcinoma of the lung (see Fig. C.25) rarely causes breathlessness as an early feature, but breathlessness in more advanced disease may be due to a lobar collapse (as discussed above), to multiple metastases in the lungs, or to lymphatic involvement producing lymphangitis carcinomatosa. This may also be due to the spread of extrapulmonary tumours, and is associated with very severe breathlessness.

Most of the generalized *connective tissue diseases* can affect the lungs. Systemic lupus erythematosus (SLE) frequently involves the pleura, with recurrent episodes of pleurisy, but can also lead to lung fibrosis. Systemic sclerosis (scleroderma) produces a diffuse interstitial pulmonary fibrosis, which can go on to produce cor pulmonale. A further cause of lung damage in this condition is recurrent aspiration if the oesophagus is also affected. Pulmonary involvement in rheumatoid disease is rare, but diffuse fibrosis or rheumatoid nodules in the lung can occasionally occur. Caplan's syndrome is a type of coalworker's pneumoconiosis that occurs in men who have the rheumatoid diathesis. Multiple rounded opacities occur on a background of scant small nodules; calcification and cavitation are quite common (Fig. D.26). The lung condition can occur without overt arthritis, but rheumatoid factor is nevertheless present in the serum.

Lung destruction as a result of infections can produce breathlessness secondary to a restrictive defect. *Tuberculosis*, with extensive cavitation, is often associated with breathlessness before adequate treatment; the breathlessness may persist after bacteriological cure due to the loss of lung tissue. *Klebsiella pneumonia* frequently destroys lung tissue, and severe cases may be left with breathlessness after recovery from the infection.

Other conditions of the lung parenchyma that can produce a restrictive ventilatory defect include schistosomiasis, fungal infections (e.g. blastomycosis

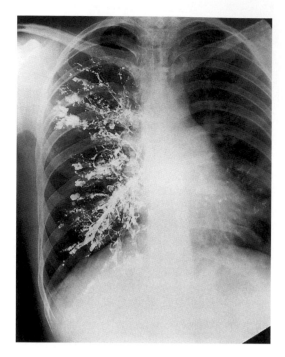

Figure D.26 Extensive bronchiectasis of right lung demonstrated by bronchogram.

and coccidioidomycosis) and alveolar proteinosis. Poisoning with the weedkiller paraquat leads to severe breathlessness due to an obliterative bronchiolitis.

One important group of conditions in which breathlessness occurs at least partially due to a restrictive ventilatory defect is that causing pulmonary oedema. Cardiac causes of pulmonary oedema include valvular lesions (e.g. mitral stenosis) and left ventricular failure. The most common cause of left ventricular failure is ischaemic heart disease; other causes are hypertensive heart disease and non-ischaemic cardiomyopathies. As the pulmonary venous and capillary pressures rise, the lungs become stiffer; the accumulation of fluid in the interstitial tissue and in the alveoli increases the lung stiffness. Thus, the work of ventilation is increased. In addition, gas transfer is impaired leading to increasingly severe arterial hypoxaemia which further drives ventilation. Breathlessness on exertion is accompanied by orthopnoea and bouts of nocturnal breathlessness (so-called 'paroxysmal nocturnal dyspnoea'). The breathlessness that is frequently the symptom which limits exercise in heart disease with left ventricular dysfunction is not fully understood. The mechanism just outlined operates in some cases, but other mechanisms – perhaps involving neurological drives to breathe – may also be important.

Acute pulmonary oedema, as every house officer knows, is a dramatic condition, with severe breathlessness developing rapidly, accompanied by a cough productive of frothy, pink sputum. There are widespread crackles in the chest, and wheezing is often a prominent feature due to oedema of the bronchial walls. It can sometimes be difficult to differentiate between acute asthma and pulmonary oedema; radiographic appearances and the finding of mitral stenosis or a cause of left ventricular failure can be helpful. It is always worth remembering that an elderly patient with severe breathlessness might be suffering from acute asthma rather than pulmonary oedema secondary to cardiac disease. The radiographic features of pulmonary venous hypertension include engorgement of the upper lobe veins and septal lymphatic lines. In acute pulmonary oedema there is enlargement of the hilar shadows and fan-shaped mid-zone opacities) (Fig. D.27).

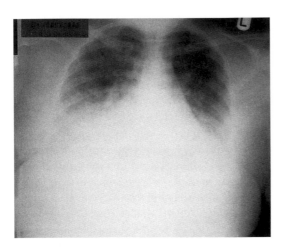

Figure D.27 Acute pulmonary oedema due to mitral stenosis.

Pulmonary oedema can be precipitated by the infusion of saline. This is unlikely to occur with a normal heart and adequate renal function, but it can readily occur in oliguric renal failure. Other non-cardiac causes of pulmonary oedema include cerebral vascular accidents, salicylate poisoning, hypersensitivity to radiographic contrast media, and adult respiratory distress syndrome when the pulmonary vasculature becomes abnormally 'leaky'. Pulmonary oedema can be caused by the inhalation of smoke or other irritant gases, such as chlorine. *Aspiration pneumonitis* (Mendelson's syndrome) is similar to pulmonary oedema. It is due to the aspiration of gastric acid, and the symptoms are virtually the same as for acute pulmonary oedema.

Conditions associated with decreased neuromuscular power

In these conditions, an increased drive to the functioning respiratory muscles is required in order to attempt to maintain ventilation. *Weakness of the respiratory muscles* may be due to primary muscle disorders, or to neurological disease. Examples include: myasthenia gravis, polyneuritis, poliomyelitis, motor neurone disease and muscular dystrophies. Despite the drive to breathe, hypoventilation is a feature of these conditions. It is also a feature of the respiratory failure associated with end-stage COPD, in particular. The hypoventilation associated with rare lesions of the respiratory centre itself is not usually associated with breathlessness, nor is the hypoventilation found in the obesity hypoventilation syndrome or Pickwickian syndrome.

Differential diagnosis of acute breathlessness

Acute severe breathlessness is a common medical emergency that is alarming for the patient and medical attendant alike. The urgency of the situation may be such that no time is available for radiographic or other investigation, and the initial diagnosis must be made on the basis of clinical examination. The differential diagnosis will be discussed in terms of the physical signs which may be elicited in such an examination.

Simple inspection can be informative. If the patient is deeply cyanosed with engorged cervical veins, struggling for breath with violent movements of the larynx, then *laryngeal* or *upper tracheal obstruction* should be considered. The stridor of upper airways obstruction is heard during both inspiration and expiration, and should be distinguished from the expiratory wheeze of ordinary bronchial obstruction. The possible causes of upper airways obstruction are discussed above. The mucosal pallor of severe *anaemia* as a cause of breathlessness may also be noted on inspection.

Examination of the arterial pulse may reveal uncontrolled *atrial fibrillation* or other arrhythmias, which can lead to sudden breathlessness, especially if there is valvular or other cardiac disease. *Cardiac tamponade* is associated with marked 'paradox' of the arterial pulse and elevation of the jugular venous pressure, with a paradoxical rise in pressure during inspiration. It may be secondary to intrapericardial haemorrhage from malignant metastases; in association with cardiac rupture from a myocardial infarction it is usually rapidly fatal. The venous pressure is also markedly elevated following a massive *pulmonary embolus*, another cause of acute severe breathlessness.

Mediastinal displacement, as indicated by lateral displacement of the trachea, can be a valuable physical sign in acute breathlessness. In *massive collapse* of a lung, for example postoperatively, the trachea is displaced towards the affected side. The trachea is deviated away from the side of the lesion in *pleural effusion* and *tension pneumothorax*. The most likely fluid to accumulate rapidly enough in the pleural space to cause acute breathlessness is blood; *haemothorax* may follow chest trauma, or even occur after pleural aspiration.

In acute *pulmonary oedema*, the venous pressure is usually also elevated and there may be signs on examination of the heart, such as a murmur of *mitral stenosis* or a gallop rhythm in *left ventricular failure*. Auscultation of the lungs usually reveals widespread crackles in pulmonary oedema and expiratory wheezes in *acute asthma*; in very severe asthma the wheeze can disappear because of gross reduction of air movement. If acute breathlessness is due to severe pulmonary infection, features such as pyrexia, purulent sputum and signs of consolidation in the lungs can be helpful diagnostically. Evidence of severe immunosuppression, such as oral candidiasis, oral hairy leukoplakia, or evidence of extreme weight loss should prompt consideration of *Pneumocystis* pneumonia complicating HIV infection.

Boris Lams

DYSURIA

There is some confusion over the definition of dysuria. In the United Kingdom, dysuria is the term applied to pain or discomfort on passing urine. In other countries, dysuria may relate to difficulties in passing urine. For the purpose of this text, dysuria is synonymous with pain felt in the urethra on micturition. The pain occurs in the urethra during voiding, may occur in the prostate in the male, and may refer to the bladder. Dysuria is often described as a feeling of 'passing broken glass', which is something a patient can easily relate to if this symptom has been experienced.

Concentrated urine in association with dehydration may cause dysuria, but the symptoms are slight and resolve when fluid intake returns to normal. An otherwise normal individual may experience dysuria when concentrated or acid urine is passed. Examples are when the patient is dehydrated from the excessive fluid loss associated with exercise or hot climate, or from an inability to drink enough fluid, perhaps during an intercontinental flight. Dysuria under these circumstances is rarely severe, and felt more as a tingling or slight stinging as urine is passed.

True dysuria is a consequence of inflammation in the urinary tract. The infection may be in the kidney (pyelitis or pyelonephritis) or in the bladder (cystitis). Urethral pain on voiding may also be experienced with urethritis in both sexes, and the urethral syndrome in women (symptoms of frequency/ dysuria without cultured infection; abacterial cystitis). *Urethritis* is a common symptom of some sexually transmitted infections, predominantly in men. Gonorrhoea typically produces a purulent urethral discharge associated with urethral pain on micturition; nongonococcal urethritis may be caused by a variety of infections, particularly *Chlamydia*, and may also cause dysuria with or without a urethral discharge. Intrameatal infection with herpes simplex virus may cause extreme pain on micturition, and primary genital infections with this virus commonly produce dysuria (Fig. D.28). Urethral syndrome is not uncommon in women in middle age. The symptoms tend to be recurrent. Urine cultures are negative, but the symptoms suggest infection. Some of these urethras are catheter-sensitive. If a urethral catheter is passed, the urethra is tender (hypersensitive), whereas

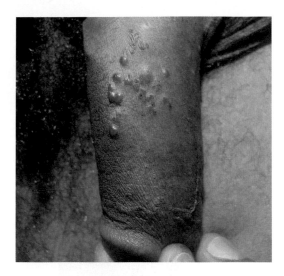

Figure D.28 Penile herpes simplex.

the normal female urethra is not usually painful during catheterization. Urethral syndrome does not require treatment with antibiotics, but does respond to urethral dilatation.

Urethral pain during micturition may be due to acute or chronic cystitis and acute or chronic prostatitis. *Acute prostatitis* is a relatively rare condition that presents in younger men with symptoms of a febrile acute urinary infection. The diagnosis is made on clinical examination of the prostate when the prostate is swollen and exquisitely painful, making the examination difficult. The prostate should not be massaged in acute prostatitis. *Chronic prostatitis* is an intractable condition in which pain is felt in the perineum and/or the base of the penis, and may be felt on micturition. The prostate is tender on examination. Prostatic massage should be used to obtain fluid for culture of the prostatic fluid and microscopy for inflammatory cells. Tuberculous cystitis may cause dysuria; though rare, it should be considered when there is a sterile cystitis.

When a bladder calculus comes into contact with the trigone and bladder neck, pain may be referred into the urethra. Urethral pain may be felt when a ureteric stone is passing down the ureter, particularly when the stone is close to the bladder – that is, in the intra-mural ureter or when the stone is passed after a bout of ureteric colic. If a stone becomes stuck in the urethra – as may happen when a ureteric or bladder stone is passed – urethral pain will occur with the sudden onset of obstruction and then retention of urine. As the meatus is the narrowest portion of the urethra, a stone may lodge in the meatus and may be felt in the distal urethra, or felt and seen at the meatus. A bladder tumour close to the bladder neck may cause discomfort on voiding or obstruction. Blood clot, which has developed from bleeding in the bladder or upper urinary tract, may cause discomfort when passed.

Pain in the perineum is caused by prostatitis. It may occur in infiltrating prostate cancer and urethritis caused by urethral infection.

Meatal pain may be caused by genital warts or distal urethritis caused by sexually transmitted diseases. Pain in the foreskin may be seen in phimosis or balanitis.

Pain felt in the bladder area is not true dysuria, but may also be present during an acute episode of cystitis. Bladder pain can also be experienced in the presence of a bladder stone, when the stone bounces up and down on the trigone during the act of micturition. The trigone is a particularly sensitive area of the bladder, and can therefore cause pain when involved by bladder or prostatic carcinoma and in acute and chronic prostatitis.

Dysuria in children

Acute cystitis will cause severe voiding pain and the child or infant will cry when voiding occurs. In the male infant, meatal ulceration and acute balanitis will also cause pain on micturition.

Julian Shah

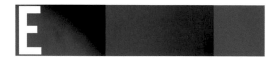

EARACHE

Earache (otalgia) may be caused by a number of conditions that affect the external and middle ear. Pain may also be referred to the ear as a result of disease processes at distant sites. These sites share sensory innervation from the same cranial nerves and spinal roots that supply the ear. Possible causes of earache are listed in Table E.1.

Table E.1 Causes of earache

Local	Referred
Auricle	■ Otitis media with effusion (rarely)
■ Trauma	■ Mastoiditis
◆ Direct	■ Malignant disease
◆ Haematoma	**Referred**
■ Furunculosis	Dental
■ Sebaceous cyst	■ Caries
■ Perichondritis	■ Abscess
■ Erysipelas	■ Pericoronitis (impacted wisdom tooth)
■ Chondrodermatitis nodularis	■ Costen's syndrome
■ Malignant disease	Pharynx
External auditory meatus	■ Tonsillitis
■ Diffuse otitis externa	■ Pharyngitis
◆ Infective	■ Postoperative pain
◆ Bacterial	■ Peritonsillar abscess (quinsy)
◆ Fungal	■ Foreign body
◆ Viral	■ Malignant disease
■ Reactive	Cervical spine
◆ Eczemateous	■ Osteoarthritis
◆ Seborrhoeic dermatitis	■ Spondylosis
◆ Neurodermatitis	Abdominal
■ Malignant otitis externa	■ Mesenteric adenitis
■ Benign necrotizing osteitis	Neurological
■ Wax impaction	■ Herpes zoster (Ramsay–Hunt syndrome)
■ Keratosis obturans	■ Glossopharyngeal neuralgia
■ Foreign bodies-impacted	■ Trigeminal neuralgia (occasional)
■ Trauma	
■ Malignant disease	
Middle ear	
■ Acute otitis media	
■ Advanced chronic otitis media	

Auricle

Causes of earache in the auricle are usually visible, and include direct trauma, haematoma, furuncles, erysipelas and perichondritis. The distinction between erysipelas and perichondritis can be made by inspection of the lobule, as this is not affected in perichondritis. The infectious causes respond to systemic antibiotics. Haematomas need to be drained as soon as possible to avoid permanent damage.

Chondrodermatitis nodularis chronicis helices is a benign nodular lesion of unknown aetiology which affects the lateral edge of the pinna. It is extremely painful, and sometimes needs to be excised. Malignant disease, squamous or basal cell carcinoma, are frequently seen in the elderly and, when advanced, become painful (Fig. E.1). Most can be successfully treated by either surgery, radiotherapy, or a combination of the two.

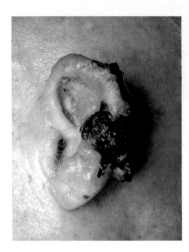

Figure E.1 Extensive and painful carcinoma of the pinna that has been neglected.

Meatus

The external auditory meatus is highly sensitive, and even mild inflammation in the confined space of the meatus can lead to considerable pain.

Foreign bodies may cause pain, usually after ineffective attempts at removal. Local infection of the skin and small furuncles may be extremely painful, the amount of pain bearing little relationship to the size of the furuncle which may be only the size of a pin's head. Impacted ear wax (or cerumen) is probably the most common ear problem in the general population. It may cause considerable pain and discomfort, especially following swimming and ineffective attempts at removal by syringing. Water may cause swelling of the wax, and sudden deafness follows complete occlusion of the meatus. Further attempts at cleaning the ears lead to trauma, and a secondary otitis externa may develop.

Diffuse otitis externa can arise as an acute episode, or it may run a more chronic course. The auricle – and specifically the tragus – is tender on movement, and this is a valuable sign to differentiate the condition from other causes. In many cases there is great swelling of the meatal skin and it may not be possible to see the eardrum. The cause of otitis externa is often multifactorial. General conditions such as eczema, seborrhoeic dermatitis and neurodermatitis may predispose to infection with bacteria (most commonly *Pseudomonas, Staphylococcus, Escherichia coli*), fungus (*Candida, Aspergillus*) or virus.

Malignant otitis externa, though not a neoplastic condition, may be a lethal condition in diabetic and immunocompromised patients. It is caused by spreading infection to bone, thereby producing an osteitis or osteomyelitis of the skull base. Long-term antibiotic therapy is required, together with meticulous attention to correction of the predisposing condition.

Middle ear

Acute otitis media is one of the commonest infections in childhood – hardly a child escapes one or more attacks. The infection usually accompanies upper respiratory tract infection, and the pain may develop within a matter of hours. It ceases abruptly when the eardrum ruptures and drainage is effected. The perforation usually closes spontaneously. Young children do not localize pain accurately, and earache for which there is no obvious local cause should prompt a wider search. Particularly aggressive acute otitis media may develop into acute mastoiditis. In this condition, the patient has an extremely high temperature (usually at least 39°C), and there is severe pain and tenderness behind and above the ear canal. Swelling and erythema develops in the postauricular sulcus, the pinna becomes proptosed, and the superior meatal skin sags. Early diagnosis and treatment is imperative as intracranial complications develop in those that are missed. Severe infection of the petrous apex may produce pain in the distribution of the ophthalmic division of the trigeminal nerve and a lateral rectus palsy caused by inflammation of the abducens nerve (Gradenigo's syndrome).

Chronic otitis media is usually painless, but becomes painful during acute exacerbations of infection. The onset of pain in patients with pre-existing attico-antral or tubo-tympanic disease should cause concern as it often heralds spreading infection and imminent complications. Such complications include facial palsy, meningitis, brain abscess and sinus thrombosis.

Poor Eustachian tube function can be unmasked by the development of pain following rapid changes in atmospheric pressure. Most commonly, this is seen after diving or a prolonged air flight in a poorly pressurized cabin.

Secretory otitis media, which is so common in children, is usually characterized by a symptomless deafness. Dull aching pain or, rarely, stabs of acute pain may be a symptom.

Malignant neoplasia of the middle ear and external canal is extremely uncommon, but when present is extremely painful. Other middle-ear tumours (e.g. glomus tumours) are not associated with pain.

Referred pain

Referred pain affecting the ear is very common. Pain is referred through the Vth, VIIth, IXth and Xth cranial nerves, the upper cervical roots and the autonomic nerve supply. Despite careful examination, no abnormality is found in the ear.

Dental causes

Caries, dental abscess and impacted wisdom teeth are all common causes of earache. Malocclusion may give rise to dysfunction of the temporo-mandibular joint (Costen's syndrome). These patients often have a history of dental extractions or a badly fitting denture, and tenderness will be found over the joint, especially on opening the jaw – a movement that may well be limited.

Pharynx

Tonsillitis and *pharyngitis* are both sometimes accompanied by earache. Severe earache is almost always experienced about 1 week after tonsillectomy, and should be controlled by non-steroidal anti-inflammatory analgesics. Frequent causes of referred pain from the pharynx are peritonsillar abscess, ulceration of the mucosa caused by trauma and aphthae. The most important group of conditions from a diagnostic point of view are *malignant lesions* of the oro-pharynx and laryngo-pharynx. Earache is found very consistently in these conditions, and may be the first symptom. Any patient who has been a heavy smoker and has otalgia for which there is no obvious local cause should have their pharynx examined very carefully.

Cervical spine

Cervical spondylosis affecting the C2 and C3 nerve roots may lead to referred pain around the ear.

Neurological causes

Herpes zoster infection of the geniculate ganglion (Ramsay–Hunt syndrome) gives rise to intense otalgia associated with vesicular lesions of the external auditory canal and pinna. Facial palsy develops quickly and may be permanent in up to 50 per cent of cases. The vesicular rash may also be seen on the palate and fauces. Rarely, hearing loss accompanies this condition.

In *glossopharyngeal neuralgia*, extremely severe, sharp pain is precipitated by swallowing. Pain that radiates from the throat to the ear may be due to glossopharyngeal neuralgia. Less severe variants can be associated with an elongated styloid process, which irritates the glossopharyngeal nerve when swallowing (Eagle's syndrome).

Michael Gleeson

EATING, DISORDERS OF

Disorders of eating are common and very numerous. Both reduced and increased oral intake have a very wide differential diagnosis indeed. This section is confined to a discussion of eating disorders as the term is generally used by psychiatrists and physicians – that is, to a discussion of anorexia nervosa and bulimia nervosa and the differential diagnosis relevant to each (Table E.2).

Anorexia nervosa is defined as a body weight maintained at least 15 per cent below that expected (or a body mass index of 17.5, or less), amenorrhoea in females, self-induced weight loss, distorted body image and a dread of fatness. Low body weight is usually achieved through a combination of reduced calorie intake and excessive exercise, though other strategies may be used. Anorexia nervosa is ten times more common in females than in males, and the age of onset is typically in the mid teens. It is increasingly appreciated that those people reaching these criteria represent the tip of an iceberg of subclinical anorexia. Some 20 per cent of 9-year-old girls in the UK have already tried dieting. Such subclinical presentations are sometimes dubbed 'the anorexic stance'. Anorexia nervosa is over-represented in the higher social classes,

Table E.2 Causes of eating disorders

Common disorders	■ Kleine–Levin syndrome
Anorexia nervosa	■ Kluver–Bucy syndrome
Bulimia nervosa	
	Self-induced vomiting
Rare disorders	■ Pyloric stenosis
Unexplained severe wasting	■ Post-gastrectomy
■ Hypopituitarism	■ Habit disorder
■ Diabetes mellitus	
■ Thyrotoxicosis	*Psychiatric disorders*
■ Malignant disease	■ Depression
■ Tuberculosis	■ Schizophrenia
■ Malabsorption	■ Obsessive–compulsive disorder
Bingeing	
■ Cerebral damage	
■ Cerebral tumour	

and in risk occupations such as modelling and the performing arts.

Anorexia nervosa most commonly presents as unexplained weight loss in a young female. Other presentations include expressions of concern from relatives, primary or secondary amenorrhoea and abdominal pain. On examination, the severe anorectic has marked wasting, lanugo hair, slow pulse, low blood pressure and cold extremities. Pubic and axillary hair are retained, thus differentiating anorexia nervosa from hypopituitarism, where the patient also tends to be less emaciated. Other readily excluded causes of severe wasting are diabetes mellitus and thyrotoxicosis, but more difficulty may occur in distinguishing a malignancy, occult tuberculosis and malabsorption syndromes.

Bulimia nervosa is characterized by frequent episodes of eating large quantities of high-calorie food in a manner that feels subjectively out of control. Such 'binges' are usually conducted in secret. The binge is usually followed by efforts to purge the body of the 'forbidden' food, and so to control the body weight despite the binge. Techniques include self-induced vomiting, laxative misuse, diuretics, appetite-suppressant drugs, thyroxine and periods of starvation. Bulimia nervosa has an older age of onset (perhaps 19 or 20 years of age) than anorexia nervosa, but again is more common in females. In contrast to anorexia, bulimia has a number of associated psychiatric problems including depression, self-mutilation and binge substance misuse.

Bulimic patients may seek help directly, but it is useful to be aware of the physical signs and complications that can occur. Complications of repeated self-induced vomiting include swelling of the parotid glands, erosion of the dental enamel, hoarseness of voice and, rarely but potentially fatally, hypokalaemia.

It is important to note that *bingeing* may occur in hypothalamic damage or tumour, Klein–Levin syndrome and Kluver–Bucy syndrome, all of which are very rare. *Self-induced vomiting* can develop in patients who have pyloric stenosis or following partial/total gastrectomy, while some individuals practise vomiting either to relieve stress (with no intention of controlling weight), or to titillate or disgust observers. *Purging* by laxative abuse is a common phenomenon, especially in older obsessional or hypochondriacal patients who require regulated bowels to lead a regulated life.

Psychiatric disorders enter the differential diagnosis, particularly depressive anorexia. The distinction can sometimes be difficult with marked weight loss, amenorrhoea, loss of energy, interests and concentration, sleep disturbance, obsessional ruminations and even suicidal ideation and over-eating being potentially shared features. However, there are differences. Appetite is typically diminished in depression but is either normal or increased in eating disorders; more importantly, preoccupation with food and its caloric content, disturbance of body image and a phobia of normal weight are not features of a primary depressive illness. Similarly, these features distinguish an eating disorder from schizophrenia and obsessive–compulsive disorder, which may occasionally present with superficial resemblances through bizarre eating habits or food/weight-related rituals and over-valued ideas.

Indeed, the distinction between an eating disorder and all the physical and psychiatric conditions that enter the differential diagnosis rests not with weight loss, dieting or any particular form of eating abuse, but with the constellation of fears, urges and attitudes that always form the psychological backdrop in both male and female patients. There is a cardinal *morbid fear of becoming fat* which persists, even when grossly underweight or losing weight. Any weight gain or eating provokes anxiety that is relieved only by losing weight either by not eating or by elimination through vomiting, purgation or exercise. Food becomes an enemy, calories an obsession; life becomes dominated by the need to control this aspect of living.

However, there may be great difficulty encountered in penetrating the patient's resistance to elicit the information that is necessary to confirm the diagnosis. Failure to establish this psychological driving force after careful, repeated assessment should alert the physician to the possibility of one of the rare, cryptic presentations in the differential diagnosis.

Andrew Hodgkiss

ELBOW, PAIN IN

See UPPER LIMB, PAIN IN (p. 745).

ENCOPRESIS

(See also FAECES, INCONTINENCE OF, p. 209)
Encopresis is often defined as the passage of faeces in socially unacceptable places; however, it is more accurate to restrict this term to the passage of normal stools in this way. Encopresis is therefore one of the forms of faecal incontinence in children, others being overflow soiling in association with a faecally loaded rectum (in children with non-Hirschsprung's megarectum) or the incontinence associated with diarrhoea (especially if the stools are persistently loose, as in Toddler diarrhoea).

Encopresis is normal in the first 3 years of life. Persistence of encopresis occurs with developmental delay, chaotic training or neglect, or neurogenic rectum (spina bifida, sacral agenesis, spinal tumours or idiopathic). Secondary encopresis (occurring after bowel control has been acquired) is most frequently a response to emotional stress, especially associated with anxiety or suppressed anger. Child physical or sexual abuse may present in this way.

The development of a neurogenic rectum due to spinal tumours, cord damage from trauma or infection will lead to secondary encopresis.

Harold Ellis

ENOPHTHALMOS (OR RETRACTION OF THE EYEBALL)

Enophthalmos is defined as abnormal retrodisplacement of the eyeball. It may be a subtle clinical sign where the palpebral aperture is narrower and the upper eyelid may droop.

This may occur in fractures of the orbital floor, where necrosis of incarcerated orbital fat results in progressive enophthalmos. The enophthalmos that occurs in *wasting diseases* is due to the absorption of orbital fat, and the diagnosis as regards the eye presents no difficulty.

Paralysis of the cervical sympathetic nerves, Horner's syndrome, can give rise to a mild degree of enophthalmos. It is always associated with the other well-defined symptoms of this lesion, namely, diminution in the size of the palpebral aperture, constriction of the pupil, absence of sweating and blushing on the para-lysed side. Occasionally, it may be noticed that the hair over the affected side of the head is behaving differently from that on the unaffected side – that is, it may lie flatter, or may lack lustre to a degree that the patient observes. The pupil is constricted owing to the paralysis of the dilator fibres.

In certain *congenital cases* there is well-marked retraction, associated with defective or irregular movements of the affected eyeball. Rarely, the condition is simulated by a maldevelopment of the globe, which has remained small and is usually extremely hypermetropic and poor-sighted.

Causes of enophthalmos

- Congenital (e.g. microphthalmus; also known as nanophthalmus): this is due to abnormal development resulting in a small eye with abnormal function.
- Phthisis bulbi is a description given to an atrophied eyeball with blindness and decreased intraocular pressure, which has occurred as a result of end-stage ocular disease (e.g. chronic endophthalmitis).
- Fracture of the orbital floor: the soft tissue of the orbit prolapses, causing the eye to sink back into the orbit.
- Atrophy of the orbital contents: secondary to irradiation of the orbit for malignant tumours, scleroderma, or trauma.
- Wasting diseases: HIV infection, malignancy.
- Horner's syndrome, cicatrizing orbital lesions (e.g. metastatic scirrhous carcinoma, any chronic sclerosing inflammatory disease of the orbit).

Sharon O'Byrne

diurnal. Children vary in the age at which they become reliably continent of urine. The majority of children are continent during the day by the age of 3 years, and by night by the age of 5 years. The prevalence of wetting diminishes with age, and approximately 15 per cent of 5-year-olds, and 3 per cent of 10-year-olds, will wet the bed once a week or more. The problem is more common in boys than girls (ratio of 2:1). There is a genetically determined delay in acquiring sphincter continence, with most children having a first-degree relative who was affected.

The commonest organic disease to lead to enuresis is urinary tract infection, especially in girls. Enuretic girls have a four-fold increased likelihood of having a urinary tract infection compared to non-enuretics. Secondary enuresis (having previously been reliably continent) should be considered suspicious of a urinary tract infection, especially when associated with other symptoms such as urinary frequency, abdominal pain, dysuria and wetting in the daytime. Faecal retention can also reduce bladder volume and bladder neck dysfunction. Secondary enuresis can also be caused by neurological problems such as neurogenic bladder (associated with spina bifida or other cord lesions such as tumours). Dribbling urinary incontinence may be the presenting sign of an ectopic ureter draining below the sphincter, or overflow from an obstructed bladder. Polyuria often leads to enuresis in children, and so diseases such as diabetes mellitus or insipidus, or chronic renal failure must be considered. Although most children with enuresis are psychologically and physically normal, emotional problems can sometimes lead to enuresis which compounds the psychological difficulties because of parental reaction (similar to encopresis). Secondary enuresis is common following family break-up or bereavement, and it is important to note that child sexual abuse may also present in this way.

Dipak Kanabar

ENURESIS

(See also URINE, INCONTINENCE OF, p. 763)
Enuresis means incontinence of urine in children, and is usually nocturnal, though it can also be

EPIPHORA

Epiphora is the overflow of tears on to the cheek, and may be due either to increased production of tears or inadequate drainage of tears (Table E.3).

Table E.3 Causes of epiphora

Increased tear secretion
Corneal foreign bodies
Corneal irritation
Corneal inflammation
Nasal irritation

Inadequate drainage of tears
Obstructions in lacrimal pathway
Strictures in lacrimal pathway
Tumours in lacrimal pathway
Punctal or eyelid malpositions
Weakness of orbicularis muscle – ectropion
Nasal obstruction with normal lacrimal pathway

Increased production of tears

Psychic lacrimation is normally associated with pain or emotional upset. Reflex stimulation of lacrimation causing epiphora is commonly associated with irritative conditions or corneal disease. Corneal injury, a blast of air or foreign body on the surface of the eye causes irritation of the trigeminal nerve that excites lacrimation. Even strong light, yawning, vomiting and laughing are associated with reflex lacrimation.

Inadequate drainage of tears

This may be due to malposition of the lacrimal puncta, which should normally be closely applied to the eye in order to attract tears by capillary action. Such malposition may occur in ectropion associated with laxity of the lids which may occur with age, or paralysis of the eyelid muscles which are responsible for blinking in facial palsy or cicatricial lid disease, which pulls the punctum out of its correct position. Obstruction of the lacrimal drainage apparatus (common canaliculus and nasolacrimal duct) will also cause epiphora.

Reginald Daniel

EPISTAXIS

It is important to realize that epistaxis (bleeding from the nose) is a sign, not a disease. Possible causes of the condition are shown in Table E.4.

Table E.4 Causes of epistaxis

Local causes
Trauma to Little's area
Dryness of nasal mucosa
Abnormal anatomy (e.g. septal deviations, spurs)
Ulceration and excoriation
Nasal fracture
Nasal infections
Tumours of the nose and sinuses (e.g. juvenile angiofibroma, squamous cell carcinoma)
Septal granulomas and perforations
Foreign bodies

Systemic causes
Drugs, anticoagulants, NSAIDs, cytotoxic drugs
Hypertension
Atherosclerosis
Coagulopathies: haemophilia, Christmas disease, von Willebrand's disease
Dyscrasias: purpura, leukaemia
Hereditary haemorrhagic telangiectasis
Vitamin deficiency – vitamin C, vitamin K
Renal dialysis

Epistaxis often arises from the anterior part of the nasal septum (Little's area). It is usually of a minor nature, and self-limiting. Bleeding from other parts of the nose may be extremely serious and, on occasion, life-threatening.

The nose receives its blood supply from branches of both the internal and external carotid arteries. The upper part of the nose is supplied by the anterior and posterior ethmoid arteries, branches of the ophthalmic artery (derived from the internal carotid), which enter it through the medial wall of the orbit. The rest of the nose receives its blood supply through the sphenopalatine branch of the maxillary artery and septal branches of the facial artery.

Very often, epistaxis can be controlled by simple measures, for example, compression of the nostrils and application of cold packs. In childhood, when bleeding is almost always from Little's area, these measures are usually effective. If this fails and the site of haemorrhage can be seen, bleeding can often be arrested by cauterization. Otherwise, the nose has to be packed with nasal tampons that expand when irrigated with water. When packing with tampons is ineffective, 1-cm ribbon gauze impregnated with an antiseptic such as bismuth-iodoform paraffin paste (BIPP) may be used instead.

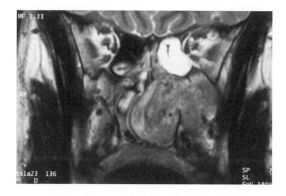

Figure E.2 Magnetic resonance scan of a juvenile angioma. The patient, an adolescent male, presented with progressive, left-sided, nasal obstruction and torrential epistaxes.

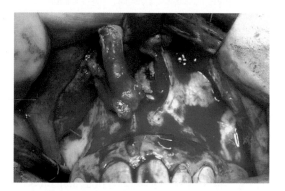

Figure E.3 At operation, the anterior end of the tumour is visible in the left nasal aperture.

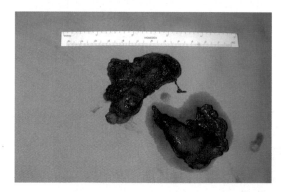

Figure E.4 The operative specimen. The tumour has been completely removed, albeit in two pieces.

All nasal packs should be carefully secured lest they fall backwards into the airway.

Continued bleeding despite local measures may require surgical or radiological intervention. Nowadays, endonasal-endoscopic ligation of the sphenopalatine artery is possible, and often effective. Other more radical approaches include intra-arterial embolization, ligation of the external carotid artery in the neck, maxillary artery behind the maxillary antrum, and ethmoid arteries in the orbit.

Once the bleeding has been stopped and the patient's condition is stable, attention must be devoted to identification of the cause. This is particularly indicated in patients with severe or recurrent minor bleeds. A number of patients will be taking NSAIDs, and these need to be stopped. Others may be anticoagulated, and this may need temporary adjustment. Blood film, indices and coagulation studies should be carefully examined, to eliminate blood discrasias and coagulopathies. Hypertension alone rarely causes nose bleeds, but it is often an accompanying and exacerbating feature and should be controlled in the recovery phase.

It should be remembered that recurrent unilateral nose bleeds may be the first sign of a nasal tumour, and if seen in an adolescent boy should alert one to the possibility of a juvenile angiofibroma (Figs E.2–E.4).

Michael Gleeson

ERYTHEMA

Erythema – redness of the skin – is, along with swelling, heat and pain, one of the four cardinal signs of inflammation, and is the result of vasodilatation caused by release of inflammatory mediators. There are many causes, both local and general (Table E.5).

Local erythema

A localized area of tender erythema may be the initial manifestation of an infection, such as a boil, or of cellulitis. The diagnosis usually becomes evident over the following hours, as the skin becomes rapidly hotter and more tender. Local infections in a limb may be associated with an *ascending lymphangitis*, manifested with a line streak of erythema moving towards the regional lymph nodes. Occasionally, malignant infiltration of the cutaneous lymphatics may present with linear erythematous streaks mimicking an infective lymphangitis, the so-called *lymphangitis carcinomatosa*. In herpetic infections, the initial

Table E.5 Causes of erythema

Localized erythema

Internal

- Boil, herpes simplex, herpes zoster, impetigo, erysipelas, gout, thrombophlebitis, lymphangitis

External

- Irritant (thermal, caustic, traumatic)
- Allergic (allergic contact dermatitis)
- Fixed drug eruption

Localized patterns of erythema (Figs E.5–E.9)

Rosacea
Palmar erythema
Psoriasis
Contact dermatitis
Erythema ab igne
Livedo reticularis
Erythema annulare centrifugum (Lyme disease)
Erythema induratum (Bazin's disease)

Generalized erythema (Figs E.10–E.12)

Toxic erythema
Exanthems

- Measles, rubella, scarlet fever, erythema infectiosum,
- HIV infection

Erythema multiforme
Erythema nodosum
Lupus erythematosus
Dermatomyositis

presentation may be with a local patch of erythema, the hallmark vesicles only becoming evident some hours later. Local erythema over a joint may suggest the diagnosis of gout. Erythema associated with swelling of the skin and intense itching occurs in an acute eczema, whether irritant or allergic in cause. *Fixed drug eruption* is an unusual disorder in which exposure to a causative drug (e.g. phenolphthalein, codeine or sulphonamides) gives a violent local erythema which rapidly darkens to a magenta colour, and usually blisters. It recurs at the same skin sites at each drug exposure.

Selected localized patterns of erythema

Rosacea

The characteristic feature of rosacea is a symmetrical erythema over the cheeks and nose, and spreading onto the forehead and chin. The affected area is red and swollen, and surmounted by sterile pustules and papules. The papules and pustules resolve with oral oxytetracycline, but the erythema tends to persist.

Palmar erythema

As an isolated phenomenon, this is best known in pregnancy, but it is also seen in chronic liver disease, thyrotoxicosis, rheumatoid arthritis and high-output cardiac states. It may also occur as a familial trait.

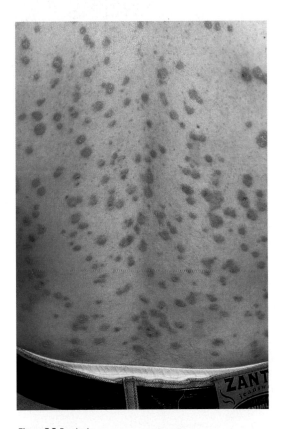

Figure E.5 Psoriasis.

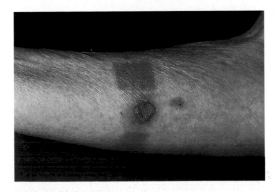

Figure E.6 Contact dermatitis.

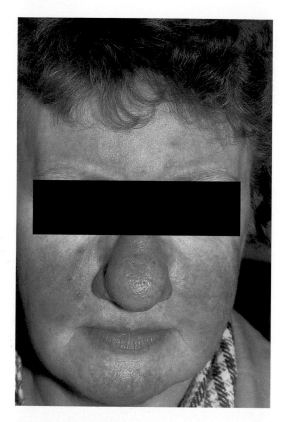

Figure E.7 Rosacea.

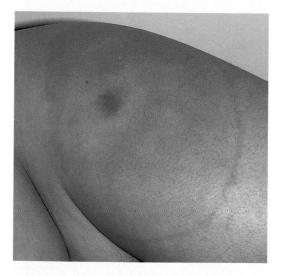

Figure E.8 Erythema chronicum migrans in a case of Lyme disease.

Erythema ab igne

This is a reticulate erythema which progresses to persistent haemosiderin pigmentation due to

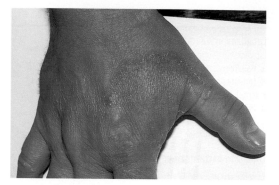

Figure E.9 Tinea manuum.

long-continued exposure to heat (infra-red radiation). It used to be seen on the legs of elderly ladies with longstanding neglected hypothyroidism who sat close to open fires, but is now most commonly encountered on the abdomen in patients with chronic pancreatitis and other painful disorders, and who have used local heat as a form of analgesia.

Erythema chronicum migrans (Lyme disease)

The slowly spreading annular erythematous margin arising at the site of a tick bite is an important manifestion of Lyme disease. This disorder is now known to be a zoonosis, caused by the spirochaete *Borrelia burgdorferi*. The reservoir of infection is in deer, and the vector is the tick *Ixodes ricinus*. The condition is so named because of an outbreak of the disorder around the town of Lyme in the north-east of the United States. A rising specific IgA titre aids clinical diagnosis. Adequate treatment with penicillin or tetracycline is very important, as a proportion of untreated patients progress to serious CNS, cardiac or rheumatological problems, sometimes *after* the erythema has resolved.

Some very rare migratory erythemas can be cutaneous markers of underlying neoplasia; examples include necrolytic migratory erythema (glucagon-secreting pancreatic tumour) and erythema gyratum repens (carcinoma or lymphoma).

Erythema induratum (Bazin's disease)

This is a rare manifestation of tuberculosis which is seen in middle-aged women. The site affected is the posterior aspect of the legs, and the condition begins as a symmetrical eruption of deep-seated painless red nodules. The surface becomes purple, and deep cold ulcers form which have undermined borders. The patients show extreme sensitivity to tuberculin on skin testing.

Generalized erythema

Erythema nodosum

In this distinctive disorder there is an acute eruption of hot, tender, erythematous nodules, usually over the extensor aspects of the lower legs, but the thighs, buttocks and extensor surfaces of the arms may also be involved. The nodules are hard and deep, with shiny red overlying skin, but they gradually soften and their colour changes to violet and finally yellow; however, they never suppurate or ulcerate. An accompanying arthralgia is common and there may be fever and malaise, whatever the underlying cause. Some cases are apparently idiopathic, but an assiduous search must be made for an underlying cause. The relative frequency of different causes will vary in different parts of the world. In Britain, the commonest cause (amongst women) is sarcoidosis, but in South Asian patients tuberculosis should be suspected. Penicillin, sulphonamides and barbiturates are the most commonly implicated drugs. Rarer causes include ulcerative colitis, Crohn's disease, histoplasmosis, coccidioidomycosis, blastomycosis, chlamydial infections and Behçet's syndrome. A leprosy conversion reaction may manifest itself as an erythema nodosum-like phenomenon.

Erythema multiforme

This disorder is characterized by a sudden eruption of erythematous lesions arising especially over the hands, feet, buttocks and genitalia, and often accompanied by lesions on the oral or genital mucosa, and the conjunctiva (Fig. E.10). The skin lesions are classically polycyclic, giving the appearance of an archery target ('target lesions'). In severe cases, the centre of the lesion may blister or become necrotic. When the mucosal lesions are severe, the condition is termed Stevens–Johnson syndrome. In some cases no specific cause is found, but it may be triggered by an infection (herpes simplex, orf, mycoplasma), a drug, or radiotherapy. Spontaneous resolution occurs, but recurrent episodes may arise.

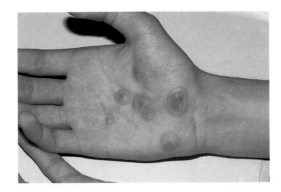

Figure E.10 Erythema multiforme.

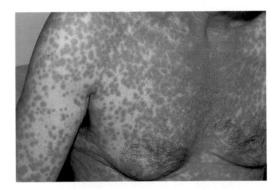

Figure E.11 Drug reaction (amoxycillin).

Toxic erythema

This is a widespread symmetrical blotchy erythema which tends to affect the trunk more than the extremities, and is often accompanied by malaise, fever and lymphadenopathy. This cutaneous reaction pattern may be provoked by many causes such as viral infections (especially glandular fever), and also drug hypersensitivity, especially to ampicillin, amoxicillin (Fig. E.11), sulphonamides and NSAIDs. Often, no cause is found. Spontaneous resolution, which usually occurs within 10–15 days, is often followed by desquamation.

Exanthems

In *measles*, the rash usually develops on the fourth day, behind the ears. It spreads to the face and downwards to the trunk and extremities on the fifth to seventh days. The eruption is usually preceded by 1 to 7 days of prodromal coryza, nasal discharge and conjunctival injection, on the second or third day of which Koplik's spots appear, as white specks surrounded by redness, on the buccal mucosa opposite the molar teeth. Koplik's spots may be lentil-sized and few in number, or salt grain-sized and very numerous. The fever, which may have been high during the prodromal stage, persists while the rash appears and usually decreases as it fades. Cough, facial puffiness and photophobia are also diagnostic pointers.

Rubella usually affects an older child or young adult, and is typically accompanied by posterior cervical and postauricular lymph node enlargement. The rash, which also begins on the face and spreads downwards to trunk and extremities, is composed of faint pink macules, and fades in 3 days. Constitutional symptoms are mild, but joint pain may be prominent in adults.

Scarlet fever usually affects children under 10 years of age, who become acutely ill with high fever and vomiting. The throat is red and oedematous, and there is characteristically a 'strawberry tongue'. The rash is lobster-red with punctate deeper red lesions (likened to small spots of red ink on red blotting paper), and appears on the second and third days behind the ears, spreading rapidly to the face, upper chest and flexor surfaces of the limbs. Purpura may develop in the skin creases. The fever persists with the rash from 2 to 5 days, and is followed by desquamation in large flakes from palms and soles.

Erythema infectiosum (*fifth disease*) affects children between 2 and 10 years of age. It begins with a 'slapped-face' erythema on the cheeks in an otherwise well child. Over the next few days a maculopapular eruption spreads, sometimes in gyrate pattern over the limbs and trunk. The illness is due to a parvovirus, and heals in 1–2 weeks, though successive bouts may occur.

A macular erythematous rash accompanies the *seroconversion illness of primary infection with HIV* in some 50 per cent of patients. Between 10 and 14 days after exposure, fever, systemic toxicity and lymphadenopathy may occur. From 5 to 8 days later, oval macular erythematous lesions may appear on the trunk and limbs, extending beyond the usual T-shirt distribution of pityriasis rosea onto the palms and soles. The oral mucosa can be affected with superficial erosions. The whole illness most closely resembles secondary syphilis or glandular fever with rash. Lymphopenia and thrombocytopenia may occur. HIV seroconversion occurs at 4–8 weeks.

Lupus erythematosus

This is an important cause of erythema. It is more common in women than men, and is usually classified into two varieties: systemic and discoid. The systemic form affects joints, kidneys and the haemopoietic, cardiovascular, respiratory and central nervous systems, as well as the skin, and occurs in a younger age group than the discoid form, which is a dermatological disorder. In the skin, both types of lupus erythematosus cause perifollicular inflammation which is followed by scarring. The classic lesion of lupus erythematosus is an atrophic red scaly plaque with follicular plugging. The histopathology is characteristic, showing epidermal thinning and basal cell liquefaction. Direct immunofluorescence microscopy demonstrates linear staining at the basement membrane in the lesions of both types.

Systemic lupus erythematosus (SLE) should be suspected in young women presenting with weakness, fever, weight loss, arthralgia and proteinuria, as well as a persistent erythematous rash on the face or areas exposed to sunlight. The so-called 'butterfly rash' over the face, whilst well-known, occurs in only a minority of patients with cutaneous manifestations of SLE. Although typical lupus erythematosus plaques may be found – particularly over the dorsa of the hands and fingers – they are less common than other erythematous rashes seen in SLE, such as urticaria, urticated plaques, livedo reticularis, photosensitivity and nailfold erythema. A diffuse telogen effluvium is not infrequent. Established cases often have tell-tale signs on the hands; as well as nailfold erythema and telangiectasia, there may be infarcts of the cuticles, finger nodules and pulp atrophy. Some 80–90 per cent of such patients will have circulating antinuclear antibodies in high titre, and raised DNA binding proteins. Different varieties of antinuclear antibodies exist and relate to differing clinical presentations, and this is the subject of current clinical research. The antinuclear antibodies can often be demonstrated throughout the skin (e.g. by taking a biopsy of non-light-exposed normal skin). This test is negative in the discoid variety. A systemic pattern, but without renal mortality, can be induced by certain drugs, such as hydralazine, procaine amide, griseofulvin and phenytoin.

Chronic discoid lupus erythematosus (CDLE) lesions largely occur on sun-exposed sites such as the cheeks, forehead, nose and perioral skin, although the scalp is not infrequently affected. Lesions persist for many months, extending slowly, and leaving depigmented, central atrophic and hairless scars. Close examination of the erythematous active edge shows telangiectasia and follicular plugging (which can be demonstrated by detaching an adherent scale and observing downward-projecting 'tin-tack' plugs). Although the direct immunofluorescent test of such lesions will be positive, in 80 per cent of patients no circulating anti-nuclear antibodies are found. Less than 5 per cent of patients progress to the systemic form.

Dermatomyositis

The principal cutaneous signs of dermatomyositis are erythema and oedema (Fig. E.12). The proximal myopathy is described in detail elsewhere. There is often marked discordance between the severity of skin and muscle disease in any individual patient. The dermatological hallmark is a particular periorbital bluish-red oedema ('heliotrope' erythema): periungual changes identical to SLE (see above) may be seen, often with papules over the dorsa of the fingers (Gottron's papules). A diffuse scaling erythema of sun-exposed areas can occur, as well as psoriasiform lesions over elbows and knees. In common with SLE, there is histological basal cell liquefaction and follicular plugging. A patient over 40 years of age with dermatomyositis should be investigated for underlying neoplasia, which will be present in some 40 per cent of cases. Childhood dermatomyositis is almost never associated with malignancy, but can be responsible for considerable and disabling soft tissue calcification.

Barry Monk

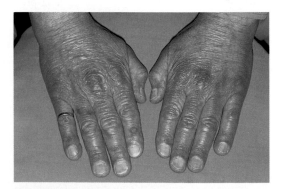

Figure E.12 Dermatomyositis.

EUPHORIA

Euphoria describes an elevation of a person's mood. It is frequently the presenting symptom of manic depressive (bipolar) illness or schizophrenia, but these diagnoses should not be made before drug-induced mania and organic mood syndromes have been ruled out. The causes of euphoria are listed in Table E.6. Mania is one of the commonest and most clearly identified causes of euphoria, but the diagnosis is frequently missed or delayed until the patient and their family has come to harm through a combination of grandiosity and poor judgement. Diagnosis is based on the presence of either elated or irritable mood associated with some or all of the following features: over-activity; pressure of speech; racing thoughts or flight of ideas; distractability; grandiose ideas which

Table E.6 Causes of euphoria

Common causes
Alcohol
Mania
Schizophrenia and schizoaffective disorder
Cyclothymic personality
Early dementia (Alzheimer's type dementia, multi-infarct)
Frontal lobe syndrome
Frontal tumours (meningioma)
Head injury
Therapeutic drugs
- Corticosteroids
- L-dopa
- Bromocriptine
- Benzhexol
- Proclidine
- Antidepressants (e.g. tricyclics, SSRIs and MAOIs)
Substance abuse
- Amphetamines and other sympathomimetics
- Cannabis
- Cocaine
- Hallucinogens (e.g. LSD, psilocybins, mescaline)
- Phencyclidine and related compounds
- Opioids (heroin, morphine, codeine, etc.)
- Inhalants (many solvents and spray-can propellants)
- Sedatives, hypnotics, anxiolytics (benzodiazepines, barbiturates)

Less common causes
Temporal lobe epilepsy
Multiple sclerosis
Hyperthyroidism
Pick's disease
Neurosyphilis
Mild hypoxia (e.g. high altitude)

may be delusional; decreased sleep; increased appetite; and behaviour which indicates poor judgement. The patient may become sexually disinhibited, spend too much money, or drive recklessly thereby endangering life. The mood can have the quality of infectious good humour, but irritability is also common, and at interview euphoria may be quickly and dramatically replaced by tearfulness, feelings of depression and remorse lasting for a few minutes before euphoria once again dominates the picture (labile mood).

In *bipolar illness* bouts of euphoria lasting more than a week or so may be preceded or followed by periods of depression. *Cyclothymia* describes a milder chronic form of bipolar illness in which the subject is prone to constant swings between mood elevation and depression, with only brief stretches of normality. In such cases a moderate level of euphoria persisting for weeks or even months serves the subject well by increasing drive and enthusiasm, leading to increased sociability and greater involvement in sexual, political, religious or occupational activities. When a patient's mood is significantly elevated it can be a difficult judgement for the clinician to decide when to try to intervene. Mania sometimes presents for the first time in the puerperium, and in some depressed patients it is precipitated by the use of treatments including antidepressants or electroconvulsant therapy (ECT). The acute phase of a severe manic illness may be impossible to distinguish from schizophrenia, and the diagnosis will only be clarified by follow-up. In schizophrenia itself, states of excitement with increased activity and euphoria are quite common, although often there is a bizarre quality to the thoughts and incongruity of affect that distinguishes the schizophrenic states from manic illness. *Schizoaffective disorder* describes those conditions which have features both of schizophrenia and depression or mania.

Many organic conditions may present with an elevated mood resembling a manic episode and these include causes of *delirium*, where there will be impairment of consciousness. Hyperthyroidism may produce a manic syndrome, and the use of corticosteroids, L-dopa, bromocriptine, and the anticholinergic drugs procyclidine and benzhexol, may cause euphoria.

Damage to the frontal lobes is sometimes associated with mild euphoria out of keeping with the patient's situation. The mood is often facile or facetious and accompanied by changes in personality, including disinhibition, deteriorating social behaviour and a loss of spontaneity and volition. Slow-growing frontal tumours (e.g. meningiomas), multiple sclerosis and dementia (Alzheimer's and Pick's disease) may cause a *frontal lobe syndrome. Temporal lobe epilepsy* may be associated with a psychosis resembling manic illness. Rarely, neurosyphilis and porphyria can cause euphoric or grandiose states.

Many drugs are taken because of their ability to cause euphoria, the most common being alcohol. The list of compounds used to obtain a 'high' include sympathomimetics (amphetamine, dextroamphetamine, methamphetamine, methylphenadate and appetite suppressants); cannabis; cocaine; hallucinogens (e.g. LSD, mescaline, magic mushrooms); inhalants, including the aliphatic and aromatic hydrocarbons found in petrol, glue, paint and typewriter correction fluid; spray-can propellants; anaesthetic gases (e.g. nitrous oxide and ether); short-acting vasodilators such as amyl or butyl nitrite; opioids (heroin, morphine), many compounds prescribed as analgesics, anaesthetics or cough suppressants (e.g. codeine, methadone); sedatives, hypnotics and anxiolytics (e.g. benzodiazepines and barbiturates).

The diagnosis of a drug-induced euphoric state is made from the history and circumstances of the admission, and by urine drug screening for substances. Typically, the altered mood state is relatively brief. Diagnostic difficulties can arise in patients with a history of prolonged drug abuse, for example with cocaine, which may trigger a psychosis that is indistinguishable from mania or schizophrenia. The picture is further complicated because patients with bipolar disorder or schizophrenia may be heavy drinkers or drug misusers and may experience an exacerbation of their underlying condition through the drugs they are using.

Andrew Hodgkiss

EXOPHTHALMOS (OR PROPTOSIS)

This condition may be either bilateral or unilateral.

Bilateral exophthalmos

The commonest cause of this condition is *Graves' disease*, in which the exophthalmos is associated with thyroid gland swelling, and other general symptoms such as tachycardia, fine tremors and general nervousness. The degree of prominence of the eyes is variable, in some cases being so great that there is inadequate lid coverage of the cornea on attempted eye closure. A protrusion causes retraction of the upper eye lid; consequently the eyes look wide open, giving the patient an expression of alarm or astonishment (Stellwag's sign; Fig. E.13). When the eyes are lowered, the upper lids lag behind the downward excursion of the eye, leaving a broad portion of the sclera visible above the cornea (von Graefe's sign). The extent of exophthalmos may be asymmetrical, with minimal involvement of the other eye. The condition sometimes appears to be unilateral. Increasing oedema of the lids along with inflammation of the conjunctiva and dilatation of the vessels over the insertion, particularly of the lateral rectus, are significant findings. The myopathy of Graves' disease most frequently involves the vertically acting muscles, with limitation of upward eye movement.

Bilateral exophthalmos is also associated with:

- Chronic obstructive pulmonary disease
- Superior vena cava syndrome
- Cushing's syndrome.

Other uncommon causes of bilateral exophthalmos are septic thrombosis of the cavernous sinus historically associated with skin infection at the inner angle of the eye or ethmoidal sinus suppuration; bilateral lymphomatous deposits; pseudotumour and, in children, the craniodysostoses.

Unilateral exophthalmos

Unilateral exophthalmos may be due to:

- Orbital cellulitis
- Orbital neoplasms
- Meningioma
- Lymphoma
- Lacrimal gland tumour
- Optic nerve glioma
- Pseudotumour (a space-filling lesion with the characteristics of a chronic infiltrating inflammatory process)
- Carotid–cavernous sinus fistulae
- Cavernous sinus thrombosis
- Cavernous haemangioma
- Mucocele
- Infiltrative disorders (e.g. sarcoid, Wegener's granulomatosis, xanthogranuloma).

Orbital cellulitis can begin as a primary inflammatory process in front of the orbital septum, thereafter extending backwards or rising from direct orbital extension of a paranasal sinus infection (Fig. E.14). The dire complication of further progression is septic cavernous sinus thrombosis. The general signs and symptoms of cavernous sinus thrombosis are more serious than in uncomplicated orbital cellulitis. Headache, nausea, vomiting and altered consciousness are early signs. Venous congestion produces gross chemosis and proptosis with a bluish discoloration of the eyelids. There is early onset of pan-ocular motor paresis. Bilateral involvement is virtually diagnostic of cavernous sinus thrombosis. Pseudotumour involvement of the orbit usually first appears above, but may also be found in, the inferior retrobulbar tissues. Another area of involvement is at the apex of the

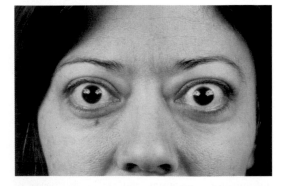

Figure E.13 Stellwag's sign. Reproduced with kind permission of the patient.

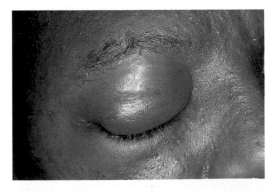

Figure E.14 Acute orbital cellulitis.

orbit when visual loss may be of early onset. A pseudotumour along the superior orbital fissure causes a painful external ophthalmoplegia (Tolosa–Hunt syndrome).

Capillary haemangioma is the commonest cause of unilateral proptosis in childhood. Adult cavernous haemangioma causes a slowly progressive exophthalmos.

Orbital lymphomas usually occur in the anterior orbit and involve the conjunctiva and eyelids. However, posterior orbital involvement may occur, and it is important to exclude a primary systemic lymphoma. Lacrimal gland tumours occur characteristically at the upper lateral portion of the orbit, causing painless downward and medial displacement of the globe and irregular enlargement of the lacrimal fossa.

Dermoid cysts specifically appear in childhood at the upper lateral quadrant of the orbit. Superior and medial swellings are more suggestive of mucocoeles of the frontal or ethmoidal sinus. Teratomas may occur congenitally or in very early life. Rhabdomyosarcoma is the commonest intra-orbital malignant tumour of childhood, presenting within the first decade of life. The development of proptosis is rapid, occurring within 1–3 weeks. The rapidity of progression is more or less pathognomonic of this tumour.

Optic nerve gliomas usually manifest before the age of 5 years, and result in a downwards nasal and forward proptosis. Meningiomas usually occur in older women, but can occur in childhood, where their course is much more rapid. Orbital haemorrhage may arise from trauma or sudden extreme physical effort and cause bleeding from orbital varices, leading to alarming, progressive orbital swelling. Arteriovenous fistula can occur following fracture of the base of the skull, with rupture of the internal carotid artery as it passes through the cavernous sinus. The carotid–cavernous sinus fistula causes a pulsatile proptosis of the eyeball associated with a bruit which is synchronous with the pulse. Gross dilatation of the conjunctival vessels is visible, with arterialization of the conjunctival veins. Intermittent unilateral exophthalmos in children following coughing or crying is nearly always associated with a deep cavernous haemangioma.

Ultrasound scanning, CT, MRI and biopsy are all useful in assessing cases of exophthalmos.

Sharon O'Byrne

EYE, BLINDNESS OF

(See also VISION, DEFECTS OF, p. 776)
The World Health Organization defines blindness as a central visual acuity of less than 3/60 (1/20), or a visual field of less than 10 degrees. An alternative functional definition is loss of vision sufficient to prevent one from being self-supporting in an occupation, making the individual dependent on other persons, agencies and devices in order to live.

Colour blindness is a genetically determined disorder which is a minor handicap and is not true blindness.

The causes and prevalence of blindness through the world vary from country to country. It is estimated that 75 per cent of blindness in the world is avoidable.

The leading causes of blindness are trachoma, leprosy, onchocerciasis, xerophthalmia and cataract. In Western countries, age-related macular degeneration, diabetic retinopathy and glaucoma are the most common problems.

Different categories of the blind have different needs, and the agencies for the blind access the individual blind person's requirements and provide a variety of services, including mobility training, visual magnifying aids, talking books, training of Braille, educational assessment, job rehabilitation and psychological counselling.

Reginald Daniel

EYE, INFLAMMATION OF (RED EYE)

Inflammation of the eye may involve the conjunctiva (as a conjunctivitis), the cornea (keratitis, usually in the form of a corneal ulcer) and, less commonly, the uvea (uveitis) and sclera (scleritis). Localized patches of episcleritis may superficially resemble conjunctivitis, and the dusky circumcorneal congestion in an acute glaucoma may simulate that from an acute anterior uveitis. The character of the inflammation varies with the type of the disease, but certain symptoms such as pain, photophobia and lacrimation are common to all inflammatory conditions, and are by themselves of little value in the differential diagnosis.

Conjunctivitis

In conjunctivitis the conjunctival vessels are dilated; they are freely movable over the subjacent sclera, and the conjunctival injection is most evident at a little distance from the corneal margin. The circumcorneal portion of the conjunctiva, owing to its firmer attachment to the sclera in this region, is relatively less injected. If the condition is purely conjunctival, the cornea is clear and bright, the anterior chamber and iris are normal in appearance, and the pupil is black with normal reactions. Purulent discharge may occur and there is often a feeling of grittiness as of sand or dust in the eye. Hyperaemia of the conjunctiva may be secondary to a foreign body on the cornea or on the conjunctiva itself, particularly underneath the upper lid.

Inturning of the eyelid (entropion) allows the eyelashes to rub against the cornea and conjunctiva (trichiasis), producing conjunctival hyperaemia and predisposing to conjunctivitis.

The use of topical drugs may produce an allergic conjunctivitis which is often associated with signs of allergy of the skin of the lids. Strong ultraviolet irradiation damages the conjunctival corneal epithelium, when using a sun-lamp or arc-welder without eye protection, producing conjunctival hyperaemia with considerable irritation or pain.

Conjunctivitis may be associated with a mucopurulent ocular discharge (Fig. E.15). The lids may be stuck together after sleep, the pain is generally slight, and allayed by closing the eyes. Mucopurulent conjunctivitis is characterized by more profuse discharge and is frequently due to infection by *Staphylococcus* or *Streptococcus* and *Haemophilus* species.

Some particular forms of conjunctivitis deserve special mention. In *ophthalmia neonatorum* (acute conjunctivitis of the newborn), caused by infection from the birth canal (*Chlamydia, Staphylococcus* or *Gonococcus*), there is often profuse mucopurulent discharge. The condition is differentiated from imperfect canalization of the nasolacrimal ducts by the fact that in the latter the discharge is present without the accompanying inflammation. Untreated cases are at grave risk of secondary corneal ulceration and require identification and early antibiotic therapy.

In *trachoma* (Fig. E.16), which is a chlamydial infection (endemic in the Middle East but rare in the UK), the conjunctiva is studded with enlarged follicles, particularly on the under-surface of the upper lid and in the upper conjunctival fornix. The follicular enlargement is associated with thickening and oedema of the tissues of the upper lid, causing partial ptosis with excess lacrimation and, in the later stages, vascular infiltrate (pannus) of the upper part of the cornea. In the later stages of trachoma the infiltration is followed by scarring which may distort the tarsal plate, leading to cicatricial entropion and trichiasis.

Conjunctival allergies are characterized particularly by oedema of the conjunctiva (conjunctival chemosis) and of the skin of the lids, epiphora and itch. They include non-specific responses to a wide miscellany of drugs, cosmetics and other irritants. Three specific clinical forms are recognized:

1 Hayfever, from exogenous pollens, etc.

2 Phlyctenular conjunctivitis (due to an allergic reaction, e.g. to a *Staphylococcus* organism), featuring marked

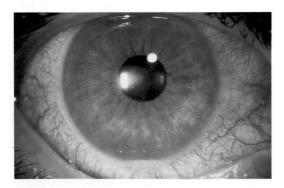

Figure E.15 Acute conjunctivitis. [Moorfields Eye Hospital.]

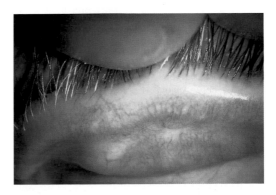

Figure E.16 Trachomatous scarring of everted upper lid. [Moorfields Eye Hospital.]

photophobia and one or more round yellowish, raised masses at the corneoscleral junction surrounded by a localized area of vascular conjunctiva. In some cases the phlycten encroach on the corneal surface, being followed by a trail or leash of conjunctival vessels.

3 Spring catarrh, which exists in palpebral and bulbar forms, the former showing polygonal flat-topped conjunctival nodules resembling cobblestones, the latter showing focal gelatinous limbal thickening.

Keratitis

Corneal ulcers produce greyish or white opacities of the corneal stroma with loss of the corneal epithelium. In more serious untreated cases, infiltrations of the cornea may lead to loss of corneal tissue and progress to perforation of the cornea. In severe cases, there may be pus in the anterior chamber – hypopyon (see Fig. C.24). The diagnosis presents no difficulty; the ulcers are obvious if the cornea is examined carefully, and stained with fluorescein.

Iritis

In iritis or 'anterior uveitis', the eye is congested and painful (in contrast to a 'posterior uveitis', or choroiditis, which simply blurs the vision). This vasodilatation differs from that in a conjunctivitis in that it is most evident in the circumcorneal region, with the tarsal conjunctiva remaining unaffected, and that the colour of the injection is brick-red rather than pink. The cornea retains its clarity, but the aqueous may be turbid due to the presence of cells and protein, and there may be punctate deposits of leucocytes on the posterior surface of the cornea (keratic precipitates), or rarely a hypopyon or pus level within the anterior chamber (see Fig. C.24). Owing to the increased vascularity of the iris, and to the exudation into iris substance, its volume is increased and its mobility impaired; hence the pupil becomes small and sluggish.

The presence of blood and exudate in the substance of the iris also changes its apparent colour – a blue iris becomes greenish, and the fine detail of the iris structure is blurred and obliterated. Adhesions are apt to occur between the iris and the lens at the point of their immediate contact, the edge of the pupil; in the constricted state of the pupil these may not be seen. On dilatation with cyclopentolate or atropine, these adhesions or posterior synechiae prevent the enlargement

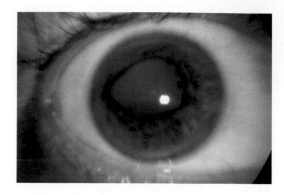

Figure E.17 Iridocyclitis synechiae. [Moorfields Eye Hospital.]

of the pupil at certain points, and it therefore becomes irregular in shape (Fig. E.17). Small masses of iris pigment may also be seen on the anterior surface of the lens where the mydriatic may have broken down some of the weaker adhesions. An exudate into the pupillary aperture may form a fibrinous membrane, completely or partially blocking the pupil.

An important form of iritis (or, more properly, of uveitis, since the ciliary body and choroid are also involved) may occur in the second eye following a perforating injury in the first – this is 'sympathetic ophthalmitis'. This possibility must always be borne in mind in cases of previous perforation of the globe, as it relentlessly leads to blindness unless suppressed by steroid treatment at an early stage.

Glaucoma

Acute-angle closure glaucoma is a disease of the later years of life, and of hypermetropes rather than myopes. It is precipitated by any of the factors that may provoke dilatation of the pupil.

At first, the chief complaint in subacute attacks is of temporary obscuring of vision and the appearance of haloes or rainbows around light sources. There is also often a feeling of tension in the eye and a dull frontal headache in addition to the loss of vision. In acute attacks, the pain is severe, radiates from the eye to the head, the ears and teeth, and is associated with nausea – a symptom which may lead to the mistaken diagnosis of migraine. The lids may be oedematous and the conjunctiva injected (Fig. E.18). The cornea is hazy due to oedema, the anterior chamber shallow, the iris appears discoloured, and the pupil mid-dilated and fixed. The eye is hard to the touch

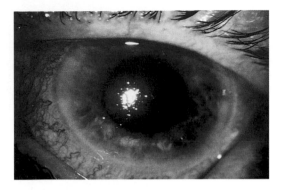

Figure E.18 Acute glaucoma. [Moorfields Eye Hospital.]

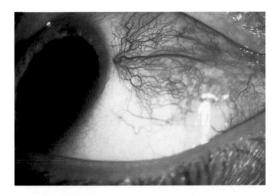

Figure E.19 Episcleritis. [Moorfields Eye Hospital.]

Table E.7 A summary of the points of distinction between conjunctivitis, iritis, acute glaucoma and keratitis

	Conjunctivitis	**Iritis**	**Acute glaucoma**	**Keratitis**
Conjunctiva	Conjunctival vessels bright red and injected; movable over subjacent sclera; injection most marked away from corneoscleral margin; colour fades on pressure	Ciliary vessels injected, deep-red; most marked at corneoscleral margin; colour does not fade on pressure	Both conjunctival and ciliary vessels injected but dusky in colour	Conjunctival vessels red and injected. Injection most marked near the corneoscleral margin
Cornea	Clear, sensitive	Clear, sensitive	Steamy, hazy, insensitive	Irregular reflex, corneal opacity
Anterior	Clear; normal depth	Aqueous may be turbid	Very shallow	Normal, hypopyon
Iris	Normal	Swollen, adherent to lens and muddy coloured	Injected	Normal
Pupil	Black, active (normal)	Small and fixed, later festooned after adhesions form to lens	Mid-dilated, fixed, oval	Black active (normal)
Intraocular	Normal	Normal	Raised	Normal tension

and very tender. Vision fails rapidly, even down to bare perception of light, within a few hours.

The distinction between subacute or acute glaucoma (as just described) and chronic simple glaucoma is easily made. Chronic simple glaucoma is an asymptomatic disease, and is usually discovered in the course of routine examination. No pain, blurring of vision, haloes or feeling of tension are complained of, and the visual field loss which characterizes this disease is rarely noticed by the patient in the early stages.

The importance of discriminating between iritis and acute-angle closure glaucoma cannot be overemphasized; the use of atropine or some similar mydriatic is a basic treatment of iritis, while in acute glaucoma it is disastrous (Table E.7).

Acute inflammation of the eye may be seen in episcleritis and scleritis (Fig. E.19). Episcleritis may be either simple or nodular, producing localized injection of the episcleral vessels. In either type the condition is normally idiopathic and asymptomatic, with the patient merely complaining of redness of the eye. Scleritis is a more serious condition, often associated with the connective tissue disorders. In contrast to episcleritis, the eye is painful and tender, with a deep-seated bluish injection. Recurrent episodes of inflammation of the sclera may produce progressive scleral thinning. Early treatment with systemic anti-inflammatory drugs or corticosteroids is mandatory.

Reginald Daniel

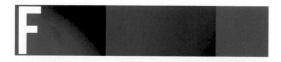

FACE, ABNORMALITIES OF APPEARANCE AND MOVEMENT

The patient's features, expression and facial movements can in many cases suggest an instant diagnosis. While such 'spot' diagnoses may often be wildly inaccurate, in many cases they prove more telling than many investigative procedures performed later to prove or disprove a diagnosis. Experience alone can teach the student to detect all that is to be learned from the patient's facies. The more subtle abnormalities of expression, the play of the emotions, and the response of the features to questioning and intellectual and emotional challenge are transient and fleeting, and cannot be recorded or reproduced. Indeed, they are sometimes so intangible as to defy any attempt to describe them. The passive vacant aspect of a chronic alcoholic, the tremor of his or her mouth when they open it to protest their temperance, are clinical observations which cannot be reproduced visually, except by a television camera. The shifty eyes of the drug addict, the fatuous placidity of the patient with advanced multiple sclerosis, the anxious look of those within a few days of death, the explosive suddenness with which the victim of multiple sclerosis or brain damage bursts into laughter or tears, the vacant stare of the mentally defective child, the unsmiling sad appearance of the depressed, the distant removed look of the schizoid personality, the excessive vivaciousness of the hypomanic – these are a few of the many familiar and striking lessons of the face which must be seen in real life if they are to be learned and utilized. It is upon the appearance of the face that people most rely for the judgement of general health and well-being, for this is the only part of the body which everybody is habitually accustomed to see – plumpness or wasting, the complexion, the expression, the carriage of the head, the way the eyes, brows, cheeks and mouth move, for example, may all suggest certain disorders. Appearances may be deceptive however. Pallor is by no means the same thing as anaemia; a ruddy complexion is not necessarily a sign of rude health; it is often far from easy to distinguish the appearance of illness from the expression of unhappiness; it is all too easy to mistake for aggression what is really shyness.

Cretinoid facies

Compared with the general stunted growth of the rest of the body, the head of the child hypothyroid from birth is relatively large. The expression is dull or stolid. The face is broad, and remarkable for thick eyelids, broad flat nose, thick lips and widely spaced eyes. The mouth is usually open, the tongue may be more or less constantly protruded, and the chin is poorly developed. The hair is scanty and brittle, the skin coarse, dry or muddy, and often almost yellow.

Myxoedematous facies

The dulled intelligence of the patient is betrayed by the apathetic physiognomy (Fig. F.1). The skin of the myxoedematous face is coarse, dry, sallow, pale and waxy, with occasionally a tinted rose-purple flush over each cheek. The puffiness of the eyelids may suggest acute glomerulonephritis, but the subcutaneous tissue everywhere is of firm consistence, and doughy rather than oedematous. The tongue is enlarged. The nose is broadened, the ears are thickened and the lips swollen. The hair is scanty, receding from the forehead, the eyebrows are thin and sparse (although the scantiness of the outer half often regarded as a

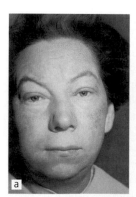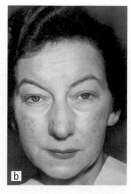

Figure F.1 Facies in myxoedema (a) before and (b) after treatment. [Dr P. M. F. Bishop.]

diagnostic feature occurs too frequently in normal subjects for this to be reliable), the nails brittle and striated. Masses of fatty tissue may be found in the neck and trunk. The slow, husky speech, the expressionless face, and the general attitude of the patient may superficially suggest parkinsonism, but the diagnosis may be made by paying attention to other clinical features. In hypopituitarism, the eyelids and nose – in contrast to myxoedema – are unaffected, and show no undue thickening. Another point of differentiation is that in pituitary disease complete loss of axillary and pubic hair is common – a feature that does not always occur in myxoedema. In hypopituitarism, the face is hairless in males or females and unduly wrinkled. The features are those of a middle-aged Peter (or Pauline) Pan. In contrast, the patient with myxoedema looks like a wax doll who has been left in a sunlit shop window for too long. In hypopituitarism the skin is soft and smooth and the hair of soft texture, whilst in myxoedema hairs and skin are of coarser quality. The voice in myxoedema is a husky croak, but in hypopituitarism it is normal.

Congenital syphilitic facies

The victims of congenital syphilis, now an extreme rarity, after 10–12 years of age, may present a facies which is unmistakable – an overhanging forehead, perhaps frontal bosses, a depressed nasal bridge, striated scars radiating from the corners and other parts of the lips, with a sallow, earthy complexion. Closer observation of the eyes and teeth may detect the opacities of old keratitis, and the changes in the upper incisors which were stated by Jonathan Hutchinson to be pathognomonic. These teeth are wide-gapped, irregular, and so deficient in enamel over the anterior and median parts of their cutting edges that the resulting crescentic notch imparts a striking appearance.

Myopathic facies

Many cases of myopathy show no characteristic facies; in *facioscapulohumeral dystrophy* the face is always involved, the muscles around the mouth being affected most with a loose pout of the lips at rest and 'transverse' smile (*tire en travers*). These features are due to defective facial musculature, particularly to

weakness of the orbicularis oris. Paresis of the orbiculares palpebrarum is only evident when an attempt is made to close the eyes, although it may sometimes lead to prominent and perhaps staring eyeballs. An inability of the patient to whistle or to blow out their cheeks demonstrates the weakness of the orbicularis oris, which is often rendered obvious by the large amount of labial mucous membrane exposed while the mouth is at rest.

In *dystrophia myotonica* (*myotonia atrophica, Steinert's disease*), ptosis, facial weakness and dysarthria occur. There is a characteristic weakness and diminution in the size of the sternomastoids and the masticatory muscles are poorly developed or waste early, giving a long lean facial appearance. In males, frontal baldness is common. In the rare *ocular myopathy* there is progressive ptosis of the eyelids and immobility of the eyes.

Myasthenic facies

In patients suffering from myasthenia gravis there are two types of facies. The first is the patient whose lids lag with fatigue. The second depends on the characteristic myasthenic smile, almost a sneer. This unfortunate and misleading facial expression is the result of deficient action on the part of the zygomatic and risorius muscles, and exemplifies the curious way in which in this disease some muscles are affected and others escape, even when they derive their innervation from the same source. In patients with this disorder, facial weakness is worsened by repeated movement, but it responds rapidly (though transiently) to anticholinesterase drugs such as intravenous edrophonium, which acts more rapidly than neostigmine. In ocular myasthenia only the extra-ocular muscles are involved.

Hyperthyroidism

The *facies of hyperthyroidism* depends chiefly upon the 'stare' (see Fig. T.11). Surprise or terror is suggested by the prominence of the eyeballs and the retraction of the eyelids. The degree of exophthalmos varies greatly, and it may be completely absent; it is sometimes unilateral. The sclera is visible between the edge of the iris and the eyelids; the usual harmony of movement between the eyeball and the eyelid is lacking; normal blinking is much diminished or entirely in abeyance. The surface of the conjunctiva may be abnormally bright and glistening, and the secretion of tears may be excessive. In contrast with the white of the eyeballs, there is often considerable dark pigmentation of the eyelids, which may also be the site of some oedema. The size of the pupils varies, with undue dilatation occurring only in exceptional cases. The upper eyelid lags as the eye follows the examiner's finger downwards. Eye movements are often diminished in range due to intrinsic muscle weakness, and the muscles of the brow are wasted, giving diminished wrinkling on raising the eyebrows (Joffroy's sign). A moist skin and a readiness to flush may often be noted in the face.

The facies of parkinsonism

In this disease a cardinal symptom is muscular rigidity which affects the skeletal muscles generally, as well as those of the face. However, the ocular muscles escape and, as a consequence, while the face as a whole is expressionless or 'mask-like', the eyes appear to move with natural or even abnormal rapidity. For instance, they will turn in the direction to which the patient desires to look before the head has assumed a corresponding position. The face often has a staring expression, the eyelids being retracted by the tonic spasm of the orbiculares palpebrarum. An absence of normal blinking has been ascribed to the same cause. In contrast with the slow development of facial expression, under the influence of emotion there may be marked want of control over the fully developed emotional movement, and the patient protests that the exuberance of their laughter or tears is entirely out of proportion to their feelings of merriment or sorrow. The poverty of facial and general movement may falsely suggest a lack of intelligence and mental activity.

Parkinsonism may occur in patients who are suffering or have suffered from an attack of *encephalitis*. This syndrome, which is now very rare, may often be distinguished from primary Parkinson's disease by the presence of disturbances in pupillary and other reflexes, tics, localized spasms and the so-called 'oculogyric crises' in which the eyes are suddenly deviated upwards, downwards or sideways so that only the white of the eye is visible to the observer. These crises which are highly unpleasant for the patient – usually

last for several minutes, and occasionally for hours. The facies of parkinsonism may also be caused by certain drugs which interfere with the action of dopamine within the basal ganglia; these include chlorpromazine, phenothiazines, butyrophenones and reserpine in large doses. In most cases, the abnormalities disappear after stopping the drug, except for tardive dyskinesia which may become permanent. This serious variety of drug-induced extrapyramidal disease consists of involuntary 'mouthing' movements of the lips, lip-smacking and protrusion of the tongue. Neuroleptic drugs with anticholinergic activity (e.g. haloperidol) produce the larger number of cases of drug-induced parkinsonism. Thioridazine has potent anticholinergic activity and does not have this side effect, although use of this drug is now limited by cardiac rhythm side effects. Less common causes of parkinsonism include carbon monoxide and manganese poisoning.

Tabetic facies

In a considerable number of the few remaining cases of tabes dorsalis the appearance of the face is sufficiently striking to afford a clue to diagnosis. The small size or the inequality of the pupils reacting to accommodation but not to light (Argyll Robertson pupils) may first attract attention. The drooping of the upper eyelids, combined with some wrinkling of the forehead produced by a compensating effort on the part of the frontalis muscle, imparts a sad expression. This drooping of the eyelid is not due to any paresis of the levator palpebrae superioris – as may be shown by the raising of the lid when the patient is looking upwards. Rather, it depends on the fact that this muscle – like most muscles of the body – is in a condition of hypotonia so that under the influence of gravity the lid hangs like a half-raised curtain in front of the eyeball. In other respects the face may be normal, but the majority of tabetics have a sallow complexion and very little subcutaneous fat – two conditions which contribute to their generally unhealthy appearance. Many victims of this disease exhibit a deficiency of the emotional reflex movements of the facial muscles; during conversation the play of the features appropriate to the subject of their talking is not so noticeable as in the case of healthy individuals.

Facies of acromegaly

In acromegaly, changes in appearance frequently take place to such a degree that the patient becomes unrecognizable to friends, who have known him or her only before the onset of the disease. These are the result of abnormal growth of the bony and subcutaneous tissues, especially in the skull and extremities. The characteristic facies is brought about by osseous hyperplasia of the frontal ridges, the mastoid, zygomatic, malar and nasal processes, while the lower jaw is usually enlarged in all directions. The prominent, arched brows, with retreating and wrinkled forehead, the massive nose, the long, thick upper lip and the heavy chin (Fig. F.2) form the most conspicuous features. The lower teeth are unduly wide apart, and may project some distance in front of the upper. The tongue may be so enlarged as to keep the mouth open and to display many fissures and indentations as the result of its pressure against the teeth. In some cases the lower jaw is not affected, and the face may be described as abnormally square (*type carree*).

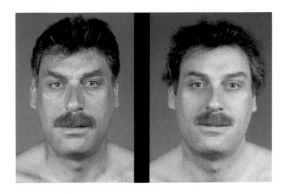

Figure F.2 A case of acromegaly, exemplifying the heavy enlargement of the front lower jaw. Before and after treatment. Reproduced with kind permission of the patient.

Down's syndrome

This facies is so distinctive that the diagnosis may usually be made at a glance. The head is brachycephalic; the palpebral fissures slant obliquely inwards and downwards towards a broad flat nose, rendered even broader by the presence of epicanthus; the eyelids show signs of chronic blepharitis; the ears are large and pitcher-shaped; the lips are fissured and often left open to allow a coarse tongue to protrude; the forehead is downy, and the hair of the scalp scanty, wiry and frequently mouse-coloured; the complexion is florid and mottled. The almond-shaped eyes, the presence of epicanthus, the florid complexion and the absence of fatty masses serve to distinguish Down's syndrome from cretinism.

The adenoid facies

This used to be described in the child sufferer with a wide open mouth resulting in the oral breathing demanded by nasal obstruction, and the over-slung lower jaw and dental occlusion with consequent incomplete musculature of the mouth and receding cheeks.

Facies of hepatolenticular degeneration (Wilson's disease)

The characteristic facies of this disease is seen only in advanced cases, and may be described as one of 'fixed emotion'. The slightest attempt to engage in conversation may evoke a sustained expression of exaggerated mirth, which is quite unlike that seen in other diseases of the nervous system. There is also a tendency to fall to one side when in the sitting position. The illness is associated with bilateral degenerative changes in the lenticular nuclei, together with cirrhosis of the liver, due to the excessive amounts of copper in the tissues. The most remarkable feature of the disease is the Kayser–Fleischer ring, which is present in about 50 per cent of patients; this is a ring of rusty-brown pigment at the periphery of the cornea. Radiating brownish spokes of copper carbonate on the anterior or posterior lens capsule less often cause the characteristic 'sunflower' cataract.

Facies of mitral stenosis

It is occasionally possible to suspect mitral stenosis at sight, on account of the remarkable malar hyperaemia and dark-crimson lips contrasting with the yellowish pallor of the forehead, peri-oral and perinasal skin. If one covers the malar regions and the lips, the face looks sallow, yet the malar flush and the dark-crimson lips give a look almost of plethora. When cardiac failure occurs and the liver becomes engorged, an element of icterus may be added.

Facies of primary polycythaemia

The coloration of the nose, lips, ears and palpebral conjunctiva is the chief feature of the facies in this malady, presenting an appearance which may be described as a combination of exposure to weather, of plethora and of cyanosis. The diagnosis depends on discovering pronounced polycythaemia, and generally a large, firm spleen. Polycythaemia may also be secondary to other conditions, cardiac, pulmonary or malignant disease.

Facies of cirrhosis of the liver

There is nothing characteristic in the facies when cirrhosis of the liver is at an early stage. Nor can one diagnose the existence of cirrhosis with certainty even when the facies is that of chronic alcoholism, with its telangiectases over the cheeks, coarsening of the tissues (especially on and around the nose and mouth), and with purplish reddening in general. However, in the later stages of cirrhosis the sallow, dull, diffusely pigmented facies is often distinctive, though the actual peculiarities are not easily described.

Facies of Addisonian pernicious anaemia

Though rarely seen today, the facies in untreated Addisonian pernicious anaemia may be absolutely characteristic in the later stages. There is no emaciation, but the colour is remarkable. Often described as 'lemon yellow', it is more often a pale primrose yellow, with a peculiar delicacy in the yellowish tint that is unmistakable when it is fully developed.

Facies of acute glomerulonephritis

The generally swollen, half-bloated look, the partial closing-up of the eyes by oedema, are usually unmistakable, but a somewhat similar appearance may be presented by the effects of insect bites, of angioneurotic oedema, or after the administration of aspirin or other drugs to which the patient is allergic. In the nephrotic syndrome (Fig. F.3), kwashiorkor and many other conditions with extensive oedema, this may extend to involve the face, but not usually in cardiac or starvation oedema which affects the dependent parts. In leprosy, a similar puffy appearance of the face may be seen, particularly around the eyes; a variety of skin lesions may occur with nodules, plaques and thickening of the skin. The ear lobes may enlarge

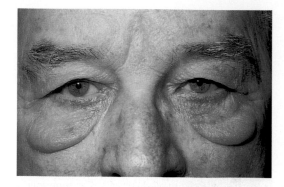

Figure F.3 Facies due to nephrotic syndrome due to cancer.

and the lines of the face may coarsen and become deeper, giving the so-called 'leonine facies'. Patches of depigmentation may occur or there is bronzed hyperpigmentation. The eyebrows and eyelashes may fall out, and the lips swell. Nasal blockage may occur and a saddle-nose deformity may develop.

Facies of arthritis and connective tissue disorders

In dermatomyositis the most characteristic rash consists of a dusky red eruption on the face, over the nose and cheeks, periorbital regions, occasionally on the forehead and on the neck, shoulders, front and back of the chest and on the arms. The erythema may be mottled or diffuse, and either intensely red or cyanotic, or a mixture of both. Sometimes, a dusky lilac hue is seen on the upper eyelids – the so-called 'heliotrope rash' which is to be typical of dermatomyositis. Telangiectasia may be present, as it may in systemic lupus erythematosus and scleroderma.

A common skin lesion of *lupus erythematosus* has a 'butterfly' distribution over the bridge of the nose and the cheeks (Fig. F.4). The facial skin lesion of *sarcoidosis* may have the same distribution, but the eyelids and ears may be infiltrated with brownish nodules.

In *scleroderma*, the parchment-like skin may be so tightly drawn over the underlying muscles that the face becomes completely expressionless (Fig. F.5) and the mouth cannot open widely.

In *giant cell (temporal) arteritis*, the inflamed temporal arteries are tender to touch and become thrombosed. Vision may be affected if the retinal arteries become involved. Tophi in the ears indicate the presence of *gout*.

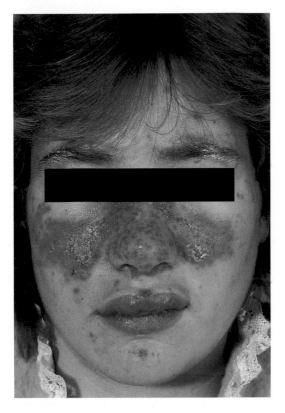

Figure F.4 Young female with systemic lupus erythematosus facial rash.

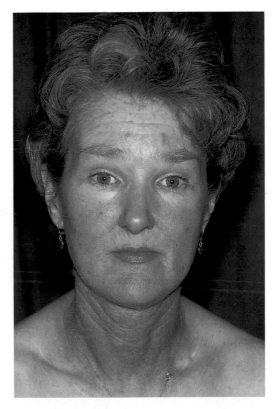

Figure F.5 Scleroderma: the skin is pigmented, the mouth is small, and on palpation the facial skin feels thickened. The patient's hands are shown in Fig. F.21.

Facies of acanthosis nigricans

The outstanding feature of this disease is the extreme pigmentation which develops in various parts of the body, as in the axillae, groin, nipples and umbilicus, but also in the neck or face. The degree may be described as what would, more or less, result if a collier's hands were stroked over the skin, producing massive darkening, almost blackening, in the areas affected. Although rarely generalized, it is usually bilateral and symmetrical, blending into adjacent normal skin. Although the disease usually indicates abdominal carcinoma (especially carcinoma of the stomach), the patient may present for treatment on account of the pigmentation only, without any suggestion at the time that there is malignant disease anywhere. It is probably an extreme degree of the liability to diffuse pigmentation of the skin that malignant disease in general tends to produce. It may precede malignant disease or follow it, but usually appears at the same time. It may also occur in

Cushing's syndrome, acromegaly, the Stein–Leventhal syndrome, adrenal insufficiency, pituitary or hypothalamic tumours or other lesions at the base of the brain. When associated with a malignant process these tend to be aggressive, and rapidly fatal. Neither clinically nor histologically can acanthosis nigricans associated with a malignant process be differentiated from the disease without this association.

Other colorations of diagnostic significance are those of *haemochromatosis*, where over 90 per cent of patients show bronzing of the skin from melanin deposition, about half having haemosiderin deposition also causing a slate-grey colour. The bluish tinge of the cartilage of the ears and sclerae in *ochronosis* appears usually between the age of 20 and 30 years. The cartilages of the ears may be slate-blue or grey, and are often thickened and irregular. Pigmentation of the sclera is usually localized to a small area halfway between the cornea and the inner or outer canthus.

The skin over the malar areas and nose is often darker than usual. Other abnormal colours which may be seen in the face include the patchy pigmentation of the chloasma of pregnancy, or that of vitiligo or albinism, and that resulting from prolonged administration of arsenic.

Facies of Addison's disease

Generalized darkening of the skin of the face may be the first thing to attract attention in a case of Addison's disease, but the distinctive character of the pigmentation is that it occurs in the mucous membranes within the mouth (Fig. F.6), where it tends to be grey, as well as on the skin of the face and other parts of the body, where it is dark brown.

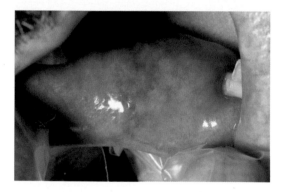

Figure F.6 Buccal pigmentation in untreated Addison's disease. Under treatment with cortisone all pigmentation disappeared within a few weeks.

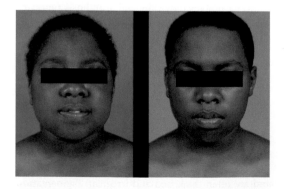

Figure F.7 The Cushingoid picture of corticosteroid therapy. Before and after treatment.

Facies in Cushing's syndrome

The red 'moon face' and hirsutism (q.v.) are characteristic, and are often seen as the result of corticosteroid therapy. Although the features look plethoric, there is no true polycythaemia. This is one point of differentiation from the features of simple obesity, others being the presence of bruising (ecchymoses), muscle weakness, wide purple red striae (those in simple obesity being more narrow and pink) and hypertension. In Cushing's syndrome the cheeks may become so chubby that when full-face, they obscure the ears (Fig. F.7).

Facies of argyria

This condition is rare nowadays, but it may still be met with amongst workers in silver. The coloration is even and uniform; there is a blue-grey appearance which persists when pressure is applied to the skin, which does not blanch as does a cyanotic skin. It is a subcutaneous rather than a dermal pigmentation.

The features in *pachydermoperiostosis*, a rare familial condition associated with pseudohypertrophic osteoarthropathy (with finger clubbing), are typical with thickening and furrowing of the face, deep nasolabial folds, greasy skin of face and scalp, and often excessive sweating. The condition appears to be transmitted by an autosomal dominant gene with variable expression.

Facies of acute illness

Erysipelas, measles, scarlatina and mumps often permit an immediate facial diagnosis. Cellulitis also is self-evident. In lobar pneumonia the bright eyes, flushed cheeks, active alae nasi and labial herpes constitute what may fairly be termed a 'typical picture'. Respiratory distress advertises itself by expression of anxiety and fear in pulmonary and cardiac disease, although alterations in colour due to cyanosis contribute to the appearance. Labial herpes (herpes febrilis) may also accompany many other febrile diseases, even a simple coryza, and may be due to sun sensitivity. Herpes zoster may affect the face and the periorbital region (Fig. F.8) and, when the nasociliary nerve is involved, lesions appear on the end of the nose and on the cornea.

Alterations in contour

Slight facial asymmetry is very common. Marked asymmetry occurs in patients with lipodystrophy,

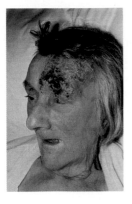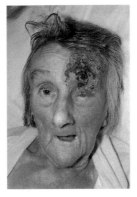

Figure F.8 Severe herpes zoster affecting the brow and sclera. Not only may scarring interfere with vision, but at this age post-herpetic neuralgia is common, subsequently causing persistent pain in the area.

hemi-atrophy or hemi-hypertrophy, or congenital absence of the condyle of the mandible. Lack of teeth or bad dentures may contribute to asymmetry, as may swelling of the parotid or other salivary glands or of the lymph nodes. Some rarer conditions may be mentioned as generally identifiable at sight. In osteitis deformans (Paget's disease), the face has the shape of an inverted triangle and, in consequence of the prominence of the forehead, appears to be toppling forwards (Fig. F.9). In leontiasis ossea there is progressive irregular enlargement of the bones of the cranium and face, with consequent asymmetry; the superior maxilla is particularly prominent. The rare condition of oxycephaly ('steeple head') need to be seen only once to be subsequently recognizable.

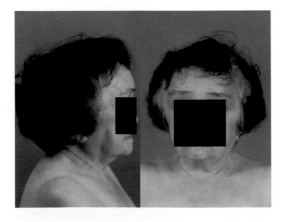

Figure F.9 Typical Paget's disease.

The eyes

The eyes alone often provide diagnostic evidence of general as well as local disease. Pigmentation, oedema of the lids and exophthalmos have been mentioned. A squint may demand a detailed consideration of the central nervous system, as will spontaneous nystagmus. Icterus of the conjunctiva may be evidence of hepatic disease, and the comparatively rare but striking appearance of blue sclerotics points to fragilitas ossium. 'Bags under the eyes' are generally devoid of any significance, but may possibly point to lack of sleep or over-indulgence in alcohol.

Voluntary movements

Weakness of the facial muscles is discussed in FACE, PARALYSIS OF (p. 200).

Abnormal movement of the jaw may be due to any painful condition of the temporomandibular joint.

Involuntary movements

Besides the tremor of the head of old age and parkinsonism, tremor may be due to alcohol, tobacco or other drugs. There is also a familial tremor of the hands, face and/or head affecting several members of the same family, usually commencing before the age of 25 years. The head-nodding of children may be mentioned in this connection. Other involuntary movements point to chorea, which may be hereditary (Huntington's), rheumatic or (rarely) senile, to habit spasms, or to tics (see p. 719). In aortic regurgitation there may be a constant jerking of the head which is synchronous with the heart beat (De Musser's sign). Facial paralysis and the peculiar condition of facial hemi-atrophy or hemi-hypertrophy are sometimes obvious, but sometimes evident only on careful examination.

Expression

The patient's expression at interview may provide an indication of their attitude not only to their illness but also to their physician and what is expected of him/her. Differentiation of the emotional from the physical factors may be very difficult. There may be an expression of melancholy or depression, of anxiety, nervous tension, or querulousness. In some cases, depression hangs over the patient like a black cloud, the face being dull, without hope for the future, expressionless, and uninterested in what is going on around.

Mark Kinirons

FACE, PAIN IN

Pain in the face may be due to:

- Local disorders of sinuses, soft tissues, joints and teeth.
- Neurological or neurovascular causes.
- Atypical facial pain.

Table F.1 Causes of facial pain

Ears, nose and throat disease
Sinus disease
Teeth disorders
Local diseases (muscles, ligaments, soft tissues, sinuses)
- Temporomandibular joint pathology
- Muscle tension (myofascial syndromes)
- Salivary gland disease
Neurological/neurovascular
- Trigeminal neuralgia
- Glossopharyngeal neuralgia
- Cluster headache
- SUNCT (short-lasting unilateral neuralgiform headache attacks with conjunctival injection and tearing)
- Paroxysmal hemicrania
- Migraine
- Temporal arteritis
- Post-herpetic neuralgia
- Ramsay–Hunt syndrome
- Tolosa–Hunt syndrome
Atypical facial pain

Here, the emphasis will be placed on neurological and neurovascular causes, although other causes will also be discussed briefly.

Local disorders

Ears, nose, sinuses and teeth

Sinusitis causes pain and tenderness which is localized to the frontal or maxillary sinuses, and percussion over the affected area worsens the pain. Blowing the nose and bending forward also worsen the discomfort. The nose will often be blocked. If simple measures

including decongestants and postural drainage are ineffective, then referral to an ear, nose and throat specialist is recommended. Nasopharyngeal carcinoma frequently infiltrates cranial nerves, especially the trigeminal nerve, causing facial pain. Disease of the petrous temporal bone from infection or neoplasm causes pain in the first trigeminal division and ipsilateral abducens palsy (*Gradenigo's syndrome*). Dental caries or root canal sepsis can cause pain in the first and second divisions of the trigeminal nerve, which is worsened by hot or cold liquids. Malocclusion of the teeth has been reported to cause trigeminal neuralgia type pain (see below).

Temporomandibular joint disease

Dysfunction of the temporomandibular joint – also termed facial arthromyalgia – is poorly understood. It has been suggested to be due to malocclusion or loss of molar teeth. The main clinical findings are tenderness of the temporomandibular joint and muscles of mastication, trismus (jaw spasm), limited or jerky jaw movements, and evidence of bruxism (tooth grinding) or frictional damage to the buccal mucosa and the tongue. Signs of subluxation of the joint include clicking noises and lateral displacement of the meniscus. Pain in the temple, face and neck with a sensation of ear fullness constitute the rather doubtful nosological entity of *Costen's syndrome*.

Neurological and neurovascular causes

Trigeminal neuralgia

Trigeminal neuralgia almost always begins after the age of 40 years, except when associated with multiple sclerosis. It is more common in women than men (ratio 3:2). Trigeminal neuralgia is characterized by paroxysmal facial pain that is intense and described as 'shooting', 'jabbing', 'stabbing' or 'like an electric shock'. Each paroxysm lasts under 30 seconds, with less than 1 minute between each successive pain. Each series of paroxysms lasts from a few seconds to a few minutes. The pain usually starts in either the maxillary or mandibular divisions (or both), rarely in the ophthalmic division to which it may later spread, and is provoked by stimulation of a trigger point in the same division as the pain. Contact with the trigger point may occur during washing, shaving, combing the hair, blowing the nose, by talking or eating, or even a slight draught on the face. Patients typically describe techniques to avoid touching the face, by contrast with other causes of facial pain in which massage is typically helpful. The pain is nearly always unilateral. The severity of the pain often causes the patient to screw up the affected side of the face in a grimace – hence the name 'tic douloureux'. Before effective treatments were available, suicide was said to be common. The pain tends in the early stages of the illness to occur in bouts lasting for days or weeks. The periods of pain subsequently become longer with shorter remissions so that eventually, although still intermittent, the pain will occur on most days. On examination, there are no abnormal signs in the nervous system, except in association with multiple sclerosis where sensory loss in the trigeminal distribution may be found. Trigeminal neuralgia occurs in about 3 per cent of patients with multiple sclerosis.

The pain may be relieved in more than half the patients by the drug of first choice, carbamazepine. Baclofen, lamotrigine, phenytoin or gabapentin are also effective, though randomized trial efficacy data for the last two agents are scarce. If carbamazepine alone is ineffective, then a second agent should be added, such as phenytoin or baclofen. If a third drug is added without response, as occurs in between 25 and 50 per cent of patients, and the symptoms are distressing, then surgery should be considered. The type of surgical procedure offered varies widely in different hospitals, and few high-quality data are available on efficacy. Radiofrequency or glycerol ablation of the Gasserian ganglion can be performed, though the 5-year recurrence rate is over 50 per cent. Microvascular compression of the trigeminal nerve by an aberrant vascular loop is now recognized as a cause of trigeminal neuralgia with the increasing use of magnetic resonance imaging, and in these cases surgical decompression can be effective. Gamma knife treatment to the trigeminal nerve has also been used recently. Relapse may occur following medical or surgical treatments, and the prognosis is difficult to predict with any certainty. Spontaneous remissions frequently occur early in the illness.

Glossopharyngeal neuralgia

This condition is much less common than trigeminal neuralgia, and causes pain that has a similar lancinating character, but which is localized instead to the ear, base of tongue or jaw angle. Pharyngeal and otalgic variants have been described depending on where the pain occurs. Glossopharyngeal neuralgia is triggered by talking, swallowing or coughing. It may be idiopathic or secondary to compression of the nerve by tumour, infection or aberrant blood vessels. Glossopharyngeal and trigeminal neuralgias may co-exist, and the medical treatments are similar.

Cluster headache, migraine and cranial arteritis

Cluster headache and the other trigeminal autonomic cephalagias, migraine and temporal arteritis, are conventionally considered to be mainly headache disorders (see HEADACHE, p. 278).

Migraine

Migraine is fully considered in the section on HEADACHE (p. 279).

Post-herpetic neuralgia and Ramsay–Hunt syndrome

Herpes zoster is caused by reactivation of the varicella zoster virus, which lies dormant in the trigeminal, geniculate and dorsal root ganglia following chickenpox infection in infancy or childhood. The vesicular rash is commonly in the trigeminal distribution, most often the ophthalmic division (see Fig. F.8). Less commonly, the external auditory meatus or upper cervical roots are affected. A herpetic rash in the external auditory meatus and a facial palsy constitute the *Ramsay–Hunt syndrome*, and are due to involvement of the geniculate ganglion. Pain in the ear or trigeminal distribution may precede the rash, or appear without any rash, causing diagnostic difficulty. Post-herpetic neuralgia is pain persisting beyond a month after the rash has crusted over. The pain may be burning and distressing, with misperception of light touch stimuli as painful over the affected area (*allodynia*). Symptomatic treatment with standard neuropathic pain drugs (e.g. carbamazepine, gabapentin) may be helpful.

Atypical facial pain

Atypical facial pain is not a clear diagnostic entity, but refers to a poorly understood group of conditions that are quite common in both medical and surgical practice. Atypical facial pain is commonly considered a diagnosis of exclusion. Nevertheless, there do seem to be some characteristic features. The pain is often poorly localized to a deep, non-muscular, non-neuralgic distribution in the face. It is usually deep, boring, aching, dragging or nagging in quality, and is long-lasting – from weeks to years without relief. It quite often starts following one or more dental procedures, and patients may subsequently be referred to a number of specialties (ear, nose and throat, maxillo-facial, neurology) in the course of their illness. The pain may be worsened by fatigue or stress. It may be associated with symptoms of anxiety or depression, and may respond to antidepressant treatment, particularly with tricyclic drugs. Examination is normal, and there are no helpful investigations.

David Werring

FACE, PARALYSIS OF

Facial paralysis is seen in three clinical forms:

- Upper motor neurone paralysis (also termed supranuclear), in which the lower half of the face is affected, and the upper half relatively spared.
- Lower motor neurone paralysis, in which there is loss of movement in all the muscles on the affected side.
- Muscle or neuromuscular junction disorders.

Upper motor neurone paralysis (supranuclear)

This condition is due to a lesion of the corticofacial projection fibres of the descending pyramidal tract anywhere between the cortex and the facial nucleus in the pons. The frontalis and orbicularis occuli muscles are relatively spared, but the teeth cannot be bared on the affected side and there is weakness of mouth closure. This is because the upper face has bilateral corticopontine innervation, whereas the lower face is predominantly (though not entirely) innervated by the contralateral cerebral cortex (*Broadbent's law*). In some cases involuntary emotional movements remain normal, despite loss of volitional movements. This may be because subcortical projections from limbic regions to the facial nucleus mediate emotional facial movements, and are preserved despite damage to

corticofacial projections in some cerebral lesions. In bilateral corticopontine lesions the upper part of the face is paralysed as well as the lower, and emotional movements are also involved. Rarely, emotional movements are lost and voluntary movements retained; this is occasionally seen in tumours or other lesions of the temporal lobe or pons.

Upper motor neurone facial paralysis occurs in any condition affecting the corticofacial projections in the cerebral hemisphere. In practice, stroke, cerebral mass lesions and inflammatory conditions (e.g. multiple sclerosis) are the most likely causes. Because the descending corticospinal motor fibres become closely packed together as they descend, in lesions involving the lower corona radiata or internal capsule facial weakness is usually associated with arm or leg weakness. Facial weakness may be associated with aphasia in dominant hemisphere lesions. Isolated upper motor neurone facial weakness has been reported with very small lacunar infarctions in the internal capsule or corona radiata.

Lower motor neurone paralysis (peripheral facial palsy)

This condition occurs as a result of a lesion of the VIIth nerve nucleus or of the nerve itself (Fig. F.10). The upper and lower halves of the face are affected equally, and there is no dissociation of emotional and voluntary movements. If there is no recovery, contractures may occur, the corners of the mouth being drawn to the affected side, thereby giving a false impression of weakness on the normal side. *Facial*

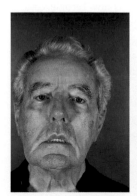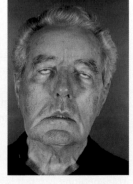

Figure F.10 Bilateral lower VIIth nerve palsy.

myokymia is a fine rippling movement of all muscles on one side of the face. It is an important physical sign, as it is most often seen in cases of multiple sclerosis and brainstem glioma, and if noted makes brain imaging (ideally with MRI) mandatory. The causes of lower motor neurone facial palsy are listed in Table F.2.

Table F.2 Causes of lower motor neurone facial weakness

Bell's palsy
Infectious
- Lyme disease*
- Guillain–Barré syndrome* (*Polyneuritis cranialis* is probably a Guillain–Barré variant)
- HIV
- Sarcoidosis*
- Chickenpox (children)
- Mycobacterial (tuberculosis, leprosy)
- Herpes zoster of the geniculate ganglion (*Ramsay–Hunt syndrome*)
- Infectious mononucleosis
- Meningeal syphilis
Inherited
- Mobius syndrome*
- Melkersson–Rosenthal syndrome
Trauma
- Penetrating wounds
- Parotid surgery
- Fracture of petrous temporal bone
Tumours
- Parotid
- Carotid body
- Cholesteatoma
- Cerebellopontine angle (acoustic neuroma, meningioma, neurofibroma)
- Glomus jugulare
- Pontine glioma
Vascular
- Pontine infarction
- Vertebral or basilar aneurysm
Inflammatory
- Brainstem demyelination (multiple sclerosis)
Muscular
- Myotonic dystrophy*
- Facioscapulohumeral dystrophy*
- Myasthenia gravis* (neuromuscular junction)

*Denotes likely to cause bilateral facial weakness.

By far the most common form of peripheral facial palsy is *Bell's palsy*, described by and named after the British surgeon Charles Bell in 1821. The onset is rapid, and the patient often awakens in the morning to find the face paralysed on one side; in other cases the condition takes a day or two to develop. In about one-half of patients there is a dull pain or numbness just below the mastoid and behind or in front of the ear at the onset. The majority will have a change in auditory acuity (hyperacusis; sounds seem louder) due to involvement of the nerve to stapedius. Some patients will have disturbed taste in the anterior two-thirds of the tongue, or impaired salivary flow due to involvement of the chorda tympani. There may be decreased lacrimation (tearing) ipsilateral to the lesion if it is proximal to the geniculate ganglion. The eye cannot be closed fully, and is liable to injury by dust. On examination there is weakness of the facial muscles and platysma, so that the face is pulled away from the affected side on smiling, etc. On attempted eye closure the globe deviates upward and inward (Bell's phenomenon). A careful search should be made for vesicles in the external auditory meatus (which suggests herpes zoster of the geniculate ganglion; Ramsay–Hunt syndrome) and for facial myokymia (which suggests pontine glioma or demyelination).

The cause of Bell's palsy is not known, though 60 per cent of patients have a preceding viral infection, and there is increasing evidence that herpes simplex virus type 1 infection of the nerve is the main pathogenic agent. An immune mechanism is possible, given the association of Bell's palsy with interferon alpha 2b treatment and the lymphocytic infiltrate seen on histology. The prognosis for recovery is excellent; 80–90 per cent of patients recover fully by 4–6 months. The elderly, and those with poorly controlled hypertension, seem to have a less favourable prognosis. The main long-term complications, occurring at 3–4 months, are contractures and synkinesis of the face.

Treatment involves careful eye protection (lubricating drops, taping at night and consideration of an eye patch if there are signs of corneal damage). Corticosteroids are probably helpful, but must be given within 7 days, before irreversible neuronal denervation has occurred. A dose of 1 mg/kg for 5 days, followed by a 5-day taper in incomplete palsy, extended to 10 days with a 5-day taper in complete palsy, is a suggested regimen. High-dose steroids should not be stopped abruptly as rebound worsening may occur.

Other causes of lower motor neurone facial paralysis are less common than Bell's palsy, and are listed in Table F.2. Most of these are associated with other symptoms and physical signs, which should provide clues to the correct diagnosis. For example, in Lyme disease a history of visiting endemic areas (e.g. the New Forest in the United Kingdom) and a migrating erythematous rash may be found, whilst Guillain–Barré syndrome in its full form includes limb paralysis, glove and stocking sensory symptoms and areflexia. In cases of tumours at the cerebellopontine angle, ipsilateral deafness, limb ataxia and an absent corneal reflex may be present. Facial myokymia suggests pontine demyelination or glioma. If both sides of the face are affected (facial diplegia), then Guillain–Barré syndrome, neurosarcoidosis (in this context also called uveo-parotid fever), Lyme disease and myasthenia gravis should be considered. Myasthenia gravis causes ptosis, diplopia and limb weakness, which are worse in the evening and fatiguable.

David Werring

FACE, SWELLING OF

In this section are included only swellings of the skin and subcutaneous tissues. Malignant and other diseases of the facial bones, etc., are considered under JAW, SWELLING OF (p. 338) and SALIVARY GLANDS, SWELLING OF (p. 627). It is necessary therefore to determine the anatomical site of the lesion before considering the pathology. For example, swelling of the parotid gland will lie below and in front of the ear, or in the anterior prolongation of the gland, lying on the outer surface of the masseter. Swelling of the sublingual gland will be seen in the floor of the mouth close to the fraenum, while lateral to this will be felt the submandibular salivary gland, which is also palpable from outside in the submandibular fossa.

Occasionally, a patient may present him/herself with painless symmetrical *oedema of the face*, commonly of the eyelids where the tissues are loosest. This will almost certainly be of renal origin, since cardiac oedema causes oedema primarily in the dependent parts. Another form of oedema which may involve the whole face, but chiefly the eyelids and lips, is *angioneurotic oedema*. The recurrent attacks, each of sudden onset, the familial history, the associated symptoms of burning and irritation and the presence of similar areas of other parts of the body should clinch the diagnosis.

Swelling of the face and neck is seen in Cushing's syndrome, whether primary or secondary to corticosteroid therapy, and when there is obstruction to the venous return to the heart from the head and neck, as is seen with mediastinal and bronchial neoplasms. In trichiniasis, oedema of the eyelids is common, though more diffuse oedema of the face may occur.

A well-defined *cystic swelling* on the face is most commonly a *sebaceous cyst*, a structure which is freely movable on the deeper tissues but attached to the skin. *Dermoid cyst* is much rarer, and occurs only at lines of suture, the commonest site being above the outer canthus of the eye (*external angular dermoid*). A cyst in this situation is strongly suggestive of dermoid origin; the diagnosis is confirmed if there is attachment to bone but not to skin, and particularly if depression of the bone has occurred (as it does in long-standing cases), the edge of the depressed area being palpable. *Meningocele* may occur occasionally as a translucent swelling at the root of the nose. It will be present at birth and will exhibit an impulse on coughing or straining. *Haemangiomas* are frequently found on the face, and may appear cystic on palpation; however, their dusky colour and surrounding dilated vessels will give the clue to their identity. They also empty on pressure. Pigmented naevi will be recognized on sight.

Solid tumours of the face are *lipomas* and *fibromas*. The latter are fairly common and include an important variety, the neurofibromas. These tumours vary in size from being quite minute to 2–3 cm or more in diameter, and they may be hard or soft. Other stigmas of von Recklinghausen's disease such as pigmentation (either diffuse or in multiple café-au-lait spots), or a profusion of soft, fleshy neurofibromas in other parts of the body (chiefly the trunk) help in the diagnosis. The condition sometimes runs in families.

Rodent ulcer is particularly common on the face and eyelids; it is the exception to find it elsewhere. It starts as a small nodule, often with a 'pearly' appearance, but soon breaks down to form the characteristic indurated ulcer with hard, rolled edges (Fig. F.11). *Epithelioma*, with its raised everted margin and indurated base, and possibly secondary enlargement of regional nodes, is another malignant condition found on the face, particularly the lips (Fig. F.12). Confusion may arise in distinguishing epithelioma from the innocent condition *molluscum sebaceum*. However, molluscum runs a short course and the centre sloughs leaving an unsightly scar.

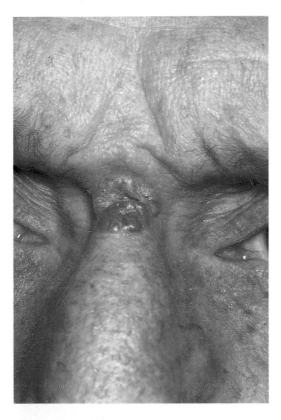

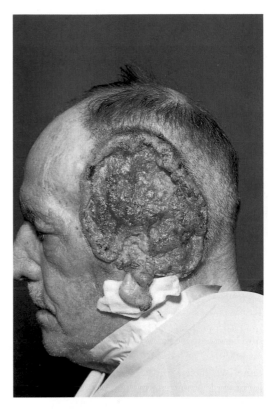

Figure F.11 Rodent ulcer.

Figure F.12 Extensive epithelioma (squamous cell carcinoma) of the scalp and pinna.

Biopsy must be performed early in any suspicious lesion.

Various inflammatory swellings are found on the face, of which the following are some of the most important:

- *Boils and carbuncles* are common, particularly around the lips. They have the same character as elsewhere, except that oedema is more marked.
- *Erysipelas* is prone to occur on the face. It is marked by a vivid red oedematous swelling associated with fever. The redness tends to spread, the edges being raised and well defined from the healthy skin. The oedema may be continuous, or it may disappear in one place and reappear in another. In very severe cases the fever is high, rigours occur, the cuticle may be raised in blebs, and sloughing may ensue.
- *Alveolar abscess* and *dental caries* are fertile sources of facial swelling, as is abscess in the nasal sinuses (see JAW, SWELLING OF, p. 338).

- *Anthrax* chiefly affects operatives in wool and horse-hair factories and workers of raw hides. The disease is characterized by the formation of a vesicle, which bursts, forms a scab, and then becomes surrounded by a ring of vesicles around which is an area of oedema. The diagnosis is confirmed by discovering anthrax bacilli in the discharge; a fluid prepared from a drop of fluid from one of the vesicles contains long chains of large, square-ended, Gram-positive bacilli, which have a characteristic growth on culture media.
- *Vaccinia.* An accidental infection about the face may be mistaken for anthrax pustule. If inquiry into the attendant circumstances is not sufficient to exclude the graver disorder, a bacteriological examination should be made.
- *Primary syphilitic sore*, if found on the face, is generally situated on the upper lip, though it may also occur upon an eyelid, the nose or elsewhere. It is not so indurated as when on the glans penis, but the surrounding oedema is more marked, and the neighbouring lymph nodes become enlarged. The condition is often missed because it is not

expected. An absolute diagnosis can be made by finding the spirochaetes in the serum discharges from the ulcer, and by serological tests, though the latter may not yet be positive if the facial chancre is of recent date.

- *Insect bites or stings* – from mosquitoes, gnats, bees, etc. – often cause large, lumpy, irritating swellings. The only difficulty in diagnosis is when the original bite or sting has become indistinguishable owing to infection with pyogenic organisms.

The various skin diseases which may be associated with swelling of the face are considered under VESICLES (p. 85).

Harold Ellis

FACE, ULCERATION OF

Any persistent ulcerated lesion on the face requires investigation, by biopsy if necessary to determine the cause (see Table F.3). Ulceration may be traumatic, for example in the habitual, and often subconscious, phenomenon of *acne excoriee.* Self-inflicted injury to the skin may be denied by the patient suffering from *dermatitis artefacta,* but the rather shallow history and the unnatural appearance of the lesions usually give a clue to the cause; there is invariably a history of psychological disturbance. Anaesthetic skin is soon traumatized and often prevented from healing by recurrent excoriation, and this can lead to extensive ulceration, as seen following surgery to the Gasserian ganglion for trigeminal neuralgia (Figs F.13 and F.14).

A similar situation obtains in other causes of facial anaesthesia, including posterior inferior cerebellar artery thrombosis and syringobulbia.

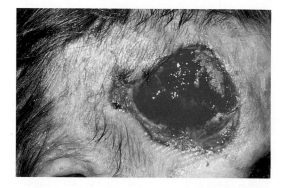

Figure F.13 Temporal arteritis.

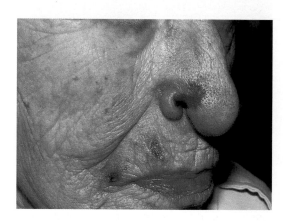

Figure F.14 Trigeminal anaesthesia.

Table F.3 Causes of face ulceration

Benign	Infection
Excoriation	Syphilitic chancre
Trauma	Gumma
Artefacta	Yaws
Anaesthetic areas (trigeminal nerve ablation)	Leishmaniasis
	Lupus vulgaris
Tumours	**Other**
Basal-cell carcinoma	Pyoderma gangrenosum
Squamous-cell carcinoma	Cancrum oris
Keratoacanthoma	Dental sinus
Malignant melanoma	
Lentigo maligna	

Facial ulceration always raises the possibility of malignancy. Perhaps the best-known malignant ulcer on the face is the *rodent ulcer* (basal-cell carcinoma; see Fig. F.11), seen chiefly on exposed white skin. There is usually a background of solar skin damage. The hallmark of a rodent ulcer is its edge, which is raised and rolled with a pearly colour and crossed by multiple telangiectatic capillaries. Usually, there is central ulceration, but some lesions remain nodular or cystic for many months before ulcerating. Rodent ulcers can be deeply pigmented, making the true diagnosis less obvious, with simulation of a banal seborrhoeic wart or malignant melanoma. *Squamous cell* carcinoma is also common on sun-damaged skin, especially the lower lip, and may ulcerate. Lesions begin as firm fleshy tumours, and grow slowly and asymmetrically. A *keratoacanthoma* is also a fleshy papular tumour on sun-damaged skin, but the lesion is too symmetrical and grows too rapidly to be a malignancy. There is a central keratin plug which may extrude, the whole lesion then having an ulcerated appearance. If not surgically removed, such lesions involute spontaneously within 3 months, leaving depressed scars. Ulcerating *malignant melanoma,* both melanotic and amelanotic, are also seen on the face. *Lentigo maligna* (Hutchinson's freckle) is an indolent black patch on elderly exposed skin. Pigmentation within the patch is variegate, and histology shows stage I malignant change of melanocytes. Later, fleshy pink nodules and/or ulceration indicate change to a more aggressive and vertical growth phase; despite this, lethal distant spread is unusual.

Infectious causes of facial ulceration are also usually serious. A primary *syphilitic chancre* may occur anywhere on the face, but especially on the lips. It develops rapidly from a small nodule to an indurated, painless ulcer with associated marked lymphadenopathy. Its rapid growth should distinguish it from neoplasms (save keratoacanthoma), and *Treponema pallidum* can be found in large numbers on dark-field examination of the serous exudate. Serological tests will be positive 10–14 days from the onset of the chancre. A tertiary *syphilitic gumma* tends to ulcerate rapidly, extending at the margins, and healing centrally. A primary *yaws ulcer* is rare on the face; in the secondary phase there are exudative nodules around the mouth, but tertiary gummatous ulcers can cause facial ulcers as well as destruction of the nasal septum or palate, as seen in syphilis. Cutaneous *leishmaniasis* may also cause a facial ulcer. The lesion begins at the site of a sandfly (*Phlebotomus*) bite, usually on a visit to South America or the Mediterranean littoral. Within a few weeks a livid papule develops and grows to 1–2 cm in size before ulcerating. The smear at this stage will be positive for Leishman–Donovan bodies. If untreated, most such ulcers heal with scaring in 12–18 months. In *lupus vulgaris* (cutaneous tuberculosis), which is now very rare, the ulceration is chronic. It begins with deep-seated nodules which, after a time, break down to form a granulomatous ulcer, covered with crusts. Around the edge the characteristic 'apple-jelly' nodules may be seen. Necrosis of cartilage of the nose and pinna is not uncommon, but bone is never attacked (in contrast to

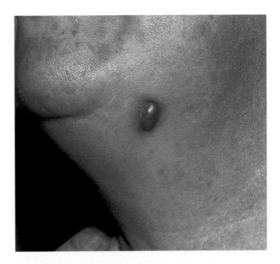

Figure F.15 Chronic dental sinus.

syphilis and malignancy). Lupus vulgaris usually begins in childhood. Other mycobacteria can produce granulomatous ulcers on the face – for example, *swimming pool granuloma* and *Buruli ulcer* in Uganda (*Mycobacterium ulcerans*). Rare causes of facial ulceration include *pyoderma gangrenosum, cancrum oris* and *ulcerating dental sinus* (Fig. F.15).

Barry Monk

FACTITIOUS DISORDERS

Factitious disorders are conditions in which *illnesses are simulated or induced*, with *deliberate deceit*, but with no *obvious motive or goal*. Their prevalence is uncertain, but likely to be seriously underestimated as recognition is difficult unless the presentation is characteristic, persistent, repeated or closely observed – and suspected (Table F.4).

Broadly, there are three types of presentation:

1   The fabrication of symptoms or signs of illness.
2   Self-inflicted injuries to induce or simulate illness.
3   The aggravation or elaboration of established disease.

Any physical or psychiatric condition can be feigned – even cases of feigned AIDS were reported within a

Table F.4 Causes of factitious disorder

Commonest	Rare
Personality disorder	Schizophrenia
Antisocial	Schizoaffective disorder
Inadequate/dependent	Anorexia nervosa
Adjustment reaction to illness	
Stress reaction	

Less common
Depression
Anxiety
Mental impairment
Brain damage

year or two of its emergence. There seems to be no limitation to the ingenuity or self-inflicted suffering of some patients; and particularly among people with a medical background or training, the application of drugs, medical equipment or pathology samples to devise illness can be scarcely credible.

The first and greatest problem facing the doctor is to recognize that the presentation is not a bona fide illness. There are usually clues in the history which may be dramatic, though this is more frequently vague, inconsistent and 'hollow', and pressing for better information can provoke resentment or anger. Detailed medical knowledge or excessive interest in the investigations or treatment may be evident. The rapid development of 'complications' or fresh, unrelated symptoms as the investigations undertaken begin to report negative results is most characteristic.

There are few readily identifiable presentations, but dermatitis artefacta is both common and may have a classically geometrical pattern to the lesions with sharply demarcated edges. The surgical wound or ulcer that repeatedly breaks down is another suspicious scenario, with tampering sometimes apparent. Fever is frequently simulated, usually by interference with the thermometer, but has been induced by injecting pyrogenic material. Bleeding from any orifice can be especially dramatic, although sometimes identifiable as self-inflicted upon careful examination. Surreptitious anticoagulant ingestion or the addition of blood to samples can prove harder to identify, while occasionally the patient may induce anaemia before presenting. Gastrointestinal and endocrine disturbances are well documented, often involving drugs. Psychosis and bereavement are commonly feigned psychological presentations.

The diagnosis becomes even more difficult when the factitious behaviour is superimposed upon a genuine illness or abnormal test result, such as chest pain in the setting of ECG evidence of an old infarct, or when the patient accepts treatment knowing that they should not have the treatment, such as with an established anaphylactic response to penicillin.

Finally, manufacturing factitious disorders in others is a rare but recognized phenomenon which occurs very occasionally, with health staff fabricating abnormalities in patients and, more often, in parents inducing or simulating illness in their child or children. This form of the disorder, *Munchausen's syndrome by proxy*, is associated with factitious illness or somatization disorder in the mother, and differs from typical child abuse in that the parents usually make no attempt to disguise their children's disorders nor give patently inadequate explanations. Thus, the spectre of non-accidental injury is rarely raised first by the parents' behaviour and attitudes. When a factitious condition is uncovered in an adult, it is always worthwhile reviewing the medical histories of any children.

The differential diagnosis of factitious disorder is relatively straightforward compared with the problems usually encountered in establishing the nature of the condition (Table F.5).

Table F.5 Differential diagnosis of factitious disorder

	Behaviour is evident and admitted	Behaviour is under voluntary control	Behaviour is directed towards an obvious goal
Factitious disorder	No	Yes	No
Deliberate self-harm	Usually	Yes	Sometimes
Hysteria	No	No	Yes
Malingering	No	Yes	Yes

Deliberate self-harm is also self-injurious behaviour, but is overt and does not entail deception in the sense of intentionally mimicking other diseases. *Conversion disorder* involves functional complaints and signs, but these are not under conscious control and have identifiable gain. *Malingering* is self-induced and consciously operated, but is directed towards an understandable goal (such as cash benefits) which, once achieved, ends the behaviour. In effect, a factitious disorder is malingering without a sensible purpose: the presentation resolves nothing.

The best-known presentation of factitious disorder is *Munchausen's syndrome*. Typically, the patient is a young or middle-aged male, has repeated presentations, and must wander. Their bizarre and multiple presentations, disruptive demanding behaviour, maladjusted unstable background and rootless existence are all hallmarks of severe personality disorder. It is because they are caricatures of the disorder that they are readily recognized and their importance, numerically and in the literature, has undoubtedly become exaggerated.

In fact, the patient with factitious disorder is more likely to be female than male, to be undramatic, not to be admitted to hospital, and to behave in a compliant manner. She tends to be a young adult, socially conforming, in employment, and with an apparently stable family background. Pre-existing disease, ready access to drugs, medical knowledge gained from training or working in healthcare or having a close relative in the health profession are all surprisingly common. The personality is characterized as passive, dependent, sensitive, introverted, obsessional, and with low self-esteem; sexual difficulties are common.

The condition sometimes represents a means of coping with an illness, a stress or relationship problem in an individual who cannot articulate or assert, or it may be the expression of an underlying depressive illness. In acute cases the outcome is favourable given appropriate management of the presentation and resolution of the primary problem. For those patients in whom the behaviour is repeated and arises in a more fundamental disorder of personality, themes of masochism and self-destruction figure persistently and prominently, self-injury is compelling and suicide a risk.

Finally, the doctor who establishes that his or her patient is simulating illness is invariably faced with a key question – to confront, or not to confront? The answer is almost always *to confront* but to approach the denouement gently, dispassionately, gradually and as part of a management plan, and not in a hot-tempered, accusatory way. When confronted, the Munchausen patient will get up, go and materialize elsewhere; but the remainder – the majority – will usually either respond positively to the suggestion of psychological help or will desist from their behaviour, even if hotly denying that the problem was self-induced. It helps if this is carried out by the physician who assessed the patient and has made the diagnosis after careful evaluation: the psychiatrist is also freed from implication in the detection process and can be seen as a helper after the event. Revealment can come as considerable relief for some patients who dislike their dishonesty as much as their doctor does, but no matter how skilfully and sensitively handled, these cases seldom prove satisfying, and very rarely conclude with the doctor–patient relationship unscathed.

Andrew Hodgkiss

FAECES, COLOUR, CONTENTS AND MORPHOLOGY

Gazing at stools and determining consistency, shape, colour and content can provide some clue as to a patient's underlying diagnosis, but findings are more often than not inconsistent and usually can only be put into context after a diagnosis has been made.

To make a broad generalization, in the presence of diarrhoea, stools of large and small volume represent small- and large-bowel pathologies, respectively. Malabsorptive states (exocrine pancreas impairment: chronic pancreatitis, pancreatic cancer, cystic fibrosis and, to a lesser degree, mucosal disease: coeliac disease, tropical sprue, lymphoma, lymphangiectasia, Whipple's disease, amyloid, scleroderma) are associated with the passage of bulky, pale stools. Pellet or sheep-like stools are common in constipation-predominant irritable bowel syndrome (IBS). Ribbon-shaped stools rarely are due to conditions causing narrowing of the distal colon (diverticular disease, tumour, Crohn's disease, anal stenosis).

The stools of bile salt malabsorption (rapid gut transport, vipoma and resection, Crohn's disease, lymphoma, neuroendocrine tumour, tuberculosis or *Yersinia* infection of the terminal ileum) are often watery. Cholera is associated with 'rice-water' stools.

Stool pallor, whether white or putty coloured, is a sign of biliary obstruction resulting in decreased levels of stercobilinogen. Such stools may accompany choledocholithiasis, ductal worms, haemobilia, cholangiocarcinoma, primary sclerosing cholangitis, ampullary adenoma/carcinoma, pancreatic head carcinoma, pancreatic cystadenoma/carcinoma, biliary atresia, surgical duct injury and anastomotic stricture. 'Silver-wire' stools have been described with ampullary carcinoma. Steatorrhoeic stools are often described as being both pale and bulky. When biliary obstruction is relieved, normal stool colour is rapidly restored.

Black bowel motions are frequently incorrectly labelled as being melaena. This term is reserved for altered blood that gives the stool a consistency of sticky black tar, with a characteristic pungent odour. Melaena may be due to both upper (peptic ulcer disease, Dieulafoy's lesion, cancer, vascular ectasia, varices) and lower (proximal colonic tumour, adenomatous polyp or vascular anomaly) gastrointestinal haemorrhage. Iron supplements will give stools a black appearance, but the stools may be solid and will have a slight dark-green tinge. Porter beer and liquorice may blacken stools.

Poorly digested foods such as tomato skins may be mistaken for blood, or during colonoscopy for being an adenomatous polyp. Mucus, which is a normal constituent of stools, can be over-produced by large colonic adenomatous polyps. Excessive mucus is also a feature of IBS. When whitish, strands of mucus can be mistaken for worms.

Worms

Several types of *worm* may appear in the stool: these include tapeworms, roundworms, threadworms and pinworms.

A common indication of *tapeworm infestation* is the passage per rectum of detached segments in either long or short tape-like strips. Close examination reveals the regular segmentation of a tapeworm, and examination with a lens reveals the glandular structure of the uterus in tapeworm segments. Patients may be symptomless or may complain of abdominal discomfort or diarrhoea; anaemia and eosinophilia may be present. The four forms of tapeworm which occur in the human intestine are *Taenia solium* (pork tapeworm), *T. saginata* (beef tapeworm), *Hymenolepis nana* (dwarf tapeworm) and *Diphyllobothrium latum* (fish tapeworm). *T. saginata* is the commonest tapeworm found in Britain. Microscopic examination of the faeces will show the characteristic eggs. Identification of the species is generally possible by the gravid proglottides. Tapeworms may also be seen on a straight X-ray film of the abdomen, or occasionally on barium meal examination.

The only *roundworm* which infests man in Britain is *Ascaris lumbricoides*. Symptoms of intestinal colic or biliary obstruction, particularly in children, may occur together with pneumonitis, urticaria and eosinophilia. There may be no symptoms until a worm is found in the stool; typical ova may be discovered in faeces. They are of relatively large size and of oval shape.

The threadworm *Oxyuris vermicularis*, if present, generally occurs in large numbers. They can be detected by naked eye examination of the faeces. Each parasite is 3–10 mm in length and is colourless. They may be associated with frequency of micturition, pruritus ani, irritability and restlessness.

Other worm infections include hookworm (*Ankylostoma duodenale* and *Necator americanus*). The ova are oval with a clear transparent shell detected on a direct faecal film or a slide mounted in saline or iodine solution, and are commonly associated with iron-deficiency anaemia. *Trichuris trichuria* (whipworm) is very common worldwide, and presents with nocturnal pruritus ani. The worm is visible to the naked eye in the stool or perianal area.

Blood in stools

Blood-stained stools are most commonly due to haemorrhoids or tiny friable vessels in the anal canal. It is important, however, to exclude more significant pathologies such as cancer of the anus, rectum or colon as well as colorectal polyps and inflammatory bowel disease (Crohn's colitis, ulcerative colitis). Uncomplicated diverticular disease may give rise to massive fresh rectal bleeding, but never passage of intermittent small-volume blood unless it is accompanied by a degree of non-specific colitis. Colonic angiodysplasia (usually proximal colon) and rectal varices will cause varying quantities of rectal bleeding. Colonic ischaemia, often of the splenic flexure, presents as abdominal pain and bloody diarrhoea in an elderly patient who may have suffered from recent hypotension (sepsis, major surgery).

It is often suggested that blood mixed in with, or coating, the stool might be indicative of proximal and distal lesions, respectively. The identification of dark and bright red blood has similarly been used to suggest the site of pathology; however, none of these generalizations is helpful, and should never be relied upon. Proximal colonic cancers may present with stools coated in bright red blood. Porphyria and beetroot ingestion can give stools a red-brown or red discoloration, respectively. Intussusception is classically associated with the combination of abdominal pain and the passage of 'redcurrant jelly'-like stools.

Investigations

The investigation of altered stools is guided by the above-mentioned features and their associations. The most direct tests are those of colonoscopy and upper gastrointestinal endoscopy. These procedures are superior to barium studies as they permit mucosal biopsy of the colon/terminal ileum and proximal small bowel (second part of the duodenum), respectively.

Blood tests will help to define associated nutritional deficiencies (ferritin, vitamin B_{12} and serum/red cell folate) and, possibly, the underlying cause (anti-endomysial or tissue transglutaminase antibodies for coeliac disease, CA19.9 and CA125 for pancreatic cancer). Prolonged stool collection to assess fat content (normal, <20 mmol with diet of 100–150 g fat per day) can define steatorrhoea, but are eschewed by many laboratories. Functional studies include the bentiromide test (BT-PABA), pancreolauryl test or direct (intravenous secretin)/indirect (Lundh meal) stimulation and duodenal aspirate enzyme/bicarbonate measurement for the pancreas and D-xylose absorption for the small bowel. Breath tests will identify primary and secondary lactase deficiency (lactose tolerance test) or bacterial overgrowth (^{14}C-labelled glycocholic breath test).

John Meenan

FAECES, INCONTINENCE OF

The individual who is affected by the inadvertent voiding of rectal contents per anum exists in a state of social alienation and professional isolation.

Anorectal control is maintained under normal conditions by a combination of several factors, the most important of which include: (i) the internal anal sphincter; (ii) the external anal sphincter; (iii) the puborectalis muscle; and (iv) anorectal sensation. The role of the internal (involuntary) anal sphincter appears to be largely one of support, providing a 'fine-tuning' mechanism. Weakness of this muscle (e.g. following manual dilation of the anus or sphincterotomy) leads to incontinence of flatus and soiling in the presence of diarrhoea, but not to major functional disturbance. The external (voluntary) anal sphincter can contract vigorously for approximately 60 seconds before fatiguing. This is probably a mechanism to prevent soiling (for a short period) should the anal sphincters become 'threatened' by the presence of loose stool in the rectum. A major contribution to anorectal control is provided by the contraction of the puborectalis muscle which creates an angle between the lower rectum and upper anal canal (the anorectal angle). Sharp angulation permits a flap-valve mechanism to operate such that increases in intra-abdominal pressure cause the anterior rectal wall to close over the top of the anal canal, excluding it from rectal contents. The sensation of a full rectum is probably caused by tension on pressure receptors situated in the pelvic floor rather than within the rectum itself. The discrimination of the nature of rectal contents is achieved by a simple locally mediated reflex whereby rectal distension (from flatus or faeces) initiates internal anal sphincter relaxation. A sample of rectal contents thereby intrudes into the anal canal and makes contact with the sensory-rich anoderm at the dentate line where it is perceived.

A complete classification of the causes of faecal incontinence is provided in Table F.6. At the outset, it is of importance to establish the degree of disability, since clearly the management of the patient with partial soiling secondary to a prolapsed haemorrhoid will differ from that in a patient with frequent and incapacitating incontinence of formed stool. In all patients a full clinical examination with special reference to the anorectum should be carried out. Digital examination of the anorectum will provide a subjective assessment of anorectal function which ought to be supported, wherever possible: by (i) proctography; (ii) anal canal manometry; and (iii) electromyography of the external anal sphincter and puborectalis muscles.

Table F.6 Classification of the causes of faecal incontinence

---

Normal sphincters and pelvic floor
Faecal impaction
Causes of diarrhoea (e.g. infection, inflammatory bowel disease)
Faecal fistula/colostomy

Abnormal sphincters and/or pelvic floor
Minor incontinence
Internal sphincter deficiency
■ Previous surgery (e.g. anal dilatation, sphincterotomy)
■ Rectal prolapse
■ Third-degree haemorrhoids
■ Idiopathic
Minor denervation of external sphincter and pelvic floor

Major incontinence
Congenital anomalies of the anorectum
Trauma
■ Iatrogenic
■ Obstetric
■ Fractures of the pelvis
■ Impalement
Denervation
■ Obstetric
■ Rectal prolapse
■ Peripheral neuropathy (e.g. diabetes mellitus)
■ Cauda equina lesion (tumour or trauma)
■ Tabes dorsalis
■ Lumbar meningomyelocoele (spina bifida)
Upper motor neurone lesion
■ Cerebral
    ◆ Multiple stroke
    ◆ Metastases and other tumours
    ◆ Trauma
    ◆ Dementia and other degenerative disorders
Spinal
■ Multiple sclerosis
■ Metastases and other tumours
■ Degenerative diseases (e.g. vitamin B_{12} deficiency)
Rectal carcinoma
Anorectal infection (e.g. lymphogranuloma)
Drug intoxication (particularly in the elderly)

Faecal incontinence in the presence of normal anal sphincters and pelvic floor

It is important to stress that the symptom of faecal incontinence need not necessarily imply deficiency of the anal sphincters or pelvic floor. Hence, any patient experiencing severe diarrhoea will frequently develop soiling of varying degree. The commonest cause of faecal incontinence therefore is probably *gastroenteritis*. Patients with severe *inflammatory bowel disease*

frequently state that the urgency and frank faecal incontinence is the most distressing aspect of the disease and this, rather than the bleeding, may militate towards a surgical approach to management. Elderly patients and those who have *depressed cortical awareness* of rectal filling (e.g. following cerebrovascular accident [CVA] or spinal cord section) may develop faecal impaction. Incontinence in these patients probably results from over-activation of a visceral reflex whereby the internal sphincter relaxes in response to rectal distension. A wide-open internal sphincter then permits the leakage of stool of looser consistency.

Minor faecal incontinence

This is defined as the inadvertent loss of flatus or liquid stool per anum, and is usually the consequence of a weak internal anal sphincter. This situation may arise secondary to some *surgical procedures* (e.g. manual dilatation of the anus) or be caused by a stretch effect in patients with a full-thickness *rectal prolapse* (Fig. F.16) or with third-degree *haemorrhoids* (Fig. F.17). In some patients, internal sphincter dysfunction is observed *without any underlying cause* apparent; in these patients there may be disease affecting the autonomic supply to this muscle. Finally, minor degrees of incontinence may result from *denervation* and other *injuries* affecting the external anal sphincter and pelvic floor; these are discussed below.

Major faecal incontinence

This is defined as the inadvertent and frequent loss of fully formed stool per rectum and, as such, represents the most severe degree of functional impairment of the anorectum. *Congenital abnormalities* of the lower gut may be associated with anorectal incontinence, particularly in some forms of rectal atresia where there has been total failure of development of the pelvic floor musculature. *Traumatic damage* may be inflicted on the external sphincter during vaginal delivery, in which case the damage sustained is usually confined to the anterior section of the sphincter (third-degree perineal tear) or by the surgeon during treatment of anal fistula when perhaps the puborectalis muscle or too much external sphincter muscle has been inappropriately divided. The pelvic floor can be damaged by 'shearing' forces when there has been complete disruption of the bony pelvis following

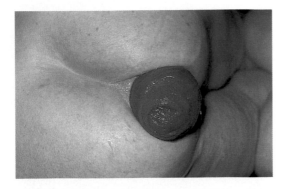

Figure F.16 Complete rectal prolapse.

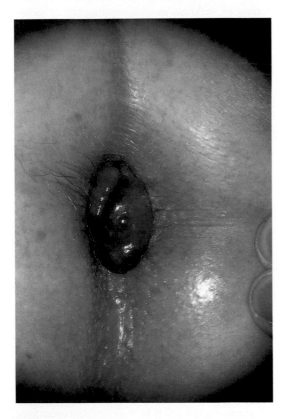

Figure F.17 Long-standing, completely prolapsed third-degree haemorrhoids.

compression injury to the pelvis. Rarely, impalement injuries to the anal sphincters and pelvic floor can lead to severe functional loss.

The greatest number of patients presenting for treatment of major faecal incontinence are found to have *denervation of the striated component of the anal sphincter musculature.* The source of nerve damage seems to be local (i.e. pudendal) in the majority, and a major factor would appear to be traumatic childbirth where the nerves are subjected to undue compression and stretching forces. Damage may also be sustained in patients who strain excessively with defaecation, and less commonly in patients with peripheral neuropathies, particularly diabetes mellitus. Finally, very rarely, lower motor neurone lesions can be the consequence of cauda equina tumours. If there is a history of severe perineal pain and the history of incontinence is brief, this diagnosis should be considered and a spinal MRI obtained.

Upper motor neurone lesions cause faecal incontinence for imprecise reasons. There is little doubt that interruption of suprasegmental control causes incontinence, partly as a consequence of a motor deficit and partly because of sensory loss which in turn leads to impaction.

Rarely, *rectal carcinoma and infection* (specifically by lymphogranuloma venereum) can give rise to extensive destruction of the pelvic floor such that faecal incontinence might develop.

Harold Ellis

FAINTS

(See also CONVULSIONS AND FITS, p. 222; VERTIGO, p. 773).

Attacks of transient loss of consciousness are common, and the causes range from simple vasovagal attacks to epilepsy. Furthermore, a complaint of 'fainting' may not always imply actual loss of consciousness; some patients may mean no more than a feeling of unsteadiness or 'light-headedness'. It is important, as always, to obtain from the patient and, whenever possible, from a witness a precise description of the nature of the attacks. The term 'syncope' has a more exact connotation, and can be defined as 'transient loss of consciousness due to a reduction in the cerebral blood flow'. It is this condition with which this discussion will be mainly concerned.

The common causes of syncope are summarized in Table F.7.

Table F.7 Causes of syncope

Vasomotor
Vasovagal attacks
Postural hypotension
Carotid sinus syncope

Cardiac syncope
Stokes–Adams attacks in atrioventricular block
Paroxysmal dysrhythmias
Central circulatory obstruction (e.g. aortic stenosis)
Cyanotic attacks in congenital heart disease

Cerebrovascular disease

Miscellaneous
Cough syncope
Micturition syncope
Breath-holding attacks

Vasomotor syncope

This rather imprecise term will be taken to include the large group of conditions in which the cardiac output and blood pressure fall as a result of a sudden fall in peripheral resistance and in the central venous pressure.

Vasovagal attacks

These are extremely common, and are almost always of no serious significance. Many predisposing factors are known, including emotion, fatigue, prolonged standing and chronic illness of almost any kind. There are other, more serious, conditions of which an apparently simple faint may be a manifestation. Haemorrhage causes syncope as a direct result of the fall in central venous pressure. If the bleeding is external, no diagnostic difficulty arises, but with internal bleeding (e.g. into the gastrointestinal tract) syncope may occur before there is any direct evidence such as haematemesis or melaena. The mechanism whereby haemorrhage causes syncope can also operate in a few patients with very large varicose veins or angiomatous malformations in the legs in which the blood accumulates in the upright posture. Severe pain can also cause syncope, as in dissecting aneurysm or myocardial infarction although, in the latter condition, there may also be a fall in cardiac output sufficient on its own to cause syncope. In elderly patients especially, syncope is quite commonly the presenting symptom of myocardial infarction; on recovering consciousness, the patient may not complain of chest pain, being perhaps more preoccupied with any trauma they may have suffered in their fall.

The clinical picture is well known – not least to the many medical students who have fainted at their first operation. The patient is nearly always in the upright position; indeed, a 'faint' occurring in the recumbent position is good evidence of some cause other than a vasovagal attack. A minor exception to this rule is the syncope experienced by some pregnant women while lying on their backs; this is probably due to pressure by the uterus on the inferior vena cava producing a fall in venous return. Prodromal symptoms include a feeling of weakness, nausea, sweating and epigastric discomfort; within a few seconds or minutes the patient falls unconscious. The pulse is of small volume and slow and the blood pressure is very low; the face is pale and the skin cold and sweating. Incontinence of urine and muscular twitching are rare, but can occur in transient loss of consciousness from any cause and do not necessarily imply that the attack is epileptic. Recovery is rapid as the cerebral blood flow increases in the recumbent posture, unless the patient is prevented from falling as in a crowd or by well-meaning bystanders. Weakness and nausea may persist for some time after recovery of consciousness.

The term 'vasovagal', which has been used to denote this type of vasomotor syncope, is now widely accepted. However, in the past it was used, originally by Sir William Gowers, to describe curious 'seizures' which resembled the attacks described above in most respects. They differed only in that loss of consciousness was rare and, usually, no precipitating cause could be found. A theory that they represented a specific entity and were possibly epileptic in nature has now been discredited, and it seems certain that these attacks were no more than a mild form of vasomotor syncope occurring in unusually susceptible subjects. All practising physicians have seen patients who faint not only from venepuncture but from a tourniquet or sphygmomanometer cuff being put around an arm.

Postural hypotension

This condition overlaps with vasovagal syncope which, as has been said, almost always occurs when the patient is upright. It is, however, worth distinguishing a group of patients who have a steep fall in blood pressure whenever they stand upright. In some of these patients a neurological cause for the failure of vasoconstriction and other compensatory mechanisms can be identified. To others, the label 'idiopathic' has been applied but, in many of these, it is probable that detailed investigation would localize a neurological lesion.

Many drugs can cause a marked postural fall in blood pressure. Among these are hypotensive agents such as guanethidine and bethanidine; nitrites, phenothiazine derivatives, monoamine oxidase inhibitors, imipramine, barbiturates, amitriptyline and other psychotherapeutic agents have also been incriminated. The hypotensive agent prazosin seems to be unusually liable to cause sudden loss of consciousness for periods of time ranging up to 1 hour. It is not known whether this is always due to postural hypotension, and it may be a specific side effect of this drug. Lesions of peripheral nervous pathways can produce a similar effect by interruption of the afferent or efferent pathways of reflex arcs. Thus, postural hypotension is well known in tabes, diabetes and acute polyneuritis, and has been described in alcoholic and carcinomatous neuropathy and in porphyria. Lesions of the central pathways are less easy to demonstrate, but degeneration of the intermediolateral column in the spinal cord, vascular lesions of the brainstem and craniopharyngioma, and other parasellar tumours, possibly involving the hypothalamus, have been demonstrated in some cases. Many of these neurological conditions have in common an abnormal response to the Valsalva manoeuvre in that the blood pressure continues to fall throughout the period of strain and no overshoot or reflex bradycardia occurs.

Carotid-sinus syncope

In many subjects, massage of a carotid sinus can cause bradycardia with some fall in blood pressure. In some, mostly elderly patients, these changes may be more marked and this increased sensitivity of the carotid-sinus reflex can be produced by neoplastic or inflammatory lesions in the neck or by digitalis intoxication. In a few patients the haemodynamic changes may be so profound and the reflexes so easily elicited, as by a tight collar, shaving or turning the head, that recurrent syncope occurs. Various types of carotid-sinus syncope have been described with or without bradycardia in addition to the hypotension, but the distinction is largely of academic interest. The carotid sinus is innervated by the glossopharyngeal nerve, and a rare condition which may be related to carotid-sinus syncope is the fainting sometimes associated with glossopharyngeal neuralgia, a condition similar to trigeminal neuralgia but causing pain in the tongue, pharynx and ear.

Cardiac syncope

In this group of conditions the cardiac output falls as a result of a primary cardiac lesion. It differs from vasomotor syncope in that attacks are much less closely related to the upright posture.

Stokes–Adams attacks

These are due to cardiac arrest, usually in asystole but occasionally in ventricular fibrillation, on a basis of atrioventricular block. Loss of consciousness can occur in any posture, and is abrupt. The patient is pale and pulseless; respiration continues. After about 15–20 seconds twitching may begin due to cerebral anoxia. The attack usually lasts for about 30 seconds, but may last longer and death may result. On recovery the patient becomes flushed; this is due to well-oxygenated blood which has been in the pulmonary capillaries during the period of circulatory arrest being flung into systemic capillaries which are widely dilated as a result of the accumulation of vasodilator metabolites. Occasionally, if the attacks occur when the patient is asleep, the only complaint may be of waking with the face feeling hot and flushed.

Paroxysmal dysrhythmias

A paroxysm of tachycardia with a heart rate much in excess of 200 beats per minute may cause syncope as diastolic filling of the heart is markedly reduced at these heart rates.

Central circulatory obstruction

Syncope on effort and (more seriously) at rest is a well-recognized feature of aortic stenosis. The mechanism is not clear as this valve lesion is not associated with a low cardiac output unless failure has occurred. It may be that baroceptors within the left ventricular wall, stimulated by the very high pressure, are in some way responsible. Effort syncope is also not uncommon in other obstructive lesions such as pulmonary stenosis and severe pulmonary hypertension, but it is rare in mitral stenosis. The acute circulatory obstruction produced by massive pulmonary embolism or by the impaction of a left atrial thrombus or myxoma in the mitral orifice may also cause syncope. Obstruction to cardiac filling due to cardiac tamponade and constrictive pericarditis can have the same effect.

Cyanotic attacks

Syncope in Fallot's tetralogy and other types of cyanotic congenital heart disease is due not so much to a fall in cardiac output as to a sudden increase in the veno-arterial shunt. This can be due to a fall in systemic resistance or to an increase in the severity of a muscular infundibular stenosis. There is little change in blood pressure, but the patient becomes deeply cyanosed and the murmur of pulmonary stenosis becomes much softer as the greater part of the systemic venous return is shunted into the aorta via the ventricular septal defect.

Ischaemic heart disease

Syncope due to acute myocardial infarction has already been discussed under 'vasomotor syncope' (see above).

Syncope due to cerebral vascular disease

Fainting is rare as a symptom of disease of the carotid arteries and their branches, but is more common with stenosis or occlusion of the vertebral arterial system. Atherosclerosis of the vertebral or basilar arteries and external compression of the vertebral arteries by cervical spondylosis or in the Klippel–Feil syndrome, can be responsible for syncopal attacks which may be induced by sudden rotatory movements of the neck.

Miscellaneous

There is a group of conditions in which syncope is associated with a rise in intrathoracic and intra-abdominal pressure. This includes *cough syncope*, in which loss of consciousness occurs at the end of a violent paroxysm of coughing. A series of coughs produces the same circulatory effects as a Valsalva manoeuvre, and a marked fall in cardiac output and blood pressure – probably combined with some degree of arterial hypoxaemia – is the mechanism of the syncope. The *breath-holding attacks* of early childhood

producing syncope and cyanosis probably have a similar mechanism. The mechanism of *micturition syncope* is not fully understood. It occurs typically when, after heavy beer-drinking, the subject rises in the middle of the night to pass urine. The sudden assumption of the upright posture and the vasodilatory action of alcohol are certainly relevant factors, and this condition may be nothing more than a vasomotor syncope. However, it is possible that afferent impulses from the bladder may play some part.

Differential diagnosis

The most important condition from which syncope must be distinguished is *epilepsy*. This can be very difficult, but a careful history will usually resolve the problem. Epileptic attacks are characteristically stereotyped in their nature and duration, and often occur without warning. Even if there is an aura it bears little resemblance to the prodromal symptoms of syncope except, possibly, in the case of complex partial seizures. Most varieties of syncope – with the notable exception of cardiac syncope – occur almost exclusively in the upright posture, whereas the onset of an epileptic fit is unrelated to posture. The typical tonic and clonic phases of major epilepsy should not be confused with the minor twitches which may occur in syncope if a history can be obtained from a reliable eye-witness. Urinary incontinence, a very common feature of epilepsy, is not a major differentiating factor as it can occur in severe or prolonged syncope. Electro-encephalography is certainly of value in some cases but, even with this aid, some doubt may remain.

Consciousness is not lost in *vertigo*, so that a history from the patient him/herself should elicit an account of the typical sensation of rotation. However, the use by the patient of such terms as 'giddiness' to describe the premonitory symptoms of vasomotor syncope, together with the nausea which is common to both conditions, may confuse the unwary.

Hysterical attacks are nearly always described by the patients as 'faints', but the gracefully dramatic fall into a convenient armchair bears no resemblance to syncope in which the patient collapses like a house of cards. Swoons are out of fashion, unless one includes the hysterical faints of teenage girls at 'pop' sessions. It is possible that the so-called 'Toronto blessing' experienced in some charismatic church services is of the same nature.

Hyperventilation is usually a hysterical phenomenon, and the feeling of light-headedness induced may be described as faintness. Here, as always, a careful history will resolve the issue, but it is worth recalling that hyperventilation followed by a Valsalva manoeuvre will infallibly cause loss of consciousness. This is known variously as the 'mess trick' or the 'fainting lark'.

Mark Kinirons

FALLS

Elderly people are liable to fall for many reasons other than 'drop attacks', and causes such as *postural hypotension*, *lack of concentration*, the *effects of sedating medicines*, *disturbances of vision*, *tripping* and *postural instability* must be excluded from the diagnosis.

Risk factors for falls in older people include:

- Muscle weakness
- History of falls
- Gait deficit
- Balance deficit
- Use of assistive device
- Visual deficit
- Arthritis
- Depression
- Cognitive impairment
- Age >80 years

The major causes of falls include:

- Accident/environment 31%
- Gait/balance/weakness 17%
- Dizzy/vertigo 13%
- Drop attack 9%
- Confusion: acute/chronic 5%
- Postural blood pressure 3%
- Visual disturbance 2%
- Syncope 0.3%
- Other 15%
- Unknown 5%

Falls are common. They increase with age and dependency (they occur most frequently in nursing homes). There are many risk factors for falls, and they have many causes (see above). It is essential to make an accurate diagnosis, and this is possible in up to 95 per cent of all falls. This allows treatments to prevent further falls. In addition, consideration should also be given to preventing fractures due to falls. This includes treatment for osteoporosis.

Mark Kinirons

FASCICULATION (MUSCLE TWITCHING)

Fasciculation is one of the classical features of a lower motor neurone lesion. It is observed clinically as an intermittent twitching movement due to the contraction of groups of muscle fibres supplied by the affected nerve. The term 'fibrillation' is applied to the contraction of single muscle fibres. Fibrillation is recorded electrically rather than observed clinically. Fasciculation can occur when only part of the lower motor nerve is affected.

Whilst fasciculation can occur with inflammatory or compressive lesions of peripheral nerves, it is in chronic degeneration of anterior horn cells that it is most conspicuous. It is thus a common and an important diagnostic feature of motor neurone disease, where the lower motor nerve is affected. Intermittent flickering movements, often around the shoulder girdle or in the thenar muscles, and sometimes felt by the patient, may be an early sign of the disease. Inspection over 2–3 minutes may be necessary before the tell-tale movement is detected. Sometimes, it can be provoked by a light tap over the muscles with a tendon hammer or flick of the finger.

It is important to note that fasciculation can also be benign. Transitory twitching of facial muscles, particularly the orbicularis oculi, is common experience in normal people; so too is fasciculation in calf muscles, sometimes after unaccustomed exercise. Such benign fasciculation, particularly when it is prolonged or extensive as it occasionally is, can be a cause of major anxiety in doctors and others unfamiliar with the features of motor neurone disease.

Mark Kinirons

FATIGUE

Fatigue is a normal reaction to exertion, but it may be produced excessively by minor exertion in any condition of ill-health, whether it be organic, psychogenic, or both. Fatigue may be caused by malignant disease, infections and their sequelae, anaemia and states of low cardiac output, endocrine and metabolic disorders and malnutrition. It may be due to lack of sleep, boredom, stress or overwork. The so-called 'combat fatigue' seen in the troops in the Second World War resulted more from the mental than the physical stress of active service. Fatigue on waking in the morning is more commonly due to mental rather than physical factors, but it may be due to either or both. Depending on the cause, fatigue may be constant or episodic and in some cases, as in myasthenia gravis, may be anticipated so that physical effort is avoided to prevent the later onset of fatigue.

Fatigue is at least as often psychological in origin as due to organic disease, but many cases are multifactorial in origin. The following list, although inevitably incomplete, includes most of the common causes.

Emotional and psychological causes

These include continued unhappiness, boredom, disappointment, overwork, lack of sleep, anxiety and depression. Neurasthenia, a nineteenth-century diagnosis, is undergoing something of a revival.

Malignant disease

Any neoplastic disease can be associated with fatigue, which may be a very early symptom – sometimes earlier than loss of weight.

Chronic infection

Tuberculosis, brucellosis, infective endocarditis and toxoplasmosis are examples of conditions of which the most obvious manifestation may be fatigue.

Human immunodeficiency virus

Fatigue is a significant problem for patients suffering from HIV disease, and is often under-reported by patients and therefore under-treated by physicians. It tends to be unpredictable and cyclical in nature, although there are some who suffer unrelenting fatigue.

The degree of fatigue can be quite debilitating, interfering considerably with requirements for daily living and, without a patient carer, leads to inability to wash, shop, eat and to comply fully with complex medical regimens. The fatigue is often explained by just having the HIV disease itself, though it can be quite severe in patients who do not have a significant viral load. There are specific conditions that may make the fatigue worse, and these should be sought out since therapeutic intervention may be of benefit. Hypogonadism associated with decreased testosterone level, adrenal insufficiency, methaemoglobinaemia secondary to dapsone treatment, anaemia, depression and malnutrition are among the associated conditions contributing to fatigue, and should all respond to therapy. Appropriate exercise programmes have also been shown to be of benefit in improving energy levels.

Post-viral fatigue syndrome

Many viral infections, of which infectious mononucleosis is the best-known example, may be followed, sometimes for many months, by profound fatigue; this may be curiously episodic. The status of myalgic encephalomyelitis (ME)/chronic fatigue syndrome (CFS) as a specific entity is unclear. Some believe that it is a severe variety of the post-viral syndrome. Others maintain that it is a different condition; in particular, it has been suggested that graded exercise, which is usually beneficial in most cases of the post-viral syndrome, causes deterioration in ME.

Tissue hypoxia

Anaemia of any type is a common cause of fatigue, as are conditions in which the cardiac output is chronically low. These include cardiac failure, severe pulmonary hypertension, valvular heart disease (e.g. aortic and mitral stenosis), Addison's disease and excessive diuretic therapy.

Connective tissue diseases

These include rheumatoid arthritis, systemic lupus erythematosus, polyarteritis nodosa, polymyalgia rheumatica, giant-cell arteritis and polymyositis.

Endocrine and metabolic disorders

Apart from Addison's disease (see above), many conditions in this category, such as hypothyroidism, mast cell disorders, renal or hepatic failure and diabetes mellitus, can present with fatigue.

Malnutrition

Whether this is due to dietary deficiency or to conditions associated with chronic diarrhoea such as coeliac disease, ulcerative colitis or Crohn's disease, fatigue is likely to be present.

Chronic pain

Fatigue can be due to persistent chronic pain causing discomfort by day, as in osteoarthritis, or lack of sleep at night, as in some cases of Paget's disease or metastatic disease of bone.

Muscular weakness

Chronic neurological disorders, such as multiple sclerosis, motor neurone disease and, especially, myasthenia gravis, in addition to the myopathies, are typically associated with excessive fatiguability.

Chronic drug intoxication

The long-term administration of beta-adrenergic blocking agents is an important cause of fatigue. Alcohol abuse and the chronic administration of benzodiazepines have a similar, but less specific, effect.

Drug withdrawal syndromes

Fatigue may be a consequence of the withdrawal of addictive drugs such as morphine and diamorphine. It can also occur after the withdrawal of corticosteroids, benzodiazepines, alcohol and antidepressants.

Sharon O'Byrne

FINGERS, CLUBBED

The four features of finger clubbing are: loss of nail bed angle; increased nail curvature (Fig. F.18); fluctuation of the nail bed; and drumstick-like swelling of the terminal phalanx. Identification is easy when all four features are present, but dispute is common when only some occur. The first two criteria must be present for finger clubbing to be diagnosed; thus, nail

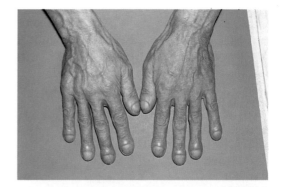

Figure F.18 Clubbing of fingers of both hands due to bronchiectasis.

bed fluctuation on its own does not constitute clubbing. The first two criteria combine to increase the hyponychial angle, subtended at the nail base by the skin crease at the dorsum of the distal interphalangeal joint and the skin immediately below the free edge of the nail (Fig. F.19). This angle, which is best measured from a shadowgram, is usually less than 190° in normal subjects, but exceeds 195° in individuals with clubbing. Clubbing may affect the toes as well as the fingers, but is usually more obvious in the hands. Clubbing is usually bilateral, but occasionally it may be unilateral in the presence of local vascular abnormalities, such as a subclavian aneurysm, an arteriovenous fistula or disruption of the cervical sympathetic nerves. The pathophysiology of finger clubbing is not understood.

Finger clubbing is an important physical sign, and may be the first and only sign of serious organic disease. The relative frequencies of causes will vary between countries; typical causes in the UK are listed in Table F.8.

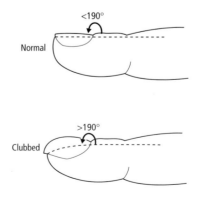

Figure F.19 Measurement of the hyponychial angle.

Table F.8 Causes of finger clubbing (United Kingdom data)

Common causes	Pulmonary
Bronchial carcinoma	■ Lung abscess
	■ Fibrotic tuberculosis
Less common causes	■ Pleural fibroma
Cardiac	■ Arteriovenous malformation
■ Cyanotic congenital heart disease	■ Metastatic deposits
■ Infective endocarditis	*Mediastinal*
Pulmonary	■ Lymphoma
■ Bronchiectasis	■ Thymoma
■ Cystic fibrosis	■ Chronic granulocytic leukaemia
■ Empyema	■ Oesophageal carcinoma
■ Mesothelioma	■ Oesophageal leiomyoma
■ Idiopathic pulmonary fibrosis	■ Peptic oesophagitis
Extra-thoracic	■ Achalasia of oesophagus
■ Idiopathic/familial/congenital	*Extra-thoracic*
■ Cirrhosis of liver	■ Nasopharyngeal carcinoma
■ Coeliac disease	■ Thyroid carcinoma
■ Crohn's disease	■ Purgative abuse
■ Ulcerative colitis	■ Repeated pregnancies
■ Thyrotoxicosis	■ Pachydermoperiostosis
Uncommon causes	
Cardiac	
■ Atrial myxoma	

Among *pulmonary diseases*, lung carcinoma is the most common cause of finger clubbing, and it is wise always to consider this diagnosis. Other intrathoracic malignancies including mesothelioma, lymphomas (and rarely secondary carcinomas or sarcomas) can cause finger clubbing. Intrathoracic sepsis is associated with clubbing, although this is now an unusual cause in Britain. Chronic bronchitis and emphysema do not cause clubbing. Diffuse pulmonary fibrosis may be associated with clubbing, but different causes vary markedly in the frequency of this association. Clubbing is common in idiopathic pulmonary fibrosis, but rare in extrinsic allergic alveolitis and sarcoidosis. Pulmonary asbestosis is the only pneumoconiosis directly associated with clubbing.

Among *diseases of the cardiovascular system*, cyanotic congenital heart disease is almost always associated with finger clubbing in those surviving beyond infancy. However, clubbing does not occur in non-cyanotic congenital heart disease such as uncomplicated atrial or ventricular septal defects or persistent ductus arteriosus. Clubbing is a well-recognized, but rather uncommon, feature of infective endocarditis; its absence must not be regarded as important evidence against the diagnosis. It usually appears 6 weeks or more after the onset of the illness, but can occasionally develop within a month. Mild finger clubbing develops late in some cases of cirrhosis of the liver, especially in biliary cirrhosis, in coeliac disease, and, rarely, in ulcerative colitis and Crohn's disease.

Clubbing due to any cause may progress to hypertrophic pulmonary osteoarthropathy, although this is almost always due to lung carcinoma. Periosteal new bone formation will then be evident, especially at the distal ends of long bones at the affected joints. Familial forms of clubbing and of hypertrophic osteoarthropathy are rare. The presence in family members and the absence of associated disease provide clues to the diagnosis. Hereditary osteoarthropathy is associated with thickening of the skin of the hands and face, the latter giving rise to a characteristic appearance of large features with coarse deeply creased skin. This rare familial condition is called 'pachydermoperiostosis'.

Patients are rarely aware of their clubbed forgers. Thus, statements that there has been no recent change in their fingers should not be taken to indicate congenital clubbing.

Boris Lams

FINGERS, CONDITIONS AFFECTING

See UPPER LIMB, PAIN IN (p. 754).

FINGERS, DEAD (WHITE, COLD)

Raynaud's phenomenon

The digital arteries of the fingers serve two purposes: (i) to supply blood for nutrition of the finger; and (ii) by controlling blood flow through the skin of the fingers, they vary the heat loss and assist in regulating the core temperature of the body. Thus, on exposure of the body to cold, these arteries normally constrict, reducing blood flow through – and heat loss from – the fingers. In subjects with Raynaud's phenomenon this reflex appears to be excessive and the digital arteries close completely such that the finger becomes 'dead', white and numb. With rewarming, the arteries open up again and blood flushes vigorously through the fingers, often causing throbbing discomfort ('rewarming pain'). During severe episodes, pallor of the digits may be followed by cyanosis and numbness prior to rewarming. In such instances the classical progression of triphasic digital colour changes is observed: white-blue-red. Other sites including the toes, tongue, nose, ears and nipples can also be affected.

Raynaud's phenomenon occurs on a worldwide basis, although it is more prevalent in cold climates. It occurs in about 3–5 per cent of healthy young females in Britain, and is far less common in males. Primary Raynaud's phenomenon occurs in the absence of underlying disease, whereas secondary Raynaud's phenomenon is associated with numerous disorders.

Primary Raynaud's phenomenon

Primary Raynaud's phenomenon has an earlier age of onset than secondary – typically between the ages of 10 and 30 years – with a milder disease course. The nail-fold capillaries and fingers remain healthy and normal in appearance, and digital ulcers or gangrene rarely develop. In addition to these clinical features, a normal erythrocyte sedimentation rate and a negative test for antinuclear antibody help to distinguish it from secondary Raynaud's. A family history is common and noted in up to 25 per cent of first-degree relatives of patients with primary Raynaud's phenomenon.

Secondary Raynaud's phenomenon

Much less common is Raynaud's phenomenon secondary to some underlying disease. In these patients the phenomenon usually appears later in life – often in middle age – though it can occur in younger patients. Men are affected more often than women in primary Raynaud's phenomenon. From the beginning, the digital ischaemia tends to be more severe, and is often at first asymmetrical. Recurrent and prolonged digital ischaemia eventually causes the fingers to change in appearance, becoming shrunken with tight skin and loss of subcutaneous tissue. Ulcers commonly appear under the fingernails (Fig. F.20) and, when healed, leave puckered scars. Repeated attacks lead to loss of tissue of the terminal phalanx with resorption of the phalanx and curved overhanging nails. Causes of secondary Raynaud's phenomenon are listed in Table F.9.

Scleroderma is the commonest cause of secondary Raynaud's phenomenon. It is usually the variety of

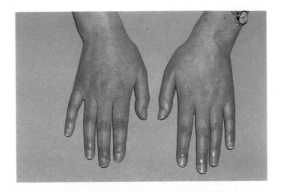

Figure F.20 Raynaud's disease in a woman aged 23 years. The hands are blue and feel cold to palpation, even at normal room temperature.

Table F.9 Causes of secondary Raynaud's phenomenon

Common causes
Rheumatological diseases
- Scleroderma
- Systemic lupus erythematosus
- Thromboangiitis obliterans (Buerger's disease)
- Rheumatoid arthritis
- Mixed connective tissue disease, dermatomyositis or polymyositis

Environmental agents and injury
- Vibration (hand–arm vibration syndrome)
- Frostbite

Less common causes
Drugs and toxins
Beta-blockers, chemotherapeutic agents, interferon, ergotamines, polyvinyl chloride

Abnormal blood elements
Cryoglobulins, cold agglutinins, cryofibrinogenaemia, paraproteinaemia

scleroderma known as the CRST syndrome (calcinosis, Raynaud's phenomenon, sclerodactyly, telangiectases). Initially, only one or two of these four components of the syndrome will be present – usually the Raynaud's and the telangiectases. The telangiectases are first seen on the nail bed, but later larger ones appear on the fingers and face. Subcutaneous calcification eventually appears, which at first is felt as tender nodules under the skin of the fingers but eventually this extrudes through the skin (Fig. F.21). Although severe involvement of the fingers often leads to a loss of digits, it does not usually affect vital organs and does not normally shorten life expectancy. Progressive systemic sclerosis with widespread skin involvement and involvement of vital organs is a rare cause of Raynaud's phenomenon, and ulceration and gangrene of digits is unusual.

Systemic lupus erythematosus (SLE) may cause severe digital arthritis with Raynaud's phenomenon and repeated attacks of digital gangrene causing extensive loss of digits. *Rheumatoid arthritis* can similarly affect the fingers with digital gangrene. *Vibration injury*, as seen in foundry workers using pneumatic-powered, hand-held buffers and grinders, caulkers and welders in the shipbuilding industry and forestry workers using hand-held, power-driven saws, can cause severe Raynaud's phenomenon. The disorder may appear within a few months in foundry workers, but takes longer to appear in shipyard and forestry workers. In addition to the white fingers, these patients develop numbness and tingling of the fingers. Although the Raynaud's phenomenon can be very severe and a considerable nuisance during cold weather, ulcers and gangrene generally do not occur.

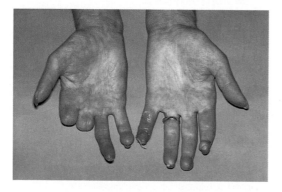

Figure F.21 Raynaud's phenomenon in a patient with scleroderma (see Fig. F.5). She has already lost two fingers of the left hand, and the tips of the remaining digits show early gangrene.

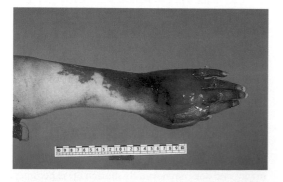

Figure F.22 Gangrene of the hand in a 78-year-old man with severe arteriosclerosis, atrial fibrillation and a brachial embolus.

Beta-blocking drugs used in the treatment of angina and hypertension commonly cause cold hands, but do not seem to induce classic Raynaud's phenomenon (i.e. digital vasoconstriction) in patients who would not otherwise have Raynaud's. However, these drugs may make Raynaud's worse in those already suffering from the condition.

Persistent digital ischaemia

Sudden onset of ischaemia of one or more digits persisting for days, weeks or months (persistent digital ischaemia) is not uncommon in the middle-aged and elderly. On examination, the finger is usually blue and cold, but capillary circulation is present and the finger usually survives. In younger patients this condition is usually due to some form of arteritis (e.g. *SLE* or *rheumatoid disease*), but in older patients investigation usually fails to reveal any abnormality except for the presence of atheroma. In these patients the ischaemia is due to rupture of an atheromatous plaque higher in the arterial tree with plaque debris embolizing the digit (Fig. F.22).

Frostbite

Apart from provoking Raynaud's phenomenon in predisposed individuals, prolonged exposure of the fingers to cold (e.g. in hill walkers or outdoor workers in winter) may result in the patient complaining of cold, dead, numb fingers due to freezing of the superficial layers of the skin. In the early stages there are white and dead patches of skin on the fingers, but later and in more severe cases, gangrene of the skin appears and may envelop the whole digit. Although it appears alarming at first, the gangrene is limited in most cases to the superficial layers of the skin, and the skin will eventually peel off, leaving a normal digit beneath.

Melvin Lobo

FINGERS, SKIN AFFECTIONS OF

The skin of the fingers is particularly prone to those dermatoses that are influenced by environmental exposure such as cold, ionizing radiation or chemicals.

The fingers are often the site of inoculation of infectious skin conditions. A comprehensive list of conditions that can be seen on fingers, divided into morphological types, is provided in Table F.10. The conditions, listed by anatomical site, are detailed in Table F.11. Some examples are shown in Figs F.23–F.26.

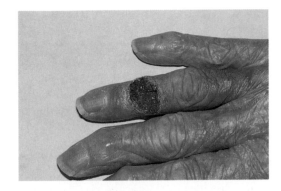

Figure F.23 Squamous-cell carcinoma.

Table F.10 Skin affections of the fingers

Erythematous
Chilblains, perniosis
Actinic dermatitis
Erythema multiforme
Lupus erythematosus
Dermatomyositis

Leprosy
Syphilitic chancre/gumma
Chrome ulcer
Trophic ulcer
Basal-cell carcinoma
Squamous-cell carcinoma
Lupus vulgaris

Papular/nodular
Warts
Cellular naevi
Actinic dermatitis
Chilblains
Granuloma annulare
Keratoacanthoma
Basal-cell carcinoma
Squamous-cell carcinoma
Lichen planus
Papular syphilide
Mucous cyst
Fish-tank granuloma
Periungual fibroma

Macular
Lentigo
Junctional naevi
Telangiectases
Scleroderma
Liver disease
Hereditary
Vitiligo

Pustular
Scabies
Boils
Whitlow
Impetigo

Vesico-bullous
Contact dermatitis
Actinic dermatitis
Erythema multiforme
Pompholyx
Scabies
Epidermolysis bullosa
Pemphigoid
Herpes simplex

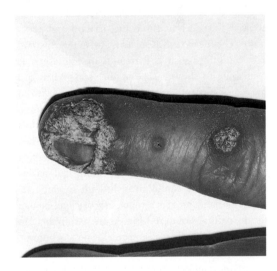

Figure F.24 Viral warts.

Scaly
Atopic eczema
Chronic dermatitis
Dermatophytosis
Psoriasis

Ulcers
Chilblains
Frostbite
Lupus erythematosus
Scleroderma

Table F.11 Anatomical sites of skin affections (fingers)

Finger webs
Irritant dermatitis
Contact dermatitis
Scabies
Candidiasis

Peri-ungual
Whitlow (bacterial or herpetic)
Warts
Mucous cysts
Herpetic whitlow
Chronic paronychia
Fibroma (tuberous sclerosis)
Chancre

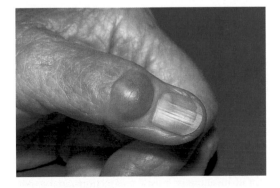

Figure F.25 Myxoid cyst.

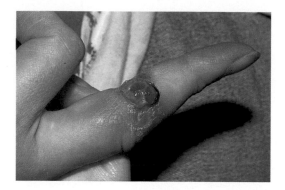

Figure F.26 Pyogenic granuloma.

One condition peculiar to the finger is that of paronychia. The most important precipitating factor is loss of the 'seal' at the nail quick. Age, wear and tear, abrasive jobs such as gardening, irritant and penetrating chemicals such as solvents and detergents, and skin conditions such as dermatitis or psoriasis may contribute to the breakage of this seal. When seal breakage has occurred, a pocket tends to form between the nail and skin which eventually becomes colonized with moisture-loving organisms such as *Candida albicans*, *Pseudomonas* or *Staphylococcus aureus*. When this occurs, an *acute* paronychia develops with swelling and considerable pain. Either side of any nail may be affected, and the condition is difficult to eliminate unless the hands are kept scrupulously dry long enough for the natural seal to re-form. Acute paronychia can also be caused by *herpes simplex* (herpetic whitlow), and the presence of a painless ulcer at the lateral margin of the nailfold, frequently of the index finger, should arouse suspicion of a *syphilitic chancre*. Positive serological tests after the 10th to 14th day, or the development of a secondary rash after 2–3 weeks, will clinch the diagnosis.

Barry Monk

FITS AND CONVULSIONS

See also TETANY (p. 708); TICS (p. 719); and VERTIGO (p. 776)

Epilepsy is derived from the Greek words for 'taking hold of'. 'Convulsion' refers to an intense paroxysm of involuntary muscle contractions, and is not synonymous with 'fit' or 'seizure', both of which can describe epileptic events involving only alteration of sensation or consciousness. Epilepsy is defined by recurrent epileptic seizures; by definition, a single seizure does not constitute epilepsy. In this section only epileptic seizures will be discussed, although it should be remembered that other phenomena can mimic epilepsy. In particular, post-syncopal myoclonic jerks following a cardiogenic or vasovagal faint, rigors and tetany can resemble convulsive seizures, so that all episodes of convulsive movements are not necessarily due to epilepsy. Non-epileptic attack disorders (sometimes called 'pseudoseizures' or 'psychogenic seizures') should also be considered in the differential diagnosis. In describing seizures, 'tonic' means sustained muscle contraction, while 'clonic' refers to repetitive brief muscle jerks. The cornerstone of the diagnosis of epilepsy remains an accurate witnessed account of the attacks.

Hughlings Jackson, a British neurologist, postulated that epilepsy is due to intermittent dysfunction of the nervous system due to '…an excessive and disorderly discharge of cerebral nervous tissue [on muscles]'. This postulate has not been seriously challenged by increasingly sophisticated electrophysiological techniques, which have confirmed the role of hyperexcitable or hypersynchronous cerebral cortex neuronal activity in seizures.

Epilepsy is a common chronic condition; indeed, in neurology clinics throughout the UK one in five referrals are because of epilepsy or suspected epilepsy. Over two-thirds of seizures begin in childhood, with a reduction in incidence after this age, and another increase after the age of 60. In childhood, epilepsy most often has a presently unknown pathological basis and is called 'primary', although many cases are likely ultimately to be attributed to a genetic predisposition (e.g. neuronal ion channel dysfunction). Adult-onset seizures are more likely to be due to an identifiable neurological disease (e.g. a brain tumour, neurodegenerative condition, hippocampal sclerosis). Seizures may be secondary to an intercurrent medical illness (as in sepsis or febrile convulsions, alcohol withdrawal or head trauma).

Seizures may be classified on the above basis (primary or secondary), but can also be classified on the basis of their clinical form (or semiology) that reflects their presumed origin in the brain (generalized – from both hemispheres; or focal – from within one hemisphere) (see Table F.12). The major distinction is

Table F.12 Classification of epileptic seizures

Generalized (bilateral symmetrical, no focal symptoms at onset)
Tonic, clonic or tonic–clonic
Absence
■ Simple – only loss of consciousness
■ Complex – plus brief tonic, clonic or automatic movements
Myoclonic seizures
Atonic (astatic) seizures with or without myoclonic jerks

Partial (focal onset)
Simple (no loss or alteration of consciousness)
■ Motor – frontal origin (tonic–clonic, Jacksonian, Rolandic, epilepsia partialis continua)
■ Sensory (somatosensory, visual, auditory, olfactory, gustatory, vertiginous)
■ Autonomic
■ Psychic
Complex (with impaired consciousness)
Other
■ Reflex (e.g. photosensitive, reading epilepsies)
■ Febrile seizures of infancy and childhood
Hysterical seizures

---

between partial and generalized seizures. Partial seizures are subdivided into simple (consciousness undisturbed) and complex (consciousness disturbed). Simple partial seizures can be subdivided according to their principal manifestations. Some partial seizures begin with a focal neurological disturbance reflecting the function of the part of the cortex in which the seizure discharge begins (see AURA, p. 48). Partial seizures may also be associated with a transient post-ictal focal disturbance, for example a hemiparesis (Todd's phenomenon). Generalized seizures may be either convulsive or non-convulsive. The most common convulsive generalized seizure is the tonic–clonic (grand mal) seizure. The prototype non-convulsive generalized seizure is the brief loss of consciousness in childhood absence (petit mal). Any partial seizure may generalize to a secondary tonic–clonic seizure.

Generalized seizures

Tonic–clonic seizures (grand mal)

This is the most common form of generalized seizure. There is, by definition, no preliminary focal (partial) aura, although there may be general prodromal symptoms such as fatigue or ill-defined malaise. As the seizure begins, the patient typically cries out during a tonic phase of contraction of extensor muscles of the trunk, limbs and neck (opisthotonus), with subsequent respiratory impairment, laboured breathing noises and cyanosis. There is often reflex emptying of the bladder, and occasionally also of the bowel. The patient then enters a clonic phase of generalized symmetric limb jerking which lasts for a variable length of time (usually several minutes), followed by deep coma and then a gradual return of consciousness, with post-ictal confusion and disorientation lasting several hours. There may occasionally be automatic behaviour afterwards.

Simple absence (petit mal)

The classic form of childhood generalized seizure is the petit mal seizure. This is a brief absence (usually 10 seconds or less) in which a child loses contact with his or her surroundings. There may be minor myoclonic activity around the eyelids. The attacks start and stop suddenly, they may be very frequent, and the child may not be aware of them. They may present as problems with learning at school. The EEG in classical absence shows characteristic 3-per-second spike-and-wave activity.

Myoclonic jerks

(See myoclonus, p. 110)
Brief myoclonic jerks occur in numerous epileptic syndromes. They may be associated with an absence, but more commonly they occur without impairment of consciousness. The arms are more frequently involved than the legs.

Partial seizures

Simple partial seizures

Frontal lobe

Frontal lobe seizures are commonly manifest as 'adversive' attacks in which there is tonic or clonic deviation of the head and eyes away from the side of the cerebral focus of origin. This is sometimes associated with jerking of the arm or the adoption of a raised flexed posture of the arm on the side to which the head turns. This form of frontal lobe seizure is more common than the classical Jacksonian motor seizure, in which there is a march of movement beginning distally in a digit and spreading up a limb.

Both of these forms of motor seizure may be followed by a Todd's paresis, and involvement of the frontal speech areas may cause speech arrest. There may be progression to altered or lost awareness, or secondary generalization into a tonic–clonic generalized seizure. The use of continuous electroencephalographic monitoring during seizures (EEG telemetry) has shown that some frontal lobe seizures cause dramatic motor phenomena including repetitive 'bicycling' movements of the legs, sometimes associated with disinhibited behaviour. Unless suspected, these seizure types are easily misclassified as being psychogenic.

Temporal lobe

Seizures beginning in the medial temporal lobe may create sensations of taste or smell (usually unpleasant), epigastric disturbances and pallor, flushing or changes in the heart rate. In addition, there may be psychic phenomena such as déjà-vu and jamais-vu. Seizures originating in the lateral temporal neocortex cause auditory or visual hallucinations, which are often described as having a cinematic playback quality. These focal symptoms often progress to altered or lost awareness (complex partial seizure, see below).

Parietal lobe

These seizures are less common, and may be associated with positive sensory disturbance such as pins and needles, or with distortions of light and colour, often confined to the contralateral half of the visual field. Occipital seizures cause simple, unformed colourful shapes, whilst more anterior (parietal) sites of origin produce more complex visual phenomena such as patterns or objects.

Complex partial seizures

Complex partial seizures – previously termed psychomotor or temporal lobe seizures – are differentiated from simple seizures by the impairment of consciousness. Such disturbance of consciousness may be preceded by symptoms of simple partial type, as above. There may also be contralateral dystonic posturing of the upper limb. Automatic behaviour (automatisms) may occur. Chewing or lip-smacking movements may be seen, as may repetitive fiddling with buttons or clothing. Occasionally, seizures are associated with more complex automatisms, which can lead to problems such as exposure to risk (e.g. climbing out of windows). Very rarely, criminal activity may result, especially in prolonged complex partial status (e.g. shoplifting, vandalism or indecent exposure).

Status epilepticus

Most epileptic seizures are self-limiting, but on rare occasions they follow one another in close succession, resulting in convulsive status epilepticus. This is described as a state of recurrent tonic–clonic seizures without recovery of consciousness. The duration most commonly used in defining status epilepticus is 30 minutes, but some experts have suggested a defining period as brief as 5 minutes. It is a medical emergency with a high morbidity and mortality, especially in the elderly. As a first presentation it is seen in those with symptomatic seizures (e.g. haemorrhagic stroke, electrolyte disturbance or meningo-encephalitis). In patients with a previous diagnosis of epilepsy, status epilepticus is most often seen in severe symptomatic epilepsies and in poorly compliant patients. Most treatment regimens involve early intravenous benzodiazepines (e.g. lorazepam), followed by intravenous phenytoin. If these standard measures fail, then anaesthetic agents and intensive monitoring should be considered at an early stage. It should be noted that non-epileptic attacks constitute a significant proportion of patients admitted to intensive treatment units, and if suspected require prompt specialist assessment. Absence status is occasionally seen in children, who present with confused behaviour, blinking or small myoclonic jerks. Complex partial status may cause confusion and disorientation, sometimes with automatic behaviour (see above). *Epilepsia partialis continua* is a repetitive rhythmic jerking of a group of muscles (see CLONUS, p. 111). It is most commonly seen in association with frontal lobe cerebrovascular disease.

Investigation of the epilepsies

The cornerstone in the diagnosis of epilepsy is a history obtained from the patient and, perhaps more importantly, from witnesses. Epileptic attacks are stereotyped, and on occasion time is required to obtain accounts of several attacks in order to make an accurate diagnosis. An electroencephalogram may add weight to a clinical diagnosis, but can never prove nor disprove epilepsy. The value of inter-ictal recordings is limited, since mild non-specific abnormalities are found in up to 10 per cent of the normal population, whilst 10–20 per cent of patients with epilepsy do not demonstrate epileptiform abnormalities. The sensitivity of the EEG increases with repeated testing and sleep recordings. Despite its limitations, the EEG remains the most useful single paraclinical diagnostic test for epilepsy. The pattern and location of inter-ictal epileptiform abnormalities not only help to make a diagnosis but also assist in classification of the epileptic syndrome, which is important in determining the prognosis and optimizing treatment. Interpretation of the EEG requires specialized expertise and liaison between the treating physician and neurophysiologist to avoid over- and under-diagnosis of epilepsy.

A definitive diagnosis of epilepsy can occasionally be made if EEG discharges can be correlated with the patient's habitual seizures clinically. Continuous long-term EEG recording with video monitoring (EEG telemetry) is expensive and not widely available, but is the most effective way to evaluate frequent habitual seizures, particularly if a non-epileptic or psychogenic component is suspected. EEG telemetry is used not only for differential diagnosis, but also for selecting patients for surgical treatment. Very precise localization of a resectable epileptogenic region is possible with the use of intracranial depth or cortical surface electrodes.

Unless an unequivocal diagnosis of a primary epilepsy is made on clinical and EEG grounds, the use of CT or MRI is appropriate to look for a treatable structural cerebral lesion, but this will depend on local availability. Imaging where available is mandatory in adult-onset patients with focal origin.

Once a diagnosis of epilepsy is made, an attempt should be made to classify the syndrome in terms of seizure type and underlying cause. The number of epilepsy syndromes and causes is formidable, but the fundamental distinctions are between primary and symptomatic epilepsy, and between generalized and partial epilepsy. The primary generalized epilepsies include childhood absence seizures, juvenile myoclonic epilepsy and generalized tonic–clonic seizures in the young adult. Primary partial epilepsies include benign focal motor epilepsy of childhood (*Rolandic epilepsy*), and benign occipital epilepsy of childhood. Symptomatic seizures may be due to a systemic disturbance such as sepsis with fever, hypoxia, hypoglycaemia, electrolyte imbalance, renal, hepatic or respiratory failure. They may be due to toxins, such as drugs (particularly tricyclic antidepressants), alcohol or heavy metals. Pyridoxine deficiency, porphyria, some inborn errors of metabolism and drug withdrawal are other possible (but rare) causes of symptomatic seizures.

Almost any central nervous system disease may cause symptomatic epilepsy. A brief selection includes: congenital disorders (e.g. tuberose sclerosis, lipid storage diseases, leucodystrophies, Down's syndrome, microcephaly and hydrocephalus); infective conditions (e.g. meningo-encephalitis, especially herpes simplex encephalitis, cerebral abscess, fungal, HIV); trauma, due to diffuse brain injury or penetrating brain injury; cerebral tumours, particularly gliomas, meningiomas and secondary metastases; stroke (infarction, intracerebral or subarachnoid haemorrhage); and degenerative conditions such as Alzheimer's disease and Pick's disease. Rarely, multiple sclerosis may present with seizures when a plaque is close to the grey matter of the cortex. Seizures may follow any craniotomy procedure.

The investigations of the various causes of symptomatic seizures may include biochemical and haematological investigation, imaging with CT or MRI, and possibly CSF examination. The clinical situation will dictate which tests are needed.

Non-epileptic attack disorders (which may also be termed pseudo-seizures, psychogenic or hysterical seizures) are increasingly recognized as an important consideration in the differential diagnosis of convulsions. There are some features that raise the possibility of non-epileptic attacks. Even when generalized they will not typically involve self-injury or incontinence. It is usually possible to demonstrate normal pupillary responses, and no focal neurological signs; the heart rate and blood pressure may remain normal, and plantar responses remain flexor. Forced eye closure during the seizure is also a useful pointer towards non-epileptic attacks. Epileptic seizures are stereotyped and usually brief (<5 minutes), whereas non-epileptic attacks may change in character and last much longer. An elevation of serum prolactin above 1000 IU on a venous sample taken within 30 minutes of an event (with a normal baseline level) supports the diagnosis of seizure disorder, but is not diagnostic. Capture of an event during EEG telemetry is the optimal method of clarifying the diagnosis of non-epileptic attacks, though it must be remembered that epileptic and non-epileptic attacks may co-exist. The management of the patient with non-epileptic seizures is challenging, and involves referral to specialist neuropsychiatric services where available. Techniques including cognitive–behavioural therapy may be very helpful, at least in the short term.

David Werring

FLATULENCE

Wind, abdominal bloating and excessive belching or flatus are common complaints for which defining a cause and treatment plan is often less than satisfactory.

Intermittent belching or eructation is commonly caused by eating onions, cabbage or fatty foods. Recurrent, prolonged episodes, however, are nearly always caused by the acquired habit of air swallowing, of which the patient is usually unaware and denies. Chronic obstruction of the oesophagogastric junction (achalasia, pseudo-achalasia), gastric outlet obstruction (peptic ulcer disease, tumour) with proximal viscous dilatation, or gastroparesis (diabetes, sepsis, viral infection and retroperitoneal cancer) may often be associated with belching. Post-prandial gastric bloating due to trapped gas is a recognized complication of anti-reflux surgery.

Abdominal day-time bloating is a feature of *irritable bowel syndrome* (IBS). Whereas IBS is often associated with altered bowel habit, the Rome II criteria recognize a bloating-predominant form. Demonstrable increases in the production of hydrogen and methane and altered transit times exist in patients with IBS. Premenstrual lower abdominal bloating is a common complaint, and ought not to be labelled as IBS. The condition of post-infectious IBS is important to recognize as it can be profound and long-lasting.

The treatment of IBS-related bloating is usually dietary, and involves the avoidance of fruit and vegetables such as apples, broccoli, cabbage, sprouts, pulses and onion as well as reducing the amount of fermentable fibre (wholemeal bread, bran, oats) consumed. Many patients are helped by avoiding gluten (wheat, barley, rye). The use of laxatives may improve bloating in those also troubled by constipation. Cognitive–behavioural therapy has been tried with good success. Pro-biotic medications, used to alter the gut flora, or the use of non-absorbable antibiotics (e.g. rifaximin) are championed, but there is no conclusive proof of efficacy and any changes to the gut flora are short-term. The use of smooth muscle relaxants and anti-depressants (e.g. low-dose paroxetine) has met with variable success. It is possible that serotonin receptor antagonists/agonists or opiate receptor agonists may be of value.

Many pathological states can give rise to bloating, but they are relatively uncommon, particularly in comparison with IBS. They include: infections (giardiasis, *Cryptosporidium parvum*, *Blastocystis hominis*, helminths), coeliac disease, disaccharidase deficiency, pancreatic insufficiency, bacterial overgrowth (blind-loop syndrome, strictures), cirrhosis, diverticular disease and, very rarely, tumours such as hepatocellular or colonic carcinoma. Medications such as lactulose, bisphosphonates and statins may be implicated in the onset of abdominal bloating.

In the acute setting, the onset of a distended abdomen may be due to toxic megacolon (colitis), volvulus (particularly of the sigmoid colon in the elderly) and pseudo-obstruction (postoperative, hypokalaemia, sepsis, abdominal cancer). Treatment of the underlying cause, for example endoscopic/radiological reduction of a volvulus or correction of an electrolyte imbalance, is of paramount importance. Other measures such as regularly altering posture (decubitus knee-chin position, upright posture, etc.) or the use of intravenous neostigmine may help in toxic megacolon and pseudo-obstruction, respectively.

John Meenan

FLUSHING

Flushing is a slowly spreading erythema of the skin due to a temporary dilatation of the capillaries, and is conventionally differentiated from emotional blushing only by severity, duration and extent. The skin of the face, neck and upper anterior chest may be involved. Depending on the underlying condition, flushing may be accompanied by light-headedness, a sense of suffocation, tremors, tinnitus and sometimes nausea and vomiting.

Menopausal flushing ('hot flushes') is extremely common in women at and just after the menopause, but it may occur earlier following bilateral oophorectomy. The flushes, which can last 15 minutes, may be accompanied by sweating and develop spontaneously, sometimes even during sleep. The mechanism is still unknown, though presumably it is neurohormonal. Interestingly, one-third of men aged 55–75 years report hot flushes; these men often have other symptoms suggestive of low testosterone concentration such as decreased muscle strength, lack of energy, and low mood. Men receiving hormonal treatment for prostate cancer may suffer from hot flushes.

Alcohol-induced flushing can be related to the quantity or variety of drink consumed. Large amounts of histamine are found in sherry and some red wines, though none in distilled spirits. Histamine causes flushing, and certain drugs and foods may release enough from mast cells to cause a blush. *Drugs* that cause flushing (particularly in combination with alcohol) are chlorpropamide, disulfiram, metronidazole, and percutaneous absorption of the anti-scabetic Tetmosol (monosulfiram).

Paroxysmal flushing is the commonest clinical feature of the *carcinoid* syndrome, and may be associated with migrating wheals. The carcinoid syndrome is due to hepatic involvement by an argentaffin cell tumour, with the production of 5-hydroxytryptamine (5-HT). Other symptoms are diarrhoea, abdominal pain, and right-sided heart failure. In *systemic mastocytosis* severe flushing attacks, often accompanied by headache, may occur spontaneously or after trauma to skin lesions. Episodes of flushing and diarrhoea may accompany the *Zollinger–Ellison syndrome,* and fainting with flushing can occur with an adrenaline-secreting *phaeochromocytoma*. It may also occur in insulin-dependent *diabetics* with both hypo- and hyperglycaemia. It may be part of an *epileptic* aura.

Post-prandial flushing of the face, especially of the nose and adjacent skin, is a characteristic of *rosacea*. In this disease, reddening later becomes permanent with telangiectasia, as well as papules and pustules (see Fig. E.7). A flushed facial appearance is seen in patients with Cushing's syndrome, polycythemia rubra vera and ACTH-secreting bronchogenic tumour.

Danielle Harari

FOOT, DEFORMITIES OF

See LOWER LIMB, PAIN IN (p. 419).

FOOT, PAIN IN

See LOWER LIMB, PAIN IN (p. 416).

FOOT, ULCERATION OF

Perforating ulcers of the foot usually occur under the ball of the great toe, but may affect any pressure area.

Ulcers can form under hard *calluses*. Anaesthesia appears to be an important precipitating factor, and such lesions are seen in patients with *sensory neuropathy* of any cause (e.g. *diabetes, leprosy, alcoholism, poliomyelitis*). Pressure ulcers are also seen in paraplegics. Aggravating factors include foot deformities and ill-fitting footwear that give rise to pressure areas.

Chronic ulceration of the sole can be the presentation of *ischaemia* (Fig. F.27), and occurs in those with

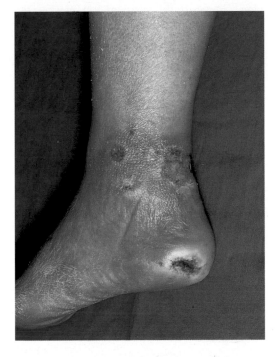

Figure F.27 Ischaemic foot ulcer in severe arteriosclerosis.

arteriosclerosis, in *heavy smokers* and in patients with *familial hyperlipidaemia*. Vasospasm of the digital arteries occurs in *Raynaud's phenomenon*, which can lead to digital ulceration of both the hands and feet. Raynaud's is characterized by a triphasic reaction of pallor, cyanosis and hyperaemia in response to cold or emotional stress. Cholesterol emboli to the small digital arterioles can present as digital ulceration on the feet, and should be suspected if the patient has recently had angiographical studies/intervention performed. Ulceration of the feet can be the presenting feature of *cryoproteinaemia*, *haemoglobinopathies* and *hereditary spherocytosis*. Intravascular thrombosis possibly plays a role in the development of the ulceration, and the lesions are more common in patients with severe anaemia. In addition, other autoimmune conditions such as systemic lupus erythematosus (SLE), the antiphospholipid syndrome, scleroderma and other connective tissue disorders should be considered when patients present with ulceration of the lower extremities. Deep skin infections can cause foot ulceration, including fungal (*blastomycosis*, *sporotrichosis* and *maduromycosis*) and bacterial (streptococci, both aerobic and anaerobic; the latter when colonizing an ulcerating expansion of a wound, either traumatic or surgical, is known as Meleney's ulcer). Mycobacterial infections can present with ulceration of the extremities including the feet (e.g. *M. marinum* found in water and *M. ulcerans*, responsible for the Buruli/Bairnsdale ulcer, found on grass

and introduced into the skin via grass cuts). Rare causes include *syphilitic gumma* and neoplasms, for example *carcinoma cunniculatum*, *squamous cell carcinoma*, malignant melanoma and Kaposi's sarcoma.

Causes of foot ulceration are listed in Table F.13.

Sharon O'Byrne

FRIGIDITY (ANORGASMIA)

Frigidity, or *anorgasmia* (a less pejorative term), like impotence (see p. 311), is due to a wide variety of causes, by far the most important of which are psychogenic. However, severe physical malformations of the genital tract whether congenital or acquired can, of course, interfere with sexual intercourse or lead to a failure to achieve orgasm. The same may also be an outcome of *dyspareunia*, which is due also to some physical lesion.

A proportion of women appear to be *constitutionally anorgasmic*. This implies that there seems to be no good physical or psychological reason for their inability to achieve orgasm, however hard or long they try. This may, however, be more apparent than real and, in the case of many women, be related to lack of knowledge of what is to be expected from sexual intercourse. However, with increasing sophistication, in part the outcome of better sex education, the level of expectation among women appears to be rising, which in turn may have led to a fall in the number of those who might once have been regarded as constitutionally anorgasmic. None the less, there remains an unknown number of women who, while they insist (on superficial questioning) that their sex lives are satisfactory, may – when pressed – reveal that they have never actually obtained full sexual satisfaction. Such women have often been brought up to believe that sexual intercourse is something to be endured rather than enjoyed.

Before considering what may be pathological, two other relevant factors need consideration. The first factor is that the achievement of sexual satisfaction by women appears to be more closely bound up with an affectionate or loving relationship than is the case with men, to whom mere physical attraction may be sufficient. The second factor is that women are slower to arouse sexually than are men. This

Table F.13 Causes of foot ulceration

Ischaemic	Atheroma, diabetes mellitus, Raynaud's phenomenon, cholesterol emboli
Neuropathic	Diabetes mellitus, leprosy, alcoholism, poliomyelitis
Vasculitides/ Intravascular thrombosis	Systemic lupus erythematosus (SLE), antiphospholipid syndrome, scleroderma, cryoproteinaemia, haemoglobinopathies (e.g. sickle cell disease), hereditary spherocytosis
Infections	Fungal: blastomycosis, sporotrichosis, maduromycosis Bacterial: streptococcal Mycobacterial: *M. marinum, M. ulcerans* Syphilis
Malignancies	Carcinoma cunniculatum, squamous cell carcinoma, malignant melanoma, Kaposi's sarcoma

means that if the male partner lacks technique, hurries the proceedings unduly, or, being partially impotent, suffers from premature ejaculation, with loss of tumescence, the woman concerned may not have sufficient time in which to achieve orgasm. If she is herself inexperienced and does not understand the reason for this, she may come to regard herself as frigid.

This type of difficulty may be regarded as *pseudofrigidity*, a state in which a potential ability to achieve orgasm is present but, owing to unpropitious circumstances, may not be realized. Other circumstances which may likewise lead to failure of orgasm may be *fear of pregnancy* – some women deliberately suppress orgasm in the belief that this may prevent pregnancy occurring; examples include sleeping in the same house as the parents or in-laws, or sharing a bedroom with children. *Alcoholism* in the marital partner may also be a source of difficulty, the inconsideration of a partly intoxicated spouse tending in due course to bring about an intense revulsion for sexual intercourse.

Like impotence, anorgasmia may arise out of *inexperience* or be due to *simple anxiety*. It may also be an outcome of *emotional immaturity,* a state often reflected by the inability of a young bride to live a separate existence independent of her parents. *Sexual interference* in childhood or adolescence by a male relative or some other person may also later impair a normal capacity for satisfactory intercourse.

The other main sexual problem leading to anorgasmia is *vaginismus.* This is an intense spasm of the muscles surrounding the introitus, leading to it remaining tightly shut and thereby interfering with penetration by the male penis. Once such spasm occurs, further attempts at penetration are painful enough to reinforce reflex closure of the introitus, creating thereby a vicious cycle. Vaginismus may be severe enough to lead to non-consummation of marriage, although in milder cases initial introital pain and spasm which may be largely the outcome of inexperience and apprehension may lessen as intercourse proceeds. Many instances of *dyspareunia* are in fact cases of vaginismus. However, in all cases of female sexual dysfunction gynaecological causes must be excluded. It may be necessary to carry out an examination under anaesthesia to exclude this.

In the case of *female homosexuals (lesbians)*, frigidity in a heterosexual relationship is common, though not apparently invariable. Some basically homosexual women marry and make a success of it sometimes by arranging a *menage à trois*. Many professional *prostitutes* are said to be frigid, and many are probably homosexual also. The same, paradoxically, applies to *nymphomania* in which state, although there is an apparently intense desire for sexual relationships – sometimes with any available male partner – satisfaction is never achieved. It has also been suggested that nymphomania represents an attempt by the female to denigrate male sexuality.

Certain matters pertaining to childbirth may be important. In some women an *abortion* may occasionally give rise to frigidity, though the vast majority remain unaffected by this event. Fear of pregnancy has already been mentioned, but, even in the absence of this and where satisfactory contraceptive methods are employed, some women tend to become anorgasmic after the birth of a second or third child when no more children are desired. This may be a reflection of the more intimate relationship between childbearing and sex which exists in women as opposed to their partners. Likewise – and sometimes surprisingly – a loss of libido quite often appears to follow sterilization, for whatever reason. Loss of sexual desire is not necessarily a sequel to the menopause; indeed, a capacity to enjoy sexual relationships may persist in some women to a relatively advanced age, although there is naturally a wide variation.

As in the case of the male, loss of libido may occur in women due to a *depressive illness*. Following treatment and satisfactory resolution of the illness sexual function may be restored once again to normal.

Mark Kinirons

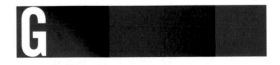

GAIT, ABNORMALITIES OF

Gait may be disturbed by:

1 Mechanical defects in the lower limbs and pelvis.

2 Pain in the legs, pelvis and lower lumbar spine.

3 Disease of muscles.

4 Disease of the nervous system:
- increased tone, either basal ganglial or pyramidal;
- weakness, either pyramidal or peripheral;
- ataxia, either sensory or cerebellar; and
- cortical.

5 Disease of the vestibular apparatus.

6 Hysteria.

Mechanical defects

Inequality in the length of the legs, congenital dislocation of the hips, ankylosis of the knee or hip joints and deformities of the feet give rise to a characteristic bold, painless limp, the source of which is readily found on examination of the limbs.

Coxa vary and coxa vatga may lead to characteristic gaits. Painless ankylosis of both hips leads to all movements being made at knees, ankles and feet, giving a short-stepping smooth gait, almost as if the patient were on roller-skates. This is seen, for instance, in some cases of ankylosing spondylitis.

Painful limp, due to pain in the pelvis or lower limb, is easily recognized by the manner in which the patient puts the weight on the sound leg and hurries off the affected one. The source of the pain may be in the limb itself, or it may be referred from disease in the pelvis, lumbar spine or cauda equina. Localized pain usually means localized disease at that site, referred pain tending to have a more diffuse and linear distribution, but many exceptions occur. The pain referred from a diseased hip may be felt only in the knee – this is an important feature in children with tuberculosis of the hip – and occasionally a root pain is limited to a small area in the foot (S1) or the lateral border of the leg (L5). Local tenderness at the site of the pain often indicates local disease, but it may equally well be present in referred pain. On the other hand, local deformity or swelling always means disease at that point. The more important causes of a painful limp are detailed in Table G.1.

Diseases of muscles

Diseases of muscles, although rare, can cause characteristic disturbances of gait. In the heredofamilial *myopathies*, usually seen in early life, the gait is

Table G.1 Causes of painful limp

The joints
Injuries
Arthritis or arthrosis of lumbar spine, or of hip, knee, ankle and/or foot on one or both sides

The bones
Injuries
Neoplastic, congenital or metabolic disease
Inflammatory infective or degenerative disease

The lumbosacral roots
Prolapse of intervertebral disc
Lesions of cauda equina
Lesions of lumbar vertebrae
Pelvic masses

Other tissues
Foreign body in foot (children)
Bursitis (gluteal, patellar and tendo Achilles)
Corns and bunions
Flat feet
Chilblains

waddling, the muscles weak and either hypertrophied or atrophied, and sensation is normal. In muscular dystrophy (MD) the muscles weaken, leading to an abnormal gait. The severity depends on the type of MD, with Duchennes being the worst and leading to death prematurely in early adult life. In *myotonia congenita*, members of affected families experience from birth a peculiar difficulty in relaxing muscles after voluntary contraction. Thus, on attempting to walk the muscles go into a tonic spasm, but this can be worked off by continued exercise. Diagnosis is made on the family history, the presence of prolonged contraction after voluntary effort, the production of a persistent localized contraction on percussion of the affected muscles, and high-frequency discharges in the electromyogram, likened on the loudspeaker to the noise of a dive-bomber. A similar myotonia is seen in *dystrophia myotonica*, a familial disease usually of adult life but occurring also in children; the gait is disturbed by myotonia, but weakness and atrophy of the quadriceps and of the dorsiflexors of the feet are a further embarrassment to walking. The presence of wasting and myotonia in the face, sternomastoids and forearm, and the frequent presence of premature baldness, cataracts and testicular atrophy, indicate the correct diagnosis.

In *myasthenia gravis*, the legs – in common with the rest of the musculature – may fatigue rapidly: the gait is normal after rest, but as fatigue supervenes it becomes shuffling, unsteady and weak. The weakness and extreme hypotonia of the muscles in *amyotonia congenita* interfere with gait in those children who survive the first critical years of infancy. They learn to walk later, and they then present the unsteadiness of weakness, but even this incapacity may be outgrown.

Disease of the nervous system

Increased tone

Spasticity due to bilateral pyramidal disease will affect both legs, as in congenital spastic diplegia, spinal cord compression, multiple sclerosis, subacute combined degeneration of the cord in the early stages, intramedullary tumours and syringomyelia. Tone is increased in the extensors and adductors, so that the limb is held in extension, with plantar flexion of the foot, and some degree of adduction. The gait is stiff, the toes scrape the ground, and if the adduction and spasticity are severe, there is a 'scissors gait'. Weakness increases the disability. A unilateral pyramidal lesion gives rise to a similar stiff, extended limb, which is dragged around its normal fellow by tilting the pelvis, thus overcoming the adduction and allowing the flexed foot to clear the ground.

The rigidity of *extrapyramidal disease* affects extensors and flexors equally, but the legs are held slightly flexed at the hip and knee because the flexors are more powerful than the extensors. The steps are short and shuffling. The patient tends to walk faster and faster, as if chasing their centre of gravity. If pushed backwards, they tend to run backwards with short, hasty steps. Fixity of expression, flexion of the neck and trunk, adduction of the arm with flexion of the elbows and the characteristic rhythmic tremor of the forearms, hands and fingers afford diagnostic assistance when the extrapyramidal lesions are due to Parkinson's disease, one of the earliest signs being a failure to swing the arm on walking. A similar gait results from extrapyramidal lesions due to parkinsonism. Parkinsonism is seen with drug-induced, arteriopathic cerebral degeneration, carbon monoxide poisoning, hepatolenticular degeneration, encephalitis lethargica and (rarely) after severe head injuries (e.g. boxing).

Weakness

Weakness plays a part in pyramidal lesions, but it is often difficult to distinguish the relative importance of this weakness and the associated spasticity in the disturbances of gait which are described above. On the other hand, weakness due to disease of the anterior horn cells or of the peripheral nerves to the legs gives rise to abnormal gaits, the features of which depend on the distribution of the weak or paralysed muscles. Where there is foot-drop, as in any form of polyneuritis, injuries to the common peroneal nerve, poliomyelitis or a lesion of the cauda equina, there is a high-stepping gait, in which the foot is lifted high and then slapped down onto the ground. If the calf muscles are paralysed, as in a lesion of the posterior tibial nerve, the gait loses its natural spring. Furthermore, disease affecting the motor fibres often also attacks the sensory fibres; proprioceptive sensory loss then adds a sensory ataxic element to the gait, which becomes clumsy, unsteady, irregular and broad-based as in tabes, many types of polyneuritis and gross disease of the cauda equina. When sensory ataxia thus complicates muscular weakness, balance is worse in the dark or when the eyes are shut.

Ataxia

Sensory ataxia has been mentioned as a factor in the clumsy, incoordinated, noisy, wide-based gait of polyneuritis, tabes, lesions of the cauda equina and some cases of subacute combined degeneration of the cord. A second form of ataxic gait is seen as a result of disease or injury of the cerebellum or its connections. The gait is wide-based and clumsy, but it is little aggravated by darkness or by closing the eyes. There is a tendency to deviate towards the side of the lesion, but over-compensation may occur, with consequent deviation to both sides in an irregular, staggering and drunken manner. The normal 'swing' of the arm on the affected side may be diminished or lost, but this feature is often absent. 'Cerebellar ataxia' is seen in multiple sclerosis, the heredofamilial ataxias, occasional cases of tabes without proprioceptive sensory loss, and in inflammatory, neoplastic, degenerative, traumatic and vascular lesions of the cerebellum.

Cortical disease

Cortical disease that affects the cortex can frequently cause abnormal gait. 'Marche à petite pas' is used to describe a gait pattern due to multiple cortical infarcts. A form of disconnection seems to impair higher cortical connections. Advanced dementia frequently impairs gait, but the diagnosis is obvious by then.

Vestibular disease

Disease of the labyrinth, the vestibular nerve or the vestibular nucleus in the pons can give rise to disturbances of gait. Vertigo makes the patient feel disorientated; the gait is unsteady, and there is a tendency to deviate to the affected side. This occurs in acute phases of Menière's disease, acute labyrinthitis and vascular lesions of the pons.

Hysteria

Hysteria is sometimes responsible for abnormal gaits. There is no set pattern, but, however bizarre hysterical gaits may be, they have in common a certain improbability and flamboyance; a tendency to subside gracefully and safely on the floor, and to stagger in the direction of objects upon which to lean. 'Astasia abasia' is a term which was formerly used for an inability to stand or walk despite normal movements of the limbs when recumbent. However, it is desirable to recall that in hereditary spinocerebellar ataxia, and in affections of the flocculonodular lobe and the vermis of the cerebellum, a gross ataxia of gait may be found despite good performance in all tests of coordination when in bed. This is due to the fact that these functions, of balance and coordination, are subserved by different regions of the cerebellum which can be involved separately in disease processes, coordination depending on the integrity of the lateral lobes of the cerebellum and balance on the midline structures. Hysterical gaits are recognized by their inconsistencies, and by a quality which can best be described as insincerity; confirmation is to be found in the presence of psychoneurosis and the absence of organic disease. Unlike organic disorders of gait, they can sometimes be cured by suggestion.

Mark Kinirons

GALL BLADDER, PALPABLE

Physical signs

On occasion, a grossly distended gall bladder in a thin subject may be visible as a distinct globular swelling in the right upper abdomen. However, palpation is the physical method of examination in detecting enlargement of the gall bladder. One may feel an oval, smooth swelling moving downward close behind the anterior abdominal wall when the patient inspires, descending either from beneath the right costal margin near the tip of the 9th rib, or attached to the undersurface of a palpable liver in the right nipple line. As it enlarges, the tumour generally extends inwards as well as downwards so that it may ultimately cross the midline below the level of the umbilicus. It may be large enough to be palpable bimanually in a thin patient, but it does not fill out the loin in a way that a renal tumour may do. It may or may not be tender, depending on whether the cause of the enlargement is or is not associated with inflammation. It feels firm and tense rather than hard. An impaired but not quite dull note is obtained on percussion.

Diagnosis from other swellings

Palpable gall bladder must be distinguished particularly from four groups of conditions:

- From carcinoma arising in the bile ducts or gall bladder itself.
- From tumours in or attached to the liver in the neighbourhood of the gall bladder – secondary new growth, primary hepatoma or more rarely gumma, abscess or hydatid cyst.
- From mobile kidney, hydronephrosis or renal tumour.
- From tumours in the neighbouring organs, such as carcinoma of the pyloric antrum or the right suprarenal.

Clinical features, as described below, will often enable an accurate diagnosis to be made. These may be supplemented by appropriate radiological studies and by ultrasound or percutaneous transhepatic cholangiography (PTC) (Fig. G.1) and, if necessary, with fine-needle aspiration.

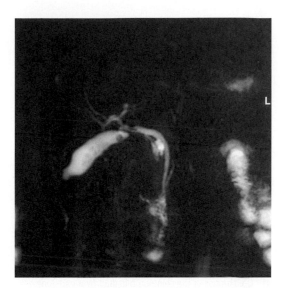

Figure G.1 Percutaneous transhepatic cholangiography (PTC). The bile ducts are dilated, and the filling defect caused by a stone can be seen at the lower end of the common bile duct.

Carcinoma of the gall bladder

It is often difficult to decide whether a tumour is merely an enlarged gall bladder or a growth infiltrating and replacing it, since in either case there may be a history extending over years of gallstones, with biliary colic, pyrexia and even jaundice, and primary new growth of the gall bladder is usually associated with gallstones. The rapidity of the enlargement in the absence of any definite cause will suggest growth, particularly in a person of the cancer age. Careful palpation may show that the mass is not smooth, as in the case of most simple gallbladder enlargements, but more or less nodulated or covered with bosses or irregularities, which in themselves suggest new growth. In some cases there may be secondary deposits in the liver, ascites, and sometimes the enlargement of the left supraclavicular lymph nodes points to malignant disease with metastasis. Notwithstanding these points, the differential diagnosis may be so difficult that further special investigations will be necessary for decision.

Tumours attached to or in the liver

Those most likely to be mistaken for enlargement of the gall bladder are Riedel's lobe, secondary carcinoma of the liver and, much more rarely, hepatoma, gumma,

abscess or hydatid cyst. It may, by physical examination, be impossible to distinguish a Riedel's lobe from an enlarged gall bladder or from a mobile kidney. Speaking generally, a Riedel's lobe usually descends from the liver farther to the right than does a gall bladder, and it is more apt to simulate an enlarged or a mobile kidney.

Metastatic deposits in the liver nearly always cause considerable (and sometimes enormous) enlargement and great hardness of the organ, not infrequently associated with jaundice. The diagnosis depends, first upon the discovery of a primary growth, which in the case of carcinoma is likely to be in the large bowel, stomach, pancreas or breast, or, in the case of melanoma, the eye; and second, on the discovery in the liver of several separate nodules, some of which may be felt to be umbilicated, that is to say depressed in their central part and raised around the edges.

Hepatoma, although rare in the UK, occasionally occurs in cirrhotics and may be multifocal. In the Far East and in eastern Africa it is far more common and, in patients from those areas, is an important condition to consider in differential diagnosis.

Gumma of the liver is rarely encountered nowadays, and when it occurs is usually mistaken for new growth, unless there is a convincing history of syphilis or the effects of tertiary lesions are visible elsewhere – especially gummatous lesions of the skin or leucoplakia of the tongue. The diagnosis may be confirmed by obtaining a positive serological reaction, or by the beneficial effects of anti-syphilitic treatment, though this does not always lead to rapid disappearance of a gumma of the liver. Even when the liver is inspected at laparotomy, the diagnosis between gumma and new growth is not always easy.

Abscess of the liver, if it is to simulate an enlargement of the gall bladder, is likely to be a single large abscess which, if it has not arisen in some pre-existent mass (such as gumma, new growth or hydatid cyst), is almost certain to have been acquired in a tropical country where the patient has suffered from amoebic dysentery. The diagnosis may not be evident until the mass is punctured with an exploring needle, yielding the typical 'anchovy sauce' pus.

Hydatid cyst of the liver is seldom situated in such a position as to cause difficulty of diagnosis for gallbladder enlargement. More usually, the cyst is embedded in the liver substance, or projects from its upper surface. The diagnosis might be entertained if the patient were known to have hydatid cysts elsewhere, or came from an area where this disease is endemic. However, in most cases it is suggested by ultrasonography or CT of the liver and sometimes determined only when laparotomy has been performed. It might have been suggested by the discovery of eosinophilia, and also by the specific hydatid serum reaction if the hydatid cyst is alive and active. But latent or calcified hydatid cysts cause no symptoms, do not produce an eosinophilia, and are not associated with a positive hydatid blood–serum reaction. Their walls, if calcified, can be seen on radiographs of the region.

Distinction between an enlarged gall bladder and a mobile kidney or hydronephrosis

There may be no jaundice to suggest gallbladder trouble, nor need there be any urinary changes to suggest kidney, so that the diagnosis may have to be made chiefly by palpation. Facts to stress are that a gall bladder is more easily felt anteriorly than posteriorly, whilst the reverse is the case with the kidney; that the kidney is, as a rule, the more freely movable of the two; that it is seldom possible to demarcate the upper pole of an enlarged gall bladder in the way that the top of a movable kidney can sometimes be defined; that with kidney tumour the loin is dull, whilst with gallbladder enlargement it is resonant; and that, on rather firm bimanual palpation, the patient may experience a peculiar sickening sensation which is characteristic of kidney. In cases of doubt, ultrasound or an intravenous pyelogram will demonstrate whether or not the right kidney is normal (see also KIDNEY, PALPABLE, p. 360).

Tumours of other organs simulating enlargement of the gall bladder

These may be distinguished to some extent by the fact that new growths of the pylorus, transverse colon or suprarenal that are big enough to stimulate an enlargement of the gall bladder seldom have the smooth oval outline that the gall bladder nearly always possesses. In addition, there may have been symptoms attributable to the primary growth, such as dilatation of the stomach, coffee-grounds vomit, or evidence of secondary deposits in the liver, in the left supraclavicular lymph nodes, or elsewhere, to indicate the diagnosis.

Modern imaging techniques (ultrasound and computed axial tomography) can usually provide anatomical delineation of an enlarged gall bladder and differentiate the other masses enumerated above. Nevertheless, in some of these cases it is impossible to exclude enlargement of the gall bladder without resorting to laparotomy.

Causes of gallbladder enlargement

These include the following:

- Empyema of the gall bladder
- Chronic pancreatitis
- Carcinoma of the head of the pancreas
- Cholecystitis as a result of:
  - gallstones
  - new growth
- Typhoid fever
- Obstruction of the common bile duct by a gallstone
- Obstruction of the cystic duct by a gallstone
- Simple mucocele

It is noteworthy that gallstones comparatively seldom lead to enlargement of the gall bladder. If the associated inflammation does not progress to empyema, the gallbladder usually becomes thick-walled, contracted and embedded in dense adhesions which prevent it from dilating, even when the cystic or common bile ducts become obstructed by a stone. Indeed, in a middle-aged patient in whom there has not been any very definite attack of biliary colic, the occurrence of progressive and considerable enlargement of the gall bladder, associated with deepening jaundice and without ascites, arouses serious suspicion of a lesion of the head of the pancreas which has extended along the pancreatic duct so as gradually to occlude the common bile duct. The most common cause of these symptoms is either chronic pancreatitis or carcinoma of the head of the pancreas or of the ampulla of Vater. In obstruction of the common bile duct due to gallstones, the gall bladder is as a rule not palpable; in obstruction due to carcinoma of the head of the pancreas, it is usually distended and is palpable in about 50 per cent of patients (Courvoisier's law, which states 'In the presence of jaundice, a palpably enlarged gall bladder is unlikely to be due to stone'.) (Fig. G.2). Painless progressive jaundice suggests a carcinoma arising at the ampulla of Vater and, if this ulcerates, the stools may be positive for occult blood. Jaundice preceded by epigastric or upper lumbar pain is more likely to be due to carcinoma or chronic pancreatitis of the body of the pancreas. Sometimes, rupturing spontaneously and causing general peritonitis. In less severe cases, the inflammatory products discharge themselves naturally by the bile passages.

Simple mucocele of the gall bladder is a relatively unusual event which results from the impaction of a gallstone at the outlet of the gall bladder when it happens to be empty. The walls of this organ continue to secrete mucus so that it becomes greatly distended with perfectly colourless mucoid liquid, free from bile pigment. The fluid is sterile. There are usually no symptoms. Such a mucocele may be mistaken for a mobile kidney. Usually, the differential diagnosis can be established by radiological examination (cholecystography or intravenous urography) or by ultrasound or computed tomography. However, the diagnosis of the nature of the mass is sometimes obscure until revealed by operation.

Harold Ellis

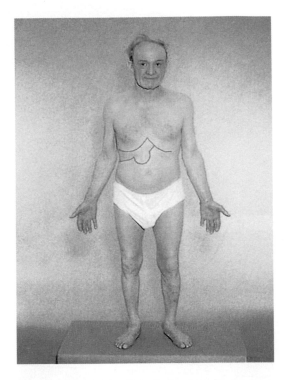

Figure G.2 Courvoisier's law. Obstructive jaundice due to a carcinoma of the head of the pancreas. The liver is smoothly enlarged due to biliary obstruction. The gall bladder forms a globular, palpable mass at its lower border.

sloughing of part of the tumour allows the pent-up bile to escape into the duodenum, with puzzling temporary remission or even disappearance of the jaundice.

In cases where gallstones are the cause of the enlargement there is nearly always tenderness over the gallbladder and pain when it is palpated firmly, associated with a rise in temperature, possibly with rigors, especially if the inflammation has spread to the bile ducts (infective or suppurative cholangitis). Leucocytosis, with a relative increase in the polymorphonuclear cells, would indicate that in addition to gallstones there is empyema of the gall bladder demanding urgent surgical treatment.

Another cause of empyema of the gall bladder, albeit rare, is typhoid fever. The diagnosis is not difficult as a rule, for in most of the cases there will be no question of new growth or of gallstones and the patient will have been suffering from a prolonged asthenic fever that has already been diagnosed serologically. In some typhoid patients bacillary infection of the gall bladder causes it to enlarge rapidly, even to the extent of

GANGRENE, PERIPHERAL

Gangrene results from death of a part of the body or an organ as a result of it being deprived of its blood supply (Fig. G.3), and with superadded bacterial infection of the resultant dead tissues. Ischaemia without infection results in a sterile infarction.

In this section, we consider gangrene of the limbs, which is seen much more frequently in the toes and foot than in the fingers and hand, although the same pathological conditions apply, in general, to both. The list of possible aetiologies is extensive, but in the great majority of patients encountered in the Western World with this condition the cause is arteriosclerotic disease, which may or may not be complicated by diabetes mellitus.

Causes of peripheral gangrene

These are listed in Table G.2.

Trauma

The diagnosis of traumatic gangrene can rarely give rise to any difficulty, in that the clinical features of history and examination will betray the cause. Inadvertent intra-arterial injection of a barbiturate or other irritant drug is a rare anaesthetic accident, but is seen more

Table G.2 Causes of peripheral gangrene

Trauma
- Injury to major limb arteries
  - ◆ Pressure from splints, tight plaster, tourniquet
  - ◆ Intra-arterial injection of barbiturate, etc.
  - ◆ Burns
  - ◆ Intense cold – frostbite

Infection
- Gas gangrene
  - ◆ Synergistic gangrene

Arterial disease
- Arteriosclerosis
- Thrombo-angiitis obliterans (Buerger's disease)
- Peripheral embolism
- Diabetes mellitus (diabetic micro-angiopathy)
- Raynaud's phenomenon
- Ergot poisoning

Venous disease
- Massive venous thrombosis

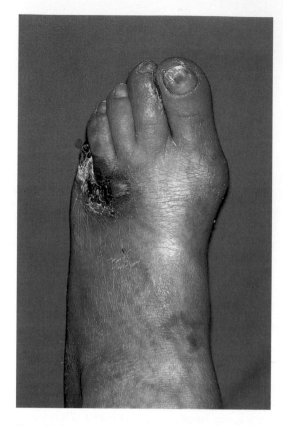

Figure G.3 Gangrene of foot due to peripheral vascular disease.

frequently in drug addicts; the additional factor in the latter cases is that the injected material is often also contaminated with bacteria.

Frostbite

Frostbite affects subjects exposed to intense cold without adequate protection, and results from ice crystals forming in the tissues, followed by capillary sludging and thrombosis in the small vessels.

The affected skin of the fingers or toes becomes first cold, white, immobile and anaesthetic. As the tissues rewarm, the affected skin becomes red and painful, blisters develop and minor trauma allows ingress of bacteria, with resultant gangrene of the dead tissues.

Infection

Gas gangrene

Gas gangrene results from *Clostridium perfringens* (*welchii*) and other *Clostridium* species. The organism is a Gram-positive, spore-forming bacillus which is an obligatory anaerobe and produces powerful exotoxins. The organisms are found in soil and faeces. Typically, gas gangrene is an infection of deep penetrating wounds where there is extensive devascularized muscle, which acts as a perfect culture medium for the organism. It is particularly seen in war wounds, but sometimes involvement of the abdominal wall or cavity may follow operations upon the alimentary tract.

Gas gangrene may complicate the amputation of an ischaemic limb.

The incubation period is about 24 hours. The patient becomes severely toxaemic, with rapid pulse, shock and vomiting. The temperature is first elevated and then becomes subnormal. The affected tissues are swollen, and crepitus is palpable due to liberated gas from protein destruction. The overlying skin becomes gangrenous and infection spreads along the muscle planes, producing first dark red, swollen muscle and then frank gangrene of the infected muscle from origin to insertion.

Synergistic gangrene

This condition, also known as progressive bacterial gangrene, is caused by the synergistic action of two or more organisms, commonly aerobic haemolytic *Staphylococcus* and micro-aerophilic non-haemolytic *Streptococcus*. When this occurs around the perineum, buttocks, or following abdominal surgery, coliform bacteria may also be present. It is more common in diabetics and immunosuppressed patients, and is often related to recent trauma or surgery (where it was previously termed progressive postoperative gangrene) or infection, for example, an ischio-anal abscess. Where it affects the scrotum it has been termed Fournier's gangrene.

Around the wound or infection, an area of cellulitis appears, which spreads rapidly. The area is exquisitely tender, the subcutaneous tissues slough with an offensive odour and most often the presence of gas (which can be mistaken for gas gangrene). The overlying skin becomes gangrenous, and the patient becomes profoundly septic.

There is a high mortality rate, and the condition can only be treated by a combination of high-dose, broad-spectrum antibiotics together with radical excision of the affected area (which may often have to be repeated on several occasions).

Arterial disease

Arteriosclerosis

This is by far the most common cause of peripheral gangrene of the toes and foot (but occasionally the fingers) in the Western World. The patient is more often male than female, usually over the age of 50, and invariably a long-standing and heavy cigarette smoker. There is a history of progressively deteriorating claudication leading to rest pain, with cramping calf pain experienced even at rest in bed. There is then some incident of minor trauma which may require direct questioning to elicit, such as nicking the toe while cutting the nail, or a minor blow to the foot, or pressure of a tight shoe, which enabled organisms to invade the ischaemic tissues through an often negligible wound. A gangrenous patch on the heel or over the lateral malleolus may result from pressure on these areas from a hard mattress.

Clinical examination of the leg, apart from the obvious area of gangrene, reveals that the peripheral skin is cold and pale or cyanosed. Elevation of the leg increases the pallor, while depression of the leg over the side of the bed usually produces a deep cyanosis (Buerger's test). The peripheral pulses are absent.

A general assessment of the patient is, of course, mandatory and often reveals features of general ischaemic disease, such as a history of angina or of previous coronary ischaemic episodes, a previous stroke or transient ischaemic attacks.

It is important to investigate the presence of co-existing diabetes mellitus. This will exacerbate the seriousness of the condition (see Diabetic gangrene, below).

The important radiological investigation is arteriography, which defines the extent of the disease and also enables the surgeon to decide if vascular reconstruction is possible by surgery or balloon angioplasty. Duplex sonography is now replacing arteriography in many centres. This technique takes longer to perform and is more subjective, but it is non-invasive and can provide better information as to the significance of stenoses.

Thrombo-angiitis obliterans (Buerger's disease)

This condition, which some regard as a variant of arteriosclerotic disease of the limbs ('juvenile arteriosclerosis'), but which the majority of experts consider a special entity, is almost confined to men in their twenties and thirties who are very heavy cigarette smokers. It was originally thought to occur only in Jews of eastern European extraction, but it is now known to be widely distributed and is seen, for example, quite commonly in Chinese, Arabs and men from the Indian sub-continent.

The distal arteries of the lower (and often the upper) limbs are affected, and show round cell infiltration and intimal proliferation with intraluminal thrombosis. Adjacent veins and nerves become involved in this inflammatory process, and there may be associated superficial venous thrombosis. The gangrenous process, which usually affects both feet (and often the fingers), is preceded by a history of claudication, eventually with rest pain, and sometimes by episodes of superficial or deep vein thrombosis in the legs. Unlike arteriosclerosis, the femoral (and often also the popliteal) pulses are usually present, although the dorsalis pedis and posterior tibial pulses are lost. Late cases of this condition are pitiful; progressive gangrene may have led to serial amputations of all four limbs.

Arteriography shows a fairly typical appearance of relatively normal arteries down to the proximal part of the brachial or popliteal, with distal vessel obliteration. Biopsy of an occluded artery or vein may provide histological confirmation of the disease.

Embolus

Gangrene due to embolism will be sudden in its inception, and rapid in its onset.

Potential sources of emboli include:

- Left atrium; atrial fibrillation with mitral stenosis, atrial myxoma.
- Heart valves; endocarditis affecting diseased valves.
- Left ventricular wall; mural thrombus after myocardial infarction or from ventricular aneurysm.
- Aorta; from aneurysm or arteriosclerosis.
- Interventricular septum; paradoxical embolus via a septal defect originating in the systemic veins (rare).

Among this list, the most common causes of arterial emboli are dislodgement of a mural clot from a myocardial infarct, often occurring around 10 days previously, and from clot in the left atrium in atrial fibrillation.

The history is usually one of sudden pain in the limb, which soon becomes white and cold. Sensation may disappear, and the muscles become rapidly paralysed. Over the next few hours the limb becomes anaesthetic, and skin staining appears which does not blanch on pressure. If untreated, peripheral gangrene will ensue. Pulses below the block, which usually takes place at a major vessel bifurcation, including that of the aorta, are absent.

Paradoxical emboli are uncommon. In patients with a patent foramen ovale or other septal defects, a clot originating in the deep veins of the leg or pelvis may not only impact in the pulmonary arterial tree but may also pass across the septal defect and lodge in the arterial system. This is particularly likely to occur after a pulmonary embolus, as the raised pulmonary artery pressure results in increased shunting across a septal defect if this is present.

A limb embolism must be differentiated from acute thrombosis occluding an arteriosclerotic artery, where there is more likely to be a history of preceding claudication. Both may require urgent surgery, but an embolus is treated by balloon embolectomy whereas acute thrombosis in arteriosclerosis may necessitate urgent endarterectomy or a bypass procedure. An arteriogram is necessary to differentiate between the two, the filling defect in an embolism showing a smooth rounded outline like a cigar butt, whereas that of acute thrombosis is irregular and merging indefinitely with the jagged outline of the locally diseased vessels.

Diabetic gangrene

Diabetes mellitus, if severe and poorly controlled, may result in infective gangrene of the foot (Fig. G.4). This

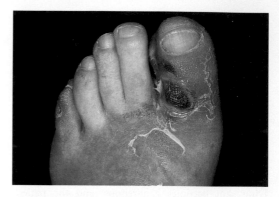

Figure G.4 Gangrene of foot due to diabetes mellitus.

results from a combination of diabetic micro-angiopathy, with subintimal arteriolar thickening producing vascular impairment, an increased susceptibility to tissue infection as a result of reduced host defences, and an associated peripheral neuropathy (often of 'glove and stocking' distribution) which renders the soft tissues more likely to trauma. Osteomyelitis of the bones of the foot is a common complication of this combination of infection and neuropathy. Since this is a disease of small vessels, the peripheral pulses are palpable. Those at the ankle may be difficult to detect because of oedema of the tissues, but their patency can be confirmed by means of a Doppler probe.

In young patients, this may well be the only pathology producing the gangrene. In older subjects, however, with co-existent arteriosclerotic disease, the presence of diabetes adds to these additional factors listed above to produce a much poorer prognosis than in patients with otherwise uncomplicated arteriosclerotic occlusive disease in the limb.

Raynaud's disease and Raynaud's phenomenon

Raynaud's disease is caused by spasm of the small arteries in the digits in the hands (and often the feet) of unknown aetiology, which was described by Maurice Raynaud, a physician in Paris, in 1862. It is almost confined to young females in their teens and twenties. As a result of exposure to cold, the fingers become white, and later slate-blue. As the hands warm, they change from livid purple to deep red, and this cycle can be precipitated by plunging the hands first into a basin full of cold and then into one of hot water. Many attacks do not pass through all these colour changes, with either pallor or cyanosis being the predominant feature.

Because the disease affects only the terminal vessels, the radial pulse is normal and, in those cases where the toes are affected, the ankle pulses are not lost. As might be expected, the disease is subject to exacerbations in the winter and remissions in the summer, but with gradual progression. With more advanced cases, chronic paronychia, with ulceration and gangrene of the fingertips may be seen, although this is much less common than in Raynaud's phenomenon (see below).

Raynaud's phenomenon – sometimes termed Raynaud's syndrome or secondary Raynaud's disease – is the term applied to a similar clinical picture affecting the fingers, but in which there is an underlining organic disease of the arteries of the upper limb (Fig. G.5). The list of such diseases is extensive and includes:

- Trauma
  - ◆ penetrating or closed arterial injury
  - ◆ frostbite
  - ◆ persistent use of vibrating tools
  - ◆ arterial thrombosis following inadvertent intra-arterial injection of barbiturate, etc.
- Arterial disease
  - ◆ arteriosclerosis
  - ◆ thromboangiitis obliterans (Buerger's disease)
  - ◆ cervical rib with embolism.
- Connective tissue disease
  - ◆ scleroderma (systemic sclerosis)
  - ◆ systemic lupus erythematosus
  - ◆ rheumatoid arthritis
- Drugs
  - ◆ beta-blockers
  - ◆ ergotism.

Among this list, patients with scleroderma are particularly likely to progress to digital gangrene (see also FINGERS, DEAD, COLD, p. 218).

Ergotism

Long ago, epidemics of painful digital gangrene were seen called 'Saint Anthony's Fire'. This is now known to be due to the ingestion over a long period of rye bread contaminated with *Claviceps purpura*, which produces ergot, which causes small arterial spasms and eventual intimal proliferation. Today, ergotism is seen occasionally in patients with severe migraine who take excessive amounts of ergotamine tartrate. The author has seen only one example of this, in an elderly lady.

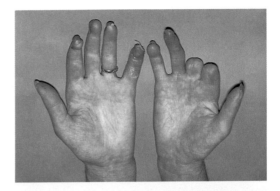

Figure G.5 Gangrene and loss of finger tips in scleroderma.

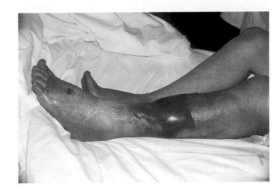

Figure G.6 Gangrene due to extensive venous thrombosis may involve an extensive area of the limb.

Venous gangrene

Gangrene is an unusual complication of thrombosis of the deep veins of the leg. This has to be extremely extensive, involving the femoral, iliac and pelvic veins. The legs are grossly swollen, oedematous and cyanosed. Gangrene may be limited to the toes, but may spread to the feet and even to involve an extensive area of the limb (Fig. G.6).

Harold Ellis

GRIP, DISTURBANCES OF

Man's privileged position in the animal kingdom is attributable to his prehensile upper limbs as well as to his superior brain. Our capacity to grip enables us to lift, carry, climb and handle tools. In terms of functional anatomy, grip depends primarily on the long flexor muscles of the fingers and the opposition of the thumb to the other digits. The latter movement is possible because the metacarpal bone of the thumb lies in a plane at right-angles to that of the other metacarpals, and because the carpo-metacarpal joint of the thumb has such a wide range of movement. Flexion thus carries the thumb medially across the palm in opposition to the other fingers.

Grip is impaired by any lesion affecting the motor supply of muscles of the forearm and hand. Thus, upper motor neurone lesions in corticospinal pathways, radicular lesions affecting C7, C8 and T1 roots, and peripheral nerve lesions, may all result in weakness of grip (see MONOPLEGIA, p. 442). As regards single peripheral nerve lesions, it is noteworthy that whilst median or ulnar nerve palsies can affect grip, the greatest disability results from an isolated radial nerve palsy. This is because without fixation of the wrist in extension, the grip becomes ineffectual.

Apart from purely motor lesions, grip can obviously be impaired also by severe incoordination, dystonia, involuntary movement or sensory deprivation. It may also be affected by disease of the joints or muscles although, in general, muscle disease tends to be of proximal rather than distal distribution. Myotonia dystrophia is characterized by normal grip but delayed relaxation of the grip.

Mark Kinirons

GROIN, SWELLING IN

Swellings in the groin are a common clinical problem, and examples are likely to be encountered in every general surgical outpatient clinic, as well as being found on routine examination of patients in other departments. The great majority can be diagnosed accurately by careful history and clinical examination.

Anatomy

The groin is not a well-defined anatomical zone, but may be divided into the inguinal and femoral regions by the inguinal ligament (not the groin skin crease) (Fig. G.7). The inguinal ligament runs from the easily defined anterior superior iliac spine to the pubic tubercle at the lateral extremity of the pubic crest. The pubic tubercle can be felt with relative ease in the

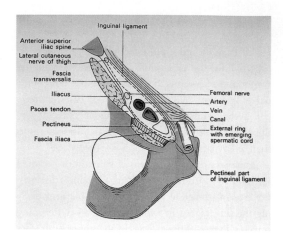

Figure G.7 Anatomy of the groin.

thin subject; in the more obese, it can be defined as the bony prominence which can be felt at the apex of the tendon of adductor longus with the hip in the flexed and abducted position. Swellings above the medial part of the inguinal ligament can be described as inguinal, those below as femoral.

Classification

As there are numerous potential causes of a swelling in the groin, a two-stage mental process is required in making a differential diagnosis: first, what anatomical structure is involved; and, second, what pathological entities may arise therefrom (Table G.3).

By far the most common are: inguinal hernia in male adults and children; inguinal and femoral hernia in adult females; inguinal lymphadenopathies; and saphena varix.

Skin and subcutaneous tissues

Sebaceous cysts occur in the groin, but are less common than on the scrotal skin.

Lipomas represent by far the most common swellings arising from the subcutaneous tissue, and may be found in the inguinal canal (lipoma of the cord), although these latter usually merely represent herniating extraperitoneal fat. Lipomas show the classical features of a soft, lobulated, mobile, fluctuant and transilluminable mass. The much rarer liposarcoma is rapidly growing, vascular and invasive.

Neurofibroma may occur unusually as a solitary swelling, and is suggested by accompanying *café au*

Table G.3 Classification of groin swellings according to tissues of origin

The skin and subcutaneous tissues
- Sebaceous cyst
- Lipoma
- Neurofibroma

Lymph nodes
- Lymphadenopathy due to infection, secondary neoplasm, lymphoma

Blood vessels
- Femoral artery – aneurysm
- Great saphenous vein – saphena varix

The hernial orifices
- Inguinal hernia – indirect and direct
- Femoral hernia

The testicular apparatus
- Ectopic testis
- Hydrocele of the spermatic cord
- Lipoma of the cord
- Hydrocele of the canal of Nück in the female

Psoas sheath
- Psoas abscess

Table G.4 Causes of groin lymphadenopathy

Inflammatory
- Acute – from septic focus in area drained by groin nodes
- Part of generalized inflammatory lymphadenopathy (viral) (e.g. glandular fever, AIDS)

Neoplastic
- Metastatic from squamous carcinoma or melanoma in area drained by groin nodes
- Lymphoma

lait pigmented areas of skin. More often, multiple lesions are found here and elsewhere as part of Von Recklinghausen's disease.

Lymph nodes (see also LYMPHADENOPATHY, p. 423)

Lymphadenopathy

The groin lymph nodes drain the lower limb, the external genitalia (scrotum and penis in the male, labia and vulva in the female), the lower anal canal, the buttock and the abdominal wall below the level of the umbilicus. All of these areas must be searched carefully for a primary focus of sepsis of neoplasm in a patient with groin lymphadenopathy.

Groin lymphadenopathy is usually multiple, but a large single node in the region of the femoral canal (Cloquet's node) may mimic an irreducible or strangulated femoral hernia. The common causes of groin lymphadenopathy are listed in Table G.4.

Inflammatory lymphadenopathy

There is usually a history of an inflammatory lesion involving the tissue drained by the lymph nodes. A search is made for a septic focus on the foot, toenails, between the toes, the leg, buttock, external genitalia,

lower abdomen and anal canal. This may appear trivial, and the lymphadenopathy may continue for up to 3–4 weeks following resolution of the initial cause. In the early phase the node may feel indurated and tender, after which it becomes firm and softens as it resolves. Reactive lymphadenopathy may be single or multiple, but the nodes usually feel discrete. Should resolution fail to occur over 3–4 weeks, then biopsy becomes important to identify specific infections or malignancy.

The inguinal lymph nodes enlarge bilaterally with a penile or vulval syphilitic chancre. They remain discrete and do not suppurate. This is in contrast to the groin lymphadenopathy in chancroid, where the enlarged groin nodes have a marked tendency to ulcerate (see PENILE SORES, p. 529).

A range of *viral infections* will cause generalized lymphadenopathy, but when sustained over weeks with ill-health and malaise, the Paul Bunnell antibody reaction may be requested where infectious mononucleosis is suspected. In modern practice toxoplasmosis and other causes of lymphadenopathy related to AIDS should be considered. In these cases the appearance and feel of the lymph nodes are similar to that with other reactive lymphadenopathies, but in AIDS lymphadenopathy is more common in the neck and axillae.

Metastatic carcinoma or melanoma

Firm, hard nodes that grow into a confluent fixed mass as the disease progresses are typical of metastatic carcinoma, which may be confirmed by either biopsy or needle aspiration cytology. If the primary has not been identified, then a careful search must be performed for primary lesions in the territory drained by the relevant lymphatics. This includes a rectal examination with proctoscopy and sigmoidoscopy, careful examination of the perineum and scrotum, and a thorough search of the legs, feet and between the toes. Occasionally, in melanoma the primary lesion may resolve despite rapidly progressive metastatic melanoma in the regional lymph nodes.

Lymphoma

The clinical features of both Hodgkin's and non-Hodgkin's lymphomas are similar, but in the latter condition the nodes may be hard and more closely resemble those of metastatic carcinoma. In Hodgkin's lymphoma the nodes often have a typical rubbery feel and may be matted together such that a clinical diagnosis can be quite confident. The diagnosis is confirmed by biopsy, which should include an intact node taken (if possible) from a region other than the groin. Once the diagnosis has been confirmed, the extent of the disease should be fully identified (staging) by further investigations which include chest X-ray and CT scanning of the chest and abdomen.

Vascular swellings

Vascular swellings in the groin should be easily recognized, and yet the saphena varix is often mistaken for a femoral hernia. Aneurysms of the common femoral artery are relatively rare and most frequently are seen following previous arterial surgery as a pseudoaneurysm (Fig. G.8). Occasionally, an inflamed pseudoaneurysm or mycotic aneurysm may present in a drug addict who has used the femoral artery for vascular access. The diagnostic importance of this is that it may be mistaken for an abscess, with catastrophic results when drainage is attempted.

Saphena varix

Anatomy

The saphena varix develops when there is incompetence of the sapheno-femoral junction and saphenous system. The proximal part of the saphenous system becomes dilated where reflux of turbulent blood impinges on the anterior wall of the vein. It lies in the upper femoral triangle just below the usual location for a femoral hernia, and just medial to the femoral pulse.

Clinical features

A saphena varix is only visible or palpable when the patient stands, as it disappears when they lay down. A cough impulse is pronounced and is usually associated with a fluid thrill, which clearly feels different from the impulse in a hernia. On compression, the swelling

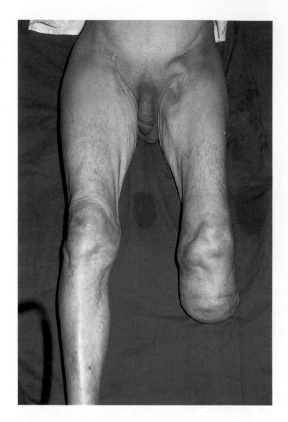

Figure G.8 Pseudoaneurysm of the left femoral artery following an aorto-bifemoral bypass using a Dacron graft. The earlier left below-knee amputation was performed for extensive gangrene of the foot.

collapses completely, but reappears immediately the finger is withdrawn. Almost invariably there are varicose veins in the distribution of the long saphenous vein from which a tap impulse may be transmitted into the saphena varix.

Femoral aneurysm

Aneurysms of the femoral artery are not common, but usually involve the common femoral just above its bifurcation. Atherosclerotic aneurysms rarely cause symptoms but occasionally thrombose spontaneously with resultant acute ischaemia or claudication. More worrying are pseudoaneurysms following bypass to the groin using prosthetic grafts such as Dacron, as these may expand rapidly and rupture. Needle puncture (often iatrogenic during arteriography) may result in pseudoaneurysm formation or, in drug addicts, mycotic aneurysm.

Anatomy

The common femoral artery lies immediately below the mid-point between the anterior superior iliac spine and the mid-point of the pubic symphysis. Aneurysms rarely extend into the profunda or superficial femoral artery, and the resultant bleeding tends to involve the groin tissues, spreading up and down in the line of the inguinal canal and promoting swelling and bruising of the scrotum or labia.

Clinical features

In the absence of inflammation the diagnosis is obvious, with easily palpated expansile pulsation. A thrill may be palpable, and auscultation often demonstrates a bruit, indicating turbulent blood flow within the aneurysmal sac. A rapidly expanding pseudoaneurysm or, more particularly mycotic aneurysm, may be mistaken for an abscess. Gentle palpation through the induration will always reveal substantial and abnormal pulsation. Occasionally, there may be the swelling of the distal limb due to compression of the vein or lymphatics.

The hernial orifices

Body wall

Groin hernias are the most frequent type of hernia, and may give rise to a number of acute complications. They are distinguished by simple clinical features readily identified on examination.

Inguinal hernia

The inguinal hernia is by far the most common variety of hernia. Approximately 3–5 per cent of the population have some variety of hernia, and 70–75 per cent of these are inguinal. Inguinal hernias are very much more common in men, and represent over 90 per cent of all hernias in men. In women, inguinal hernias are also nearly twice as common as femoral hernias, although there is a misconception that as femoral hernias commonly occur in women they are also more common than inguinal hernias.

Most groin hernias present as a soft lump in the groin that may be associated with local pain or discomfort on standing, lifting, or after heavy work. The clinical features of an inguinal hernia are of a lump arising just superior to the lower one-third of the inguinal ligament. Most hernias are reducible, in which case there

will be an impulse on coughing. In small hernias the sensation of reduction is perhaps the most reliable clinical sign confirming the presence of a hernia.

Anatomy

The inguinal canal is formed by the descent of the testis from the posterior abdominal wall during early development. During fetal development it passes obliquely through the anterior abdominal wall, extending from the internal inguinal ring at the mid-point of the inguinal ligament to the external inguinal ring just above the pubic tubercle. The anterior wall is formed by the external oblique aponeurosis and incorporates the lower-most fibres of the internal oblique at the internal ring. Inferiorly, there is the inguinal ligament and posteriorly the transversalis fascia, reinforced medially by the fibres of the conjoint tendon. The internal oblique and transversus muscles arch over the canal superiorly. Indirect inguinal herniae arise through the internal ring, passing into what is probably a congenital sac consisting of a persistent patent processus vaginalis. Direct inguinal herniae occur as a result of weakness in the posterior wall of the inguinal canal medial to the inferior epigastric artery, which passes in the medial border of the internal ring.

Clinical features

The vast majority of patients notice a lump in the groin, which may be asymptomatic or cause an aching or dragging sensation (Fig. G.9). Occasionally, the presenting symptoms are those of small-bowel obstruction when the bowel herniates and then becomes stuck in the sac, with oedema and obstruction at the hernia ring. A local, irreducible and acutely inflamed lump

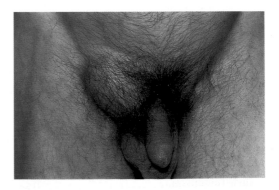

Figure G.9 Right inguinal hernia.

implies strangulation of the hernial contents, which may be extraperitoneal fat, omentum or intestine.

Inguinal herniae in infants and children

These are almost invariably indirect, with 90 per cent occurring in boys. The lump may be noticed by the mother while bathing the child, or when the child is straining, coughing or upset. It may also be detected either during the post-natal examination or as the child first starts to walk. It is frequently difficult to demonstrate the hernia in the clinic, but a clear history from the mother is sufficient to make a confident diagnosis. As there is a definite risk of strangulation, the surgeon should not refrain from exploring the affected side where an appropriate and reliable history can be obtained. The differential diagnosis consists of a hydrocele of the cord, undescended testis or torsion of the testis. Careful examination of the scrotum is therefore mandatory.

Inguinal hernia in adults

Essentially, adults may have either indirect or direct inguinal hernias, with sliding hernias representing a variety (usually indirect) in which an adjacent partly peritonealized organ herniates as part of the hernia sac wall. This usually involves the caecum, the sigmoid colon or the bladder.

Indirect inguinal hernias

These arise from the internal ring lateral to the inferior epigastric vessels and pass down the inguinal canal within the cord. Frequently, they pass down into the scrotum and may reach a substantial size (Fig. G.10). This variety of hernia occurs ten times more frequently in men than in women, and is more common than the direct variety. It is identified by an impulse passing obliquely from lateral to medial as the hernia is produced on coughing, and by the sensation of reduction in the line of the inguinal canal on gentle pressure. Once the hernia is reduced, it can be controlled by digital pressure over the internal ring, even with the patient standing or coughing.

Direct inguinal hernia

This variety of hernia is extremely rare under the age of 40 years, and typically presents in the elderly. A bulge is identified over the most medial part of the inguinal ligament which may reach sizeable proportions but very

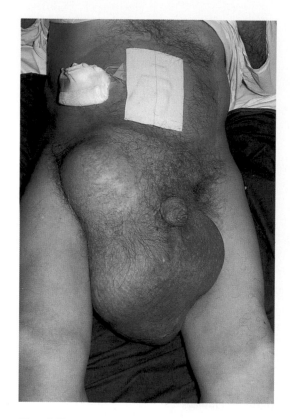

Figure G.10 A massive irreducible indirect right inguinal hernia.

rarely descends into the scrotum. It is uncommon for direct hernias to obstruct, and they usually have an obvious and prominent cough impulse which appears to come directly out through the body wall rather than obliquely in the line of the inguinal canal.

The differential diagnosis of inguinal herniae include hydrocele of the cord, herniated extraperitoneal fat or lipoma of the cord, inguinal lymphadenopathy, ectopic testis and femoral hernia. The inguinal hernia is best distinguished from the femoral hernia by carefully identifying the pubic tubercle where the insertion of the inguinal ligament can usually be felt. The inguinal hernia arises above the inguinal ligament, passing over this point towards the medial side. The femoral hernia, which may appear to fold over the inguinal ligament, can be felt to arise in its deeper part from the femoral canal below and lateral to a finger on the pubic tubercle.

Femoral hernia

Although relatively common as a cause of small-bowel obstruction, femoral hernias are less common than inguinal, incisional and paraumbilical hernias, representing only 3–5 per cent of all hernias. They are two to three times more common in women than men, so that femoral hernias represent over 20 per cent of all hernias in women. They occur more frequently on the right side, and over 30 per cent present with a complication such as obstruction or strangulation.

Anatomy

The femoral hernia descends through the femoral canal bordered medially by the lacunar ligament, posteriorly by the iliopectineal band, and anteriorly by the inguinal ligament. As these three rigid walls limit femoral canal expansion, which can only occur by displacing the femoral vein laterally, there is a definite risk that the hernia will become irreducible or strangulate. The sac then descends to the sapheno-femoral junction, where the least resistance turns the hernia forwards and upwards to lie anterior and sometimes even extended above the inguinal ligament (Fig. G.11).

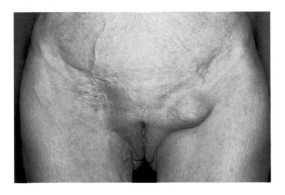

Figure G.11 An irreducible left femoral hernia.

Clinical features

Femoral herniation is rare before late adult life. It may present as a firm or even rubbery lump in the groin which often represents no more than herniated extraperitoneal fat, together with the tissue accumulated around the sac as it descends through the femoral canal and up through the cribriform fascia. As a result, the hernial sac can almost invariably be palpated in the upper medial femoral triangle, even when the contents are reduced. It is unusual to feel a cough impulse in a femoral hernia unless it contains omentum or gut which is freely reducible. An irreducible hernia, particularly in the presence of strangulation, will be tender, tense and often inflamed. On careful palpation of the

pubic tubercle the neck of the sac may be felt below and lateral as it passes under the inguinal ligament.

The testicular apparatus

An *ectopic testis* may be palpated in the region of the external inguinal ring, superficial to the inguinal ligament, or rarely at the root of the penis. It is the size and consistency of the testis, and gives a testicular-type sensation on compression. The important clue to the diagnosis, of course, is that the testis on the side of the swelling is absent from the scrotum.

A *hydrocele of the cord* presents as a cystic swelling at the external inguinal ring. Traction on the testis draws the swelling downwards with the cord – a diagnostic physical sign.

A *lipoma of the cord* as it emerges from the inguinal canal does not demonstrate a cough impulse. However, it frequently co-exists with an indirect inguinal hernia sac, representing merely a collection of extraperitoneal fatty tissue on the sac wall.

In the female, a hydrocele of the canal of Nück (a cyst of the processus vaginalis along the round ligament) is a common differential diagnosis of an irreducible inguinal hernia. It is smooth, painless, fixed in position, fluctuant, and transilluminates brilliantly.

The psoas sheath

Pus within the psoas sheath, originating from advanced tuberculous disease of the lumbar spine or from fistulating Crohn's disease or, rarely, from an appendix abscess, may track beneath the inguinal ligament and present in the groin.

Harold Ellis

GUMS, BLEEDING

Bleeding from the gums is a common complaint, the predominant underlying local cause being infection, both bacterial and viral. The induced inflammatory response renders the mucosa very susceptible to minor trauma. The co-existence of systemic disease can exacerbate this gingival inflammation, or may even initiate it through a reduced resistance to infection or a defect in blood coagulation.

Dental diseases

Periodontal disease is almost endemic within the human race. The most significant factor is poor oral hygiene, leading to the accumulation of food debris and bacteria in the supporting tissues, which subsequently becomes organized into dental plaque and calculus. Bacterial toxins cause destruction of the periodontal ligament supporting the teeth; pockets form, where further bacteria may accumulate. Slow progressive destruction and infection of the supporting tissues follows. The gingival mucosa becomes swollen and hyperaemic, leading to a reluctance to clean the teeth, which aids further infection. Any minor trauma to this swollen and inflamed mucosa, such as mastication or tooth brushing, causes bleeding. There may also be a purulent discharge from the necks of the teeth and the breath smells unpleasant (Fig. G.12).

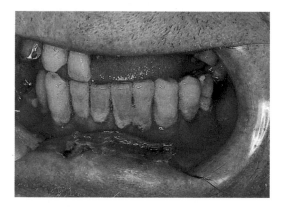

Figure G.12 Gingival erythema due to chronic periodontal disease.

Dental caries, when present, may be obvious to the naked eye, or less conspicuously between the teeth or beneath the gingival mucosa. This also allows an accumulation of bacteria leading to localized infection and, again, gingival hyperaemia and haemorrhage. If both of these conditions are left untreated, then eventually abscess formation will occur which is discussed elsewhere (see JAW, SWELLING OF, p. 338).

Blood dyscrasias

Abnormal or defective bone marrow activity as in aplastic anaemia, or neoplastic infiltration, will cause bleeding of the gums due to a reduced resistance to infection, and in turn a reduction in the number of circulating platelets. The gingival mucosa becomes acutely inflamed, swollen, and bleeds readily. In acute leukaemia the swelling is also due to the local accumulation of leukaemic cells in the gingival tissues. Thrombocytopenia also occurs as part of marrow disorders, any of which may give rise to purpura in the oral cavity. Purpuric spots may best be seen in the hard and soft palates, and haemorrhage from the gums occurs readily. In the mucosal tissues of the cheeks and lips, where the surface epithelium is not so tightly bound down to the underlying supporting connective tissue, large ecchymoses may be found.

The coagulation defect in haemophilia and von Willebrand's disease may cause spontaneous haemorrhage within the oral tissues, and may be particularly troublesome after dental extraction unless appropriate measures are taken.

Disorders of blood vessels

Scurvy can be conveniently discussed under this heading, as the main defect is one of abnormal collagen production leading to capillary fragility. There is also a general lack of tissue resistance which, in the gingival mucosa, may lead to superimposed infection. It is probably this latter aspect which produces the majority of the gingival enlargement characteristic of the disease, as in the presence of good oral hygiene the swelling is far less marked. Whilst scurvy in the developed world is now an uncommon disease, it can still be found amongst old and neglected people with a restricted diet, and also in people who for dietary reasons reduce their input of food containing ascorbic acid. It may also be found in alcoholics and patients with peptic ulceration existing on a milk diet.

Hereditary haemorrhagic telangiectasia (Fig. G.13) is caused by a capillary abnormality, and the head and

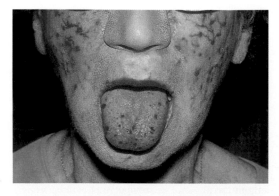

Figure G.13 Hereditary haemorrhagic telangiectasia.

neck region is a common site. In the mouth these abnormal vessels are visible through the mucous membrane, and minor trauma may produce a persistent haemorrhage, which is difficult to control. Both von Willebrand's disease and Henoch–Scholein purpura may occur in the oral cavity, but these are not a predominant feature of the disease.

Chemical poisoning

Mercury was previously used in the treatment of syphilis, and frequently produced a severe acute stomatitis with profuse salivation, halitosis and painful swellings of the lips, gums, tongue and cheeks. The patient suffered a metallic taste, and the regional lymph nodes could be involved. This method of treatment has long been discontinued, but poisoning can still occasionally occur from industrial exposure. The gums become hyperaemic and tend to bleed which, as always, is aggravated by poor oral hygiene. Eventually, necrosis of the gingival mucosa may occur.

Phosphorus was at one time responsible for severe stomatitis, going on to necrosis of the jaw ('phossy jaw'), not infrequently ending in death as the result of fatty degeneration of the liver and heart. Since restrictions are now laid upon the use of crude yellow phosphorus in the manufacture of matches, this condition is now almost unknown. Apart from occupation, the patient may, with suicidal intent, have been taking a rat poison or other vermin-killer containing phosphorus.

Arsenic and *lead* are rare causes of gingival bleeding and usually arise from industrial contamination. The gingivae are again inflamed, swollen and bleed easily and, in the case of lead, there is a characteristic blue line at the gingival margin known as the Burtonian line. Other signs of poisoning may be present, particularly pigmentation of the skin, vomiting, diarrhoea, hyperkeratosis of the soles of the feet and the palms of the hands. Generalized peripheral neuritis may be found in the case of arsenic, and the symptoms given under anaemia in the case of lead. Arsenic may be found in excess in the hair, or lead may be detected in the faeces, or in the urine.

Pregnancy

The hormonal changes that take place during pregnancy may have the effect of exacerbating a pre-existing gingivitis. Generalized swelling of the gingival mucosa may occur, or it may be confined to one inter-dental papilla, giving rise to a pregnancy tumour (Fig. G.14). Histologically, this tissue consists of immature granulation tissue and is extremely vascular. Haemorrhage readily occurs and, provided that the diagnosis is certain, all that is necessary are oral hygiene measures, as once the pregnancy is completed the vascular tissue will recede. However, isolated lesions which remain should be excised.

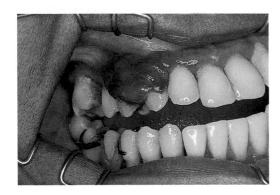

Figure G.14 Pregnancy tumour.

Malabsorption

Patients with malabsorption may show signs of anaemia in the mouth, with a red and swollen tongue and pallor of the mucosa. In addition to this, the gingival mucosa may haemorrhage readily.

Iatrogenic

Overdose with the drug warfarin may produce spontaneous bleeding of the oral mucosa, and will require vitamin K preparations or transfusion of fresh-frozen plasma to arrest the haemorrhage. In the mouth with pre-existing gingivitis, phenytoin (used to control epilepsy) and other drugs may cause hypertrophy of the gingival mucosa. This hypertrophy, however, involves predominantly the interdental papillae to give a uniform appearance which is different from the hypertrophy caused only by poor cleaning (Fig. G.15). Regular maintenance of good oral hygiene becomes very difficult, and further secondary infection supervenes. At this stage, the gingival mucosa becomes inflamed and is associated with local haemorrhage. Treatment is through scaling and polishing of the teeth and the maintenance of good oral hygiene, but in some cases it may be necessary to withdraw the drug or excise the hyperplastic tissue.

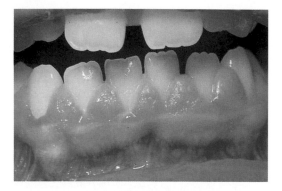

Figure G.15 Gingival hypertrophy as a result of phenytoin therapy.

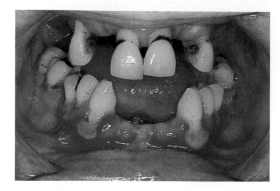

Figure G.16 Gingival recession due to chronic periodontal disease.

Radiotherapy

Radiation to the oral cavity in the management of malignant tumours induces a severe mucositis of the oral mucosa, which is characterized by erythema, superficial ulceration and pain. Good oral hygiene is difficult to maintain, and supra-infection – especially with *Candida* – may ensue. Spontaneous haemorrhage of the mucosa during mastication and tooth cleaning is not uncommon. Regular assistance with oral hygiene should be given during this difficult time, and dental disease eliminated prior to treatment.

Chemotherapy

Because of their toxic effect on the bone marrow, cytotoxic agents may produce changes in the oral cavity similar to those seen with the blood dyscrasias.

Infection

The oral cavity is commonly involved in bacterial infection due to dental causes. However, generalized infection of the oral mucous membrane due to bacteria is rare, the majority being caused by viruses.

Bacterial infection

The most important example of bacterial infection is acute ulcerative gingivitis, which is characterized by a proliferation of Vincent's organisms, *Treponema vincentii* and *Fusiformis fusiformis*. The predominant features are bleeding of the gums, soreness and halitosis (Fig. G.16). There is a characteristic ulceration and blunting of the interdental papillae with considerable debris and slough in the gingival crevice. There

may be an associated fever, malaise and regional lymphadenitis.

This infection may be associated with pre-existing poor oral hygiene, and stress has also been implicated. It may also be a feature of patients with a reduced resistance to infection as in acute leukaemia, agranulocytosis and those undergoing cytotoxic chemotherapy.

In the African continent, the association with measles and suppression of the immune system by malnutrition leading to cancrum oris is well described. Here, small areas of dark necrosis occur in the cheeks or lips, which rapidly progress to produce widespread necrosis and destruction of the circum-oral and oral structures.

Viral infection

Acute inflammation of the oral cavity occurs with viral infections, the most common being herpes simplex and herpes varicella-zoster. The primary infection with herpes simplex may often be subclinical, but if not then acute herpetic gingivostomatitis is encountered. This is characterized by severe inflammation and vesicle formation, leading to ulceration of the entire oral mucous membrane with constitutional symptoms of fever, malaise and enlargement of the regional lymph nodes. The gingivae are acutely inflamed, swollen and bleed easily. The disease is usually self-limiting after a few days, and only symptomatic relief is required and the maintenance of oral hygiene. Secondary infection of the vesicles may be prevented by chlorhexidine or tetracycline mouthwashes.

Reactivation of the herpes zoster virus (shingles) in the distribution of the trigeminal nerve may cause severe erythema, ulceration and haemorrhage of the oral mucosa in the exact distribution of the branch involved, usually the maxillary branch. The condition is again self-limiting, and the intraoral lesions require only symptomatic relief, although an antiviral agent may be valuable in the protracted case.

The Epstein–Barr virus (infectious mononucleosis) may cause a gingivostomatitis where the gingivae are characteristically red, swollen and haemorrhagic, similar to the appearance found in acute leukaemia or scurvy. Acute bacterial ulcerative gingivitis may follow. A high proportion of patients show petechiae in the soft palate which, because of its characteristic appearance, is of diagnostic importance.

Patients with HIV infection may develop significant inflammation of the gingival tissues not commensurate with the level of oral hygiene and periodontal disease. They are also prone to acute necrotizing ulcerative gingivitis and acute necrotizing periodontitis.

Autoimmune disease

The oral mucous membrane is frequently involved by autoimmune conditions whereby the mucosa under goes superficial bullous formation followed by ulceration. This is invariably associated with inflammation, a degree of secondary infection and possibly haemorrhage. The most common disease is aphthous ulceration of the minor or major type, but the mouth is also not infrequently involved by systemic lupus erythematosus, pemphigus, mucous membrane pemphigoid, bullous erythema multiforme and epidermolysis bullosa. The autoimmune condition lichen planus is a common finding in the mouth, and the erosive type is associated with widespread ulceration, soreness and haemorrhage. The majority of cases are not associated with cutaneous lichen planus. Good oral hygiene may be difficult, but is essential if the symptoms are to be controlled. Water irrigation with a 'water pik' is a useful adjunct to normal tooth-cleaning methods. Treatment involves the use of chlorhexidine mouthwashes and topical steroids. Severe cases may require systemic steroids.

Neoplastic disease

The commonest malignant tumour of the oral cavity is the squamous cell carcinoma, although primary involvement of the dental structures is not the most common presentation. The tumour may undergo central necrosis, causing ulceration and secondary infection with loosening of the teeth. This may be associated with intermittent haemorrhage, especially if the tumour erodes an adjacent blood vessel.

Developmental lesions

The oral cavity may be involved by capillary or cavernous haemangiomas and, on occasion, lymphangiomas. All of these lesions are liable to bleed with trauma, and are particularly hazardous following dental extractions, should these involve the bone of the mandible or the maxilla.

Inflammation

The fibrous epulis, denture granuloma, pyogenic granuloma and the giant-cell epulis have a similar clinical and histological appearance. These soft-tissue swellings arise within the oral or gingival mucosa and consist of a fibrous tissue stroma, which may be vascular and covered by squamous epithelium. These swellings when subjected to trauma will be a source of haemorrhage within the oral cavity.

Peter Blenkinsopp

GUMS, HYPERTROPHY OF

True hypertrophy of the gingival mucosa is relatively rare, and accordingly enlargement can conveniently be classified into that caused by predominantly fibrous tissue and that caused by a cellular infiltration. It should be remembered that the most common cause of gingival enlargement is infection associated with the dental structures [for discussions, see GUMS, BLEEDING (p. 245) and JAW, SWELLING OF (p. 338)].

Fibrous infiltration

Hereditary gingival fibromatosis is a rare autosomal dominant condition in which all the gingival tissues become enlarged to such an extent that the teeth may become almost buried, and in the child will interfere with tooth eruption. Mucosal inflammation is not always a feature, and treatment is by surgical reduction and the maintenance of good oral hygiene. There may, in addition, be hirsutism and thickening of the facial features, associated epilepsy and mental retardation.

A proportion of patients taking the anticonvulsant drug phenytoin or ciclosporins over a long period of time will develop fibrous hyperplasia of the gingival tissues, but this predominantly affects the interdental papillae (see Fig. G.15) Again, the enlargement may be such as partially to obscure the teeth from view, and the situation is made worse by the presence of chronic infection. In severe cases, it may be necessary to consider substituting a different drug; local measures consist of improving the oral hygiene and gingivectomy.

Vascular or inflammatory enlargement

Pregnancy gingivitis, acute leukaemia and scurvy were discussed previously (see GUMS, BLEEDING, p. 245). Wegener's granulomatosis is a disease of focal necrotizing vasculitis which affects the upper and lower respiratory tracts. Occasionally, a proliferative gingivitis may occur which arises interdentally and spreads mainly along the buccal gingivae. Extensive periodontal destruction may occur, and the diagnosis can only be obtained by biopsy.

Infiltration of the gingivae by angiomatous tissue occurs as part of a haemangioma (see JAW, SWELLING OF, p. 338), and should be distinguished from a localized proliferation of capillaries due to chronic irritation, such as that which is caused by a carious tooth or a retained dental root. The latter will resolve with removal of the irritant stimulus, while the former is usually part of a more extensive proliferation involving adjacent structures.

Peter Blenkinsopp

GUMS, RETRACTION OF

Retraction of the gingival mucosa is mostly associated with chronic periodontal disease (see Fig. G.16). The accumulation of dental plaque causes progressive destruction of the alveolar bone supporting the teeth such that the mucous membrane – if not swollen by inflammation – retracts with the bone. So common is this process with age that it is often referred to as 'getting long in the tooth'. Vigorous attention to the periodontal tissues will limit the rate of bone loss, but in some patients the condition is progressive, with little evidence of infection.

Retraction of the gingivae may also be associated with intra-oral scarring, as occurs in epidermolysis

bullosa, submucous fibrosis and various connective tissue disorders. Occasionally, high muscle attachments will cause localized recession due to recurrent traction during function.

Peter Blenkinsopp

GYNAECOMASTIA

Gynaecomastia is enlargement of the male breast due to an increase in the duct tissue and in the periductal stroma. It is thought to arise from a disturbance of oestrogen physiology. If the condition lasts for longer than a year, the stroma becomes fibrous and the gynaecomastia tends to persist. The condition should not be confused with fat in the mammary region; in this case no glandular tissue is palpable behind the areola. Other conditions that cause swelling in the breast should be excluded, such as carcinoma, lipoma or neurofibroma. Mammography and breast ultrasound are useful in investigation.

Gynaecomastia is common in neonates and at puberty. When it occurs in older age-groups a pathological cause is more likely, though in the elderly it may be a physiological accompaniment of declining testicular function.

The pathophysiology of gynaecomastia is poorly understood. In some cases, a decreased ratio of free androgens to free oestrogens has been shown. In other cases, the cause may be an undue sensitivity of breast tissue to normal circulating hormones; sometimes the enlargement is unilateral. The causes of gynaecomastia are detailed in Table G.5.

Neonatal gynaecomastia

Approximately 70 per cent of male neonates have some breast enlargement. In just over half of these cases, fluid ('witch's milk') can be expressed on squeezing. The breast enlargement is probably due to the effect of placental oestrogens and human chorionic gonadotrophin stimulating the Leydig cells of the baby's testes to produce oestrogen. The witch's milk may possibly be the result of maternal prolactin. Histological examination shows the typical features of a lactating breast.

Table G.5 Causes of gynaecomastia

Physiological
Neonatal
Pubertal
Senescent

Familial

Endocrine pathology
Hypogonadism
■ Prepubertal testicular failure
 ◆ Agenesis
 ◆ Bilateral torsion of the testes
 ◆ Klinefelter's syndrome
 ◆ Reifenstein's syndrome
 ◆ Noonan's syndrome
 ◆ Cryptorchidism
■ Destructive lesions of the testes
 ◆ Trauma
 ◆ Castration
 ◆ Mumps, orchitis
 ◆ Tuberculous orchitis
 ◆ Leprous orchitis
 ◆ External radiation
■ Defects in testosterone synthesis

Testicular tumours
Leydig-cell tumour
Sertoli-cell tumour
Chorion carcinoma
Teratoma
Seminoma

Other tumours
Bronchogenic carcinoma

Thyroid
Hyperthyroidism
Hypothyroidism

Adrenal
Adrenocortical carcinoma or adenoma

Pituitary
Acromegaly
Chromophobe adenoma

Hypothalamic lesions

Disorders of sex differentiation
Male pseudohermaphroditism
True hermaphroditism

Liver dysfunction
Hepatitis
Cirrhosis
Haemochromatosis
Hepatic carcinoma

Neurological disorders
Traumatic paraplegia
Dystrophia myotonica
Friedreich's ataxia
Syringomyelia

Respiratory disorders
Carcinoma of the bronchus
Chronic suppurative lung disease

Renal disorders
Chronic renal failure
During maintenance haemodialysis
Hypernephroma

Gastrointestinal disorders
Chronic ulcerative colitis
Following extensive gut surgery

Polyostotic fibrous dysplasia (McCune–Albright syndrome)

Renutrition following starvation and malnutrition

Drugs
Hormones
■ Oestrogens
■ Human chorionic gonadotrophin
■ Methyl testosterone
■ Desoxycorticosterone
Androgen antagonists
■ Spironolactone
■ Progestogens
■ Cyproterone
■ Cannabis
■ Cimetidine
■ Griseofulvin
■ Digitalis glycosides
■ Flutamide
Unknown mechanism
■ Busulfan
■ Calcium channel-blocking agents
■ Diazepam
■ Isoniazid
■ Methyldopa
■ Omeprazole
■ Penicillamine
■ Tricyclic antidepressants

Pubertal gynaecomastia

The vast majority of boys develop a minor degree of gynaecomastia at the time of puberty (Fig. G.17). Before the gynaecomastia appears, there is a rise in plasma oestradiol which anticipates the expected pubertal rise in plasma testosterone. Along with the increased oestradiol there is an increase in prolactin, but the levels fall as the gynaecomastia develops. In boys

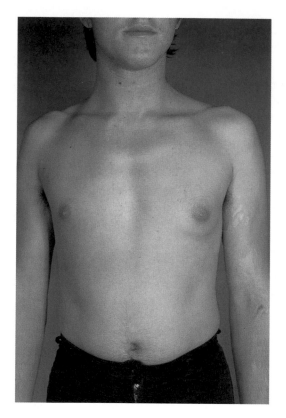

Figure G.17 Bilateral gynaecomastia in a boy at puberty.

examine the testicles carefully for the presence of a tumour. If one testis appears to be normal and the other one is small, the 'normal' testis may be harbouring a tumour. The oestrogens produced by the tumour may have suppressed pituitary gonadotrophins and caused failure of development of the contralateral testis. Testicular ultrasonography is a useful way of detecting small tumours.

Senescent gynaecomastia

Occasionally, patients in the sixth or later decades of life may develop gynaecomastia (Figs G.18 and G.19). There may be associated loss of libido and occasional hot flushes. The plasma testosterone level is reduced, while plasma oestradiol levels remain normal, though plasma oestrone levels rise due to increased conversion from androstenedione. Sex hormone-binding globulin (SHBG) levels rise, with a consequent increase in the binding of testosterone. The result is a further reduction in free testosterone and an imbalance in the ratio

in whom pubertal gynaecomastia does not occur, this sequence of hormonal events does not take place. In some boys the gynaecomastia is more marked, and may even approximate to the normal female breast. Often, the condition arises in one breast only, or develops on one side some weeks or months before it appears in the other. Occasionally, fluid can be expressed. In an appreciable number of cases there is a history of neonatal gynaecomastia, or even a family history, suggesting that there may be a constitutional sensitivity to oestrogen secreted by the Leydig cells of the testis. This sensitivity could possibly be mediated by increased numbers of oestrogen receptors in breast tissue.

Mild, early gynaecomastia usually regresses, but moderate to severe degrees tend to persist. Although, in theory, anti-oestrogens such as tamoxifen should be of value, they seem to have little effect on anything but mild gynaecomastia. The patient is best referred early for plastic surgery. A peri-areolar incision should leave a virtually invisible scar.

It is important to consider other causes of gynaecomastia in a pubertal boy, such as drug ingestion, and to

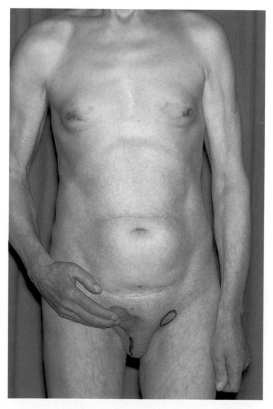

Figure G.18 Gynaecomastia in an elderly man receiving stilboestrol for carcinoma of the prostate. Note the nipple pigmentation.

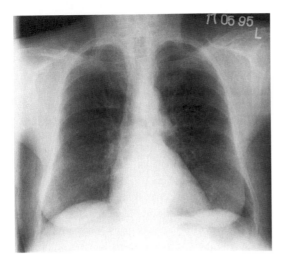

Figure G.19 Chest X-ray in an elderly man, demonstrating gynaecomastia.

of free testosterone to free oestrogens. The serum gonadotrophin levels are raised. It is important, however, in this age group to consider other causes of gynaecomastia, such as bronchogenic carcinoma, drug ingestion, liver disease, etc.

Pathological gynaecomastia is found in men where there is a disturbance in the normal balance between testosterone and oestrogen function. This results from conditions where there may be a decrease in testosterone production; a decrease in testosterone action; an increase in oestrogen production; or an increase in oestrogen activity. It should be noted that gynaecomastia is not usually a feature of hypogonadism secondary to pituitary or hypothalamic disease.

Conditions associated with decreased testosterone production

Congenital

Klinefelter's syndrome describes a phenotypical male with 47,XXY sex chromosome genotype. The condition presents in adolescence, with seminiferous tubule dysgenesis giving rise to primary hypogonadism and male infertility. There is clinical evidence of gynaecomastia in a significant number of cases, along with small atrophic testes and aspermatogenesis. There is a decrease in testicular production of testosterone, with a consequent increase in the oestrogen:androgen ratio.

Congenital anorchia describes phenotypically normal 46,XY males with failure to locate testes on surgical

exploration. Some 50 per cent of these patients develop gynaecomastia due to low production of testosterone.

Defects in testosterone synthesis due to enzyme deficiencies in the metabolic pathway from cholesterol to testosterone results in incomplete virilization of the male fetus during embryogenesis. 'Male pseudohermaphroditism' is a term used to describe individuals who have testes and an XY chromosomal constitution but ambiguous external genitalia. Examples of enzyme deficiencies include congenital adrenal hyperplasia (20,22-desmolase deficiency, 3-*R*-hydroxysteroid dehydrogenase deficiency; 17-α-hydroxylase deficiency); failure of conversion of testosterone to dihydrotestosterone because of 5-α-reductase deficiency or failure of testosterone production because of 17-β-hydroxysteroid dehydrogenase deficiency. The clinical manifestations vary widely from hypospadias to grossly abnormal appearances with a small penis exhibiting chordee, a bifid scrotum, a persistent urogenital sinus, and a vagina opening into the posterior urethra. A rudimentary uterus and Fallopian tubes may be present. The testes are undescended or present in the labioscrotal folds. Gynaecomastia may appear at puberty.

Acquired

Bilateral testicular atrophy is associated with decreased production of testosterone. This occurs in the presence of normal production of oestrogens (oestradiol and oestrone) from extraglandular sources resulting in a reduction in the androgen:oestrogen ratio. Gynaecomastia is a common feature.

The most common causes of testicular atrophy acquired after puberty are the following: (i) viral orchitis due to mumps virus, echovirus, group B arbovirus; (ii) trauma; (iii) neurological disease (e.g. myotonic dytrophy, traumatic paraplegia, syringomyelia, Friedreich's ataxia); (iv) granulomatous disease involving the testis (e.g. leprosy); and (v) renal failure – gynaecomastia is present in approximately 50 per cent of patients receiving haemodialysis.

Conditions associated with resistance to testosterone action

Congenital

Androgen resistance describes either testicular feminization syndrome or Reifenstein's syndrome. In these conditions the underlying pathology is a resistance at the androgen receptor to endogenous and exogenous androgens. The result is a range of incomplete virilization in a 46,XY sex chromosome genotype, resulting in:

- Phenotypic women with testicular feminization (male pseudohermaphrodite) associated with complete resistance at the androgen receptor. The appearance is female, there is absent pubic and axillary hair, the external genitalia resemble those of a normal female, but there is a blind vagina. The testes are usually intra-abdominal, but may lie in the inguinal canal or in the labia majora. The breasts are those of a normal female, except that the nipples and areolae are often small.
- Incomplete resistance at the androgen receptor, examples of which include phenotypic men with hypospadias and gynaecomastia (Reifenstein's syndrome) and infertile male syndrome.

Conditions associated with increased oestrogen production

Testicular tumours

Testicular tumours such as those of the stromal cells (e.g. Leydig cells and Sertoli cells) produce gynaecomastia because of increased oestrogen secretion. The other germ cell tumours (e.g. chorion carcinoma, embryonal carcinomas, teratomas) do so because human chorionic gonadotrophin (hCG), produced by the tumour, stimulates testicular tissue to secrete oestrogens. In the early stages, germ cell tumours of the testis may be impalpable, so estimations of serum hCG are important, particularly since chorion carcinoma is the most common testicular tumour to cause gynaecomastia. Ultrasound of the testis can detect the presence of a small tumour.

Leydig cell tumours are rare before puberty, but should be considered as a cause of gynaecomastia in adult males. Seminomas may cause gynaecomastia but this is rare. The rarest testicular tumour of all, the Sertoli cell tumour, frequently presents with gynaecomastia and loss of libido.

Thyroid disorders

Some 80 per cent of male thyrotoxics have histological evidence of gynaecomastia. Plasma oestradiol levels are elevated. This is thought to be due to increased androstenedione production and increased oestrogen production in extraglandular sites. Increased oestrogen levels and excess thyroid hormones both lead to a rise

in SHBG levels, so that more testosterone is bound and the ratio of free testosterone to free oestradiol falls.

Gynaecomastia occurs rarely in patients with hypothyroidism – the mechanism is uncertain.

Suprarenal tumours

Adrenocortical carcinoma and, more rarely, adenoma may produce oestrogens and lead to the development of gynaecomastia. However, most adrenal tumours produce large amounts of adrenal androgens (e.g. androstenedione and dehydroepiandrosterone). These androgens are metabolized by aromatization (aromatase enzyme), producing large amounts of oestrogen. Plasma or urinary oestrogen levels are therefore raised, and gonadotrophin levels may be suppressed. Urinary 17-oxo-steroid levels can be increased or normal. The testes are small and aspermia is present. Testicular biopsy may show hypoplasia of Leydig cells. CT scanning of the adrenals should be carried out to localize the tumour.

Similarly, in congenital suprarenal hyperplasia the increased oestrogen production is due to increased production of androstenedione, which is metabolized by extraglandular aromatase to oestrogen.

Pituitary tumours

Acidophil or chromophobe tumours of the pituitary causing acromegaly, or chromophobe tumours not producing excess growth hormone, may secrete large amounts of prolactin (Fig. G.20). However, prolactin

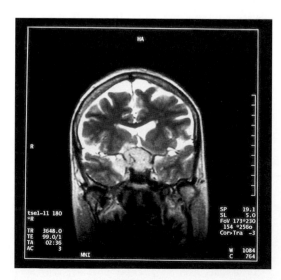

Figure G.20 Pituitary tumour (prolactinoma).

does not promote growth or development of breast tissue and is therefore believed not to play a direct role in the development of gynaecomastia. If gynaecomastia develops in association with a prolactin-secreting tumour it is thought to be the result of secondary hypogonadism and an alteration in the ratio of free testosterone to free oestradiol. Some pituitary tumours have caused gynaecomastia because of the secretion of luteinizing hormone.

Hypothalamic disorders

Lesions in the hypothalamus may give rise to precocious puberty and gynaecomastia.

Liver dysfunction

In chronic liver disease (e.g. cirrhosis) there is a decline in testosterone production. In addition, there is a decreased clearance of androstenedione by the liver, and therefore more is available for extraglandular aromatization to oestrogen. The SHBG levels rise, and this reduces further the level of free testosterone. The resultant decrease in the androgen:oestrogen ratio produces the feminization and gynaecomastia associated with chronic liver disease.

Nutrition

Refeeding after a period of starvation or malnutrition is associated with gynaecomastia which eventually regresses once nutrition is maintained. The mechanism of feminization is not well understood, but it may have a similar pathogenesis to that associated with chronic liver disease – that is, decreased clearance of androgens by the liver, making them available for extraglandular aromatization to oestrogen.

Another interesting theory regarding poor nutrition was noted in starving ex-prisoners of war when they were re-fed. Gonadotrophin levels, which are depressed during the period of starvation, rise following the receipt of food. The testes become stimulated again and the individual goes through what is, in effect, a second puberty.

Respiratory disorders

Carcinoma of the bronchus may secrete hCG which, by stimulating the testes, leads to increased oestrogen production. In most cases where bronchial carcinoma has caused gynaecomastia there has been associated hypertrophic pulmonary osteoarthropathy.

Drugs

Drugs are an important cause of gynaecomastia, especially in adults. Oestrogen therapy invariably produces gynaecomastia, and when stilboestrol is used a deep brown pigmentation of the nipple and areola develops (see Fig. G.18). Gynaecomastia has been described in pharmaceutical industry workers involved in the manufacture of oestrogens. In particular, young men and boys are very sensitive to the effects of oestrogen. Exposure may occur through contact with oestrogen-containing creams, or oestrogen present in meat and dairy products from oestrogen-treated animals. hCG administration may cause gynaecomastia when used for the treatment of undescended testes. Methyl testosterone can occasionally lead to breast enlargement, possibly because of peripheral conversion to oestrogens. Any drug which is an androgen antagonist (see Table G.5) may cause gynaecomastia by allowing the unopposed action of oestrogens on breast tissue. Digoxin is associated with gynaecomastia in approximately 10 per cent of treated men, though the underlying mechanism is not fully understood. Although digoxin does not cause a rise in plasma oestrogen, it does bind to the human oestrogen receptor, and may promote gynaecomastia by enhancing the action of endogenous oestrogens. Antiretroviral therapy for HIV infection (particularly with the drug efavirenz) has been associated with gynaecomastia, although the mechanism is currently obscure. Clomiphene acts as an anti-oestrogen by blocking oestrogen receptors, and is used to treat gynaecomastia in boys. It induces gonadotrophin release by interfering with the negative feedback effects of oestrogen on the hypothalamus and, therefore, may cause gynaecomastia on discontinuation of treatment due to luteinizing hormone (LH) effects on oestrogen production by the testes.

Any drugs that interfere with the synthesis of testosterone by the testes for sufficient time will produce feminization and gynaecomastia by lowering the androgen:oestrogen ratio. Examples include drugs from the imidazole group (e.g. ketoconazole, metronidazole, etomidate) which interfere with steroid hormone synthesis in Leydig cells, and antineoplastic drugs through long-lasting toxic effects on Leydig cells (e.g. alkylating agents used for systemic or testicular neoplasms).

Spironolactone affects testosterone activity by interfering with testosterone synthesis (high dose) and blocking androgen receptors (low dose). Gynaecomastia is found in 50 per cent of men who receive 150 mg spironolactone per day. When the active metabolite canrenoate is used instead of the parent drug, gynaecomastia does not develop.

Anti-androgens, by inhibiting testosterone binding to the androgen receptor, cause gynaecomastia. Examples of anti-androgens include cyproterone acetate, flutamide, zanoterone and bicalutamide. Cimetidine, and far less commonly ranitidine, cause gynaecomastia by blocking the androgen receptor. Cimetidine may also prevent the breakdown of oestradiol.

Sharon O'Byrne

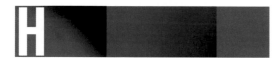

HAEMATEMESIS

Causes of haematemesis

Gastrointestinal haemorrhage commonly presents as vomiting of blood or blood-stained gastric content; this is defined as haematemesis. Causes of haematemesis are listed in Table H.1.

The most common causes of profuse haematemesis are acute gastric erosions, gastric ulcer, duodenal ulcer and cirrhosis of the liver. A long history of typical peptic ulcer symptoms may be present in patients bleeding from gastric or duodenal ulcer, but this may not always be present. Acute erosions are particularly common in patients taking aspirin or other NSAIDs, or they may follow acute alcohol ingestion. A history of alcoholism may point to cirrhosis of the liver, and may be accompanied by jaundice, palmar erythema, spider naevi and ascites; the liver may be enlarged and the spleen may also be palpable. Absence of these features does not exclude the diagnosis. Endoscopic examination of the oesophagus, stomach and duodenum is essential in all cases of significant haematemesis.

Table H.1 Causes of haematemesis

Swallowed blood
Epistaxis
Haemoptysis
Bleeding from mouth or throat
Spurious

Diseases of the oesophagus
Hiatus hernia and reflux oesophagitis
Oesophageal varices
Mallory–Weiss syndrome
Oesophageal ulcer
Mediastinal tumour perforating oesophagus and aorta
Foreign body perforating oesophagus and aorta

Diseases of the stomach
Gastric ulcer
Acute gastritis and haemorrhagic erosions
Tumours, carcinoma, haemangioma, leiomyosarcoma
Pseudoxanthoma elasticum
Hereditary haemorrhagic telangiectasia (Osier–Rendu–Weber syndrome)

Diseases of the duodenum
Duodenal ulcer
Diverticula
Tumours, primary or invasion from pancreas
Gallstones ulcerating into duodenum

Portal obstruction
Hepatic cirrhosis
Portal vein thrombosis

Disordered haemostasis
Thrombocytopenia and non-thrombocytopenic purpura
Polycythaemia purpura
Leukaemia and related disorders
Aplastic anaemia
Haemophilia and related disorders
Von Willebrand's disease
Scurvy
Chronic liver disease

Drugs
Anticoagulant and antiplatelet therapy
Non-steroidal anti-inflammatory drugs (NSAIDs), aspirin, phenylbutazone, indomethacin and many others

Miscellaneous
Abdominal aneurysm opening into stomach or duodenum
Uraemia
Abdominal surgery, trauma or burns (Curling's ulcer)
Polyarteritis nodosa, systemic lupus erythematosus
Malignant hypertension
Acute febrile disorders, variola, scarlet fever, measles, malaria, yellow fever, Dengue, infective endocarditis

Swallowed blood

Epistaxis

Bleeding from the nose may be followed by haematemesis when blood has been swallowed and then vomited; this may occur at night when blood has been swallowed during sleep.

Haemoptysis

Blood coming from the lungs may be swallowed, especially if haemorrhage occurs during sleep. The patient may cough up blood, which is subsequently swallowed.

Bleeding from the mouth and throat

Bleeding may occur from the gums, tongue and fauces, and blood from these sources may be swallowed and subsequently vomited. Bleeding from the gums may occur in scurvy or mercurial stomatitis.

Spurious

Some patients suffering from a variant of the Munchausen syndrome may swallow blood in secret, and subsequently vomit this with an intent to deceive.

Diseases of the oesophagus

Hiatus hernia and reflux oesophagitis

Hiatus hernia is common, but is mostly associated with the symptoms of acid reflux and oesophagitis than with gastrointestinal bleeding. Blood loss in oesophagitis and hiatus hernia is usually chronic, presenting as iron-deficiency anaemia, but occasionally haematemesis does occur. This most often occurs from the gastric side of the oesophagogastric junction, and is more common with a paraoesophageal rather than a sliding hiatus hernia. Haematemesis may be associated with Barrett's syndrome, in which ulceration of gastric mucosa may occur in the lower oesophagus.

Oesophageal varices

Varices developing at the lower end of the oesophagus or the upper end of the stomach as a result of portal hypertension are generally associated with cirrhosis of the liver, and may be the cause of profuse haematemesis if rupture occurs. Stigmata of chronic liver disease may be present such as jaundice, ascites, palmar erythema or spider naevi. The absence of these features does not exclude the presence of portal hypertension and varices.

Mallory–Weiss syndrome

Rupture of the gastric mucosa at the oesophagogastric junction may result in haematemesis. This may follow vomiting, and is particularly common in alcoholics. Such tears are generally linear, at or just below the mucosal junction, and may extend into a submucosal plexus of thin-walled vessels. The characteristic clinical picture of retching and vomiting followed by haemorrhage is not the only way the Mallory–Weiss syndrome presents, as early endoscopy in patients has shown this to be a relatively common cause of haematemesis.

Oesophageal ulcer

Such ulcers may be either benign or malignant, and may be associated with hiatus hernia and reflux oesophagitis. Although a relatively uncommon cause of haematemesis, significant bleeding may occur, the diagnosis being confirmed by endoscopy with biopsy.

Mediastinal tumour perforating oesophagus and aorta

This is an infrequent complication of such tumours, but it may occur if the tumour erodes into the oesophagus. It may be associated with compression and invasion of large veins, leading to oedema of the neck and extremities, cyanosis and dilated superficial veins.

Foreign body perforating oesophagus and aorta

This rare cause of haematemesis may be induced by a fish bone, pin or dental plate perforating both the oesophagus and a large vessel or aorta. A history of a foreign body being swallowed, followed by a feeling of discomfort in the oesophagus, suggests the condition which is generally confirmed by radiology or endoscopy.

Diseases of the stomach

Gastric ulcer

Haematemesis may occur in acute or chronic gastric ulcer. Gradual loss of blood may allow sufficient time for acid gastric juice to convert haemoglobin into haematin, which gives the vomit a dark brown or 'coffee-grounds' appearance. Severe bleeding may occur if a medium-sized or large vessel is eroded.

Profuse haemorrhage causes a feeling of faintness, restlessness, syncope and a rapid feeble pulse. There may be abdominal pain, nausea, vomiting and associated melaena. The pain is generally epigastric, but many haematemeses from ulcers are associated with no abdominal discomfort.

Endoscopy is the most important investigation in determining gastric ulcer as a cause of haematemesis; the site of the ulcer can be positively identified, the severity of the bleeding assessed, and biopsy obtained to determine if the ulcer is benign or malignant. Usually, a biopsy is not taken from bleeding ulcers, the endoscopy being repeated in a few days for the purpose of obtaining suitable biopsies. It is current convention to repeat endoscopy to ensure ulcer healing after 6–8 weeks because of the strong association with gastric cancer.

Acute gastritis and haemorrhagic erosions

In acute gastritis the mucosa is congested and small haemorrhages and erosions are identified at endoscopy. Generally slight haemorrhage occurs, although it may be *occasionally* profuse. Haemorrhagic erosions are small or minute ulcers, the differences between these and multiple small gastric ulcers being that of degree rather than of kind.

Acute gastritis and haemorrhagic erosions may be associated with the ingestion of irritating foods, alcohol, or corrosive and irritant poisons. There may be a feeling of discomfort and tenderness in the epigastrium, nausea and vomiting.

NSAIDs are now perhaps the most common cause of bleeding from erosive gastritis.

Other causes of bleeding from such lesions are very severe acute infections such as variola, infective endocarditis, yellow fever, black water fever and Dengue fever.

Gastritis and haematemesis may also be due to corrosive poisons, strong acids or alkalis destroying the surface membranes of mouth, throat, oesophagus or stomach, causing intense pain, dysphagia, retrosternal discomfort, abdominal distension, collapse and haematemesis. In arsenic poisoning, the mucous membrane of the stomach is red, inflamed, partly detached and covered with blood-stained mucus. The principal symptoms are nausea, severe sickness, burning epigastric pain and diarrhoea. The vomitus is usually a brown, turbid fluid mixed with mucus and streaked with blood in which arsenic may be detected by appropriate tests; severe diarrhoea may come later.

Tumours

Severe haematemesis is relatively rare in *carcinoma of the stomach*, accounting for less than 5 per cent of all haematemeses. The patient may have epigastric discomfort, nausea, vomiting, anorexia and weight loss. Pyrexia, anaemia, cachexia and an abdominal mass may also be present. Sometimes, no preceding symptoms occur and the patient presents with haematemesis. Pain is variable, but when present is generally central, occasionally being referred to the back. If narrowing at the pyloric area has occurred, the patient may have regular vomiting streaked with blood of 'coffee-grounds' appearance. If the tumour is at the cardia, regurgitation of food may occur rather than true vomiting, and this may happen a few minutes after eating. Troisier's sign – enlargement of the left supraclavicular lymph node – is a rare finding, but if present it strongly suggests malignant disease.

Gastric tumours are best diagnosed by endoscopy, through which adequate biopsies can be obtained under direct vision.

Other tumours of the stomach may rarely occur; these include haemangioma, a benign tumour comprising newly formed blood vessels; and leiomyoma, a sarcoma containing large spindle cells of unstriped muscle. These are rare tumours, but they are likely to ulcerate and bleed.

Pseudoxanthoma elasticum (Grondblad–Strandberg syndrome)

This is a hereditary disease characterized by widespread abiotrophy of elastic tissue throughout the body. Disintegration of the submucosal artery elastica leads to severe haemorrhage from the stomach and is an uncommon cause of haematemesis. Characteristic appearances of the skin of head, neck and body may suggest the diagnosis; these have been termed the 'plucked chicken' appearance. Angiod breaks in the retina are also seen; these can lead to visual loss (Fig. H.1).

Hereditary haemorrhagic telangiectasia (Osler–Rendu–Weber syndrome)

This is caused by focal dilatation of post-capillary venules which have excessive layers of smooth muscle

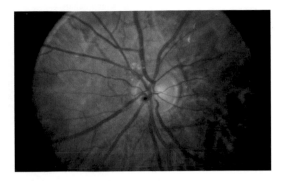

Figure H.1 Angiod streaks (seen as irregular greyish lines radiating from around the optic nerve) in a patient with pseudoxanthoma elasticum.

devoid of elastin. There are multiple telangiectasia which are commonly found on the lips and mucous membranes of the mouth and nose and throughout the gastrointestinal tract. There may also be arteriovenous fistulae in the lungs, liver and brain. The condition is inherited in an autosomal dominant manner. The most common presentations are gastrointestinal tract bleeding, often haematemesis, sometimes melaena, or epistaxis. Endoscopic examination of the stomach generally identifies such lesions, but milder bleeding distal to the stomach is often difficult to diagnose.

Diseases of the duodenum

Duodenal ulcer

Haematemesis occurs when a duodenal ulcer erodes a blood vessel, some of the blood regurgitating through the pylorus into the stomach to be vomited, the rest passing down the gastrointestinal tract to cause melaena. If bleeding is severe, red blood may be passed per rectum. It is common for duodenal ulcer and haematemesis to have little pain. If pain is present it is central, upper abdominal and possibly radiating to the back. There may be a dyspeptic history with pain occurring some hours after food, often at night, with symptoms showing periodicity. Generally, endoscopy can rapidly identify the presence and site of a bleeding duodenal ulcer.

Diverticula

Duodenal diverticula are fairly commonly seen on radiological examination, but are generally asymptomatic. If inflammation occurs within a diverticulum the symptoms may resemble those of duodenal ulcer, although there is generally not the classical regular food relationship. A co-existing ulcer may be present. Haematemesis is rare in association with duodenal diverticula.

Tumours

Duodenal tumours are rare, mostly arising from the ampulla of Vater, and being associated with jaundice and pale or silvery stools. Occasionally, invasion of the duodenum occurs from tumour in the head of the pancreas, resulting in haematemesis.

Gallstones ulcerating into the duodenum

This is a rare cause of haematemesis, and is generally associated with previous attacks of colicky abdominal pain, classically under the right costal margin, and sometimes associated with jaundice. The diagnosis is generally confirmed by plain abdominal X-ray showing air in the biliary tree, ultrasound examination, or the passage of stone in the faeces, or endoscopy.

Portal hypertension

Chronic liver disease

Chronic liver disease may be associated with disordered haemostasis in the form of thrombocytopenia associated with portal hypertension, or coagulation abnormalities. Thus, any other cause of bleeding such as peptic ulceration or oesophageal varices may lead to a major haematemesis because of the abnormal haemostatic mechanisms.

Portal vein obstruction

Extrahepatic portal vein thrombosis usually occurs in infants and early childhood. The cause is usually unknown, and infection is rare. The patient presents with haematemesis from oesophageal varices, or splenomegaly. There is rarely evidence of liver dysfunction clinically or biochemically. The outlook is good. Surgery should be avoided, but if bleeding is a problem then some form of portal systemic shunt surgery is required.

In adults, portal vein thrombosis is usually due to thrombosis, trauma or neoplastic invasion.

Disordered haemostasis

A large number of conditions may be associated with disordered haemostasis. These may cause gastrointestinal haemorrhage with haematemesis. Often, another lesion in the stomach or duodenum (e.g. a small erosion or ulcer) may start to bleed, but the bleeding may become significant in the presence of such conditions, and this leads to abnormal haemostasis.

Thrombocytopenia

A number of conditions may be associated with thrombocytopenia, including hepatic cirrhosis with portal hypertension, side effects of drugs, or reticuloses. Any of these conditions may be associated with bleeding, becoming significant and leading to haematemesis.

Polycythaemia

Patients with polycythaemia rubra vera may develop thrombotic episodes leading to ulceration and followed by bleeding from the stomach or duodenum.

Purpura

Purpuric conditions may be associated with haemorrhage from any mucous membranes, anywhere in the gastrointestinal tract. The underlying cause of the purpura should be investigated.

Leukaemia and related disorders

Leukaemia and other associated conditions such as Hodgkin's disease, lymphomas and other reticuloses may develop haemorrhages from any part of the gastrointestinal tract, leading to haematemesis. Enlargement of the spleen may indicate the underlying condition. The diagnosis is established by blood or bone marrow examination.

Aplastic anaemia

Aplastic anaemias may be related to a range of conditions, including viral infection and the side effects of drugs. They may rarely be associated with gastrointestinal haemorrhage and haematemesis. The diagnosis is again established by blood or bone marrow examination.

Haemophilia and related disorders

Excessive bleeding from many sites may be associated with haemophilia and other disorders of coagulation.

Gastrointestinal bleeding presenting as haematemesis is relatively common in these conditions; the diagnosis has generally been made before such bleeding occurs. Haemorrhage into joints may be present.

Von Willebrand's disease

A deficiency of von Willebrand factor leads to ineffective platelet adhesion. Bleeding may result, although the defect is generally mild. Sometimes there may be an associated haematemesis.

Scurvy

Haematemesis may occur in severe cases of scurvy. The patient may also have swollen, spongy gums, anaemia, cutaneous haemorrhages and subcutaneous indurations. The patient may give a history of a diet deficient in fresh vegetables, or there may be underlying conditions such as Crohn's disease or coeliac disease leading to malabsorption and malnutrition. Measurement of ascorbic acid levels in blood and in tissues will give the diagnosis.

Drugs

A number of drugs may be associated with haematemesis, the cause being suspected by an accurate and detailed drug history from the patient, or the presence of a disorder such as arthropathy, suggesting that the patient may be having – or has had – drugs such as NSAIDS which may lead to gastrointestinal haemorrhage.

Anticoagulant and antiplatelet therapy

Anticoagulants may be indicated in various conditions, including deep venous thrombosis or pulmonary thromboembolism, and patients on long-term anticoagulant therapy may have significant gastrointestinal haemorrhage from relatively minor lesions in the stomach or duodenum such as small ulcers or erosions. Antiplatelet medications are used in a variety of vascular diseases, in particular the acute coronary syndromes, and increase the risk of gastrointestinal haemorrhage. These include well-established drugs such as aspirin and dipyridamole. Newer drugs now being more commonly prescribed include clopidogrel, and the intravenous glycoprotein IIb/IIIa receptor inhibitors abciximab, tirofiban and eptifibatide.

NSAIDs

These drugs are widely used in all forms of arthropathy, and may lead to the development of haemorrhagic erosions or erosive gastritis in the stomach or duodenum, with haematemesis. They are widely used, especially in elderly patients. An accurate drug history should provide the clue to the cause, but endoscopy will localize the site and assess the severity of the lesion.

Miscellaneous

A number of rarer conditions may be associated with gastrointestinal haemorrhage and haematemesis. These include: severe bleeding from an abdominal aneurysm opening into the stomach or duodenum; uraemia associated with chronic nephritis (in which the presence of high blood pressure, cardiac hypertrophy, retinopathy, polyuria and urine of low specific gravity with albumin or blood present may point to the diagnosis); abdominal surgery; trauma or burns (Curling's ulcer); and autoimmune disorders such as polyarteritis nodosa or systemic lupus erythematosus. Gastrointestinal bleeding may be associated rarely with malignant hypertension and acute febrile disorders.

Melvin Lobo

HAEMATURIA

Haematuria means the presence of red blood cells in the urine and, although free haemoglobin may be present in the urine as a result of lysis of cells in the urinary tract, it should not be confused with haemoglobinuria in which the pigment alone is filtered through the glomeruli. In clinical practice, there are two main ways in which haematuria may pose a diagnostic problem. Macroscopic haematuria may be a presenting feature, with or without other symptoms, or blood may be found in the urine only by 'dipstick' testing or microscopy. In the former case, the remainder of the history and examination – together with special investigations – will be aimed at finding the site and cause of the bleeding. In the latter, the finding of microscopic haematuria will either support a diagnosis already made or suspected, or will prompt specific investigations. The only reason for ignoring

this finding, temporarily, is when blood is found on routine urine testing in a woman who is menstruating.

Frank haematuria – in other words, macroscopic or visible haematuria – may be painful or painless. The colour of the blood may be of some slight significance as, if it is bright red, it is more likely to have come from the bladder or urethra. Initial haematuria is when bleeding occurs at the start of micturition and implies that the bleeding may be coming from the urethra, prostate or bladder neck area. Blood which is mixed with the urinary stream may have a source in the kidneys, ureters or the bladder. The amount of blood present is also of diagnostic importance; in the absence of trauma, a large quantity of blood is suggestive of a tumour of the urinary tract, although profuse bleeding is quite common in several other conditions, for example benign prostatic hypertrophy. Painless haematuria is more likely to be due to neoplasia – bladder tumours most commonly present with this symptom. Painful haematuria is more common where there is associated bladder infection, but tumours cannot be excluded on the basis of clinical history alone.

The history should include an enquiry into the urological symptoms along with the patient's past and family history, together with details of his or her occupation and of any drugs being taken. Loin pain may be associated with a renal lesion and can occur in renal tumours and obstruction. Loin pain that radiates to the groin, and which is colicky in nature, suggests renal colic due to the passage of a stone. Increased urinary frequency or penile pain immediately after micturition suggests bladder disease. Pain in the pelvic or sacral area with haematuria suggests malignant disease in the bladder or prostate. The site of associated symptoms may, however, be misleading. For example, a tumour in the bladder may, by occluding the ureter, cause unilateral hydronephrosis with loin pain; likewise, tuberculosis of the kidney and ureter can cause increased frequency of micturition in the absence of bladder infection.

The physical examination in a patient with haematuria is usually unremarkable. There are no specific signs of haematuria except for blood at the external meatus, which may be seen in association with urethral trauma (as a result of catheterization or pelvic fracture injury). The kidneys should be palpated to determine their size and to elicit any tenderness. Kidneys are not normally palpable except in very thin subjects, and this requires experience. Suprapubic palpation may detect a distended bladder due to retention. A bladder mass is rare except when large tumours are present. Rectal and vaginal examinations will allow the palpation of pelvic viscera. On rectal examination, the uniform, elastic and movable prostate affected by benign hypertrophy can be distinguished from the hard, nodular, often immovable gland without a median groove characteristic of carcinoma. Lymphatic spread from a carcinoma of the bladder or prostate may be palpable as thickening in the lateral pelvic space. A vaginal examination will also allow palpation of the bladder base and lateral pelvic space as well as of the other pelvic organs; in the fornices, the lower end of each ureter can sometimes be felt if it is diseased or contains a calculus. The testes should be examined, particularly for evidence of tuberculosis of the epididymis.

The urine itself should be examined, both by using dipsticks and by sending urine for microscopy and culture. Macroscopic inspection may reveal clots, the shape of which may suggest the source of bleeding. Thus, clots formed in a renal pelvis may be triangular in shape, while those formed in a ureter are likely to be thin and 'worm-like'. Microscopy of the urine is more revealing, but it must be carried out on a fresh specimen. The presence of red cell casts is pathognomonic of glomerular bleeding. Large numbers of oxalate crystals may indicate a tendency to oxalate stone formation; the much rarer crystals of cystine are diagnostic of cystinuria, with its strong tendency to the formation of calculi. The finding of clumps of transitional epithelial cells is suggestive of carcinoma or papilloma of the bladder, and is an indication for formal cytological examination of the urine. Rarely, fragments of renal papillae may be seen, sometimes with the naked eye, in papillary necrosis associated with chronic interstitial nephritis. The presence of leucocytes is not very helpful as they are likely to be found not only in bacterial infections but also in tuberculosis, tumours and benign prostatic hypertrophy.

Further investigation of haematuria should usually include a plain supine X-ray of the abdomen (to look for stones or the shadow of a renal mass) and ultrasound scanning of the urinary tract. Intravenous urography (IVU) is less commonly performed nowadays as ultrasonography provides useful information and will pick up urinary tract tumours in the bladder and kidneys. Where transitional cell carcinoma or ureteric stone are suspected, IVU should be performed. A CT scan of the abdomen and pelvis will be used when a renal tumour is demonstrated on ultrasonography, or in the staging of renal, bladder and prostatic cancer.

The main causes of haematuria are summarized in Table H.2.

Table H.2 Causes of haematuria

Renal	Vesical
Trauma	Trauma
Tumours	Tumours
Calculus	Prostatic enlargement
Glomerulonephritis	Tuberculosis
Polycystic kidneys	Calculus
Tuberculosis	Cystitis
Pyelonephritis	Foreign body
Infarction	Disease of adjacent organs
Polyarteritis nodosa	
Chronic interstitial nephritis	**Urethral**
Hydronephrosis	Urethritis
Irradiation nephritis	Calculus
Hydatid disease	Tumours
Medullary sponge kidney	Foreign body
Relief of tension	Caruncle
Ureteric	**General**
Calculus	Drugs
Tumours	Bleeding disorders

Renal causes of haematuria

Haematuria can follow *trauma* of any degree of severity. A history of an accident or a blow or kick to the lumbar region, which is associated with haematuria, suggests damage to the kidneys. Even slight injury to the loin, of which there may be no recollection or external sign, can cause haematuria, especially if there is a pre-existing renal lesion. The kidney may be palpable, but this may be due to extravasation of blood in the perinephric tissues.

Trauma to the urinary tract may give rise to haematuria, and the site of injury usually indicates the likely source of bleeding. Thus, pelvic fracture may be accompanied by haematuria due to urethral injury. Urethral injury may be contusion or rupture. Blood at the external meatus, although signifying a likely urethral injury, does not mean that the urethra has been completely ruptured. Thus, the gentle passage of a urethral catheter under aseptic conditions may be tried without causing further damage. Traumatic bladder injury may give rise to extravasation. However, the signs may be masked by the associated pelvic injury. A CT scan will help in making the diagnosis.

Renal tumours are important causes of haematuria. The commonest presenting symptom in *carcinoma of the kidney* is profuse intermittent haematuria. A mass may be felt in the loin, and there may be pain in that region resulting from increasing tension or colic from the passage of clots. Unexplained fever, polycythaemia and hypercalcaemia may be present, and hypertension is present in about 30 per cent of cases. An ultrasound scan will demonstrate a mass with mixed echogenicity. When a tumour is suspected on ultrasound scanning, a CT scan will usually confirm the diagnosis. Renal arteriography is not usually performed in the investigation of renal tumours, except when a partial nephrectomy (renal conservation) is proposed so that the vascular anatomy of the kidney can be studied prior to surgery.

In children with *nephroblastoma* (Wilms' tumour), the presenting feature is commonly abdominal distension and a mass is almost always palpable; haematuria occurs later.

An *angiomyolipoma* of the kidney may present with visible bleeding, but is more likely to present with pain in which bleeding has occurred into the perinephric tissues. CT scanning is necessary to diagnose this specifically.

Transitional cell carcinoma of the renal pelvis is uncommon, and may cause profuse haematuria. Ultrasonography may show a filling defect in the renal pelvis. *Squamous cell carcinoma* of the renal pelvis is a very rare cause of slight or moderate haematuria.

Renal calculus seldom causes profuse bleeding. Haematuria (macroscopic or microscopic) and often pyuria, may occur. An ache in the loin is common while the stone remains in the kidney, and may be followed by renal colic if a smaller stone passes down the ureter. This typically very severe pain passes from the loin downwards and forwards to the groin, upper part of the thigh and testicle and is accompanied by urinary frequency. The radiographic diagnosis of ureteric calculus is discussed below (see p. 265). A renal calculus may become too large to pass into the ureter, and may then cause hydronephrosis or pyonephrosis with corresponding symptoms which may include haematuria (Fig. H.2).

Glomerular disease is a common and important cause of haematuria, both macroscopic and microscopic.

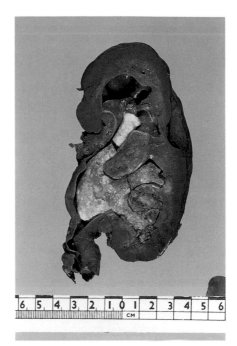

Figure H.2 A large staghorn calcium phosphate stone; operative specimen.

Post-streptococcal glomerulonephritis is now rare in the Western world, but is still common in developing countries where it often follows streptococcal skin infections. The characteristic features are haematuria, producing the typical 'smoky' appearance, and proteinuria, generalized oedema and hypertension. A similar lesion is a common complication of *infective endocarditis*, in which the glomerular changes are focal and segmental. The examination of a fresh specimen of urine will show red cells in a majority of cases of endocarditis, and thus it is an important diagnostic procedure. In both of these conditions the glomerulitis is due to deposition of immune complexes, as it is in *shunt nephritis* associated with infection of shunts used to drain hydrocephalus and in the nephritis occasionally associated with *chronic sepsis*. *Rapidly progressive glomerulonephritis* is a cause of macroscopic haematuria with loin pain; it causes rapid deterioration and can lead to acute renal failure within a few days. It can occur in Henoch–Schönlein syndrome, cryoglobulinaemia, microscopic polyarteritis, Wegener's granulomatosis and the nephritis associated with the development of antibodies to glomerular basement membrane (*anti-GBM nephritis*). The latter is often associated with pulmonary haemorrhage

(*Goodpasture's syndrome*). Another cause of recurrent macroscopic or microscopic haematuria is *Berger's nephritis* (*IgA disease*). The aetiology is unknown, but the episodes of haematuria commonly follow upper respiratory tract infections; the characteristic histological feature is the deposition of IgA in the glomeruli. This condition predominantly affects children and young adults; when it was first described the prognosis was thought to be good, but it is now known to account for cases of chronic renal failure. Nephritis is also a common feature of *Henoch–Schönlein syndrome* which, although occasionally severe (see above), is more often a relatively benign condition characterized by haematuria with typical purpuric and oedematous skin lesions, arthritis and abdominal pain with intestinal bleeding. A number of hereditary varieties of nephritis can also cause haematuria; of these the most common is *Alport's syndrome* in which a renal lesion which is often severe (but less so in females) is associated with nerve deafness; the differential diagnosis, which can be made by renal biopsy, includes *familial benign haematuria* in which proteinuria and deafness do not occur, and intermittent or persistent microscopic haematuria which continues for many years without any deterioration in renal function. Nephritis with haematuria is also a feature of several systemic diseases, of which the most important is *systemic lupus erythematosus* (SLE); of the numerous manifestations of this disease, arthritis, cutaneous lesions and hypertension are those most often associated with nephritis. Haematuria is not one of the typical features of the nephrotic syndrome, but some of the causes of the latter (including SLE) produce sufficient glomerular inflammation to cause haemorrhage. Apart from this, *renal vein thrombosis*, which is a recognized complication of the nephrotic syndrome, causes sudden deterioration in renal function together with haematuria, which is often macroscopic. *Postural proteinuria* – that is, proteinuria occurring *only* in the erect position – is occasionally associated with slight haematuria which does not affect the generally good prognosis; haematuria may also occur with the proteinuria associated with *vigorous* exercise – the so-called 'jogger's nephritis'.

Adult polycystic disease of the kidneys is frequently associated with haematuria, either painless or with clot colic; it can be precipitated by mild trauma. Both kidneys are usually palpable, and hypertension is common. The differential diagnosis includes bilateral hydronephrosis; in the latter situation haematuria is uncommon, and there will usually be evidence of a lesion of the bladder, prostate or urethra causing obstruction. The pyelographic appearances are quite different; in polycystic disease the calyces are narrow and elongated, quite unlike the dilated pelvis in hydronephrosis.

Haematuria in *renal tuberculosis* is usually slight and is associated with pyuria; occasionally, an episode of gross haematuria is the presenting feature. The patients affected are usually young adults who may complain of a dull ache in one loin with occasional exacerbations resembling renal colic. Once the tuberculous focus has ruptured into the renal pelvis, the characteristic symptom is increased frequency of micturition both by day and by night, even without any involvement of the bladder. The bleeding is rarely increased by exertion, unlike with renal calculus. The thickened lower end of the ureter may be palpable on rectal or vaginal examination, and in males nodules may be felt in the prostate or seminal vesicles. The cystoscopic appearance of the ureteric orifice may be distinctive. Hydronephrosis may develop in the affected kidney, and intravenous urography will reveal characteristic changes. The diagnosis can be confirmed by special bacteriological culture of early morning specimens of urine. Other infections of the kidney, such as *acute pyelonephritis*, occasionally cause haematuria.

Vascular lesions of the kidneys can cause haematuria. *Infarction* is usually due to an embolus arising, for example, from a fibrillating left atrium, mural thrombus following myocardial infarction, a large vegetation in infective endocarditis or, very rarely, left atrial myxoma. Infarction can also occur in *macroscopic polyarteritis nodosa*. *Sickle cell disease* may cause haematuria as a consequence of vascular damage, while *aneurysm of the renal artery* and *intrarenal arteriovenous fistula* are also rare causes of haematuria. *Accelerated* ('*malignant*') *hypertension* can cause haematuria which is usually microscopic but occasionally macroscopic.

Less common causes of haematuria include *chronic interstitial nephritis* due to analgesics; bleeding may be profuse when there has been recent papillary necrosis. Recurrent bleeding in such a case should, however, prompt a search for transitional cell carcinoma of the renal pelvis, which is a recognized complication of this condition. In *hydronephrosis*, haematuria is more likely to be due to an obstructive lesion than to the hydronephrosis itself. *Irradiation nephritis* is a rare cause of haematuria. *Medullary sponge kidney* is usually symptomatic, but haematuria and renal colic may occur as a result of calculus formation. The sudden emptying of the bladder in a case of chronic urinary retention may cause bleeding, which usually comes from vessels within the bladder wall or occasionally from the kidney. Slow release of urinary retention does not prevent this, and has no place in the modern management of chronic urinary retention.

Ureteric causes of haematuria

Some 90 per cent of ureteric calculi will be associated with haematuria, which is usually identified with urine dipstick or microscopy, and is unusually macroscopic.

Transitional cell carcinoma of the ureter is rare; it can be diagnosed by finding a filling defect in the ureter with dilatation above on an ultrasound scan of the dilated ureter, an IVU or retrograde ureterography. The differential diagnosis of the negative shadow produced by a tumour in the ureterogram includes a non-opaque calculus or an air bubble.

Vesical causes of haematuria

Intermittent profuse painless haematuria is characteristic of transitional cell carcinoma of the bladder. Other symptoms include urinary frequency and urgency. Cystoscopy is the essential diagnostic procedure. *Bladder tumours* may occur at any age, but are rare below the age of 25, and most commonly occur in the 60s and 70s. Tumours may be either single or multiple. Adenocarcinoma and squamous cell carcinoma of the bladder are rare tumours, as is sarcoma of the bladder. The latter occurs in children and, occasionally, in adults and forms a rapidly growing mass, sometimes resembling a bunch of grapes (sarcoma botryoides). Profuse haematuria may occur in patients with benign or malignant prostatic enlargement. *Vesical tuberculosis* occurs most commonly in young adults. Persistent frequency, slight haematuria and pyuria are suggestive features although, as indicated above, such symptoms can occur in renal tuberculosis before bladder infection has occurred. Evidence of tuberculosis elsewhere, in the lungs or the genital organs, may be found.

A *bladder stone* may produce haematuria due to direct trauma to the bladder from the stone or in association with urinary tract infection.

Acute cystitis is often accompanied by haematuria; the diagnosis will usually be obvious on other grounds.

There is, however, a form of haemorrhagic cystitis in which bleeding predominates over other symptoms; a similar form of haemorrhagic cystitis is a complication of treatment with cyclophosphamide.

Chronic interstitial cystitis more commonly in the female may be accompanied by painful haematuria and an increase in frequency of micturition due to reduced bladder capacity.

Radiation cystitis is characterized by multiple telangiectases in the vesical mucosa which may bleed. Vesical *schistosomiasis* causes slight haematuria and other symptoms similar to those of vesical tuberculosis. There is likely to be a history of residence in an endemic area such as Egypt and the neighbouring countries. The typical ova of *Schistosoma haematobium* may be found in the urine, and at cystoscopy so-called 'sandy patches' may be seen; these consist of numerous ova without any inflammatory reaction.

Foreign bodies may be introduced into the bladder by accident or design and cause bleeding; their presence will be revealed by cystoscopy or radiography.

Haematuria may occur as a result of spread of *disease of neighbouring viscera* to the bladder. Carcinoma of the uterus, vagina, rectum or pelvic colon can all invade the bladder, usually at a late stage of the disease. Haematuria which may result from the contact of an acutely inflamed appendix with the bladder wall and cause localized cystitis. This may be a source of diagnostic confusion, but the other symptoms of acute appendicitis are likely to be present. Rectal examination will reveal the inflammatory process in the right side of the pelvis. More rarely, acute salpingitis or pelvic abscess can cause haematuria by a similar mechanism. Haematuria can also be caused by direct spread of inflammation from tuberculosis or dysenteric ulceration of the intestines or from diverticulitis of the colon; the latter is particularly likely to lead to a vesicocolic fistula with pneumaturia as well as haematuria.

Urethral causes of haematuria

Lesions of the urethra can cause blood to appear spontaneously at the meatus, as well as haematuria. Such conditions include *acute urethritis, calculus, papilloma* and *carcinoma. Angiomas* are rare but can bleed heavily; there may be other similar lesions elsewhere in the body. *Foreign bodies* may be introduced into the urethra as a form of sexual excitement and, in females, a *caruncle* at the urethral orifice.

General causes of haematuria

Several drugs have been implicated as causes of haematuria, but *anticoagulants* are the only ones of practical importance. Haematuria is common if control is poor, but it must be remembered that in such a patient the fact that he or she is receiving anticoagulants does not exclude other causes of haematuria; bleeding apparently induced by anticoagulant therapy can be the first sign of renal, bladder or prostatic carcinoma. Finally, *thrombocytopenia* and disorders of platelet function can cause haematuria, as can *haemophilia, Christmas disease* and, occasionally, *scurvy*. In these conditions the diagnosis will usually be clear on other grounds.

Harold Ellis

HAEMOPTYSIS

The coughing up of blood is defined as haemoptysis, a term generally accepted to refer specifically to expectoration of blood resulting from bleeding in the lungs or bronchi. The amount of expectorated blood may vary widely from slight streaking of the sputum to massive exsanguinating haemorrhage. Blood – either alone or mixed with sputum – is nearly always produced by coughing, but rarely may trickle past the larynx to 'well up in the throat'. For this reason, some patients with *true haemoptysis* present to an otolaryngologist. Blood from the nasopharynx or larynx may lead to spitting of blood or blood-stained secretions. This is sometimes called *spurious haemoptysis* since the blood does not in the strict sense arise from the lungs.

In the assessment of haemoptysis it is important to establish whether the bleeding has arisen from the chest, from the nasopharynx, or the upper gastrointestinal tract. Although examination of the nasopharynx should never be omitted, it is unusual to find bleeding lesions in the upper respiratory tract. Bleeding of oesophageal, gastric or duodenal origin can usually be differentiated from haemoptysis by the presence of gastrointestinal symptoms, such as nausea or vomiting, or a history of oesophageal varices or peptic ulcer disease. Prompt upper gastrointestinal tract endoscopy will settle the issue in doubtful cases. Distinguishing features that might help differentiate between haemoptysis and haematemesis are listed in Table H.3.

Patients usually regard the presence of blood in the sputum as a sinister sign of serious lung disease. Haemoptysis may be a single event, and of little prognostic importance if a slight blood-staining of the sputum follows a repeated violent bout of coughing. An effortless haemoptysis of 1–2 ml of blood is much more likely to be of importance, especially if it is followed by the production of further blood-stained sputum. The history and physical examination, with special attention to the respiratory and cardiovascular systems (including the leg veins) and to the nasopharynx, may provide clues to the underlying cause of haemoptysis, but are seldom diagnostic. A technically satisfactory chest X-ray is mandatory, and may reveal evidence of old or new inflammatory lesions, probable malignancies, or vascular abnormalities. Routine laboratory tests should include a full blood count and tests to exclude a bleeding diathesis. Virtually every patient with significant haemoptysis should undergo bronchoscopy to determine the site of bleeding and its cause, although the timing of the procedure is controversial. Whilst it is desirable to determine the site of bleeding, this can be difficult if all the airways contain fresh blood. Sputum cytology may be of value. If routine investigations are

Table H.3 Haemoptysis and haematemesis: distinguishing features

Suggesting haemoptysis	*Suggesting haematemesis*
Respiratory symptoms	Dyspepsia
Tickle or gurgle in the throat; cough	Faintness; abdominal pain; nausea
Blood produced by repeated acts of coughing; may be mixed with sputum; blood-stained sputum may be produced for several days	Blood produced by isolated acts of vomiting; may be mixed with food debris
Usually bright red; may be frothy; reaction on alkaline side	Usually dark in colour; may resemble coffee-grounds; usually acid in reaction
Rapid bleeding either from lung or from upper alimentary tract produces only slightly altered blood, with or without clots	
Stools usually normal in appearance; may contain occult blood	Stools often dark and tarry (melaena) and always give positive test for occult blood

normal but haemoptysis persists, then further imaging of the chest by CT scanning may be helpful to exclude the possibility of localized bronchiectasis and to assist in identifying the presence of arteriovenous fistulae.

Haemoptysis, especially isolated instances of blood-staining of sputum, often remains unexplained even after extensive investigations. Up to one-fifth of patients are in this category, and it is conventional to follow them with further chest radiography after an interval of about 2 months, with the view also of obtaining the results of culture for mycobacteria and repeating investigations as necessary.

The causes of haemoptysis according to appearances on chest radiography are listed in Table H.4.

Table H.4 Causes of haemoptysis on chest radiography

Radiological abnormality which is readily diagnosed
Pulmonary tuberculosis
Tumours of the lung – carcinoma, adenoma, etc.
Pneumonia
Pulmonary infarction
Aspergilloma
Contused lung due to trauma
Mitral stenosis
Large arteriovenous malformation

Radiological abnormality, the nature of which is not immediately obvious
Pulmonary infarction
Pulmonary haemosiderosis
   Childhood haemosiderosis
   Adult haemosiderosis
Goodpasture's syndrome
Associated with systemic lupus erythematosus
Associated with pulmonary vasculitis

With no gross radiological abnormality
Mitral stenosis
Pulmonary embolism
Essential hypertension
Bronchitis and/or bronchiectasis
Tumours of the larynx, trachea or larger bronchi not yet blocking
   the lumen
Hereditary haemorrhagic telangiectasia and other pulmonary
   arteriovenous malformations

Bleeding diathesis
The primary disease is virtually always obvious from its other
   manifestations. Puzzling haemoptysis is rarely due to an
   unrecognized bleeding disorder

Iatrogenic
Needle lung biopsy
Transbronchial lung biopsy

Spurious haemoptysis

Bleeding from the upper respiratory tract usually presents as obvious bleeding from the gums or from the nose (see EPISTAXIS, p. 177). As noted above, it may give rise to 'haemoptysis', because blood can be aspirated into the lungs during sleep and subsequently expectorated on awakening, possibly mixed with bronchial secretions. The nasopharynx should be examined in all cases of haemoptysis.

True haemoptysis

The patient's age and environment are of importance. Where tuberculosis is a common disease, haemoptysis must always give rise to a suspicion of pulmonary tuberculosis, especially in younger patients. Bronchial carcinoma is a frequent cause of haemoptysis in middle-aged or older patients who smoke cigarettes. With either of these diseases there may be a history of ill health with non-specific respiratory symptoms preceding haemoptysis by a few weeks or months; however, the haemoptysis is often the first event to alert the patient to seek medical advice.

Pulmonary tuberculosis

Haemoptysis is often an early symptom of pulmonary tuberculosis. At this stage, physical examination is seldom abnormal, but radiographic changes are to be expected with localized mottled shadowing or consolidation, possibly with cavitation. Rarely, haemoptysis may arise from radiographically obscure disease, with localized shadowing concealed by the overlying skeleton, hilar or mediastinal shadows. Lateral, apical, tomographic or CT scanning views may then be required for diagnosis. Haemoptysis in patients with active tuberculosis varies in severity from streaky staining of the sputum to profuse life-threatening bleeding. Severe haemoptysis may arise in chronic cavitated disease from rupture of aneurysmal dilatation of an artery, exceptionally remaining patent in a strand of tissue traversing a cavity – the so-called 'aneurysm of Rasmussen'. Old calcified tuberculous lesions may also be sufficient cause for haemoptysis simply due to local bronchiectasis, though reactivation of tuberculosis must be considered. Investigation of all cases in which there is radiological evidence suggesting active or inactive tuberculosis must include examination of the sputum for tubercle bacilli.

Fungal infections

When more common diseases such as tuberculosis have been excluded, histoplasmosis, coccidioidomycosis and blastomycosis must be considered in the differential diagnosis of haemoptysis associated with abnormal appearances in the lung, especially in areas where these diseases are prevalent. Diagnosis depends upon isolation of the causal organism, and may be aided by serological tests. Other rare infections that must be similarly considered when tuberculosis has been excluded include actinomycosis, nocardiosis and cryptococcosis; diagnosis of these depends upon isolation of the causal organism.

Bronchial carcinoma

Haemoptysis, an early symptom of bronchial carcinoma, usually takes the form of blood-streaking of sputum and possibly small free haemoptysis, often repeated over days or weeks. Later, more severe bleeding may occur from the erosion of larger vessels, either by the tumour or by the suppuration, which often results from bacterial infection beyond it. Bronchial carcinoma must be suspected especially in cigarette smokers at or past middle-age, but may occur in younger individuals. There is usually an obvious abnormality on the chest X-ray; the more common findings are of two sorts. The first abnormality is associated with tumours originating in large bronchi, and consists of air-absorption collapse or consolidation of a segment, a lobe (Fig. H.3) or even a whole lung beyond a complete obstruction, or patchy inflammatory consolidation beyond a partial obstruction. The second abnormality consists of localized (usually rounded) shadows in the lung fields, produced by tumours originating more peripherally. In some cases of squamous cell carcinoma, a rounded shadow of this sort may show a central transradiant area, due to necrosis of the central part of the tumour. Such appearances must lead to a provisional diagnosis of bronchial carcinoma. In occasional cases, a bronchial carcinoma arising in a large bronchus causes haemoptysis before it has obstructed the bronchus and before there is any abnormality on the ordinary chest X-ray taken in full inspiration. In such patients there is likely to be a wheeze that may be mistaken for an asthmatic or bronchitic wheeze of expiratory airflow obstruction. Wheezes due to partial obstruction of larger airways differ in two respects.

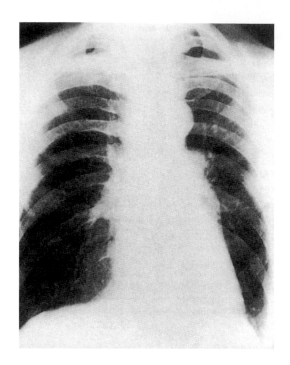

Figure H.3 Radiograph of the chest showing collapse of the left lower lobe due to carcinoma of the bronchus. Note the displacement of the heart to the left, the slight raising of the diaphragm, and slight narrowing of the spaces between the left lower ribs; the displaced heart almost hides the characteristic triangular shadow of the collapsed lung itself.

First, they may be localized and 'fixed' – that is, they do not clear on coughing. Second, they are as apparent in inspiration as in expiration – a fact that can be confirmed on spirometry; inspiratory flow rates are decreased as much as expiratory flow rates, resulting in characteristic changes in the volume–flow loops. Another way of recognizing partial obstruction of one of the lobar or main bronchi is to take a chest X-ray on full expiration. This may result in air trapping in the affected lobe or lung.

In all cases of suspected bronchial carcinoma, at least three specimens of sputum should be examined for malignant cells. These will yield about 70 per cent true positive and 30 per cent false negative results on patients who have bronchial carcinoma. The tumour cell type can be predicted as accurately by sputum cytology as by a specimen obtained at bronchoscopy. Hence, if the sputum cytology is positive, then bronchoscopy is unnecessary in patients who are clearly inoperable by reason of general frailty or the spread of the tumour. When sputum cytology yields negative results, fibre-optic bronchoscopy is indicated to obtain histological specimens by brush biopsy, forceps biopsy and bronchial washings. In the case of peripheral tumours that cannot be reached by fibre-optic bronchoscopy, even under fluoroscopic control, transthoracic biopsy with a thin needle may be indicated. As transthoracic needle biopsy is a 'rule in' test (i.e. whilst a positive result is diagnostic, a negative result does not rule out carcinoma), patients should not be exposed unnecessarily to the risks of this when thoracotomy will be indicated, whatever the result.

Bronchial adenoma

Haemoptysis is an important symptom in *bronchial adenoma*; these tumours may be highly vascular. Episodes of haemoptysis may occur over several years, and there may also be a history of recurrent attacks of pneumonia always involving the same lobe. There may be clinical and radiological evidence of lobar collapse or consolidation, possibly with abscess formation; an adenoma in a central bronchus may present with the manifestations of partial obstruction of a large airway, as described above for bronchial carcinoma. Since most of the tumours arise in the large bronchi, a bronchoscopic diagnosis is straightforward.

Pneumonia

Bacterial pneumonias usually present as an acute illness with chest pain, dyspnoea, cough, fever and even rigors. The characteristic clinical features and the results of the blood count and direct examination of the Gram-stained smear of sputum that indicate the likely organism (for initiation of therapy), before the results of sputum cultures become available, are listed in Table H5. Haemoptysis rarely amounts to more than bloodstaining; the rusty sputum associated especially with *pneumococcal pneumonia* usually does not appear until several days after the beginning of the illness. If the sputum is (or becomes) frankly purulent, the possibility of a *suppurative pneumonia* or *lung abscess* must be considered. Haemoptysis associated with lung abscess may be secondary to bronchial obstruction (e.g. by carcinoma), especially in middle-aged or older smokers, but more rarely by an adenoma in younger adults, or a foreign body in children.

Pulmonary infarction

This diagnosis is simple if haemoptysis is preceded or accompanied by pleuritic pain of sudden onset, and possibly by slight fever with or without dyspnoea, in a

Table H.5 Acute pneumonia in previously healthy adults and children

Causes of pneumonia	Initial clinical features	Age	Blood count	Gram-stained sputum smear
Streptococcus pneumoniae Staphylococcus aureus	Sudden onset with fever, cough and pleuritic chest pain	All ages especially adults	Leucocytosis >12 000/mm³	Smear shows bacteria and large numbers of leucocytes
Haemophilus influenzae		Children		
Legionella pneumophila	Onset with 'flu'-like symptoms and chest pain, confusion, diarrhoea and abdominal pain	Middle aged or elderly males	Leucocytosis <15 000/mm³ Lymphocytopenia <1000/mm³	
Mycoplasma pneumoniae	More gradual onset with general symptoms of malaise, body pains and headache, with symptoms of upper respiratory tract infection	Young adults and children		Sputum mucoid Few leucocytes No significant pathogens seen
Chlamydia psittaci		Adults		
Coxiella burnetti		Adults		
Influenza viruses		All ages		
Adenovirus		Young adults and children	Normal or a leucopenia	
RS virus				
		Children 3–5 years old		
Measles	Rash, etc.	Children		
Varicella	Rash, etc.	Adults		

patient with heart disease (especially if there is atrial fibrillation), or if the patient has present evidence of deep leg vein thrombosis providing an obvious origin for a *pulmonary embolus*. However, in many patients, signs of pelvic or leg vein thrombosis do not become clinically manifest until days or weeks after an episode of pulmonary embolism, and sometimes never at all. Disorders known to increase the risk of venous thromboembolism – which, if present, should raise the diagnostic suspicion of *pulmonary infarction* as the cause of haemoptysis – are listed in Table H.6.

Table H.6 Factors predisposing to increased risk of venous thromboembolism

Disease process	*General*
Surgery – especially pelvic	Increasing age
Myocardial infarction	Previous thromboembolism
Congestive cardiac failure	Varicose veins
Trauma	Obesity
Stroke	Pregnancy
Malignant disease – especially pancreatic	Oral contraceptive use
Lower limb fracture – especially the hip	Immobility
	Bed rest
	Air and bus travel

Bronchiectasis

Haemoptysis in a patient with a long history of cough and persistently or intermittently purulent sputum, possibly with episodes of increased volume and purulence associated with fever, suggests *bronchiectasis* (see Fig. D.26). Localized crackles may be found persistently over the affected part of the lung, and clubbing of the fingers may be present, particularly in those with long-standing persistently purulent infection. Bleeding probably arises from the large pulmonary–systemic arterial anastomoses that develop in long-standing cases; it may be the principal symptom and may be severe, even with bronchiectasis of limited extent. CT scanning of the thorax may help to establish the diagnosis. Bronchography may be performed prior to surgical resection of bronchiectasis, but is seldom required for diagnosis.

Chronic bronchitis

Patients with chronic bronchitis not uncommonly cough up blood-streaked sputum, especially during an exacerbation of their condition; expectoration of pure blood is much less common. In either case some explanation for the haemoptysis, other than chronic bronchitis, should always be considered. Chronic bronchitics are nearly always cigarette-smokers, and they are also candidates for carcinoma of the lung. (For a discussion of the recognition of chronic bronchitis, see p. 270.)

Aspergilloma

The fungus *Aspergillus fumigatus* particularly colonizes not only open healed tuberculous cavities, but also any previously damaged lung tissue, such as occurs in bronchiectasis, sarcoidosis and pneumoconiosis, diffuse fibrosis and localized fibrosis of the lung (as associated with ankylosing spondylitis). The mycelia grow into a ball that almost fills the cavity but leaves a crescent of air above the opacity. This results in the characteristic radiological appearances.

Aspergillomas are usually discovered on a routine chest X-ray, but recurrent haemoptysis is a characteristic feature and may herald a massive pulmonary haemorrhage.

A sputum examination for aspergilli is unhelpful because the organisms may be present in healthy persons and are, in any case, not often identified in the sputum of patients with aspergilloma. There is a useful precipitin test which is almost always strongly positive, whereas the aspergillin skin test is positive only in about 20 per cent of cases.

Foreign bodies in the tracheobronchial tree

These can give rise to haemoptysis in two ways. Soon after lodgement, a hard foreign body with sharp edges may lacerate the mucosa, cause local ulceration and lead to bleeding which is usually slight, with no more than blood-streaked sputum. Later, infection beyond a foreign body obstructing a bronchus can cause pneumonia, abscess formation and, if neglected, eventually bronchiectasis – all of which are possible causes of haemoptysis. If it is not radio-opaque, or if it is lodged centrally where it may be hidden in the mediastinal shadow, a foreign body will be radiologically inapparent, and provide no radiological evidence of its presence until the secondary changes arising from bronchial obstruction appear. A non-occluding foreign body of metal, bone or plastic material often produces no immediate irritative symptoms, and haemoptysis may be the first symptom to draw attention to its presence. The diagnosis will be made or confirmed at bronchoscopy.

Hydatid cyst

Infection with *Echinococcus granulosus* is particularly prevalent in the Middle East, Mediterranean coastal countries, South America, South Africa and Australia. Haemoptysis is the most common single symptom of an intact hydatid cyst, and is possibly due to the size of the cyst causing congestion and blood vessel erosion; indeed, it often precedes cyst rupture. When a cyst has ruptured, infection often complicates the picture, with all the possible consequences of pulmonary suppuration, including severe haemoptysis. The diagnosis will be suggested by the chest X-ray, which will show one or more rounded shadows. The rupture of cysts and added infection will, of course, affect the appearances. Complement fixation and Casoni skin tests may be helpful in diagnosis.

Paragonimiasis

Haemoptysis is a leading feature of infection with the lung fluke, *Paragonimus westermani*. This occurs endemically in Japan, China, Korea and Taiwan; it also occurs in Africa, particularly in the Cameroons. In addition to haemoptysis, cough and chest pain are apparent. The chest X-ray shows characteristic air-containing cysts, usually 1–2 mm in diameter with a thickened base, scattered throughout the lungs. These cysts may be mistaken for tuberculous cavities, particularly if the changes are limited to the subclavicular zones as frequently happens. The diagnosis finally depends upon the finding of ova in sputum or stool.

Other parasitic infestations

Haemoptysis may occur either as parasites pass through the lungs, or when they finally settle in the lungs. Most of these parasites have fairly well-defined geographic distributions, and are only likely to affect those patients who are (or have been) resident in endemic areas. Among parasites which may cause haemoptysis by their passage through the lungs are included:

- *Ascaris lumbricoides*, which has a worldwide distribution.
- *Schistosoma*, of which various species have different, mainly tropical, distributions. These cause haemoptysis during the passage of larvae through the lungs, though the principal pulmonary manifestation – obliterative

arteriolitis with granuloma formation – arises later and is not especially associated with haemoptysis.
- *Dirofilaria immitis*, the heart-worm of dogs in Australia, which may cause haemoptysis and radiologically detectable lesions in the lungs of humans.

Pulmonary haemosiderosis

Pulmonary haemosiderosis is a condition which is characterized by episodic bleeding into the lungs, and this results in the deposition of haemosiderin in intra-alveolar macrophages and in interstitial histiocytes, together with a variable degree of alveolar wall fibrosis in the more chronic forms of the disease. The disorder presents in different ways at different ages.

In *childhood haemosiderosis*, acute episodes of pulmonary haemorrhage with fever, cough, haemoptysis and breathlessness occur, and the child is found to be anaemic. The individual episodes are often self-limiting and clear rapidly, but they can be life-threatening. The sputum characteristically contains iron-laden macrophages between the episodes of haemorrhage. Physical signs in the chest are unimpressive; crackles are sometimes heard. The chest X-ray shows large bilateral confluent lesions which appear and disappear rapidly. Antibasement membrane (ABM) antibodies are not found.

In *adult idiopathic haemosiderosis*, there is a gradually increasing breathlessness accompanied by small 'fleck' haemoptyses, which occurs repeatedly over a prolonged period. The chest X-ray shows widespread fine stippling, often of pinhead size, and most densely distributed at the bases. Areas of acute confluent shadowing are rarely seen. The appearances may remain unaltered over many years. A physical examination of the chest usually reveals little in the way of abnormal signs unless alveolar wall fibrosis is marked, when finger clubbing may develop. The diagnosis is made by finding haemosiderin-laden macrophages in the sputum between episodes of haemoptysis. If there is no sputum for examination, macrophages can be obtained by bronchoalveolar lavage using the fibre-optic bronchoscope. Large numbers of these iron-laden cells are obtained, sometimes rendering the lavage fluid almost black. Some patients have air-flow obstruction as well as a restrictive defect; the explanation for this is not known, but the finding does not negate the diagnosis.

Goodpasture's syndrome occurs most frequently (but not exclusively) in young male cigarette smokers (male:female ratio, 6:1). The pulmonary lesions usually develop first; there is episodic haemoptysis which is sometimes severe enough to be life-threatening, and the chest X-ray shows confluent or widespread fine shadows related to the severity of the bleeding. Within about a year renal impairment develops, with fairly rapid progression to renal failure and death.

The features that distinguish this form of pulmonary haemosiderosis from the others is the presence in the serum of ABM antibodies. These antibodies are believed to cross-react with the basement membranes of both the lungs and the kidneys. Renal and lung biopsies demonstrate a pattern of linear fluorescence, both in the glomeruli and along the capillaries in the alveolar walls. Typically, the disorder affects cigarette smokers who present with cough, dyspnoea and haemoptysis which may be streaky and intermittent, or sometimes severe enough to be life-threatening. The lungs are usually spared in non-smokers.

Systemic lupus erythematosus (SLE) may be associated with recurrent haemoptyses. The chest X-ray usually shows widespread confluent patchy shadows, and the patient has other clinical features of SLE; immunological tests confirm this diagnosis. The lesion in the lung is believed to be due to a pulmonary vasculitis. In contrast to some other types of haemosiderosis, resolution with corticosteroids is often dramatic.

Diffuse lymphangioleiomyomatosis

This exceedingly rare condition is diagnosed by histological examination of a lung biopsy from patients who present with a diffuse lung disorder, haemoptysis and slowly increasing breathlessness. Obstructive distortion of the pulmonary veins by hypertrophic muscle leads to capillary haemorrhage and resulting siderosis. Other clinical features are recurrent pneumothoraces and chylothorax. The aetiology has not been established, but the condition is probably a hamartomatous malformation of lymphatic and perilymphatic tissue.

Systemic vasculitides

In the rare cases of *polyarteritis nodosa* in which the pulmonary arteries are involved with consequent small infarctions of the lung, haemoptysis may occur. Suspicion of the diagnosis depends on the other systemic features of polyarteritis nodosa. Confirmation of the diagnosis may be by tissue biopsy or the demonstration of multiple intraparenchymal aneurysms on visceral angiography.

In the *Churg–Strauss syndrome* (*eosinophilic granulomatosis, allergic angiitis and granulomatosis*), there is usually a long history of asthma with eosinophilia and eventually the patient develops other manifestations of generalized vasculitis. Haemoptysis, though not a particular feature, may occur; the chest X-ray may be normal or show transient or 'fixed infiltrations' or nodules.

Haemoptysis is more likely to be a clinical symptom in *Wegener's granulomatosis*. This condition is characterized by necrotizing granulomas in the respiratory tract, including the nose and sinuses. There is also widespread vasculitis which usually affects the kidney. The chest X-ray shows multiple, usually bilateral nodular shadows which may vary in size from time to time and may cavitate; when they do so, the cavities often have thick irregular walls. Diagnosis is made by biopsy of a lesion in the nose, sinuses or lung.

Arteriovenous fistula of the lung

This usually causes symptoms and signs arising from shunting of mixed venous blood directly from pulmonary artery into pulmonary vein – effectively a 'right-to-left' shunt. Haemoptysis occurs in only a minority of cases. About half of these are associated with *hereditary haemorrhagic telangiectasia*, of which epistaxis is a frequent symptom.

Trauma

Haemoptysis occurs not only when the lung is directly penetrated, or lacerated by fractured ribs, but also in non-penetrating injuries. These may be associated with contusion of the lung, even without rib fractures. Exposure to blast from explosions may cause haemorrhagic consolidation of the lung (blast injury) with haemoptysis.

Mitral stenosis

The heart should be carefully auscultated for signs of mitral stenosis in all cases of haemoptysis. Rheumatic heart disease is less often encountered in Western countries. The cause of the haemoptysis may be the high pulmonary venous pressure or pulmonary embolism and infarction, particularly in patients with atrial fibrillation and/or cardiac failure. Pulmonary embolism leading to infarcts, especially in patients with atrial fibrillation, is a frequent cause. Less severe bleeding leading to blood-stained sputum may be associated with the high pulmonary venous pressure.

Left ventricular failure

The thin, frothy sputum produced in pulmonary oedema is frequently tinged pink with blood. Diagnosis depends upon the recognition of the underlying cardiac disease.

Aortic aneurysm

An aortic aneurysm may erode into a bronchus, leading to rapidly fatal haemorrhage with massive haemoptysis. Most aneurysms of the thoracic aorta seen now arise as a result of traumatic dissection following a road traffic accident. The classic syphilitic aortic aneurysm has become a rarity.

Bleeding diathesis

In disease associated with disturbances of haemostasis and clotting, such as *thrombocytopenia, Henoch–Schönlein purpura, scurvy, leukaemias* and *aplastic anaemia*, haemoptysis may occur, but as a minor feature of a generalized bleeding tendency in which epistaxis and bleeding from the gums are more prominent. These may be accompanied by bleeding from the alimentary or urinary tracts, or by purpura, leading to appropriate haematological investigations. Haemoptysis is virtually never the sole clinically evident presenting feature of these diseases.

Factitious 'haemoptysis'

When a patient presents with a history of haemoptysis as the sole symptom, and investigation has shown no evidence of its source, nor of any organic disease, it must be remembered that single episodes of unexplained haemoptysis are not uncommon. Moreover, the patient may have come for investigation because they sought reassurance; for instance, they may have a friend who has been found to be suffering from tuberculosis or bronchial carcinoma with haemoptysis as an initial symptom, and have become alarmed lest the streaks of blood they notice after cleaning their teeth are the first sign of the same thing in themselves. Very occasionally, a patient returns with recurrent complaints of haemoptyses, the blood being deliberately produced by various forms of trauma in the mouth or pharynx.

Boris Lams

HALLUCINATIONS

Hallucinations may most simply be defined as *percepts without objects*. They need to be distinguished from illusions, which are *misperceived objects*.

It has been known for well over a century now that certain types of hallucinations are found in normal mental health. For example, hearing one's name called in the street or hearing a phone ring is not unusual. States of expectancy, exhaustion, sensory deprivation or sleep deprivation will certainly provoke hallucinations in people with good mental health. In such instances, a degree of insight into the hallucinatory nature of the perception is generally maintained, and some authorities call such phenomena 'pseudohallucinations'. Bereavement is another state in which hallucinations commonly occur, typically auditory or visual hallucinations of the deceased. Brief hallucinations on falling asleep (hypnogogic) or upon waking from sleep (hypnopompic) are also reported in the general population, and this can also be prominent in narcoleptic patients.

However, the sensory modality, duration and other detailed features of hallucinations can be of great diagnostic value. For example, if a general hospital in-patient describes visual hallucinations they are best initially considered delirious until proven otherwise. Intoxication or withdrawal from drugs or alcohol must be immediately considered. Delirium tremens, an acute confusional state complicating the early days of withdrawal from alcohol, typically includes visual hallucinations of insects or rodents scuttling along floors and walls. Prescribed medication with atropine-like actions is a potent cause of visual hallucinosis and disorientation in the elderly. If the visual hallucination recurs sporadically over several weeks, but is always the same in form and content, the possibility of an epileptic focus or space-occupying lesion is raised. Sustained Lilliputian visual hallucinations are almost pathognomic of the rare Charles Bonnet syndrome.

About 20 per cent of patients with schizophrenia report visual hallucinations, and these can be quite complex tableaux connected to delusional beliefs. Visual hallucinations in psychotic depression are rare and tend to be mood-congruent pictures of morbid scenes such as coffins and corpses. Finally, the classical visual hallucinations of LSD intoxication (and subsequent flashbacks) deserve mention. These tend

Table H.7 Causes of hallucinations

Sleep and sensory deprivation
Extreme fatigue
Bereavement
Narcolepsy
Delirium
Alcoholic hallucinosis
Drugs
- Amphetamine
- Cocaine, LSD, mescaline, magic mushrooms, dimethyltryptamine, anticholinergics, bromocriptine, inhaled solvents
Schizophrenia
Mania
Depression
Post-concussional states
Temporal lobe epilepsy
Intracranial space-occupying lesions

to involve shifting geometric patterns or surreally altered figures (e.g. a man with the head of a tortoise).

Auditory hallucinations can also be of great diagnostic value. Patients who hear their own thoughts spoken out loud in external space, or their thoughts echoed by voices, or their behaviour discussed by others in the third person as a running commentary, are most likely to suffer from schizophrenia. In the acute, early phase of the disorder this can be an extremely distressing experience, while over a period of years many patients gain a degree of acceptance or even mastery of the problem. It should be added that auditory hallucinations of this form are also found in 20 per cent of manic patients. The auditory hallucinations of patients with psychotic depression or mania tend to be briefer, mood-congruent phenomena in the second person (for example 'Why don't you just kill yourself', or 'You are the Messiah'). Auditory hallucinations do occur in delirium, and musical hallucinations in particular should prompt a serious investigation for an organic aetiology.

Olfactory hallucinations, typically of unpleasant smells, occur commonly in schizophrenia but also as an aura to temporal lobe epilepsy. Tactile hallucinations, particularly formication (the feeling of ants crawling under the skin), point to cocaine misuse or alcohol withdrawal. Bizarre somatic hallucinations, such as the feeling of being impregnated, do occur in schizophrenia.

The common causes of hallucinations are summarized in Table H.7.

Andrew Hodgkiss

HANDS, CONDITIONS AFFECTING

See UPPER LIMB, PAIN IN (p. 754).

HEAD, RETRACTION OF

The common causes of head retraction (and stiffness) are listed in Table H.8. At its most dramatic (as in meningitis), it is possible to lift the whole body by lifting the head up. Stiffness due to disease of the cervical spine and paraspinal tissues is dealt with elsewhere (see p. 476).

Table H.8 Causes of retraction of the head

Meningism
Meningitis
- Bacterial
- Viral
- Spirochaetal
- Fungal
- Carcinomatous
- Sarcoid
Subarachnoid haemorrhage
Pressure cones
Asphyxia
Intermittent retraction
- Spasmodic torticollis
- Torsion spasm
- Tetanus
- Rabies
- Strychnine poisoning
Spinal and paraspinal disease

The term *meningism* is applied to the headache, photophobia and stiff neck which occur, as a rule, in children, in the course of general infections such as tonsillitis, pneumonia and pyelitis. The pressure of the spinal fluid is raised, but its contents are normal.

Meningitis causes resistance to forward flexion of the neck, but this may be absent in very mild cases and also in fulminating infections. Actual retraction of the head is best seen in tuberculous meningitis and in meningococcal meningitis. Inflammation of the leptomeninges is caused by many organisms – bacteria, viruses, spirochaetes and yeasts – and a low-grade 'meningitis' can occur when the meninges are invaded by secondary carcinomatosis and sarcoidosis.

Features common to most cases of meningitis are headache, photophobia, vomiting, giddiness and fever.

There may be a rigor, or a convulsion, at the onset of the more virulent types, especially in children. There is stiffness of the neck, spinal muscles and hamstrings. Thus, forward flexion of the neck is resisted, and it may evoke flexion of the hips and knees (Brudzinski's sign). There is resistance to extension of the knee on the flexed thigh (Kernig's sign), because this movement pulls on the roots of the cauda equina. There may or may not be evidence of focal damage to the brain and cranial nerves. The latter are involved as they traverse the subarachnoid space, and the brain itself can be damaged by spread of the infection along the meningeal sheaths which cover the vessels as they penetrate the surface of the brain. Moreover, thrombosis both of arteries and of veins can occur, with infarction, oedema or brain abscess as a result.

Infection can gain access to the meninges by several routes. In most cases it is blood-borne, and in an important minority it spreads from local infections in the ear, accessory nasal sinuses, face and scalp. The existence of this second group emphasizes the need to seek for evidence in the history and on physical examination as to the possibility of local infection in every case. Points to be looked for are the presence of otitis, mastoiditis or sinusitis. Moreover, a history of head injury, whether recent or remote, may mean that there is a fracture and a dural tear leading into an air sinus, thereby providing a path for the entry of microorganisms. In such cases, meningitis is apt to be associated with an abscess, whether extradural, intradural or intracerebral, along the track of entry. Sepsis in the face or scalp, such as furunculosis, erysipelas, infected scalp wounds or herpes, can lead to meningitis in debilitated persons. Infection may also enter via a meningocele, or a congenital dermal sinus at the base of the spine, and these must be looked for in unexplained meningitis in infants. Yet another manner of infection is following lumbar puncture or spinal anaesthesia, fortunately rare; in such cases low-grade infection is usual (e.g. by *Bacillus pyocyaneus*).

Meningococcal meningitis (syn. spotted fever, cerebrospinal fever) usually occurs in epidemics which are initiated by droplet infection from healthy carriers. A bacteraemia precedes the meningitis by hours, days or even weeks. Occasionally, there is a *chronic meningococcal septicaemia* with fever, purpura and transient pain, and swelling in the joints, and a proportion of such cases will end up with meningitis. In another small group, the patient is overwhelmed by a fulminating septicaemia within a few hours of the onset; some pass rapidly into coma, without a significant fall in blood pressure, while others remain clear in mind but suffer a drastic fall in blood pressure due to circulatory collapse, and these cases usually present a diffuse purpuric rash on the skin (the *Waterhouse–Friderichsen syndrome*, which is also seen in other severe infections). In the usual type of meningococcal meningitis, however, there is fever, meningeal irritation, severe headache and sometimes a purpuric or macular rash. Convulsions may occur at the onset. Transient cranial nerve palsies and papilloedema may be found, and delirium is common. Tendon reflexes are reduced, and extensor plantar responses are common in the more severe cases. The spinal fluid in meningitis usually contains a polymorph pleocytosis, with a rise of protein and a fall of glucose. Both intracellular and extracellular diplococci are found.

In some cases of *meningococcal meningitis*, the exudate is largely confined to the base of the brain, thereby leading to an obstructive hydrocephalus. There is mild fever, vomiting, papilloedema and head retraction. In infants (the usual victims), the head enlarges and there is a slow downward course with emaciation, vomiting and increasing stupor. During the first few days of the illness the changes in the spinal fluid are the same as in the ordinary type of meningococcal meningitis, but thereafter the meningococci disappear and there is merely a lymphocytic pleocytosis, a rise of protein, and rather a low sugar content. In such cases ventricular tap may produce the diplococcus.

Further sequels of meningococcal meningitis are the subdural hygroma referred to above, cranial nerve palsies, and disabilities arising from the formation of scar tissue around the spinal cord. These include a lower motor neurone paralysis of muscles in the limbs, and occasionally an incomplete transverse lesion of the cord with paraplegia, sensory impairment and sphincter disturbances.

Other forms of pyogenic meningitis are sporadic rather than epidemic in incidence, do not as a rule produce a rash, and are usually derived from a more or less obvious source of infection. Thus, *pneumococcal cases* commonly arise from infection in the ears or sinuses, or from pneumococcal pneumonia. *Streptococcal meningitis* is rarer than the pneumococcal form, but occurs in similar circumstances; in a proportion of cases, however, there is a cerebral abscess in addition to the meningitis, and this must always be looked for, if necessary by CT scanning. *Haemophilus influenzae* (Pfeiffer) is an important cause of meningitis in infants, and may cause the disease in adults; it may or may not be preceded by upper respiratory infection or by pneumonia. The signs of meningeal irritation may be slight. Other bacterial causes of meningitis are relatively rare, and they will be identified by culture of the spinal fluid.

Meningitis with a predominantly lymphocytic response in the cerebrospinal fluid (CSF) occurs in infection by tuberculosis, viruses, yeasts and spirochaetes. Of these, tuberculosis is the most important. The meningitis is secondary to tuberculosis elsewhere, although the source may not be clinically apparent. It rarely occurs before the age of 6 months, and is most common in children and young adults. The onset is commonly insidious, with malaise and occasional headaches which may precede the signs of meningitis for days, weeks or even months. The meningeal phase includes headaches, signs of meningeal irritation and retraction of the head. Epileptic attacks – whether focal or general – and sudden hemiplegia or monoplegia, aphasia or cranial nerve palsies, mental changes, and papilloedema with visual loss, are common; hydrocephalus tends to increase, leading in untreated cases to stupor, incontinence, a rise in pulse and medullary failure. Choroidal tubercles may be found on examination of the retina, and the Mantoux test is positive in the majority of cases. The spinal fluid is under increased pressure, and may be either clear or opalescent; a fibrin clot forms on standing for some hours. There is an excess of lymphocytes and there may be a few polymorphs. The protein is raised, and the sugar content falls at an early stage. The definitive test is the demonstration of the organism in the fluid by direct smear with Ziehl–Neelson staining; if the evidence in favour of the disease is good, treatment should not be withheld until the organism is found. In the early stages of the disease the conditions which may cause difficulty in diagnosis are acute lymphocytic choriomeningitis and other virus infections of the meninges in which, however, the sugar and chloride content of the CSF are normal, and the clinical course quite different, with rapid recovery in most cases. In acute syphilitic meningitis the VDRL reaction is positive, while in meningitis associated with aural and sinus infections there may be both lymphocytes and polymorphs present, with negative culture and a normal sugar content in some cases (*aseptic meningitis*).

Meningitis can complicate Weil's disease (*spirochaetosis icterohaemorrhagica*), but an acute and predominantly lymphocytic meningitis can also occur without jaundice, renal damage or haemorrhagic symptoms – a syndrome complex that is strongly suggestive of this spirochete.

Weil's disease occurs in persons who have been in contact with rats (e.g. canal bathers, sewage workers, etc.), and the CSF is sterile if ordinary culture media are used. Sugar and chloride contents are normal. A benign meningitis can also be caused by *Leptospirosis canicola*, which is carried by dogs. There may be conjunctival suffusion, and a rash which may resemble erythema nodosum. The CSF contains an excess of lymphocytes, while the sugar content is normal, and the fluid is sterile in ordinary culture media. Diagnosis is confirmed, as in Weil's disease, by guinea-pig inoculation and by the detection of antibodies in the blood.

Lymphocytic meningitis may also occur with *tick-borne relapsing fever* (*T. recurrentis*), either during the first attack of fever, or more often in subsequent bouts. There is severe headache, neck stiffness and slight papilloedema. Cranial nerve palsies, notably the VIIth, are not uncommon. There is increase of protein and lymphocytes in the CSF, and the organism can be identified by dark-ground illumination, or by inoculation of the CSF into a suitable animal. A similar syndrome occurs with Lyme's disease due to *Borrelia bergdorferi* with the addition of a skin rash typically.

A well-marked lymphocytic meningitis can be caused by the viruses of acute choriomeningitis, mumps and glandular fever, whereas the meningeal reaction of poliomyelitis, zoster and arthropod-borne encephalitis is usually less obtrusive. A specific virus is responsible for *acute lymphocytic aboriomeningitis*, a benign disease characterized by a prodromal period of malaise, headaches, muscle pains, pyrexia and upper respiratory catarrh; this is followed after a week or two by severe headache, photophobia, neck stiffness and a positive Kernig sign. In a minority of cases, transverse myelitis, facial palsy or temporary mental and emotional changes may occur. The protein level is raised in the CSF, and there may be from 50 to 3000 cells/ml of CSF, of which at least 95 per cent are usually lymphocytes. Sugar is normal, and the virus can sometimes be isolated from the CSF. *Mumps meningitis* usually starts on the fifth to tenth day of the illness, but meningeal symptoms may precede the parotitis, or they may occur with orchitis but without parotitis. The meningitis may be accompanied by encephalitis with disturbances of consciousness and, rarely, focal cerebral and cerebellar signs. Cranial nerve palsies and myelitis have been described. Sudden permanent deafness, in one or both ears, and with or without vertigo and vomiting, may occur in mumps without evidence of meningoencephalitis. In *glandular fever* there may be a well-marked lymphocytic meningitis of sudden onset, with enlargement of glands, increase of the mononuclear lymphocytes in the blood, and an increasing titre in the Paul–Bunnell test. Acute polyneuritis may complicate the disease, or it may occur in glandular fever without meningitis. *Japanese B encephalitis* occurs in Japan and China. The virus is spread by mosquitoes. There are meningeal signs, drowsiness, stupor, signs of diffuse cerebral involvement, convulsions and tremors. There is a lymphocytosis in the CSF, while the sugar remains normal. The mortality in this disease can be over 50 per cent.

Infection by yeasts has been uncommon in the past, but it appears to be on the increase since the advent of antibiotics. *Cryptococcosis* (*Torula histolytica*) involves the subcutaneous tissues, the lungs, and the central nervous system, either alone or in combination, or in series. Subcutaneous granulomas break down to form abscesses and ulcers. Pulmonary lesions may mimic either chronic tuberculosis or carcinoma. The cerebral type usually starts insidiously with headaches, dizziness and stiffness of the neck, but it may commence suddenly. There is little or no fever, but gradually the CSF pressure rises, producing papilloedema, and there may be cranial nerve palsies, hemiparesis or ataxia. Large granulomas may, in fact, cause symptoms of a cerebral tumour. The patient eventually sinks into coma. There is a marked mononuclear pleocytosis in the CSF, and the protein is raised. The glucose content is reduced, and cryptococci, which are readily mistaken for erythrocytes or lymphocytes, can be found in small numbers in the CSF.

Sarcoidosis, which causes uveoparotid polyneuritis, can also give rise to a low-grade meningitis with headaches, slight stiffness of the neck, and a rise in lymphocytes and protein in the CSF. It can pass on to cause an obstructive hydrocephalus, with papilloedema and optic atrophy. Cranial nerve palsies and diabetes insipidus have been described. The diagnosis can only be inferred by the presence of typical lesions in other areas (e.g. skin, liver, lungs and eyes).

Subarachnoid haemorrhage (SAH) is usually due to rupture of a saccular aneurysm, or of an atheromatous aneurysm. Less common causes are hypertension, angiomatous malformations, mycotic and syphilitic aneurysms, and purpura. An abrupt onset, early loss of consciousness in most cases, and the presence of blood in the CSF distinguish the average case from meningitis. When the leak is slow, however, the severe headache, stiffness of the neck, slight pyrexia, ocular palsies and positive Kernig sign may simulate meningitis, and it is only the blood in the CSF which clinches the diagnosis. If the lumbar puncture is delayed for a day or two, the CSF may be found to be yellowish in colour (xanthochromia), and not blood-stained. Therefore, xanthochromia should be sought if SAH is suspected. Rarely, pain starts in the lumbar region and gradually spreads down the back of the legs and up to the neck. Another unusual form presents as sudden coma, and there may, in such a case, be a history of former attacks of unexplained coma with neck stiffness.

Pressure cones at the tentorial hiatus and at the foramen magnum can cause stiffness of the neck. They occur as a result of space-occupying lesions and, occasionally, from cerebral oedema. The local rise of pressure from an expanding mass in the head, or from hydrocephalus, dislocates and displaces brain substance. Thus, a mass in the middle fossa (e.g. tumour or extradural haematoma) can dislocate part of the temporal lobe into the posterior fossa, with the result that the mid-brain and the displaced tissue are tightly wedged in the dural ring. This may obstruct the aqueduct, thus aggravating the situation by causing internal hydrocephalus. In posterior fossa tumours, the reverse is seen: the oedematous brainstem and cerebellar tissue is displaced upwards through the tentorial notch. Downward herniation of the medulla and cerebellar tonsils through the foramen also occurs, and will also give rise to rigidity of the neck.

Pressure cones can arise as the result of intracranial space-occupying lesions: tumour, abscess, haematoma, internal hydrocephalus and occasionally from cerebral oedema due to vascular lesions. All of these conditions may therefore cause stiffness of the neck.

It is important to recognize the presence of a pressure cone, because the removal of even a small quantity of CSF by lumbar puncture may cause collapse and death.

Asphyxia can cause retraction of the head, or stiffness of the neck. The more striking examples are usually seen in children with bronchopneumonia, bronchiolitis, or foreign body in the larynx. Asphyxia has also sometimes been noted in retropharyngeal abscess. Even in adults with severe bronchopneumonia there may be stiffness of the neck, though retraction is rare. That asphyxia without cerebral oedema can cause retraction of the head is well illustrated by the retraction seen during the administration of pure nitrous oxide (e.g. for dental extraction), but this may not be the whole explanation in the diseases mentioned.

Mark Kinirons

HEADACHE

Headache (cephalgia) is one of the most frequent reasons for visiting a doctor. It is not known why headache so common, but the face, scalp, nasal passages, eye and ear contain many pain receptors, and humans are concerned about pain in the head due to the possibility of a serious cause (e.g. a brain tumour). In the United Kingdom, about 80 per cent of the population will experience a headache in a given year. About 1–2 per cent of the population will consult their GP, and about 0.3 per cent will be referred on to a hospital specialist, usually a neurologist. The vast majority of headaches seen in primary care (>95%) are not due to a serious intracranial cause. There are many possible causes of headache (Table H.9), and the first priority is to make sure that serious or treatable intracranial pathology are not missed. In general, the length of the history is a useful guide: headache with a short history requires prompt diagnosis, and possibly urgent investigations. Other features indicating the possibility of serious intracranial pathology are: *sudden* onset of pain (possible intracranial haemorrhage); fever or neck stiffness (possible intracranial infection); focal neurological symptoms or signs (possible mass lesion); temporal artery tenderness (possible giant cell arteritis).

Although the clinician must be alert to serious causes of headache, it should be remembered that in primary care less than 5 per cent of headaches are due to serious intracranial pathology. Migraine and tension-type headache are by far the most common causes seen in clinical practice. A detailed history should allow accurate diagnosis of these types of headache, but this often requires considerable patience in allowing the history to unfold. It should be evident that because headache can be due to serious pathology, symptomatic treatment should never precede a

Table H.9 Causes of headache

Migraine
- Migraine with aura
- Migraine without aura
- Special forms (ophthalmoplegic migraine, retinal migraine, acephalagic migraine)

Tension-type

Trigeminal autonomic cephalgias
- Cluster headache
- SUNCT (short-lasting unilateral neuralgiform headache with conjunctival injection and tearing)
- Paroxysmal hemicrania

Vascular disorders
- Acute ischaemic stroke
- Acute haemorrhagic stroke (subarachnoid or intracranial haemorrhage)
- Temporal arteritis
- Hypertension
- Venous sinus thrombosis

Non-vascular intracranial pathology
- Abnormal cerebrospinal fluid pressure (high or low)
- Infection (meningitis, meningoencephalitis, abscess)
- Tumours
- Systemic infection (viral, bacterial, others) or metabolic disturbance

Head and face pain arising from other structures
- Cranial bones, neck, eyes, ears, nose, sinuses, teeth, jaws, temporomandibular joints

Craniofacial neuralgias
- Trigeminal neuralgia
- Glossopharyngeal neuralgia

Specific headache syndromes
- Idiopathic stabbing headache
- Coital cephalgia
- Cold stimulus headache (ice-cream)
- Benign exertional and cough headache

Trauma

Substance use

Substance withdrawal

careful history, adequate physical examination, and consideration of further investigation. As in all types of pain, when assessing headache, the quality, location, severity, time course and exacerbating and relieving factors should be determined. The head should be examined for signs of temporal arteritis (pulseless, thickened, tender temporal arteries). The blood pressure should be measured and the optic fundi examined for papilloedema, which *usually* indicates raised intracranial pressure (papilloedema can also be caused by local pathology at the optic nerve head; see OPTIC FUNDUS, ABNORMALITIES IN, p. 501). Raised intracranial pressure may be due to a structural lesion, or to obstruction of normal cerebrospinal fluid (CSF) circulation, as in idiopathic intracranial hypertension or cerebral venous sinus thrombosis. A neurological screening examination should be performed, to include pupils (including looking for Horner's syndrome), visual fields, extraocular movements, drift of outstretched hands, co-ordination testing (finger–nose test), reflexes and plantar responses, and heel–toe walking; recent-onset headache with focal neurological signs is an indication for urgent brain imaging.

The differential diagnosis of headache is shifted at different ages; for example, cranial arteritis is almost exclusively seen in the elderly (aged 60 years and above), whilst in children posterior fossa tumours must be considered with any refractory recent-onset headache. In this discussion the common causes of headache (migraine and tension-type) will be considered first and in detail, before dealing with headache due to vascular causes (intracranial and extracranial), non-vascular intracranial pathology including tumour, infection (systemic or intracranial), and finally some rare but distinctive headache syndromes and headaches due to systemic disease. Pain which is mainly limited to the face (craniofacial neuralgias; head or face pain due to disorders of teeth, sinuses, ear, nose and other structures) are considered elsewhere (see FACE, PAIN IN, p. 198).

Migraine

Pathophysiology

A useful pathophysiological model of migraine is that of an inherited disorder causing increased sensitivity to afferent stimuli; during attacks stimuli including light, sound and movement exacerbate the headache. Migraine attacks are thought to result from increased neuronal activity in midline brainstem structures, including the periaqueductal grey matter, the dorsal raphe nuclei, reticular formation and locus coeruleus. Functional imaging studies show increased cerebral blood flow in these areas during an attack. These brainstem nuclei, together with the trigeminal nuclei, can influence extracranial blood flow by reflex connections with the parasympathetic part of the facial nerve. This link between neural and vascular systems is termed the *trigeminovascular system*. The same brainstem nuclei can also modulate cortical activity and blood flow, as well as central pain control mechanisms. The migraine 'aura' is thought to involve a wave of neuronal depression spreading across the cortex, associated with reduced cerebral blood flow (oligaemia) and neurological symptoms corresponding to the brain region affected. Thus, the visual aura may propagate across the visual field as the wave of cortical spreading depression moves across the occipital cortex. The pain is thought to result from neurogenic inflammation resulting from the release of neuropeptides (by trigeminal nerve endings) and other pain-inducing compounds including histamine, serotonin, prostaglandins and nitric oxide (from plasma, platelets, and mast cells). These agents induce cranial vasodilatation and extravasation of plasma proteins, as well as the sensitization of trigeminal nociceptive nerve endings. Most current treatments for migraine act on the serotonergic system.

Clinical features

Migraine causes severe episodic headaches that last from several hours to several days, and are absent more than they are present. The periodicity is important: attacks typically occur about once per month, and if headaches occur more than twice a week, then episodic migraine (on its own) is unlikely to be the diagnosis. In migraine with aura (see AURA, p. 48) – which affects about one-fifth of patients – the aura evolves over minutes and usually lasts under 30 minutes, almost always under an hour. The aura most often arises from the occipital cortex and so is commonly visual, involving positive phenomena such as photopsia (unformed flashing lights) or fortification spectra (tessellated structures resembling zigzag lines). Fortification spectra are so named because they resemble the fortifications of a medieval town. Teichopsia is an equivalent term derived from the Greek word *teichos* (meaning 'wall'). Negative phenomena (scotomata) may be reported, sometimes following the teichopsia as it propagates across the visual field. Auras may also affect sensation, movement, cognitive, or vestibular functions. Illusions of body image may be reported (*'Alice in Wonderland'* syndrome). The headache typically follows the aura, but less commonly can come first or coincide with it.

The headache in migraine is usually (but not always) unilateral and throbbing. It is severe, and made worse by moving around, by loud noises, or bright light. The patient typically describes wanting to lay down in a quiet, darkened room; they often feel nauseous and may vomit. In migraine without aura (formerly termed *common migraine*, affecting about 75% of patients), the headache is similar in character to migraine with aura, but fewer specific accompanying symptoms occur than in classical migraine. There may be gastrointestinal symptoms or heightened sensory perception.

Treatment of migraine is of two types: (i) the symptomatic treatment of acute attacks; and (ii) prophylactic agents, which are usually recommended if more than three attacks occur per month. First-line acute treatments include high-dose aspirin with antiemetic (e.g. domperidone), and the triptans (e.g. sumatriptan) given by the oral or subcutaneous routes. Prophylactic treatments include propranolol and other beta-blockers, and amitriptyline.

Differential diagnosis

The main differential diagnoses are tension-type headache, cluster headache and other trigeminal autonomic cephalgias, and medication over-use headache. The main distinguishing feature from tension-type headache is in periodicity. Migraine is generally episodic and rarely more frequent than twice a week, whereas tension-type headache is present on most days. It should be noted, however, that migraine and tension-type headache often co-exist, causing so-called *mixed chronic daily headache*. Furthermore, it is now appreciated that there is a frequent form of migraine (chronic migraine).

The main difference between migraine and the trigeminal autonomic cephalgias (including cluster headache) is that autonomic features (e.g. nasal congestion, conjunctival injection, ptosis, lacrimation) are more prominent in the latter group. Medication over-use headache is more difficult to diagnose; it often results in the context of migraine with regular high-dose analgesics use, with subsequent transformation into a mixed migraine and chronic tension-type headache disorder.

Tension-type headache

As discussed above, the traditional classification of the most common recurrent headache syndromes into migraine and tension-type headache has been questioned recently, and it has been suggested that they are different expressions of the same pathophysiological process. At present, the distinction between them is useful in that different management strategies are effective for each group. Tension-type headache – also referred to as chronic daily headache – is common, accounting for 70 per cent of referrals to a headache clinic. In comparison to migraine it has no defining characteristics: the headaches are rather featureless, with no photophobia, phonophobia, nausea or vomiting. In tension-type headache, pain is described in many different ways; it is often diffuse, but may localize to the vertex, forehead or the neck. It is more often bilateral than unilateral. The classic description is of a 'tight band around the head' or 'like the head being in a vice'. Patients will sometimes report that 'my head feels as if it is bursting', or that 'sharp knives are being driven in'. The headache is worse in the evenings, and with fatigue or stress. Because the headache is chronic, often occurring for years, analgesic misuse is a frequent problem. The most effective drug treatment for recurrent tension-type headache is with tricyclic agents (e.g. amitriptyline). Relaxation exercises may also be helpful.

Cluster headache and the trigeminal autonomic cephalgias

Cluster headache

Cluster headache is one of the trigeminal autonomic cephalgias, a group of primary headache disorders linked by their trigeminal distribution, short duration and prominent ipsilateral cranial autonomic features. Cluster headache is characterized by a severe, distressing unilateral head or face pain lasting from about 15 minutes to 3 hours. The localization is usually orbital or temporal, and the onset and offset are rapid. The pain is described as burning, piercing, throbbing or pulsing. The full syndrome includes conjunctival injection, forehead sweating, meiosis, ptosis, lacrimation, eyelid oedema and nasal congestion. The pain occurs once or more than once daily for weeks to months, with pain-free intervals of 2 weeks or more. Alcohol may precipitate an attack. During an attack the patient will often pace around the room, grasping the affected eye in an attempt to relieve the pain. This is in contrast to the patient with migraine who will usually wish to lie still in a quiet, dark environment. Sumatriptan subcutaneously is the drug of choice in the treatment of acute attacks; inhalation of 100 per cent oxygen can also be very helpful. For short-term prophylaxis, oral corticosteroids, methysergide or ergotamine may be helpful, whilst for longer-term prophylaxis verapamil is a first-line treatment. About 10–20 per cent of patients do not have remissions (or remissions less than 2 weeks) and are classified as having chronic cluster headache.

Short-lasting unilateral neuralgiform headache attacks with conjunctival injection and tearing (SUNCT)

This is another trigeminal autonomic cephalgia syndrome, distinguished from cluster headache by brief (average 50 seconds), frequent attacks (up to 30 per hour) with prominent autonomic features in the majority of patients. The treatment of SUNCT is challenging. Some response has been seen with carbamazepine, and more recently lamotrigine, which is a promising potential first-line treatment. Further data from randomized trials are awaited.

Paroxysmal hemicrania

This is also a short-duration unilateral headache syndrome with pain in the maxillary, orbital, frontal or temporal regions and associated autonomic features. The characteristic and distinguishing feature is the excellent response to indomethacin treatment. Unlike cluster headache, only half of the patients tend to pace around when the pain occurs.

Vascular disorders

A mild headache occurs at the onset of about one-quarter of *ischaemic stroke* or *transient ischaemic attacks*. It has been reported to be more common with vertebrobasilar territory events than with carotid territory events, and is rarer still in lacunar syndromes. If head pain is lateralized and severe, and followed by fixed neurological deficit, then *arterial dissection* must be considered. Carotid dissection typically causes unilateral pain localized to the face, fontal region or eye, whilst vertebral dissection may cause unilateral or bilateral occipital pain. Headache of raised intracranial pressure-type (i.e. headache worse on waking, exacerbated by coughing, sneezing or straining) may be a feature of cerebral venous sinus thrombosis, in which focal signs including seizures are often found. The usual presentation of venous sinus thrombosis is with a subacute raised pressure headache rather than an acute headache.

Sudden, severe headache is the most important symptom of *subarachnoid haemorrhage*, and may be the only complaint in one-third of patients. It occurs at some stage in the illness in between 85 and 100 per cent of cases. The cardinal feature of this type of headache is its exceptionally rapid onset. It may be described as being 'like a hammer blow to the head', or 'like an explosion in the head', and most patients will volunteer that it is the worst headache that they have ever experienced. It reaches a maximum in a split second or within a few seconds. A history like this makes CT scanning mandatory to seek evidence of acute subarachnoid blood, which appears as high attenuation (bright). If the CT scan is negative, then a lumbar puncture must be performed to look for red cells or their breakdown products. The most common focal neurological sign in subarachnoid haemorrhage is of a IIIrd nerve palsy. *Pituitary apoplexy* can cause a similar sudden severe headache, classically in association with sudden bilateral visual loss. *Intraventricular haemorrhage* can also mimic the headache of subarachnoid haemorrhage.

Primary intracerebral haemorrhage, especially in a peripheral lobar distribution, is preceded by headache in one-half of patients. Focal neurological deficit is almost always found.

It is rare for unruptured intracranial *aneurysms* to cause significant headache, but occasionally a large posterior communicating artery aneurysm may cause pain localized to behind the eye.

Temporal arteritis must be remembered because it is a preventable cause of blindness. It usually occurs in patients aged over 50 years, and the prevalence increases with increasing age. Head or face pain is found at presentation in 50 per cent of cases. One-quarter of patients have systemic symptoms at presentation (arthralgia, myalgia, low-grade pyrexia). Pain in the temporal or masseter muscles on chewing (jaw claudication) is highly characteristic, and virtually diagnostic. Blindness occurs due to involvement of the posterior ciliary artery, which supplies the optic disc. On examination, the temporal artery may be palpable and tender. The erythrocyte sedimentation rate is usually markedly elevated (up to 140 mm/h). The acute treatment is high-dose oral or intravenous corticosteroids.

Cerebral venous sinus thrombosis often presents with headache, but is only of sudden onset in about 15 per cent of patients. Most patients will have symptoms and signs suggesting raised intracranial pressure, and about one-third will experience seizures or focal neurological signs (e.g. hemiparesis).

Non-vascular intacranial pathology

Raised intracranial pressure

High intracranial cerebrospinal fluid (CSF) pressure causes a characteristic headache that has already been mentioned briefly. The headache is typically aching or throbbing, exacerbated by coughing, bending over or straining, worse in the morning, and may cause wakening from sleep. It may be worse after exertion or on lying flat. As the headache worsens, then vomiting, diplopia and papilloedema develop. The raised intracranial pressure may be due to obstruction of normal CSF flow by an intracranial tumour, or by another mechanism affecting CSF dynamics. The first clinical priority if high intracranial pressure is suspected is to exclude an intracranial mass lesion by imaging – with CT or ideally magnetic resonance imaging (MRI) (better quality images of the posterior fossa). If there is no mass lesion, then raised pressure must be due to another mechanism (Table H.10).

Table H.10 Causes of raised intracranial pressure

Cerebral, dural or extradural mass causing impaired CSF flow
- Tumour
- Abscess
- Haematoma

Generalized brain swelling
- Hypoxia
- Metabolic disturbance
- Hypertensive encephalopathy

Increase in cerebral venous pressure
- Heart failure
- Obstruction of superior mediastinal or jugular veins
- Cerebral venous sinus thrombosis

Obstruction to CSF resorption or flow
- Meningitis (granulomatous, carcinomatous, haemorrhagic)
- Subarachnoid haemorrhage

Expansion of CSF volume
- CSF secreting tumour (choroids plexus tumour) – rare

Unknown mechanism
- Idiopathic intracranial hypertension

Raised pressure may also be due to impaired CSF re-absorption; this may result from current or previous meningitis (acute, subacute or chronic, e.g. granulomatous or carcinomatous) or from subarachnoid haemorrhage; both of these processes block the arachnoid granulations. Thus, once a mass lesion is excluded by imaging, the CSF should be examined by lumbar puncture to seek red or white cells and to determine the protein concentration. If the CSF is normal and there is no mass lesion, and the patient has focal hemisphere signs or seizures, then cerebral venous sinus thrombosis must be considered and excluded by either formal or magnetic resonance venography studies.

If CSF pressure is elevated but focal neurological signs are minimal or absent, and both imaging (including venography) and CSF analysis are normal, then the patient has a syndrome of idiopathic intracranial hypertension (formerly called benign intracranial hypertension or pseudotumour cerebri). In its classical form this syndrome occurs in women who are overweight and often with menstrual irregularities. As well as a raised pressure headache, patients will often complain of transient visual loss on changing posture (e.g. bending over), termed visual obscurations. Diplopia or unilateral facial numbness may also be present. A number of associations exist with this syndrome, including the use of tetracycline antibiotic, lead poisoning, vitamin A toxicity, and metabolic disturbance (hypothyroidism).

Some conditions cause raised intracranial pressure by raising the CSF protein dramatically (Guillain–Barré syndrome, spinal oligodendroglioma, SLE).

Low CSF pressure headache

Low CSF pressure can also cause a distinctive headache syndrome. This type of headache may follow lumbar puncture. The pain is not usually present on waking, is worse on sitting up or standing, and is rapidly relieved by laying flat. The presumed mechanism is of persistent CSF leakage through a dural tear. The management of post-lumbar puncture headache is bed rest, fluids and analgesia; it may take several weeks to resolve, and in severe cases epidural blood patches have been used. Sometimes, low-pressure headache can occur spontaneously or following head, neck or spinal trauma. In other cases there may be an index Valsalva event such as coughing, straining, lifting, etc. In low-pressure headache, MRI with contrast demonstrates striking meningeal enhancement. The management is similar to that of post-lumbar puncture headache. Intravenous caffeine or theophylline have been effective in some cases.

Intracranial infection

Meningitis is inflammation of the pia and arachnoid, caused by bacterial, viral, fungal or other infections. The clinical syndrome of meningeal irritation must be recognized quickly so that appropriate treatment can be commenced. Untreated bacterial meningitis can be very rapidly fatal. The headache in acute meningeal irritation is of rapid onset (less than 48 hours), and severe. There are accompanying symptoms of photophobia, and drowsiness, vomiting, irritability and seizures may develop. The important physical signs are fever, neck stiffness, *Kernig's sign* (pain and resistance when the examiner extends the knee with the hip fully flexed) and *Brudzinski's sign* (hips flex when the head is flexed forward towards the chest). Lumbar puncture must be performed rapidly to confirm the diagnosis and the organism, unless there is drowsiness, suspicion of raised intracranial pressure or focal neurological signs, in which case CT must be performed first, and empirical antibiotics commenced. The most common organisms in adults are *Meningococcus* and *Pneumococcus*, but in the immunocompromised or elderly *Listeria*, fungi (including *Cryptococcus*) and tuberculosis must also be considered. In the immunocompromised, some of the typical features of meningitis, such as neck stiffness and a positive Kernig's sign, may be absent. *Aseptic meningitis* may give an identical clinical syndrome, but no organisms are identified in the CSF. *Chronic meningitis* may be due to granulomatous or carcinomatous meningeal irritation, and will have a less acute onset and often associated cranial nerve palsies. In patients with HIV infection and advanced disease, headache may be due to infection with *Toxoplasma gondii*. This characteristically produces multiple ring-enhancing intracerebral lesions on CT or MRI scans; the diagnosis is confirmed by a response to empirical therapy, or much less often by brain biopsy.

Encephalitis is inflammation of the brain parenchyma, although a variable degree of meningeal involvement usually occurs as well. The patient will often have similar symptoms to those of meningitis, but there may be a subacute history of personality change, and seizures with focal signs (e.g. hemiparesis) are common. Viruses are the most common cause (e.g. herpes simplex, coxsackie, echovirus, rabies) and

if the diagnosis is suspected then treatment with acyclovir should be started empirically.

Cerebral tumour

Although headache is an early symptom in about one-third of brain tumours, the vast majority of headaches are *not* due to tumours. There are no specific features, though the features of raised intracranial pressure (see above) may develop if the tumour is impeding the CSF circulation. Tumours may cause headache without raised CSF pressure; the presumed mechanism is the distension of local pain-sensitive structures (blood vessels, dura). If lateralized headache is present, it is very often on the side of the tumour. It is self-evident that a tumour may produce focal neurological symptoms and signs depending on its location, though some present with only subtle cognitive disturbance. New-onset seizures in an adult should always raise the suspicion of cerebral tumour. Any headache of recent onset with focal neurological symptoms or signs (especially seizures), or papilloedema, requires urgent neuroimaging. Pupillary abnormalities and reduced conscious level are usually late symptoms reflecting tentorial herniation or rapidly rising intracranial pressure.

Headache associated with systemic infection

Many infectious illnesses are associated with headache, for example viral infections. There will be other symptoms to indicate the systemic nature of the illness.

Specific headache syndromes

It is helpful to be able to recognize these syndromes, as doing so will allow a firm diagnosis to be made, and reassurance or appropriate treatment to be offered.

- *Idiopathic stabbing headache*: This describes sharp, stabbing pain in the head that may occur once or in recurrent volleys. The pain is usually in the first trigeminal division, lasts only a split second, and recurs irregularly (hours to days apart). It is more common in women, and tends to be spontaneous rather than triggered. There are no autonomic features, and indomethacin is an effective treatment.
- *Coital cephalgia*: This is a severe, throbbing explosive headache occurring at the point of orgasm, and persisting for minute to hours. It typically occurs on several consecutive episodes of sexual activity and then spontaneously remits. Although this is a benign syndrome, every

new-onset case must be investigated for possible ruptured aneurysm and subarachnoid haemorrhage, which
can also occur during sexual activity.

- *Cold stimulus headache*: This condition, also called 'ice-
cream headache', is reported to occur in about one-third
of the population. Cold stimulation of the pharynx or
palate induces pain shortly afterwards (10–20 seconds)
that is often lateralized and is of short duration
(seconds), but it can be longer. The pain may be referred
to the forehead or temple by the trigeminal nerve, or to the
ears by the glossopharyngeal nerve. In recent studies, ice-
cream headache has been reported to be less common in
patients with migraine than in the general population.

- *Benign cough and exertional headache*: Some patients
report severe, transient head pain on coughing, sneezing, laughing vigorously or lifting heavy weights, bending over or straining. The pain is typically frontal or
occipital, follows the action by 1–2 seconds, and lasts for
only a few seconds. It may be described as 'explosive' or
'bursting'. It often occurs recurrently for months to a year or
two, and then remits. This is a benign syndrome, but serious pathology can cause identical symptoms, for example
posterior fossa tumours, so investigations may be needed.
Runners and other athletes often get headaches on exertion. These headaches may have associated features
suggesting that they are a form of migraine. Exertional
and cough headaches may respond to indomethacin.

Headache associated with head trauma

Headaches affect most symptomatic patients after mild
head injury. Post-traumatic headaches usually begin
hours or days after the injury, but they may be delayed
for weeks. Headaches may paradoxically occur more
often and for longer in patients with mild compared
to severe trauma. Commonly associated symptoms
include dizziness, irritability, lack of concentration and
intolerance to alcohol. Vertigo, hearing disturbance,
apathy and tiredness may also occur as part of the 'post-
head injury syndrome'. Headaches after trauma may be
localized or diffuse, episodic or daily. They most often
resemble chronic tension-type headaches, but may be
migrainous. Neuralgic or trigeminal autonomic cephal-
gia-type pains less commonly occur. If the dura has
been damaged, low-pressure headaches may result.

Headache associated with substance use

Some substances reliably induce headaches during
acute use in some individuals. Nitrates, found in
preserved, processed or cured meats, cause so-called
'hot-dog headache' which is usually bitemporal and
associated with facial flushing. Monosodium gluata-
mate causes what has been termed 'Chinese restau-
rant headache', where associated features include
chest tightness, and burning in the head and upper
trunk. Carbon monoxide is an important cause of
headache, but there will usually be associated features
including reduced consciousness level. Hyperbaric
oxygen treatment can be rapidly effective. Alcohol-
induced headache occurs within hours of ingestion
(unlike typical 'hangover' headache, which is delayed)
and is most commonly migrainous. Chocolate and
cheese have long been thought to be important triggers for migraine, but they can also cause headaches
in non-migraineurs.

Headache associated with substance misuse

Headache from substance misuse can occur with
central nervous system stimulants (amphetamines,
cocaine, designer drugs), barbiturates and sedatives,
or opiates. The headaches may be associated with
acute or 'binge' use, or may occur during withdrawal
from these substances.

David Werring

HEART IMPULSE, DISPLACED

The position of the cardiac apex is defined as the fur-
thest outward and downward point at which a cardiac impulse can be felt in the supine, unrotated
patient. This point usually lies in the 5th or 6th left
intercostal space in the midclavicular line. Displacement of the apex may be due to a congenitally abnormal position of the heart, to cardiac enlargement, or
to cardiac displacement resulting from chest wall or
intrathoracic abnormalities.

Congenital dextrocardia may involve simple mirror-
image inversion of the heart and other viscera (situs
inversus), or may be associated with a variety of complex congenital cardiac defects. In adults, simple dextrocardia without associated defects is more common,
and is benign (Fig. H.4).

Displacement of the cardiac apex resulting from
cardiac enlargement can usually be suspected on the
basis of the patient's symptoms of heart disease, or

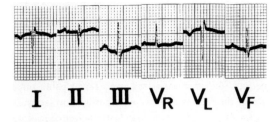

I   II   III   V_R   V_L   V_F

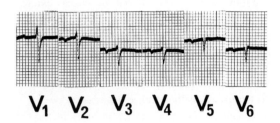

V₁   V₂   V₃   V₄   V₅   V₆

Figure H.4 ECG in subject with dextracardia, demonstrating R wave progression across the chest leads and bizarre cardiac axis.

Table H.11 Displacement of the cardiac apex

Lung and pleura
- Pleural effusion
- Pneumonectomy
- Tension pneumothorax

Diaphragm
- Congenital diaphragmatic hernia
- Hiatus hernia

Pericardium
- Clearwater cyst of pericardium
- Pericardial tumour

Oesophagus
- Achalasia of the cardia/megaoesophagus
- Foregut duplication cyst

Aorta
- Aneurysm of descending aorta

the presence of murmurs or abnormal heart sounds. Confirmation can be made by chest radiography, ECG and echocardiography. The differential diagnosis is discussed more elsewhere (see HEART, ENLARGEMENT OF, p. 288).

Displacement of the cardiac apex from *abnormalities of the chest wall* is usually apparent on inspection of the patient; these abnormalities include pectus excavatum (funnel chest), pectus carinatum (pigeon chest), kyphoscoliosis and thoracoplasty.

An exception is sometimes a 'compensated' thoracic kyphoscoliosis, which may be more easily appreciated on a chest X-ray. Conversely, pectus excavatum is obvious clinically, but is sometimes missed on cursory inspection of a posteroanterior chest radiograph.

Displacements of the cardiac apex as a result of intrathoracic abnormalities are listed in Table H.11, according to the organ or tissue involved. Pulmonary or diaphragmatic causes are common, the remainder are rare.

Lymphoid tissue and thymus

Enlargement of thoracic lymph nodes is common, but seldom causes cardiac displacement. Rarely, enlargement of para-aortic nodes or aberrant thymus tissues may do so.

The differential diagnosis can often be clarified by radiography in the posteroanterior and lateral projections, with the help of a barium swallow to outline the oesophagus. In more difficult cases, CT scanning and echocardiography – particularly transoesophageal echocardiography – are useful.

Melvin Lobo

HEART SOUNDS

Tradition describes four heart sounds. The first and second are almost always audible, the third and fourth occur only in specific circumstances. There is also a medley of *added sounds*, mainly described as 'clicks', 'snaps' or 'plops', which can be heard in patients with particular conditions – these are distinguished from murmurs and rubs (see HEART, MURMURS IN, p. 291; and RUB, PERICARDIAL, p. 622) by their short duration.

First sound

The first heart sound is due to the closure of the mitral and tricuspid valves. Closure is normally simultaneous, but occasionally one valve closes slightly before the other, causing splitting of the first sound. This may be associated with right bundle branch block, but is seldom of clinical importance.

The first sound is usually readily recognized as the 'lub' in the traditional 'lubdup' cadence of heart sounds. It is the sound which immediately precedes the upstroke of the carotid pulse. A *loud first heart sound* is most commonly associated with a hyperdynamic circulation (e.g. in pregnancy, febrile illness, thyrotoxicosis). Echocardiography has shown that the mitral cusps are still wide apart at the onset of systole as a consequence of the atrial augmentation of ventricular filling, and it is this, together with the increased rate of rise of ventricular pressure (dp/dt) as a result of sympathetic stimulation and a low peripheral resistance, which increases the force of valve closure. A loud first sound is not a feature of paroxysmal tachycardia, where ventricular stroke volume is reduced and the synchrony of atrial and ventricular contraction may be disturbed. *Mitral stenosis* is the other common cause of an abnormally loud first sound. In rheumatic mitral stenosis the mitral cusps are fused together laterally to form a diaphragm which bulges into the left ventricle during diastole, and is propelled sharply back towards the left atrium in systole. The latter movement produces a loud, ringing first sound, often palpable as well as audible. A loud first sound is best heard in patients with a stenosed but still mobile valve in sinus rhythm. Progressive calcification restricts valve movement, and the sound becomes quieter. A loud first sound alone does not make the diagnosis of mitral stenosis, but should prompt a careful search for a mid-diastolic murmur. A much rarer cause of a loud first heart sound is left atrial myxoma. Tricuspid stenosis may also cause a loud first sound, but this is rare. Apparently increased loudness of the first heart sound may simply be due to a relative lack of soft tissue between heart and stethoscope, as in fit thin young subjects or patients who have had a mastectomy. Conversely, obesity or emphysema may muffle the heart sounds.

Varying intensity of the first sound occurs in three common conditions: (i) atrial fibrillation; (ii) extrasystoles; and (iii) complete heart block. In atrial fibrillation, the varying length of diastole causes the mitral cusps to be in varying positions at the onset of systole, and ventricular stroke volume also varies with the length of diastole. To some extent these effects cancel out, so the variation in first sound intensity may be less than in complete heart block, where stroke volume is relatively constant but where the varying relationship of atrial to ventricular systole causes the position of the mitral cusps to vary from beat to beat

at the onset of systole. With extrasystoles, the fast sound of the premature beat is invariably softer. Coupled extrasystoles cause a characteristic cadence of loud first, normal second sound, soft first and second sound, pause. This is often misinterpreted because the premature beat gives no palpable pulse and all the sounds are ascribed to a single cardiac cycle.

An *abnormally quiet first heart sound*, unless an artefact of obesity or emphysema, is usually due to a reduced cardiac output. In left ventricular failure a small increase in left ventricular volume during diastole causes a large rise in pressure, and echocardiography shows that the mitral cusps have virtually drifted together before the onset of systole. In these circumstances a quiet first heart sound frequently accompanies a third or fourth sound, as described below.

A sudden *diminution in the intensity* of the first sound may occur in acute mitral regurgitation, when it will be associated with the appearance of a pansystolic murmur. Even more rarely, an endocarditic vegetation or an atrial myxoma (see below) may interfere with mitral valve closure and cause a sudden reduction in the first sound.

The changes in intensity of the first heart sound can be summarized as follows:

- **Loud**
  - ◆ Thin chest wall
  - ◆ Hyperdynamic circulation
  - ◆ Mitral stenosis
  - ◆ Atrial myxoma
- **Soft**
  - ◆ Obesity/emphysema
  - ◆ Cardiac failure
  - ◆ Acute mitral regurgitation
  - ◆ Endocarditis/myxoma
- **Variable**
  - ◆ Atrial fibrillation
  - ◆ Extrasystoles
  - ◆ Complete heart block
  - ◆ Atrial myxoma

Second sound

The second heart sound is due to closure of the aortic and pulmonary valves. In expiration, their closure is normally synchronous, but in inspiration there is a tendency for the aortic valve to close slightly earlier, the negative intrathoracic pressure causing blood to pool in the pulmonary veins, and the pulmonary valve slightly later, as venous return to the right side of the heart is increased. *Inspiratory splitting of the second heart sound* is the result – a normal finding in children and in some adults. It is best appreciated with the stethoscope diaphragm applied at the left of the sternum in the second or third intercostal space.

Fixed splitting of the second heart sound is virtually pathognomonic of atrial septal defect. The second sound is split because of the increased volume load on the right ventricle, and the split is fixed because the septal defect equalizes right and left atrial pressure throughout the cardiac cycle. Fixed splitting is not a feature of ventricular septal defect (VSD) or persistent ductus arteriosus.

Fixed splitting must be distinguished from *wide splitting* of the second sound, where the split is audible in both inspiration and expiration but wider in inspiration. This occurs in right bundle branch block and in pulmonary stenosis. There is a direct relationship between the width of the expiratory split and the pulmonary gradient. In severe pulmonary stenosis or Fallot's tetralogy the pulmonary component of the second sound may be so quiet as to be inaudible. Wide splitting of the second sound is not usually found in pulmonary hypertension.

Reversed splitting of the second sound occurs when left ventricular ejection is prolonged or delayed so that pulmonary closure precedes aortic valve closure. Inspiration now causes the sounds to move together, so wider splitting is heard in expiration. In practice, reversed splitting is uncommon, and is mainly associated with left bundle branch block, hypertrophic obstructive cardiomyopathy and some cases of congenital aortic stenosis. In most adult cases of aortic stenosis the valve cusps are so rigid that the aortic second sound is inaudible.

An *abnormally loud second heart sound* is most commonly due to systemic hypertension. The second sound may also be loud in patients with a dilated or aneurysmal ascending aorta. Because the pulmonary artery lies closer to the surface than the ascending aorta, pulmonary hypertension can cause a very loud second heart sound which may be palpable as well as audible. In patients with transposition of the aorta and pulmonary arteries a loud second sound is heard for the same reason.

The characteristics of the second heart sound in various conditions can be summarized as follows:

- **Loud**
  - Thin chest wall
  - Hyperdynamic circulation
  - Pulmonary hypertension
  - Transposition of great arteries
- **Soft**
  - Obesity
  - Low cardiac output
  - Severe aortic or pulmonary stenosis
- **Normal split**
  - Healthy children, some adults
- **Wide split**
  - Pulmonary stenosis
  - Right bundle branch block
- **Fixed split**
  - Atrial septal defect
- **Reversed split**
  - Hypertrophic cardiomyopathy
  - Left bundle branch block

Third sound

The third heart sound is a low-pitched sound, like a thump or a thud, which occurs in mid-diastole. It is 'physiological' in athletes, some children, and in association with a hyperdynamic circulation (e.g. during pregnancy). In other patients it is associated with a dilated, poorly contracting left ventricle with a high end-diastolic pressure. The precise mechanism of the third heart sound is controversial. Its timing has been shown to coincide with the end of the phase of rapid diastolic ventricular filling.

A third sound in a fit patient with a resting bradycardia is nearly always physiological. Likewise, when there is evidence of a hyperdynamic circulation such as loud first and second heart sounds, peripheral vasodilatation and a good pulse volume, a third sound is little cause for worry. A third sound is also often heard in severe mitral regurgitation, even in the absence of heart failure.

A pathological third sound is usually part of a characteristic cadence described as a 'gallop rhythm'. There is a tachycardia, a soft first heart sound quickly followed by a soft second sound, and then a loud third sound: da-da-dum, da-da-dum. The patient often looks ill, and the cardiac apex is displaced and has a diffuse or dyskinetic feel. A chest X-ray will confirm cardiac enlargement, and the best way to confirm impaired ventricular function is by echocardiography.

Fourth sound

The fourth heart sound is associated with a hypertrophied atrium emptying into a rather stiff left ventricle.

It is only heard in sinus rhythm, and precedes the first sound by about 0.15 seconds: da-lub-dup, da-lub-dup. It is characteristically heard in hypertension and in hypertrophic cardiomyopathy, and occasionally in patients with ischaemic heart disease, especially soon after myocardial infarction, or aortic stenosis. In severe hypertension or hypertrophic cardiomyopathy there is often a separate palpable and visible component to the apex beat which coincides with the fourth heart sound. A fourth sound is not a feature of mitral stenosis (where the stenosed valve prevents rapid atrial emptying) or of mitral regurgitation where the atrium is too distended to contract forcefully. Some authorities describe patients with a fourth sound as having a 'presystolic gallop rhythm'.

Added or extra sounds

The *opening snap* is a feature of mitral (more rarely tricuspid) stenosis. It coincides with the bulging of the mitral valve 'diaphragm' into the ventricle in early diastole. It is a sharp, high-pitched sound best heard with the stethoscope diaphragm in the third or fourth left intercostal space about 3 cm from the left sternal edge, and is apt to be confused with a widely split second sound. The presence of an opening snap indicates that the valve, though stenosed, is still mobile. The interval between the second sound and opening snap reflects left atrial pressure – a high pressure, and thus severe stenosis, causing an early opening snap.

An *ejection click* is a short, loud, ringing sound immediately following the first heart sound ('as the l follows c in click'). It is a feature of valvar aortic stenosis with a mobile aortic valve, bicuspid aortic valve, or valvar pulmonary stenosis, and it is usually followed by an ejection systolic murmur. It is best heard in the aortic or pulmonary 'areas' depending on its cause. The mechanism is thought to be tensing of the aortic or pulmonary cusps just prior to ejection. An ejection click without a murmur sometimes occurs in idiopathic dilatation of the pulmonary artery.

Midsystolic clicks are usually associated with mitral valve prolapse (see HEART, MURMURS IN, p. 293), and are due to sudden tensing of parts of the mitral valve apparatus during systole. There may or may not be an associated systolic murmur. Both clicks and murmur may vary with posture and phase of respiration.

A *clicking pneumothorax* occurs when a small left pneumothorax causes a clicking sound, often loud and audible to the patient, in phase with the cardiac cycle. It is benign and self-limiting, but may recur.

Prosthetic valve sounds are heard in patients who have undergone valve replacement with mechanical prostheses (e.g. Starr–Edwards, Björk–Shiley or St. Jude Medical valves). Each valve has an opening sound analogous to the opening snap or ejection click, and a closing sound analogous to the first or second heart sound. The closing sound is usually much the louder – if it accompanies the first sound the patient has had a mitral valve replacement, and conversely for aortic valve replacement. The sound and cadence of the clicks are fairly constant for an individual patient, and sudden muffling of one or other prosthetic sound usually indicates prosthetic malfunction, perhaps due to thrombosis.

Melvin Lobo

HEART, ENLARGEMENT OF

Cardiac enlargement may be detected or suspected on the basis of clinical examination (see HEART IMPULSE, DISPLACED, p. 284), a chest radiograph or an electrocardiogram. Full assessment usually requires the combination of these three forms of investigation, plus echocardiography. When considering a patient with apparent cardiac enlargement, it is necessary to decide: (i) whether the enlargement is genuine or spurious; (ii) if genuine, whether it is physiological or pathological; and (iii) if pathological, whether it is due primarily to a myocardial disorder or a haemodynamic lesion.

The identification of genuine cardiac enlargement

The clinical diagnosis of cardiac enlargement is usually made because of displacement of the cardiac impulse. With left ventricular hypertrophy due to hypertension, aortic stenosis or hypertrophic cardiomyopathy, the apex may not be displaced but has a heaving, sustained character quite different from the normal. *Radiographic* cardiac enlargement is diagnosed when the cardiothoracic ratio is greater than 0.5 in a posteroanterior chest radiograph, with a tube-to-film distance of at least 2 m, taken in full inspiration. The cardiothoracic ratio is the ratio of the widest part of the cardiac shadow to the widest part of the lung fields. A spurious impression of cardiomegaly is caused by anteroposterior projections, portable apparatus with a reduced tube–film distance, and a poor inspiratory effort. In pectus excavation (funnel chest), a false impression of cardiac enlargement may be obtained from a posteroanterior film, but a lateral film will clarify the issue.

Radiological enlargement of the cardiac shadow may be due to a pericardial effusion. This is more likely if the enlargement is rapid (and previous films are available for comparison). Clinically, there will usually be elevation of the jugular venous pressure; there may be a pericardial friction rub, and an increased area of cardiac dullness. The ECG usually shows low voltages and there may be electrical alternans (alternating large and small QRS complexes in the same lead). Echocardiography is diagnostic.

An electrocardiographic diagnosis of cardiac enlargement is usually based on large QRS voltages, and is felt to be a relatively insensitive method for detection of cardiac hypertrophy. By convention, a sum of the S wave in lead V2 and the R wave in V5 of greater than 3.5 mV is one of the criteria for left ventricular hypertrophy. However, this criterion is sometimes met in fit muscular young men with thin chest walls, and echocardiography is commonly used definitively to diagnose cardiac chamber enlargement/ hypertrophy.

The identification of a pathological process

Athletes tend to have enlarged hearts, a slow resting pulse rate, and often a soft ejection systolic murmur related to a large resting stroke volume. In 'duration' sports (e.g. running or swimming) there is chamber enlargement without disproportionate hypertrophy of the ventricular walls. In 'power' sports (e.g. weightlifting) there may also be ventricular hypertrophy. If left ventricular hypertrophy is marked on electrocardiography or echocardiography it is worth asking about – and warning against – the abuse of anabolic steroids.

Cardiac enlargement is sometimes found in patients with congenital heart block, as an adaptive response to a slow pulse rate. It is usually present in acromegaly – sometimes as part of a general process of soft tissue hypertrophy, but sometimes as a feature of acromegalic heart muscle disease.

The distinction between myocardial and haemodynamic disorders

Cardiac enlargement, without a murmur but with an added third or fourth heart sound, is more likely to be due to a myocardial disorder and, with a murmur, to a haemodynamic lesion; the distinction is not absolute, however. The best diagnostic tool is duplex ultrasound (echocardiography plus Doppler cardiography) which gives information about both valve performance and ventricular function.

Myocardial problems

The principal heart muscle problems (in order of frequency, in 'Western' practice) are ischaemic heart disease, dilated cardiomyopathy, hypertrophic cardiomyopathy and the 'specific heart muscle diseases' which mimic dilated cardiomyopathy.

Ischaemic heart disease

Myocardial infarction can lead to left ventricular aneurysm formation. This is more frequent after anterior infarction. The cardiac impulse is displaced and has a diffuse 'dyskinetic' or 'hypokinetic' feel. The ECG shows evidence of old infarction, sometimes with persistent ST segment elevation. The chest X-ray usually shows cardiomegaly, occasionally with calcification in the aneurysm. Echocardiography is diagnostic. Ischaemic heart disease can also cause global left ventricular dilatation that is indistinguishable clinically from a dilated cardiomyopathy, though symptoms of angina or a history of myocardial infarction may provide clues.

Dilated cardiomyopathy

Dilated cardiomyopathy is the consequence of diffuse damage to cardiac muscle. By definition, the cause of 'cardiomyopathy' is unknown, but a similar clinical pattern is found in acute myocarditis and in association with a number of 'specific heart muscle diseases' (Table H.12). (Note: This is not an exhaustive list of specific heart muscle diseases, but emphasizes those which may present with cardiac enlargement.)

The heart is clinically and radiologically enlarged, and there are usually features of cardiac failure. There is a tachycardia and often a gallop rhythm with a loud third heart sound. The apex is displaced, and there may be soft systolic murmurs from functional mitral or tricuspid regurgitation. The electrocardiogram is

Table H.12 Specific heart muscle diseases

Connective tissue diseases
Sarcoidosis
Systemic lupus erythematosus
Polyarteritis nodosa
Rheumatoid arthritis (+pericardial effusion)

Infections
Chagas' disease
Viral myocarditis
Rickettsial myocarditis

Neurological/neuromuscular disorders
Duchenne's progressive muscular dystrophy
Friedreich's ataxia (mimics hypertrophic cardiomyopathy)
Dystrophia myotonica (+heart block)
X-linked humeroperoneal neuromuscular disease (mainly heart block)

Neoplastic disease (primary or metastatic)
Leukaemia, lymphomas

Metabolic disease
Amyloidosis
Haemochromatosis
Cardiac glycogenosis
Polysaccharide storage disease
Tay–Sachs disease
Fabry's disease
Gout
Oxalosis
Mucopolysaccharidoses (Hurler's syndrome)
Refsum's disease

Endocrine
Diabetes (+ischaemic heart disease)
Phaeochromocytoma
Thyrotoxicosis
Myxoedema (+pericardial effusion)
Acromegaly
Cushing's syndrome (+hypertension)

Nutritional
Beri-beri
Kwashiorkor

Toxic chemical and drug effects
Alcohol
Cobalt
Emetine and chloroquine
Daunorubicin and doxorubicin

usually abnormal, but the changes are non-specific. Echocardiography shows a characteristic pattern with dilatation of all four cardiac chambers and very poor ventricular contraction. Myocardial biopsy has a limited role, largely in excluding myocarditis or a specific cause. The prognosis is best when there is a remediable cause such as alcohol abuse, or where acute myocarditis is followed by spontaneous recovery.

Acute myocarditis is probably the most common cause of a dilated cardiomyopathy pattern in younger adults. There is often a preceding acute febrile illness or respiratory tract infection. Many viruses have been implicated, but the most consistent link is with the Coxsackie B group. The vast majority of cases of myocarditis probably goes unrecognized, but the prognosis in cases which present with cardiac failure is poor.

Alcoholic heart disease is probably the most common of the specific heart muscle diseases in middle-aged Western males, and there is some evidence that it may be reversible. Amyloid heart disease is unusual, among the specific heart muscle diseases, in that ventricular dilatation is not a prominent feature, although ventricular function is impaired.

Hypertrophic cardiomyopathy

Hypertrophic cardiomyopathy is characterized by abnormal hypertrophy of all or part of the ventricular muscle in the absence of an obvious stimulus. Different forms of the disease are increasingly recognized, including one which is usually inherited as an autosomal dominant trait and tends to present in adolescence and may cause sudden death, usually after physical exertion. Multiple mutations have now been identified (in sarcomeric genes) as the cause of this disorder in a substantial proportion of affected adults.

There is usually clinical cardiac enlargement. The apex is displaced and often has a 'double beat' character from a palpable atrial impulse, as well as the sustained lift of ventricular hypertrophy. There is usually a systolic murmur, which becomes louder during a Valsalva manoeuvre. There may be reversed splitting of the second heart sound, and the peripheral pulses are 'jerky'. The electrocardiogram is abnormal, sometimes showing left ventricular hypertrophy with marked T-wave changes, and sometimes mimicking an inferior infarct. Echocardiography is diagnostic. Patients with the hereditary neurological disorder of Friedreich's ataxia and those with Noonan's syndrome frequently have cardiac lesions similar to those of hypertrophic cardiomyopathy.

Haemodynamic problems

Haemodynamic problems causing cardiac enlargement can be divided into those causing a *volume load* and those causing a *pressure load* (Tables H.13 and H.14). The initial response to a volume load is an

Table H.13 Causes of pressure load

Left-sided

Common
- Systemic hypertension
- Aortic stenosis

Less common
- Coarctation of the aorta

Rare
- Phaeochromocytoma

Right-sided

Common
- Cor pulmonale
- Reactive pulmonary hypertension from left-sided problem

Less common
- Chronic thromboembolic pulmonary hypertension
- Pulmonary stenosis
- Eisenmenger's syndrome

Rare
- Primary pulmonary hypertension
- Carcinoid syndrome
- Appetite suppressants

Table H.14 Causes of volume load

Left-sided

Common
- Mitral regurgitation
- Aortic regurgitation

Less common
- Systemic arteriovenous fistula
- Severe anaemia
- Congenital heart disease: persistent ductus arteriosus, VSD

Rare
- Paget's disease of bone
- Erythroderma (in both cases via arteriovenous shunts)

Right-sided
- Atrial septal defect
- Other complex congenital heart disease
- Tricuspid regurgitation

increase in stroke volume, with enlargement of the cardiac chambers concerned, but with preservation of vigorous contraction. The response to a pressure load is hypertrophy, without dilatation, of the chambers involved. If either a volume or a pressure load persists beyond the capacity of the heart to compensate, then the chambers will dilate and contraction will become impaired. Chronic failure of the 'left side'

of the heart, from mitral valve disease, or left ventricular impairment, may be accompanied by reactive pulmonary vasoconstriction and secondary pulmonary hypertension, with ensuing dilatation of the right heart chambers as well.

Systemic hypertension is by far the most common 'pressure load' cause of cardiac enlargement. Most cases are due to 'essential' hypertension, but renal and endocrine causes should be remembered. Aortic coarctation causes delayed femoral pulses, and there is often a systolic murmur. A phaeochromocytoma can cause severe, but intermittent, hypertension. Murmurs should lead to the diagnosis of aortic or pulmonary stenosis. Aortic stenosis is frequently severe even when there is little or no radiological cardiac enlargement, but the presence of post-stenotic dilatation of the ascending aorta may give a clue. The diagnosis of pulmonary hypertension is often missed. The circumstances may be suggestive, and clinically the combination of a pronounced right parasternal impulse with changes of right ventricular hypertrophy in the electrocardiogram should lead it to be suspected.

Mitral and aortic regurgitation are detected through their distinctive murmurs. Selective enlargement of the different cardiac chambers may give a characteristic radiographic appearance. However, in some cases the radiographic appearance is non-specific and further aid must be sought from ultrasound scanning. 'Extracardiac' causes of an increased volume load are often difficult to detect, and require careful clinical assessment, possibly backed by objective measurement of cardiac output at rest by echocardiography, dye dilution or radionuclide techniques.

Melvin Lobo

HEART, MURMURS IN

A heart murmur is the audible sign of turbulent blood flow within the heart. The site of maximum intensity of the murmur should be noted, together with the direction in which it radiates – as a rule, this is the direction in which the turbulent blood is flowing. Other clues such as cardiac enlargement or abnormal pulsation in the precordium or neck vessels should also be sought. A *thrill* is a palpable vibration and, for practical purposes, precordial thrills can be regarded as 'palpable' murmurs. High-pitched vibration is usually more easily heard than felt and the significance of a thrill is simply that of a loud murmur. With low-frequency vibrations, some observers claim to find a thrill easier to feel than a low-pitched murmur is to hear.

Heart murmurs can be classified as either *systolic* or *diastolic* (the continuous murmur of persistent ductus arteriosus is, strictly speaking, exocardiac), though a single lesion can sometimes cause both. Systolic murmurs accompany the upstroke of the carotid pulse, diastolic murmurs precede or follow it.

Systolic murmurs

These are further classified as *ejection systolic murmurs*, which increase to a crescendo in midsystole and then die away before the second sound, and *pansystolic murmurs*, which remain at a more or less constant amplitude throughout systole. Late systolic murmurs are a variant of the latter, appearing in mid or late systole and continuing to the second sound (Fig. H.5).

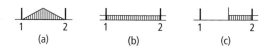

Figure H.5 Diagrammatic representation of ejection systolic (a), pansystolic (b) and late systolic murmurs (c).

Ejection systolic murmurs

The causes of these are listed in Table H.15.

Table H.15 Causes of ejection systolic murmurs

Most common
Innocent murmur
Flow murmur of high cardiac output
Mild aortic stenosis; bicuspid aortic valve
Mild pulmonary stenosis

Common
More severe aortic stenosis
Flow murmur of aortic regurgitation
Pulmonary stenosis
Pulmonary flow murmur of atrial septal defect
Hypertrophic cardiomyopathy

Uncommon
Supra- or subvalvar aortic stenosis
Severe hypercholesterolaemia

Innocent systolic murmurs

An ejection systolic murmur is commonly heard in fit children or young adults, particularly after exercise or vasodilatation, for example during pregnancy. Characteristically, the murmur is soft, best heard in the second left intercostal space, and becomes louder on inspiration; the second sound is normally split (see HEART SOUNDS, p. 286), and there are no other abnormal signs. Further investigation of these patients is almost always negative, and the long-term prognosis is excellent.

Aortic and pulmonary stenosis

The murmurs of mild aortic or pulmonary stenosis differ from innocent murmurs, principally in that they tend to be louder and the murmur is often preceded by an ejection click. Most patients with mild congenital aortic stenosis have bicuspid valves. Eventually, the abnormal valve tends to calcify and a mild stenosis may become severe. In elderly patients a soft ejection systolic murmur is usually due to calcific infiltration of the aortic valve and an ejection click is absent. The murmur of aortic stenosis can usually be heard all over the precordium, and tends to radiate to the upper right sternal edge and the neck. The murmur of pulmonary stenosis is loudest at the left sternal edge and may radiate to the back. In aortic coarctation, an ejection murmur may be heard beneath the left scapula; other signs such as delayed femoral pulses are also present. In young patients, the murmurs of severe pulmonary or aortic stenosis tend to be loud and harsh, but loudness is a poor guide to the severity of aortic stenosis in the elderly or when the cardiac output is low. Other features of severe aortic stenosis include clinical evidence of left ventricular hypertrophy and a slow-rising carotid pulse. In severe pulmonary stenosis the second sound is widely split. Duplex ultrasound scanning (two-dimensional echocardiography plus Doppler studies) is the most useful investigation.

Flow murmurs

Ejection systolic murmurs may be due to turbulence caused by a normal blood flow through a stenotic valve orifice, as in aortic stenosis, or by an increased blood flow through a non-stenotic valve. The latter mechanism accounts for most innocent murmurs, and for the pulmonary ejection systolic murmur of atrial septal defect, in which the flow through the pulmonary valve orifice may be increased two- or three-fold above normal. These patients have an 'active' feel to the precordium, there is fixed splitting of the second sound, and there may be a tricuspid diastolic flow murmur. Similarly, patients with marked aortic regurgitation may have a systolic murmur, despite the absence of anatomical stenosis.

Hypertrophic cardiomyopathy

Patients with this condition usually have an ejection systolic murmur, clinical evidence of left ventricular hypertrophy, and often a characteristically 'jerky' pulse. In these patients, the murmur paradoxically tends to become softer in inspiration and louder during expiration or in a Valsalva manoeuvre. Echocardiography is usually diagnostic.

Pansystolic murmurs

The causes of such murmurs are listed in Table H.16.

Table H.16 Causes of pansystolic murmurs

Most common
Mitral regurgitation (in adults)
■ Rheumatic
■ Mitral valve prolapse
■ Ischaemic
■ Due to endocarditis
■ Secondary to dilatation of mitral annulus
Ventricular septal defect (in children)

Common
Tricuspid regurgitation
■ Secondary
■ Rheumatic
■ Due to endocarditis
Post-infarction VSD

Uncommon
Pneumomediastinum 'pseudomurmur' or 'pericardial crunch'

Mitral regurgitation

The murmur of mitral regurgitation is usually loudest at the apex and radiates to the axilla. Loudness is some indication of severity, but there are exceptions. Torrential mitral regurgitation from papillary muscle rupture may be almost silent, while some patients with mitral valve prolapse and haemodynamically mild regurgitation may occasionally emit exceedingly loud 'honks' or 'whoops' that are audible across the room. The severity can be assessed from the patient's general condition, cardiac enlargement, the presence of cardiac failure, and the radiographic appearances as well as from the murmur. The term 'mitral valve prolapse' is used, confusingly, to describe either a diverse group of causes of non-rheumatic mitral regurgitation which have in common excessive elongation of the chordae tendineae, or a clinical syndrome which includes both the consequences of mitral regurgitation and also other features such as a predisposition to arrhythmias and, possibly, sudden death. Echocardiography is sometimes able to distinguish patients who simply have thin, stretched chordae tendineae (pellucid valve syndrome) from those with thickened, redundant, myxomatous valve tissue. It is in the latter group that most of the 'extra-valvar' events occur.

Clinically, patients with mitral valve prolapse are sometimes indistinguishable from those with other causes of regurgitation. The murmur of prolapse tends, however, to be mid- or late-systolic rather than pansystolic, at least in the early stages, and there may be one or more mid-systolic 'clicks' which are due to tensing of the chordae.

Congenital VSD

This is the most common cause of a pansystolic murmur in children and young adults. Large VSDs can cause cardiac failure within the first 3 months of life and, if untreated, sometimes induce reactive pulmonary hypertension with diminution (and eventual reversal) of shunt blood flow, cyanosis and disappearance of the murmur. Most pansystolic murmurs in older children are due to small defects with a loud murmur but a small shunt (*maladie de Roger*). The murmur is heard all over the precordium, but maximally at the upper left sternal edge. Duplex ultrasound scanning is the investigation of choice. An accurate knowledge of the size and position of a defect helps to predict whether it is likely to close spontaneously.

Acquired VSD

In adults, this may follow stab wounds or, more commonly, acute myocardial infarction. Clinical distinction between post-infarction septal defect and mitral regurgitation is difficult, but ultrasound is diagnostic.

Tricuspid regurgitation

This may be primary, from rheumatic heart disease or endocarditis, or secondary to right ventricular dilatation in response to pulmonary hypertension. The murmur is loudest at the lower left sternal edge, and is accompanied by pathognomonic 'v' waves in the jugular venous pulse. This lesion is seen much more often in conjunction with other cardiac lesions than on its own.

Pericardial 'crunch'

Patients with acute rupture of the oesophagus may develop a noise in the chest, synchronous with the heart beat, which is virtually indistinguishable from a loud pansystolic murmur. It is presumably a consequence of surgical emphysema in the mediastinum being 'crunched' with each systole.

Diastolic murmurs

These can be divided into early diastolic and mid-diastolic. Early diastolic murmurs are usually soft, decrescendo, high-pitched – 'like the letter R whispered', and best heard with the diaphragm of the stethoscope. They immediately follow the second heart sound, or the downstroke of the carotid pulse, and tend to be best heard at the left (sometimes right) sternal border with the patient sitting up, leaning forward and breathing out. Mid-diastolic murmurs are usually low-pitched, rumbling and best heard with the stethoscope bell (Fig. H.6).

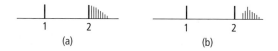

Figure H.6 Diagrammatic representation of (a) early diastolic and (b) mid-diastolic murmurs.

There are only two important causes of such murmurs – *aortic* and *pulmonary regurgitation*. The causes of these lesions are listed in Table H.17.

Aortic regurgitation

Unless this lesion is mild, it is usually accompanied by a wide pulse pressure and a collapsing arterial

Table H.17 Causes of early diastolic murmurs

Aortic regurgitation due to
Most common
Bicuspid aortic valve
Chronic rheumatic heart disease

Common
Chronic hypertension
Dissecting aneurysm of aorta
Infective endocarditis
Failing aortic prosthesis

Uncommon
Acute rheumatic fever
Rheumatoid heart disease
Ankylosing spondylitis
Reiter's syndrome
Chronic renal failure

Pulmonary regurgitation due to
Common
Secondary pulmonary hypertension (e.g. in mitral valve disease)
Following pulmonary valvotomy or valvuloplasty

Uncommon
Primary pulmonary hypertension
Thromboembolic pulmonary hypertension
Eisenmenger's syndrome

pulse. Features such as exaggerated carotid pulsation (Corrigan's sign), 'pistol shot' femoral bruits and capillary pulsation (Quincke's sign) are 'makeweights' to be sought when the diagnosis is already firm. The murmur of *acute* aortic regurgitation, as in acute endocarditis, is similar in timing to the more usual early diastolic murmur but may be quite different in quality, being loud and harsh and apt to be confused with a systolic murmur, unless it is timed against the pulse.

Pulmonary regurgitation

This is usually secondary to pulmonary hypertension; the murmur of pulmonary regurgitation secondary to chronic rheumatic mitral stenosis was described by Graham Steell. Pulmonary regurgitation may also be due to a damaged pulmonary valve resulting from a previous valvotomy or balloon valvuloplasty; in the absence of pulmonary hypertension, pulmonary regurgitation seems to be very well tolerated. Distinction from aortic regurgitation is usually easy from the clinical circumstances and the absence of other features of aortic regurgitation. Confirmation is possible by Doppler cardiography.

Mid-diastolic murmurs

The causes of these murmurs are listed in Table H.18.

Table H.18 Causes of mid-diastolic murmurs

Common
Rheumatic mitral stenosis

Uncommon
Austin Flint murmur in aortic regurgitation
Tricuspid flow murmur in atrial septal defect
Tricuspid stenosis
Carey Coombs murmur in acute rheumatic fever
Left or right atrial myxoma
Mitral flow murmur in VSD or persistent ductus arteriosus with
 large shunt

Mitral stenosis

This is by far the most common cause of a mid-diastolic murmur, which is best heard at the cardiac apex. There is often an audible or palpable opening snap in addition. The murmur of mitral stenosis is often accentuated just before the first sound (presystolic accentuation). This is most often recognized in sinus rhythm, and attributed to an increased flow during atrial systole, but it is sometimes heard in atrial fibrillation.

Carey Coombs murmur

A soft, low-pitched mid-diastolic murmur is sometimes heard in acute rheumatic fever, and is called after the physician who first described it. It is not due to mitral stenosis, but probably represents turbulence from minute vegetations on the mitral valve surface and from stiffening of the valve itself.

Austin Flint murmur

This murmur is due to fluttering of the anterior leaflet of the mitral valve, as a result of turbulence caused by aortic regurgitation. There is invariably an early diastolic murmur of aortic regurgitation and the opening snap of mitral stenosis is absent. Echocardiography is diagnostic.

Mid-diastolic flow murmurs

The mid-diastolic murmur of increased tricuspid flow in atrial septal defect is usually heard only in children and adolescents. It tends to be higher pitched than the murmur of mitral stenosis, and is best heard at the lower left sternal edge. A similar murmur may be heard at the apex in patients with a large VSD or persistent ductus arteriosus.

Tricuspid stenosis

The murmurs of tricuspid stenosis are similar to those of mitral stenosis, but the condition is much less common. The jugular venous pressure is elevated and the venous pulse has a characteristic waveform (see NECK, ENGORGED VEINS IN, p. 469).

Atrial myxoma

Left atrial myxomas are more common than right, though both are rare. They may cause murmurs mimicking mitral stenosis but, often, the murmurs vary with posture as the myxoma prolapses in or out of the valve orifice. The first sound is loud and there may be an extra sound, called a 'tumour plop', from movement of the myxoma.

Melvin Lobo

HEARTBURN

Retrosternal burning, rising from the epigastrium towards the throat, lies within the spectrum of dyspeptic symptoms. It is commonly ascribed to the reflux of acid or bile into the lower oesophagus secondary to inappropriate relaxation of the lower oesophageal sphincter or mechanical disruption of this mechanism (hiatus hernia, previous surgery or the presence of a stent). There is usually a co-existing element of oesophageal dysmotility impairing acid/bile clearance. Symptoms are classically exacerbated by lying flat or by stooping. Such heartburn may also occur paradoxically in patients with achalasia. Cancer of the gastro-oesophageal junction and gallstones may present with this complaint.

Gastroscopic findings with reflux are usually unremarkable; commonly a normal mucosa is seen. Barrett's oesophagus (intestinal metaplasia of the oesophageal squamous epithelium) is found in approximately 5 per cent of patients complaining of reflux, and is equally as likely to be found in those with epigastric pain alone. The development of such metaplasia may be associated with a disappearance of reflux symptoms, a testament to the protective nature of intestinal-type mucosa. Barrett's oesophagus is of malignant potential, with 0.5 per cent of Barrett's cases developing adenocarcinoma per year; those found to have high-grade dysplasia on biopsy have foci of intra-mucosal cancer in 50 per cent of cases.

Acid reflux has been implicated in the marked rise in the incidence of adenocarcinoma of the gastro-oesophageal junction reported from developed countries. The majority of people with significant acid reflux, however, do not have any symptoms; those with heartburn are no more likely than those with epigastric pain alone to have acid reflux on investigation. This is of clinical importance in patient management, as targeting those patients with reflux symptoms for cancer prevention would yield little benefit to a population.

A diagnosis of acid/bile reflux and associated dysmotility is made by oesophageal manometry and pH studies. An acid-sensitive oesophagus may also be detected at this test through the blinded introduction of dilute acid (Bernstein test). Patients over the age of 55 years with recent-onset reflux-like symptoms, and particularly those with alarm features (dysphagia, odynophagia, anaemia, weight loss), must undergo gastroscopy or barium studies to exclude cancer. A clinical response to medical therapy does not mean that cancer is any less likely to be present.

Patients who display an acid-sensitive oesophagus without detectable gross acid reflux, and those with dysmotility, respond poorly to surgical intervention. Proton-pump inhibitors offer the best initial therapy for reflux, being superior to H_2-receptor antagonists, simple antacids or motility agents alone. Life-style alterations, including weight reduction, avoidance of alcohol, cigarettes and fatty foods and raising the head of the bed, generally have limited impact in symptom control. There is no definite link between the presence of *Helicobacter pylori* and reflux; indeed, it has been suggested that eradication of this gastric antral dwelling bacterium may induce acid reflux.

Endoscopic treatments for reflux include submucosal injection or insertion of implants at the oesophagogastric junction, application of radiofrequency energy, or the suturing/stapling of this area. The results of long-term studies for these techniques are not available.

Guidance on the management of heartburn is offered by many national gastroenterological societies, but must be adapted to take into account local variation in pathology (UK, www.bsg.org; USA, www.gastro.org).

John Meenan

HEMIANOPIA

Hemianopia means an inability to see objects in one-half of the visual field. An understanding of the different types of hemianopia requires an understanding of the anatomy of the visual pathways (Fig. H.7).

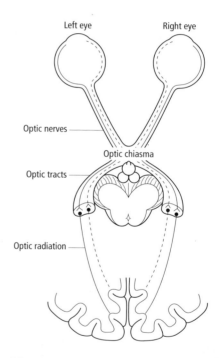

Figure H.7 Diagram illustrating the connections of the optic nerves and tracts, and the occipital cortex. The left occipital cortex sees objects in the right half of the field of vision, while the right occipital cortex sees objects in the left half of the field of vision.

Monocular hemianopia

The loss of half of the visual field in one eye usually indicates optic nerve pathology, but may occasionally result from retinal damage. Monocular hemianopia may be either temporal or nasal, depending on which fibres in the optic nerve have been damaged. A monocular quandrantanopia indicates loss of one-quarter of one field.

Compression of the optic nerve from a tumour may result in a monocular hemianopia, but optic neuritis – such as frequently occurs in multiple sclerosis – more commonly produces a central field defect in the form of a scotoma. The commonest cause of monocular hemianopia is ischaemic damage to the optic nerve.

Bitemporal hemianopia

This most commonly results from damage to the optic chiasma, usually from a pituitary tumour. Less common causes are suprasellar cysts, aneurysms, meningiomas of the tuberculum sellae or craniopharyngiomas.

When the pressure upon the chiasma begins from below, the visual field defect typically begins in the upper part of the temporal fields, leading initially to a bitemporal quandrantanopia. Pressure from above the chiasma produces initially a lower bitemporal defect. By the time all the crossing fibres in the optic chiasm are compressed, a complete bitemporal hemianopia will have developed.

Skull X-rays will usually show an enlarged pituitary fossa when a bitemporal hemianopia has resulted from a pituitary tumour. When bitemporal hemianopia is due to other causes, the skull X-ray may be normal. The investigation of choice is CT scanning or MRI (Fig. H.8).

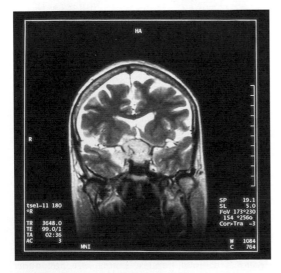

Figure H.8 Pituitary tumour (prolactinoma).

Homonymous hemianopia

In homonymous hemianopia the visual loss affects the right or left half of each visual field, and usually results from damage to the optic radiation or visual cortex. Optic tract damage or damage to the lateral geniculate body may produce a homonymous hemianopia, but such cases are rare. Homonymous hemianopia may be either congruous or incongruous. Congruous defects are those that are identical in shape and degree in each field; incongruous defects are asymmetrical.

In the optic tracts the intermingling of fibres from the homonymous halves of the two retinas is not as complete as in the optic radiation. Consequently, a lesion of the tract tends to lead to an incongruous homonymous hemianopia, whereas a lesion of the optic radiation is more likely to produce a congruous field defect.

Damage to the visual cortex may spare the area responsible for the macular vision, resulting in homonymous hemianopia with macular sparing. Lesions of the parietal lobe typically produce a hemianopia which begins with loss of vision in the lower parts of the field, whereas a temporal lobe lesion characteristically affects the upper parts of the visual field (homonymous quandrantanopias). Associated signs may assist in localization.

The visual field defect, when plotted using the Bjerrum screen, may be the same for different sized objects, and is then said to have 'sharp edges'. A visual field defect which varies depending on the size of the object presented is said to have 'sloping edges'. The former is more typical of a vascular cause, whereas the latter is said to be more often encountered when the optic pathway is compressed by tumour.

In testing the visual fields clinically, it is customary to present an object – usually a finger or coloured pinhead – first to the temporal field of one eye, and then to that of the other eye. It is also useful to present a wagging finger to both temporal fields simultaneously. Occasionally, there is a failure in this test to pick up the finger in one field, although it is perceived when presented singly. This is the phenomenon of visual inattention (or extinction) and it is encountered in some parietal lobe lesions.

Reginald Daniel

HEMIPLEGIA

Hemiplegia refers to complete paralysis of one side of the body affecting both upper and lower limbs; hemiparesis refers to partial paralysis, though in practice the terms tend to be used interchangeably. The terms are usually applied in cases in which the paralysis is of upper motor neurone type, though it is possible to see unilateral weakness affecting both the arm and leg in lower motor neurone disorders, such as poliomyelitis, motor neurone disease or combined cervical and lumbar radiculopathy. Hemiplegia is most commonly seen in damage to the upper motor neurone above the level of the foramen magnum. A discrete lesion of the spinal cord in the upper cervical region may produce a hemiplegia, but this is rare.

Hemiplegia occurs most commonly as a result of ischaemic (Fig. H.9) or haemorrhagic (Fig. H.10) stroke affecting the motor cortex, internal capsule or, occasionally, the brainstem. The widely used Oxfordshire Community Stroke project classification of stroke which is predominantly clinical but refined by neuroimaging is shown in Table H.19. Intracranial mass lesions such as tumour or subdural haematoma (Fig. H.11) may also present with hemiplegia, though usually of gradual onset. Typically, the so-called 'physiological' flexors are weaker than the extensors. This results in more profound weakness of shoulder abduction, elbow extension, wrist extension, finger

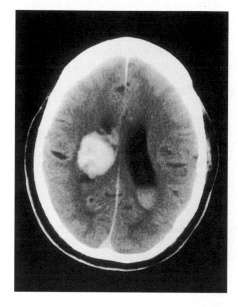

Figure H.10 Computed tomogram showing left subcortical haemorrhage with intraventricular rupture and mass effect.

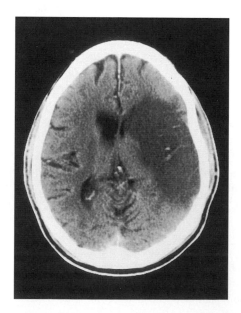

Figure H.9 Computed tomogram showing extensive left middle cerebral artery territory infarction with mass effect.

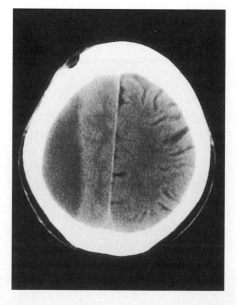

Figure H.11 Computed tomogram showing large right chronic subdural haematoma.

Table H.19 The Oxfordshire Community Stroke project classification of stroke

Primary intracerebral haemorrhage

Subarachnoid haemorrhage

Lacunar infarction (LACI): Requires one of the classical lacunar syndromes:
- Isolated hemiparesis
- Isolated hemianaesthesia
- Hemiparesis + hemianaesthesia
- Ataxic hemiparesis
- Dysarthria – clumsy hand syndrome

Plus imaging showing a deep infarct <1.5 cm in diameter or a normal CT scan. The diagnosis is excluded by the presence of cortical signs or features that clearly localized the lesion in the vertebrobasilar distribution.

Total anterior circulation infarction (TACI): evidence of higher cerebral dysfunction (e.g. dysphasia, dyscalculia, visuospatial disorders), homonymous visual field defect, and ipsilateral motor and/or sensory deficits of at least two areas of the face, arm and leg. If consciousness is impaired so that formal testing of higher cerebral function or visual fields is not possible, then a deficit was assumed.

Partial anterior circulation infarction (PACI): two of the three components of the TACI syndrome, higher cerebral dysfunction alone, or with a motor/sensory deficit more restricted than those classified as LACI (e.g. confined to one limb, or to face and hand, but not the whole arm).

Posterior circulation infarction (POCI): patients presenting with any of the following: ipsilateral cranial nerve palsy with contralateral motor and/or sensory deficit; disorder of conjugate eye movement; cerebellar dysfunction without ipsilateral long tract deficit (i.e. ataxic hemiparesis); or isolated homonymous visual field defect.

Table H.20 The causes of hemiplegia

Congenital	Porencephaly, cerebral agenesis, cerebral angioma, Sturge–Weber syndrome (cerebral palsy)
Head injury	Birth injury, cerebral contusion, traumatic cerebral haemorrhage, subdural haematoma, extradural haematoma
Cerebrovascular accidents	Cerebral thrombosis, hypertensive encephalopathy, cerebral haemorrhage, subarachnoid haemorrhage, cerebral embolism
Neoplasms	Primary neoplasms, secondary neoplasms
Infection	Meningitis (various), cerebral abscess, cortical thrombophlebitis, encephalitis, hydatid cyst
Demyelinating conditions	Multiple sclerosis, Schilder's disease, acute disseminated encephalomyelitis
Degenerative conditions	Motor neurone disease
Miscellaneous conditions	Pick's disease, epiloia
Hysteria	

extension and finger abduction in the arm, and hip flexion, knee flexion and ankle dorsiflexion in the leg. The opposing muscles tend to be those which are associated with spasticity, and this results in the typical hemiplegic posture of an abducted flexed arm and an extended leg. Associated signs include hyper-reflexia, extensor plantar responses and ankle and knee clonus. The abdominal and cremasteric reflexes are lost on the side of the hemiplegia. In cases of chronic hemiplegia there may be some slight loss of muscle bulk, and contractures may become prominent. Paralysis occurring in childhood before bone growth ceases may be associated with hemi-atrophy.

The pathological causes of hemiplegia are listed in Table H.20.

James Kelly

HICCUP

Hiccup is very common, and is only significant if persistent. It is caused by sudden involuntary contraction of both the diaphragm and external intercostal muscles in association with rapid glottic closure. Hiccups may be induced by stimulating a variety of sensory nerves, particularly the vagus and phrenic. Hiccups usually occur with a frequency of between 4 and 60 per minute.

The commonest cause of hiccup is gastric distension after rapid ingestion of food, alcohol or air. Other common causes include excitement and a sudden change in temperature, either of the environment or of the stomach induced by a hot or very cold meal. However, in persistent cases, the following causes should be considered.

Intrathoracic

Mediastinal

Irritation of a phrenic nerve may cause recurrent attacks of intractable hiccup. In an adult, this may be due to malignant lymphadenopathy due to tumours of the lung or oesophagus or to a lymphoma. An aortic aneurysm may rarely cause hiccup. Hiccup may also follow mediastinal surgery or mediastinitis.

Diaphragmatic

Hiccup may occur in pneumonia and empyema due to diaphragmatic pleurisy, and may also occur in myocardial infarction and pericarditis.

Intra-abdominal disease

Hiccup of intra-abdominal cause often results from diaphragmatic irritation due, for example, to diaphragmatic hernia, subphrenic abscess, peritonitis, pancreatitis, liver metastases, liver abscess, splenic infarct and carcinoma of the stomach. However, other conditions such as carcinoma of the sigmoid colon and carcinoma of the uterus have been associated with hiccup, even without any obvious diaphragmatic involvement. Hiccup may occur after abdominal or pelvic operations, and is seen in association with acute postoperative dilatation of the stomach and with intestinal obstruction.

Central

Epidemic encephalitis

This rare cause of hiccup was probably a variety of encephalitis lethargica in which there was inflammation affecting the third and fourth segments of the cervical cord, those from which the phrenic nerve originates. Hiccup may also follow lesions of the medulla.

Intracranial

Hiccup may rarely result from intracranial tumours, intracranial haemorrhage, brain abscess or meningitis, especially when the brainstem or basal meninges are involved.

Toxic

Uraemic hiccups are uncommon, but may be persistent. Acute severe fevers including typhoid, malaria and cholera may also be accompanied by hiccups.

Hysterical hiccup

This occasional cause of hiccup usually affects young women, who may hiccup persistently during wakefulness. However, the hiccup stops during sleep.

Drugs

Benzodiazepines and short-acting barbiturates can also cause hiccup. Chlorpromazine is an effective treatment.

Boris Lams

HIP, PAIN IN

See LOWER LIMB, PAIN IN (p. 381).

HIRSUTISM

Hirsutism is said to be present when a female has excessive growth of hair in androgen-sensitive areas where hair growth is normally minimal or absent. Hirsutism in isolation (i.e. without other signs of virilization) is usually benign, and the majority of patients are suffering from polycystic ovary syndrome (PCOS). However, it is worthwhile looking for evidence of virilization (clitoral enlargement, deepening of the voice, temporal balding, decreased breast size and loss of the female body contour), which makes a pathological cause much more likely. The cause of hirsutism is an increased secretion of androgens from the ovary or adrenal glands. Normally, testosterone is produced directly from the ovary and by extraglandular conversion of androstenedione secreted from both the ovaries and adrenal glands. The adrenal gland produces only minimal amounts of testosterone, but it is the main source of the pro-androgen dehydroepiandrosterone (DHEA) and its sulphate (DHEAS). Serum testosterone is markedly elevated in ovarian causes of virilization, and DHEAS is elevated in cases of virilization due to adrenal pathology.

Types of hair growth

Lanugo

This is the very fine, silky – but sometimes quite long – hair which covers the entire skin surface of the fetus;

it is usually shed by the seventh or eighth month of intrauterine life.

Vellus

Males and females are born with the same number of hair follicles. In childhood, the follicles produce vellus hair which is fine and non-pigmented. This type of hair persists into adult life in the areas of skin which are not producing terminal hair (see below). Occasionally, a woman may notice vellus hair, particularly on the face, when looking into a mirror with the sun or light behind her head. She may then look for them elsewhere and be horrified to find them on her chest, arms and legs. This, of course, is not hirsutism but 'pseudohirsutism'. Non-androgenic causes of hirsutism usually result in increased vellus hair formation.

Intermediate hair

This hair is soft and silky, but may grow long and become pigmented. It then becomes a source of embarrassment. A combination of vellus and intermediate hair over the face and shoulders is characteristic of Cushing's syndrome.

Terminal hair

Terminal hair is coarse and pigmented and is of three types:

- *Non-sexual hair*, which is present on the scalp, eyebrows, arms and legs.
- *Ambosexual hair*, which is initiated by low levels of androgens and is present in the axillae, lower pubic triangle and limbs.
- *Sexual hair*, which is produced by male levels of androgens and is present in the upper pubic triangle as the 'male escutcheon', on the face, nose, ears, trunk and limbs, where it is present in more profusion than ambosexual hair. When this type of sexual hair is present in a woman she is deemed to be suffering from 'hirsutism'.

However, it is important to realize that there is an overlap between what can be considered to be normal and that which is regarded as 'hirsute'. In a study of 400 consecutive Welsh and English women students at the University of Wales, 26 per cent had terminal hair on the face, 17 per cent on the chest or breasts, 35 per cent on the lower abdomen (mainly linea alba) and 84 per cent on the lower arm and leg. Of these latter 84 per cent, nearly three-quarters also had terminal

hair on the thighs and upper arms. As mentioned earlier, Mediterranean (and some Indian) women tend to grow more terminal hair than Nordic women, whereas women of the Mongolian races (Japanese, Chinese, American Indians, etc.) grow much less. These racial factors must therefore be taken into account when assessing hirsutism. The presence of oligomenorrhoea, amenorrhoea, seborrhoea and acne in a hirsute woman are factors indicating the necessity for investigation.

Hirsutism and virilization

Virilism may accompany hirsutism, and is characterized by clitoral enlargement, breast atrophy, temporal hair recession, frontal baldness and loss of normal female contours due to increased muscularity. Deepening of the voice often occurs, and there is usually amenorrhoea. The presence of virilization should draw attention to the possibility of one of the conditions marked by asterisks in Table H.21.

Table H.21 Causes of hirsutism (in order of frequency)

Polycystic ovary syndrome[*]
Idiopathic (often familial)
Menopause

Drugs
Menopausal preparations (containing methyltestosterone)
Androgens[*]
Anabolic steroids[*]
Synthetic 17-nor-progestogens; ACTH
Phenytoin[†]
Diazoxide[†]
Minoxidil[†]
Glucocorticoids[†]

Metabolic disorders
Anorexia nervosa[†]
Porphyria cutanea tarda[†]

Miscellaneous disorders
Cornelia de Lange syndrome[†]
Hypertrichosis lanuginosa[†]

Endocrine disorders
Acromegaly
Cushing's syndrome[*†]
Congenital and juvenile hypothyroidism[†]
Congenital adrenal hyperplasia[*]
Adrenal carcinoma or adenoma[*]
Ovarian tumours[*]
Arrhenoblastoma
Hilus cell tumour (and hyperplasia)
Luteoma

[*]May be associated also with virilization.
[†]Associated with vellus rather than with terminal hair production.

Polycystic ovary syndrome (PCOS)

This is the most common cause of hirsutism in clinical practice. The classic features originally described by Stein and Leventhal are hirsutism, obesity, oligomenorrhoea or amenorrhoea, and enlarged cystic ovaries with thickened capsules. On microscopic examination, numerous small atretic follicles are found, surrounded by hyperplastic theca interna. In most cases the menstrual disturbance starts shortly after puberty and tends to become progressively worse. Anovulation is invariable. Hirsutism is present in about 50 per cent of cases, and occasionally virilization is seen. The ovary produces excess androstenedione, which is converted into testosterone. In addition, the androstenedione undergoes conversion to oestrone in fatty tissue. Thus, there is not only androgenization but also continuous oestrogen production. The result is continuous high luteinizing hormone (LH) production by the pituitary, which tends to perpetuate the situation. Follicle-stimulating hormone (FSH) levels are in the low normal range, while 17-keto-steroids are usually in the high normal range.

The classic syndrome may not always be present. Obesity may be absent, hirsutism is not a feature in 50 per cent of patients, and some patients may have normal-sized ovaries with a solitary atretic follicle. In contrast, the triad of hyperandrogenism, insulin resistance and acanthosis nigricans forms a specific subset of women with PCOS (HAIR-AN syndrome). In these women the hirsutism is severe.

Idiopathic hirsutism

This is the second most common type of hirsutism, and may reflect an increased sensitivity of the pilosebaceous unit to relatively normal plasma levels of androgen. The diagnosis should only be reached after excluding all of the other possible causes listed above. If there is a history of hirsutism in other close female relatives, or a history of baldness in father or brothers, the diagnosis of idiopathic hirsutism is more certain. Although the condition is called 'idiopathic', minor hormonal abnormalities are frequently found. In normal women small amounts of the pro-androgens androstenedione and DHEA are secreted mainly by the adrenal gland. These are then converted into testosterone and its derivative, the more powerful hormone dihydrotestosterone. In women with hirsutism there may be an increased production of androstenedione by the ovary as well as the adrenal and this leads to increased conversion to testosterone and dihydrotestosterone. The rise in active androgens lowers the concentration of sex hormone-binding globulin (SHBG); the net effect is to decrease the amount of bound androgen and to increase the amount of free androgen, thus amplifying its biological action. In idiopathic hirsutism the usual finding is either a slightly raised or a normal plasma testosterone level. If the SHBG is reduced, then the free testosterone may be elevated. Urinary 17-keto-steroid levels are usually normal because they are only increased when very large amounts of androstenedione and DHEA are being produced.

Menopause

At the time of the menopause there tends to be an increase in the growth of terminal hair in the moustache and beard areas, whereas, paradoxically, body hair gradually becomes less. This is physiological because of the change in the oestrogen:androgen ratio.

Drugs

Menopausal preparations containing methyltestosterone, androgens in general, anabolic steroids, the synthetic 17-nor-progestogens and adrenocorticotrophic hormone (ACTH) may all cause an increased growth of terminal hair. Androgens and anabolic steroids may even cause some degree of virilization.

Other drugs (phenytoin, diazoxide, minoxidil and glucocorticoids) cause stimulation of vellus hair growth.

Metabolic and miscellaneous disorders

Vellus hair growth is seen as a feature of anorexia nervosa and porphyria cutanea tarda. In the condition known as 'hypertrichosis lanuginosa', the lanugo hair which was shed *in utero* at the seventh or eighth month suddenly regrows and completely covers the face so that the features become unrecognizable. In the Cornelia de Lange syndrome (see p. 678), which is associated with short stature ('Amsterdam dwarfism'), the scalp hair reaches down to the bushy and confluent eyebrows, and there is also generalized hirsutism of a mixed vellus and intermediate type.

Endocrine disorders

Acromegaly

The incidence of this disease is about three newly diagnosed cases per million of the population each year, whereas the prevalence of previously diagnosed cases is approximately 40 per million of the population. Just over half the women with acromegaly complain of hirsutism, and in them urinary 17-keto-steroid levels may be slightly raised. The mechanism for the increase in 17-keto-steroids is unknown. The hair is of the terminal type.

Cushing's syndrome

Apart from iatrogenic disease caused by the administration of glucocorticoids, Cushing's syndrome is rare, occurring in only one to two people per million of the population each year. The condition is relatively more common in women, when it is usually associated with hirsutism. There is conspicuous hair growth in the beard and moustache areas, but the characteristic feature is a rather widespread, vellus hirsutism on the face and over the shoulders. The plethoric moon-shaped face, buffalo hump, supraclavicular puffiness, livid cutaneous striae, central obesity, thin limbs and subcutaneous bruising of the classic case make the diagnosis easy. However, mild or early cases of Cushing's syndrome may not be easy to recognize, and it is a diagnosis always worth bearing in mind in a woman with hirsutism. The best screening tests to use are a 24-hour urine collection for free cortisol, or a 9 a.m. plasma cortisol following 1 mg of oral dexamethasone taken the previous night before retiring. A normal urinary free cortisol and a suppressed 9 a.m. plasma cortisol will exclude the diagnosis.

Congenital and juvenile hypothyroidism

Congenital hypothyroidism occurs in approximately one per 5000 births in the United Kingdom. With the increasing use of neonatal thyroid-stimulating hormone (TSH) screening, most cases should be diagnosed shortly after birth, and treatment initiated. In cases diagnosed later on, the babies may develop a coat of vellus or intermediate hair over the back and extensor surfaces of the skin. A similar picture is sometimes seen in patients with juvenile hypothyroidism.

Congenital adrenal hyperplasia

Congenital adrenal hyperplasia results from excessive ACTH stimulation. This is caused by an inherited deficiency of an enzyme necessary for the synthesis of cortisol. Five different types of enzyme deficiency have been recognized, but 21-hydroxylase deficiency is by far the most common. This occurs with a frequency of one per 5000 live births. In the female, the condition is usually recognized at birth because of genital abnormalities such as enlargement of the clitoris and fusion of the labia. In girls with less severe enzyme defects, 21-hydroxylase may present at a later age with premature false puberty (see p. 566) and hirsutism. Occasionally, the condition becomes apparent after puberty; in addition to hirsutism there may be clitoromegaly and either oligomenorrhoea or amenorrhoea.

The increase in adrenal androgens is caused by an ACTH-stimulated build-up of the precursors of cortisol. These can be measured as 17-keto-steroids in the urine.

In 21-hydroxylase deficiency, raised levels of 17-hydroxyprogesterone are found in the blood, while levels of its metabolite, pregnanetriol, are increased in the urine.

A few women with hirsutism are carriers for 21-hydroxylase deficiency, and show marked rises in 17-hydroxyprogesterone when given ACTH.

Adrenal carcinoma or adenoma

Adrenal tumours producing hirsutism and virilization are rare, and symptoms and signs develop abruptly. There are usually very high levels of urinary 17-keto-steroids that cannot be suppressed to 50 per cent of the original levels by 0.5 mg of dexamethasone given 6-hourly for 3 days. Some 40 per cent of carcinomas are palpable, whilst adenomas may be very small. Calcification in a carcinoma may sometimes be seen on X-ray. CT scanning is usually informative but, if not, then isotope scanning or selective venous sampling for adrenal androgens may localize the tumour.

Ovarian tumours

These are exceedingly rare as a cause of hirsutism and virilism, and symptoms and signs develop abruptly. They usually give rise to extreme degrees of virilism because the androgen that they produce, testosterone, is very potent. Levels of testosterone are high in the blood, but urinary 17-keto-steroids, which only measure 25 per cent of all testosterone secreted, may be within the normal range. The tumour may be palpable on pelvic examination, and the enlargement can be confirmed by ultrasound.

Sharon O'Byrne

HYPERVENTILATION

Hyperventilation is over-breathing or ventilation in excess of metabolic requirements, with symptoms arising from respiratory alkalosis and hypocapnia (Table H.22).

Table H.22 Causes of acute hyperventilation

Commonest	Rare
Stress reaction	Acidotic disorders
Anxiety	■ Biguanide intolerance
Phobia	■ Intestinal fistula
Panic	■ Surgical relocation of ureters in ileum or colon
Less common	Psychiatric disorders
Acidotic disorders	■ Hysteria
■ Diabetic ketoacidosis	■ Malingering
■ Salicylate poisoning	Others
■ Renal failure	■ Epilepsy
Pulmonary disorders	■ Acute porphyria
■ Asthma	■ Phaeochromocytoma
■ Pulmonary oedema	■ Hepatic cirrhosis
■ Pulmonary embolism	■ Pyloric stenosis
■ Pleural effusion	
■ Spontaneous pneumothorax	
Vasovagal attacks	
Following childbirth or abdominal surgery	

Acute hyperventilation

This condition is easily recognized because over-breathing is apparent. The characteristic patient is a young woman, and the presentation has a readily identified precipitant which may have aroused anxiety, fear, distress, excitement, adulation or other powerful feelings. Occasionally, the respiratory alkalosis is compensation for a metabolic acidosis, and especially in the young, diabetic ketoacidosis and salicylate poisoning can present occultly and ought to be

excluded. Asthma, which has been identified as both a cause and a consequence of hyperventilation, may also present as stress-induced dyspnoea, although it is usually distinguishable by evident expiratory difficulty. In hospital, acute hyperventilation is not uncommonly precipitated by abdominal surgery or childbirth, when anxiety is accompanied by an avoidance of abdominal breathing as a protective mechanism against pain or fear of re-opening the wound. The differential diagnosis of acute breathlessness in these circumstances is pulmonary embolism, which may also provoke as well as mimic acute hyperventilation.

Chronic hyperventilation

Chronic hyperventilation syndrome is much more difficult to recognize because, once established, the disorder can be maintained by occasional deep breaths or sighs. Chronic hyperventilation accounts for 6–10 per cent of medical referrals, but it is frequently unconsidered, with the patient's multiple unexplained somatic and psychological complaints leading all too readily to a label of 'functional disorder'.

Even when chronic hyperventilation syndrome is contemplated, the clinician faces difficulty establishing the disorder's presence because there is no satisfactorily reliable sign or test. The diagnosis rests upon a combination of typical symptoms and signs, clinical tests and investigations of respiratory function. The central symptom is breathlessness, an air hunger which is associated with gasping, sighing and a feeling of suffocating. Breathlessness tends to be worse at rest, following exercise or on awakening, and it may be associated with a particular setting, such as shops or buses, or be triggered by emotions. Common physical symptoms include fatigue, dizziness, faintness, headaches, tremors, sweating, palpitations, chest pain, dysphagia, nausea, heartburn, diarrhoea, flatulence. Common psychological symptoms are anxiety, depression, poor concentration and memory and depersonalization. Any of these may be the presenting complaint, but it is the sheer number and range of symptoms that provide the clue. A more characteristic pointer is paraesthesiae in the hands, fingers and around the mouth, while tetany is strong (but rare) evidence. In susceptible individuals hyperventilation may present with fits.

At interview, gasping, sighing and a rapid, uneven respiratory pattern may be noted. The frequent interruption of speech by the need to breathe can be an important sign. Excessive thoracic movement during breathing is characteristic, while forced, voluntary over-breathing may rapidly provoke the re-experience of presenting symptoms; re-breathing into a paper bag may abolish these. Assessment of respiratory function helps to establish the diagnosis (Table H.23).

Table H.23 Causes of chronic hyperventilation

Commonest
Anxiety

Less common
Pulmonary disorders
■ Asthma
■ Pulmonary embolism
■ Bronchial neoplasm
■ Diffuse pulmonary fibrosis
Renal failure
Psychiatric disorders
■ Phobia
■ Panic
■ Depression
■ Briquet's syndrome (somatization disorder)
■ Hypochondriasis
■ Primary habit disorder

Rare
Neurological disorders
■ Damage to respiratory pathways
■ Raised intracranial pressure

Metabolic disorders
■ Congestive cardiac failure
■ Persistent hypoxaemia
■ Liver failure
Psychiatric disorders
■ Schizophrenia
■ Malingering

It cannot be assumed that chronic hyperventilation invariably arises from a disturbed emotional state. Physical causes include disorders of ventilation– perfusion: asthma, pulmonary embolism, parenchymatous lung disease and, rarely, neurological damage to the respiratory pathways, usually in the brainstem. However, the most common causes are *psychological disorders*, especially anxiety, phobias and panic disorder. Paradoxically it is now evident that chronic over-breathing may induce these conditions as well as result from them. This interaction is complex, and best understood

as a feedback loop (Fig. H.12), although the implication is that treatment can be focused upon either the breathing abnormality or the emotional disorder with the expectation of ameliorating both aspects.

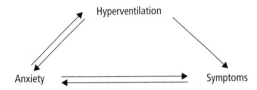

Figure H.12 The relationship between hyperventilation and anxiety.

Finally, a substantial minority have no evidence of underlying physical or psychological disorder. In these patients, chronic hyperventilation syndrome is probably a *primary habit disorder*, although the predisposing biological and psychosocial mechanisms are still unknown. All habits tend to be exaggerated when under pressure, so it should be anticipated that such individuals become symptomatic on stressful occasions: without considering this, it is easy to mislabel these patients as pathologically anxious.

Andrew Hodgkiss

HYPOCHONDRIASIS

The characteristics of hypochondriasis are:

■ Concern with health or disease in oneself, present most of the time.
■ Preoccupation not justified by the amount of organic pathology.
■ Does not respond adequately to reassurance, given after a careful physical assessment.

The abnormal health beliefs lie on a spectrum ranging from a preoccupation to an over-valued idea to a delusion. Hypochondriacal delusions have a different differential diagnosis and require different treatment to non-delusional hypochondriasis.

When faced with a hypochondriacal patient, the first and most essential step is to defer reaching this conclusion until physical conditions are excluded.

Suspicions that the presentation is not hypochondriacal are raised if: (i) the presentation is acute; (ii) there is no past history of medically unexplained disorders; (iii) there are no stressors evident; and (iv) there is no psychological disturbance beyond the anxiety/apprehension appropriate in the circumstances (Table H.24).

Table H.24 Causes of hypochondriasis

Commonest
Stress reaction
Adjustment reaction (especially to illness)
Anxiety
Depression
Early or otherwise undetected physical illness

Less common
Panic
Phobia
Obsessive–compulsive disorder
Schizophrenia
Primary hypochondriasis

Rare
Dementia
Mental impairment
Schizoaffective disorder
Monosymptomatic hypochondriacal delusional state
Post-traumatic stress disorder
Hysteria
Briquet's syndrome (somatization disorder)

Hypochondriacal presentations are usefully divided into *primary* and *secondary*. The distinction is made more important by the poor prognosis found in primary hypochondriasis contrasting with the favourable outcome generally attained when hypochondriasis is in the setting of another psychological disorder. *Transient hypochondriacal reactions* are common, usually responding well to explanation and reassurance, but occasionally developing and persisting. Any stress or situation may be the trigger in a vulnerable individual, but there are some common circumstances in which personal vulnerability is less crucial. Recovering from serious illness may precipitate this response as part of an adjustment reaction; similarly, serious illness in a close friend or relative may lead to concerns about having the same disease, the mental mechanism being identification with the loved one and sharing their suffering, or as part of a grief reaction

when death has occurred. Hypochondriacal reactions are more common in the elderly, particularly if the patient has an established painful condition, and in this group the loss of work, outside interests and friends may conspire to focus attention and interest on the functioning of the 'inner world'.

Hypochondriacal *delusions* are uncommon and may take easily recognizable, bizarre forms in schizophrenia, dementia and monosymptomatic hypochondriacal psychosis (a rare condition in which the delusions are not accompanied by features which would permit classification as a primary organic or functional psychosis). Among the more common presentations are beliefs of infestation, emitting odours and changes in size, and the shape or function of organs. In major depression the delusions may be more subtle and difficult to detect, although detection is the more important because these phenomena are associated with a substantial risk of suicide. Generally, depressive hypochondriacal delusions are understandable in the context of other depressive changes. For example, delusions of venereal disease arise from depressive guilt and sometimes impotence, while delusions of cancer can be the outcome of morbid, pessimistic thinking accompanied by constipation, impaired appetite and weight loss.

Hypochondriacal *preoccupations*, *worries* and *fears* occur commonly in the setting of neurotic disorders. In anxiety, agoraphobia, panic disorder and depressive neurosis hypochondriacal features can usually be easily established as one element in a constellation of symptoms and signs that typify the underlying disorder. Physical symptoms may be the presenting feature of any of these conditions, and these may be perceived with enhanced alarm or dread by a patient who has an abnormal mood state. The presenting complaint is usually a typical feature of anxiety or depression, such as musculoskeletal pain, cardiovascular, gastrointestinal or neurological symptoms, which basically become magnified and misinterpreted.

Primary hypochondriasis is rare, but its existence as an entity is now widely accepted. It is essentially a diagnosis by exclusion of the causes already outlined, but the condition has some characteristic features: (i) first and foremost, persistent complaining; (ii) detailed accounts: 'the organ recital'; (iii) matter-of-fact presentation; and (iv) less interest in the response than in the narrating. Such patients are usually obsessional and often anxiety-prone. These characteristics of style and personality aid in distinguishing primary hypochondriasis from somatization disorder (Briquet's syndrome), where patients have persistent unexplained physical complaints but tend to be inarticulate, poor historians who give highly dramatic accounts of events but sketchy information about their symptoms, with the emphasis upon extraordinariness rather than detail.

Finally, it should be borne in mind that patients with primary hypochondriasis are not immune to physical illnesses and are indeed vulnerable to mental disorders. Exaggeration in hypochondriacal complaining may indicate a superimposed depressive illness or anxiety state. On the other hand, repeated specialist referrals and investigations reinforce this behaviour! Hence, the doctor has a delicate balance to strike over when to investigate and treat, and unfortunately his or her decision-making is frequently hindered by the antipathy and alienation that tends to develop in the doctor–patient relationship.

Latterly, there has been increasing optimism about the treatability of primary hypochondriasis, specifically with cognitive–behavioural psychotherapy. Elements of this treatment include the banning of reassurance, self-monitoring and challenging abnormal health beliefs.

Andrew Hodgkiss

HYPOTHERMIA

Hypothermia is defined as a core temperature of below 35°C (95.8°F). Normally protected parts (e.g. the abdomen) are cold to the touch. When hypothermia is suspected, the deep rectal temperature should be measured with a low-reading thermometer. It is important to have a low threshold of suspicion in older people who will not feel the cold, and therefore neither complain of it, nor make concerted attempts to rewarm themselves.

Mild hypothermia down to 32°C (90°F) may be characterized by confusion, slow responses, slurred husky speech, ataxia and involuntary movements resembling cerebellar incoordination. Skin pallor, shivering and some degree of tachycardia and mild hypertension are often noted.

Moderate to severe hypothermia is characterized by drowsiness, stupor or overt coma. Some patients may

be comatose at 31°C, others may still be conscious at 27°C. The pupils are usually constricted and unresponsive to light (mimicking opium poisoning or pontine haemorrhage). Occasionally, fixed dilated pupils are noted in those with severe, protracted hypothermia and then may mimic closed head injury. The skin may show cyanotic or pink blotches, and sometimes purpuric lesions, skin haemorrhages or pressure lesions. Fluid shifts give the skin a typical puffy or oedematous consistency. At very low core temperatures, fine muscle tremors and muscle rigidity have replaced shivering. Tendon jerks, if still present, show slow contraction and relaxation phases. The knee jerk is the last to be lost. The plantar responses may be bilaterally extensor or absent; a unilateral extensor response usually indicates an underlying cerebrovascular catastrophe. Severe bradycardia or atrial fibrillation may be present. Tachycardia is inappropriate in hypothermia and suggests internal haemorrhage, for example from severe gastric erosions. Any intra-abdominal catastrophe may not be detectable until after re-warming. Coarse pulmonary crepitations indicate oedematous and often infected lungs, but respiration may be too poor for these features to be recognized. An ECG is likely to show characteristic J waves (Fig. H.13).

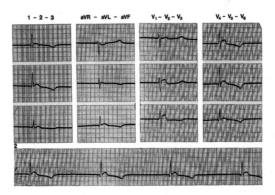

Figure H.13 ECG showing characteristic J waves in a 67-year-old male with myxoedema (temperature 25°C rectal).

Severely hypothermic patients lack easily detectable vital signs, with imperceptible peripheral pulses, inaudible heart sounds, unrecordable blood pressure, and slow, shallow respiration; the pupils may be widely dilated and unresponsive. An ECG will exclude death, but even ventricular fibrillation may reverse

Table H.25 Causes of hypothermia

Decreased heat production
Inactivity and immobility (e.g. lying on floor after a stroke or fractured femur)
Hypoglycaemia
Impaired shivering capacity (elderly)
Myxoedema
Starvation and malnutrition
Hypopituitarism

Increased heat loss
Outdoors cold/wet exposure or cold-water immersion
Low ambient home temperatures due to poor heating and housing
Reduced awareness to cold due to dementia or delirium
Ethanol
Vasoconstriction failure (e.g. elderly survivors of previous accidental hypothermia)
Malnutrition (e.g. kwashiorkor)
Erythroderma (e.g. generalized psoriasis, exfoliative dermatitis, Paget's disease of bone)

Central thermoregulatory failure
Uraemia
Cerebrovascular injury or cerebral trauma
Drugs (including self-poisoning) (e.g. phenothiazine tranquillizers, tricyclic antidepressants, barbiturates)
Diabetic ketoacidosis
Wernicke's encephalopathy
CO poisoning/anoxic brain injury (e.g. after cardiac arrest, organophosphate poisoning)
Blood transfusion reaction

Peripheral thermoregulatory failure
Spinal cord lesions, especially cervical
Autonomic neuropathy (e.g. diabetes mellitus, Parkinson's disease)

Mechanism(s) uncertain
Severe chronic or debilitating disease (preterminal) (e.g. malignancy, hepatic cirrhosis)
Overwhelming infection (e.g. severe bronchopneumonia, overwhelming TB, falciparum malaria)
Severe congestive heart failure
Shock after multiple injury, major operation, severe coronary thrombosis or pulmonary embolism
Collapse due to severe dehydration (e.g. severe diarrhoea, including cholera)
Pancreatitis

with re-warming. The diagnosis of death should not be made until re-warming has been achieved, and vigorous resuscitation attempts made.

Many elderly hypothermic patients have complex physical signs, either because of complications of the hypothermia (e.g. pulmonary crepitations) or because the risk of developing hypothermia is greater with concomitant medical disease. It should be remembered that while hypothermia is more common during cold weather in older people, the condition is by no means confined to the colder winter months.

The important causes of hypothermia are listed in Table H.25.

Danielle Harari

HYSTERIA

The term *hysteria* has been dropped in ICD10, to be replaced by conversion disorder. However, *hysteria* will be used in this section of the Index.

Before describing hysterical presentations and their differential diagnosis, the topic should be prefaced by some comments about related aspects that can lead to confusion. The terms 'hysteria' and 'hysterical' have different connotations when applied to behaviour and personality. Hysterical *behaviour* refers to histrionic, attention-seeking behaviour, while hysterical *personality* describes a shallow, flamboyant, self-absorbed, 'showbiz' individual. However, both terms tend to denote disapproval. Hysteria in its proper sense is a presentation of neurosis in which a psychological stress or conflict, and the anxiety that this engenders, are avoided through the defence mechanism of conversion. Although embracing these disorders under one umbrella has passed out of fashion in the United States, where the term hysteria has largely been dropped, hysteria or hysterical neurosis remains an accepted unitary concept elsewhere.

The justification for delimiting hysteria lies in the features common to all presentations (Table H.26), and without all three characteristics being present the diagnosis is erroneous.

Table H.26 Characteristics of hysteria

---
1 The presentation corresponds to an idea in the patient's mind of how the disorder should present, i.e. (a) physical or sensory changes do not obey anatomical and physiological rules; (b) psychological changes do not adhere to accepted psychological principles.

2 The disability must be apparent and definable in terms of positive findings. Clinical examination usually reveals obvious inconsistencies or anomalies, particularly the preservation of functions that ought to be lost or the absence of abnormalities that ought to be present.

3 Primary gain. The disorder resolves an emotional conflict or personal problem, which is kept out of consciousness.

There are other features linked to hysterical symptoms, none of which is invariable. The most important is *secondary gain(s)* – that is, the spin-off benefits arising from being ill which may perpetuate the condition when the primary cause has been resolved. *Suggestibility* is a useful clinical sign (and a potent tool in therapy); this ability to influence site, characteristics and severity as well as inducing or removing symptoms altogether may sometimes be enhanced by hypnosis, or abreaction using diazepam or amytal, when the underlying conflict may also be explored if necessary. *La belle indifference* describes a bland lack of concern towards what is manifestly a serious condition – it is also frequently found in stoical, physically ill patients, and its presence in hysteria is usually confined to acute presentations as opposed to chronic states where high levels of anxiety are the rule. *Symbolism*, or what the symptom means, is an important concept in psychoanalysis, sometimes being interpreted as a precise communication and representation of the nature of the underlying conflict. Finally, failure to respond to conventional, physical interventions or drugs is characteristic, and should alert the doctor's suspicions before proceeding to more invasive techniques – while a sustained response to a physical treatment mitigates against a hysterical aetiology.

Perhaps surprisingly, appreciable hysterical personality traits are found in only 15 per cent of cases. The breeding ground for hysteria is much more frequently a passive, dependent, inarticulate individual who is in a submissive role and cannot express him/herself freely, either through inability or fear of the consequences. Through illness, hysteria generates control without confrontation – hence its links with other conditions in which sick role behaviour is prominent such as chronic pain and factitious disorder.

Conversion disorders can mimic any physical condition, but by far the most common presentations are neurological, involving mobility, sensory modalities (including pain and the special senses) and pseudoseizures, while less common presentations include vomiting, urinary retention and pseudocyesis. There are numerous signs and tests that aid in identifying a presentation as a conversion disorder, all of which are derived from the themes in the first and second requirements in Table H.26. The features of hysteria evolve and there is an impression that the more bizarre and obviously functional presentations such as glove and stocking anaesthesia are diminishing in frequency to be replaced by disorders that can be more difficult to distinguish clinically – hysterical epilepsy being a good example (Table H.27).

Table H.27 Causes of a hysterical presentation

Common
Hysteria–hysterical neurosis (conversion disorder/dissociative state)

Less common
Neurological disorders
Systemic disorders with CNS effects
Depression

Rare
Schizophrenia
Alcoholism

Before establishing the diagnosis of hysteria, it is essential to exclude a primary physical or psychiatric explanation for the symptom. *Neurological disorders* of all types and systemic diseases with CNS effects must be ruled out, by extensive investigation if neces-sary. Even if all investigations are negative and the presentation bears the unequivocal physical charac-teristics of a conversion disorder, the diagnosis of hysteria must not be made unless the psychodynamic requirement is met (i.e. primary gain is identified), because follow-up studies have demonstrated that these patients may proceed to develop neurological disorders such as tumour, multiple sclerosis and dementing processes. A conversion sign developing in a patient aged over 40 years and with no psycho-logical explanation and no past history of hysteria or other mental illness is a sinister occurrence which merits careful review. Indeed, it was by maintaining an open mind in such circumstances that the physical basis has been established for conditions such as globus hystericus, torticollis, paroxysmal hemicrania, thoracic outlet syndrome and the syndrome of painful legs and moving toes.

Hysterical presentations also occur in the set-ting of *psychiatric disorders*, particularly depression, but also dementia, schizophrenia and alcoholism. Occasionally, the mental disorder only becomes apparent on follow-up after the hysterical presenta-tion has resolved, but the possibility of an underlying depressive illness should be actively considered in older patients and in those with a personal or family history of affective disorder.

Differentiating hysteria from *factitious disorder* rarely presents problems (Table H.28), because the former – as by definition – is obviously produced to secure gain through the resolution of an emotional conflict, whilst the gains obtained from factitious dis-order are, at best, obscure. In practice, neurological symptoms apart from epilepsy are rarely simulated in factitious conditions, whilst in hysteria self-injury sel-dom occurs intentionally. An interesting distinction in presentation between the two conditions is that the hysteric knows and cares little about health issues, whilst the patient with factitious disorder is often immersed in all aspects of illnesses and hospitals.

Table H.28 Differential diagnosis of hysteria

Physical/mental illness
Hypochondriasis
Factitious disorder
Malingering

Differentiating hysteria from *malingering* is a much harder task because both conditions involve evident gains, and the sole point of distinction is whether the patient's behaviour is consciously or unconsciously motivated. The only time when a definite diagnosis can be made with confidence is during the early stages of the first, acute presentation before the dis-order has been elaborated by factors such as suggestion and illness experiences. Here, the nature of the pri-mary gain frequently aids diagnosis, malingering being particularly linked to obvious environmental advantage such as compensation or avoiding military service.

In almost all chronic cases, which includes all compensation cases, as well as in some acute cases, the distinction between hysteria and malingering is spurious, and irrelevant for clinical purposes. The problem is that insight is neither fixed nor dichot-omous, it comes and it goes – hence the apposite maxim 'in time all malingerers become hysterics and all hysterics become malingerers'. It is also possible for both diagnoses to be present; for example, pseu-doseizures sometimes being used consciously for obvious gain while on other occasions being uncon-sciously motivated. This phenomenon is particu-larly evident in protracted compensation cases where many patients with functional disorders fail to improve even after a satisfactory financial settlement. This is because secondary gains have superseded money as the basis for maintaining symptoms, and have developed imperceptibly as part of the patient's and their family's adjustment. In these cases it is typ-ical for there to be a number of gains understood with varying degrees of insight by the patient, and these gains and insights change as circumstances unfold.

It is an understanding of the gains and the psycho-dynamics, what makes the patient tick, and what are the circumstances including the nature and roles of close friends and relatives that matter in clinical prac-tice. The malingering versus hysteria debate is irrele-vant in tipping the scales in the direction of shedding symptoms rather than maintaining them, or in encouraging the patient to get well through a combin-ation of suggestion, problem-solving and reward whilst avoiding reward and reinforcement of illness behaviour.

Andrew Hodgkiss

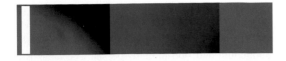

IMPOTENCE

Erectile dysfunction (ED), otherwise known as impotence, may be defined as the failure to achieve a personally satisfying level of sexual performance. This may be classified into mild, moderate and complete failure based on a number of criteria including the level of sexual activity, frequency of full erections, and the frequency of early morning erections on awakening. Ejaculatory insufficiency describes absent or reduced seminal emission. This may be because of a lack of external ejaculation or premature ejaculation, and may be accompanied by lack of orgasm (Table I.1).

Table I.1 Causes of erectile dysfunction

Vascular	Arterial: atheroma Venous: veno-occlusive incompetence – ageing, diabetes mellitus
Neurogenic	CNS/PNS: cerebrovascular disease, multiple sclerosis, spinal-cord compression and paraplegia, tabes dorsalis Autonomic dysfunction: diabetes mellitus, Shy–Drager syndrome, pelvic irradiation Surgery: interruption of pelvic nerve pathways after surgery (e.g. abdominoperineal resection, post-chemotherapy lymph node dissection for testicular tumours) Psychogenic: depression
Endocrine	Testicular failure Hypothalamic–pituitary disease Prolactinoma Oestrogen excess Hypo/hyperthyroidism
Drugs	Methyldopa, atenolol, bendrofluazide, spironolactone, cimetidine, ranitidine, ketoconazole, chronic ethanol abuse, oestrogens, progestagens, nicotine, etc.
Local	Peyronie's disease (scarring disorder of the tunica albuginea) Intersinusoidal fibrosis, diabetes mellitus, ageing Penile trauma Pudendal nerve trauma: bicycle rider's palsy
HIV infection	Most probably due to a mixture of testicular failure and hypogonadotrophic hypogonadism

There is a progressive decline in sexual activity in association with a mild degree of hypogonadism in men with ageing. This decline is accelerated in the presence of ill health. If hypogonadism is severe, usually associated with pathology, there is loss of libido and erectile function and a decrease in ejaculate volume. The majority of secondary cases of ED are caused by arterial occlusive disease. In subjects with diabetes mellitus, vascular abnormalities dominate in patients with type 2 diabetes; however, neurogenic factors play an important role in addition to vascular abnormalities in type 1 diabetes. The onset of ED in patients with hypertension is very frequently associated with the start of antihypertensive therapy. ED is a side effect of many of the commonly used antihypertensive agents including thiazide diuretics, beta blockers, angiotensin-converting enzyme inhibitors and calcium-channel blockers. This side effect covers many classes of antihypertensive agents, which have varying mechanisms of action for lowering blood pressure. Therefore, the end result of lowering systemic blood pressure, which may interfere with maximal penile-filling capacity, rather than any individual effect unique to the class of antihypertensive, may be the causative factor in ED. Uraemia is associated with raised luteinizing hormone (LH), oestrogen and prolactin levels and low levels of testosterone. Approximately 50 per cent of males with uraemia suffer from ED. The use of erythropoietin in these patients has been shown to improve sexual function, which may be related to a reduction in prolactin and an improvement in the gonadotrophin plasma profile. There is a high prevalence of ED amongst chronic alcoholics who invariably have liver damage. The associated hypogonadism, feminization and neuropathy exacerbate the problem. Heavy cigarette smoking, in addition to its deleterious effects on peripheral vascular disease, is also associated with ED by the action of nicotine, which reduces corporeal blood flow and inhibits cavernosal venoconstriction. Peyronie's disease, which starts off as an inflammatory process with cellular infiltrates followed by collagen deposition, is a cause of ED. The scars formed in this condition may distort the shape of the erect penis. The tunica albuginea is stiffened due to a depletion of elastic fibres and disables veno-occlusion. The plaque formation found at the periphery of the penis and in the midline interferes with arterial inflow. Both abnormalities of blood flow impair the tumescent and full erection phase for normal erectile function.

The prevalence of psychogenic ED is unclear. In many studies, psychogenic ED has been attributed to less than a third of cases. The measurement of this condition is compounded by the fact that complete vascular, neurological and psychological assessments are difficult to make in the non-erotic setting. In addition, abnormalities of nocturnal penile tumescence as a marker of ED is not a valid means of distinguishing among causes.

Ejaculatory insufficiency

This condition is usually organic, and is relatively common in neurological disease such as diabetic autonomic neuropathy, multiple sclerosis, paraplegia, etc. In the absence of any overt disorder, the two main causes of failure of ejaculation are retrograde ejaculation and anejaculation. The former can be diagnosed by the finding of many sperm in the post-coital urine sample. The latter may be difficult to diagnose, but there may be an absence of one or both vas deferens and an absent or very small prostate.

A common problem is premature ejaculation. This may occur in younger men where the response to sexual stimuli may be very rapid. With reassurance from the doctor and familiarity with sexual stimuli the problem usually resolves.

Sharon O'Byrne

INDIGESTION

Indigestion and dyspepsia are equally vague umbrella terms that refer to a constellation of symptoms including upper abdominal discomfort or bloating, retrosternal or epigastric pain, nausea, loss of appetite and early satiety. Dyspepsia affects 20–40 per cent of the Western populations, of whom 25 per cent seek medical attention. Symptoms alone are a poor indicator of underlying pathology, and so other factors must be taken into account when formulating a management plan; in particular, the presence of 'alarm' features. These include associated dysphagia, odynophagia, weight loss, anaemia or iron deficiency, haematemesis, pernicious anaemia, previous gastric surgery and, in particular, recent onset when over 55 years of age. Gastro-oesophageal cancer in the absence of an alarm feature under this age is rare.

Many conditions may give rise to dyspepsia. The commonest are peptic ulcer disease, comprising ulceration or inflammation of the oesophagus, stomach or duodenum and non-ulcer dyspepsia. The latter is a variant of irritable bowel syndrome. Other conditions to be considered are reflux oesophagitis, gallstones, neuropathic gastropathy (diabetes mellitus), viral or drug-induced gastropathy, infiltrating conditions (lymphoma, scleroderma), pyloric outlet obstruction, Crohn's disease, giardiasis, gluten enteropathy, pancreatitis, achalasia and space-occupying lesions of the upper gastrointestinal tract (adenocarcinoma, squamous cell carcinoma, mucosa-associated lymphoid tissue lymphoma, metastatic cancer, Kaposi's sarcoma, stromal cell tumours, submucosal cysts, ectopic pancreas and lipomata). Systemic disease and its therapy, or pathology in the distal gastrointestinal tract, may cause marked nausea. Many of the conditions mentioned are intimated at by the clinical setting or are only diagnosed following investigation.

The main focus of investigating dyspepsia is to exclude cancer. The mainstays of investigation are gastroscopy and barium studies. It is not feasible to perform such tests, however, on all people presenting with this symptom. Many national gastroenterological organizations, including the British Society of Gastroenterology (www.bsg.org.uk) and the American Gastroenterology Association (www.gastro.org), have made recommendations with respect to the best course of approach, but such guidelines must be adapted to suit local populations. The presence or absence of alarm features and the association of *Helicobacter pylori* with gastroduodenal pathology, consequently, is used to stratify patients to an appropriate course of management. Guidelines for one patient population may not, however, translate well to those of other regions.

H. pylori is a Gram-negative anaerobe that colonizes the gastric antrum in a variable proportion of the population, being more common in the elderly and those from poorer socioeconomic groups. Its presence is associated with more than 90 per cent of duodenal ulcers, 60–70 per cent of gastric ulcers, and an increased risk for the development of gastric mucosa-associated lymphoid tissue lymphoma and distal gastric adenocarcinoma (Fig. I.1). Those infected are more susceptible to non-steroidal anti-inflammatory drug-induced gastric injury than the general population. The association between *H. pylori* and reflux oesophagitis or non-ulcer dyspepsia, importantly, is uncertain but probably weak.

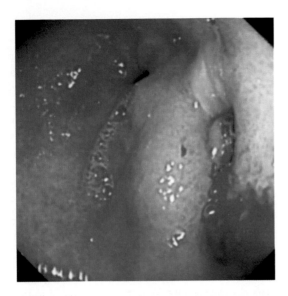

Figure I.1 Acute pre-pyloric antral ulcer with some oozing of fresh blood.

The antigenic properties of *H. pylori* and its ability to split urea are used to diagnose its presence through serology, stool sampling, ^{13}C- or ^{14}C-labelled urea breath test, or gastric mucosal biopsy.

Patients under the age of 55 years with dyspepsia, but no alarm features, ought to undergo testing for *H. pylori*, the most convenient test being serology. If the test is positive, 'triple' therapy with a proton-pump inhibitor and two antibiotics may be given for 7–10 days. A common regimen is a proton-pump inhibitor with clarithromycin and amoxicillin for 7 days. Metronidazole may be used in place of clarithromycin, but levels of resistance are high. There is little value in such patients undergoing subsequent gastroscopy prior to therapy. Eradication cannot be accurately assessed by serology as antibodies are slow to be cleared. A ^{13}C/^{14}C-labelled urea breath test is the most appropriate follow-up investigation.

Those patients having a negative initial test for *H. pylori* are most likely to have non-ulcer dyspepsia. There is perhaps little advantage in these patients undergoing gastroscopy, other than for personal reassurance, as such endoscopies are invariably normal. An upper abdominal ultrasound may be justified, however, to exclude other pathology such as gallstones. The optimal treatment for non-ulcer dyspepsia is unknown, but acid suppression is helpful for many.

Patients of any age with alarm features or presenting with recent-onset dyspepsia when over the age of 55 years must be investigated with either gastroscopy or barium studies. The testing and treating of *H. pylori* or trial therapy with acid suppression, even if successful, may mask the presence of a cancer.

John Meenan

INFERTILITY

Infertility or subfertility is defined as the failure to conceive within 12 months of commencing unprotected regular intercourse. After one year, 80 per cent of women have managed to conceive, and a further 5–10 per cent of pregnancies will have been successful by the end of the 18 months. It is estimated that approximately 12 per cent of couples will have infertility and require investigation. Infertility can be divided into:

- Primary infertility, when the woman has never been pregnant.
- Secondary infertility, when the woman has had a previous pregnancy, whatever the outcome.

It is essential that both partners be investigated.

The causes of infertility can be summarized as:

- Tubal problem (15%)
- Anovulation (20%)
- Other female factors including mucus hostility, endometriosis (10%)
- Male factor (25%)
- Sexual problems (5%)
- Unexplained (25%)

These figures are approximate, and in some cases there may be more than one problem. It is always important to explore the frequency of sexual intercourse, as after ejaculation the sperm will last for approximately 72 hours, during which time it can fertilize the ovum, which is fertilizable for approximately 24 hours. Therefore, timing may be a significant factor in some couples. In many patients the failure is due to a number of minor 'infertility factors' which are unimportant in themselves but which, in aggregate, may result in an inability to conceive.

Investigations are aimed at answering three main questions:

1 Is the woman producing eggs? This can be answered by checking a mid-luteal phase serum progesterone which should be >30 nmol/l, or follicle tracking by ultrasound scanning. In the latter, the follicle should grow to 18–25 mm in diameter.

2 Are the Fallopian tubes and passageways sufficiently patent that they will allow the sperm to access the egg? To check this, either an X-ray in the form of a hysterosalpingogram (HSG) (Fig. I.2) can be performed, or dye laparoscopy. Both techniques should show whether the tubes are patent. The HSG does not require general anaesthesia, and must be carried out after menstruation has finished, whereupon it will outline the cavity of the uterus. The dye laparoscopy will show the tubes and any spillage of dye, but must be performed under a general anaesthetic. It will not provide any information about the uterine cavity, but will demonstrate if there are adhesions present, and whether the patient would be amenable to tubal surgery.

3 What is the number and quality of the sperm? Spermatogenesis takes 74 days to complete, and consequently the sperm count may reflect the health of the individual when that process commenced. A routine semen analysis will examine the following factors:
   - Volume 2–6 ml
   - Liquefaction complete in 30 minutes
   - Sperm count >20 million/ml
   - Sperm motility 60 per cent forward progressive
   - Sperm morphology ⩾70 per cent normal forms
   - Mixed antibody reaction test negative.

As the sperm count varies within the ejaculate, if an initial count is low it should be repeated at least once. The ejaculate should be fresh, and be passed to the laboratory within 12 hours of ejaculation. Provided that there are some spermatozoa in the ejaculate, it is not possible to say that a man is infertile, no matter how low the semen count. Pregnancies seem to occur in the face of very low counts.

Male factors

The causes of male infertility fall into the following broad categories which may lead to oligospermia, necrospermia and azoospermia.

- *Occupation*: If the male is exposed to toxins or irradiation, or is sedentary, then the sperm count may be compromised. Over-work of a mental nature can also affect sperm production.
- *Illnesses/operations*: Constitutional diseases associated with infertility include: (i) tuberculosis, diabetes mellitus, anaemia, cystic fibrosis, syphilis, alcoholism and dietary deficiencies; (ii) endocrine factors such as hypothyroidism or hyperthyroidism; (iii) hypopituitarism, as suggested by under-development of the penis, and obesity; (iv) febrile illnesses may affect the sperm count and take some months to normalize; and (v) bladder neck surgery may also affect the situation.
- *Infections*: The most common cause of complete sterility in the male is blockage of the epididymis due to gonorrhoea or other infection. Atrophy of the testes following orchitis as a complication of mumps (about 10% of males contracting mumps develop orchitis) may be responsible.
- *Drugs* less commonly cause infertility, but they include sulphasalazine, chemotherapy, antimicrobials, antihypertensives, alcohol, nicotine and marijuana.

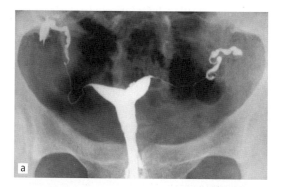

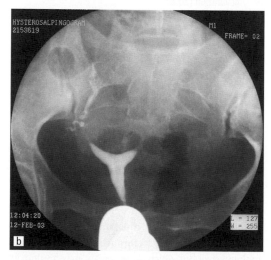

Figure I.2 Two illustrations of a hysterosalpingogram. (a) Normal; (b) showing a blocked left Fallopian tube.

- *Sexual function*: Failure of the male to ejaculate during coitus is a not infrequent cause when both partners are found to be normally fertile. This may be due to coital frequency, premature ejaculation and maintenance of an erection.
- *Trauma and stress.*
- *Constitutional problems*: Men suffering from the chromosomal anomaly, Klinefelter's syndrome (XXY), have undeveloped genitalia with small soft testes, and are infertile. Between 3–5 per cent of men are infertile because of autoimmunization with circulating antibodies to their own spermatozoa. Cryptorchidism may affect the function of the testis and make it more likely to develop a malignancy within it. The testis in this case is almost certainly sterile. The presence of a varicocele may affect sperm production and may warrant removal.

Female factors

In females, fertility problems occur in a number of areas:

- *Sexual dysfunction* includes dyspareunia or vaginismus.
- *Cervical factor*: Cervical lesions include abnormalities of cervical secretion and stenosis of the cervix following treatment for premalignant disease.
- *Uterine and/or tubal problems*: Gross pelvic lesions which include absence of uterus, vagina, Fallopian tubes or ovaries, closure of the hymen or vagina, fibroids, polyps, carcinoma, tuberculosis of the endometrium, endometriosis. Tubal lesions include inflammatory disease including *Chlamydia*, tuberculosis. Occasionally, the tubes may be rudimentary.
- *Endocrine problems*: These include ovarian failure either primary or secondary. Generalized endocrine disorders such as hypo- or hyperthyroidism, adrenocortical hypo- or hyperfunction and uncontrolled diabetes may result in infertility. Bilaterally enlarged polycystic ovaries, secondary amenorrhoea or oligomenorrhoea and infertility characterize polycystic ovarian disease. About half of the patients are hirsute, and many are obese. Infertility is due to failure of ovulation. The enlarged ovaries may be palpable on bimanual vaginal examination, but are best diagnosed on ultrasonography or laparoscopy. Blood levels of luteinizing hormone (LH) are raised, and there may be an increased urinary excretion of androstenedione or dehydroepiandrosterone.
- *Previous obstetric history.*
- *Contraception*: Use of the oral contraceptive pill (OCP) and intra-uterine contraceptive device (IUCD).

- *Constitutional chromosomal anomalies*: These include Turner's syndrome (XO) and super-female (XXX).
- *Anxiety.*
- *Anaemia and age*: Fertility is problematic with increasing age of the woman.

Combined male and female factors

- Subnormal sperm count with abnormal cervical secretion in the female.
- Incomplete penetration.
- Lack of seminal plasma.
- Defective germ plasma.

The above lists show that some causes of infertility are primary, others secondary. Thus, an absence of the uterus or infantile uterus means primary sterility, whilst failure to ovulate, salpingitis, etc. may occur in women who have had children, and consequently cause secondary infertility or sterility.

Congenital anomalies

Some of the congenital lesions are diagnosed easily, such as imperforate hymen, absence of the vagina, or stenosis of the cervix, whilst absence of the essential organs often requires an anaesthetic in order that a bimanual examination may be made satisfactorily, or for a laparoscopic examination to be undertaken.

Patients with gonadal agenesis suffer from too-short stature, sexual infantilism and primary amenorrhoea. Two-thirds of these patients have an XO chromosome complement and other features of Turner's syndrome. Laparoscopy reveals small elongated ovarian streaks of fibrous tissue in place of the ovaries. Male pseudohermaphrodites with testicular feminization and a 46, XY chromosome karyotype have the appearance of a female of normal height and often well-developed breasts. They have absent or scanty axillary and pubic hair, a short, blind vagina, absent uterus and tubes, and they suffer from primary amenorrhoea. Bilateral testes may be present in the abdomen or in the inguinal canal. The cause is end-organ resistance to testosterone or androgen insensitivity. Other members of the family are liable to have the condition.

Post-coital test

When the man's sperm count is adequate and the woman's Fallopian tubes are patent, attention should

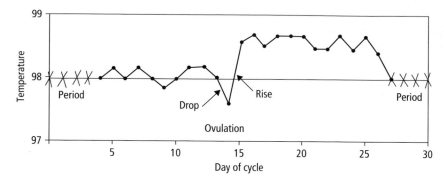

Figure I.3 A typical basal temperature chart.

be paid to the Simms–Hiihner post-coital test. Mucus is aspirated from the cervical canal at the time of ovulation following intercourse the night before or on the morning of the test. The mucus is placed on a slide, covered with a coverslip and examined under a high-power microscope. There should be at least two (and normally five or more) motile spermatozoa progressing in straight lines across the high-power field. A negative post-coital test may be due to abnormal sperm production, inadequate intercourse, failure to ejaculate or hostile cervical mucus.

Endocrine causes

Endocrine causes of infertility are common. Pregnancy is not possible during periods of amenorrhoea because of failure to ovulate. Women who suffer from oligomenorrhoea have their fertility reduced. It is rare for women who menstruate regularly at monthly intervals not to ovulate, although some of them do have a defective corpus luteum and a poor or short luteal phase of the menstrual cycle. If an early menopause is suspected, the serum FSH level will be >30 u/l. The occurrence and timing of ovulation can be verified by taking the temperature (by mouth) first thing on waking before moving or getting out of bed. The basal temperature in the first half of the cycle is slightly lower than it is in the second half. A characteristic drop, followed by a rise at mid-cycle, indicates ovulation which, in most women, takes place about 14 days before the onset of the next period (Fig. I.3). Ovulation is followed by the formation of a corpus luteum, and this can be diagnosed by a raised serum level of progesterone (>30 nmol/l)

usually carried out on the 21st day of a normal 28-day cycle. Following ovulation, the uterine endometrium undergoes the histological changes of the secretory (or progestational) phase, which become increasingly marked up to the time of the onset of menstruation. The stromal cells enlarge and the glands become tortuous with deep serrations in their walls and secretion in their lumina. A biopsy of the endometrium towards the end of the cycle will show these changes if ovulation has taken place. The finding in the cervix of the typical clear elastic mucus in mid-cycle is further proof that ovulation has occurred. Mid-cycle cervical mucus can be drawn into threads up to 10 cm in length; this is known as 'spinnbarkeit', and is an indication of high oestrogen secretion by the ovary. 'Ferning' is another effect of high mid-cycle oestrogen. The mid-cycle cervical mucus is spread thickly on a glass slide, rinsed in distilled water and allowed to dry. A characteristic pattern resembling a fern leaf forms on the slide. Later in the cycle an absence of spinnbarkeit and ferning indicates a progesterone effect and functioning corpus luteum.

In practice, it is important during the history taking to ask for the length of the menstrual cycle. Ovulation usually takes place 14 days prior to a period, so by having intercourse on alternate days around this time one increases the chances of conception. Currently, ovulation kits looking for the LH surge just prior to ovulation are available commercially, and these help the couple to identify the most fertile part of the month.

Antony Hollingworth

JAUNDICE

Types

Jaundice may be caused by a raised conjugated or unconjugated bilirubin. Unconjugated hyperbilirubinaemia may be due to excessive production of bilirubin (haemolysis), reduced uptake of bilirubin, or a failure of conjugation by the liver. Conjugated hyperbilirubinaemia results from hepatocellular damage or obstruction of the bile ducts, either within the liver (intrahepatic cholestasis) or of a major bile duct (extrahepatic obstruction jaundice). Jaundice is also often classified into pre-hepatic (haemolysis), hepatic and extra-hepatic types. Clues as to the cause of jaundice may be obtained from the history and physical examination (Tables J.1 and J.2).

Investigations of jaundice

The simplest investigations are liver function tests and urine examinations; typical abnormalities are shown in Table J.3. The liver enzymes, aspartate transaminase (AST) and alanine transaminase (ALT), are normally contained within the liver cells, and are released during hepatocellular necrosis, whereas alkaline phosphatase is excreted into the biliary system and rises in situations of intra-hepatic or extra-hepatic biliary stasis.

There is no bilirubin present in the urine of patients with pre-hepatic (haemolytic) jaundice because unconjugated bilirubin is tightly bound to albumin and is not filtered at the glomerulus. On the other hand, conjugated bilirubin is water-soluble and stains the urine dark in hepatocellular and obstructive jaundice. Urobilinogen is produced by bacteria in the gut, and is normally partially reabsorbed into the portal vein, taken up by hepatocytes and re-excreted in bile. When the liver is damaged, hepatic extraction is less efficient and the concentration of urobilinogen in plasma, and hence in the urine, rises. The presence of urobilinogen in the urine is thus a test of liver

Table J.1 History of jaundice

Haemolytic	Hepatic		Obstructive
Family history	Flu symptoms		Abdominal
Racial origin	Rashes		pain
Drug history	Joint pains	Viral	Pale stools
Symptoms of	Contact with jaundice		Dark urine
anaemia	Blood transfusions		Itching
	Infections		
	Drug history		
	Alcoholic intake		
	Previous jaundice		

Table J.2 Physical signs associated with jaundice

Haemolytic	Hepatic		Obstructive	
Splenomegaly, reduced stature	Dupuytren's contractures Parotid enlargement		Alcohol	Scratch marks Mass in abdomen
	Spider naevi Gynaecomastia Testicular atrophy Loss of hair Red hands		Endocrine	Gall bladder In a patient with obstructive jaundice, if the gall bladder is palpable the cause is unlikely to be gallstones – Courvoisier's law
	White nails Ascites and oedema		Hypoproteinaemia	
	Bruising		Prothrombin time prolonged	
	Splenomegaly Veins around umbilicus		Portal hypertension	

Table J.3 Liver function tests and urinalysis in jaundice

	Unconjugated bilirubinaemia (haemolytic)	Hepatocellular jaundice	Obstructive jaundice
Liver function tests	Direct bilirubin ↑ AST ALT ALK-P	Indirect bilirubin ↑ AST↑↑ ALT↑↑ ALK-P↑	Indirect bilirubin ↑↑ AST↑ ALT↑ ALK-P↑↑
Urine tests	Bilirubin 0 Urobilinogen Normally not raised	Bilirubin + Urobilinogen + +	Bilirubin + + + Urobilinogen→

function, and one of the earliest signs of recovery from hepatocellular jaundice is the disappearance of urobilinogen from the urine as it is again removed by the liver. In complete obstructive jaundice, urobilinogen is absent from the urine as there is no bilirubin in the gut.

All patients presenting with cholestatic jaundice should undergo ultrasound examination of the liver. This examination is cheap, without complication and, in experienced hands, accurate at determining whether or not there is obstruction to the biliary tree. If equivocal, the ultrasound should be repeated as jaundice deepens, and it may then be obvious that there is indeed an obstructive cause. In addition to demonstrating dilated ducts, expert ultrasonographers can often show the cause of obstruction, but this is unreliable and definitive cholangiography should be performed in all circumstances. The radiologist may also show dilatation of the gall bladder, cholelithiasis and secondary deposits within the liver. Furthermore, the pancreas, portal and hepatic veins and the spleen can be visualized. Once the diagnosis of extra-hepatic biliary obstruction has been made, the bile ducts should be outlined by cholangiography. This is best done by using endoscopic retrograde cholangiopancreatography (ERCP), in which a side-viewing endoscope is passed into the second part of the duodenum (Fig. J.1). The ampulla of Vater is first seen, and ampullary tumours can be identified and biopsied. The bile duct and pancreas are cannulated and opacified using radiological contrast material. The procedure is successful in approximately 90 per cent of patients in expert hands and, as well as defining the cause of the obstruction, the endoscopist

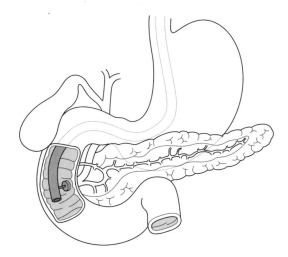

Figure J.1 Cannulation of the ampulla of Vater.

has the capacity to relieve obstruction by extracting calculi or placing stents within strictures. When the endoscopist fails to achieve a diagnosis, the alternative approach to ERCP is to perform either a percutaneous transhepatic cholangiogram (PTC) using a 'skinny' needle or a CT scan of the abdomen. PTC is a technically easier procedure in patients with a dilated biliary tract, but is also successful in approximately 60 per cent of patients with non-dilated bile ducts.

A rational approach to the investigation of jaundice is illustrated in Figure J.2. Liver biopsy confirms the presence of hepatocellular damage, but the differentiation of large duct obstruction from intrahepatic cholestasis may be difficult (see later).

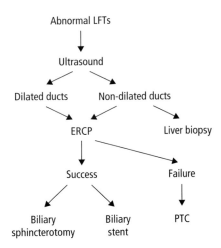

Figure J.2 Investigation of cholestatic jaundice.

Unconjugated hyperbilirubinaemia

This condition is due to:

1 An increased production of bilirubin:
   ■ Inefficient marrow production
   ■ Increased breakdown (haemolysis)
      ◆ Haemoglobinopathies
      ◆ Antibody-mediated
      ◆ Drug-induced
2 Decreased uptake of bilirubin into the liver: Gilbert's disease.
3 Decreased conjugation of bilirubin in the liver:
   ■ Crigler–Najjar syndrome
   ■ Neonatal jaundice
   ■ Drugs
   ■ Lucey–Driscoll syndrome

Increased production of bilirubin without haemolysis (shunt hyperbilirubinaemia)

Very rarely, inefficient marrow production of haemoglobin results in increased amounts of unconjugated bilirubin being released into the circulation ('early label' bilirubin). The red cells manufactured, however, have a normal life span. This is a rare primary condition and also occurs in a number of other causes of inefficient erythropoiesis, for example anaemia.

Increased production of bilirubin due to haemolysis

Most commonly, unconjugated hyperbilirubinaemia results from haemolysis, either caused by an intrinsic abnormality of the red cells or due to the development of an abnormal mechanism of destruction (extrinsic). The general investigation of patients with a haemolytic anaemia is summarized below.

■ Evidence of intravascular haemolysis:
   ◆ Haptoglobins
   ◆ Haemoglobinaemia
   ◆ Haemoglobinuria
   ◆ Haemosiderinuria
   ◆ Methaemalbuminaemia
■ Evidence of increased marrow production:
   ◆ Reticulocytosis
   ◆ Skeletal changes
   ◆ Marrow hyperplasia
■ Evidence of red cell damage:
   ◆ Fragmented forms
■ Evidence of shortened red cell life span:
   ◆ Radioactive labelling of red cells

Evidence of intravascular haemolysis

Haemoglobin released during intravascular haemolysis is normally attached to haptoglobin, the levels of which are usually reduced in chronic haemolytic states. However, levels may also be reduced by chronic liver disease and increased non-specifically in a number of connective tissue disorders. Haemoglobinaemia (associated sometimes with methaemalbuminaemia), haemoglobinuria and haemosiderinuria provide incontrovertible evidence of intravascular haemolysis, but are frequently absent in chronic haemolytic anaemias.

Evidence of increased marrow production

In a compensated anaemia, reticulocytosis with a raised mean corpuscular volume (MCV) is common. Increased marrow activity results in skeletal changes which are frequent in thalassaemia and sickle-cell disease, but rare in other conditions. The skull of such patients demonstrates a thickened vault and the diploe are widened. Bony trabeculae arising at right-angles to the dipole may produce a 'hair-on-end' appearance.

The bones of the limbs have a widened narrow cavity with a coarse trabecular pattern.

Evidence of red cell damage

Fragmented forms may provide evidence of increased red cell destruction.

Evidence of shortened red cell life span

The standard clinical test to detect shortened red cell survival is to tag the patient's cells with radioactive chromium and to measure the decline in plasma radioactivity.

Intrinsic defects of the red cells leading to increased haemolysis

These include:

- Spherocytosis
- Elliptocytosis
- Enzyme defects
- Haemoglobinopathies
  - ◆ Sickle-cell disease
  - ◆ HbSC disease
  - ◆ Thalassaemia
- Paroxysmal nocturnal haemoglobinuria

Congenital spherocytosis

This is a dominantly inherited defect which probably affects the red cell membrane, rendering it more permeable to sodium. The red cells are spherical rather than the usual biconcave shape, and are more readily haemolysed in hypotonic saline (red cell fragility test). The patient usually presents in early childhood, even though jaundice may have been noticed in early childhood; often, jaundice is first identified in the teens. Splenomegaly is common; bile pigment stones are frequently formed, and patients occasionally present with obstructive jaundice. The disease is characterized by crises of worsening anaemia and jaundice caused by increased haemolysis due to infection. The diagnosis is usually straightforward with splenomegaly, a family history and a typical blood film, but it must be remembered that spherocytes may be a feature of a number of different types of haemolytic anaemia, and that occasional mild cases of congenital spherocytosis do not present until adulthood. Splenectomy is usually followed by long-term remission of symptoms.

Congenital elliptocytosis

This is another Mendelian dominant disorder and it is usually asymptomatic, without haemolysis. Occasionally, a compensated haemolytic anaemia occurs, but anaemia sufficient to produce jaundice is extremely rare.

Enzyme defects

A wide variety of enzyme defects in the red cells have been described which produce a haemolytic anaemia and jaundice. These are usually recessively inherited. Suspicion of this type of disorder is always aroused if haemoglobin electrophoresis and osmotic fragility are normal in a patient with haemolytic anaemia. Splenectomy in these patients is not beneficial. The commonest of these disorders is pyruvate kinase deficiency, the clinical features of which are more variable in severity, but similar to congenital spherocytosis.

Haemoglobinopathies

The primary structure of haemoglobin is four polypeptide chains attached to a haem molecule. Normal adult haemoglobin has two identical alpha and two identical beta polypeptide chains attached to the haem. In the fetus, the haemoglobin has two gamma chains replacing the beta chain (fetal haemoglobin), and a small proportion of adult haemoglobin has two delta chains instead of two beta chains (A2 haemoglobin).

A2 and fetal haemoglobins will increase in disease affecting the beta chains. There are two basic types of haemoglobinopathies. One involves qualitative defects affecting one of the polypeptide chains (usually a single amino acid substitution). The other is a quantitative defect affecting the production of the whole of one long chain.

Qualitative defects of haemoglobin

Single amino acid substitution in the polypeptide chain of haemoglobin commonly produces no disease. Occasionally, an amino acid substitution produces a haemolytic anaemia, and sickle-cell anaemia provides the model for such an illness. Patients who inherit one abnormal gene only (heterozygous or sickle-cell trait) are usually only mildly affected and do not become jaundiced. Patients who inherit two sickle-cell genes have sickle-cell disease. An amino acid substitution in the beta chain produces an unstable haemoglobin molecule, which polymerizes into the reduced state, producing long chains that distort the red cells into a sickle shape. Sickle-cell disease affects Africans predominantly, and is characterized by jaundice, anaemia and skeletal changes. Although the clinical manifestations are variable, life for the patient is frequently punctuated by crises of spontaneous sickling in the circulation which produces severe abdominal and bone pain and a high fever. Although splenomegaly is common in children, repeated infarcts of the spleen usually lead to atrophy in adulthood. Gallstones are again common, which may produce obstructive jaundice. The prognosis is serious, with many patients still dying either as children or in young adult life.

The diagnosis is made by haemoglobin electrophoresis, which will show increased amounts of fetal and A2 haemoglobin, and by demonstrating in-vitro sickling of cells by addition of a reducing agent to the blood (sickle-cell test).

Sickle-cell HbC disease

Although heterozygous sickle-cell disease is usually asymptomatic, if another abnormal haemoglobin (e.g. HbC) is inherited from the other parent, haemolysis and jaundice may result, although the disease is usually milder than homozygous sickle-cell disease. Similar clinical symptoms may occur with the inheritance of one thalassaemia gene and one sickle-cell gene.

Qualitative defects of haemoglobin can lead to increased haemolysis (thalassaemia). The homozygous inheritance of defective production of alpha chains of haemoglobin is not compatible with life. The heterozygous inheritance of defective production of alpha or beta chains (alpha or beta thalassaemia minor) produces a mild abnormality that rarely gives rise to jaundice. Beta-thalassaemia major is the only homozygous thalassaemia syndrome which may occasionally result in jaundice. This condition is found most commonly in patients originating from the Mediterranean littoral, and anaemia dominates the clinical picture. Hepatosplenomegaly and marked skeletal changes may also occur. The blood picture is similar to that of iron-deficiency anaemia, and the diagnosis is made by an increased amount of circulating fetal haemoglobin on haemoglobin electrophoresis. For reasons that are unknown, A2 haemoglobin is not usually increased. There is often an *increased* resistance to haemolysis in hypotonic saline (osmotic fragility test).

Paroxysmal nocturnal haemoglobinuria

Episodes of haemolysis may be accompanied by slight jaundice in this rare condition. Diagnosis can be made by the characteristic history of red urine, which contains haemoglobin, following sleeping. The abnormal haemolysis of the red cells can be demonstrated if the plasma is acidified (Ham's test).

Extrinsic factors leading to increased haemolysis

These include:

- Autoimmune haemolytic anaemia
- Cold haemoglobinuria
- Drugs and chemicals
- Glucose-6-phosphate dehydrogenase deficiency
- Miscellaneous

Warm antibody autoimmune haemolytic anaemia

In this condition, antibody coats the patient's red cells at 37°C, and this results in increased extravascular destruction. The antibody is usually of the IgG class and incomplete (i.e. does not directly cause agglutination or haemolysis). This antibody can be detected by the direct Coombs' test, where the addition of antibody to IgG *in vitro* causes the red cells to agglutinate. Spherocytes are often present in the blood film, the white count may be raised, and occasionally the platelets are low, producing purpura. In acute acquired haemolytic anaemia the patient is usually a child with a palpable spleen, jaundice, anaemia and the constitutional symptoms of fever, vomiting and prostration. In the chronic form the onset is insidious, usually in adults, but again the patient is usually jaundiced (in 75% of cases) and has a palpable spleen. In half the patients with acquired haemolytic anaemia no cause for the antibody formation is found, but in the remainder it is secondary to a number of diseases, most importantly systemic lupus erythematosus (SLE), but also recticuloendothelial malignancy, leukaemia and sarcoidosis. Resolution of the symptoms usually occurs following treatment with corticosteroids or, occasionally, splenectomy.

Cold antibody autoimmune anaemia

Occasionally, antibody is produced which reacts with the patient's red cells at low temperatures. Depending on the thermal range of the antibody, a continuous mild haemolytic anaemia may occur which is punctuated by paroxysms of intravenous haemolysis with abdominal pain, rigors, transient jaundice and splenomegaly, that may be provoked by exposure to the cold. Cold antibody haemolytic anaemia is frequently secondary to viral infections and malignancy.

Drug and chemical-induced haemolysis

Some chemicals (e.g. arsenic and naphthalene in moth-balls) produce haemolysis and jaundice which is directly dose-related. Haemolysis may occur with other drugs; this is unrelated to the dose, and occurs only in a few susceptible individuals (Table J.4). The two important mechanisms for producing haemolysis in this situation are an associated deficiency of glucose-6-phosphate dehydrogenase in the red cell, or the production of auto-antibodies, often directed against the drug attached to the red cell membrane, which acts as a hapten. In this type of haemolysis the blood film often shows spherocytes and red cell inclusions (Heinz bodies).

Table J.4 Drugs occasionally causing haemolysis

In glucose-6-phosphate dehydrogenase-deficient subjects

Antimalarials	Primaquine, mepacrine
Antibacterials	Chloramphenicol, sulphonamides
Nitrofurans	Nitrofurantoin
Quinines	Quinidine

Auto-immune
Penicillin
Sulphonamides
Quinine and quinidine
Methyldopa
Mefenamic acid
Sulphasalazine
Para-aminosalicylic acid

Glucose-6-phosphate dehydrogenase deficiency is common in blacks and inhabitants of the Mediterranean littoral. This enzyme helps to maintain the cell concentration of reduced glutathione, which in turn stabilizes the haemoglobin molecule.

Favism is a disorder characterized by intravascular haemolysis and jaundice occurring when a glucose-6-phosphate dehydrogenase-deficient patient – usually a child from the Mediterranean region – ingests fava beans or inhales the pollen.

Similar episodes occur when the patient is exposed to certain drugs (see Table J.4). Haemolysis ceases when the older population of red cells containing less of the enzyme is destroyed.

Autoimmune drug-induced haemolysis is particularly common with methyldopa, where the direct Coombs' test is positive in 20 per cent of patients taking the drug, but haemolysis occurs in less than 1 per cent.

Other conditions causing haemolysis

Acute haemolysis with jaundice may occur with various infections (e.g. malaria and gangrene), and more mildly with viral pneumonia (usually due to cold agglutinins). It may also follow a mismatched blood transfusion, or occur in a severely burned patient.

Excessive exercise, particularly on hard roads, may also lead to episodes of intravascular haemolysis (*march haemoglobinuria*).

Microangiopathic haemolytic anaemia is the name given to a group of conditions characterized by haemolysis in association with fragmentation of red cells as they pass through blood vessels damaged by clots. Evidence of disseminated intravascular coagulation (DIC) is common. Such haemolytic anaemias are present in thrombotic thrombocytopenic purpura, malignant hypertension, disseminated neoplasia and in association with uraemia in children (the haemolytic uraemic syndrome).

Unconjugated hyperbilirubinaemia caused by impaired uptake of bilirubin into the liver

Gilbert's disease

There is some debate as to whether this condition exists, or whether it represents the upper range of a normal population distribution of unconjugated bilirubin. However, most would accept that it is a common familial condition in which there is a mild degree of unconjugated hyperbilirubinaemia. It is probably inherited as a Mendelian dominant with variable penetrance. The degree of jaundice varies and often increases following an infection or a period of fasting. Episodes of deepening jaundice may be associated with recurrent, vague abdominal pains. Mild decreases in red cell life span and the liver's ability to conjugate bilirubin are associated with a failure of transport of unconjugated bilirubin into the liver cell. The diagnosis is made by excluding liver disease. It may be confirmed by fasting the patient or by giving an intravenous injection of nicotinic acid. Both of these manoeuvres result in an increase in serum bilirubin concentrations. They are rarely necessary however, since the diagnosis is usually obvious.

Unconjugated hyperbilirubinaemia caused by impaired conjugation in the liver

Crigler–Najjar syndrome

In this familial condition there is a deficiency of the liver enzyme, glucuronyl transferase, which conjugates bilirubin. In severely affected patients (Type 1), death occurs during the neonatal period. A partial enzyme defect with some conjugated bilirubin in the bile and a better prognosis (Type 2) also occurs.

Neonatal jaundice

Glucuronyl transferase matures shortly before birth, and newborn babies – particularly if premature – will become mildly jaundiced. This may be severe in conditions increasing the bilirubin load (e.g. haemolysis), and kernicterus may result. Occasionally, prolonged neonatal jaundice is thought to occur in breast-fed babies due to the presence of pregnanediol in the milk.

Lucey–Driscoll syndrome

Unconjugated bilirubin has rarely been described in pregnancy due to hormonal inhibition of bilirubin conjugation.

Conjugated hyperbilirubinaemia

The hepatic causes of conjugated bilirubinaemia may be divided into: (i) acute hepatocellular damage, associated with considerable increases in hepatic enzymes and a short clinical course; and (ii) chronic damage, where the course is protracted and there are lesser rises in liver enzymes:

- Acute liver damage
  - ◆ Viral hepatitis
  - ◆ Non-viral infections
  - ◆ Drug-induced
  - ◆ Poisons
  - ◆ Fatty liver of pregnancy
- Chronic liver damage
  - ◆ Cirrhosis
  - ◆ Tumours
    - Primary
    - Secondary

- Infiltrations
  - ◆ Reticuloendothelial tumours
  - ◆ Amyloidosis

Acute hepatic damage

Causes of acute hepatic damage may produce a mild clinical illness or a severe disease (fulminant hepatic failure) with encephalopathy and a high mortality, when cerebral oedema, renal failure and a bleeding diathesis are frequent causes of death.

Viral hepatitis

Although a large number of viruses occasionally cause hepatitis (including rubella, Coxsackie B, herpes simplex, yellow fever virus and cytomegalovirus), the four common ones are virus A, virus B, virus C and infectious mononucleosis. The recognition of serological markers for hepatitis A and B have revolutionized our understanding of viral hepatitis, and it is now realized that many patients with these infections do not become jaundiced.

Virus A (infectious hepatitis) This is an endemic infection that is caused by a 27 nm RNA virus with a short incubation period (15–20 days). Outbreaks usually occur in conditions of poor hygiene or overcrowding. The usual transmission is faeco-oral. Patients present with malaise, anorexia, fever and a rapid onset of jaundice. There is often a vague ache in the right upper quadrant, and the liver is enlarged and tender. The spleen may also be palpable. Complete recovery is usually within a few weeks, although relapses may occur. Occasionally, patients develop deep jaundice due to intrahepatic cholestasis during the convalescent period. The diagnosis is confirmed by the demonstration of IgM antibody to the virus.

Virus B (serum hepatitis) This infection has a longer incubation period, and arthralgias and rashes may occur in the prodromal period. It is caused by a DNA virus which has an outer coat derived from the host cells and an inner core. Originally, only blood transmission was recognized (e.g. blood transfusions, transfusions of blood products; haemophilic globulin), or by needles contaminated with blood in drug addicts and in tattooing. Outbreaks in renal dialysis units produced by blood contamination have caused great concern in the past. The disease is also venereally transmitted as the virus is present in semen. Hepatitis B is common in homosexuals, 10 per cent of whom have serological markers of past infection. Asymptomatic carriers of hepatitis B infection are very frequent in certain parts of the world (e.g. Africa, China and parts of the Mediterranean). These patients may transmit the infection vertically from mother to offspring. The diagnosis of virus B hepatitis is made by the detection of the presence of surface antigen (HbsAg) in the bloodstream. For the patient to be infectious, whole virus (Dane) particles must be present in the bloodstream, and the presence of e antigen is a marker for this.

The majority of patients develop an acute viral hepatitis, and this is associated with formation of antibodies and clearance of the virus from the liver. Other individuals fail to clear the virus, become carriers, and some of these develop chronic liver disease. Patients with persistent hepatitis B virus infection are at risk of developing primary hepatocellular carcinoma.

Hepatitis D virus is an RNA virus which replicates in patients with acute or chronic hepatitis B infection. Simultaneous infection with both B and D virus leads to an acute exacerbation of hepatitis, which may be self-limiting. When chronic infection develops with co-infection the hepatitis is frequently more severe.

Virus C The prevalence of hepatitis C is approximately 2–3 per cent worldwide, with higher prevalence in certain areas such as the Middle East, where rates may be as high as 14 per cent. Hepatitis is associated with an increased risk of cirrhosis and hepatocellular carcinoma. The mode of transmission is similar to that of hepatitis B. The hepatitis C virus is a small, enveloped RNA virus. In acute hepatitis C the clinical course may be mild, only 25 per cent of patients become jaundiced, and these patients are more likely to clear the virus. Most cases of chronic hepatitis C are not preceded by an acute illness. Serum transaminases remain elevated in 60–85 per cent of patients at 1 year after diagnosis, and there is evidence of chronic hepatitis histologically. Cirrhosis develops in approximately 10 years in 10–20 per cent of cases with chronic disease, and hepatitis C RNA persists in patients with abnormal liver enzymes.

Hepatitis E is an RNA virus of which there are many genotypes. It is endemic in Asia, Africa, the Middle East and Central America, and is associated with poor sanitation. The seroprevalence is approximately 5 per cent in children aged under 10 years, and 10–40 per cent in adults. The virus is particularly virulent in pregnant women, amongst whom there is a high fatality rate of approximately 20 per cent. In non-endemic regions, hepatitis E accounts for <1 per cent of cases of acute viral hepatitis.

Infectious mononucleosis Up to 15 per cent of patients with glandular fever develop jaundice. The clinical picture is characteristic, with malaise, sore throat, skin rashes, lymphadenopathy and splenomegaly. Atypical mononuclear cells are found in the peripheral blood, and the test for heterophile antibody (Paul–Bunnell) is usually positive.

Yellow fever This is a zoonosis and is transmitted to man from a primate pool by the mosquito in tropical Africa, the Caribbean and South America. The incubation period is short (3–4 days), with a sudden onset of rigors, jaundice and abdominal pain. Its course may be fulminant with renal failure and a bleeding diathesis.

Non-viral infections

Relapsing fever This condition is caused by a spirochaete of the *Borrelia* group of bacteria, and is characterized by jaundice and a fever of up to 40°C, which normally lasts for 4–5 days and then remits. The epidemic form of the disease is usually caused by lice, and is common during periods of famine. An endemic infection is usually transmitted by the tick and is common in the Far East, Africa and America.

Leptospirosis The spirochaete *Leptospira icterohaemorrhagica* infects a variety of small animals, and humans contract the disease by bathing in water contaminated with these infected animals' urine. The disease is biphasic, with an initial illness a few days after exposure, a temperature, meningism and prominent myalgias and conjunctivitis. Recovery may occur, or after a week the patient may develop widespread bruising, jaundice and occasionally renal failure. *L. icterohaemorrhagiae* is transmitted by rats' urine, mainly to agricultural and sewage workers, and produces a severe form of the disease where jaundice and renal failure are particularly likely to occur.

Other bacterial infections Jaundice may complicate any septicaemic illness. Occasionally, an infected thrombus in the portal vein may occur (portal pyaemia) following an acute infection in the area drained by the portal system (e.g. appendicitis). The signs of a portal pyaemia are severe prostration, a swinging pyrexia and jaundice.

Drug-induced acute hepatic damage

Drugs either produce predictable dose-related hepatic necrosis (e.g. paracetamol) or, more commonly, damage is produced unpredictably in only a few of the patients exposed to the drug and unrelated to its dosage. There are two basic patterns of liver damage: acute hepatic cellular necrosis with features identical to viral hepatitis; or intrahepatic cholestasis. It is not possible to provide an exhaustive list of drugs producing hepatocellular damage (Table J.5), and a high index of suspicion should exist in any jaundiced patient who is taking drugs. There are certain situations that will make the individual more susceptible to liver damage; for example, reactions are more likely at the extremes of age, HIV infection renders the liver more sensitive to co-trimoxazole and sulphonamides, enzyme inducers increase sensitivity to rifampicin and isoniazid, enzyme inhibitors to oestrogens, whilst in any condition that interferes with nutrition (e.g. intravenous drug or alcohol abuse, HIV infection), malabsorption increases the toxicity of paracetamol.

Table J.5 Drug-induced hepatic damage (drugs in italics are the most common causes of liver damage)

Drug	Acute hepatic necrosis	Cholestasis
Paracetamol	+	
Dextropropoxyphene	+	+
Halothane	+	
Tetracycline	+ (in pregnancy)	
Erythromycin estolate		+
Penicillin	+	
Sulphasalazine		+
Nitrofurantoin	+	
Pheniramine maleate	+	
Piperazine	+	
Isoniazid	+	
Rifampicin	+	
Para-aminosalicylic acid	+	+
Chlorpromazine		+
Monoamine oxidase inhibitor	+ (? cirrhosis)	
Methyldopa	+	
Quinidine	+ (? cirrhosis)	
Perhexiline		+
Chlorpropamide	+	
Phenytoin	+	+
Propylthiouracil		+
Oral contraceptives		+
Anabolic steroids		+

Paracetamol Paracetamol overdose is the most common cause of fulminant hepatic failure in the UK. Hepatic damage is dose-related, but death has been reported with amounts as low as 7.5 g. Following ingestion, paracetamol is metabolized to a toxic intermediate which is scavenged by glutathione. When glutathione stores are exhausted, the metabolite binds covalently to the membrane of hepatocytes, causing cell death. Chronic alcoholics whose microsomal enzymes are reduced and whose glutathione stores tend to be depressed are at increased risk following the overdose. Nausea, vomiting and abdominal pain develop within 12–36 hours, and jaundice develops 2–3 days later. In severe cases this leads to liver failure with coagulopathy and encephalopathy. A very characteristic feature of paracetamol poisoning is the development of renal failure.

Halothane Halothane is a very safe anaesthetic, but there is an undoubted small incidence (0.003%) of serious acute hepatic necrosis following the use of the drug, which may lead to fever, jaundice and death. Inadvertent repeated use in patients who were previously jaundiced following exposure to halothane results in recurrence of the patient's jaundice. Halothane hepatitis is more common after repeated exposures, particularly in obese patients. Jaundice associated with pyrexia usually occurs 2 weeks after the initial exposure, but only 10 days after subsequent administration. Halothane should not be re-used in patients who have suffered a febrile illness and abnormal liver function tests after a previous encounter with this agent.

Oral contraceptives The older oral contraceptives containing a relatively high concentration of oestrogen occasionally led to a mild cholestatic jaundice. These individuals are particularly prone to develop cholestasis in pregnancy. In addition, the older contraceptives also had a tendency to cause the Budd–Chiari syndrome and a variety of tumours within the liver, in particular benign adenomas. The newer contraceptives, which contain much lower concentrations of oestrogens, are much safer and rarely cause these complications.

Anabolic steroids The C17-alpha-alkylated-substituted testosterones (e.g. norethisterone and norethanandrolone) produce a dose-related cholestasis by a similar mechanism to the oral contraceptive.

Chlorpromazine An unpredictable cholestatic jaundice may occur in 1 per cent of patients within a month of starting treatment with this drug. Eosinophilia and mitochondrial antibodies are frequently found in the bloodstream. The patient itches, has pale stools and dark urine. Three-quarters of patients recover on withdrawal of the drug, but a few develop prolonged cholestasis resembling primary biliary cirrhosis (see below).

Antineoplastic drugs   A variety of such drugs cause jaundice and liver damage (e.g. methotrexate). However, the primary conditions for which these drugs are administered are often a cause for jaundice.

Industrial toxins

These are only rarely a cause of jaundice in humans. Most seem to act by inhibiting protein synthesis. Carbon tetrachloride and (less commonly) other volatile hydrocarbons produce acute hepatocellular necrosis and jaundice within 1–2 days of exposure. Renal failure, pancreatitis, pulmonary oedema and death may also occur. Dicophane (DDT) and trinitrotoluene (TNT) also occasionally produce hepatic necrosis.

A cholestatic jaundice has been described following accidental ingestion of flour contaminated by diaminodiphenyl methane (so-called 'Epping jaundice', named after the place where the outbreak occurred).

Amanita   Ingestion of as little as three wild mushrooms of the *Amanita* species may be fatal. Abdominal pain and diarrhoea occur within 18 hours of ingestion, followed 3 days later by the development of fulminant hepatic failure and jaundice.

Acute fatty liver of pregnancy

This condition occurs in 1 in 15 000 cases. It is common in primigravids and multiple pregnancies. It is associated with genetically determined defects of β-oxidation of fatty acids in some cases. Onset occurs in the third trimester with vomiting, upper abdominal pain, anorexia and malaise. Later, disseminated intravascular coagulation, leucocytosis, hypoglycaemia and hyperammonaemia develop and progress to fulminant hepatic failure. Mortality rates (mother and baby) are high if the condition is not recognized and allowed to progress. Treatment is by prompt delivery of the baby.

Chronic liver damage: cirrhosis

Cirrhosis is defined as diffuse fibrosis with nodular regeneration of the liver which destroys the normal spatial relationship of the lobules. It is classified as micronodular, macronodular or mixed, depending on the size of the nodules. The condition may be suspected in cases of jaundice where the liver is firm and palpable, although sometimes it is shrunken and impalpable. The stigmata of chronic liver disease (see Table J.2) are often present, and the spleen may be enlarged because of portal hypertension. Oedema and ascites are caused by a combination of portal hypertension, sodium retention and hypoalbuminaemia. Hepatic encephalopathy may occur, with a sweet musty odour to the breath (caused by mercaptans originating from gut breakdown of methionine), a flapping tremor (asterixis), disorders of the sleep rhythm, and then frank unconsciousness. A chronic form of encephalopathy with slowness and psychiatric changes may also occur. Jaundice is a relatively late complication of cirrhosis, and many patients with compensated cirrhosis have relatively normal liver function tests.

Causes of cirrhosis include the following:

- Alcoholic liver disease
  - Infections
  - Viral (HBV, HCV)
  - Bacterial (syphilis)
  - Protozoan (schistosomiasis)
- Chronic active hepatitis
  - Lupoid
  - HBV
  - Drugs
- Genetic defects
  - Haemochromatosis
  - Wilson's disease
  - Galactosaemia
  - Glycogen storage diseases
  - Alpha-1 antitrypsin deficiency
- Biliary disease
  - Long-standing extrahepatic biliary obstruction
  - Primary biliary cirrhosis
  - Sclerosing cholangitis
  - Congenital hepatic fibrosis
- Venous congestion
  - Cardiac failure
  - Constrictive pericarditis
  - Budd–Chiari syndrome
- Jejuno-ileal bypass

Alcoholic liver disease

There is a strong relationship between the national figures for consumption of alcohol and death from cirrhosis. Women are more susceptible to the effects of alcohol than men, and drinking more than 20 g a day is associated with an increased risk of cirrhosis. In men, a consumption of over 80 g a day is associated with an increased risk which rises to 25-fold normal if more than 100 g a day is consumed. It is probable that steady alcohol consumption for about 10 years is required rather than bouts of drinking. Individual susceptibility is also important as some patients never develop cirrhosis, however much they drink. There are three types of liver disease associated with alcohol:

- *Fatty infiltration* does not cause jaundice and does not lead to cirrhosis.
- *Alcoholic hepatitis* is a clinical syndrome which occurs after a bout of heavy drinking with fever, jaundice and multiple spider naevi. The aspartate transaminase is only mildly elevated, but the patient may be deeply jaundiced. The white blood cell count is often markedly increased, and the prothrombin time may be very prolonged. Such patients have a significant mortality and may later develop cirrhosis, even if they stop drinking completely. Histological changes consist of an acute inflammatory reaction at the portal tract and necrosis of liver cells, often with multiple protein inclusions (Mallory's alcoholic hyaline). These histological changes are seen quite frequently in patients who drink excessive alcohol, and are not always associated with the full clinical syndrome of alcoholic hepatitis. In Zieve's syndrome, alcoholic hepatitis is associated with haemolytic anaemia and hyperlipidaemia in addition to jaundice.
- *Cirrhosis.* Alcohol produces a micronodular cirrhosis, and the prognosis is undoubtedly worse if the patient continues to drink. It has been suggested that autoimmune mechanisms, particularly in alcoholic hepatitis, may be important. A combination of alcohol abuse and hepatitis B infection is particularly likely to lead to the development of cirrhosis and strongly predisposes to primary hepatic carcinoma.

Infections

The discovery of markers for hepatitis B and C has demonstrated that these are both important causes of cirrhosis.

Congenital syphilis may produce a pericellular fibrosis, but true cirrhosis is uncommon as regeneration nodules do not usually develop.

Schistosomiasis classically produces periportal fibrosis (pipesteam fibrosis) leading to portal hypertension,

but cirrhosis may also develop and is thought to be due to associated conditions (e.g. hepatitis B infection, which is also very common in these patients).

Chronic active hepatitis

Chronic active hepatitis is a consequence of a variety of diseases. The most common cause worldwide is chronic infection with the hepatitis B virus. A history of drug abuse, homosexuality or exposure to blood products is often elucidated in patients presenting with hepatitis B in the Western hemisphere. Autoimmune chronic active hepatitis (lupoid hepatitis) is an autoimmune disease of women which is characterized by the presence of circulating smooth muscle antibodies, antinuclear factor and high titres of immunoglobulins (IgG). Chronic active hepatitis may also be due to ingestion of drugs including oxyphenacetin, methyldopa, antituberculous agents or anticonvulsants. Very similar appearances may also be seen in patients presenting with Wilson's disease, and the appearances may be indistinguishable from conditions as apparently distinct as primary sclerosing cholangitis.

Chronic active hepatitis presents with malaise, jaundice and eventually with hepatic decompensation. The spleen is frequently enlarged, and patients with the autoimmune type commonly have associated arthralgia.

The diagnosis is made by demonstrating abnormal liver function tests, particularly hypertransaminasaemia, which must persist for at least 6 months. There may be evidence of chronic hepatitis B infection, circulating smooth muscle antibodies or antinuclear factor. Liver biopsy reveals an inflammatory infiltrate radiating from the portal tracts and broaching the limiting plates. Fibrosis is almost invariable and may encircle groups of hepatocytes, resulting in the formation of rosettes. Frank cirrhosis may be present at the time of diagnosis.

Genetic defects

Haemochromatosis

This is an autosomal recessive disease characterized by increased intestinal iron absorption. The disease is rare in premenopausal women, and most patients also abuse alcohol, which further increases iron intake. Slate-grey pigmentation develops because of melanin and iron deposition in the skin. Cirrhosis occurs; the liver is invariably enlarged and there is evidence of portal hypertension and hepatic decomposition. Iron deposition in the pancreas causes diabetes mellitus ('bronze diabetes'). Accumulation in other endocrine glands leads to testicular atrophy, gynaecomastia and loss of body hair; hypopituitarism can occur. The diagnosis is suggested by a high serum ferritin concentration and confirmed by liver biopsy. Primary hepatocellular carcinoma is a relatively common complication and cause of death.

Wilson's disease

Wilson's disease is a recessively inherited disease of impaired copper metabolism. Copper accumulates in the liver, causing cirrhosis, and also in the basal ganglia of the brain, causing an extrapyramidal neurological syndrome. Patients usually present between the ages of 5 and 25 years with either or both liver and neurological disease. The hepatic presentation may be insidious with jaundice and ascites. The liver is usually small and fibrosed. The presentation may alternatively be acute with fulminant hepatic failure and severe haemolytic anaemia.

The diagnosis is made by slit-lamp examination of the eyes, when Kayser–Fleischer rings can be demonstrated. Urinary 24-hour copper excretion is increased, and this increases further with penicillamine therapy. In addition, serum copper concentrations are increased and caeruloplasmin levels are low. Liver biopsy shows cirrhosis. Copper stains are positive.

Other metabolic errors

All the other metabolic errors leading to cirrhosis and jaundice mentioned above are exceedingly rare. Among the glycogen storage diseases, only type IV leads to cirrhosis and jaundice.

Alpha-1 antitrypsin deficiency

This autosomally recessively inherited disease may present as a severe neonatal hepatitis or as established cirrhosis in patients below the age of 20 years. There may be associated lung disease which characteristically presents as emphysema, pulmonary fibrosis and respiratory failure. Liver biopsy shows periodic acid–Schiff (PAS)-positive-stained inclusion bodies within hepatocytes.

Biliary disease

Disease affecting the extra-hepatic biliary tract, intra-hepatic ductules or canaliculi can lead to cirrhosis.

Extra-hepatic biliary obstruction following trauma to the bile ducts can occasionally cause a secondary biliary cirrhosis; extra-hepatic biliary obstruction is considered below. The most important causes of intra-hepatic cholestasis are drugs and primary biliary cirrhosis.

Primary biliary cirrhosis predominantly affects middle-aged females, and is due to destruction of bile ductules by a cell-mediated autoimmune process. The disease progresses extremely slowly in the majority of patients, and usually presents with a cholestatic syndrome comprising itching, pale stools and dark urine. Hypercholesterolaemia is common and may lead to the development of xanthelasmas. The disease is associated with other autoimmune diseases, including hypothyroidism, Addison's disease, systemic sclerosis, diabetes and renal tubular acidosis. Other patients present with bleeding oesophageal varices or ascites, without any previous history of itching. A physical examination may reveal stigmata of chronic liver disease, jaundice, pigmentation and xanthelasmas. The liver is enlarged and firm; the spleen may be palpable, and ascites develop because of portal hypertension.

Primary biliary cirrhosis should be considered in women presenting with cholestatic liver function tests. The mitochondrial antibody is positive in more than 98 per cent of patients. Serum IgM concentrations are increased. A liver biopsy shows chronic inflammatory infiltrate in the portal tract, with destruction and paucity of bile ductules. Granulomas may be seen within portal tracts.

Sclerosing cholangitis

Secondary sclerosing cholangitis is a condition in which progressive fibrosis and narrowing of the intra-hepatic and extra-hepatic biliary tree occurs as a consequence of biliary sepsis. It follows bile duct injury. Primary sclerosing cholangitis is a disease that is strongly associated with ulcerative colitis. Many individuals are asymptomatic and merely have cholestatic liver function tests, whereas others present with fluctuating jaundice. In advanced disease this leads to secondary biliary cirrhosis. It is likely that the condition predisposes to the development of cholangiocarcinoma.

Hepatic congestion

True cirrhosis due to heart failure is very uncommon, although jaundice may occur in association with heart failure.

Budd–Chiari syndrome

This syndrome is a rare condition in which the main hepatic veins are occluded (for a discussion, see LIVER, ENLARGEMENT OF, p. 376). The liver scan often shows a central area of uptake which is due to the enlargement of the caudate lobe of the liver, the veins of which drain separately into the inferior vena cava.

Chronic liver damage: infiltrations

Amyloidosis

The liver may be involved by infiltration with amyloid, both in the primary disease and where it is secondary to chronic suppuration, myelomatosis or rheumatoid arthritis. Amyloid is an antigen–antibody complex which stains metachromatically with crystal violet and shows birefringence with Congo red staining. The liver is enlarged and rubbery, and the patient may show other features of amyloidosis such as nephrotic syndrome, cardiac failure and malabsorption. Hepatocellular failure – and hence jaundice – is rare in this condition, and the diagnosis may be made by liver or rectal biopsy.

Chronic liver damage: tumours

The liver may be affected by benign or malignant tumours, but only the latter will produce jaundice. Secondary deposits are 25-fold more common than a primary malignant growth.

Primary hepatocellular carcinoma

Primary tumours of the liver are a frequent accompaniment of cirrhosis, and are said to be found in between 50–60 per cent of post-mortem examinations in cirrhotic patients. Hepatocellular cancer is particularly common in certain parts of the world, especially Africa and China, where hepatitis B is the important aetiological agent. Hepatitis C is an important cause in the West. Aflatoxin, which is produced by a fungus growing on grain stored in humid conditions, and the now obsolete radiocontrast material Thorotrast (thorium dioxide), are often associated with the development of the tumour.

Primary hepatocellular carcinoma tumours may occur at any age, are five-fold more common in males than females, and should be suspected in any patient with cirrhosis who deteriorates or who develops a lump in the liver. A friction sound is occasionally heard over the tumour, and arterial murmurs may be present. The diagnosis is made by finding elevated alpha-fetoprotein concentrations, and by liver biopsy.

Primary sarcoma of the liver and malignant haemangiosarcoma

These are extremely rare tumours, which may cause jaundice in their terminal stages. Malignant haemangiosarcoma is associated with exposure to Thorotrast and vinyl chloride.

Secondary tumours

The liver is the most frequent site of blood-borne metastatic tumours, whether drained by systemic or portal veins. It is involved in about one-third of all cancers, including half of those in the stomach, large bowel, breast and lung. The liver may be either normal in size or grossly enlarged, with palpable hard deposits. Jaundice may be absent and is usually mild. The serum alkaline phosphatase level is often markedly raised.

Reticuloendothelial diseases in the liver

The reticuloendothelial cells of the liver may be involved by any malignant process involving this system. Jaundice is usually mild, and may occasionally be due to haemolysis.

Intrahepatic cholestasis

Causes of this condition include:

- Drugs
- Viral hepatitis
- Cirrhosis (occasionally)
- Dubin–Johnson syndrome
- Pregnancy
- Sclerosing cholangitis
- Biliary atresia
- Recurrent idiopathic cholestasis

In this group of conditions the patient presents with an obstructive jaundice, usually with pale stools, dark urine and itching, but investigations reveal no obstruction of the extra-hepatic bile ducts.

Dubin–Johnson and Rotor syndromes

These are rare familial benign intermittent conditions that produce jaundice with conjugated hyperbilirubinaemia. In the Dubin–Johnson type, the liver is greenish black and contains brown pigment. Jaundice is rarely deep, and the alkaline phosphatase remains normal. The diagnosis may be made using a bromsulphthalein (BSP) retention test in which, after an initial fall, the serum level of BSP rises after 2 hours and remains detectable for 48 hours. The condition is thought to be due to poor transport of conjugated bilirubin into the biliary canaliculi. The Rotor syndrome resembles Dubin–Johnson both clinically and biochemically, the main difference being the absence of brown pigment in the liver.

Pregnancy

Some women develop intrahepatic cholestasis during the last trimester of pregnancy; it is associated with itching, pale stools or dark urine. The mechanism seems similar to that of oral contraceptive-induced cholestasis.

Extra-hepatic biliary obstruction

Extra-hepatic biliary obstruction can be classified as being due to diseases within the lumen of the bile ducts, those affecting the wall of the ducts, or diseases compressing the duct from outside (Table J.6).

Obstruction is usually followed by dilatation of the common bile duct, although this may take some time to develop. The architecture of the liver is usually

Table J.6 Causes of obstruction to the bile ducts

Causes within the lumen of the bile ducts
Gallstones
Parasites

Causes affecting the wall of the ducts
Accidental division
Acute pancreatitis
Chronic pancreatitis
Carcinoma of the bile duct
Congenital obliteration of the bile duct

Causes compressing the bile duct or invading it from the outside
Tumours of the pancreas
Peritoneal adhesions
Enlarged portal lymph nodes
Aneurysm of the hepatic artery
Hydatid cysts
Retroperitoneal cysts
Duodenal diverticulum

normal, but biopsies show pigmentation, bile plugs and infarcts. Cirrhosis can rarely develop in extremely long-standing obstruction. The patient is clinically jaundiced, and the degree of jaundice may be very deep, resulting in a greenish tinge. The urine is dark because of an excess of bilirubin. The stools are pale, clay-coloured and bulky because of their increased fat content. Biochemical investigations reveal a raised serum alkaline phosphatase concentration, prolonged prothrombin time because of vitamin K malabsorption, and hypocalcaemia because of vitamin D malabsorption. The serum albumin concentration is usually maintained until the late stages.

The investigation of obstructive jaundice has already been alluded to. The steps involved are ultrasound followed by either endoscopic, percutaneous cholangiography, and CT scanning of the abdomen or liver biopsy.

Causes due to obstruction of the bile duct lumen

Gallstones

This is the most common cause of extra-hepatic biliary obstruction in the UK. The gallstones are mixed and usually originate from the gall bladder, although it is likely that primary bile duct stones may also occur.

The patient presenting with choledocholithiasis and obstructive jaundice may or may not have had a previous cholecystectomy. Severe right upper quadrant pain radiating through to the back usually occurs. Fever associated with rigors is common. The jaundice fluctuates and may disappear completely, presumably because the calculus either passes into the duodenum, or disimpacts from the ampulla, and returns into the lumen of the duct. Another important consequence is gallstone pancreatitis. Occasional patients (usually elderly) present with painless progressive jaundice simulating a carcinoma of the pancreas. Some patients with bile duct calculi have no symptoms and present incidentally with abnormal liver function tests. Examination usually reveals mild jaundice. There may be tenderness of the liver and pyrexia. The gall bladder is usually impalpable.

Investigations reveal cholestatic liver function tests and leucocytosis. Calcified gallstones may be seen on plain abdominal X-ray in 20 per cent of patients with cholelithiasis. An ultrasound examination may or may not reveal a dilated biliary tree. Stones may be seen within the bile duct, although they are often overlooked. Calculi may be identified within the gall bladder, but this is uncommon in patients in whom jaundice is not caused by choledocholithiasis.

Percutaneous transhepatic cholangiography (Fig. J.3) and ERCP reveal filling defects within the common bile duct. Gallstones may also be demonstrated by CT scanning.

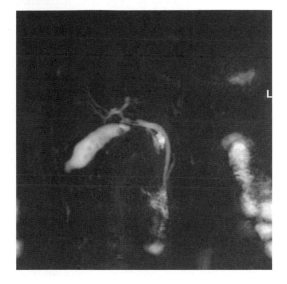

Figure J.3 Percutaneous transhepatic cholangiography (PTC). The bile ducts are dilated, and the filling defect caused by a stone can be seen at the lower end of the common bile duct. Multiple stones are also seen in the gall bladder.

Parasites

The most important of these is the worm *Ascaris lumbricoides*, which is released from an ovum in the duodenum and migrates into the intestinal wall and hence the portal circulation. Worms enter the liver, heart and lungs, migrate into the pharynx, and are swallowed. Patients present with haemoptysis, bronchitis and pneumonia; occasionally, a worm blocks the bile duct to cause jaundice or to act as a nidus for the development of a calculus. Roundworm jaundice is a common cause of icterus in African children.

Causes affecting the wall of the bile duct

Bile duct trauma

This is usually a consequence of division at operation, and is more likely to occur if the surgeon is inexperienced, in patients who have had previous biliary operations or who have an inflammatory mass around the bile duct.

Cholangiocarcinoma

These are epithelial tumours of the bile duct, and arise at any point within the biliary tree. Patients present with painless obstructive jaundice, and it may be impossible to differentiate the lesion from tumours of the pancreas – either clinically or by investigation. One important variant is a tumour arising at the bifurcation of the main left and right hepatic duct (Klatskin tumour). This is an extremely hard, fibrous, but slow-growing tumour which carries a better prognosis than tumours arising elsewhere in the biliary tree.

Carcinoma of the ampulla

Tumours arising from the ampulla are uncommon and present with painless obstructive jaundice. They are more slowly growing than carcinoma of the pancreas, and should be considered for Whipple's operation.

Biliary atresia

This presents as deepening obstructive jaundice within 2–3 days of birth. Liver failure develops by the age of 3–6 months. The diagnosis is made by HIDA scanning, followed by cholangiography.

Sclerosing cholangitis

This is an autoimmune condition leading to inflammation of the biliary system, with a typical patchy pattern seen on ERCP.

Causes compressing the bile duct from outside

Carcinoma of the pancreas

The most important cause is carcinoma of the pancreas, which invades the common bile duct as it passes through the head of the gland. The patient presents with painless obstructive jaundice, although others complain of progressive and continuous pain in the back due to invasion of the coeliac plexus and other retroperitoneal structures. Jaundice is progressive and associated with weight loss. Rigors are unusual.

Examination reveals cachexia, deep jaundice, hepatomegaly and a palpable gall bladder (Fig. J.4; see also Fig. G.2). There may be evidence of metastatic spread; in particular there may be supraclavicular lymphadenopathy or tumour nodules in the umbilicus (Sister Joseph's nodule).

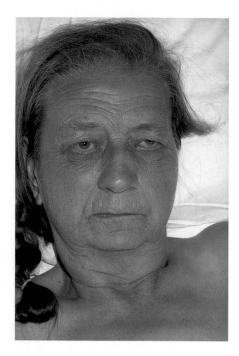

Figure J.4 Severe jaundice in a patient with extensive hepatic metastases from a carcinoma of the colon.

Most tumours arise from ductular epithelium and carry a very poor prognosis. It is important, however, to remember that some tumours are more amenable to therapy; these include cystadenocarcinoma, a tumour of relatively young women, and apudomas. Ultrasonography reveals dilated intra-hepatic and extra-hepatic bile ducts. It may also show a mass within the pancreatic head. Endoscopy may demonstrate invasion of the duodenum by tumour, and the diagnosis can then be confirmed by biopsy. ERCP reveals a stricture within the lead of the pancreas corresponding to a low bile duct malignant stenosis.

Malignant obstruction of the extra-hepatic bile duct may also be due to enlarged lymph nodes in the region of the porta hepatis, and this is usually encountered in patients with breast carcinoma or secondary carcinoma from gastrointestinal origin. Occasionally, true secondary deposits occur within the bile duct, usually from melanoma or carcinoma of the breast.

Mirizzi's syndrome

This is a rare entity in which a stone impacts in Hartmann's pouch, causing compression and obstruction of the common hepatic duct.

Aneurysm of the hepatic artery

This is a rare cause of obstructive jaundice diagnosed by arteriography.

Cysts

Hydatid cyst is a rare cause of obstructive jaundice; far more commonly these are found incidentally by plain X-ray. Simple cysts or choledochal cysts may also cause obstructive jaundice.

Sharon O'Byrne

JAW, DEFORMITY OF

The jaws may become deformed by congenital or acquired disease; for a discussion of the latter condition, see JAW, SWELLING OF (p. 338). The reader should refer to this section for details of pathological conditions causing jaw deformity. Trauma to the jaws may cause deformity due to bone fragment displacement, and this will be maintained if inadequate treatment results in non-union or malunion of the fracture. The majority of conditions, however, to be considered here are of a developmental nature occurring before birth or during the growth period:

Congenital conditions:

- Cleft palate
- Pierre Robin's syndrome
- First arch syndrome
- Treacher–Collins syndrome

Acquired conditions:

- Premature synostoses
- Achondroplasia
- Diseases of the temporomandibular joint
- Acromegaly

Growth of the facial skeleton takes place by sutural growth, surface deposition and remodelling, and cartilaginous growth with secondary ossification. The main stimulus for growth of the maxilla is the growth of the brain, causing an increase in size of the cranial vault and the cranial base to which the maxilla is joined. The cranial base also increases in length by cartilaginous growth at the spheno-occipital synchrondrosis. Growth within the maxilla is stimulated by the development of the nasal capsule and the eyes.

The mandible forms *in utero* around a rod of cartilage known as Meckel's cartilage, which is subsequently replaced by bone, leaving only the condylar cartilage at the temporomandibular joint. Subsequent elongation of the mandible occurs by the growth of this cartilage with secondary ossification, and development is completed by surface deposition of bone and remodelling.

There is an inherent genetic potential for growth of the facial skeleton, but this is aided by eruption of the dentition and by the muscular forces placed upon it by the muscles of mastication. A defect in one or more of these mechanisms of growth will produce jaw deformity. However, the majority of cases of jaw deformity arise from a simple imbalance between the growth of the maxilla and the mandible to produce a dental malocclusion (Fig. J.5).

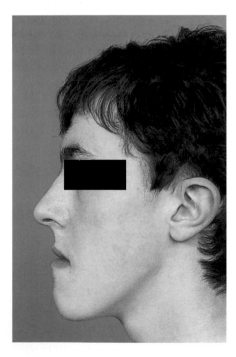

Figure J.5 Patient exhibiting growth imbalance of the maxilla and mandible.

Congenital jaw deformities

Cleft palate

Cleft palate occurs in approximately one in every 700 live births, and is due to a failure of growth and fusion of the palatal shelves in the embryo. Females are affected more than males, and there may be an associated cleft of the lip (Fig. J.6). There is a genetic disposition to this deformity with a strong family history, but other exogenous factors have been implicated. These are drugs such as retinoids, phenytoin, methotrexate and other anti-folate agents. As folic acid deficiency is implicated with this abnormality, all mothers should be given folic acid supplements at conception. Some 5 per cent of cases of cleft lip and palate are associated with other congenital abnormalities.

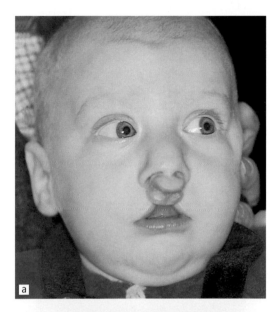

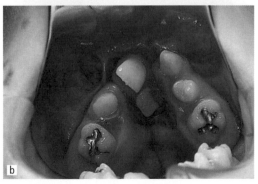

Figure J.6 (a,b) Bilateral cleft lip, and palate with rotation of the premaxilla.

Pierre Robin's syndrome

This syndrome is thought to be caused by hypoplasia of the mandible, preventing the normal descent of the tongue and thus preventing fusion of the embryonic palatal shelves. The syndrome is, therefore, characterized by a small mandible, cleft palate and protruding tongue. The baby may present with feeding and respiratory problems, which can be corrected by the construction of a small dental plate and nursing in the supine position.

Normal growth of the mandible can be anticipated after a few years, once any palatal defect has been closed.

First arch syndrome

This syndrome characteristically exhibits a deformed or absent ear, macrostomia and an under-development of the mandibular ramus and condyle. The masticatory muscles on that side are also deficient, and there is hypoplasia of the orbit and zygoma on the ipsilateral side (Fig. J.7). Other associated abnormalities may be present, particularly of the vertebrae. According to Poswillo, haemorrhage of the stapedial artery in the region of the otic ganglion during uterine development is proposed as the cause.

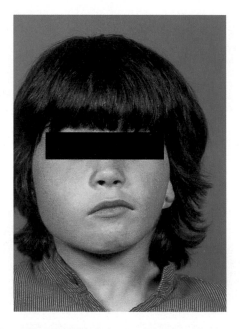

Figure J.7 Patient with the first arch syndrome.

Treacher–Collins syndrome

This is an inherited autosomal dominant condition affecting the facial skeleton in a similar way to the first arch syndrome, but the abnormalities are bilateral and symmetrical. Due to the poor development of the zygomatic arches, prominent nose, and small jaw, many of the patients have a fish-like appearance.

Acquired jaw deformities

Premature synostosis

Premature fusion of the cranial sutures are a feature of Cruzon's and Apert's syndrome, producing deformities of the cranial vault. Because of an associated lack of growth of the cranial base, patients also exhibit extreme under-development of the mid-third of the face.

Achondroplasia

This rare condition usually represents a sporadic mutation; less than 20 per cent will be of a familial nature. The aetiology is not completely understood, but there is a defect of endochondral ossification. Failure of growth at the spheno-occipital synchondrosis and lack of growth in the maxilla produces the characteristic under-development of the mid-third of the face. Curiously, growth of the mandible is unaffected, leading to relative mandibular prognathism.

Disorders of the temporomandibular joint

The mandibular condyle may be affected by trauma, infection from the middle ear or juvenile arthritis, all of which will damage the condylar growth centre. The result is under-development of one side of the mandible with compensatory growth on the contralateral side. This produces a facial asymmetry and under-development of the ipsilateral side of the face in the vertical plane. Fractures of the temporomandibular joint may, on occasions, be followed by ankylosis and this, too, will prevent normal development of the affected side of the face (Fig. J.8). Treatment of all these conditions is by surgical correction.

In some patients there may be excessive growth of the condyle known as *condylar hyperplasia*, resulting in asymmetry of the facial skeleton with over-growth of the affected site. Asymmetry may also be caused by hemifacial hypertrophy or hemifacial atrophy. In the latter case there is slow progressive atrophy of the soft tissues of one side of the face with secondary deformity of the facial skeleton. Patients may also exhibit contralateral Jacksonian epilepsy and trigeminal neuralgia. This condition is thought to be due to an

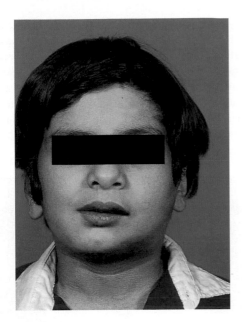

Figure J.8 Facial deformity due to ankylosis of the right temporomandibular joint.

abnormality of the sympathetic system, and is often associated with scleroderma.

Acromegaly

Acromegaly follows autonomous hypersecretion of growth hormone caused by hyperplasia or an adenoma of the pituitary acidophil cells. The face is invariably affected by this condition, with over-growth of the mandible to produce prognathism with malocclusion, enlargement of the tongue and deposition of bone at the supraorbital ridges and zygomas.

The facial skin also becomes thickened, as does the subcutaneous tissue, producing an accentuation of the normal skin folds. The nose becomes enlarged, especially at the tip, as do the lips. Treatment should be for the underlying pituitary problem and corrective jaw surgery should only be undertaken following stabilization of the condition. Many of these patients have a cardiomyopathy, and there may be serious complications during anaesthesia.

Management of jaw deformity

The facial appearance and jaw function of these patients with jaw deformity can be improved by combined orthodontic and surgical correction. Minor deformity can be corrected by movement through

osteotomy procedures, while the more severe cases with significant abnormalities of the soft tissues should be treated by distraction osteogenesis techniques.

Peter T. Blenkinsopp

JAW, PAIN IN

Pain in the jaw mostly arises from the dental structures and their supporting bone, the temporomandibular joint and the associated muscles of mastication. In the upper jaw, infections of the nose and paranasal sinuses may additionally cause pain in the maxilla. Disorders of the trigeminal nerve are a relatively rare cause of facial pain, but atypical facial pain, which is part of a psychological illness (usually depression), is quite common.

Dental pain

Inflammation in the pulp chamber of a tooth caused by dental caries, inadequately insulated restorations or occlusal trauma characteristically causes pain with thermal stimulation or pressure. This then progresses to an ache, which lasts for increasing periods of time or may be worse at night when the patient lies down.

As the inflammation progresses, the pain becomes very severe and constant until such time as remedial therapy is carried out, or gangrene of the pulp occurs. At this stage, the pain diminishes but is replaced by an ache within the alveolar bone should a dental alveolar abscess develop (Fig. J.9).

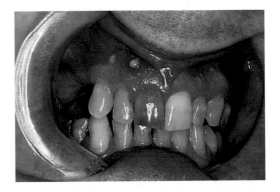

Figure J.9 Upper right central incisor with gangrene of the dental pulp and pus discharging through the alveolar bone.

With increasing infection, the visible signs of inflammation become apparent and a swelling develops in the mucous membrane or associated soft tissues (see JAW, SWELLING OF, p. 338). At any stage this pain may be worsened by occlusal trauma to the tooth during mastication, or when the teeth are percussed. The pain associated with a periodontal abscess or pericoronal infection is similar to the pain associated with an alveolar abscess; that is, the pain is moderate to severe and throbbing in nature.

Any of the conditions developing within the jaw (e.g. dental cysts, ameloblastoma; see JAW, SWELLING OF, p. 338) may become infected and, again, the pain is similar to abscess formation of dental origin. The diagnosis is usually readily apparent following a careful recording of the history followed by clinical and radiographical examination. Should the abscess formation involve the masticatory muscles, then trismus will also be present as well as signs of acute infection.

Acute post-extraction osteitis

This pain commences 2–3 days after the extraction of a tooth, and is due to bacterial contamination of the bone lining the tooth socket, should the normal healing blood clot break down. The pain is severe, dull, throbbing or gnawing in character. It is usually associated with a bad taste in the mouth, and examination will demonstrate an empty tooth socket (dry socket) in which food has collected. Treatment is by local cleansing of the socket and instillation of local antiseptic agents. Antibiotics are not normally required.

Acute maxillary sinusitis

Pain arising in the acutely infected maxillary sinus may be confused with pain of dental origin as the tooth roots of the upper teeth have a very close relationship to this structure. Maxillary sinusitis normally follows an upper respiratory tract infection, especially if the normal drainage of the antrum through the ostium is reduced, for example, by a deviated nasal septum. However, maxillary sinusitis can arise from dental infection should the abscess present in the maxillary antrum rather than in the oral cavity. Infection of the maxillary sinus may also follow the creation of an oro-antral fistula after dental extraction.

In maxillary sinusitis, the patient suffers from a throbbing pain in the cheek with radiation towards the eye, but there is never any swelling of the face. The teeth may be tender to percussion, and the pain is aggravated by bending forward or lying down. Intranasal examination may demonstrate a mucopurulent discharge through the normal ostium. The healthy maxillary sinuses are translucent on X-ray examination. Opacification is indicative of disease and, while unilateral opacification may be due to obstruction of the natural drainage into the nose, dental infection or a tumour must be eliminated as the cause (Fig. J.10).

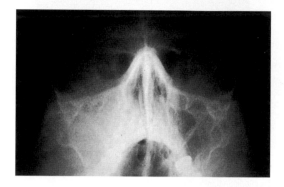

Figure J.10 Acute right maxillary sinusitis. The sinus is radiologically opaque.

A neoplastic process of the maxillary antrum should be suspected if the pain does not respond to normal measures, or if there is swelling of the face or oral cavity associated with bone destruction and displacement of the teeth. A tumour of the maxillary antrum may also cause epistaxis and sensory loss in the maxillary division of the trigeminal nerve. If these signs are present, then a biopsy should be obtained either endoscopically through the nose or via a Caldwell–Luc approach.

Temporomandibular joint

The temporomandibular joint may be affected by any of the conditions which afflict the other joints, for example rheumatoid arthritis, osteoarthritis and septic arthritis. In this case, pain and swelling in the acute phase are present in the pre-auricular region, with limitation of jaw movements. An acute effusion in the temporomandibular joint may arise as a result of a blow to the jaw or a fracture involving the joint. This again will cause pain and swelling anterior to the ear.

The most common cause of pain arising in the temporomandibular joint is, however, associated with the temporomandibular joint pain dysfunction syndrome.

This is an extremely common and much-written about condition, without the aetiology being universally recognized. It is a physical problem caused by excessive load being placed on the temporomandibular joint, which is not a load-bearing joint. The upper and lower teeth should never really make positive contact, with food only being emulsified during mastication by close approximation of the upper and lower teeth. As a habit or a response to stress, the individual holds their teeth in contact. This causes undue load on the temporomandibular joint, and inflammation can follow within the joint. The muscles of mastication are contracted for long periods of time when they should be relaxed, and muscle spasm and pain follows. Prolonged contraction of the muscles may induce muscular hypertrophy, especially of the masseter muscle, which produces a characteristic swelling at the angle of the jaw. Pain may be experienced in the temple region from the temporalis muscle, radiating behind the eye, which is interpreted as a headache. Pain is also experienced within the ear and in the pre-auricular region radiating forwards into both jaws, especially the upper jaw. Advice is commonly sought wrongly for a potential ear problem. Tenderness may be elicited intra-orally at the upper insertion on the masseter muscle and at the anterior margin of the medial pterygoid muscle.

Fibres of the lateral pterygoid muscle are inserted into the meniscus of the temporomandibular joint, and sustained contraction causes anterior displacement producing a click on movement of the jaw and further displacement causes locking of the joint with significantly reduced mouth opening. This may improve within a short period of time, or it may become permanent.

Dental malocclusion is often put forward as an aetiological cause, but as the teeth normally do not meet this postulation is difficult to understand. A significant dental interference during mastication may, however, be a cause, but this is not commonly found in the majority of patients.

Many patients find this concept difficult to accept, but unless these clenching habits for whatever reason are eliminated, improvement in the symptoms will not occur.

Chewing 'chewing gum' is a further potent cause of temporomandibular joint problems. Lecturers, singers and musicians playing instruments in the mouth may also be prone to these problems.

Primary neuralgias

Primary neuralgias may be defined as the disturbed function of a nerve without there necessarily being any recognized aetiological factor or pathological process acting at some point along the nerve pathway or its central connections. In the jaws, the trigeminal nerve is affected, and very occasionally also the glossopharyngeal nerve. There are no associated signs, and the diagnosis is made from the history.

The pain characteristically affects almost always only one branch of the trigeminal nerve initially, although later on in the disease it may spread to affect two or occasionally three divisions. The disease most commonly affects patients aged over 50 years, and the incidence is twice as common in women as in men.

The pain is very severe, and is described as sharp, or similar to an electric shock. It is paroxysmal in nature, lasting for only a few seconds with intervals of a few minutes or a few hours. The pain may be felt spontaneously or in response to stimulation within a trigger area on the face. This trigger area may be activated by a cold wind, shaving, washing, eating or cleaning the teeth. Natural remission is fairly common.

The main differential diagnosis is between causes of dental pain, and these should be excluded before a diagnosis of trigeminal neuralgia is made. Treatment is with antispasmodic drugs, such as carbamazepine, epanutin or gabapentin. Response to these drugs assists in the diagnosis. The drug carbamazepine occasionally causes agranulocytosis, and therefore regular monitoring of the white blood cell count is essential. In every case, a careful examination of the central nervous system should be made, which often includes an MRI scan to exclude a neoplasm or pulsatile intracranial aneurysm as the cause. In the younger age group multiple sclerosis needs to be excluded, which can mimic trigeminal neuralgia in the early stages of the disease. Should medical treatment fail, then a surgical approach should be considered.

Secondary neuralgias

Here, an identifiable pathological process is acting at some point along the trigeminal nerve or its central connections, producing pain at the periphery. The symptoms may be similar to trigeminal neuralgia or it may be a duller, more continuous pain. Neoplasms are the most significant cause, other examples being aneurysms or compression of the nerve in the bony canal in Paget's disease.

Exact testing of the function of the cranial nerves is essential, followed by a full clinical and radiographical examination, including CT or MRI scans to establish the diagnosis.

Post-herpetic neuralgia

Involvement of one of the branches of the trigeminal nerve with the herpes zoster virus will produce pain and vesiculation in the anatomical distribution of that nerve. Once this attack has resolved, scarring of the involved nerve may leave the patient with post-herpetic neuralgia and possibly sensory disturbance. This pain can be severe and very resistant to treatment.

Migraine

Migraine and migrainous neuralgia may occasionally involve the upper jaw, although the predominant features are manifested as headache. The diagnosis is normally made from the history when an intense pain is associated with visual disturbance, nausea and constitutional symptoms. In migrainous neuralgia, the pain is predominantly behind the eye and patients may also experience pain in the maxilla and temple regions. There may be watering of the eye and flushing of the facial skin.

Referred pain

The only important example of referred pain to the jaws is that of coronary artery insufficiency which may produce pain in the left side of the mandible.

Atypical facial pain

Large numbers of patients present with atypical facial pain, which is symptomatic of a psychological illness. The pain is described as being very severe, but it does not produce any restriction upon the normal function of the jaws and oral cavity. It does not have an anatomical distribution, commonly involves both sides of the face and jaws, and moves from one part of the facial skeleton to another. It does not respond to analgesics and usually there are many other associated symptoms such as a dry mouth, burning tongue, and other complaints throughout the body.

There can be some overlap between this condition, and temporomandibular joint dysfunction caused by stress but, in every case, it is essential to exclude pain due to any one of the other causes just described. Therefore, atypical facial pain is often a diagnosis of exclusion and, once made, any underlying depression should be treated by medication or referral for psychiatric help. (See also FACE, PAIN IN, p. 198.)

Peter T. Blenkinsopp

JAW, SWELLING OF

Swellings of the jaw, once they have reached a certain size, will be obvious as a facial swelling or swelling in the submandibular region. The true nature will, however, only be ascertained by an intra-oral examination and, in many cases, the taking of radiographs. Smaller swellings may only be visible on examination of the oral cavity, or will have been discovered by the patient during normal oral function. Testing of the trigeminal cranial nerve should always be carried out as a change in sensation may have very significant consequences. Swellings of the jaws can, to the inexperienced clinician, be incorrectly diagnosed as swellings of the submandibular salivary gland, submandibular lymph nodes or swellings of the parotid gland.

Infection associated with the dental structures

Bacterial infection associated with the dental structures is by far the most common cause of swellings of the jaw. An alveolar abscess arises when gangrene of the dental pulp occurs following dental caries, extensive dental restorations or trauma (Fig. J.11). This infection then spreads to the alveolar bone to cause a

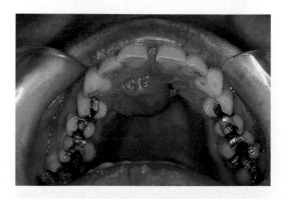

Figure J.11 Intraoral dental abscess in the palate.

localized osteitis but remarkably, in the majority of cases, does not cause osteomyelitis. Instead, the abscess as it enlarges becomes localized and perforates either the lateral or medial plate of the outer compact alveolar bone. It is at this stage that it presents as a swelling of the jaw, which is tender and covered by inflamed mucosa. Occasionally, an alveolar abscess is associated with sensory loss of the mandibular branch of the trigeminal nerve.

A periodontal abscess arises from bacterial infection within the periodontal membrane of the tooth, which is usually associated with previous chronic periodontal disease. A pericoronal abscess arises in the mucous membrane surrounding the crown of an erupting or impacted tooth; the majority being associated with wisdom teeth. At this stage the swelling is largely confined to the region of the jaws and may discharge intra-orally. However, should the bacteria gain access to the adjacent soft-tissue compartments, then facial cellulitis or soft-tissue abscess formation will follow. Depending upon the anatomical position of the infection, the submandibular area may become swollen, or the cheek (buccal space) or more posteriorly the submasseteric space, which may be misdiagnosed as a parotid swelling (Fig. J.12).

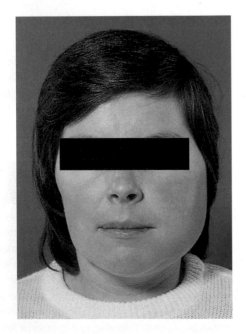

Figure J.12 Facial swelling due to infection from an impacted wisdom tooth.

On the medial aspect of the jaw, swelling in the sublingual space may occur or more posteriorly in the pterygoid, lateral pharyngeal or peritonsillar space. Diagnosis of these latter space infections may be difficult and, if beneath a muscle compartment, are associated with severe trismus.

An orthopantomogram X-ray is required in all cases of facial swelling to establish or eliminate a dental cause. The majority of swellings will respond to antibiotic treatment of an underlying dental cause and surgical drainage where necessary.

The medial swellings are potentially very serious, as respiratory obstruction may follow unless the neck is decompressed in severe cases. Ludwig's angina is an acute emergency in which both sublingual and submandibular spaces are involved in acute infection. Again, urgent surgical decompression of the neck is required to prevent respiratory obstruction.

Persistent recurrent infection causing chronic swelling and discharge may be due to an opportunistic infection with actinomycosis.

Osteomyelitis

True osteomyelitis of the jaws is now relatively rare following the improvement in general dental health and the use of antibiotics. However, when established, severe pain with loosening of the adjacent teeth is encountered, and usually there is sensory loss of the mandibular branch of the trigeminal nerve. The overlying mucosa becomes swollen and hyperaemic and, indeed, sinuses may develop through which there is a discharge of pus and bony sequestra. In the acute phase, it is invariably associated with significant soft tissue swelling. The radiographic changes take some time to develop, but show diffuse rarefaction and sequestrum formation. Subperiosteal woven bone may also be a feature and the infected bone may be subjected to a pathological fracture.

Management of all these infections is by antibiotics and drainage in the acute phase. This is then followed by the appropriate treatment to the causative dental structure, which may require extraction, and the removal of any sequestrum.

Trauma

Fractures of the mandible are relatively common and are associated with swelling caused by haematoma formation from the bleeding marrow spaces and periosteum. The swelling may be made worse by a protruding bone fragment or the presence of a foreign body. The injury may not be sufficient to cause a fracture, but may nevertheless produce a haematoma in the soft tissue. This normally resolves without treatment but, occasionally, requires aspiration. The diagnosis of a fracture is normally easy to make from the history, the abnormal mobility of the fragments and the irregularity of the dental arches. In many fractures, a laceration of the oral mucosa is also present. The diagnosis is confirmed by radiographic examination.

Swellings associated with benign dental pathology

Unerupted teeth are a frequent cause of jaw swelling which, commonly, are the canine and premolar teeth in the palate and the premolars in the lower jaw. In the elderly, when the molar teeth have been lost, an erupting wisdom tooth may produce a swelling in the posterior area of the alveolus.

The follicle of unerupted teeth may undergo dentigerous cyst formation, which is an epithelial-lined sac embracing the crown of the tooth (Fig. J.13). This slowly enlarges and may cause displacement of the involved tooth or the adjacent teeth. As the expansion continues, the alveolus enlarges and, just before perforation, exhibits the phenomenon of 'eggshell crackling'. Once perforated, the swelling is naturally fluctuant. The cyst may slowly enlarge or, should it become infected, acute swelling with inflammation occurs. Other cysts, which have a similar clinical presentation, are dental cysts, residual dental cysts and keratocysts. Keratocysts, however, tend to be multilocular and have a greater tendency to recur after removal.

Odontomes, which are developmental abnormalities of the dental lamina, may give rise to a swelling of the jaw and the diagnosis is confirmed by X-ray. *Osteomas* of the jaw present as hard, round, bony swellings which may be endosteal (central) or subperiosteal (peripheral). Multiple osteomas of the facial bones are found in Gardner's syndrome, the other main feature being polyps of the large intestine, which have a tendency to become malignant. Radiologically, osteomas may be composed of dense radio-opaque bone or may have a high cancellous component, in which case they are relatively radiolucent. Torus palatinus is a developmental abnormality of the midline of the hard palate characterized by a cylindrical enlargement in the region of the midline palatal suture (Fig. J.14). Torus mandibularis is a similar, slowly enlarging developmental abnormality, but it arises on the lingual aspect of the mandible in the premolar region. All these osteomas are simply removed if they prove troublesome as a result of trauma to the overlying mucosa.

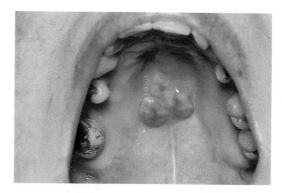

Figure J.14 Torus palatinus.

Fibrous dysplasia

This condition of bone of unknown origin is characterized by replacement with fibrous tissue and enlargement in all three dimensions. At this stage the abnormal bone is very vascular, but subsequently ossification occurs to produce an amorphous radio-opaque appearance on the radiograph. The process tends to cease at skeletal maturity. The jaws are frequently affected in monostotic fibrous dysplasia and may also be involved in polyostotic fibrous dysplasia and Albright's syndrome. This facial deformity is usually corrected by surgical sculpturing.

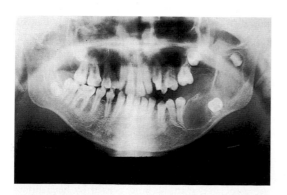

Figure J.13 Extensive dentigerous cyst formation, left mandible.

Ossifying fibroma

This is a benign fibro-osseous lesion, which causes a well-circumscribed mass of fibrous tissue showing areas of speckled calcification. It normally arises within the substance of the bone and slowly expands in all directions to produce a sclerotic margin. With time, the lesion becomes more calcified and can cause loosening of the adjacent teeth. Treatment is by surgical excision.

Cementifying fibroma

This condition is similar in some ways to ossifying fibroma in that an area of bone is replaced by fibrous tissue, but subsequent calcification resembles dental cementum. Periapical cemental dysplasia is similar to cementifying fibroma but produces multiple sites of ossification with cementum. The diagnosis is usually easy to make from the radiographic appearances but may, in some patients, produce a bony hard irregularity of the dental alveolus. Surgical removal is rarely required.

Cherubism (familial fibrous dysplasia)

Symmetrical enlargement of the facial skeleton occurs in this inherited condition, which is usually apparent in early life and then arrests at puberty. Radiographs show symmetrical multilocular radiolucent areas of the jaws and, histologically, the bone is replaced by fibrous tissue with multinucleated giant cells as a predominant feature. The giant cells, in some cases, make the differential diagnosis difficult from giant-cell granuloma or hyperparathyroidism. The blood chemistry is, however, usually normal.

Paget's disease

This disease of bone of unknown aetiology found in patients in middle to late life may affect the mandible but, more commonly, the maxilla. According to some studies, approximately 15 per cent of cases show involvement of the facial skeleton. Enlargement of the facial bones may produce the characteristic 'leonine facies' and, intra-orally, expansion of the dental alveolus occurs with displacement of the teeth. Pain may occur due to entrapment of the trigeminal nerve, and the radiograph shows the typical areas of patchy sclerosis. Extraction of the teeth can be difficult due to hypercementosis, and post-extraction bleeding may be severe. In the active phase of the disease, the serum alkaline phosphatase is raised, which will aid the diagnosis of the condition. Sarcomatous change in long-standing Paget's disease occurs, but is relatively rare.

Epulis

This term denotes a swelling arising from the gum of which the majority are either pyogenic granulomas, fibroepithelial polyps or peripheral giant-cell granulomas. They may be sessile or pedunculated in shape and covered by pink or red mucosa (Fig. J.15). Histologically they exhibit a core of granulation or fibrous tissue covered by epithelium.

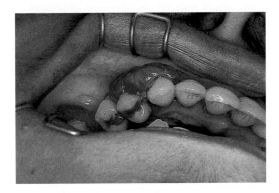

Figure J.15 Epulis of the gum (pyogenic granuloma).

The pyogenic granuloma and fibroepithelial polyp represent an exaggerated soft-tissue response to minor trauma, and are treated by simple excision and curettage. Pyogenic granulomas are common in pregnancy (see GUMS, BLEEDING, p. 245).

Denture granulomas are histologically similar to the fibroepithelial polyp, but arise from low-grade persistent denture trauma. Pseudofolds of mucous membrane with a fibrous tissue stroma are formed in the region of a traumatic denture flange. Treatment is again by excision, with attention to the prosthesis.

Papilloma

This benign tumour of epithelium is uncommon in the mouth and, when present, is usually found towards the back of the mouth in the soft palate or on the pillars of the fauces. It is pedunculated with an irregular surface or pale filiform projections. Many of these papillomas are viral in origin. The lesion should be excised with its base.

Giant-cell granuloma

The aetiology of this lesion is again unknown. It arises in the young age group, and is confined to the tooth-bearing areas of the jaws, with the mandible as the most frequent location. Radiographs show a radiolucent area, and histologically, the tissue is vascular fibrous tissue with multinucleated giant cells. The lesion can grow rapidly. The central giant-cell granuloma develops within the jaw, later perforating the alveolar bone to present in the mouth as a spherical purple swelling. Confusion can arise with the brown tumour of hyper-parathyroidism, but here the occurrence in the older age group with raised serum calcium and parathormone levels would indicate the diagnosis. Additionally, radiographs in hyperparathyroidism show multiple osteolytic lesions, osteitis fibrosa cystica, on skeletal survey. The peripheral giant-cell granuloma is similar in every respect to the central, except that it arises from the gingival margin as a localized fleshy mass, which bleeds easily. The treatment of both types is by surgical excision.

Ameloblastoma

Ameloblastoma is a tumour that is peculiar to the jaws, and is a locally invasive neoplasm of odontogenic epithelium. Unless infection supervenes, the tumour is quite painless as it slowly enlarges. In under-developed countries the lesions may reach enormous proportions before assistance is sought. Radiographs usually show a multilocular radiolucency, but unilocular variants may present. Spacing of the teeth may occur, but sensory disturbance of the trigeminal nerve is not usually a feature. Treatment is by resection with a margin of healthy bone and bone graft reconstruction.

Eosinophilic granuloma

The solitary eosinophilic granuloma produces an area of bone loss in the jaw, and there is an associated soft tissue swelling with gingival ulceration. The condition may first come to be noticed because of loosening of the teeth, the failure of a tooth extraction site to heal, or a pathological fracture. The jaws may also be affected by multifocal eosinophilic granuloma where, with loosening of the teeth, there is also generalized inflammation of the oral cavity and gingival enlargement. Single lesions are not neoplastic and should be excised, while multiple lesions require a systemic approach.

Myxoma

Another benign tumour to affect the jaws and cause expansion is the myxoma, which is a rare benign neoplasm arising from odontogenic mesenchyme. It produces a multilocular radiolucent appearance with multiple criss-crossing septi in the defect. Treatment is by surgical excision and bone graft reconstruction.

Haemangioma

The endosteal haemangioma is more common in the mandible than the maxilla and, if truly endosteal, presents as a hard, non-tender, painless swelling. Haemorrhage may occur around the necks of the teeth, which may become loosened, and severe haemorrhage follows dental extraction.

Minor salivary glands

The minor salivary glands are distributed widely throughout the oral mucosa, but are found in abundance at the junction of the hard and soft palate. The important benign causes of enlargement are mucous extravasation cysts and pleomorphic adenomas (Fig. J.16). Mucous extravasation cysts commonly occur in the lower lip.

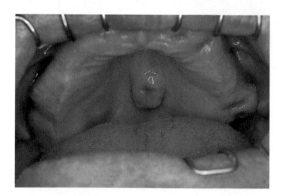

Figure J.16 Pleomorphic adenoma arising from a minor salivary gland in the palate.

Malignant tumours

Sarcomas of the jaw are rare, with the mandible being affected more often than the maxilla. The tumour presents as a rapidly enlarging swelling with drifting and loosening of the teeth and sensory disturbance of the involved trigeminal nerve. Radiographs demonstrate irregular destruction of the jaw, but in the osteogenic sarcoma there are, in addition, radiating trabeculae of new bone formation to give the characteristic 'sun ray' appearance. Treatment is by wide resection, and blood-borne metastases do not normally occur as rapidly as in osteosarcomas found elsewhere in the skeleton. More rarely, a chondrosarcoma may involve the jaws with similar clinical signs to the osteosarcoma. Treatment is again by wide resection and chemotherapy.

Intrabony squamous cell carcinoma is rare, but when present it causes a destructive lesion within the mandible on X-ray, sensory disturbance of the trigeminal nerve and expansion of the bone with loosening of the teeth. The more common squamous cell carcinoma arising in the oral mucous membrane produces swelling of the soft tissue overlying the jaw, usually with central ulceration and underlying bone destruction (Fig. J.17).

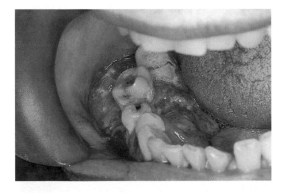

Figure J.17 Squamous cell carcinoma of the mandibular alveolus.

Lymphoma affecting the oral cavity is not common, but should be suspected in an adult presenting with a painless, nondescript soft swelling. The soft tissues of the cheek, palate, gingivae and fauces can all be affected, but the regional lymph nodes are not necessarily enlarged. Secondary ulceration of the lesion can occur. The instance of oral lymphoma is significantly raised in patients with HIV infection. The adult lymphoma needs to be distinguished from Burkitt's lymphoma, which is commonly found in children in East Africa and is associated with the Epstein–Barr virus. Involvement of the jaw is the predominant site, with secondary spread into the adjacent tissues. This tumour responds well to chemotherapy.

The *Kaposi sarcoma* was relatively uncommon in the oral cavity until the advent of AIDS and HIV infection. This is a vascular tumour with a nodular, purplish

appearance. The palate is the most frequent site in the oral cavity. It is particularly associated with homosexual males with HIV infection, and in this group has become almost pathognomonic of AIDS, unless the individual is immunosuppressed for another reason. The lesion is thought to be caused by the herpes virus. Treatment is by surgical excision, radiotherapy or chemotherapy.

Carcinoma of the maxillary antrum, and malignant tumours of the minor salivary glands contained within the mucosa of the palate, will eventually cause intra-oral swelling of the upper jaw, leading to ulceration. A malignant lesion should be suspected if growth is rapid and is associated with bone destruction, loosening of the teeth, haemorrhage, and sensory disturbance of the trigeminal nerve. The diagnosis is confirmed by biopsy. The important malignant tumours affecting the upper jaw in addition to carcinoma of the antrum are adenocystic carcinoma, adenocarcinoma, malignant pleomorphic adenoma and lymphoma.

Metastatic tumours of the jaws

Secondary deposits of tumours rarely affect the jaws, with the mandible as the more common site. Tumours of the bronchus, breast, kidney and thyroid produce osteolytic lesions, while carcinoma of the prostate tends to form an osteosclerotic deposit. The clinical signs are similar to other intrabony malignant tumours with swelling, pain, loosening of the teeth and sensory disturbance. Eventually, pathological fracture occurs.

Secondary deposits may also develop in the overlying soft tissue of the jaws, especially at the gingival margin, and may be confused with a benign epulis. Rapid growth usually occurs to produce a fleshy mass, which may be friable and haemorrhagic. These lesions should be excised and submitted for histological examination lest the diagnosis be missed.

Peter T. Blenkinsopp

JOINTS, AFFECTIONS OF

Joint affections may be acute, as in rheumatic fever, gout or traumatic hydrarthrosis; acute relapsing becoming chronic, as in rheumatoid arthritis or Reiter's disease; chronic with acute onset, as in some cases of generalized osteoarthritis; or insidious and chronic as in most cases of osteoarthritis. The affection may be of one joint – a monarthritis – as may be seen in tuberculous arthritis; or it may be the start of a polyarthritis, as is seen not infrequently in psoriatic arthropathy, in which a number of joints are eventually affected. The pattern of joint involvement may be important: rheumatoid arthritis affects initially and chiefly peripheral joints; ankylosing spondylitis affects the sacroiliacs and spine; polymyalgia rheumatica affects the girdle joints, pelvis and shoulders. The terminal interphalangeal joints are affected commonly in osteoarthritis (Heberden's nodes) and psoriatic arthropathy, occasionally in adolescent rheumatoid arthritis, but rarely in adult rheumatoid arthritis. Interphalangeal involvement of the toes is rare in rheumatoid arthritis but more common in the arthritis associated with ulcerative colitis or Reiter's disease. Joint involvement may be in the form of a flitting and transient polyarthritis, as in rheumatic fever, some cases of SLE and in a number of other conditions or in a recurring or palindromic pattern subsiding completely between episodes, as in some cases of rheumatoid arthritis. Joints may be swollen because of:

- Bony enlargement, as in osteoarthritis or Charcot's joints in tabes dorsalis or syringomyelia.
- New periosteal bone deposition as in hypertrophic pulmonary osteoarthropathy or thyroid acropachy.
- Synovial effusion. The joint fluid may be: clear and acellular in association with serious injury; inflammatory and cellular, as in rheumatoid arthritis; bloodstained, as in traumatic haemarthrosis and bleeding disorders; purulent, as in pyogenic infection or acute crystal synovitis; milky, as in chylous arthritis associated with filiariasis.
- Synovial proliferation, as in rheumatoid arthritis.
- Rarely, because of malignant changes, as in sarcoma and secondary carcinoma.

Not infrequently, joints are swollen from a combination of two or more of these factors. Swelling of synovial tendon sheaths or bursae alongside joints may also contribute greatly to the clinical picture. Symmetrical involvement of extensor sheaths on the dorsum of the wrists are very typical of rheumatoid arthritis. Subacromial and semi-membranosus bursal involvement may contribute much swelling when shoulders or knees are affected by an inflammatory arthritis. If there is doubt regarding the presence of infecting organisms, then aspiration should be performed. This will often

contribute useful information in non-infective conditions such as gout, chondrocalcinosis or haemarthrosis if the diagnosis is in doubt.

Joints affected by any disease process may show a variable blend of five factors: swelling; pain; stiffness; tenderness; and weakness. These five factors in variable combinations cause the dysfunction typical of the particular arthritic disease in question. In progressive systemic sclerosis (scleroderma), stiffness is the dominant component, whereas in gout it is swelling, tenderness and pain. The joints in rheumatoid arthritis vary and differ depending on activity and stage of the disease process; stiffness in early rheumatoid disease is largely due to joint swelling, in advanced disease to irreversible change, even in some patients, to the point of bony or fibrous ankylosis. In many instances chronic joint swelling produces excessive joint laxity allowing reversible deformity or subluxation. In other cases the destruction of joint tissue in rheumatoid arthritis causes gross hypermobility, the so-called 'lorgnette' or 'telescopic fingers' being extreme examples of this.

Two of the cardinal signs of inflammation – heat and redness – are often absent in inflammatory arthritis, whilst in acute pyarthrosis the joint is hot, and in gout it is hot and red. In most patients with rheumatoid arthritis the joints tend to be cold and moist without erythema, though swollen, painful and tender. Palmar erythema is common in rheumatoid arthritis and in SLE, the palms and fingertips being often a bright pink. Inflammatory arthropathies usually cause most discomfort in the early morning, the tissues becoming 'gelled' with disuse in the night. This early morning increase in pain and stiffness of fingers, wrists and shoulders in particular is characteristic of rheumatoid and similar arthropathies; in ankylosing spondylitis a similar increase in stiffness and pain occurs in the spine, hips and shoulders. Painful morning stiffness is also seen characteristically in polymyalgia rheumatica in the shoulders and hips.

There are very many possible causes of joint involvement in systemic disease, and these are listed in Table J.7. Not all can be discussed and described in the present text; thus, the following account deals only with the more common and distinctive causes.

Congenital arthropathies

In *classical achondroplasia* bony growth is abnormal but epiphysial development is normal; premature

Table J.7 Arthropathies in systemic disease

Congenital
Achondroplasia and pseudoachondroplasia
Angiokeratoma corporis diffusum (Fabry's disease)
Arthrogryposis multiplex congenita
Camptodactyly
Chondrodysplasia punctata (Conradi's syndrome)
Congenital indifference to pain
Down's syndrome
Dysplasia epiphysalis multiplex
Ehlers–Danlos syndrome
Familial dysautonomia (Riley–Day syndrome)
Hereditary progressive arthro-ophthalmopathy
Hypermobility syndrome
Marfan's syndrome
Morquio–Brailsford syndrome
Osteodysplasty
Osteogenesis imperfecta
Spondyloepiphysial dysplasia

Degenerative, traumatic and occupational
Ankylosing vertebral hyperostosis (Forrestier's disease,
   diffuse interstitial spinal hyperostosis (DISH))
Occupational syndromes (e.g. porter's neck, wicket-
   keeper's fingers)
Osteoarthritis
Traumatic syndromes (e.g. traumatic haemarthrosis)

Dietetic
Fluorosis
Kashin–Beck disease
Rickets
Scurvy

Endocrine
Acromegaly
Cretinous and myxoedematous arthropathy
Diabetic cheiroarthropathy
Hyperparathyroidism
Hypoparathyroidism
Thyroid acropachy

Gut-associated
Acute gastrointestinal bacterial infection
Antibiotic-induced (pseudomembranous) colitis
Crohn's disease
Jejuno-ileal bypass arthritis–dermatitis syndrome
Ulcerative colitis
Whipple's disease

Idiopathic inflammatory
Acne fulminans arthritis
Behçet's syndrome
Erythema multiforme
Dermatomyositis and polymyositis
Dressier's syndrome
Erythema nodosum
Familial Mediterranean fever
Henoch—Schönlein syndrome (anaphylactoid purpura)

Intermittent hydrarthrosis
Juvenile chronic arthritis (pauciarticular, polyarticular,
   systemic)
Mixed connective tissue disease
Palindromic rheumatism
Pigmented villonodular synovitis
Progressive systemic sclerosis (scleroderma)
Relapsing polychondritis
Rheumatoid arthritis, including Felty's syndrome,
   Caplan's syndrome
Sarcoidosis
Spondyloarthropathy (e.g. ankylosing spondylitis,
   psoriatic arthritis, reactive arthritis, Reiter's
   syndrome, enteropathic arthritis (Crohn's disease,
   ulcerative arthritis)
SAPHO syndrome
Sjögren's syndrome
Systemic lupus erythematosus

Idiopathic non-inflammatory
Osteochondritis dissecans
Osteochondrosis

Haematological
Agammaglobulinaemia
Haemophilia and allied disorders
Leukaemia
Sickle-cell disease
Thalassaemia

Infective
*Bacterial infections (including spirochaetes and
mycoplasma)*
- Anthrax
- *Brucella abortus* and *B. melitensis* arthritis
- Cat-scratch fever
- Glutton's joints
- Diphtheria
- Erysipelas
- Glanders
- Haverhill fever
- Infective endocarditis
- Jaccoud's arthropathy
- Leprosy
- Lyme arthritis
- Lymphogranuloma venereum
- Meningococcal fever
- *Mycoplasma pneumoniae*
- Poncet's disease
- *Pseudomonas pseudomallei* (melioidosis)
- Pyogenic (staphylococcal, psittacosis, gonococcal,
   pneumococcal, etc.)
- Rat-bite fever
- Rheumatic fever
- Secondary syphilis
- Streptococcal reactive arthritis
- Tuberculosis

(continued)

Table J.7 *(continued)*

- Typhoid and paratyphoid fever
- Weil's disease (*Leptospirosis icterohaemorrhagica*)
- Yaws

Viral infections
- Chikungunya
- Dengue
- Echo virus infection
- Glandular fever (infectious mononucleosis)
- Influenza
- Measles
- Mumps
- O'Nyong-Nyong fever
- Parvovirus (human)
- Poliomyelitis
- Ross River virus arthritis
- Rubella
- Viral hepatitis (mainly 'B')

Fungal infections
- Actinomycosis
- Aspergillosis
- Blastomycosis
- Coccidioidomycosis
- Cryptococcosis (torulosis)
- Histoplasmosis
- Madura foot (mycetoma pedis)
- Sporotrichosis
- Infections due to protozoa
- Amoebiasis
- Giardiasis

Worm infections
- Chylous arthritis
- Dracunculosis (Guinea-worm arthritis)
- Filariasis
- Trichiniasis
- Schistosomiasis
- Strongyloidiasis

Metabolic
Amyloidosis
Biliary and alcoholic cirrhosis
Calcinosis circumscripta (pyrophosphate arthropathy)
Calcinosis uraemica
Chondrocalcinosis
Disseminated lipogranulomatosis (Farber's disease)
Familial hypercholesterolaemia
Familial lipochrome pigmentary arthritis
Gaucher's disease
Gout
Haemochromatosis
Hunter's syndrome
Hurler's syndrome (gargoylism)
Multicentric reticulohistiocytosis (lipoid
  dermato-arthritis)

Myositis ossificans
Ochronosis
Renal transplant and haemodialysis syndrome
Wilson's disease

Vascular
Avascular necrosis (fat emboli, caisson, etc.)
Polyarteritis nodosa
Polymyalgia arteritica (giant-cell arteritis and
  polymyalgia rheumatica)
Takayasu's (pulseless) disease
Wegener's granulomatosis

Neoplastic
Chondrosarcoma
Haemangioma
Hypertrophic pulmonary osteoarthropathy
Left atrial myxoma
Lymphoma
Metastatic malignant disease
Multiple myeloma
Osteoid osteoma
Paget's sarcoma
Hypertrophic pulmonary osteoarthropathy
Synovioma

Neuropathic
Algodystrophy (shoulder-hand syndrome, transient
  osteoporosis, Sudek's atrophy)
Charcot's joints, tabetic or syringomyelic
Diabetic arthopathy (neuropathic and infective)
Paraplegia syndrome
Ulcero-osteolytic neuropathy

Drug-induced
Anticoagulants
Barbiturates
Corticosteroid arthropathy
Hydralazine syndrome (procaine amide, oral
  contraceptives, etc.)
Isoniazid shoulder–hand syndrome
Quinidine
Serum sickness

Miscellaneous
Acro-osteolysis syndrome
Dupuytren's contracture
Knuckle pads (Hale–White) (Garrod)
Paget's disease of bone
Periostitis deformans (Soriano)
Thorn synovitis
Septic focus syndrome
Subacute pancreatitis
Xiphoid syndrome

pyrophosphate dihydrate. In *idiopathic hypoparathy-roidism*, back pain and stiffness may cause a clinical picture similar to that of ankylosing spondylitis but, though ligamentous calcification is present, the sacro-iliac joints are normal. It is associated with hypo-calcaemia, cataracts, fits, tetany and rashes. In *thyroid acropachy*, subperiosteal thickening is seen in the metacarpal and phalangeal bones of the hands in patients with hyperthyroidism who have in many cases been treated and rendered euthyroid. Exophthalmos is common, and so-called 'pretibial myxoedema' may be present. The somewhat thickened hand resembles that seen in hypertrophic pulmonary osteoarthropathy, but the condition is milder and less extensive, being usu-ally confined to the hands.

Gut-associated arthropathies

The more characteristic of these are considered in the next section, under the spondyloarthropathies.

Idiopathic inflammatory arthropathies

In *dermatomyositis* and *polymyositis*, minimal or moderate transitory arthralgia or arthritis occurs in about one-third of cases. Effusions are less common. The fingers and knees are most commonly affected. The skin and muscle manifestations point to the true diagnosis, the muscles of the pelvic girdle and thighs and shoulder girdle becoming weak. The association of dermatomyositis with malignant disease in adult cases should be kept in mind.

Dressler's syndrome following myocardial infarc-tion or cardiac injury or surgery occurs at about 2–4 weeks or more after the acute episode, with pericard-itis, arthralgia and, rarely, arthritis.

The diagnosis of *erythema multiforme* probably covers several different entities, with some mild and some severe, and with the so-called 'Stevens–Johnson syndrome' being a severe variant. Arthritis or arthral-gia may occur along with other inflammatory reac-tions in the skin, eye, mouth and elsewhere.

Familial Mediterranean fever is a poorly understood disorder which is characterized by recurrent and sometimes periodic attacks of arthralgia or arthritis. It occurs predominantly in people of Mediterranean origin, Armenians, Arabs and Sephardic Jews. Onset is in childhood or adolescence, with episodes of fever recurring with polyserositis, abdominal pain, urticaria and other rashes, arthralgia and arthritis

and, later, amyloidosis. Joint manifestations occur in one-third to one-half of the cases; these are usually arthralgia, but sometimes mono- or oligoarthritis occur. The acute episodes last for only a few days (rarely weeks), and most cases show no permanent sequelae. Sacroiliac changes may occur late in the disease.

Henoch–Schönlein syndrome ('anaphylactoid pur-pura') is most common in children aged under 12 years. The outstanding feature is a maculo-petechial and sometimes a papular rash on the buttocks and extensor surfaces of the lower limbs particularly. Urti-caria and purpura may occur. Pain, swelling and stiff-ness of joints – most commonly of the ankles and knees – is usually transient and lasts for only a few days. Alimentary haemorrhage and haematuria are not uncommon, and about 10 per cent of cases develop renal failure.

Intermittent hydrarthrosis, usually in the knees, may resolve without sequelae, but approximately 50 per cent of patients eventually develop rheumatoid arth-ritis or ankylosing spondylitis. Hydrarthrosis may, how-ever, be a manifestation of infective systemic disease such as syphilis or brucellosis. There is usually com-plete or almost complete remission between attacks. It may also occur after trauma, in osteoarthritis and osteochondritis dissecans; in other words, it is a phys-ical sign and not a diagnosis. Some patients recover without showing signs of any other disorder.

Palindromic rheumatism is a name given to recur-ring episodes of arthritis due to many causes, the most common probably being the early phase of rheuma-toid arthritis.

Pigmented villonodular synovitis presents as a per-sistent but usually relatively painless synovial prolifer-ation with blood-stained joint fluid. Brown nodular masses, possibly due to haemangiomas, form in the synovia; these become traumatized, inflamed and hyperplastic, the hyperplastic synovial cells containing haemosiderin. The condition is usually monarticular, commonly of the knee, and occurs in young adults, males rather than females. The joint may lock repeat-edly. The aspirated joint fluid is characteristically blood-stained or dark brown in colour.

In *progressive systemic sclerosis* (scleroderma) the skin is stretched tight over the underlying tissues, the joints being intact but initially showing changes resembling those of rheumatoid arthritis.

Relapsing (or *atrophic*) *polychondritis* is a rare dis-order in which the cartilages of the joints, ears, nose and trachea soften and collapse; this leads to arthritis, facial changes, dyspnoea or stridor and, occasionally, death.

Rheumatoid arthritis (Fig. J.21) is sufficiently well known as to need no description. It is as well to remember that tendons and tendon sheaths and bursae are commonly involved by the inflammatory process, and these add to the clinical picture. *Juvenile arthritis* is, in only a small minority of cases, an early form of rheumatoid arthritis. In a few cases (particularly in boys) it may be an early form of ankylosing spondylitis, but it is usually a seronegative chronic arthritis. It differs from adult polyarthritis in that splenomegaly and lymphadenopathy are more common, tests for rheumatoid factor are usually negative, involvement of terminal interphalangeal joints of fingers and cervical spine are more common, and skin rashes of maculopapular type are more common. In the eye, iritis with band opacity in the cornea occurs, sometimes with secondary cataract formation; these are not seen in rheumatoid arthritis in adults. Growth in general may be arrested if the disease is severe, and premature fusion may occur in epiphyses adjacent to involved joints. Pericarditis is more common in juvenile arthritis than in adult rheumatoid arthritis.

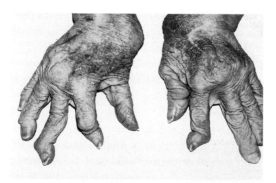
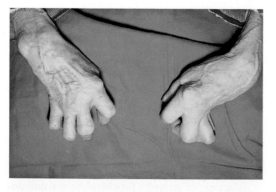

Figure J.21 Hands with severe rheumatoid arthritis.

In *Felty's syndrome*, splenomegaly, enlargement of lymph nodes, neutropenia and sometimes pigmentation of the skin are superimposed on the usual picture of rheumatoid arthritis. The only reason for maintaining the title in what is merely a variant of rheumatoid arthritis is to emphasize the importance of the neutropenia, for intercurrent infections are the rule and splenectomy may be necessary. Leg ulcers are relatively common, the usual site being the lower shin anteriorly.

The arthropathy associated with *sarcoidosis* is often accompanied by erythema nodosum; a weak or negative tuberculin reaction is usual, and the Kveim test may be positive. The arthropathy may be no more than a migratory arthralgia, or it may be a true polyarthritis with pain, fever, systemic upset and swelling of several joints, usually the larger ones. In the majority of cases, polyarthritis subsides in a few weeks. Hilar node enlargement is common in chest radiographs, and lymph nodes may be palpable in the neck and axilla in some cases. Splenomegaly may be present. Histoplasmosis may also present with hilar lymphadenopathy and joint pains ('pseudosarcoidosis').

The term *spondyloarthropathy* is applied to a family of conditions, the key features of which include: involvement of the spine and sacroiliac joints; oligoarticular lower limb arthritis; an association with iritis, psoriasis and inflammatory bowel disease; and a high prevalence of the HLA-B27 antigen.

The principal members of this group are: ankylosing spondylitis; reactive arthritis; Reiter's disease; psoriatic arthropathy; enteropathic arthritis associated with ulcerative colitis; and Crohn's disease.

Behçet's syndrome and the Stevens–Johnson syndrome share some features with this family, though their inclusion within the group is contentious.

The classical picture of ankylosing spondylitis is that of a young male adult with a stiff back and chest, and often also a stiff neck and hips. The erythrocyte sedimentation rate is elevated, anterior uveitis is present in 25 per cent of cases at some stage in the disease course, and radiographs show typical changes in sacroiliac joints and usually in the dorsolumbar spine.

Peripheral joint involvement may occur but is usually, though not always, transient. Knee effusions are not uncommon. The pattern of the disorder is essentially central, spine and girdle joints being predominantly affected, peripheral small joints rarely and transiently; this contrasts with rheumatoid arthritis.

Nodules do not occur and rheumatoid factor is not present in the serum. The histocompatibility antigen HLA-1327 is found in over 90 per cent of patients.

Reiter's disease comprises arthritis associated with genital-tract inflammation or recent gastrointestinal infection. The syndrome may be caused by either sexually transmitted infection or acute gastrointestinal infection, and in either case urethritis or cervicitis may be present. Recognized causal pathogens include *Chlamydia trachomatis*, *Salmonella enteritidis* and *S. typhimurium*, *Shigella flexneri*, *Yersinia enterocolitica* and *Y. pseudotuberculosis* and *Campylobacter jejuni*. Traditionally, arthritis, urethritis and conjunctivitis comprise the classical triad; conjunctivitis is often transient or mild, whilst genital tract symptoms may be mild, overlooked or denied. Diagnosis therefore requires a careful history and a genitourinary examination including microscopic examination of urethral and/or cervical smears. A variety of terms are used to describe this condition; commonly, the relationship between infection in the genitourinary or gastrointestinal tract with aseptic arthritis is described by the term 'reactive arthritis'. Arthritic symptoms appear a few days or up to 3 weeks after the initial symptoms of the causative infection. The distribution of affected joints, ankles, heels and knees being principally affected is characteristic, and lesions of buccal mucosa, of the glans penis or prepuce (balanitis circinata), or of skin (keratoderma blenorrhagica) suggest the correct diagnosis. Later, sacroiliac changes may occur and sometimes a clinical picture similar to that seen in ankylosing spondylitis develops. Caucasian patients with Reiter's disease usually have the tissue antigen HLA-1327, and those with the picture of ankylosing spondylitis almost 100 per cent. Rheumatoid factor is absent from the blood; nodules do not occur. When skin manifestations are present the condition may closely resemble that of psoriatic arthropathy. The interphalangeal joints of the toes, though rarely involved in rheumatoid arthritis, may be affected in Reiter's disease. Iridocyclitis and iritis, both of which are rare in rheumatoid arthritis, are not uncommon in Reiter's disease.

In *psoriatic arthropathy* (Fig. J.22) the arthritis usually – but not invariably – follows the skin disorder by several years. The seronegative, non-nodular polyarthritis tends to be more patchy and less evenly symmetrical than rheumatoid arthritis, and the terminal interphalangeal joints of the fingers are frequently affected, particularly if the nails are affected by the

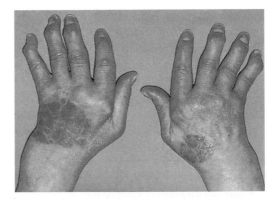

Figure J.22 Psoriatic arthropathy, showing involvement of terminal interphalangeal joints.

pitting, ridging and separation of psoriasis. When all the joints of a finger are affected by inflammatory arthritis the digit resembles a hot sausage, as was noted many years ago by French rheumatologists. In some cases the sacroiliac joints or the spine are affected, the clinical picture being that of ankylosing spondylitis.

In *Crohn's disease* and *ulcerative colitis* and, less commonly, in *Whipple's disease* (intestinal lipodystrophy), arthralgia or arthritis may occur in the spine or peripheral joints. In all of these conditions, rheumatoid factor is absent from the blood and rheumatoid nodules are not seen. In the arthropathy of ulcerative colitis, the best documented of these three disorders, onset is usually between the ages of 15 and 45 years. It is usually symmetrical and often monarticular with short exacerbations and usually complete recovery, with joint erosions being rare and minor in character. It affects both sexes in equal proportions, and usually begins acutely, affecting one knee or ankle primarily, with subsequent attacks being of similar pattern. The arthritis usually commences long after the onset of the colitis and may coincide with an exacerbation of the disease. In all three conditions – ulcerative colitis, Crohn's disease and Whipple's disease – a picture similar to that of ankylosing spondylitis may eventually appear after some years.

In *systemic lupus erythematosus*, any or all systems of the body may be involved in addition to the joints, which are not invariably involved, though arthralgia is usually present at some stage in the course of the disease. The patient (usually a female) is more ill than arthritic in most cases, though joint involvement is present in about two-thirds of cases. The finding of numerous antibodies (including antinuclear antibody) in high titre, and DNA antibody in the blood is strong confirmatory diagnostic evidence. The joint involvement may be flitting, resembling rheumatic fever, or more constant, resembling rheumatoid arthritis. The co-existence of skin lesions and visceral manifestations suggests the correct diagnosis, with the typical lupus butterfly rash over nose and cheeks being particularly characteristic. Neutropenia and anaemia are common, and thrombocytopenia is not uncommon. Asthma, proteinuria, neurological signs, splenomegaly, retinal exudates and a number of other co-existent findings in any arthritic should make one think of this disorder or a related connective tissue disease. Epileptiform fits occur in about 10 per cent of cases. Patients with neurological and renal involvement fare worst. Patients having a combination of clinical features of SLE, progressive systemic sclerosis and polymyositis with high titres of a circulating antinuclear antibody with specificity for a nuclear ribonucleoprotein are said to have 'mixed connective tissue disease'.

Idiopathic non-inflammatory arthropathies

In *osteochondritis dissecans*, flakes of articular cartilage – sometimes with a portion of the underlying bone – become detached without evident trauma, the condition manifesting itself as recurring attacks of arthritis. The most common site (85%) is the knee; the radial head is the next most common, while the hip and ankles are rarely involved. The condition may be bilateral, and X-rays are usually diagnostic.

In *osteochondrosis* the diagnosis is also essentially a radiological one. It is essentially a disturbance of epiphysial ossification seen in childhood and early adult life, possibly ischaemic in origin. Early radiographs show dense fragments in the epiphysis and a broadening of the epiphysial line with, later, areas of rarefaction and condensation so that a core of dense bone is seen in a porotic matrix. The epiphyses are affected during the periods of their greatest activity, for instance the femoral head from 4 to 12 years (Legg–Calve–Perthe's disease), and the tibial tubercle from 10 to 16 years (Osgood–Schlatter disease).

Haematological arthropathies

It is wise to perform a full blood count, erythrocyte sedimentation rate and examination of plasma proteins in obscure cases of arthritis. Approximately 25 per cent of patients with agammaglobulinaemia, either congenital or acquired, develop a non-suppurative arthritis not unlike rheumatoid arthritis, with the joints showing effusions, pain, tenderness and stiffness. The condition is usually asymmetrical, is unaccompanied by radiological changes, and may be transient, subsiding in a few weeks without sequelae, or may persist for years but with little residual change. Biopsy of synovial tissue does not distinguish between the two conditions. The erythrocyte sedimentation rate is usually normal, and tests for rheumatoid factor are negative. In some cases arthritis has been attributed to *Mycoplasma* infection, but recurrent infection with the usual pyogenic organisms is also common.

Haemarthrosis may occur in *haemophilia* (factor VIII deficiency) and allied disorders, such as Christmas disease (factor IX deficiency), and in patients receiving anticoagulant therapy, but is rare in von Willebrand's disease. In *leukaemia*, haemorrhages are common and flitting pains resembling rheumatic fever are not uncommon in acute leukaemia. This, taken in conjunction with a systolic cardiac murmur, may cause diagnostic confusion, particularly in acute aleukaemic leukaemia. Pains in bones and joints occur not infrequently in acute leukaemia in childhood and in chronic leukaemia in adults, both myeloid and lymphatic. In children, juvenile arthritis is often diagnosed in error.

In *sickle-cell anaemia* painful crises occur which are characteristic of the disorder, and these may occur not only in the abdomen but also in the bones and joints in children or adults. Although the most common symptoms are those of anaemia, some patients have no complaints except during crises. Aseptic necrosis of bone may occur, particularly in the head of the humerus or femur, radiographs showing subsequently areas of increased density and areas of necrosis. The course of the disease is that of a chronic haemolytic process punctuated by periodic painful crises. Chronic ulceration of the lower legs is relatively common, and scars are commonly to be seen around the malleoli. Another striking complication of sickle-cell disease, particularly in children, is salmonella osteomyelitis, often multifocal. In *thalassaemia major*, pains and swelling may occur in the ankles and feet.

Infective arthropathies

In the infective arthropathies the infecting organism is present in locomotor tissues; in gonococcal arthritis, for instance, gonococci can be isolated from the infected joints or joint; the condition responds to appropriate antibiotics. Any of the infections due to bacteria, spirochaetes or mycoplasma may, if there is destruction of tissue, lead to chronic changes in bones and joints, but if the correct treatment is given early there may be little or no residual disability. In these days of extensive and rapid worldwide travel, conditions previously unknown in residents of one country can occur with resulting arthralgia or arthritis.

Viral arthropathies are common throughout the world, but are usually mild and transient. Arbovirus infections including Chikungunya and O'Nyong-Nyong are common in some parts of Africa and South America. To a lesser extent, arbovirus infections also occur in Scandinavia (Ockelbo, Pogosta) and Australia (Ross River virus arthritis). In Europe and the USA, parvovirus arthritis is the commonest viral joint disease, also associated with a transient rash, upper respiratory infection and malaise (erythema infectiosum, fifth disease). Arthritis following natural rubella is uncommon because of widespread vaccination, but may follow vaccination itself. If viral arthritis is suspected, hepatitis B infection must also be excluded. Usually, joint involvement is polyarticular and symmetrical, and carpal tunnel syndrome may develop. Symptoms generally subside within 3 weeks. Post-vaccination arthritis may affect a single joint only and persist or recur. Lyme arthritis, named after the part of East Connecticut in which it was first identified, comprises a variable multisystem disease combined with transient asymmetrical oligarthritis. The causative agent is a spirochaete, *Borrelia burgdorferi*, which is transmitted by tick bites. The disease is only acquired therefore in areas where ticks of the genus *Ixodes* are endemic. The disease responds to antibiotic treatment.

Rheumatic fever is seen much less often today than previously. It is as well to remember that many other arthropathies may present in similar form, joints being successively affected and remitting rapidly, the so-called 'flitting pains' rippling round the locomotor system. Not only may rheumatoid arthritis present in this way, but also systemic lupus erythematosus, ankylosing spondylitis, Hodgkin's lymphoma, leukaemia, brucellosis and a number of other disorders. The heart is rarely seriously involved if rheumatic fever first occurs over the age of 17 years.

Jaccoud's arthritis is an extremely rare disorder following repeated attacks of rheumatic fever, characterized by ulnar deviation of the fingers and hyperextension of the proximal interphalangeal joints without bone destruction.

The arthropathy occurring after *prostatectomy*, and sometimes after gynaecological operations, affects the hips in particular, the patient lying in great pain with hips partly flexed. On rising from their bed, they may have to walk backwards as forward progression is too painful. The disorder is usually rapidly relieved by draining a pocket of fluid or infective material from behind the symphysis pubis; occasionally, true osteitis pubis is present.

Metabolic arthropathies

The most common of these is *gout*. This disorder is characterized by the sudden agonizing nature of the acute attack, which is often so severe as to make the patient – almost always an adult male – feel he must have broken a bone in his foot, but for the fact that the disorder frequently starts in bed in the early morning. There are usually clear signs of inflammation, the skin being tense, shiny, hot and red over the big toe metatarsophalangeal joint, ankle or hand, the last named being the most common (Fig. J.23). Acute attacks may also occur in the knee. Although hyperuricaemia is usually present it is not invariably so, and an elevated plasma urate concentration occurs in many other disorders and is not in itself diagnostic. The presence of tophi in the ears or elsewhere suggests the diagnosis, although the symptoms and signs are usually diagnostic. The only absolute proof is the identification of urate crystals from the affected joint under the polarizing microscope.

In some cases, suggestive of gout, intra-articular crystals turn out not to be urate but calcium pyrophosphate, the condition being *chondrocalcinosis articularis* or 'pseudogout'. This condition affects knees most commonly, but other joints are also affected – often in symmetrical fashion – with the appearance of calcification in the joint cartilages. Acute inflammatory episodes occur also in chronic renal failure with deposition of calcium salts in the soft tissues alongside, rather than in, joints. This may also be seen in patients following *renal transplantation* from cadavers or living donors other than identical twins. Polyarthritis with effusions, often in the knees, may

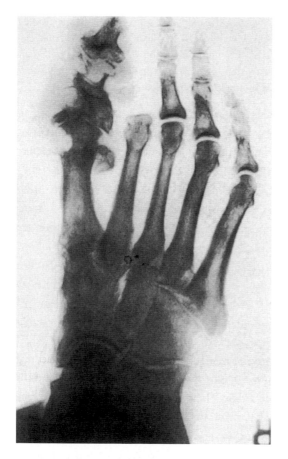

Figure J.23 Severe destructive tophaceous gout. The second toe was even more severely affected and was removed.

occur in these patients who may have rheumatoid factor in the blood.

In *calcinosis circumscripta*, calcium salts (carbonate and phosphate) may be deposited under the skin, but they are again para-articular rather than in the joint tissues, which appear normal.

Amyloidosis may be secondary to rheumatoid arthritis, ankylosing spondylitis and (more rarely) Reiter's disease, but it may also occur in primary form associated with pains and swellings in joints. When associated with multiple myeloma, it may cause the carpal tunnel syndrome.

Joint symptoms, and backache in particular, occur in ochronosis. Here, the diagnosis is made by examination of the urine for homogentisic acid, and the cartilage of the ears for pigmentation. Radiographs of the spine are typical, with heavy calcification occurring in the intervertebral cartilages.

Multicentric reticulohistiocytosis (*lipoid dermatoarthritis*) may be mistaken for rheumatoid arthritis in adults as changes in fingers and tenosynovitis occur, but the presence of yellow nodules on the ears, forehead, neck, forearms and elsewhere, with groups of purple papules, suggests the true diagnosis which can be confirmed by biopsy. In advanced cases, the erosion of phalanges leads to shortening of the fingers.

In *Wilson's disease*, characterized by accumulation of copper in the tissues, arthritic changes – most commonly in the hands, wrists and knees – may start about the age of 30. Associated features are hepatic cirrhosis, psychiatric disease, and the Kayser – Fleischer green-brown ring around the cornea is diagnostic.

Vascular arthropathies

Avascular necrosis occurs in *caisson disease* (nitrogen or air embolism), from fat embolism, and occasionally in chronic alcoholism. The hips are often bilaterally involved with destruction of parts of the heads of the femurs, but the shoulders and one or both knees may also be affected.

Giant-cell arteritis and polymyalgia rheumatica are probably two facets of the same condition occurring in the elderly as, on existing evidence, both conditions are due to an arteritis of those vessels having an internal elastic lamina. Renal and cerebral vessels are therefore usually spared. The patients, who are usually over the age of 60, are of either sex, have marked morning stiffness, erythrocyte sedimentation rates of up to 100 mm in the first hour (Westergren), and pains and stiffness of shoulder and hip girdles. When the temporal vessels are involved a severe headache is often present, and the main danger is to vision if branches of the ophthalmic artery become affected. Pulses may disappear and murmurs be heard at the points of arterial narrowing. The sternoclavicular joints may be affected, but the disorder – as far as the girdle joints in general are concerned – is one of pain and stiffness in hips and shoulders without progressive clinical or radiological change, and eventually with full recovery. Diagnosis can be confirmed by arterial biopsy.

In *polyarteritis nodosa*, arthralgia is much more common than actual arthritis, but any joint may be affected in any pattern, local or general, severe or mild, flitting or constant. The appearance of nodules clinches the diagnosis, but these occur in only a minority of cases and many biopsies may have to be carried out before the diagnosis is confirmed. Eosinophilia occurs in about 15 per cent of cases. Bronchial spasm is among the more common manifestations elsewhere, but it is the multisystem distribution of symptoms which may suggest the diagnosis. When asthma, allergic rhinitis and eosinophilia are present, the term 'Churg–Strauss vasculitis' is used.

Neoplastic arthropathies

Metastatic malignant disease or multiple myeloma usually cause bony rather than joint changes. The serum alkaline phosphatase, often elevated in the former, is usually normal in the latter as there is no osteoblastic activity in myelomatosis. Joint changes occur, however, in *hypertrophic pulmonary osteoarthropathy*, a condition mostly associated with a bronchial carcinoma, usually a peripheral one. Removal of the primary lesion leads to rapid resolution of the effusions and arthritic changes in the more commonly affected joints, the knees and ankles. Fingers and toes are clubbed, and the extremities show a thickening based on new subperiosteal bone deposition which can be seen in radiographs. Not all cases of hypertrophic osteoarthropathy are secondary to malignancy, however, some being due to cyanotic congenital heart disease, colonic and other conditions (see FINGERS, CLUBBED, p. 217). In a familial primary form, symptoms of *pachydermoperiostosis* start usually in adolescence, more commonly in males, the hands and feet enlarging with marked clubbing and cylindrical thickening of forearms and legs; recurrent joint effusions may occur. The patient's features thicken, giving a leonine appearance.

Osteoid osteoma is a benign disorder and, although not a disease of joints, it should be mentioned because of the pain it causes and the difficulties in differential diagnosis. The pain is initially intermittent, but becomes more persistent and severe and is often aggravated by movement. There are no physical signs. It affects adolescents and young adults and, although any bone except the skull may be affected, the most common to be involved are the femur and tibia, which account for half the cases. Radiographs show a characteristic central opacity surrounded by a translucent zone, surrounded in turn by a zone of sclerosis. It may affect the bones of the spine, where it is

often very difficult to diagnose and is usually not suspected. The pains are sometimes worse at night than during the day.

Neuropathic arthropathies

Although the *carpal tunnel syndrome* is not strictly a joint affection, it is so often a manifestation of rheumatoid arthritis that is should be mentioned. It is not infrequently the first sign of this disorder. Other causes are pregnancy, acromegaly, myxoedema, multiple myeloma and amyloidosis. There is also an idiopathic variety with no apparent cause. Characteristic symptoms are tingling and hot and cold electrical sensations up the arms, interfering with sleep.

Neuropathic joints (Fig. J.24) in the form of Charcot's joints in tabes dorsalis are characterized by their gross deformity, painlessness and florid X-ray appearances, where numbers of bone islands surround a grossly deformed or disorganized joint. *Syringomyelia* affects chiefly shoulder and elbow; knee, ankle, hip and spine are more commonly affected in tabes. Diabetic arthropathy is different in that clinical and radiological signs of infection are often present along with poor vascularization and signs of peripheral neuropathy; the condition is usually confined to the feet and toes. Osborne's

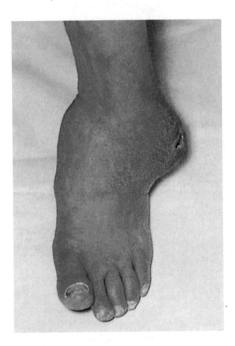

Figure J.24 Charcot's disease of the ankle, showing disorganization of the joint.

syndrome is due to ulnar nerve compression beneath the arcuate ligament just below the elbow.

In the *shoulder–hand syndrome*, which is a reflex dystrophy, trophic changes follow soon after injury to the shoulder or weeks or months after myocardial infarction. A similar syndrome has been reported in patients receiving antituberculous therapy, and in other pathological conditions. The shoulder is stiff and painful, the skin of the hand shiny and smooth and sometimes hyperaesthetic, and the muscles atrophic. There is no joint swelling, though initially there may be considerable swelling of the whole hand and fingers. X-rays show initially osteoporosis of humeral head and wrist, but later a more diffuse 'ground-glass' appearance. In many cases there is no apparent cause for the condition.

Drug-induced arthropathy

Alcoholics are especially likely to sustain injuries to bones and joints; they are also more prone to septic arthritis and avascular necrosis of bone. Prolonged corticosteroid therapy may also be associated with septic arthritis, osteoporosis and fractures. Crush fractures of lumbar or dorsal vertebrae are not uncommon. A condition very similar to SLE with LE cells present in the blood can be due to a large range of drugs, the most common being procaine amide; this is the so-called 'hydralazine syndrome'.

Symptoms disappear on stopping the drug. It has also been reported with oral contraceptives, though such cases are very rare.

Miscellaneous arthropathies

The *knuckle pads* (Garrod's pads), seen not infrequently on the dorsal aspects of the proximal interphalangeal joints of the fingers, are usually not accompanied by any symptoms and are best disregarded. They are due to fibrous thickenings the size of small orange pips, and are not part of the clinical picture of osteoarthritis or any other form of arthritis. They are not associated with any bony changes, though in some cases they occur with *Dupuytren's contracture* which, in turn, is occasionally associated with Peyronie's disease (induratio penis plastica). The palmar contractures occurring in rheumatoid arthritis may, on occasion, resemble Dupuytren's contracture (see Fig. J.21). *Thorn synovitis*

is an inflammatory condition due to a thorn or splinter of wood or a foreign body being knelt on by a child, who is hardly aware of it at the time. The *septic focus syndrome* is a rare disorder where diffuse aches and pains in and around joints are rapidly relieved by the removal of a septic focus or drainage of an abscess. No residual changes are left in the tissues. Lastly, the *xiphoid syndrome* refers to pains which stem from a displaced or mobile xiphisternum, often the result of trauma. This simple condition is only noteworthy in that it may be mistaken for more serious disorders of stomach, duodenum, gall bladder or heart.

Joint disease in young children

The following conditions should be considered when children under 5 years of age present with joint symptoms:

- *Septic arthritis*: due to staphylococci, haemolytic streptococci, *H. influenzae*, tuberculosis).
- *Associated with or following infection*: adenovirus, rubella, mumps, chickenpox, *Mycoplasma pneumoniae*, cytomegalovirus, rickettsia, Lyme arthritis, Kawasaki's syndrome.
- *Idiopathic*: chronic juvenile arthritis (Still's disease), familial Mediterranean fever.
- *Vascular and haematological*: Henoch–Schönlein syndrome, sickle-cell disease, leukaemia, haemophilia, haemangioma, hypogammaglobulinaemia.
- *Dietetic*: rickets.
- *Miscellaneous*: Farber's disease, the mucopolysaccharidoses (e.g. Hurler–Scheic syndrome), injuries (the battered child syndrome), neuroblastoma, thorn synovitis.

Infective (septic conditions)

Infection in infancy

Staphylococcal infection is common, but many organisms may be responsible. The infant is ill, often rejecting food, vomiting or convulsing, but sometimes is only mildly ill with slight fever. The hip is the most common joint to be affected, and is held flexed and adducted, with oedema appearing around the adductors.

Infection in 1–5-year age group

Haemophilus influenzae infection is common in the UK. If several joints are affected, suspect hypogammaglobulinaemia or some other immune abnormality.

Staphylococcal, haemolytic streptococcal and, more rarely, tuberculous infection should be considered.

Infections

Other infections with adenoviruses often start with pharyngitis, followed a few days later by fever, macular erythematous rash and a symmetrical arthritis which lasts for up to 6 weeks. A similar transient arthropathy may occur with rubella, mumps and chickenpox. Infection with cytomegalovirus is often associated with abnormal tests of liver function and infection with *Mycoplasma pneumoniae* with erythema multiforme. Other infections not seen in the UK (unless imported) are rickettsial infections such as Rocky Mountain Spotted Fever or Lyme arthritis, where a small red macule or papule enlarges to form a large erythematous ring followed by fever and arthritis, usually of only a few joints. In Japan and the East, Kawasaki's syndrome should be considered a possibility.

Non infective inflammatory conditions

Juvenile chronic arthritis often presents under 5 years of age (see p. 352). If of inflammatory onset, it must be distinguished from the infective conditions above.

Mark Kinirons

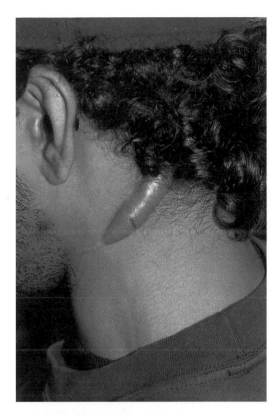

Figure K.1 Keloid following knife wound.

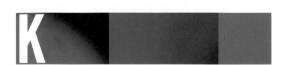

KELOID

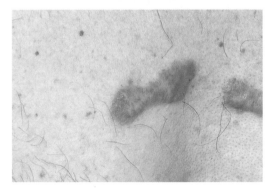

Figure K.2 Spontaneous keloid.

A keloid is a benign but uncontrolled fibrous overgrowth of the dermis in response to injury. The tendency to form keloids is a personal trait, more common in blacks, young adults and in the stretched skin of neck and chest (Fig. K.1). Usually, the antecedent damage is obvious – for example, surgical incisions, pierced ear lobes, burns and chickenpox. Keloids may follow acne and folliculitis, chiefly on the chest (Fig. K.2) and at the back of the neck, where ingrowing hairs may be a perpetuating factor. Keloids commonly recur following an excision, even if intralesional steroids are injected at the time of operation. Care must be taken to avoid unnecessary trauma (e.g. excision of benign moles) in susceptible subjects.

Barry Monk

KIDNEY, PALPABLE

The kidneys are difficult to palpate. The normal kidney can be felt by an expert, but not usually by a novice. Palpation of the kidney is easier in a thin individual but is difficult in the obese; even a considerably enlarged kidney may not be palpable in such a patient. However, the causes of an enlarged kidney that lead it to be felt on clinical examination are: renal tumours (renal cell carcinoma); large obstructed kidneys due to pelvi-ureteric junction obstruction or pyonephrosis; polycystic disease of the kidney; and solitary or multiple renal cysts.

It is usually large swellings of the kidney that are noticed by the patient, either because of an increase in girth (tight-fitting clothing) or abdominal discomfort. In bilateral polycystic kidneys the abdomen will be symmetrically enlarged. In unilateral renal disease one side of the abdomen will be distorted. For most palpable kidneys, even if asymmetrically enlarged, distinction of the features is difficult. The kidney should initially be palpated from the front, followed by an attempt to 'balot' the kidney using one examining hand behind the lower ribs pushing the kidney forward so that it can be felt with the anterior examining hand. Rough palpation of suspected renal tumours should be avoided to reduce the risk of dissemination of tumour cells. Ultrasound or CT scanning will confirm the diagnosis.

The onset of a varicocele in adult life, particularly on the right, should raise concern as to the presence of a renal cancer. Renal tumours may obstruct the testicular vein where it drains into the renal vein on the left and inferior vena cava on the right and give rise to a varicocele.

Renal tumours present most commonly with macroscopic haematuria. Suspicion of a diagnosis of renal tumour will lead to ultrasound scanning of the urinary tract, when the diagnosis will be made.

A pelvic kidney, which is found at or below the brim of the pelvis, may be felt in the iliac fossa. A renal transplant will also be easily palpable in the iliac fossa.

A *supradrenal tumour* may be sufficiently large to be palpable in its own right, or it may push the kidney down and make it palpable, or push the liver forwards such that the liver becomes palpable.

A renal swelling may be so slight that it is only found upon clinical examination, or it may be large enough to attract the patient's attention. Hydronephrosis, pyonephrosis, renal tuberculosis or abscess, new growth or cysts (single or multiple) in the kidney must be diagnosed not only one from another but also from other tumours simulating a renal swelling. The characteristic points of a renal tumour are:

- *The intestine is in front of the tumour.* When either kidney is merely slightly enlarged, both large and small intestines will be in front of it; however, when the organ is so enlarged as to reach the anterior abdominal wall, the coils of small intestine are pushed aside. The anatomical relationship of the large intestine to the kidney, and the absence of a mesentery, do not allow the same mobility for the colon, which usually retains its position in front of the kidney, although it is sometimes pushed downwards by a tumour projecting forwards from the lower pole. Hence, an area of resonance can usually be obtained in front of a renal swelling; if the colon is empty it can sometimes be felt in a thin subject and rolled by the fingers on the surface of the tumour. Bowel is almost never placed in front of a splenic tumour, and only rarely in front of a hepatic tumour.
- *The area of dullness to percussion* is continuous from the lateral aspect of the swelling to the midline posteriorly; that is, there is no area of resonance between the mass and the vertebral spines, as with a splenic or ovarian tumour.
- *A renal tumour usually retains the shape of the kidney*; it is rounded at its borders and poles, and does not possess any edge or sharp margin, as do splenic or hepatic swellings (Fig. K.3). The surface of the tumour may present rounded, smooth, raised bosses in cases of renal growths or in polycystic disease.
- *A renal tumour in the process of enlargement projects forwards and downwards.* It may fill up the natural hollow of the loin, but seldom causes any prominence posteriorly. A perinephric abscess, which often simulates a renal swelling, may cause a distinct prominence in the loin.
- *A renal tumour may be movable downwards or inwards*, unless it is fixed in the loin by preceding inflammation, or by the spread of carcinoma into the perirenal tissues. An enlarged kidney may be felt bimanually, and if grasped between the two hands can be pushed into the loin. A renal tumour rarely descends into the iliac fossa, but it may be present there in congenital ectopia or in cases of excessive mobility.

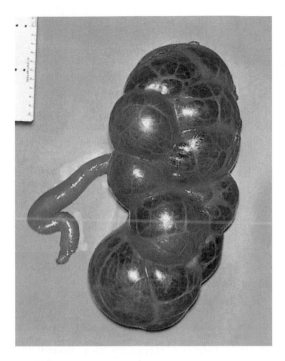

Figure K.3 Enormous hydronephrosis due to a small stone impacted in the distal ureter. The kidney was so large that it could readily be felt on rectal as well as abdominal examination, yet it has retained its reniform shape.

- When a renal tumour is large enough to reach the anterior abdominal wall it commonly comes in contact with it at the level of the umbilicus, at the same time bulging out the iliocostal space. There is usually a line of resonance between the upper margin of the tumour and the hepatic dullness.
- A varicocele may be developed on the same side as the renal tumour due to obstruction of the testicular vein as this drains into the renal vein on the left or the inferior vena cava on the right. This is especially significant on the right side, although it is a rare finding.
- With a renal tumour there may be changes in the urine pointing to renal disease. On the other hand, the urine at any one time may be normal, free from blood or pus, based on the fact that the ureter of the diseased side is blocked, or that the disease does not involve the renal pelvis.
- In exceptional cases, a tumour of the right kidney may extend upwards towards the dome of the diaphragm, rotating the liver so that the anterior margin of the latter descends below the costal margin, and preventing satisfactory palpation of the renal areas.

Differential diagnosis of renal tumours and renal swellings

Based on the above physical characters, a renal tumour should present little difficulty in diagnosis; however, a tumour possessing several of these characters may often create considerable doubt as to the nature of the organ from which it has arisen. The following points will assist in the differentiation of renal swellings from other tumours with which they may be confused.

Enlargements of the gall bladder

This is located immediately below the costal margin, so that no interval exists between the tumour and the lower margin of the liver. It is usually oval in outline, with the long axis in the line between the 9th right costal cartilage and the umbilicus, and is freely movable with respiratory movement, and movable from side to side about an axis at the costal margin. There is dullness on percussion over the swelling, and it cannot be felt in the loin or be grasped bimanually. With an enlarged gall bladder there may be attacks of colic, with or without jaundice. Ultrasonography is a particularly valuable non-invasive method of demonstrating the distended gall bladder; moreover, it will also show up gallstones, which are highly echogenic.

Enlargements of the liver

These pass downwards from beneath the costal margin so that there is no line or resonance, or any area in which the hand can be depressed, between the tumour and the costal margin. Hepatic tumours do not impair the normal resonance in the loin in the same manner as a renal tumour does. A tongue-shaped lobe of the liver (Riedel's lobe) may cause difficulty in diagnosis, but here the lower margin is seldom so rounded as that of a renal tumour, nor will the mass be felt in the loin on bimanual examination. A tumour or cyst in the concave aspect or left lobe of the liver is especially liable to cause error in diagnosis, whereas a tumour of the right kidney (which projects upwards behind the liver) may so rotate the latter that its anterior margin descends below the costal margin and completely obscures the kidney. In the case of a large carcinoma of the right kidney, the liver may in this way be so depressed as to render palpation of the kidney impossible. A pyelographic examination may reveal a normal renal picture, or it may indicate a hydronephrosis or renal growth. Ultrasonography will readily differentiate between hepatic and renal swellings.

Enlargements of the spleen

These descend from beneath the left costal margin, and have no bowel in front of them; they are therefore dull to percussion. The edge of a splenic tumour is usually well-defined and often notched, and there is resonance between the posterior aspect of the tumour and the spinal column. A splenic tumour is more movable than is a left renal tumour. A blood count may help in deciding in favour of a splenic enlargement, and a pyelogram may show a normal kidney. Ultrasonography or CT scanning readily differentiate between the two organs.

Perinephric effusions

A perinephric effusion – whether of blood, pus or urine – may form a mass in the loin which, upon physical examination, may be mistaken for a renal swelling. A perinephric effusion may arise from suppuration of the kidney, so that the previous history and examination of the urine will not assist in the differential diagnosis; or it may be due to conditions entirely distinct from renal disease. An effusion of blood around the kidney is, in nearly all cases, caused by an injury to the loin, and will be accompanied by other signs of injury. It may, however, occur from the spontaneous growth and rupture of a renal neoplasm. A perinephric abscess forms a less well-defined tumour than that caused by a renal swelling, and is more acute in its general symptoms, such as pain and temperature. The skin over the abscess may be thickened or oedematous, and fluctuation may be felt to be more superficial than in a renal swelling. A perinephric abscess may result from suppuration in association with a carcinoma or diverticulum of the large bowel, from appendiceal inflammation, or from suppuration in a perinephric haematoma due to injury; it may be a sequel to a specific blow, or be due to a haematogenous infection. Bilateral palpation and comparison of the loins may detect a perinephric swelling by the way the loin is filled out and becomes even convex on the affected side. This is best seen by laying the patient prone and carefully inspecting both sides.

Tumours arising from the pelvic organs

Tumours arising from the pelvic organs, from the ovary or uterus, may in some cases simulate renal tumours. An ovarian cyst with a long pedicle occupying the loin may be mistaken for an enlarged or movable kidney, and any sudden attacks of pain occurring from torsion of the pedicle may be looked upon as due to renal colic. The normally placed ovarian cyst or uterine fibroid will seldom be confused with a renal swelling, for it is placed in the midline of the body, can be felt to come up from the pelvis, and can be felt on bimanual vaginal examination to be attached to the uterus or its appendages. These tumours give rise to dullness anteriorly, and do not alter the normal resonance in the loin. In cases of malignant ovarian tumours associated with ascites, the lumbar resonance may be lost. However, on turning the patient over on one side the previously dull note becomes replaced by resonance in the uppermost loin. In the case of an ovarian cyst with a long pedicle, or of a uterine fibroid of pedunculated, subserous form, the position in the loin may sometimes suggest a renal tumour. The cyst will be found, however, to occupy a more anterior position in the abdomen than a renal tumour, and to possess a much greater range of movement, and it does not slip back into the loin under the costal margin in the same manner as an enlarged kidney does. There is resonance posteriorly, the kidney may be actually palpated as well as the abdominal tumour, while a distinct connection with the pelvic organs can sometimes be traced from the tumour when the latter is drawn up.

In contradistinction to the above, a very large cystic renal swelling may be mistaken for an ovarian cyst. It may occupy the greater part of the abdomen, and even be felt per vaginam to be encroaching upon the pelvis. However, on careful examination of a renal tumour of this form there will be no line of resonance between the mass and the vertebral column posteriorly, the natural hollow of the loin will be filled up, and there is frequently a distinct bulging in the lower thoracic wall, together with an increased length of the iliocostal space on the affected side. Some assistance may be obtained from the history; a hydronephrosis may have been first noted as a tumour starting under the costal margin and gradually increasing downwards towards the iliac fossa and inwards across the median line, whereas an ovarian tumour may have been noted to increase upwards from the pelvis. Ultrasonography and/or CT scanning usually enables accurate anatomical diagnosis of the pelvic mass.

Suprarenal tumours

Suprarenal tumours may occasionally be of sufficient size to form an abdominal tumour, presenting as a rounded, movable swelling in the hypochondrium.

Faecal accumulation in the colon, caecum or sigmoid flexure

These may give rise to a tumour and pain of a colicky nature in the loin, the examining fingers can some times indent the tumour. Such swellings will be distinguished from renal swellings by the general intestinal symptoms, flatulence and the changes in form consequent on the administration of large enemas. A patient with a collection of faeces in the colon may not complain of constipation, but may in fact have a small daily evacuation from the overloaded bowel.

Appendicular inflammatory mass

This will be diagnosed from renal tumours by the situation of the pain and by the swelling being in the iliac fossa rather than in the loin. In some cases, however, the pain may be referred to the lumbar region, or an appendiceal inflammatory mass may spread upwards. This is especially so when the appendix is retrocaecal in position. The onset of the trouble, the acute symptoms, and the febrile disturbance will usually distinguish these cases from renal lesions.

Malignant growth of the large intestine

Malignant growth of the large intestine, especially of the ascending or descending colon, may form a tumour in the loin, which closely resembles a renal swelling. The mass formed by the growth may be grasped bimanually, is movable in the same directions as a renal tumour, and comes forward under the costal margin. The percussion note over the front of the lump is resonant, and there is usually an aching pain in the loin. If the growth has infiltrated through the wall of the bowel uncovered by peritoneum, the perirenal tissues may be thickened, or proteinuria may be produced by direct invasion of the kidney, when the case will even more resemble a renal lesion. Carcinoma of the large intestine should be suspected if there is any irregularity

in the action of the bowels, mucus or blood in the motions, or any symptom of incipient obstruction in the intestine. The intestinal tumour may be irregular and nodular, whereas a renal tumour presents rounded margins. The occurrence of a tumour in either side, associated with discomfort or palpable distension of the caecum from the accumulation of faeces, would render a growth in the colon the more suspicious.

The diagnosis of a large-bowel tumour can usually be established by a barium enema X ray examination. Confirmation can be made by direct colonoscopic examination, at which biopsy material can usually be obtained for histological examination.

Tumours of the omentum, mesentery or pancreas

These tumours – either cystic or malignant – are more median in position, do not project into the loin, and seldom resemble a renal tumour. Retroperitoneal and perirenal tumours may closely simulate renal tumours, but will be distinguished on ultrasonography and certainly by CT or MRI scanning.

Differential diagnosis of radiographic shadows in the abdomen and pelvis

It is necessary for the true interpretation of radiographs that a clear concept be held of the various conditions which may cast a shadow on an X-ray negative. In the diagnosis of cases of urinary disease, much information may be gained by the use of X-rays, and not merely in the confirmation of the presence of calculi in some part of the urinary tract. In a good film, the outline and the size of the kidney can be seen. Likewise, after efficient alimentary preparation, the outline of a normal kidney should be visible, lying opposite the bodies of the 1st, 2nd and 3rd lumbar vertebrae (Fig. K.4), and having an excursion of 4–5 cm in forced inspiration and expiration.

The following are the most frequent causes of a shadow which may be mistaken for a calculus.

- *Intestinal contents*: These may cast a shadow in the renal area owing to inefficient preparation of the patient, or to the fact that he or she has recently taken bismuth, magnesium salts, etc. If any doubt exists, a second examination should be made after further purgation. There may be some residue in the intestine from a recent barium meal examination.
- *Calcification of the abdominal or mesenteric lymph nodes* may cause a shadow in any part of the abdominal

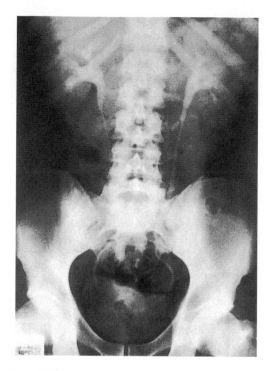

Figure K.4 Normal excretion pyelogram, 30-minute film after removal of compression. The calices are cupped, the left ureter is filled completely, and the right partially.

cavity. Although they are most frequently seen near the lower lumbar vertebrae or about the sacroiliac joint, and are therefore external to the renal shadow, they may be superimposed upon the latter and cause difficulty in diagnosis. The shadow of a calcified node is usually mottled in appearance, with small areas in the shadow showing increased density owing to the irregular deposition of lime salts. Calcareous nodes are frequently multiple, but their chief characteristic is their range of mobility. Thus, if more than one negative is taken with varying degrees of compression, the shadows of calcareous nodes may show a varying position with regard to the renal shadow, whilst in a lateral view a lymph node shadow is usually in front of the bodies of the vertebrae and not superimposed upon them. A calcified node may be placed immediately in front of the kidney and move equally with it, causing great difficulty in diagnosis; alternatively, there may be a calculus in one kidney and calcareous nodes imitating calculi on the other side. A pyelogram will show the relation of a calculus to the renal pelvis (Fig. K.5).

- *Gallstones*, on the right side, may produce a shadow in the renal area. They are frequently multiple, and may be seen to be faceted in a fusiform collection presenting the shape of the distended gall bladder (Fig. K.6). A single

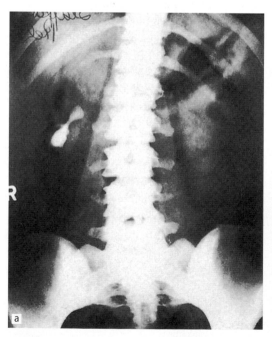

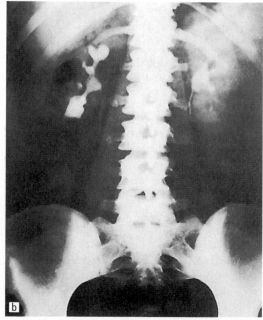

Figure K.5 (a) Radiograph showing a dumb-bell shadow in the right renal area. (b) The excretion pyelogram shows that the shadow is a stone occupying the lowest calix and pelvis of the right kidney.

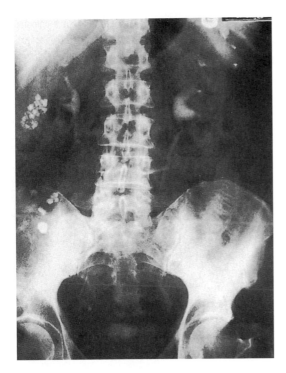

Figure K.6 Intravenous pyelogram showing also a collection of faceted stones in the gallbladder, calcified mesenteric glands in the right iliac fossa and phleboliths in the pelvis

gallstone superimposed on the renal shadow may cause difficulty; the shadow of a gallstone is less dense than is that of a renal stone, and is frequently more dense in the central than in the peripheral part. In a lateral view, a stone in the gall bladder will occupy an anterior position in the abdomen, though one impacted in the common bile duct may be seen opposite the body of the 1st or 2nd lumbar vertebra; in this case there will probably be jaundice. In a cholecystographic examination a gallstone may cause a filling defect (negative shadow) in the area of the gall bladder occupied by the dye. The distribution of stones in a horseshoe kidney may cause confusion until a pyelogram is performed (Fig. K.7).

■ *Calcification of the costal cartilages* may produce a shadow in the renal area in an anteroposterior negative. The shadows are not dense, are hazy in outline, and tend to assume a horizontal or oblique axis. In a lateral view they will be placed immediately under the anterior abdominal wall.

■ *Calcified masses in a tuberculous kidney*: The shadow in this condition is rarely so defined as is that of a calculus, is of moderate density with blurred and indistinct margins, appearing as one or more blotches in the renal area.

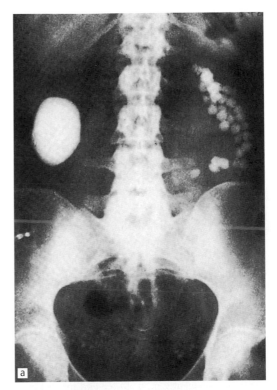

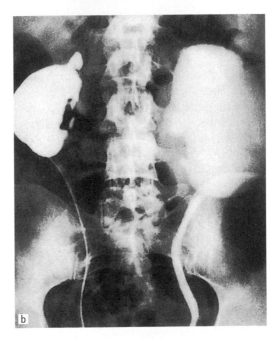

Figure K.7 (a) Single dense shadow on the right and multiple small ones on the left. (b) Pyelography shows that the shadows are enclosed in the dilated pelves of a horseshoe kidney. Note the inwardly pointing calices and the flower-vase pattern of the ureters.

However, on occasion – from the deposition of calcium salts – it may be very like the radiograph of a calculus.

- *Areas of calcification in a renal growth*: Rarely, faint ill-defined areas of calcification may be present in a renal carcinoma. There will, however, be symptoms of growth, such as haematuria and renal tumour, whilst a pyelographic examination will show a deformity of the pelvis and renal calices.
- *Foreign bodies*: A foreign body, such as shrapnel from a bullet, lying in front of or behind the kidney may mimic a calculus.

The line of the *normal ureter* lies anatomically along or just internal to the tips of the transverse processes of the 2nd to 5th lumbar vertebrae, passes with a slight curve outwards in front of the sacro-iliac articulation, and then with a marked curve forwards and inwards to the base of the bladder. A shadow in this line may be due to a calculus in the ureter, but it must be differentiated carefully from other conditions. A calculus is usually small, rounded or oval, with a long axis in the line of the ureter. It may be found in any part of the course of the ureter, but it is seen most frequently in the lower end just before it enters the bladder. The conditions which may produce a shadow that is likely to be mistaken for a ureteric calculus are:

- *Calcified lymph nodes* in the line of the ureter are placed most frequently in the angle between the last lumbar vertebra and the ala of the sacrum. They are usually multiple, forming a group in this situation in triangular form rather than in the longitudinal axis of the ureter. They are mottled in appearance, of irregular density, and are so movable that their position varies in successive radiographs.
- *A concretion in the appendix* may occasionally give rise to a shadow in the line of the right ureter, suggesting a calculus with very similar clinical symptoms. Further examination with a radio-opaque catheter in the ureter will show that the shadow is extra-ureteric.
- *Phleboliths in the pelvis* are liable to be mistaken for ureteric calculi, but they often have a characteristic ring-like appearance, which is quite diagnostic. They are usually multiple and are placed towards the peripheral areas of the pelvis, often at about the level of the ischial spine. A stereoscopic examination with an opaque catheter in the ureter will differentiate them from calculi, though it may not be possible to distinguish them from calcified

lymph nodes. It must not be forgotten that a calculus may be present in the ureter in addition to phleboliths, but the distinction can be made by excretion pyelography or radiography after the passage of a ureteric catheter. Figure K.8 shows that the shadow of the ureter does not impinge on any of the numerous phleboliths present in the pelvis.
- *Foreign bodies*, especially after periods of war, may occasionally lie near the line of the ureter. They are usually more dense than calculi.

A shadow may be present in a pelvic radiograph which must be differentiated from that of a vesical calculus. The latter is usually rounded or oval, occupies a fairly central position in the pelvis, and may show rings of varying density owing to the deposition of layers of urinary salts of different composition. Occasionally, one or more vesical calculi may form a shadow in a more lateral position in successive negatives, when a suspicion of their presence in a diverticulum in the bladder will arise. The diagnosis of this condition is discussed below.

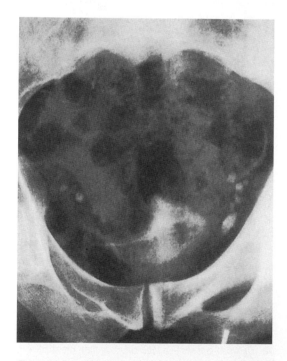

Figure K.8 Excretion pyelogram showing numerous phleboliths in the pelvis; the left ureter is seen passing between them. Note the 'bite defect' in the bladder on the right caused by a solid carcinoma.

The following conditions may give rise to radiographic shadows in the pelvis:

■ *Prostatic calculi* may be either single or multiple, but in the radiograph they occupy a position very low in

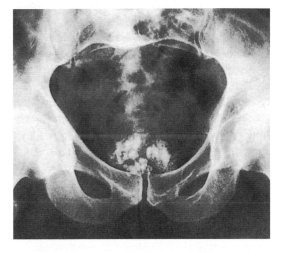

Figure K.9 Radiograph showing shadows in the pelvis due to multiple prostatic calculi.

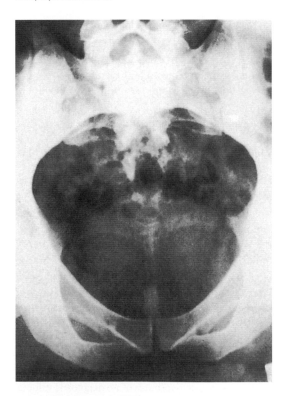

Figure K.10 Radiograph showing a shadow above the pubis due to a cystine calculus in the prostatic urethra.

the pelvis, often behind the shadow of the pubis (Fig. K.9).

■ *Calcification of a fibroid tumour of the uterus* provides a large, irregular shadow of varying degree of density. Bimanual palpation of a tumour moving with the uterus would point to the diagnosis.

■ *Ovarian dermoids* may give rise to irregular shadows in the pelvis due to the formation of bone or teeth in the cyst. They may be present in young adult life, and a tumour would be palpated on abdominal or pelvic examination.

■ *Phosphatic encrustation upon a vesical tumour* may occur in a case of growth in the presence of cystitis and give rise to faint ill-defined shadows in the pelvic radiograph. A cystoscopic examination will reveal the true nature of the lesion.

■ *Foreign bodies* in the bladder may become so encrusted with urinary salts that a shadow like that of a calculus may be present. A variety of foreign bodies have been found in the bladder, introduced either by intent or by the accidental breaking off of a piece of catheter or the like. In some cases the shadow will show a central area of different density, or even a metallic nucleus.

■ *Urethral calculi* may be retained in the canal behind a stricture and enlarge *in situ*. They form a shadow in a radiograph above or below the pubic arch (Fig. K.10).

Harold Ellis

KNEE, PAIN IN

See LOWER LIMB, PAIN IN (p. 390).

KYPHOSIS

See SPINE, DEFORMITY OF (p. 658).

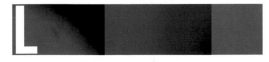

LACRIMATION

Lacrimation or tearing is a function of the lacrimal gland and the accessory lacrimal glands. Tears wet the surface of the cornea and conjunctivae, thereby protecting the surface epithelium. They also inhibit the growth of organisms, provide the cornea with nutrient substances, and make the cornea a smooth optical surface by abolishing minute surface irregularities. Basal tear production provides enough tears for these purposes, and reflex lacrimation occurs with irritative conditions or corneal disease (see EPIPHORA, p. 176). Psychic lacrimation is normally associated with pain or emotional upset.

Tear production diminishes with age, and dryness of the eyes is a common complaint of the elderly.

Reginald Daniel

LEG, OEDEMA OF

In the great majority of patients with generalized oedema, the legs, particularly the ankles, are likely to be affected (see OEDEMA, GENERALIZED, p. 494). In most of these cases both legs will be involved, but occasionally – and perhaps due to the patient's position in bed – the oedema may be somewhat asymmetrical. In most of the conditions discussed in this section, the oedema is strictly unilateral and there will, therefore, be little difficulty in distinguishing them from the causes of generalized oedema. The causes of oedema of the legs can be classified under the headings of *trauma, inflammation, venous obstruction* and *lymphatic obstruction*.

Trauma

The cause of the swelling associated with sprains and fractures, bites and stings, and burns and frostbite is likely to be obvious. There is, however, a late complication of trauma, of which oedema is a feature, which may present a diagnostic problem. This is *algodystrophy* or *Sudek's atrophy*. This rather rare condition usually follows trauma to a limb, which may be very mild, and, in the leg, most commonly affects the ankle. It is characterized by pain, which may be very severe, and the ankle is warm, red and oedematous, suggesting local inflammation; there is, however, no systemic evidence of inflammation. These changes subside after a few weeks and the skin around the joint becomes cold, cyanosed and, ultimately, atrophic. X-rays show local osteoporosis. Full recovery is usual, but this may not occur for many months. The aetiology is unknown, but

it has been suggested that abnormal autonomic reflexes may be responsible.

Inflammation

Oedema is one of the cardinal signs of inflammation. Local lesions, such as *boils* and *carbuncles*, are easily identified, but more widespread inflammatory lesions may initially cause diagnostic confusion. The bright red areas with palpable raised margins of *erysipelas* are characteristic, but oedema due to obstruction of cutaneous lymphatics may persist after the acute inflammation has subsided. *Cellulitis* causes more diffuse oedema, as does *acute osteomyelitis*; lymphangitis and lymphadenitis are commoner in the former while, in the latter, the constitutional disturbance is greater. *Chronic osteomyelitis* can cause puzzling oedema, but imaging will settle the diagnostic issue. *Acute arthritis* of any type is associated with local oedema. In most cases the swelling of the joint itself will make the diagnosis clear, but *acute gout* can cause a swelling which is widespread enough to simulate cellulitis. *Acute rheumatoid arthritis* is less likely to cause confusion, but it is worth remembering that, in this condition, more generalized oedema can occur; this is probably due to a combination of hypoalbuminaemia, stasis in an immobile patient and, perhaps, increased capillary permeability. The painful swelling of the calf with ankle oedema caused by a *ruptured Baker's cyst* is easily confused with deep venous thrombosis; a history of prior swelling of the joint, decreasing with the onset of the calf pain, is an important diagnostic feature.

Venous obstruction

Deep venous thrombosis in the calf muscles is an important cause of oedema of the ankle; the swelling will extend further up the leg if thrombus is also present in the femoral and iliac veins. Venous thrombosis is a common complication of major surgery and of prolonged recumbency for any reason; it can also often occur without any obvious cause. Long coach journeys by the elderly and, in women, the use of oestrogen-containing oral contraceptive agents increase the risk of deep venous thrombosis. In addition to the ankle oedema, the calf is typically swollen and tender on pressure from behind and from side to side. Homan's sign (pain in the calf on dorsiflexion at the ankle) may be positive, but is of no diagnostic value as it can be positive with any painful lesion of the calf. Very often, none of these signs is present; the first evidence of deep venous thrombosis may be a fatal pulmonary embolism.

Thrombus may spread upwards beyond the iliac veins to involve the *inferior vena cava* and, in that case, the other leg will become oedematous. With such a sequence of events, the diagnosis of inferior vena caval occlusion is clear. Primary occlusion of this vessel, however, will present with bilateral ankle and leg oedema, in which case the differential diagnosis includes all the causes of generalized oedema. Diagnostic assistance may be provided by investigations such as Doppler flow studies, but the definitive diagnosis of venous occlusion can be made only by venography or CT scanning. In any patient in whom venous thrombosis has occurred without obvious cause, a thorough general examination – including rectal and vaginal examination – is essential to detect pelvic or abdominal tumours causing pressure on veins.

Varicose veins, with or without previous thrombosis, commonly cause ankle oedema, usually quite mild. Although in the great majority of cases it is the veins themselves which are the seat of the trouble, it is wise, at the first presentation, to examine the patient with the possibility of external pressure on the large veins in mind, as in patients with acute venous occlusion.

Lymphatic obstruction

The oedema fluid in lymphatic obstruction contains much more protein than the fluid in other conditions causing oedema. Consequently, although initially the swelling 'pits' on pressure and disappears overnight, it later becomes firm and non-pitting ('brawny') and is present all the time. Later, the skin becomes grossly thickened and, sometimes, ulcerated. The common causes of lymphatic obstruction in Western countries include *neoplastic infiltration* of the lymphatics and lymph nodes, and scarring from *trauma*, surgical or otherwise, and from *irradiation*; recurrent *streptococcal infection* can cause similar damage. In tropical countries, *filariasis* is a common cause of lymphatic obstruction and chronic oedema of the legs known as 'elephantiasis'. The commonest form of filariasis is that due to *Wuchereria bancrofti*; this is widespread in the tropics and causes elephantiasis of the whole leg and also of the genitalia, especially in males. Another filaria, *Brugia malayi*, is found in the Far East, especially South-East Asia; the inguinal lymph nodes are affected, as in Bancroftian filariasis, but curiously the oedema

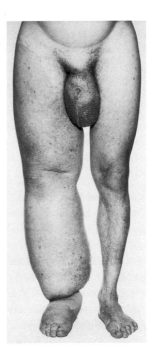

Figure L.1 Milroy's disease; unilateral lymphoedema due to congenital lymphatic hypoplasia.

and elephantiasis are confined to the lower parts of the legs. There is also a *non-filarial elephantiasis* seen in parts of Africa and Central and South America; this is due to chronic lymphangitis apparently caused by microscopic particles of silica absorbed through the skin of the feet; it usually affects the feet and lower parts of the legs. *Lymphatic hypoplasia* is a rare cause of oedema which occurs in two forms: a congenital variety presenting with oedema in early infancy; and a familial form, sometimes known as Milroy's disease. In the latter, there is an abrupt demarcation between the swollen and the normal tissue at the level of a joint – ankle, knee or hip (Fig. L.1). There is sometimes a history of attacks of pyrexia in association with the spread of the oedema which is typically episodic. Thus, the swelling – having been present at the ankle only for several years – may rather suddenly spread to reach the knee and, later, in a similar fashion, the hip.

Boris Lams

LEG, PAIN IN

See LOWER LIMB, PAIN IN (p. 413).

LEG, ULCERATION OF

Although it is true that the great majority of leg ulcers are due to venous disease – all too often called, and inaccurately labelled 'varicose ulcers' – it must be remembered that a large number of other conditions can lead to this common clinical situation.

The various aetiologies of leg ulceration can be classified into:

- Venous – following deep vein thrombosis.
- Arterial – especially arteriosclerosis (see GANGRENE, PERIPHERAL, p. 237).
- Mixed venous and arterial.
- Neuropathic – especially diabetes mellitus.
- Chronic infection (e.g. gumma, pyoderma gangrenosa).
- Complicating systemic disease (e.g. rheumatoid arthritis, haemolytic anaemias, ulcerative colitis).
- Trauma – including Munchausen's syndrome.
- Malignant disease – Marjolin's ulcer, malignant melanoma.

Venous ulcer

Venous, or gravitational, ulcer almost invariably results from a preceding episode of deep vein thrombosis. There is usually a history of a painful swollen leg following childbirth, surgical operation or a period of recumbency from any disease, manifested by an episode of slight pyrexia, calf pain and tenderness and swelling of the leg as a result of thrombosis of the deep veins of the leg. Recanalization results in damage to the venous valves. Over subsequent years, the leg becomes swollen, superficial varicose veins may form due to perforator incompetence secondary to the raised venous pressure, pigmentation of the skin occurs, particularly over the medial side of the leg just above the medial malleolus (the pigment being haemosiderin), the subcutaneous, affected skin becomes eczematous, and the subcutaneous fat becomes replaced by thick fibrous tissue. Ulceration occurs as a consequence of the poor skin nutrition, either following some minor trauma or from scratching of the eczematous skin.

The patient may well have forgotten the original episode of deep vein thrombosis, perhaps many years before, and will blame the secondary varicose veins (as may, indeed, their medical practitioner) on the consequent ulcer, although it is unlikely that primary varicose veins alone give rise to this condition.

A venous ulcer is situated on the gaiter area of the leg, has a sloping edge and a floor that may be made up of red, velvety granulations if the ulcer is uninfected, white and fibrous if it is long-standing, and purulent and smelly if it is infected (Fig. L.2). If the ulcer is large, the foot is often oedematous, so that the pedal pulses may not be palpable. It is important to exclude co-existing arterial disease (see below) and the presence or absence of these pulses must be determined with the Doppler probe.

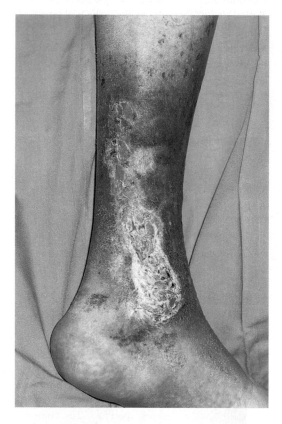

Figure L.2 Varicose (venous) ulcer. Note the extensive surrounding pigmentation due to deposition of haemosiderin.

Arterial

Arteriosclerosis and the other less common causes of arterial insufficiency may result in ulceration of the leg (see GANGRENE, PERIPHERAL, p. 237). This is particularly likely to occur over the pressure areas of the heel and malleoli rather than the gaiter area. There are the other features of peripheral arterial disease, including an absence of pulses, but it is important to remember that many elderly patients with venous ulceration of the leg have co-existing arterial disease, and this must be excluded. The use of the Doppler probe is particularly valuable in this respect (see above).

Neuropathic

Loss of sensation in the lower limb may result in trophic ulceration as a result of the pressure of the shoe, or an orthopaedic appliance, etc. Both in the industrialized world and increasingly in the Asian subcontinent, the commonest cause of neuropathic ulcers is diabetes. Typical sites are over the malleoli, the heel, or on the sole of the foot over the heads of the metatarsals. In the severe diabetic, this neuropathy may be complicated by the associated vascular impairment of diabetic micro-angiopathy and by the increased propensity of the diabetic to infection (Fig. L.3).

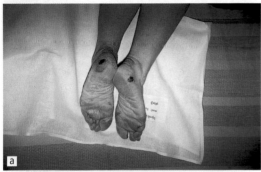

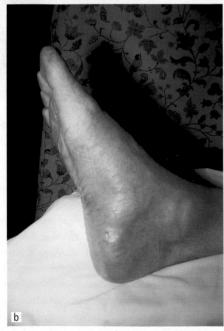

Figure L.3 (a,b) Diabetic leg ulcers due to peripheral neuropathy.

Other examples of neuropathic ulceration will be seen in conditions such as leprosy, tabes dorsalis and hemiplegia following a stroke.

Chronic infection

Syphilitic ulcers are the result of breakdown of a gumma which has formed in the subcutaneous tissues in tertiary syphilis. These ulcers occur in the upper third of the leg (in contrast to venous ulcers, which are confined to the lower third). They are almost always circular and present a punched-out appearance. They are generally multiple and tend to run into each other, forming a large ulcer with a serpiginous outline. There may be other signs of syphilis, and there will be positive serological tests for this disease. However, today it is rarely seen in the Western World.

Pyoderma gangrenosum produces multiple ulcers, which may occur anywhere in the body, but frequently affect the leg. They are multiple and have ragged blue-red overhanging edges and necrotic bases. They often start as tender infected nodules, often following minor trauma, and are usually associated with patients suffering from chronic ulcerative colitis or Crohn's disease.

Leg ulcers may be seen in amoebiasis, chancroid, diphtheria, leprosy, yaws and kala-azar, all of which might be considered in recent immigrants. Chronic sores and ulcers of the leg, as with other parts of the body, may be due to various skin fungi (e.g. blastomycosis, sporotrichosis and actinomycosis). Multiple discharging sinuses in a swollen and distorted foot may be seen in Madura foot, resulting from infection with the fungus *Nocardia madurae*.

Lupus vulgaris, a form of primary tuberculosis of the skin, is not often found on the leg, although it may occur there as in any cutaneous area.

Systemic disease

Ulcers may complicate a large variety of systemic diseases. Pyoderma gangrenosa in ulcerative colitis and Crohn's disease has already been noted. Ulcers of the leg may also occur in rheumatoid arthritis, sickle-cell anaemia, thalassaemia, polycythaemia rubra vera, thrombocytopenic purpura, hereditary spherocytosis and the leukaemias. All of these might be considered where the aetiology is not evident.

Trauma

Trauma, unless it is continuous, is not alone sufficient to cause an ulcer in healthy people. Old ladies, with thin atrophic skin, may lacerate the tissues over the shin and the poor blood supply may result in necrosis and subsequent ulceration of the damaged skin. Ulceration may result in inadvertent permeation of the subcutaneous tissues by the sclerosing fluid used in the injection treatment of varicose veins. The malingerer may rub corrosive agents into the leg or use a coin bandaged firmly against the skin (examples of the so-called Baron von Munchausen syndrome). The diagnosis is often suggested by the rectangular or other definite shape of the ulcer itself, as well as by the strange personality of the patient.

Malignant disease

A carcinoma may develop in a chronic ulcer, particularly a venous ulcer that has existed for many years (Marjolin's ulcer). The ulcer at one edge becomes heaped up, everted and indurated (Fig. L.4). The

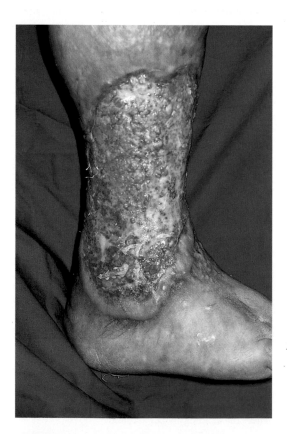

Figure L.4 Marjolin ulcer. Carcinomatous change has taken place at the lower margin of this venous ulcer, which had remained unhealed for 20 years.

inguinal lymph nodes may become enlarged. The appearance of bare bone at the base of a venous ulcer should always arouse the gravest suspicion that malignant change has taken place. A biopsy specimen at the edge of the ulcer should be removed for histological examination in any case of doubt.

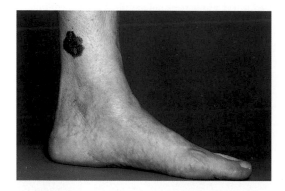

Figure L.5 Malignant melanoma of the leg with commencing ulceration.

A malignant melanoma may ulcerate and bleed (Fig. L.5). Soft tissue or bone carcinomas may, at a late stage, fungate through the skin and give rise to an irregular breaking-down mass.

Harold Ellis

LIBIDO, EXCESSIVE

The desire for sexual intercourse in humans is a biological variable which, like everything else, goes from the diminutive to the excessive. There is no doubt that some people are constitutionally extremely interested in sex and demonstrate excessive libido. The causes of excessive libido are listed in Table L.1.

Females may show excessive libido during the manic phase of a manic-depressive psychosis. Precocious puberty in a boy (see p. 563) or a girl may lead to a libido which is excessive for that individual, in that it is inappropriate for the age. A similar situation may be found in untreated congenital adrenal hyperplasia, commonly due to a 21-hydroxylase deficiency, when there is a build up of androgens in the adrenal. The result is raised testosterone levels in boys and girls, with penile and clitoral enlargement.

Table L.1 Causes of excessive libido

Male	Female
Constitutional	Constitutional
Psychological	Psychological
Rapists	Nymphomaniacs
Psychopaths	Manic phase of manic–depressive psychosis
	Menopause
Hormonal	Hormonal
Precocious puberty	Precocious puberty
Adrenogenital syndrome	Adrenogenital syndrome
	Androgen-secreting tumour of adrenal or ovary
	Polycystic ovarian disease
	Androgen therapy
Infections	Infections
Tuberculosis	Tuberculosis
Drugs	Drugs
Alcohol (in small doses)	Alcohol (in small doses)
	Following opioid or benzodiazepine withdrawal

Since androgens are important in maintaining libido in women, any situation in which a woman is exposed to excess androgens may promote excessive libido. These include androgen administration, the polycystic ovary syndrome (p. 302) or the very rare case of androgen-secreting tumour of the adrenal or ovary.

Most infections tend to reduce libido, but curiously it was noticed in both sexes, at a time when chronic tuberculosis was rife, that patients were prone to an increase in their sexuality. Whether this was a true effect of the disease is unknown.

Alcohol may stimulate libido in both sexes in small doses, but larger amounts – particularly if taken chronically – tend to depress libido. Some cases of increased libido in women have been described following opioid or benzodiazepine withdrawal.

Sharon O'Byrne

LIBIDO, LOSS OF

Libido is the desire to have sexual intercourse. It is promoted by androgens in both male and female, being derived largely from the testes in men and from the adrenal glands in women. Thus, hypothalamic or pituitary disease, which reduces gonadotrophin levels in men or adrenocorticotrophic hormone in women, will deprive each sex respectively of their main source of androgen. Similarly, testicular disease or damage in a male or Addison's disease in a female will achieve the same effect.

A reduction in gonadotrophins may occur in chronic alcoholics. In addition, cirrhosis of the liver gives rise to an increased oestrogen:testosterone (O:T) ratio in a male, which may also lead to a reduction in libido. Similarly, an increased O:T ratio is found in thyrotoxicosis. Oestrogen treatment or down-regulation of gonadotrophins by long-acting gonadotrophin-releasing hormone analogues in the treatment of carcinoma of the prostate lead to a loss of libido.

Hyperprolactinaemia may give rise to a reduction in libido in men by reducing the secretion of gonadotrophins, and by blocking the action of gonadotrophins on the testes. The cause of hyperprolactinaemia may be a pituitary tumour (prolactinoma) or other hypothalamic and pituitary disease leading to lack of prolactin inhibiting factor. Raised prolactin levels may also be found in primary hypothyroidism and renal failure and as a result of drug therapy (Table L.2). Anti-androgens used in the treatment of benign prostatic hypertrophy or carcinoma may also lead to a loss of libido.

Psychological problems are important as causes of loss of libido. Some people just have naturally low levels of libido, whilst others are anxious or depressed. The effect of childhood sexual abuse and rape on future sexual behaviour has not been fully evaluated. This may be a significant cause of loss of libido, particularly in women. Local causes of dyspareunia such as median episiotomy scar, previous pelvic surgery and relaxed vaginal outlet secondary to multiple vaginal deliveries can give rise to reduced sexual enjoyment for women and, in the latter case, for both partners. Diminished libido has been documented in women taking alpha- and beta-blockers and opiates.

Sharon O'Byrne

Table L.2 Causes of loss of libido

Condition	Mechanism	Condition	Mechanism
Male		**Female**	
Endocrine		*Endocrine*	
Hypothalamic disease	Low gonadotrophins and TSH	Hypothalamic disease	Reduced ACTH
Pituitary disease	Raised prolactin	Pituitary disease	
Thyrotoxicosis	Raised oestrogen: testosterone ratio	Hypothyroidism	Psychomotor retardation, lethargy
Hypothyroidism	Psychomotor retardation, lethargy, raised prolactin		Decreased secretion of androgens
Cushing's disease	Decreased luteinizing hormone	Addison's disease	Decreased adrenal androgens
Feminizing tumour of testis or adrenal	Oestrogen secretion	*Psychological*	
Testicular disease or castration	Reduced testosterone	Depression	?
Ageing	Reduced testosterone	Anxiety	
	Increased prolactin	*Drugs*	
		Cyproterone acetate	Anti-androgen
General disease		Alpha- and beta-blockers	
General debilitating disease (e.g. chronic infection, cancer)	? Psychological	Opiates	
Chronic alcoholism	Reduced gonadotrophins	Chronic alcohol excess	
	Testicular damage	*Systemic disease*	
Cirrhosis of the liver	Raised oestrogen: testosterone ratio	Pelvic and breast neoplasms	Raised prolactin
		Myocardial infarction	
Renal failure	General debility	Renal failure	
	Raised prolactin	Irritable bowel syndrome	
Psychological		*Infections*	
Idiopathic lack of sexual desire	?	Vaginitis:	
Depression		*Trichomonas*	
Anxiety		Yeasts	
Drugs		Bacteria	
Gonadotrophin-releasing hormone analogues	Reduced gonadotrophins	Pelvic inflammatory disease	
Oestrogens	Raised oestrogen: testosterone ratio	HIV	Advanced AIDS giving rise to ovarian failure
	Reduced gonadotrophins	*Local*	
	Increased prolactin	Dyspareunia	
Cytotoxic agents ⎫		Endometriosis	
Alcohol ⎭	Testicular damage	Menopause	Vaginal dryness secondary to oestrogen deficiency
Phenothiazines ⎫			Atrophy of urogenital tissue
Metoclopramide		Episiotomy scarring	
Haloperidol		Post-radiation vaginal atrophy	
Pimozide ⎬	Hyperprolactinaemia	Vulvitis	
Methyldopa		Infection of Bartholin's gland	
Reserpine		Hymenal obstruction	
Cimetidine ⎭		Pelvic surgery	
Spironolactone ⎫		Relaxed vaginal musculature secondary to multiple pregnancies	Reduced sexual enjoyment
Cimetidine			
Cyproterone acetate ⎬	Anti-androgens		
Flutamide			
Finasteride ⎭			

LIPS, AFFECTIONS OF

The lips form an important mucocutaneous junction, and their proper function is important for feeding and communication. They are subserved by a very large quantity of nerves, and hence inflammation can cause disproportionate irritation and pain. The lips are also of considerable cosmetic, psychological and emotional importance (see Table L.3).

Table L.3 Affections of the lips

Macules	Melkersson–Rosenthal
Flat mole (junctional naevus)	syndrome
Freckle (ephelide)	Crohn's disease
Peutz–Jegher's syndrome	
Telangiectasis	**Erosions**
■ Hereditary haemorrhagic	Impetigo
telangiectasia	Herpes simplex
■ Liver disease	Hand-foot-and-mouth disease
	Secondary syphilis
Papules	Erythema multiforme
Plane warts	Fixed drug eruption
Lichen planus	Zinc deficiency
Discoid lupus erythematosus	Acrodermatitis enteropathica
Pyogenic granuloma	Pemphigus
Venous lake	
Syphilitic chancre	**Thickening**
Actinic cheilitis	Atopic dermatitis
■ Solar keratosis	Lip-rubbing
■ Squamous-cell carcinoma	
	Cheilitis
Swollen lips	Candidiasis
Trauma, thermal insult	Contact dermatitis
Angio-oedema	Lip-licking

Macular affections (see p. 425) around the lips include flat *moles*, *freckles* and the multiple tiny dark freckles seen in *Peutz–Jegher's syndrome*. Multiple lip telangiectases are seen in *hereditary haemorrhagic telangiectasia* (see p. 32) and sometimes with severe liver disease.

The most common papules on lips are probably plane *warts*, but *lichen planus* papules have a predilection for the lips, as do plaques of *discoid lupus erythematosus*. *Pyogenic granuloma* can form at this site, and in older patients *venous lakes* are commonly seen. The lip can be the site of a primary *syphilitic* chancre. *Actinic cheilitis is* common on the lower lip, especially in seafarers and agricultural workers. The appearance

is of atrophy with greyish plaques often surmounted by crusts in cold weather. *Solar keratoses* appear and invasive *squamous-cell carcinoma* must be detected early, as metastases can quickly occur. *Molluscum contagiosum* and *viral warts* may occur on the lips in people with immunosuppression from HIV infection.

Swollen lips can follow trauma and thermal insult, or be part of an *urticaria*, as *angio-oedema* (see p. 791). The *Melkersson–Rosenthal syndrome* comprises permanently oedematous thickened lips (granulomatous cheilitis) with recurrent facial palsy and scrotal tongue. Granulomatous cheilitis is occasionally seen in Crohn's disease. Thickening of the skin around the mouth (rather than swelling) is a characteristic feature of *atopic dermatitis* due to rubbing of the lips with the backs of the hands.

Erosions on the lips occur in acute infections such as *impetigo* in children, *herpes simplex*, which may be recurrent in adults, *hand-foot-and-mouth disease* and secondary *syphilis*. Erosive dermatoses which affect the lips include *erythema multiforme* (Stevens–Johnson syndrome; see p. 181) and *fixed drug eruption* (codeine and sulphonamides). Cocaine smoking is a direct cause of lip erosions. Chronic erosions around the lips are seen in *zinc deficiency*, *acrodermatitis enteropathica* and *perrophigus* (see p. 722).

When inflammation is confined to the lips, a search should be made for occult *candidiasis*, especially in those with dentures and iron deficiency. Exfoliative cheilitis may occur in patients with HIV infection and oral candidiasis. Chronic *contact dermatitis* can occur at this site – for example, nickel dermatitis from sucking hairpins, lipstick dermatitis, toothpaste dermatitis and, rather surprisingly, nail varnish dermatitis. Irritation from excessive *lip-licking* can often be observed in patients with cheilitis, and may sometimes be the primary cause.

Danielle Harari

LIVER, ENLARGEMENT OF

The normal liver is palpable in children, in thin people with lax abdominal muscles, and in those with chronic obstructive airways disease. Palpation of the liver is an unreliable indicator of actual liver size, and the most accurate way of determining this is by percussion. Hepatic dullness extends from the 5th intercostal space in the right nipple line to the 7th intercostal space in the midaxillary line with a span of about 12 cm.

In health, the edge of the liver is firm and uniform and the surface feels smooth. If the liver is transposed, the right lobe is small and the left large. A tongue-like projection of the right lobe may protrude from its lower right-hand part. This projection, known as *Riedel's lobe*, is more common in women than in men. It may cause difficulty of diagnosis, being confused with a mobile kidney, gall bladder or tumour.

Many conditions that are unconnected with the liver cause an apparent alteration in its size. In emphysema, the liver is easily palpable but percussion will reveal that the organ is merely displaced. Deformities of the chest due to rickets or curvature of the spine may depress the liver, as may a right subphrenic abscess. It is unusual for enlargement of the liver to lead to upward extension of hepatic dullness because the weight of the liver causes it to descend. Elevation of the upper limit of hepatic dullness occurs when local hepatic disease involves the diaphragm (amoebic abscess, hydatid cyst). Loss of hepatic dullness occurs in emphysema, principally because of displacement of the liver. Free gas in the peritoneum or distension of the colon may also do this.

Hepatoptosis or *wandering liver* are terms applied to a liver which is found in an abnormal position. This is rare, but it does occur after therapeutic pneumoperitoneum at laparoscopy. It is usually an asymptomatic condition, although the patient may complain of a dragging sensation and heaviness in the right upper quadrant of the abdomen. The liver which is displaced may be thought to be enlarged.

Hepatomegaly is a feature of acute hepatitis whether of infectious (hepatitis A, B, C, E; cytomegalovirus, Epstein–Barr virus, herpes simplex, toxoplasma), toxic (alcohol, medications, plant toxins), metabolic (haemachromatosis, Wilson's disease, fatty liver of pregnancy) or auto-immune disease. Such hepatic enlargement is often tender and is associated with jaundice with fever. This common constellation of signs and symptoms can often lead to less common conditions being misdiagnosed.

Vascular causes of acute hepatomegaly are uncommon. Acute onset of jaundice, hepatomegaly and ascites are the cardinal features of Budd–Chiari syndrome, thrombosis of the hepatic veins that may occur due to a hypercoagulable state (hormonal medication, malignancy, genetic clotting abnormalities) or a vascular web at the junction of the hepatic vein/inferior vena cava.

Venous congestion secondary to right heart failure, tricuspid incompetence or constrictive pericarditis may result in tender, pulsatile hepatomegaly with peripheral oedema, ascites, jaundice and markedly raised jugular venous pressure (JVP). Ischaemic hepatitis with transaminases activities raised into the thousands of units is a well-recognized complication of heart surgery. Veno-occlusive disease of the liver is an increasingly recognized condition that is caused by ingestion of plants in the form of drinks ('bush-tea') and chewing (kava). Sickle-cell crisis and malaria-associated haemolysis are further causes of tender hepatomegaly.

Infiltration by cancer (non-Hodgkin's lymphoma, secondary deposits, sarcoma) or the onset of primary hepatoma in patients with pre-existing cirrhosis due to chronic viral hepatitis (HBV, HCV), alcohol or haemochromatosis, is often tender. The co-existence of splenomegaly or the detection of lymphadenopathy may indicate lymphoma. Metastatic neuroendocrine gut tumours (formerly known as carcinoid tumours) are associated with the symptoms of the carcinoid syndrome, namely facial flushing, asthma, diarrhoea, valvular heart disease (pulmonary stenosis) and abdominal cramps.

Infiltrative conditions such as sarcoid, amyloid and fatty liver tend to give rise to non-tender hepatomegaly. So-called 'fatty liver' (steatosis) is a common condition found particularly in those with diabetes, hyperlipidaemia, alcoholism, obesity, jejuno-ileal bypass or, paradoxically, protein malnutrition. Although usually benign, it can give rise to significant hepatitis that has been labelled non-alcoholic steatohepatitis (NASH) and non-alcoholic fatty liver (NAFL). An acute form of this condition is fatty liver of pregnancy, which occurs in the third trimester and may be fatal. Hepatic sarcoid is of little clinical consequence to the liver, but it may indicate other visceral involvement such as myocardial infiltration, particularly in Afro-Caribbean Americans, and carries a poor prognosis.

In addition to viral disease, the liver is also a target for other infections such as tuberculosis, schistosomiasis, malaria, kala-azar, hydatid disease (Fig. L.6), liver flukes and *Ascaris lumbricoides* (biliary ducts) and syphilis. In most of these conditions the hepatomegaly is firm and non-tender, while with syphilis it is nodular. Acute painful hepatomegaly occurs during the crises of malaria. With schistosomiasis, presinusoidal portal hypertension causes splenomegaly, and oesophageal varices develop. Hepatic synthetic function is maintained until a late stage, and jaundice

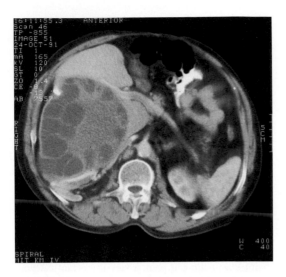

Figure L.6 Multiple cysts of the liver due to hydatid disease.

is relatively mild. Acute bacterial infections and abscesses may arise due to seeding from elsewhere, such as the appendix or diverticular disease, or from biliary obstruction (primary sclerosing cholangitis).

An amoebic abscess may be single and large. It commonly follows a history of dysentery, and the majority occur in the right lobe. Men are affected more often than women. The patient presents with swinging pyrexia, associated with rigors and tachycardia, a considerably enlarged and very tender liver, and there may also be a sympathetic pleural effusion. These abscesses can be slow to reveal themselves, and often require repeated ultrasound scans to be diagnosed. Disseminated visceral *Candida* affecting the liver is a well-recognized complication of the early post-chemotherapy period when granulocyte counts are recovering.

Large hydatid cysts can occur within the liver, but these are usually asymptomatic and cause no disturbance of liver function. The cysts may achieve considerable size, they are rounded and smooth, and there may be a thrill perceived on percussion (ballottment). The diagnosis is made by plain abdominal X-ray if the cysts are calcified. Ultrasound appearances are extremely characteristic, and daughter cysts are often seen. Needle aspiration is contraindicated because this may cause infection and spillage of cysts within the peritoneal cavity. The Casoni test is usually positive.

Simple cysts of the liver are very common and usually go undetected. They can be associated with cysts of the kidney and pancreas in polycystic disease and

Von Hippel–Lindau syndrome. Giant cysts can cause significant chronic symptoms due to their size, or rarely acute pain due to internal haemorrhage. Aspiration is of no value in treating these cysts, as they recur.

Hepatic haemangiomas are common and generally are of no clinical consequence other than for causing confusion on the interpretation of scans. Both fibro-lamellar tumours and hepatic adenomas are well recognized; adenomas are associated with pregnancy and the use of oestrogens.

A variety of metabolic, genetic and endocrine disorders are associated with the development of hepatomegaly. *Glycogen storage diseases* cause hepatomegaly from birth. Lipid storage disorders such as *Gaucher's disease* are associated with massive hepatosplenomegaly and growth retardation, while *Niemann–Pick disease* may have neurological associations, including mental retardation.

Haemochromatosis is an autosomal recessive disorder of iron metabolism. The disease is rare in premenopausal women because of menstrual blood loss. The liver is firm and considerably enlarged. There may be evidence of portal hypertension including splenomegaly and ascites, while a proportion of patients present for the first time with a variceal haemorrhage. Iron is also deposited in the skin, producing a dusky, slate-grey pigmentation. Deposition also occurs in endocrine glands, accounting for the common association with diabetes ('bronze diabetes'). Marked feminization manifests as gynaecomastia, whilst absent body hair, testicular atrophy and a decreased need for shaving are prominent features. Iron deposition in other endocrine glands (pituitary, adrenals, etc.) leads to deficiency states, and joint disease is a common finding. Although relatively unusual, the diagnosis of haemochromatosis is important because the prognosis is greatly improved by venesection. Massive hepatomegaly associated with haemochromatosis may be due to the development of hepatocellular cancer, which is a relatively common late complication.

Wilson's disease is an autosomal recessive condition leading to the accumulation of copper, particularly in the liver and brain. The golden rings of copper deposited in Descemet's membrane of the eyes seen on slit-lamp examination (Kayser–Fleischer rings) are diagnostic of central nervous system involvement. Blue lunula may be seen on examination of the hands.

Acromegaly is associated with hepatomegaly, without evidence of liver dysfunction. The liver is modestly enlarged, but soft. Thyrotoxicosis may also be associated with hepatic enlargement and deranged liver function tests.

Diagnostic investigations

The investigation of hepatomegaly usually involves an ultrasound scan with additional information being contributed by CT and MRI. In cases of hepatomegaly, the liver blood tests are rarely helpful, with most causes giving a slight rise in alkaline phosphatase and possibly gamma-glutamyl transaminase. Serum tumour markers such as carcinoembryonic antigen (colon), alpha-fetoprotein (testicular cancer, primary hepatoma) and CA19.9 (pancreas) may provide some indication of the primary site of a supposed metastatic cancer. Serum angiotensin-converting enzyme activity is raised in the case of a sarcoidosis. Specific antibody tests are available to identify infectious agents.

The introduction of genetic tests has transformed the diagnosis of haemochromatosis. Cases may be suspected on finding a raised serum ferritin or the combination of a raised serum iron with a paradoxically low total iron binding capacity. Whereas liver biopsy, with a Pearl's stain for iron, was required in the past, a blood test for carriage of the C282Y;H63D gene is now the investigation of choice. CT and MRI assessment of iron stores have been used in specialized centres. Wilson's disease is diagnosed on the basis of a low serum caeruloplasmin level (carrier protein for copper) and either raised hepatic iron, excessive urinary copper excretion or the presence of Kayser–Fleischer rings.

Neuroendocrine tumours giving rise to the carcinoid syndrome can be detected by urinary measurement of 5-hydroxy indole acetic acid (5-HIAA).

Liver biopsy is a generally safe procedure that can be carried out either 'blindly' or under ultrasound guidance. The platelet count and International Normalized Ratio (INR) must be checked prior to the procedure in order to identify possible coagulopathy. If a coagulopathy is present, then a transjugular approach may be safest.

John Meenan

LORDOSIS

See SPINE, DEFORMITY OF (p. 659).

LOWER LIMB, PAIN IN

The presenting features of disease and injury of the lower limb are pain, deformity, diminished movement, weakness, numbness, swelling, instability and limp. Of these features, pain is by far the most common. Therefore, this section is subdivided into regions according to the presentation of pain. The first section concerns radicular pain referred from the spine and the differential diagnosis from vascular pain, both of which can affect the whole leg. Other sections subsequently consider pain arising from local causes mostly of a musculoskeletal origin: buttock pain; pain in the groin and front of the thigh – classically the site of hip joint pain; knee pain; calf pain, a very important category since the differential includes causes both life- and limb-threatening deep-vein thrombosis, critical arterial ischaemia and compartment syndromes; ankle pain; and foot pain concluding with foot deformities.

Leg pain of radicular or vascular origin

This section deals specifically with the causes of pain referred into the limb arising from local lesions rather than generalized diseases. The subdivision of the section is largely anatomical, but nerve root compression ('sciatica'), ischaemia (intermittent claudication) and spinal stenosis (spinal claudication), which are responsible for a large proportion of pain in the buttock and leg, are considered separately first.

Sciatica

Sciatica is a term hallowed by common usage, both in the lay population and by doctors, but unfortunately it means a multiplicity of different things and is therefore probably a term to be avoided. Asking the question 'Is there any evidence that the patient has nerve root compression?' is much more valuable. If the term is used, it should be restricted to those cases in which there is definite evidence of involvement of the sciatic nerve or one of its component roots. For example, pain which radiates from the lower back to the buttock and down the back of the thigh to the knee is quite commonly found in patients with a spondylolisthesis, who do not show any evidence of nerve root compression. Restrict 'sciatica' to a pain that radiates from the back down through the buttock, down the back of the thigh and down to the ankle or foot, passing along either the lateral or posterior aspect of the calf and aggravated by coughing or sneezing, together with the presence of nerve root tension signs, e.g. a positive straight leg raising test. Objective motor signs, such as loss of the ankle jerk (S1) or weakness of extension of the big toe (L5; extensor hallucis longus), are much more reliable in defining which nerve root is involved than sensory loss. Unfortunately for the clinician – but fortunately for the patient – radicular pain of recent onset is usually not accompanied by any objective neurological signs.

While lumbar degenerative disc disease and spondylosis account for the vast majority of cases of backache and referred pain into the legs, other lesions can be associated with pain on coughing, a positive Laségue's straight leg raising test and a positive l'Hermitte's sign – a surge of paraesthesia down the trunk into the limbs on forward flexion of the neck. Examples include multiple sclerosis, sub-acute combined degeneration of the cord, a cervical spinal tumour and cervical spondylosis causing cord compression.

The most common cause of radicular referred pain is a *posterolateral disc protusion* at the L4/5 or L5/S1 level. Classic disc disease is episodic, and often first presents in early adult life, being frequently precipitated by a 'minor' injury such as lifting a heavy weight. With recurrent episodes, the pain radiates further down the leg and the nerve root tension signs become more evident. However, there may be no such history and symptoms from nerve root compression may be present from the first episode. The lumbar lordosis may be lost or there may be a scoliosis, which becomes more marked on forward flexion. Tenderness is often – but by no means invariably – present at the level of the lesion, and also in the region of the posterior superior iliac spine. A characteristic of mechanical backache is that a good (if not full) range is retained in at least one direction. Areas of reduced sensation to pin prick, weakness and reflex

changes associated with individual root lesions are summarized in Figure L.7 and Table L.4.

Beware of the patient who presents with referred pain into both legs or pain that alternates between the two legs as there may be a *compression of the cauda equina*. In particular, look for loss of sensation in the perianal area, and a loss of anal tone. Fortunately, cauda equina lesions due to a central disc prolapse are uncommon, but the symptoms can be vague and are frequently missed, especially when due to a slowly expanding benign tumour such as a neurofibroma.

Plain X-rays of the lumbar spine are usually unhelpful in diagnosing degenerative causes of symptoms as a

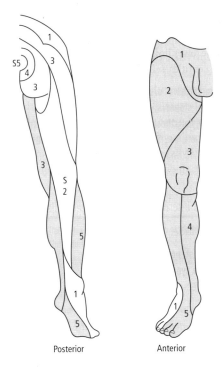

Figure L.7 Areas of reduced sensation to pinprick in lumbosacral root lesions.

Table L.4 Signs associated with common nerve root lesions affecting the legs

Root	Paraesthesiae/numbness	Muscle weakness	Reflex change
L1	Groin	—	—
L2	Front of mid thigh	Quadriceps	—
L3	Front of lower thigh	Quadriceps	Knee ↓
L4	Front of lower thigh, knee and inner aspect of shin	Quadriceps and tibialis anterior	Knee ↓
L5	Back of thigh, lateral aspect of leg, dorsum of foot to big toe	Extensor hallucis longus	—
S1	Back of leg, lateral aspect of foot and sole	Calf wasting and weakness of plantar flexors	Ankle ↓

N.B. It is uncommon to lose a knee jerk due to the dual innervation from L3, L4.

sacroiliac joint, and is an uncommon presentation of hip pathology.

Hip joint disease in children and adolescents

Congenital dislocation of the hip should be diagnosed at birth, when treatment in the majority of cases is not only straightforward but the prognosis is also good. Consequently all practitioners with responsibility for children – doctors, nurses and health visitors – should be able to make this diagnosis. It is good practice to examine the baby's hip more than once, and special care needs to be taken if there is a family history or if there has been a breech delivery. There is a high incidence in communities in which the young are swaddled whereby the hips are kept adducted, and a low incidence in communities in which babies are carried on their mothers backs with the hips abducted. The reason is obvious since the initial treatment requires the hip to be held in flexion and abduction. In unilateral cases, signs include: skin crease asymmetry and restricted abduction in flexion (Fig. L.8); Ortolani's

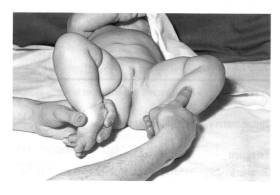

Figure L.8 Congenital dislocation of the right hip. Abduction in flexion is limited.

test demonstrates the click/clunk of reduction, while Barlow's test demonstrates the reverse (i.e. a click as the hip is dislocated). Any 'clicking hips' should be examined with ultrasound, which is the investigation of choice; X-rays are much harder to interpret as the ossific nucleus of the head is not present at birth, but appears during the first year. Bilateral dislocated hips are more difficult to diagnose as there is no asymmetry and both hips have similar restriction of movement. As a consequence, there is a higher incidence of bilateral dislocation presenting late, often when the child starts to walk and the characteristic waddling gait becomes

evident. An additional feature of bilateral dislocation is a markedly increased lumbar lordosis.

Two other conditions (both of which are rare) can produce similar physical signs in the young child. The first is *infantile coxa vara*, in which there is a stress fracture through the neck of femur and as a consequence the leg is short and the hip lacks abduction due to impingement of the greater trochanter on the ilium (Fig. L.9). The head of the femur is, of course, located in the socket. The other condition results from the destruction of the head, consequent upon infection, and is termed *acute epiphysitis of infancy* (Tom Smith's disease) (Fig. L.10). Close inspection will usually reveal a small scar often hidden in the groin, the hallmark of an old sinus, where the abscess plus the destroyed head of the femur was discharged.

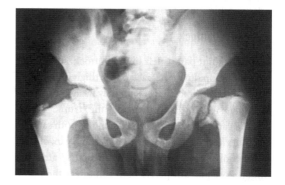

Figure L.9 Conditions with similar signs to a congenital dislocation of the hip. Infantile coxa vara. In the left hip the epiphyseal plate is vertical, a triangular bony fragment is present inferiorly in the neck, and the trochanteric ossification centre is lying proximal (i.e. the head is 'slipping off the neck' and the leg is short).

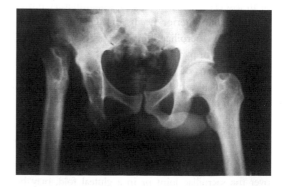

Figure L.10 Conditions with similar signs to congenital dislocation of the hip. Septic arthritis: the end result is loss of the femoral head, and consequently the hip dislocates.

Legg–Calve–Perthe's disease is usually just referred to by the name of the third describer of the condition, Perthe. There is still much dispute concerning the precipitating cause. It is probably multi-factorial, but the common final pathway causes avascular necrosis of the ossific nucleus (Fig. L.11) and consequent deformation of the hip (Fig. L.12). Severe cases are likely to lead to development of osteoarthritis in young adult life (Fig. L.13). Presenting features are a painful limp and restricted hip movement, especially abduction.

Perthe's disease accounts for only a small percentage of children presenting with an *irritable hip* (*transient synovitis*). This affects a similar age group, usually aged 6–12 years, but the symptoms settle rapidly with rest and the hip reverts to normal. Ultrasound shows an effusion within the hip only in a minority of cases. Its importance is merely to distinguish it from other serious diseases such as infection, juvenile rheumatoid arthritis and Perthe's disease.

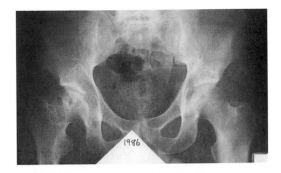

Figure L.13 Same patient as Fig. L.11. By his mid-twenties, changes of osteoarthritis are present with marked cystic changes in the femoral head.

Slipped capital femoral epiphysis occurs around the time of puberty, and therefore presents a little later in boys than in girls. In essence, it is a stress fracture occurring through the growth plate at the level of the hypertrophic cartilage cells. Many of the children are obese (Fig. L.14) or else tall and thin, and it has in the

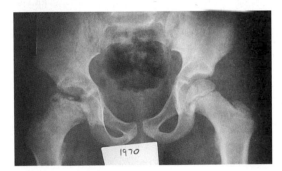

Figure L.11 Legg–Calve–Perthe's disease. Anteroposterior X-ray of the pelvis in a 10-year-old boy who presented with avascular change affecting the whole of the right capital epiphysis. Note the widened joint space, the flattened irregular epiphyseal plate and the widened metaphysis of the neck.

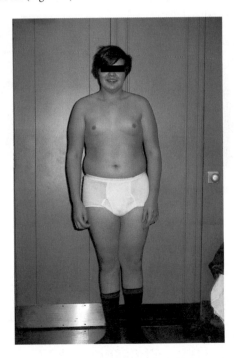

Figure L.14 Slipped capital femoral epiphysis. The typical clinical features in an overweight, sexually immature early teenage boy.

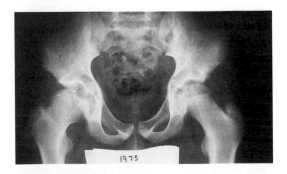

Figure L.12 Same patient as Fig. L.11. Five years later, the hip has healed but with marked deformity.

past been postulated that there could be a hormonal imbalance. However, hormone studies are normal, unless it occurs outside the age group 9–14 years in girls and 11–16 years in boys, when it may be secondary to a pituitary tumour. A slipped epiphysis may present purely with knee pain, and is easy to confuse with the common teenage anterior knee pain secondary to problems in the patellofemoral joint, so never attribute knee pain to the knee in this age group unless you have demonstrated that hip movements are normal. In the early stages, both the symptoms and signs may be subtle. The pain and the limp may only be present on activity, the external rotation deformity of the leg may be very mild as are the loss of hip movements, especially flexion, abduction and internal rotation. Look in particular for increasing external rotation as the hip is flexed. The X-ray changes are easy to miss, especially on the AP film (Figs L.15 and L.16). As the degree of the slip increases, so the signs – including shortening of the leg – become more obvious. If the diagnosis is delayed, then these children are particularly susceptible to a minor injury causing an *acute-on-chronic slip* in which the deformity at the level of epiphyseal plate suddenly increases; indeed, the head and neck can

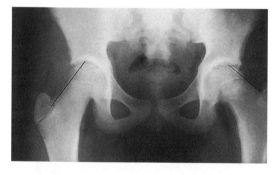

Figure L.15 Same patient as Fig. L.14. Anteroposterior X-ray of the pelvis. In the symptomatic left hip, the epiphyseal plate appears widened and the lateral prominence of the head is reduced as indicated by a line superimposed along the upper border of the femoral neck.

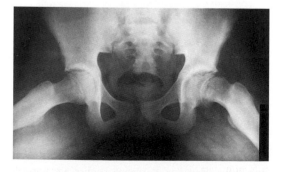

Figure L.16 Same patient as Fig. L.14. The lateral view confirms that the head is no longer centred on the neck, but has 'slipped' posteriorly.

separate as if there had been a fracture. This group is the most difficult to treat and has the highest incidence of avascular necrosis.

Septic arthritis of the hip and *osteomyelitis of the proximal femoral neck* are both important diseases to diagnose and treat before the hip joint is destroyed. Since the capsule of the hip has 'migrated' down the femoral neck, the proximal metaphysis lies within the hip joint. Consequently, pus forming from infection in this region can discharge into the hip, causing secondary septic arthritis. In the classical scenario, a child presents with a high fever and is obviously ill. In modern practice, however, the disease may be less fulminating but, while it may be less lethal, it can still be sufficient to destroy the hip. The error, which the author has seen on a number of occasions, is to mistake this scenario for juvenile rheumatoid arthritis of the hip. To prevent this error, the rule is 'treat the patient for septic arthritis and investigate to determine if it is a juvenile rheumatoid arthritis'. The child will present with pain and limp, or if the infection is severe will not move or use the leg. There is a fever and hip movements are grossly restricted; indeed, any attempt at moving the hip may be very painful. X-rays will be normal since any destruction of bone will not show for 10 days. Take blood cultures in addition to the routine Hb, WBC, differential and ESR and obtain synovial fluid for culture from the hip. With an osteomyelitis, there may merely be a sympathetic effusion in the early stages (N.B. a negative culture does not exclude infection), whereas in septic arthritis organisms will be present. Treatment with the appropriate antibiotic within 48 hours usually leads to resolution. A child presenting later, or whose fever does not settle on antibiotics, requires surgery for two reasons: first, to obtain pus for the diagnosis; and second to decompress the metaphysis by drilling up the femoral neck (under X-ray guidance to prevent damage to the growth plate); or, in the case of a primary septic arthritis, to decompress the hip joint by incising the capsule in addition to obtaining cultures.

Tuberculosis of the hip can be deceptive, and there is often a delay in making the diagnosis, particularly in Western society, now that this disease is uncommon. There is usually weight loss and often night sweats. Hip movements will be restricted in all directions and, characteristically, muscle wasting is often very marked. X-ray changes show a wide variety of patterns, primarily dependent on the initial site of the infection – that is, whether this was a tubercular synovitis, in which case

Table L.7 Causes of hip joint disease

In children and adolescents	
Age	**Disease**
0–5 years	Congenital dislocation of the hip (hip dysplasia)
	Infantile coxa vara
	Acute infective epiphysitis
5–10 years	Legg–Calve–Perthe's disease
10–15 years	Slipped capital femoral epiphysis
At any age	Infection
	■ Acute osteomyelitis of the proximal femur
	■ Septic arthritis of the hip
	■ Tuberculosis
	Inflammatory arthropathy
	■ Juvenile rheumatoid arthritis (Still's disease)

In adults

Traumatic
■ Subcapital and intertrochanteric fractures
Infective
■ Pyogenic septic arthritis
■ Sepsis complicating surgical arthroplasty (e.g. total hip replacement)
■ Tuberculous synovitis and osteomyelitis
Inflammatory arthropathy
■ Rheumatoid arthritis
■ Juvenile rheumatoid arthritis (Still's disease)
■ Ankylosing spondylitis
Degenerative arthropathy
■ Osteoarthritis
■ Osteonecrosis (avascular necrosis)

Other causes

Neurogenic
■ Lumbar root irritation
■ Obturator nerve irritation
■ Meralgia paraesthetica
Abdominal pathology
■ Hernias: inguinal, femoral, obturator
■ Retroperitoneal inflammation
Infective
■ Local abscess
■ Inflamed inguinal lymph nodes
■ Psoas abscess
Tumours
■ Metastatic disease involving the pelvis or proximal femur
■ Primary malignant bone tumours: osteosarcoma, chrondrosarcoma
■ Benign bone tumour and tumour-like conditions
■ Soft tissue tumours: pigmented villonodular synovitis
Muscle and tendon
■ Sprains (e.g. adductor tendon sprain)
■ Haematoma: myositis ossificans
Other pathology
■ Synovial chondromatosis

there may be erosions at the capsular attachment to the bones or a tubercular osteomyelitis.

Table L.7 summarizes the causes of hip joint disease in children and adolescents, and shows the causes in adults.

Hip joint disease in adults

Trauma Subcapital and intertrochanteric fractures of the femoral neck are not only common, but the age-related incidence also continues to rise. The underlying problem is bone fragility due to osteoporosis or osteomalacia, the latter being all too easy to overlook. They often occur after minimal trauma such as a fall or stumble. When the fracture is displaced the signs are obvious, as the leg is shortened and externally rotated and the patient unable to walk. Undisplaced fractures can however be deceptive, and if missed are often a cause of litigation (Figs L.17 and L.18). If the X-ray is inconclusive, obtain a technetium bone scan before discharging an elderly patient suffering groin pain after a fall.

Infection Pyogenic hip infection in an otherwise fit adult is uncommon, but is a 'silent area' for sepsis in intensive care units as it can develop secondary to a femoral artery or a femoral vein puncture; that is, the needle missed the vessel and punctured the hip which lies directly behind the vessels. Occasionally, pyogenic infection complicates an osteoarthritic joint. Adult *tubercular infection* is again on the increase. Surprisingly in the adult, it can be mistaken for

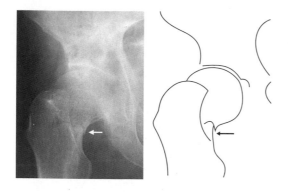

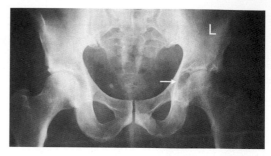

Figure L.19 Tubercular synovitis of left hip. This was initially diagnosed as a monoarticular variant of rheumatoid arthritis. In addition to joint space narrowing, there is a marked bony erosion at the synovial margins, most marked in the acetebular fossa (arrow).

Figure L.17 Sub-capital fracture of the femoral neck. This 70-year-old woman presented with mild groin pain and a limp following a fall. The AP X-ray was erroneously considered normal, though there is a suggestion of a fracture in the calcar (arrows).

Inflammatory arthropathies Whilst *rheumatoid arthritis* predominantly affects the small peripheral joints (e.g. hands, wrists, feet and ankles), the hip is by no means spared, but the diagnosis is usually obvious due to the generality of the disease. Isolated hip joint involvement does occur with other inflammatory arthropathies, especially *ankylosing spondylitis* (see also p. 58). The fixed flexion deformity of the hip is a major contributory factor to these patients' inability to stand erect and to see ahead (Figs B.3 and B.4).

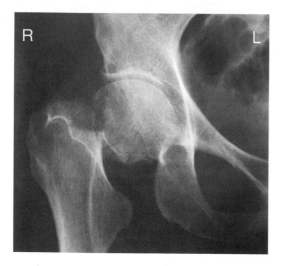

Figure L.18 Same patient as Fig. L.17. Shortly after discharge the patient stumbled and the fracture was displaced.

Degenerative arthropathy In *osteoarthritis*, typically the symptoms of pain and stiffness are slowly progressive, usually over many years. The hip joint in particular has a propensity to cause night pain, which is characteristically felt in the groin with radiation down the front of the thigh. While movements of the joint are restricted in all directions, close inspection will reveal that this is not uniform. Abduction and internal rotation are usually more restricted than adduction and external rotation, although sometimes this pattern may be reversed. A useful clinical definition of an osteoarthritic joint is that there is a free painless arc of movement terminated by painful restriction. X-ray changes are also slowly progressive (Fig. L.20). A patient with X-ray changes which could be mistaken for osteoarthritis but clinically has excessive movement is likely to have a *charcot joint* (Figs L.21 and L.22).

osteoarthritis or rheumatoid arthritis (Fig. L.19). A proper history will reveal the difference. There is often marked gluteal or quadriceps wasting as well as signs of hip irritability, weight loss and night sweats (see section above, Hip pain in children). Radiologically, tubercular synovitis can be confused with pigmented villonodular synovitis, which also causes bone erosion at the synovial margins (see Pain in and around the knee, p. 390). *Chronic infection*, often with sinus formation around a total hip replacement, is a 'new' disease of modern medicine. It is important to establish a precise bacteriological diagnosis for a wide variety of organisms have been implicated. The infection rate for primary hip arthroplasty should be 1 per cent or less.

Beware of the joint presenting with marked muscle spasm and very painful grossly restricted movements. Even if the X-rays show signs of osteoarthritis, this is not the diagnosis until proven otherwise – septic arthritis, gout, chondrocarcinosis (pseudogout) and other inflammatory arthropathies require exclusion.

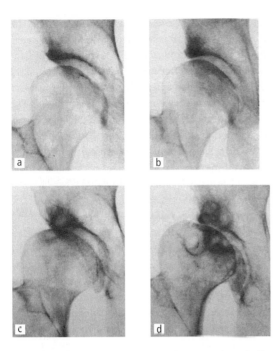

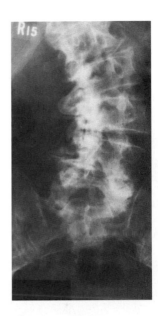

Figure L.22 Same patient as Fig. L.21. Anteroposterior X-ray of the lumbar spine and sacrum.

Figure L.20 Sequential X-ray changes of osteoarthritis of the hip. The earliest feature is an increase in the subchondral sclerosis (a), followed by joint space narrowing (b), cyst formation and osteophytes (c). Note the gradual increase in size of the osteophyte on the medial aspect of the head. (d) Finally, bone erosion, loss of congruity and lateral subluxation of the femoral head. [Pauwels (1976) Biomechanics of the Normal and Diseased Hip, Springer Verlag, Heidelberg. With kind permission of Springer Science and Business Media.]

Interestingly, osteonecrosis always affects the convex side of the joint; other sites are the capitulum, the proximal pole of the scaphoid, the dome of the talus and the navicular. Many diseases are associated with osteonecrosis of the hip, which should therefore never be regarded as a primary diagnosis. The main groups are: trauma, especially following fractures through the femoral neck; alcoholism (Figs L.23–L.25); steroids; haemoglobinopathies (especially sickle-cell disease); Caisson's disease (Fig. L.26); or iatrogenic (i.e. secondary to treatment for childhood congenital dislocation of the hip, adolescent slipped capital femoral epiphysis etc.). In the early stages osteonecrosis can be very

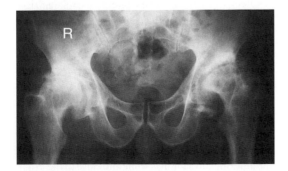

Figure L.21 Charcot joints secondary to tabes dorsalis. Anteroposterior X-ray of the pelvis. Note the wide saucer-shape acetabulum of the left hip. Bone destruction in the right hip is less pronounced, and the features are those of advanced osteoarthritis. Clinically there was, however, excessive movement of both hips.

In *avascular* (*osteonecrosis*) *necrosis* the articular cartilage is normal and the problem is in the underlying bone. The pattern of vascular supply to the head of the femur leaves the hip particularly prone to avascularity.

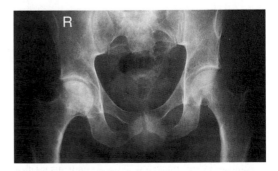

Figure L.23 Osteonecrosis of the right hip secondary to alcoholism in a 30-year-old man. Anteroposterior X-ray showing increased sclerosis of the right femoral head.

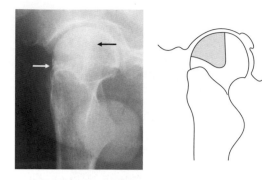

Figure L.24 Same patient as Fig. L.23. Lateral X-ray suggests sclerosis is localized to the anterior aspect of the head (shown between two arrows).

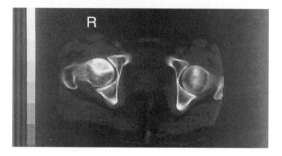

Figure L.25 Same patient as Fig. L.23. The presence of sclerosis is confirmed by a CT scan.

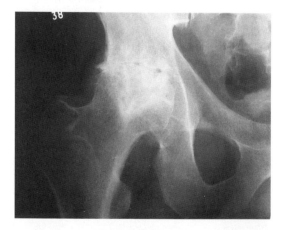

Figure L.26 Caisson's disease. Anteroposterior X-ray of the right hip showing collapse of the femoral head secondary to osteonecrosis following an attack of 'the bends' several years previously.

deceptive for the pain may be mild and atypical, that is, presenting in the thigh, the knee or with discomfort around the greater trochanter rather than groin pain. Movements may be largely preserved, but some restriction will be evident on close inspection. The X-ray in the early stages is often normal and only later does the sclerosis in the femoral head become evident (this is indicative of new bone being laid done on dead trabeculae). A technetium bone scan and an MRI scan are both sensitive investigations in the early stages. The presence of a subchondral fracture through the avascular bone (revealed as the 'crescent sign' on the lateral plain X-ray) is a poor prognostic sign, as this means that the overlying cartilage plus a slither of the subchondral bone plate has separated from the femoral head.

Other conditions causing groin and anterior thigh pain

Radicular pain arising from the nerve roots of the lumbar plexus is much less common than with the sacral plexus, since degenerative back disease is far more frequent at the L4/5 and 5S1 levels than the upper lumbar spine. Indeed, beware of attributing pain to an upper lumbar disc since this is relatively uncommon and there is, therefore, a greater chance of the patient having a more serious entity such as a benign spinal tumour or irritation of the plexus by retroperitoneal pathology with pain radiating down the femoral nerve anteriorly into the thigh. The signs are often subtle. Careful examination may find wasting of the quadriceps. The knee jerk is rarely lost as it has a dual innervation from L3 and L4 (see Table L.4, p. 379).

Obturator nerve irritation produces pain radiating along the inner side of the thigh. It is uncommon, and tends to be associated with serious disease – metastatic disease within the pelvic cavity or within the pelvic bones, especially the pubis. Physical signs are often minimal, but there may be wasting of the adductor group.

Meralgia paraesthetica is common, but frequently missed. It is due to entrapment of the lateral cutaneous nerve of the thigh, where it exits through the deep fascia, just distal to the inguinal ligament below the anterior superior iliac spine and close to the origin of the sartorius. The pain is often rather diffuse, but careful testing usually reveals an area of numbness anterolaterally and there is often a tender spot at the exit point of the nerve through the deep fascia. Long-acting local anaesthetic injections to this site will not only confirm the diagnosis but are also often curative.

Local causes of infection in the groin, including *lymphadenitis of the inguinal nodes,* usually have obvious signs. Inspect the leg for a possible primary source of infection and, if present, remember to check for diabetes. The incidence of *spinal tuberculosis* is rising rapidly due to the HIV/AIDS epidemic, and one can expect the incidence of psoas abscess will once again increase. The spinal pathology is usually at the thoracic lumbar junction with the caseous material tracking along the psoas sheath to the groin.

By far the most common *tumours* causing pain around the hip and down the thigh are metastases, destroying either part of the pelvis or the proximal femur. A useful rule states that 'if 50 per cent of the femoral cortex is involved, then there is a 50 per cent chance of fracture'. *Primary malignant tumours of bone* are very uncommon, but when they do occur the region of the hip joint is the second most common site after the knee. Chondrosarcomas in particular arise from the flat bones, the pelvis and the scapula, often from a pre-existing exostosis. Consequently, any change in size in an exostosis in adult life needs urgent investigation. Chondrosarcomas are slow growing and usually affect the 30- to 50-year age group (see Pain in and around the knee, p. 390). *Pigmented villonodular synovitis*, which is now classified as a benign soft tissue neoplasm (see Pain in and around the knee: Arthropathies, p. 395), presents as a low-grade inflammatory condition. In the hip, it can mimic rheumatoid arthritis and tuberculous synovitis due to the presence of periarticular erosions on X-ray. Eventually the repeated haemarthroses lead to severe osteoarthritis.

Muscle and tendon sprains around the hip are common, especially in athletes. Strains of the attachments of the adductors are probably the most frequent, but all muscle groups including the psoas are at risk. *Small inguinal hernias* are the main differential diagnosis. *Myositis ossificans* (Figs L.27 and L.28) results from a direct blow to the thigh and consequent ossification of a haematoma in vastus intermedius. The loss of knee flexion distinguishes it from a malignant bone tumour in which knee mobility is retained (see Pain in and around the knee, p. 390). The condition resolves over several months. Myositis ossificans is a well-recognized complication of hip surgery, especially incisions that damage the periosteum of the outer iliac wall. The abductors, gluteus medius and minimus are the most frequent sites. Minor degrees resolve, but when severe, loss of hip movement is permanent without further surgery.

The hip is the third most common joint, after the knee and elbow, to be affected by synovial

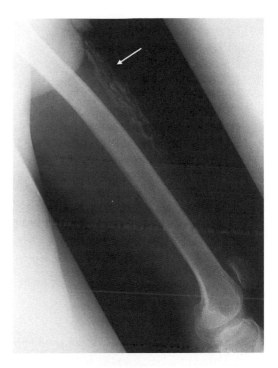

Figure L.27 Myositis ossificans of the left quadriceps femoris in a 22-year-old man. Lateral X-ray of the left thigh. There is an area of ossification lying anteriorally over the mid shaft of the femur. Note the area of separation between the myositis ossificans and the femur.

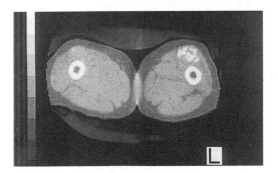

Figure L.28 Same patient as Fig. L.27. The ossification is more clearly seen on the CT scan.

chondromatosis (Figs L.29 and L.30). It usually presents as a mild synovitis, with a tendency for the hip to give way. Actual locking is uncommon. CT and MRI scans will clearly delineate loose bodies which are easy to overlook on plain X-rays.

Pain in and around the knee

The knee is a complex joint both as regards: (i) its anatomy – in practical terms, it is composed of three

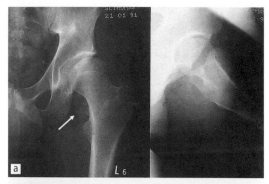

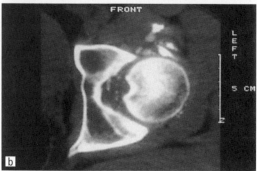

Figure L.29 (a) Synovial chondromatosis of the left hip. Anteroposterior and lateral X-rays of the left hip. Numerous loose bodies are present. (b) Loose bodies are confirmed by CT scanning; the majority appear to be lying anteriorly, but some are present deep within the joint.

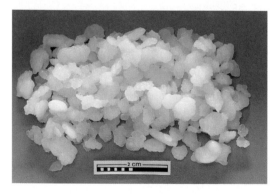

Figure L.30 Synovial chondamatosis of the knee. Numerous small cartilaginous loose bodies approximately 3–5 mm in size, found at a diagnostic arthroscopy for chronic synovitis in a 22-year-old man. The X-ray was normal.

joints, the patellofemoral joint and the medial and lateral compartments of the tibiofemoral joint; (ii) its mechanics; and (iii) the presenting diseases/injuries which together cover almost the entire range of

musculoskeletal conditions. The objective in taking the history is to narrow the options. White's schema (see Table L.8) includes the six most common categories of knee problems is a helpful practical approach. There are numerous specialized physical signs, and a good history will enable one to select the correct set. All patients should be examined standing to observe any malalignment (Figs L.31 and L.32), walking to observe the gait pattern, and then lying down on a firm couch (examining the knee on a soft bed makes it much more difficult to determine whether there is loss of extension; this is an important physical sign as full extension is a requisite for normal knee function).

Two warnings! First, the knee and the hip are supplied by the same nerves and hence hip pathology can present purely with knee pain. The classic condition in this respect is slipped capital femoral epiphysis of the teenager. It is all to easy to dismiss this as teenage anterior knee pain. Second, ensure that any pathology found on special investigations such as arthroscopy and MRI scans actually matches the patient's symptoms. Degenerative change affecting the menisci and the patellofemoral joint is almost universal over the age of 40 years, and the consequent changes on scans usually lie within the spectrum of normality.

Internal derangement (locked/locking knee)

The characteristic of these knees is that they suddenly jam and the joint cannot fully extend. The most common cause is meniscal tears, followed by loose bodies, while chondral flaps are relatively uncommon and have only been appreciated since the advent of arthroscopy. Transient episodes of 'catching', in which the fragment catches then releases, often present as 'giving way'. A locked knee needs to be distinguished from other acute causes of loss of extension such as a haemarthrosis or acute arthritis, especially gout or pseudo-gout (chondrocalcinosis). A more difficult differential is from a patellar dislocation. There are two main types of meniscal tear: vertical tears, which occur through a normal meniscus; and horizontal cleavage tears, which are found in a wearing meniscus. A third meniscal syndrome, the degenerative or immobile meniscus, presents with pain without locking.

Vertical meniscal tears (Fig. L.33), which occur more frequently in the medial than the lateral meniscus, are usually secondary to a twisting injury sustained while playing sports. As with other knee injuries, they are

Table L.8 The six categories of knee pain (after White, S., *Arthritis and Rheumatism Council for Research: Practical Problems No. 10, Series 3 'The Assessment and Management of Knee Problems'*)

1 Internal derangement/ 'locked' knee	Meniscus − vertical tears − horizontal cleavage tears − degenerate medial meniscus syndrome	Loose bodies − osteochondral fractures − osteochondritis dissecans − synovial chrondromatosis − osteoarthritis	Articular surface irregularity − chondral flaps − osteoarthritis with severe eburnation	
2 Ligament injuries	Medial collateral complete tears − partial tears	Lateral collateral − complete tears − iliotibial band avulsion	Anterior cruciate	Posterior cruciate
3 Arthropathies	Osteoarthritis: varus knee (medial compartment)	Osteoarthritis: valgus knee (lateral compartment) Haemophilia	Inflammatory arthropathies − rheumatoid arthritis − chondrocalcinosis gout	Repeated haemarthroses Pigmented villonodular synovitis Haemophilia Haemangiomas Anticoagulants and osteoarthritis
4 Patellofemoral derangement/ extensor mechanism injuries	Anterior knee pain syndrome Chondromalacia patellae Lateral hyperpressure syndrome	Patellar instability − subluxation − dislocation − acute − recurrent − habitual − permanent	Extensor mechanism injuries/ stress conditions − Osgood−Schlatter's disease − ruptured patellar tendon − Johanssen−Larsen syndrome/ jumper's knee − patellar fractures − quadriceps femoris injuries − myositis ossificans	
5 Infection/tumours/ tumour-like conditions	Pyogenic infection − septic arthritis − osteomyelitis	Chronic infection − tuberculosis − infected arthroplasty − Brodie's abscess	Tumours A. Malignant − osteosarcoma − Ewing's sarcoma − chondrosarcoma B. Benign − osteoclastoma − osteochondroma − chondromablastoma enchondroma − chondromyxoid fibroma	Tumour-like conditions − fibrous cortical defect − non-ossifying fibroma − fibrous dysplasia − osteoid osteoma − osteoblastoma − unicameral bone cyst − aneurysmal bone cyst − osteitis fibrosa cystica
6 Bursitis/cysts/tendinitis	Bursitis − prepatellar − infrapatellar, etc.	Cysts − semi- membranosus − Baker's cyst − meniscal	Tendinitis − iliotibial band insertion − pes anserinus insertion − semi-membranosis insertion − bicep's femoris insertion	

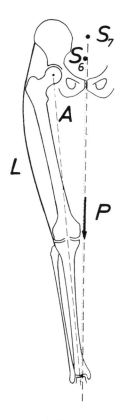

Figure L.31 Maquet diagram. In the normal lower limb, the hip, knee and ankle lie on a straight line (the mechanical axis), and the transverse plane of the knee lies parallel to the ground when standing on one leg. S6: Centre of gravity of the body. S7: Centre of gravity of the part of the body supported by the knee when standing an one leg. P: Weight of this part of the body. L: Muscle/tension band balancing P. [Maquet (1984) Biomechanics of the knee, second edition, Springer-Verlag. With kind permission of Springer Science and Business Media.]

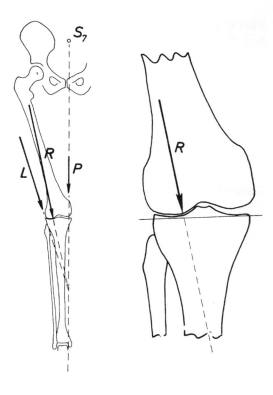

Figure L.32 If the leg deviates into varus (bow leg) or valgus (knock knee), the balance of the normal forces across the joint is lost; this results in an increased stress in the medial or lateral compartments respectively and an increased risk of developing osteoarthritis. R is the resultant force acting through the lateral compartment in this example of a valgus osteoarthritic knee.

much more common in men than women, although there is a rising incidence in the latter now that girls have started to play football and even rugby. Vertical tears usually begin on the inferior aspect of the meniscus in the posterior horn. With recurrent injuries the tear spreads, until eventually the loose fragment – the 'bucket handle' – becomes sufficiently mobile to displace into the intercondylar notch and hence lock the knee. In keeping with the pathology, the classical history is one of recurrent episodes of pain affecting the medial side of the knee precipitated by a twist and usually accompanied by a transient effusion. Symptoms settle over a few days and sports can then be resumed. As the tear enlarges, so less trauma is required to produce symptoms and patients often complain

that the joint feels insecure. Eventually giving way on minor provocation occurs, followed finally by true locking. Examination between episodes may fail to reveal any abnormality. When symptomatic, there is usually a small effusion, tenderness is present along the appropriate joint line, and tibial rotation is painful. The classical special manoeuvre is the McMurray test (tibial rotation with the joint under compression) in which the examiner endeavours to reproduce not just the pain but also a 'clunk' as the meniscal fragment dislocates. Check, in particular, the integrity of the ligaments as the meniscus is at much greater risk of being torn if the knee is unstable.

Horizontal cleavage tears occur in older age groups, generally 30–60 years. By comparison with the vertical tears, the initial trauma is less severe; indeed, the patient may have no recollection of any significant trauma. Otherwise the history is similar with recurrent episodes,

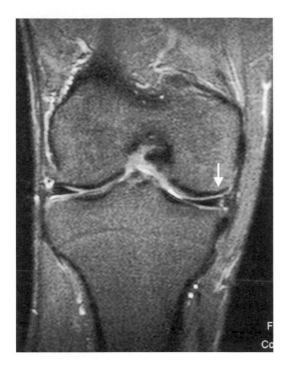

Figure L.33 MRI scan showing a peripheral undisplaced 'bucket handle' tear of the medial meniscus (arrow).

usually precipitated by a minor twist. The tear gradually increases, and eventually a 'parrot beak flap' can dislocate between the condyles causing locking or giving way.

A very different presentation of the wearing meniscus is the *immobile* or *degenerative medial meniscus syndrome*. This is also usually precipitated by a minor twisting injury in late middle age (50–65 years), but symptoms are often persistent and aggravated by the slightest twist, for example, going around a corner. If severe, it may be accompanied by giving way, but there is no mechanical history of locking. The medial joint line is markedly tender and acute pain can be precipitated by tibial rotation. Characteristically, patients are often woken at night and complain that they cannot sleep on their side as they are unable to rest one knee on top of the other. In most instances, there is a horizontal cleavage tear of the medial meniscus. This syndrome usually responds well to conservative treatment. The features reflect the sensory supply to the meniscus, which is predominantly at its attachment to the capsule. As the meniscus loses its natural pliability, so there is increased tension exerted peripherally.

The knee is the most common site for *loose bodies*. These are frequently seen on plain X-rays, but only a minority are intra-articular and therefore a cause of mechanical symptoms. Debris within a joint usually becomes attached to the synovium, the cells of which then proliferate around the loose body, not just entrapping it but extruding it into the sub-synovial layer. Even when loose bodies are theoretically intra-articular, they may be ensnared in a recess and hence are unable to float free within the joint cavity; an example is loose bodies in a Baker's cyst. There is therefore a tendency to over-diagnose loose bodies as a cause of symptoms. They precipitate locking or giving way, but are not a cause of persistent pain.

Osteochondritis dissecans affects adolescents and is always on the convex surface of a joint. For example, in the knee, it affects a femoral condyle, in the elbow the capitulum (see Fig. U.14), and in the ankle the dome of the talus. It is best regarded as a shear fracture through the subchondral plate. The important feature is that the overlying articular cartilage is normal and, as the osteochondral fragment does not separate to become a loose body until late in the course of the disease, the diagnosis is easily missed at arthroscopy since the articular surface is often still intact. Prior to separation, complaints are often of rather vague symptoms, including a feeling of insecurity. There is usually a slight but definite loss of full extension; this is a particularly helpful sign in distinguishing osteochondritis dissecans from teenage anterior knee pain. The lesion shows clearly on a technetium bone scan and MRI (Figs L.34 and L.35), but it is easy to overlook on plain X-rays.

Synovial chondromatosis is a rare condition in which a change in the synovium leads to the production of multiple lose bodies. There are two forms, the osteochondral and the cartilaginous 'rice body' types.

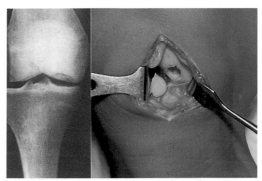

Figure L.34 Osteochondritis dissecans of the median femoral condyle. Anteroposterior X-ray and operative photograph of the loose osteochondral fragment and the defect. See also Fig. L.35.

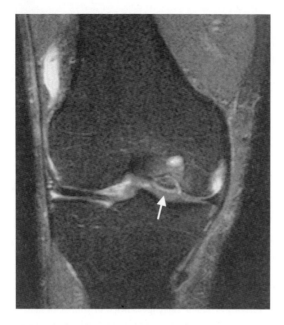

Figure L.35 Same patient as Fig. L.34. The osteochondral fragment with its clear zone of separation from the femoral condyle is clearly displayed on the T1 image on MRI. A fluid-filled reactive bone cyst is present deep to the defect.

In the former there are multiple discrete loose bodies, usually numbering between 10 and 20, and approximately the size of peas. They are visible on plain X-rays, and cause locking. In the second type, there are hundreds of small loose bodies which, being cartilaginous, are invisible on X-rays (Fig. L.30). These present with persistent aching discomfort, accompanied by an effusion and synovial thickening. They do not cause locking. Clinically, they are indistinguishable from other low-grade forms of chronic synovitis. These loose bodies usually appear as a surprise on arthroscopy!

Ligament injuries

Everything about the ligaments of the knee is complex – their anatomy, the mechanism of their injuries, the precise diagnosis of those injuries, and their treatment.

Note:

- The more serious the injury, the less pain.
- There is a high rate of popliteal artery damage associ-ated with posterior dislocations of the knee. '*Rule*': if a posterior dislocation is suspected an angiogram is mandatory.

Contrary to what one might expect, these are not all high-velocity injuries; indeed, the author can clearly recall a case in which an overweight woman aged 70

ruptured both cruciate ligaments and transected the popliteal artery by merely tripping over a small step. In the classical injury with rupture of the medial ligament, rupture of the anterior cruciate ligament and a tear of the medial meniscus, the knee has been subject to a severe valgus external rotatory force, for example, a rugby tackle. At the moment of injury, there is a severe pain often accompanied by a loud crack such that the individual may fear the leg has 'broken'. After a few minutes the pain has largely disappeared and many players then seek to carry on playing. However, the next time they receive a ball, the knee gives way as soon as they pivot or twist. When first seen, the injury does not appear serious, as there is little or no pain (the ligaments having snapped, the nerve endings do not fire since they respond to tension) and there is no haemarthrosis (the capsule has been disrupted and the blood has escaped into the soft tissues). Finally, if the athlete is fit, their muscles are strong and hence the doctor may not detect the instability. First, examine the uninjured knee and determine not just the degree of laxity in both full extension and in 30° of flexion, but in addition note the feel of the 'end point' whilst at the same time palpating the ligament; this will appear as a well-defined taut band. Repeat this on the injured knee. If on the medial side an end point cannot be felt and a taut band cannot be demonstrated, then the medial ligament must be presumed to be injured until proven otherwise. With lateral ligament injuries feel not just for the lateral ligament itself but also for the iliotibial band which inserts on to the proximal tibia just anterior to the fibula head. The anterior cruciate ligament should be examined by doing the anterior draw test in 30° of flexion whilst the posterior cruciate should be examined at 90°. When doing the latter test, ensure that the examiner's hands grip the proximal tibia with the thumbs placed over the tibial tubercle while the fingers should grip the tibia high up in the popliteal fossa in order to relax the hamstrings, or to detect if there is hamstring spasm. With posterior cruciate disruption, the tibia will fall backwards on the femur with the knee flexed to 90°. With acute major injuries always check the distal pulses and the peripheral neurology. The common peroneal nerve is particularly at risk from severe lateral ligament complex injuries.

There are a number of special tests, but these can be difficult to elicit (even by the experts) when the patient is awake, and are best demonstrated under an anaesthetic. The most important of these is the 'pivot shift' test for the anterior cruciate ligament. When ruptured, there is a rotational instability that allows the tibia to sublux off the femur in extension, causing the knee to give way. Patients with this instability can often run in a straight line, but the knee collapses when they change direction. To perform the test on the right knee, lift up the extended leg by the heel with the thumb over the lateral malleolus; exert a proximal force up the leg to replicate the ground reaction force; place the left hand behind the fibula and apply an internal rotation force; still applying these forces gently flex the knee. When positive, the tibia will relocate onto the femur with a 'jerk' at approximately 30° of flexion. This test therefore reproduces one of the common ways of sustaining the injury – when the ski bindings fail to release and the ski applies a twisting force to the knee. Two other characteristics of the acute anterior cruciate rupture are that the patient may have heard or felt a 'pop' from within the joint, and there is a rapid onset of swelling due to a haemarthrosis.

Partial tears (sprains) of the medial ligament present very differently to complete ruptures. These are never missed because they are very painful, but they are easily confused with a locked knee due to a bucket-handle tear of the medial meniscus, since the pain is felt medially and the knee lacks full extension. This, however, is 'pseudo-locking'. Anatomically, the screw-home mechanism of the knee enables one to stand without using muscle power except for slight activity in the tensor fascia lata, as tibial rotation at the extreme of extension tightens the ligaments. This mechanism is blocked by the pain from stretching the damaged medial ligament, and hence the knee lacks full extension and appears locked. The distinguishing physical sign between these two injuries is that the tenderness from a medial ligament sprain is always localized above the joint line whereas, with a bucket-handle tear, the tenderness is along the joint line. Medial ligament sprains may take several weeks to resolve. This is particularly the case if an area of calcification forms at the femoral attachment.

Arthropathies

Osteoarthritis of the knee is an extremely common condition throughout the world. It can affect the medial compartment in association with a varus deformity, the lateral compartment in association with the valgus deformity or the patellofemoral joint in association with patellofemoral mal-tracking. The history of medial or lateral compartment osteoarthritis is of slow deterioration over many years. Pain is brought on by activity and is usually localized to the affected side (for patellofemoral osteoarthritis, see Anterior knee pain, below). Night pain, unlike in the hip, is not a particular feature. Acute episodes of pain, often associated with episodes of catching or giving way followed by an effusion, can occur in advanced disease. This is due to gross eburnation and irregular ridging in the affected compartment – in effect, the femur has jumped a groove on the tibia!

On examination, first check for deformity with the patient standing (i.e. bow leg, knock knee, loss of full extension; bow legs are easy to overlook in the obese). Observe the patient walking – in advanced medial compartment disease the knee collapses into more varus. Joint line tenderness is often slight, but usually localizes to the affected side. The presence of an effusion is very variable but is often small. Movements are restricted, but this more marked in Caucasians than in Arab or Asian populations.

The confirmatory sign for osteoarthritis is to elicit bony crepitus from the affected compartment. For a varus knee, first stress the lateral compartment applying a valgus stress. Compress the surfaces together while flexing and extending the knee. This surface will be relatively intact, and the feeling elicited is normal smooth movement. Repeat this with a varus stress. Flex the knee through the complete range of flexion/extension, and if there is eburnation at some point through this arc, often between 40–60°, one not only elicits bony crepitus but also reproduces the patient's pain. Routine X-rays are misleading, particularly taken with a patient lying down. A standing AP X-ray usually tells the truth, either a narrowing or absence of the joint space. Even more useful is the AP film taken in 30° of flexion (Fig. L.36). In keeping with the physical signs of the 'agony test' described above, this can reveal total obliteration of the joint space when the standing film in extension shows only a partial loss. In summary, there is a tendency to underestimate the severity of this common condition as night pain is unusual, the signs may be subtle and difficult to elicit, while X-rays often fail to show the true extent of cartilage loss.

The knee joint is affected in many of the inflammatory arthropathies; these are considered in detail under JOINTS, AFFECTION OF (p. 343). *Rheumatoid arthritis* characteristically results in a valgus deformity with concomitant external rotation of the tibia (see Fig. 00). *Chondrocalcinosis* occurs more frequently in the knee than in any other joint. It is due to deposition of calcium pyrophosphate crystals within the menisci or

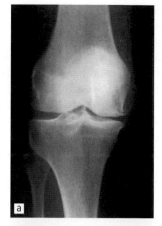

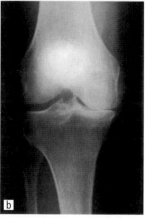

Figure L.36 Osteoarthritis of the knee. X-rays can be misleading. The AP film (a) shows only slight narrowing of the medial joint space. The standing film (b), taken at 30° flexion, reveals complete loss of articular cartilage (i.e. advanced disease).

within the articular surfaces. It is a very frequent X-ray finding and, in the majority of instances, is asymptomatic. Symptoms are precipitated when, secondary to early wear, pyrophosphate crystals 'escape' from the articular surface or from the menisci and cause an acute painful reaction within the joint. Characteristically, the knee is warm with a marked effusion and restricted mobility. Often there is a loss of 20–30° of extension, with flexion only to 90°. Attacks of *gout* affecting the knee, whilst uncommon, are all too easy to misdiagnose. Confirmation of both chondrocalcinosis and gout is by finding the crystals in a synovial aspirate.

While the diagnosis of *haemophiliac arthropathy* is usually clear from the history, it can be difficult if it is the presenting symptom especially when the extent of the bleeding is mild. The appearances are then of a

persistent synovitis with recurrent flares. Any joint can be involved, but the knees, ankles and elbows are particularly at risk. A clotting screen will elucidate the precise defect. When this is normal, a MRI scan can be very helpful in diagnosing a local cause, for example a haemangioma of the synovium or pigmented villonodular synovitis. A haemarthrosis as a complication of osteoarthritis used to be rare, but is becoming more frequent due to the increase in prescribing low-dose aspirin (see JOINTS, AFFECTIONS OF, p. 343).

Pigmented villonodular synovitis is now classified as a benign soft tissue neoplasm. It is included in this section because it presents as a low-grade synovitis with episodic acute flares due to bleeding into the joint. It therefore mimics gout, chondrocalcinosis, monoarticular rheumatoid, haemophiliac synovitis and bleeding from an arteriovenous haemangioma involving the synovium. The common sites are the knee and the hip. The knee X-rays are usually normal, but in the hip periarticular bone erosion can mimic tuberculosis. The appearances on both MRI and arthroscopy are usually diagnostic (Fig. L.37). An identical histological lesion, *giant cell tumour of tendon sheath*, occurs in the flexor tendon sheaths of the fingers. This presents as a soft tissue swelling, or occasionally as a trigger finger (see UPPER LIMB, conditions affecting hands and fingers, p. 757).

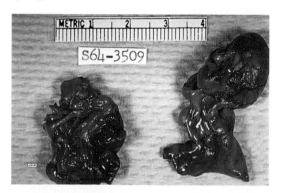

Figure L.37 Operative specimen following synovectomy of the knee for pigmented villonodular synovitis. The brown discoloration, due to haemosiderin, and florid synovitis are typical.

Pain in the front of the knee

Anterior knee pain/patellofemoral problems

The common cause of pain in the front of the knee is malfunction in the patellofemoral joint. It is important first to ensure that the pain is not referred from the hip, and second, that the patellofemoral joint is not over-looked as the source of pain as it can mimic several other conditions. Classically, pain from this joint radiates down anteriorly over the patellar tendon and the anterior proximal tibia. Frequently it spreads antero-medially, and when this is combined with episodes of giving way due to patella subluxation, it mimics a torn medial meniscus. The patellofemoral joint can reproduce locking, giving way, instability, feelings of insecurity and pain from almost any other mechanical problem in the knee. Furthermore, malfunction of the extensor mechanism is also a potent cause of chronic tendon sprains in the lower limb as other muscle groups overcompensate; for example, overactivity in the iliotibial band/gluteal muscles may precipitate pain at the tibial insertion or the greater trochanter. Other sites of secondary tendinitis are the pes anserine insertion (sartorius, gracilis, semi-tendinosus); semi-membranosus at the posteromedial corner and the biceps femoris over the fibula. With all of these tendinitidies, look closely at the quadriceps/patellofemoral mechanism for a possible primary cause. Classically, patellofemoral symptoms are aggravated by taking weight through the flexed knee (e.g. on stairs, or by squatting). Indeed, if the patient can squat and 'duck walk' (walking in the full squat position), this mechanism is probably innocent. The exception is the patella dislocation on extension since the patella stabilizes in the groove on flexion. Fortunately, dislocation in extension is one of the more obvious patellofemoral entities to diagnose, as the patella literally jumps laterally out of the femoral groove as the knee nears full extension.

On examination, look at limb alignment and patellar tracking. Tenderness is usually located along the medial border of the patella and over the anteromedial aspect of the knee in the triangle bounded by the medial femoral condyle, the medial tibial plateau and the patellar tendon. Test for patellar laxity: with the knee extended, feel particularly for the end point on lateral stressing. Feel for patellofemoral crepitus by placing a hand over the patella as the patient crouches. Elicit whether the patellofemoral pressure test reproduces the patient's symptoms (with the knee extended, press above the proximal pole of the patella with two fingers and then get the patient to contract the quadriceps whilst maintaining this downward pressure).

As indicated in White's schema, there is a variety of patellofemoral syndromes. These reflect the anatomical peculiarities of this joint. The patella: (i) being a sesamoid bone is dependent on muscular control, particularly the distal fibres of vastus medialis, to maintain its stability as it slides, tilts and rotates in spiralling down the femoral groove; (ii) has a complex shape; and (iii) has the thickest and softest articular surface of any joint.

The anterior knee pain syndrome predominantly affects teenagers, and is increasing in incidence particularly in Western society. There is a suspicion that it affects those who are athletic and those who take no exercise at all. It is the most common cause for discharge on medical grounds from the Armed Services. Fortunately, for most teenagers the condition is mild and usually settles within two years. Many factors have been implicated, but it is probably best regarded as the temporary imbalance between the muscular control of the patella, the stress to which the joint is subjected and minor abnormalities in the complex anatomical shape of both the patella and the femoral groove and the fact that the knee accounts for most of the growth in length of the lower limb.

To diagnose *chrondromalacia patellae* the articular surface of the patella must be shown to be excessively softened or disrupted (i.e. by arthroscopy or open surgery). There are important distinguishing features between chondromalacia and osteoarthritis. The former affects just one side of the joint, the convex patellar side, whereas osteoarthritis results in damage to both articular surfaces.

Chondromalacia on the medial facet is of little clinical importance; in the central area it can cause anterior knee pain while on the lateral facet it is a precursor of osteoarthritis – the *lateral hyperpressure syndrome*.

Patellofemoral osteoarthritis is a very common condition. It can be isolated or be present in conjunction with either medial or lateral compartment osteoarthritis. In the majority of cases the symptoms are either mild, or overshadowed by the tibiofemoral wear. When symptomatic, it causes anterior knee pain which is aggravated by taking weight on the bent knee, difficulty in kneeling or in rising from sitting, and giving way. On examination, the patella is often laterally placed, locally tender and there is marked bony crepitus, which is frequently audible on crouching.

The two instability syndromes of *patellar subluxation* and *patellar dislocation* are distinguished from the other patellar symptoms by one feature in particular, episodic major giving way; that is, the patient is usually unable to catch himself and consequently falls. The episodes are often precipitated by a slight twist and, if they occur whilst walking down the stairs or crossing the road, can result in lethal injury. Ligament laxity is frequently present. This can be generalized, affecting all joints, or localized just to the patella. In between episodes of dislocation, the knee usually behaves normally and the physical signs are subtle. Feel in particular for the end point on displacing the patella laterally. This manoeuvre often precipitates a positive apprehension test (i.e. the patient recognizes that the patella is about to dislocate and the quadriceps suddenly tighten). *Recurrent dislocation* may also occur in a previously normal knee that was subject to a traumatic dislocation; that is, the patella was forcibly knocked out of its groove. Often the patella relocates

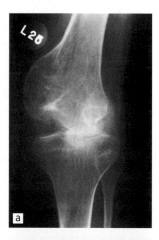

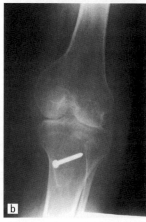

Figure L.38 Permanent dislocation of the patella accounts for this remarkable X-ray (a) in an 18-year-old with juvenile rheumatoid arthritis. When the patella was re-sited (b), the femur and tibia realigned. The knee functioned satisfactorily for a further 15 years before requiring replacement.

immediately the knee is straightened. The patient is usually unaware as to what exactly happened, and on inspection the only abnormal finding is that the knee is rather bruised and swollen. Routine AP and lateral X-rays are normal and the patient is dismissed. However, a skyline view of the patella often reveals an avulsion fracture, indicating that vastus medialis has been torn from the patella. If this is not repaired surgically there is a high incidence of recurrent dislocation. Finally, there are two other patterns of patella dislocation: *habitual dislocation*, in which the patella dislocates every time the knee is flexed, and *permanent dislocation*, which means precisely what it says – the patella is always dislocated. Remarkably, this diagnosis is frequently missed (Fig. L.38). The signs are that the knee is locked at 30° of flexion, the foot is externally rotated, and a skyline view demonstrates that the patella is not in its groove. Note that with all patterns of dislocation, the patients frequently say that the patella has dislocated medially because the deformity they notice is the uncovered prominence of the medial femoral condyle.

Other conditions and injuries of the extensor mechanism (listed from distal to proximal)

Osgood–Schlatter's disease is due to a chronic stress at the tibial apophysis, and occurs predominantly in teenage boys. The pain is localized around the tibial tubercle, which often becomes prominent (Fig. L.39). Symptoms usually settle over 6 months, but may last up to 2 years. Occasionally, symptoms persist after the end of growth due to a small fragment of the bone failing to unite on to the tibial shaft. The condition must be distinguished from an *acute traumatic avulsion of the tibial tubercle* which, if left untreated, results in a quadriceps lag and a fixed flexion deformity. Fortunately, this injury is rare.

Traumatic rupture of the patella tendon occurs in middle age. There is usually a small fragment of bone, avulsed from the distal pole of the patella. Surprisingly it can be missed, since the quadriceps expansion may still be intact and consequently close inspection is required to detect that the patella has moved proximally. Straight leg raising will be either impossible or there will be a marked lag.

Johannsen–Larsen syndrome is another cause of teenage anterior knee pain. This a chronic stress syndrome affecting the proximal attachment of the patellar tendon, the adult equivalent being *jumper's*

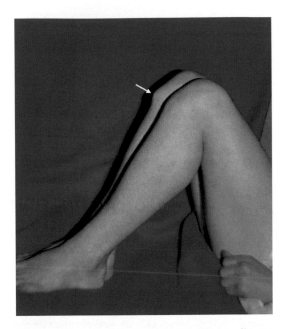

Figure L.39 Osgood–Schlatter's disease of the right knee. Note the prominence of the tibial tubercle secondary to the pull of the quadriceps muscle across the growth plate.

knee which is usually seen in fading middle-aged athletes who take up such sports as marathon running. To localize the tenderness to the distal pole of the patella, flex the knee to 90°, stabilize the foot by sitting on the toes, and ask the patient to straighten the knee (i.e. put the quadriceps into action).

There are two main types of patella fractures. *Stellate fractures* occur from a direct blow to the patella, while *transverse fractures* are caused by the patient tripping and then the quadriceps exerting a sudden reflex contraction – that is, the patella has snapped in two before the knee hits the ground. A similar mechanism causes *avulsion injuries of the quadriceps* or one of its component parts from the patella. This injury is often associated with chronic illness requiring steroids, renal dialysis, etc. *Rupture of the rectus femoris* occurs in the mid thigh region, and is an injury of athletes. When the quadriceps contracts, the rectus then rolls up like a ball. This condition must be distinguished from soft tissue tumours such as an intrafascial lipoma. *Myositis ossificans* affects the vastus intermedius. There is usually a clear history of a blow to the quadriceps. The resulting haematoma then ossifies (see Figs L.27 and L.28). The diagnosis becomes obvious with the passage of time, but it can be a confusing condition in the early stages when the thigh is merely swollen and X-rays are

normal. Evidence of calcification appears after 6 weeks. The differential diagnosis is from a tumour. The important distinguishing clinical sign is that with tumours of bone, the knee remains mobile, whereas with myositis ossificans or infection, movement is lost. With myositis ossificans the area of ossification gradually remodels and knee movements return over a period of a year to 18 months.

Infection

The knee is the most common site for pyogenic osteomyelitis. The infection begins on the metaphyseal side of the growth plate in either the distal femur or proximal tibia. The child presents with pyrexia and severe pain, and any movement of the knee is extremely painful. There is usually a small effusion present, particularly if the infection is in the distal femur. X-rays are normal in the early stages and do not become abnormal until pus, classically due to *Staphlyococcus aureus*, has formed, broken through the cortex and caused periosteal elevation. This bone destruction and periosteal reaction may not be radiologically evident for 10–12 days. In severe untreated cases the pus strips the periosteum of the shaft and the nutrient artery becomes thrombosed, resulting in infarction of diaphysis and eventual sequestrum formation. The periosteum continues to lay down new bone with the formation of an involucrum. The condition has now reached the chronic stage and the clinical picture is completed by the presence of discharging sinuses. The disease is especially devastating if the child is malnourished, when there is a significant mortality due to either overwhelming sepsis or secondary abscess formation affecting in particular the brain, lungs and other bones. In modern practice this fulminating picture is rarely seen, but if the diagnosis is delayed the condition can still cause local destruction and long-term disability. Distinguishing features between osteomyelitis and acute septic arthritis of the joint are: (i) in the latter the synovial thickening, the effusion and the warmth are more marked; and (ii) the child will not even permit a jog of movement from the joint.

The most common infecting organism of both osteomyelitis and septic arthritis is *Staphylococcus aureus*. *Streptococcal septic arthritis* can be surprisingly persistent, even though the organism is sensitive to penicillin, as antibiotics do not penetrate well into the extensive fibrinous exudate which forms in the knee. Low-grade osteomyelitis or septic arthritis must be distinguished from the inflammatory arthropathies.

A simple joint aspiration will confirm a septic arthritis, whilst a technetium bone scan can be very helpful in localizing osteomyelitis. *Gonococcal arthritis* is easy to overlook as it is a low-grade infection. The signs are not dissimilar to those of a mild haemarthrosis with an effusion, some synovial thickening and some warmth. If in any doubt about a knee effusion attributed by the patient to trauma, ask if there is a urethritis and look for a skin rash. Aspiration of the joint effusion will confirm the diagnosis. The diagnosis of tuberculous infection is frequently delayed, especially in Western medicine. Excessive quadriceps wasting is a feature of *tubercular synovitis* (Figs L.40 and L.41). The classic site for a *Brodie's abscess*, which is a localized area of chronic osteomyelitis usually due to *Staph. aureus*, is in the proximal tibial metaphysis. It causes a dull, aching, persistent pain. The differential diagnosis is from an osteoid osteoma or a benign tumour.

Tumours of bone

Malignant tumours

Primary malignant tumours of bone are rare diseases. Metastases are far more common. The *osteosarcoma*, which is the most common of this rare group, affects children, adolescents and young adults. The majority present with pain, which is unremitting, usually worse at night, and is often initially attributed by the patient to an injury. In the early stages the physical signs are very variable and there may be little to find except some local tenderness. However, this is an aggressive, rapidly expanding tumour and a mass soon becomes evident, though the bony pathology may be camouflaged by the swollen overlying soft tissues. There is often a small effusion within the knee, but movement is retained; this is the distinguishing feature from infection. X-ray features are variable, but essentially reveal destruction of the normal trabecular pattern, an indistinct margin and evidence of periosteal new bone formation – the classical 'Codman's triangle' or 'star burst' formation (Figs L.42 and L.43). A bone biopsy is required to establish the precise nature of the tumour.

Malignant transformation is a rare complication of Paget's disease, but *osteosarcoma secondary to Paget's disease* accounts for most osteosarcomas appearing in later life. This complication should be suspected in any long-standing Paget bone in which there is an alteration in the level of pain or swelling. The tumour is particularly aggressive, and many patients have

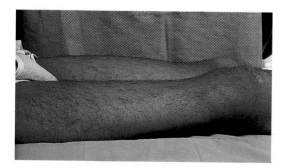

Figure L.40 Tuberculosis of the right knee. Marked muscle wasting of the thigh is a common finding, even in relatively early tuberculosis.

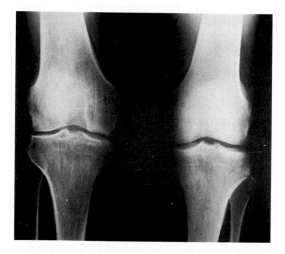

Figure L.41 Same patient as Fig. L.40. Anteroposterior X-ray of both knees. There is marked generalized osteoporosis of the right knee with 'pencilling' of the cortical margins and subchondral plates. Biopsy confirmed tuberculous synovitis.

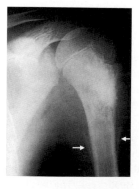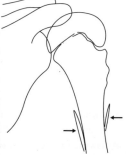

Figure L.42 Osteogenic sarcoma of the proximal humerus in a teenage boy. There is a rapidly expanding destructive lesion with the periosteal reaction shown as a Codman's triangle distally (arrowed).

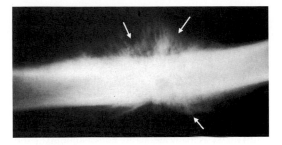

Figure L.43 Osteogenic sarcoma of the femoral shaft. The periosteal reaction is indicated by the sun-ray spicules (arrowed).

pulmonary metastases by the time of diagnosis. Plain X-rays show areas of bone destruction and soft tissue invasion, superimposed on the features of Paget's.

Ewing's sarcoma is the second most common primary malignant tumour of bone in children. It consists of islands of non-osteogenic and anaplastic small round cells closely associated with blood vessels. The precise cell of origin remains unknown, but it is probably a neural cell. The patient is usually aged between 10 and 20 years, and presents with pain and swelling accompanied by warmth and tenderness which, together with the systemic signs of pyrexia and a raised ESR, can mimic a low-grade osteomyelitis. X-rays show a permeating destructive lesion which, unlike an osteogenic sarcoma, is usually diaphyseal (Fig. L.44). The rapid expansion of the tumour produces periosteal elevation, which appears radiologically as a Codman's triangle and 'sun ray' spicules. Occasionally, this shows as the 'onion peel' effect, this being due to repeated layers of periosteal bone being laid down around the diaphysis. CT and MRI imaging reveal a large extra-osseous component. Spread is to the lungs and other bones. The differential diagnosis is from primary lymphoma of bone and osteomyelitis.

Chondrosarcomas in particular arise from the flat bones, the pelvis and the scapula, often from a preexisting exostosis (Fig. L.45). Consequently, any change in size in an exostosis in adult life needs urgent investigation. Chondrosarcomas are slow-growing lesions, and usually affect the 30- to 50-year age group.

Benign tumours

Giant cell tumour of bone (*osteoclastoma*) derives its name from the presence of large, multinucleated giant cells. The tumour is usually considered benign but locally expansive within the bone. Although 2–10 per cent of these tumours metastasize to the lungs, the

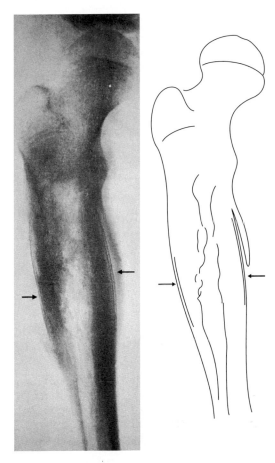

Figure L.44 Ewing's sarcoma of the upper femur. The classical but uncommon 'onion skin' periosteal reaction is present (arrowed).

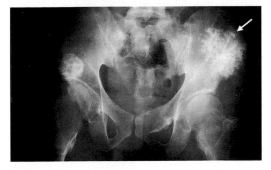

Figure L.45 Chondrosarcoma of the left ilium (arrow) arising in a previous exostosis in a 35-year-old male who had noticed an increase in lesion size over the previous 6 months.

prognosis is still quite good and far better than with other malignant bone tumours. Most patients are between 20 and 40 years. The most common site is the knee, followed by the sacrum and then the distal radius.

The presenting feature is pain and swelling around the joint which usually passes unnoticed for several months. The tumour has a unique classical appearance on X-ray as it involves the epiphyseal end of long bones and extends up to the joint margin (Fig. L.46). A delay in diagnosis increases the likelihood of a pathological fracture which, if it occurs into the joint, makes subsequent treatment more difficult.

Osteochondroma (*cartilage capped exostosis*) is the most common primary benign bone tumour. It has a bony base with a cartilage cap and occurs in the metaphyses of long bones, especially at the fast-growing joints (i.e. the knee, shoulder and wrist) (Fig. L.47).

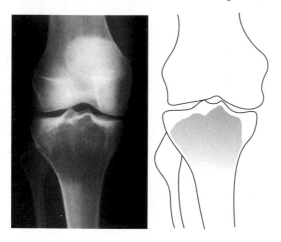

Figure L.46 Osteoclastoma (giant cell tumour) in a 20-year-old female. The lesion extends up to the subchondral plate of the knee. Distally, the tumour margin is poorly defined, indicative of aggressive local invasion.

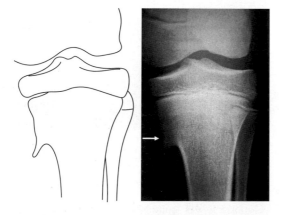

Figure L.47 Cartilage-capped exostosis of the tibia. There is a well-defined prominence of the medial aspect of the proximal tibia. Anteroposterior X-ray showing the bony stalk (arrowed). The cartilage cap is radiolucent.

However, it can also be found in any bone of cartilaginous origin. It can be either solitary or multiple, and in the latter case may be hereditary (an autosomal dominant skeletal dysplasia). This lesion is generally considered to be a failure of remodelling at the growth plate and, when multiple lesions affect a single bone, this bone will be shorter as the growth potential of the bone has been partially squandered. The true incidence is unknown, as many lesions are non-symptomatic and therefore undetected. Many are discovered purely as chance findings, often later in life. Most patients who present with either symptoms or a lump do so as teenagers or young adults. Osteochondromas are usually painless, but they can interfere mechanically with the function of tendons which catch over the bony prominence. Since they are derived from the growth plate, growth of individual osteochondromata ceases when the patient stops growing. Any alteration of size later in life should raise suspicion of malignant transformation, usually to a chondrosarcoma. Fortunately, this is rare, probably occurring in less than 1 per cent of solitary lesions, though more frequently, possibly up to 5 per cent, with multiple lesions.

Chondroblastoma is a benign tumour of cartilage, and is distinguishable by being one of the few tumours to be confined to the epiphysis. It usually presents with a constant ache in the joint and localized tenderness in the adjacent affected bone. Patients are usually in their teens or early adult life (i.e. around the end of the growth period). X-rays classically show a rounded, well-demarcated radiolucent area in the epiphysis, often with an extension into the adjacent metaphysis (Fig. L.48).

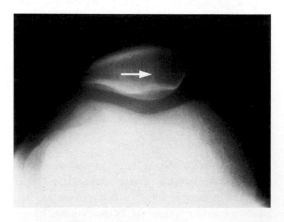

Figure L.48 Chondroblastoma classically occurs in the epiphysis of long bones, but may occur elsewhere, as in this patella of a teenage boy.

Enchondromas also affect the metaphyseal/diaphyseal region and, like fibrous dysplasia, are centrally located. They are most frequently located in the metacarpals (Fig. L.49) or metatarsals, but they can occur in long bones, especially the humerus, femur and tibia. Radiologically in children they show as well-defined cystic lesions, and it is not until the bone develops maturity that characteristic flecks of calcification show within the lucent area. Many are diagnosed incidentally, while some – particularly those in the hand – present with bony deformity.

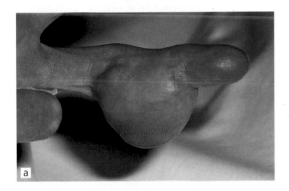

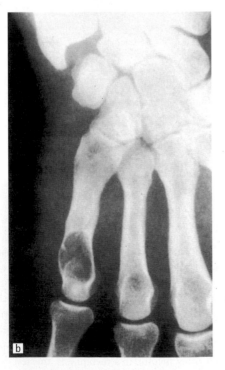

Figure L.49 (a) A large enchondroma of the middle phalanx of the ring finger. (b) Anteroposterior X-ray of enchondroma of the fifth metacarpal. Note the well-defined margin indicating its benign nature.

Do not dismiss pain as being due to a pathological fracture without good evidence, as malignant transformations to a chondrosarcoma can occur. This is rare in solitary lesions but more common in Ollier's disease (multiple enchondromas) and Maffucci's syndrome.

Chondromyxoid fibromas are rare benign tumours which also occupy the metaphyseal/diaphyseal junction. They are much more prevalent in the bones of the lower limb than the upper limb. They are eccentrically placed, and have a dense endosteal margin. They present with pain and, in a superficial bone such as the tibia, there is overlying warmth and local swelling.

Tumour-like conditions

Many authorities consider that *fibrous cortical defects/non-ossifying fibroma* are essentially the same lesion. They are probably not true neoplasms but rather developmental proliferations of fibrous tissue and histiocytes. Some 80 per cent of lesions occur in either the distal femur, the proximal tibia or the distal tibia. They are the most common bone lesion in children, being found in up to 30 per cent of children aged 4–8 years, and are usually discovered incidentally as they are asymptomatic (Fig. L.50). They may range from several millimetres to several centimetres in size. They heal spontaneously and do not require treatment unless there is a risk of a pathological fracture. Non-ossifying fibromas are merely larger and

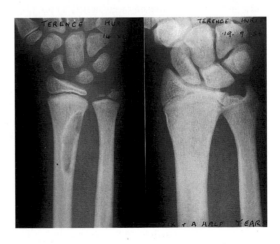

Figure L.50 Left: fibrous cortical defect of a distal radius. Histologically, this lesion is identical to a non-ossifying fibroma, but only involves the cortex and does not extend deep into the bone. It was a chance finding on an X-ray taken in the A&E department. Right: an X-ray taken 6 years later shows the lesion has healed spontaneously.

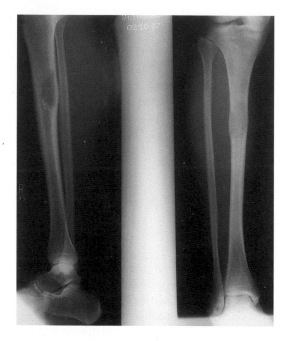

Figure L.51 Non-ossifying fibroma of the tibia. Anteroposterior and lateral X-rays.

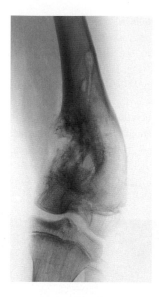

Figure L.52 Fibrous dysplasia. Anteroposterior X-ray of the distal femur, showing an extensive lesion affecting the medial half of the distal femoral metaphysis resulting in inequality of growth.

extend more deeply into the bone than the fibrous cortical defects (Fig. L.51). Consequently there is a greater risk of pathological fracture.

Fibrous dysplasia arises in the marrow and is therefore situated centrally on a plain X-ray. It is composed of fibrous tissue and immature bone and occurs in two forms, solitary (80%) or polyostotic (20%). Common sites are the ribs, cranium, facial bones, femur (Fig. L.52), tibia and humerus. They are usually discovered incidentally on plain X-rays, on which they classically give an appearance of 'ground glass'. However, appearances are very variable and fibrous dysplasia is well-recognized as being able to mimic many other bone lesions. Most solitary lesions are asymptomatic but they can present as a pathological fracture or bone deformity (Fig. L.53). The polyostotic form can be associated with a variety of endocrine disorders: hyperthyroidism, acromegaly, hyperparathyroidism, Cushing's syndrome, diabetes and Albright's syndrome – fibrous dysplasia, precocious puberty and pigmented skin lesions. Occasionally, the polyostotic form may undergo malignant transformation.

Osteoid osteoma can occur in any bone except the skull. It is a tiny, tumour-like condition which on excision appears as a dark brown or reddish nucleus surrounded by dense bone. Radiologically, lesions in

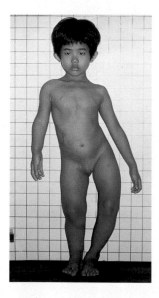

Figure L.53 Same patient as Fig. L.52. Clinically, there is a marked bowing of the left leg.

the cortex show dense sclerosis and cortical thickening which may mask the underlying small central nidus. This can be revealed either by tomography or by CT scanning (Figs L.54–L.56). A technetium bone scan is often helpful. In a metaphysis, this lesion can sometimes be difficult to distinguish from a small Brodie's abscess – an area of well-confined chronic

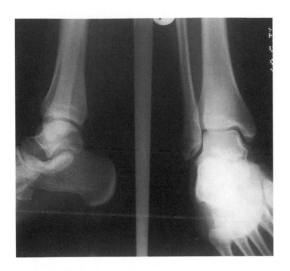

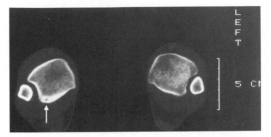

Figure L.56 Same patient as Fig. L.54. CT scanning revealed the classical lesion of sclerosis with a small lucent central nidus in the posterior cortex of the tibia adjacent to the distal tibiofibular joint (arrowed).

Figure L.54 Osteoid osteoma of distal tibia in a 17-year-old male. Although the patient gave a clear history of severe pain, well-controlled by simple analgesia, standard X-rays appeared normal.

common site. It is slow growing and presents with mild persistent backache which is relieved by analgesics. Radiologically, the lesion is variable but is usually expansile, well-circumscribed and partially calcified.

A *simple bone cyst* (*unicameral*) is a benign unilocular or partially locular fluid-filled cyst which occurs in the first two decades of life, most commonly in the proximal humerus and proximal femur. Many are found as chance findings on routine X-rays. These may never become symptomatic and appear to resolve spontaneously. Symptoms are the result of a pathological fracture through the weakened cortex (Fig. L.57).

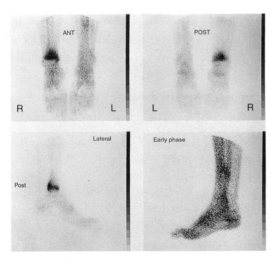

Figure L.55 Same patient as Fig. L.54. This bone scan showed an increase in uptake in the distal tibia, most marked posteriorly.

osteomyelitis. The pain from an osteoid osteoma is out of all proportion to its size. The pain is persistent and, characteristically, is dramatically relieved by aspirin. Sometimes, however, the pain may be diffuse, particularly if the lesion involves the pelvis or the spine. It is the classic cause of a painful scoliosis. The pain is immediately abolished by either excising or ablating the lesion.

Osteoblastoma (*giant osteoid osteoma*) has similarities to an osteoid osteoma, though it is now officially classified as a benign tumour. The spine is the most

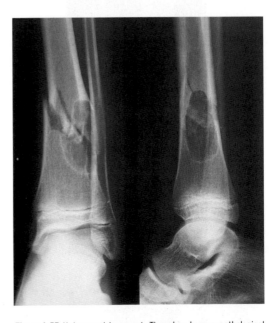

Figure L.57 Unicameral bone cyst. There has been a pathological fracture through this cyst in an 8-year-old boy. The lesion has a well-defined margin and is located in the metaphysis, having 'migrated' from the epiphyseal plate.

Plain X-rays are normally diagnostic as the cyst has a well-defined margin and never penetrates the cortex, which may be thinned and appear slightly expanded particularly when the cyst migrates down from the metaphysis into the diaphysis. This expansion is never greater than the width of the overlying epiphyseal plate.

While *aneurysmal bone cysts* are classified as reactive lesions of bone (not neoplasms), they are nonetheless locally destructive. They can arise at any age and in any bone, but are most commonly found in young adults affecting the metaphysis, especially the proximal humerus, the distal femur and the proximal tibia (Figs L.58 and L.59). They are blood-filled, expanding

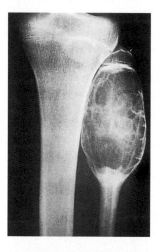

Figure L.58 Aneurysmal bone cyst. Anteroposterior X-ray showing the expansion of the proximal fibula.

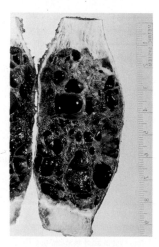

Figure L.59 Aneurysmal bone cyst. Operative specimen showing the typical vascular appearance of the lesion.

lesions, and although the overlying cortex is not destroyed it may be rendered so thin as to be almost invisible on X-ray. Radiologically, they have a 'soap bubble' appearance due to bony ridges on the wall of the cyst. There are two types: primary, arising de novo; or secondary to bleeding into some other lesion, for example a giant cell tumour. They usually present with discomfort or occasionally as a bony swelling.

Osteitis fibrosa cystica (*brown tumour*) occurs in advanced hyperparathyroidism. Although uncommon, they nonetheless remain important diagnostically. Radiologically they can be easily confused with other tumours and cysts of bone, while histologically they are indistinguishable from an osteoclastoma. (Pathologists will refuse to give an opinion on a biopsy from a lesion with a provisional diagnosis of osteoclastoma unless they have evidence that the calcium is normal). Multiple brown tumours are also easily confused with metastatic malignancy. Brown tumours are usually found in the long bones (Fig. L.60), the ribs or the skull ('pepper pot' skull). Other features include subperiosteal resorption in the phalanges, femoral neck, upper tibia and medial end of clavicle.

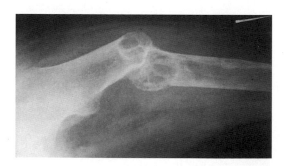

Figure L.60 Hyperparathyroidism (Brown tumour). There has been a pathological fracture through this lesion in the proximal femoral diaphysis. Histologically, it is indistinguishable from an osteoclastoma.

Apley's diagram (Fig. L.61) is a useful aide memoire for this group of 'cyst and cyst-like' conditions of bone. Remember also that metastases are by far the most common malignant tumours found in bone, and that both metastatic and primary tumours can be confused with traumatic fractures (Fig. L.62).

Bursitis and tendinitis

Prepatellar bursitis (*housemaid's knee*) is rarely seen in housemaids, but is an occupational hazard of those

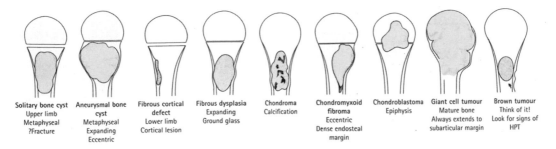

Solitary bone cyst	Aneurysmal bone	Fibrous cortical	Fibrous dysplasia	Chondroma	Chondromyxoid	Chondroblastoma	Giant cell tumour	Brown tumour
Upper limb	cyst	defect	Expanding	Calcification	fibroma	Epiphysis	Mature bone	Think of it!
Metaphyseal	Metaphyseal	Lower limb	Ground glass		Eccentric		Always extends to	Look for signs of
?Fracture	Expanding	Cortical lesion			Dense endosteal		subarticular margin	HPT
	Eccentric				margin			

Figure L.61 Cyst and cyst-like lesions of bone.

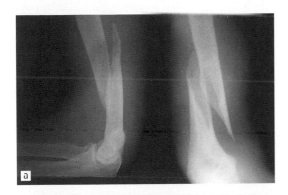

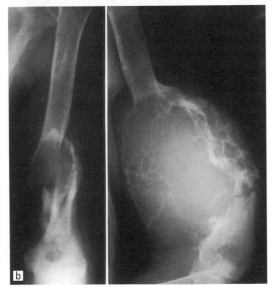

Figure L.62 (a) Pathological fracture of the distal humerus secondary to a renal carcinoma; hypernephroma. The initial X-rays were deceptive and the lesions considered to be a straightforward traumatic short spiral fracture. (b) An X-ray taken 6 weeks later shows the true destructive nature of the tumour, which is so vascular that clinically the lesion was pulsatile.

who do a lot of kneeling, for example carpet layers. When uninfected, it presents as a smooth, circumscribed swelling anterior to the patella (Fig. L.63). *Infrapatellar bursitis* (*clergyman's knee*) is more distally situated and lies over the patella tendon (Fig. L.64). When either superficial bursa becomes infected the physical signs are obvious: tenderness, warmth and surrounding superficial oedema. The knee joint is not involved. *Deep infrapatellar bursitis* involves the bursa lying behind the patella tendon, above its insertion onto the tibial tubercle. If this bursa is infected, the signs are less obvious than with the superficial bursae. The area of induration is more widespread, the tenderness is deeper and the erythema less marked. Flexion of the knee is uncomfortable and as a consequence, tends to be restricted.

The *semi-membranosus bursa* presents with a painless lump situated posteromedially; the bursa lies between the semi-membranosus and the medial head of the gastrocnemius (Fig. L.65). It is most commonly seen in children and usually resolves spontaneously. The knee joint is normal. It needs to be distinguished from a *popliteal cyst* (*Baker's cyst*). This is a herniation

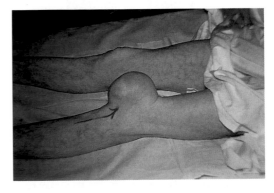

Figure L.63 Pre-patellar bursitis. A pre-patellar bursar lies directly over the patella.

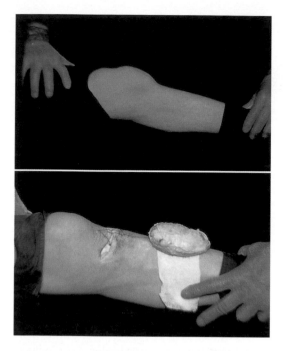

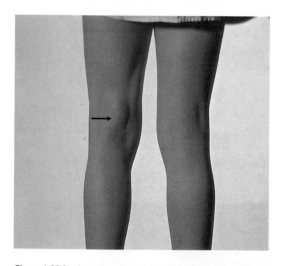

Figure L.64 An infra-patellar bursa lies distal to the patella over the patella tendon, before (upper) and after (lower) surgical excision.

Figure L.65 Semi-membranosus bursa of the knee. This presents as a painless swelling in the popliteal fossa (arrowed), usually in children or adolescents. It is most prominent when the knee is straight.

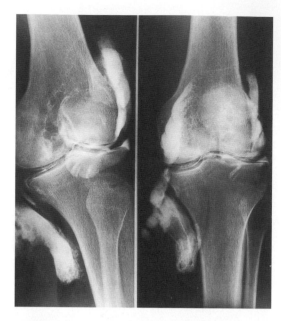

Figure L.66 Arthrogram of the knee showing the extravasation of contrast into the calf from a ruptured Baker's cyst.

tender calf. Patients need to be reassured as to the benign nature of the Baker's cyst but warned about spon-taneous rupture (Fig. L.66). Finally, do make certain that any cyst in the back of the knee is not pulsatile i.e. a *popliteal aneurysm*!

Meniscal cysts arise from the meniscus/capsular junction and are a reflection of abnormal mechanics within the meniscus, usually in association with a horizontal cleavage tear. Their pathology is identical to a ganglion of the wrist. The presentation between the two menisci is very different due to the lateral meniscal cyst being trapped under the dense iliotibial tract. *Lateral cysts* cause aching discomfort, present early when they are still small, and feel almost bony hard; indeed, they are frequently mistaken for an exostosis or an osteophyte. The lump is situated at or just below the level of the joint line, usually anterior to the collateral ligament, and is most evident with the knee slightly flexed. On full flexion they often vanish in the sense that they are no longer palpable. *Medial meniscal cysts* are much less common. The signs are very different, usually being large, clearly cystic and relatively soft (Fig. L.67). Their peculiarity is that they frequently migrate a considerable distance away from the joint line and the meniscus to which they are attached by a 'stalk'. They may be mistaken for a bursa which lies over the medial tibial

of the synovium and is a sign of pathology within the knee (usually osteoarthritis), though they can occur secondary to any pathology including tuberculosis. Their importance lies in the fact that they may rupture and, when they do so, the signs are identical to those of a deep-vein thrombosis, with a swollen

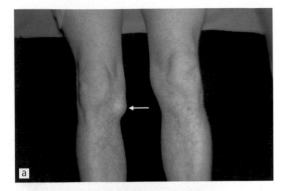

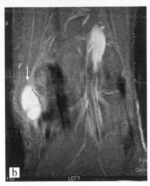

Figure L.67 Cyst of the medial meniscus of the right knee. (a) The cyst is lying over the medial tibial condyle, just below the joint line. These cysts can 'migrate' anteriorly into the fat pad, move further down the proximal tibia, or appear posteromedially in the popliteal fossa as shown on the MRI scan (b).

condyle some 5 cm below the joint line at the insertion of sartorius. They can migrate into the fat pad anteriorly, or occasionally appear at the posteromedial corner of the knee, masquerading as a semi-membranosus bursa in the wrong age group. A good quality MRI usually reveals the meniscal attachment.

Tendinitidies around the knee are common, as are muscular sprains. These may be due to acute injuries, chronic stress injuries, for example in middle-aged amateur marathon runners, or they may be secondary to an altered pattern of gait due to pathology elsewhere in the leg, for example malfunction of the quadriceps leading to overuse of the iliotibial band with pain at the insertion onto the proximal anterolateral tibia.

Pain in the calf and shin

Calf pain is a far more frequent symptom than pain affecting the anterior aspect of the lower leg.

Furthermore, pain in the calf is commonly encountered with diseases which are either life-threatening or limb-threatening. Thus, calf pain requires a precise diagnosis and should never be dismissed as a muscular sprain.

Causes of calf or shin pain include:

- Life- or limb-threatening
  - ◆ Deep-vein thrombosis
  - ◆ Arterial disease
    - Acute arterial ischaemia
    - Intermittent claudication
    - Compartment syndrome
- Less serious causes
  - ◆ Referred pain from the lumbar spine
    - sciatica
    - spinal stenosis
  - ◆ Ruptured Baker's cyst
  - ◆ Muscle and tendon ruptures
    - gastrocnemius/soleus ruptures
    - ruptured Achilles tendon
  - ◆ Varicose veins
  - ◆ Nerve entrapment
    - common peroneal nerve
    - superficial peroneal nerve
  - ◆ Peripheral neuropathies

Life- or limb-threatening causes of calf pain

The causes of the first group should never be missed. Both deep-vein thrombosis and compartment syndromes can be very deceptive.

Deep-vein thrombosis (DVT) requires permanent vigilance in most situations in which there is a known high incidence, especially postoperatively, bed rest for any illnesses, plaster splintage, air travel, etc. Postoperative prophylactic antithrombotic cover is no guarantee that this complication will not occur. Furthermore, those thrombi which are more likely to embolize often have less in the way of physical signs. For example, pulmonary embolism remains the main cause of death following routine hip replacement. Without prophylaxis, the incidence of DVT after major hip surgery is the order of 60 per cent. This complication is not confined to surgical patients, but is also common in medical patients. After myocardial infarction or cerebrovascular accidents, the incidence has been estimated to be as high as 20 per cent. It is a well-described complication of the high-oestrogen contraceptive pill. It can even occur spontaneously in otherwise healthy individuals, for example on long-haul aircraft flights. The signs are usually unilateral. However, the apparently normal leg may be the site of a major embolus, since the signs become more apparent when the embolus becomes fixed in the vein. In terms of clinical features, look in particular for slight pitting oedema around the ankle; calf pain and tenderness; and a low-grade pyrexia. Homan's test – pain on ankle dorsiflexion – is notoriously unreliable and should be discarded. In the 'medical' or outpatient setting, a low clinical probability score on the Wells criteria (see Table L.9), plus a normal D-dimer assay, makes a diagnosis of venous thrombosis most likely. In the early postoperative period, measurement of D-dimer – a fibrin degradation product – is elevated due to the surgical haematoma, and hence this assay is not diagnostic. Postoperatively – or if there is any doubt from the Wells probability/D-dimer combination – then any suspicion of a DVT requires exclusion by investigation. Ultrasonic venous imaging is now the first line, but is less specific than radiological venography. Thus, if ultrasound is negative and clinical suspicion remains high, it should either be repeated two or three days later, or alternatively a venogram should be performed. A massive proximal thrombosis affecting the iliofemoral veins can cause a very swollen white oedematous limb (phlegmasia alba dolens), but more commonly this presents as a blue leg (phlegmasia cerulea). An iliofemoral thrombosis can occasionally progress to true venous gangrene. The common long-term sequelae of DVT is venous ulceration.

Table L.9 Wells clinical probability tool

Wells explicit assessment
Active cancer
Paralysis, paresis or recent plaster, or immobilization of lower limb
Recently bedridden for more than three days or major surgery in the last four weeks or more
Localized tenderness
Entire leg swollen
Calf swelling >3 cm compared with asymptomatic leg
Pitting oedema
Collateral superficial veins
Two point deduction
Alternative diagnosis as likely or greater than deep-vein thrombosis

Each positive response is 1 point, except if an alternative diagnosis is as likely as or greater than deep-vein thrombosis, where two points are deducted. 0 or fewer points = low probability; 1–2 points = moderate probability; ≥3 points = high probability.

Intermittent claudication was discussed previously as part of the differential diagnosis of spinal stenosis (see Leg pain of radicular or vascular origin, p. 378).

Acute arterial ischaemia is classically due either to embolism – the most frequent cause is a thrombosis in the atrium secondary to atrial fibrillation – or to an acute thrombosis developing on a subintimal myocardial infarct. Other causes of acute ischaemia include an aortic dissection, thrombosis in an aneurysm (especially a popliteal aneurysm), an arteritis, or trauma. Arterial injuries in association with fractures through the proximal third of the tibia are all too easy to miss as the symptoms may be obscured by the major trauma to the limb. The effect of an embolus depends upon the extent and site of obstruction, the potential for collateral formation, and the speed at which it becomes effective. Classically, emboli produce vasospasm with occlusion of the distal vessels leading to claudication, rest pain and gangrene. Clearly if the occlusion is to a major vessel then the symptoms of pain are instant. Small peripheral emboli cause patches of cutaneous gangrene, with multiple small dark spots or blotches best seen in the foot.

Compartment syndrome is a deceptive and destructive condition due to muscle ischaemia as a result of a rise in pressure within the muscle compartment, eventually causing venous occlusion (Table L.10). A vicious

Table L.10 Causes of compartment syndrome in the leg

Acute traumatic
Soft tissue crush injuries
■ Acute severe local crush
■ Prolonged compression → ischaemia
■ Drug addicts secondary to coma
Fractures
Dislocation of knee
Haematoma

Postoperative
Vascular
■ Post embolectomy
■ Post arterial reconstruction
Orthopaedic
■ Closed reduction of tibial fractures
■ Intra-medullary nailing of tibia
■ Operations involving division of fibula (e.g. upper tibial osteotomy)
Bleeding disorders (e.g. haemophilia)

Chronic
Muscle ischaemia in athletes

*Compartment syndrome is more common in closed than open injuries.

circle is then set up in which capillary pressure rises towards arterial pressure, which results in diffusion of fluid into the extracellular compartment, causing a further rise in pressure. The more rigid the anatomical construction of the compartment, the more likely is this syndrome to occur. The forearm and the leg, which both contain two bones joined by a tough interosseous membrane and muscles contained within strong fascial compartments, account for the vast majority of cases. However, it can occur in other sites, for example the gluteal compartments in which it can be particularly lethal due to a massive release of myoglobin, precipitating renal failure. An acute compartment syndrome is a surgical emergency and requires urgent decompression. Any delay over 4 hours leads to increasing disability secondary to muscle necrosis, resulting in fibrosis and contracture.

Soft tissue crush injuries can be particularly deceptive, especially if the patient is seen shortly after the injury, before any swelling has become manifest. Never discharge a patient from the casualty department who has evidence of tyre marks across the calf! (Fig. L.68) Compartment syndrome also arises after *prolonged crush injury*, for example, when a patient is trapped in a collapsed building or a motor car and sustained arterial compression and distal ischaemia.

Finally, in this group are included *drug addicts* who have been unconscious for long periods resulting in local ischaemia. This is the most common cause of gluteal ischaemia. *Open fractures of the tibia* in which there has been wide soft tissue destruction are less likely to suffer a compartment syndrome as the compartments have already been decompressed. The deceptive injury is the apparently straightforward *closed fracture of the tibia and fibula* in which the bones

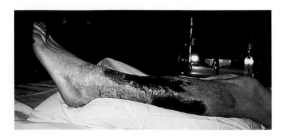

Figure L.68 Extensive skin necrosis following a crush injury. The patient was run over by a car. In casualty, the only signs of the injury were tyre marks on the skin and a fractured fibula. One week later, the full extent of the injury is apparent.

are overlapped. The chances of developing a compartment syndrome are increased by a closed reduction in which any overlap is fully corrected. The application of a plaster not only adds a further constriction to the limb but also makes compartment syndromes more difficult to diagnose as the calf is not available to examine. However, treatment with intramedullary nailing also has a high risk – the process of reaming and putting down a nail produces a surge of pressure in the muscle compartments. *Dislocation of the knee and fracture separation of the distal femoral epiphysis* (an injury which occurs in the late teens before this epiphysis fuses) can both cause either lacerations or compression of the popliteal vessels and consequently a high risk of calf compartment syndrome. Do not be deluded into believing that severe trauma is a prerequisite – the author has seen an anterolateral compartment syndrome following a kick at football causing a haematoma. In such circumstances, remember to check that the patient does not have a bleeding disorder. Compartment syndromes are well-recognized following *vascular surgery*, especially post-embolectomy and after arterial reconstruction if there has been distal ischaemia for a significant period.

The diagnosis, as with DVT, is primarily dependent upon a high level of suspicion. The most important symptom is pain. It increases in severity to become unremitting. However, eventually the pain will subside and disappear when the muscle and the nerves are dead. The most important sign is pain on passive stretching of the involved muscle. This obviously involves a knowledge of which muscle is in which compartment (Table L.11). Due to the pain, the patient will be reluctant to move the limb. Clearly, the involved muscles will eventually be 'paralysed'. In the early stages of the compression, paraesthesia can be present, but this is usually masked by the pain. The area of sensory loss is a very important sign, especially if the patient is in plaster and only the toes and the distal part of the foot can be examined. With regard to the pulse, beware! First, there may still be sufficient arterial pressure for the pulse to be transmitted through an involved compartment. Second, the pulse may have been transmitted via an unaffected normal compartment; for example, a compartment syndrome of the anterolateral compartment will not obliterate the posterior tibial or the dorsalis pedis pulses. Finally, to complete the list of signs and symptoms commencing with the letter 'P', if the diagnosis is missed, the

Table L.11 Compartments of the leg

Compartment	Muscles	Artery	Nerve	Site of sensory loss
Anterior	Tibialis anterior Extensor digitorum longus Extensor hallucis longus Peroneus tertius	Anterior Tibial	Deep peroneal	Cleft between hallux and second toe
Anterolateral	Peroneus longus Peroneus brevis	Peroneal	Superficial Peroneal	Dorsum of foot
Deep posterior	Tibialis posterior Flexor digitorium longus Flexor hallucis longus	Posterior Tibial	Tibial	Sole of foot
Superficial posterior	Gastrocnemius Soleus		Sural	Heel and lateral border of foot

muscles will perish, the limb may perish, and so may the patient if this complication is further complicated by renal failure secondary to myoglobinaemia. In an established compartment syndrome, there is characteristic feel, described as 'woody'. There are various methods of measuring intracompartmental pressure, but these can be unreliable. The old adage remains pertinent – 'depend on the symptoms and the signs and, if in any doubt, decompress' (Table L.12).

Other causes of calf pain

Referred pain from the lumbar spine, due either to radicular nerve involvement (sciatica) or to spinal stenosis, was discussed earlier (see PAIN IN THE LEG, p. 378). For a *ruptured Baker's cyst*, see CYSTS

Table L.12 Compartment syndrome: the cardinal symptoms and signs

Pain	The most important symptom
Pain on passive movement	The most important sign
Palpation	A solid 'woody feel' usually means the compartment requires decompression
Parasthesia/numbness	Very useful in localizing which compartment
Paralysis	Can be a presenting feature of compartment syndrome in drug addicts following prolonged coma
Pulse	Very misleading (see text)
Pressure studies	Several methods. Useful in the unconscious patient, but requires experience both technically and with interpretation

If the clinical signs indicate compression, then decompress

AROUND THE KNEE (p. 407). It is of course perfectly possible simultaneously to have a DVT and a Baker's cyst, so proof must be obtained either that the cyst has ruptured and leaked or that the veins are patent. *Muscle ruptures* of either the *gastrocnemius* or the *soleus* occur at their attachment to the aponeurosis of the Achilles tendon. There is a calf haematoma, the tenderness is situated proximally at the site of the rupture, and the tendon itself is intact. An *Achilles tendon rupture* normally occurs in older athletes, the 45- to 60-year age group, but can occasionally be seen in early adult life. It is easily missed, since the 'gap' is obscured by swelling and the patient is still able to plantar flex the foot due to the action of other plantar flexors (tibialis posterior, etc.). They cannot however stand on tip-toe. The best sign is Simmond's test (Fig. L.69). Here, the patient lies prone with the feet over the end of the couch; first, observe the position of the foot – if the tendon is ruptured, the foot will be lying at a right-angle. Then squeeze the calf – if the tendon is intact, the foot will move, but if it is ruptured the foot will not move.

Peripheral neuropathies can be a cause of fleeting pains in the calf, so always beware of dual pathology. That is, if a nerve is irritable due to an underlying neurological disease, then it will be much more prone to be symptomatic or will be paralysed by a superimposed mechanical disease such as disc or nerve root entrapment. *Entrapments* are uncommon in the leg, but are well described for the *common peroneal nerve* at the level of the fibula neck and the *superficial peroneal nerve* where it exits through the deep fascia at the junction of the middle and distal thirds of the leg, just anterior to the fibula. The common peroneal

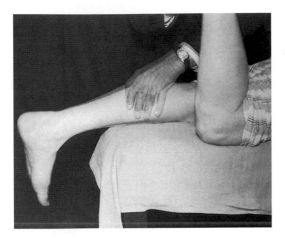

Figure L.69 Ruptured tendo-Achilles. With the patient prone and the foot over the end of the couch, the ankle assumes a right-angle. In addition, there is no passive plantar flexion of the foot on squeezing the calf (Simmond's sign).

nerve is also at risk from a direct trauma, such as a kick at football and/or from inadequate protection during obstetric or urological surgery in the lithotomy position. The author has even seen a foot drop secondary to a very tightly applied crepe bandage.

Shin pain

The common cause of pain over the anterior aspect of the proximal tibia is referred pain from the patellofemoral joint (see ANTERIOR KNEE PAIN, p. 396). *Shin splints* are a complaint of runners. In the unfit who suddenly take up 'keep fit', there may be a stress fracture of the tibia. More commonly, there is a periosteal reaction along the lateral border of the tibial shaft. In both of these conditions, technetium bone scanning shows increased uptake (Fig. L.70).

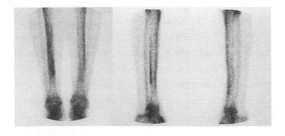

Figure L.70 Shin splints in a 20-year-old athlete. The technetium scan shows an increased uptake in both tibial diaphyses, more marked on the right than the left.

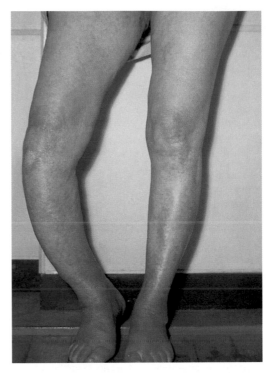

Figure L.71 Paget's disease of the right tibia. Note the typical varus deformity.

These bone changes must be distinguished from a *chronic compartment syndrome* secondary to muscle ischaemia. This particularly affects long-distance runners. There are other rare causes of pain such as the lightening pains of tabes dorsalis, while a periosteal reaction occurs in hypertrophic pulmonary osteoarthropathy. *Paget's disease*, in which there is increased bone turnover, causes tibial enlargement with anterior and lateral bowing (Fig. L.71). This can be painful early during the period of deformity when the bone is relatively soft. Pain in an established Paget's is due to: (i) a stress fracture; (ii) development of osteoarthritis in the knee or ankle; or (iii) malignant transformation to an osteogenic sarcoma.

Pain in the ankle and hindfoot

A wide variety of injuries occur around the ankle, and in many instances these involve a combination of ligamentous and bony injury. They occur sequentially according to the severity of the injury. For example, in the common inversion injury the anterior talofibular component of the lateral ligament is the initial

Table L.13 Brief summary of causes of ankle pain

Traumatic
- Fractures (often referred to as Pott's fractures)
- Ligament sprains/ruptures
- Tendinitis: acute, chronic, rupture
- Osteochrondritis dissecans

Infective
- Septic arthritis
- Osteomyelitis

Inflammatory
- Rheumatoid arthritis

Degenerative
- Osteoarthritis

Referred pain
- Lumbar disc disease with 'sciatica'

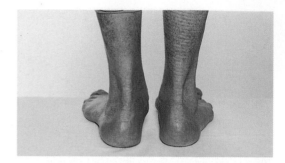

Figure L.72 Flat foot secondary to rupture of the tibialis posterior tendon. The heel is in valgus, the medial longitudinal arch has collapsed, and the foot is pronated. Viewed from behind, the toes of the left foot are visible – the 'too many toes' sign.

structure at risk. In the simplest sprain, the tenderness is therefore located anteriorly on the lateral side of the talar neck, just in front of the ankle and over the anterior distal aspect of the fibula. Pain is aggravated by inversion of the foot at the subtalar joint. With increasing severity, the injury involves the rest of the lateral ligament complex and marked swelling around the distal fibula is evident. As the force increases, a spiral fracture of the fibula results and finally an additional shear fracture of the medial malleolus occurs as the talus disrupts the ankle mortice. Other patterns of injury result from adduction, abduction and eversion injuries. The important initial assessment is to establish whether or not the talus is stable in the ankle mortice. Beware of the ankle which has marked tenderness over both malleoli, even if the X-ray shows only an undisplaced fracture of one of the malleoli, for a fracture on one side and a ligamentous injury to the other side equal 'potential instability'. If in doubt, take stress X-rays of both ankles for comparison.

Tendinitis, whether acute or chronic, is common around the ankle. The tendons involved are:

- Posteriorly: tendo-Achilles.
- Laterally: peroneus longus/brevis.
- Medially: tibialis posterior; flexor hallucis longus; and flexor digitorum longus.
- Anteriorly: tibialis anterior; extensor hallucis longus; extensor digitorum longus; and peroneus tertius.

A painful limp is the usual presenting feature, while the signs are the classical triad of local tenderness, pain on active resisted movement and pain on passive stretching. Note if there is marked swelling along the involved tendon sheath as this is often indicative of insipient tendon rupture. A common example is a *rupture of the tibialis posterior tendon*, which leads to a classical deformity with marked valgus at the heel, a fallen longitudinal arch and a flat externally rotated foot (Fig. L.72).

Osteochondritis dissecans affects the dome of the talus, usually at the superomedial corner of the articular surface. This presents with aching discomfort aggravated by use, or occasionally with locking if the fragment has separated. The fragment is often small and can be missed on routine X-rays if their quality is poor.

Septic arthritis can be difficult to diagnosis if it is low-grade or if it occurs as a complication of rheumatoid arthritis. *Tuberculous infection* can occur not only in the ankle joint but also may affect a tendon sheath. Synovial thickening and warmth from the ankle is best felt behind the malleoli, the normal concavity on either side of the tendo-Achilles being obliterated (Fig. L.73). The distal tibial metaphysis and metatarsal bones of the feet are common sites for *osteomyelitis* (Fig. L.74). Since the bone is superficial, signs of inflammation are often present in the overlying skin. It is therefore easy to confuse osteomyelitis with cellulitis; indeed, so much so that the old rule states, 'a cellulitis over a superficial bone is an osteomyelitis until proven otherwise'. Both the ankle and the subtalar joints are frequently involved in *rheumatoid disease*. This produces a characteristic valgus hindfoot deformity, which is occasionally complicated by a tarsal tunnel syndrome with compression of the plantar nerves. Any severe valgus deformity can cause localized pain at the distal end of the fibula due to

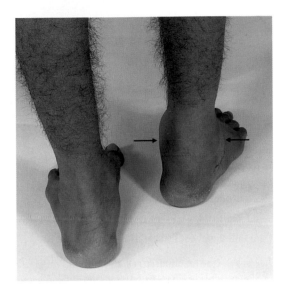

Figure L.73 Tuberculous synovitis of the right ankle in a 16-year-old boy. Note the loss of concavity on both sides of the right tendo-Achilles (arrowed).

impingement of this bone on to the calcaneus and consequent entrapment of the peroneal tendons. An acute exacerbation of pain in the hindfoot, in the absence of a flare of rheumatoid in other involved joints, should raise suspicion of a superimposed septic arthritis.

Significant symptoms due to *osteoarthritis* of the ankle are uncommon – a surprising fact considering how frequently this joint is injured. However, since the joint works in its mid range, it rarely becomes symptomatic until there has been sufficient loss of mobility to cause a fixed equinus deformity. The precipitating cause is usually obvious – malunited fracture, severe ligamentous instability, osteochondritis dissecans of the talus, previous infection, inflammatory arthropathies or bleeding disorders. Similar comments apply to osteoarthritis of the subtalar joint. The most common cause is incongruity secondary to fractures of the calcaneus. The natural history following this injury is for the pain gradually to settle over a period of 18 months to 2 years, but the joint remains stiff and the heel remains widened; this can cause problems with shoe fitting. However, it is surprising how well patients adjust to this disability given sufficient time.

Several entities present specifically with pain below or behind the heel. These are age-related. *Sever's disease* is a traction apophysitis of the Achilles tendon that most commonly affects boys aged 10–12 years.

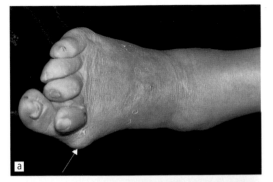

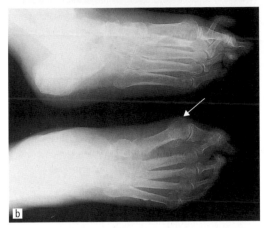

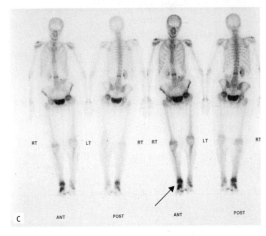

Figure L.74 Patient with acute osteomyelitis. (a) clinical photograph; (b) X-ray; (c) bone scan. Arrows point to affected anatomy that correspond to high up take on scan.

The boys present with a transient discomfort and mild tenderness localized to the posterior aspect of the calcaneus (Fig. L.75). 'Heel-Knobs' is a complaint of teenage girls, the prominence on the back of the calcaneus being aggravated by fashionable shoes.

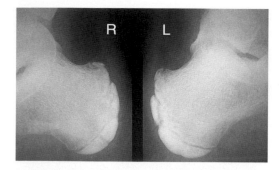

Figure L.75 Sever's disease: osteochondritis of the epiphysis of the calcaneum. Although both X-rays show similar fragmentation, only the right foot was painful.

Table L.14 Summary of causes of pain in the mid-foot

Condition	Site	Diagnostic entity
Osteochondritis/ Osteonecrosis	Navicular	Children: Kohler's disease Adults: Brailsford's disease
Bone overgrowth	Medial cuneiform/ First metatarsal	Bone knob
Tendinitis	Navicular tuberosity	Tibialis posterior
	Medial cuneiform/ First metatarsal	Tibialis anterior
	Base of fifth metatarsal	Peroneus brevis
Osteoarthritis	Talo-navicular joint Calcaneo-cuboid joint Cuneiform-metatarsal (1st, 2nd, 3rd) joints Cuboid-metatarsal (4th, 5th) joints	
Rheumatoid arthritis	Pan-tarsal involvement	
Charcot joint	Pan-tarsal involvement	Diabetes Other peripheral neuropathies Tabes dorsalis

Tight-fitting shoes or boots in young adults can result in an *Achilles bursitis* localized just above the insertion on the calcaneus. Achilles *peritendonitis* is a common problem in athletes of all ages, but it can also be precipitated by ill-fitting shoes. *Plantar fasciitis* occurs acutely in association with Reiter's disease or ankylosing spondylitis in young men. Occasionally, it may be the presenting symptom of these diseases. The common type of plantar fasciitis, 'policeman's heel', occurs in 40- to 60-year-olds. There are no signs

of overt inflammation, and the pain and tenderness are localized under the heel. Symptoms are usually worst first thing in the morning, and the first few steps taken on getting out of bed are particularly uncomfortable. If symptoms persist, check the uric acid level for gout. A bony spur is sometimes present on the lateral X-ray of the calcaneus, but this is also present in many patients who never have any symptoms of heel pain. A better indication for an X-ray is to exclude diseases of the calcaneus, for example tuberculous osteomyelitis or Paget's disease, which can masquerade as a plantar fasciitis.

Pain in the mid-foot (mid-tarsus)

Kohler's disease (in children) (Fig. L.76) *and Brailsford's disease* (middle age in women) both affect the navicular, and are both best regarded as an avascular necrosis. A bony prominence over the dorsal surface of the medial cuneiform and adjacent first metatarsal (*a bone knob*) is a common condition in the high-arch foot and can cause pressure against the shoe. *Tibialis posterior* and *tibialis anterior tendinitis* with tenderness and discomfort localized to the insertions on the medial side of the mid-foot is another common condition often associated with 'falling arches'; there is a secondary

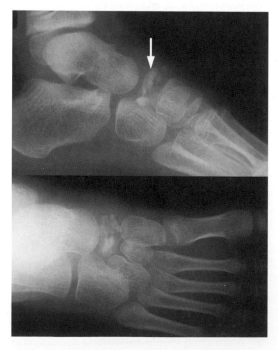

Figure L.76 Osteonecrosis of the navicular (arrow): Kohler's disease.

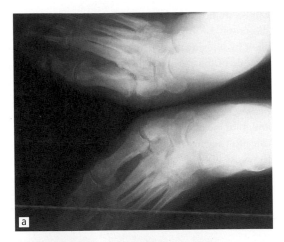

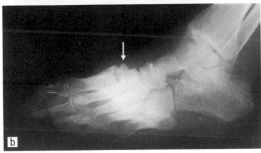

Figure L.77 Anteroposterior (a) and lateral (b) X-rays of a Charcot foot in a diabetic patient. There is dislocation and disintegration across the mid tarsus (arrow).

planovalgus mid-foot deformity. Tenderness at the base of the fifth metatarsal is usually precipitated by an inversion sprain, as both peroneus brevis and tertius tendons attach here. Quite frequently there is undisplaced avulsion fracture at the base of this bone, since normal tendons are stronger than bone. *Mid-foot osteoarthritis* is common in middle years and later life, and the symptoms are usually mild. *Charcot neuropathic joints* are often initiated by a stress fracture occurring into the articular surface, and at this stage they may be painful. Rapid destruction of the mid-foot soon occurs. The foot shortens and the joints sublux to produce the classical deformity of the 'square tarsus' (Fig. L.77).

Painful forefoot (metatarsalgia)

The causes of painful forefoot include:

■ Conditions affecting the hallux:
  ◆ Hallux rigidus
  ◆ Hallux valgus/bunion
  ◆ Rheumatoid arthritis/gout
■ Conditions affecting the metatarsals (two, three, four and five):
  ◆ Freiberg's disease (an osteonecrosis of the second metatarsal head)
  ◆ Kohler's second disease (an osteonecrosis of the third metatarsal head)
  ◆ Antebunion (a bursa over a prominent 5th metatarsal head)
  ◆ Stress fracture of the metatarsal shaft
  ◆ Morton's neuroma
■ Conditions affecting the metatarso-phalangeal joints:
  ◆ Rheumatoid arthritis
  ◆ Traumatic dislocation/subluxation
■ Other conditions:
  ◆ Plantar warts
  ◆ Peripheral neuropathy
  ◆ Erythromelalgia
  ◆ Ischaemia
  ◆ Ingrowing toenails
  ◆ Subungual exostosis
  ◆ Onchogryphosis

Hallux rigidus is a stiff great toe secondary to osteoarthritis of the first metatarsophalangeal joint. Pain is caused by the loss of movement preventing the passive hyperextension of the joint, which is required for 'toe off' at the end of the normal gait cycle. The toe is usually in good alignment, but there is bony swelling around the joint secondary to osteophyte formation. Plantar-flexion and dorsi-flexion are both markedly restricted. The pain is best reproduced by moving the joint while compressing the toe against the metatarsal. Many cases of *hallux valgus* are painless, the metatarsophalangeal joint retaining a good range of movement. Symptoms are usually due to wearing shoes that can no longer accommodate the widened splayed forefoot – the first metatarsal moves medially whilst the toe itself moves valgus (i.e. laterally), and as it does so the lesser toes are also displaced in a valgus direction or else become over-riding (Fig. L.78). A *bunion* is due to an adventitial bursa forming over the medial side of the prominent metatarsal head. This is prone to secondary infection. The severe pain of *acute gouty arthritis* accompanied by the surrounding erythema and oedema is very characteristic (Fig. L.79). *Rheumatoid disease* commonly affects the metatarsophalangeal joints, usually in a symmetrical pattern in both feet.

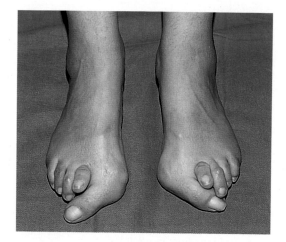

Figure L.78 A severe hallux valgus deformity in a 45-year-old woman. All her symptoms were related to the overlying second toe. The hallux retained a good range of movement at the metatarsophalangeal joint, and was painless.

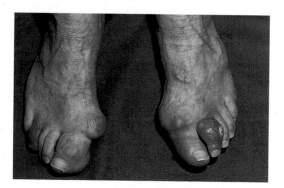

Figure L.79 Gout. There is an acute exacerbation of the left second toe. Tophi are also present over metatarsophalangeal joints of both big toes and under the distal phalanx of the right big toe.

Pain and local tenderness under the metatarsal heads is a common 'mechanical' problem, especially in a cavus foot with curly toes, a combination which drives the metatarsal heads into the sole of the shoe. During the gait cycle in the normal foot, the pressure zone moves from the heel along the lateral border of the foot, and then swings back medially across the metatarsal heads to the hallux. Any bony prominence will create a high pressure point resulting in thickening of the overlying skin, thus increasing the effect of the bony prominence and thereby establishing a vicious circle, resulting in a corn or a callosity. The pressure pattern can be studied using a pedobarograph, but sufficient diagnostic information can simply be found in the clinic by studying the pattern of callosities, the wear on the sole of the shoe, and the presence of humps and hollows in the insole.

Freiberg's and *Kohler's second disease* (Fig. L.80) are best regarded as an osteonecrosis that affects the second and third metatarsal heads, respectively. *Stress fractures* can affect any metatarsal, but most commonly occur in the necks of the second and third, usually following a prolonged period of unaccustomed activity (Fig. L.81).

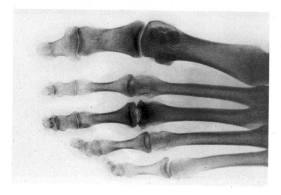

Figure L.80 Osteonecrosis of the third metatarsal head.

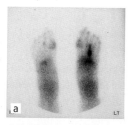

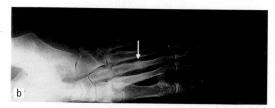

Figure L.81 Stress fracture of the third metatarsal. After a walking holiday, a 40-year-old woman complained of metatarsalgia. She was tender over the third metatarsal. (a) The initial X-ray was normal, but there was a markedly increased uptake on the technetium scan. (b) An X-ray taken after 3 weeks shows a healing callus (arrow).

Morton's neuroma is a swelling of digital nerve secondary to entrapment between the metatarsal heads. Pain is aggravated by walking and relieved by rest, particularly by removing the shoe. It is sometimes accompanied by paraesthesia of the appropriate toes. On examination there are frequently no abnormal findings. The most useful sign is to apply cross pressure to the metatarsal heads by squeezing the forefoot transversely while at the same time, with the other hand, eliciting the tenderness localized to the affected cleft; the third/fourth cleft is the most commonly involved. Demonstrable loss of sensation of the adjacent sides of the toes of the affected cleft is confirmatory but is unfortunately an infrequent finding.

A bunion, termed an *antebunion*, can also form over a prominent fifth metatarsal head often in association with a hallux valgus deformity consequent to widening of the forefoot and its entrapment in a shoe.

Plantar warts (*verrucas*) are particularly troublesome if they occur directly beneath a metatarsal head. Superficially, they can be difficult to distinguish from a corn, but paring down the skin with a scalpel blade will reveal the characteristic circular pattern of the verruca. *Bone and joint infections* in normal feet are uncommon unless there has been a penetrating injury. However, it is all too easy to overlook bone infection in an ulcerated neuropathic foot, especially in diabetes. Immunocompromised patients and those with HIV are also at risk. *Peripheral neuropathy*, particularly in the early stages, can cause burning pain in the foot. The common causes are diabetes, alcoholism, nutritional deficiencies (especially vitamin B) and HIV infection. Burning pain also occurs in the unusual condition of erythromelalgia. This is an abnormality of the superficial blood vessels found in polycythaemia, syringomyelia or the early stages of chronic arsenical poisoning. The pain is followed by cutaneous flushing and cyanosis, with the pain becoming pulsatile in character. Oedema, tenderness and hyperhydrosis may all be present. Occasionally Raynaud's phenomenon can produce similar episodic pain.

Rest pain that worsens at night is a classical symptom of *critical limb ischaemia* secondary to peripheral vascular disease. The pain is dull, severe and often requires opiate analgesics. Classically, the patient is woken with a painful cold foot that is relieved by hanging the foot over the side of the bed or walking about. In critical ischaemia, pressure at the ankle is less than 50 mmHg, or 20 mmHg at the toe in patients who are

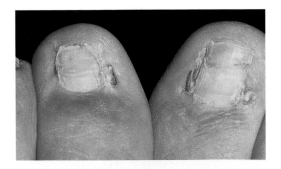

Figure L.82 Infected in-growing toe nails in a teenage boy.

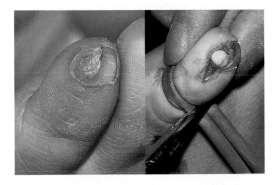

Figure L.83 Subungual exostosis. Left: preoperatively. Right: at surgery, the exostosis is a well-defined spherical nodule attached to the distal phalanx.

not diabetic. Signs of ischaemia vary from dry necrosis of the skin on the toes to gangrene. Nail-fold infection can be a presenting sign of arterial insufficiency. Do not confuse this with the *infected ingrowing toe nail of the hallux* that is most frequently seen in teenage boys (Fig. L.82).

A *subungual exostosis* (Fig. L.83) arises from the terminal phalanx of the hallux and the progressive enlargement causes deformity of the nail and pain secondary to pressure from the nail and the shoe. An *onchogryphosis* (Fig. L.84) is a disordered growth of the nail, usually secondary to trauma to the nail-bed. The nail fails to grow forward, becomes thickened and deformed, catches against the shoe, and is difficult to cut.

Deformities of the foot

The term 'talipes' denotes a foot deformity affecting the hind foot; varus describes the inverted heel; valgus the everted heel; equinus the plantar-flexed foot; and

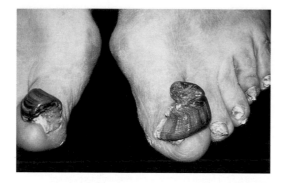

Figure L.84 Onchogryphosis of the toe nails of both big toes.

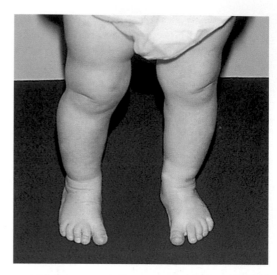

Figure L.86 Metatarsus adductors (varus). This is a common deformity in children, and rarely needs treatment apart from using suitable shoes.

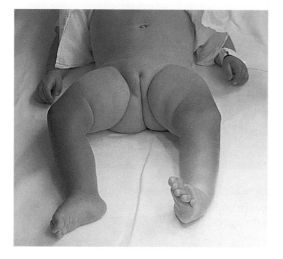

Figure L.85 Talipes equino varus (club foot) of the left foot. The heel is in varus, the foot is pronated and the forefoot is adducted.

calcaneus the dorsi-flexed foot. Mid-foot deformities are: pes cavus, the high arch foot; and pes planus, the flat foot. The metatarsals are referred to as adducted or varus, in which the metatarsal points medially; while metatarsus valgus means that the metatarsal points laterally and is an uncommon deformity usually due to a surgical over-correction of a metatarsal osteotomy for hallux valgus. If the foot is supinated then it is inverted and rotated so that the first metatarsal tends to rise off the ground, the longitudinal arch is accentuated and weight bearing occurs along the lateral border of the foot. A pronated foot is the reverse, the foot appearing flat with depression of the longitudinal arch and the first metatarsal head being forced into the ground. *With any foot deformity in childhood, it is essential to examine the peripheral neurology and also the spine.*

Talipes equino-varus (*club foot*) (Fig. L.85) describes a combined deformity of plantar-flexion and inversion of the hind foot, usually accompanied by a metatarsus adductus deformity arising at the tarso-metatarsal joint. It is classified into three groups: postural (due to intrauterine position, for example in oligohydramnios); congenital, in which the child is otherwise normal; and acquired (syndromic), in which there are other generalized abnormalities (e.g. arthrogryposis, diastrophic dwarfism) or neurological imbalance (e.g. myelomeningocoele; spinal dysraphism). There is a great variation in severity. In general, the postural-type correct relatively easily, the acquired-type are resistant, while the congenital are variable. Approximately 1 per 1000 live births are resistant, producing a 'rigid' uncorrectable structural deformity. Males are twice as commonly affected as females, but although there is a familial incidence with an increase in first-degree relatives, the precise genetics remain unknown. One-third of cases are bilateral.

Talipes calcaneo-valgus is a common mild deformity secondary to intrauterine moulding. It corrects easily with manual stretching, and the foot becomes normal.

Adduction deformities of the forefoot occur in association with a congenital club foot but also arise independently; this is *congenital metatarsus varus* (Fig. L.86). This is a common deformity in the baby and

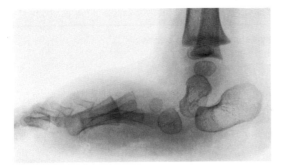

Figure L.87 Flat foot secondary to a congenital vertical talus. There is dislocation of the foot through the talo-navicular joint.

young child. The vast majority resolve spontaneously with growth, and surgical correction is rarely required.

Pes planus (sometimes referred to as pes valgus as the heel is a valgus position) describes the flat foot. This is a common, indeed almost universal, finding in young children, the normal arch only gradually appearing over the first few years. Ensure however, that the foot is mobile. *Congenital vertical talus* is a rare disorder in which there is a talo-navicular dislocation with the navicular lying on top of the neck of the talus (Fig. L.87). The foot is stiff and consequently acts in a 'rocker-bottom' manner. Occasionally, a flat foot persists into adult life when it may be associated with other causes of ligamentous laxity, for example Ehlers–Danlos syndrome or Marfan's syndrome. *Spasmodic flat foot* is a well-recognized entity, though the foot is not necessarily flat, nor is the problem necessarily spasmodic. This condition is due to a bony union of the tarsal bones, a talo-calcaneal bar being the most common type. The foot is held rigidly everted secondary to muscle spasm. The peroneal and extensor tendons stand out prominently (Figs L.88 and L.89). Subtalar movements are grossly restricted and often painful. Mid tarsal movements are diminished, but ankle movements are usually normal. Special oblique X-ray views are required to demonstrate a bar or an abnormal joint. Technetium bone scanning can be helpful in pin-pointing the site of the anatomical problem, which is usually best shown by a CT scan. Inflammatory conditions affecting the subtalar–mid-tarsal joints can also cause this deformity. A pes planus is common in *paralytic disorders*. In the elderly, it can be associated with a general muscular

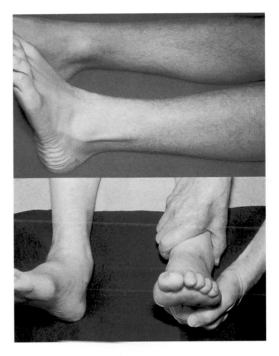

Figure L.88 Spasmodic flat foot. Upper: the peroneal tendons stand out sharply in spasm. Lower: the examiner is unable to invert the hind foot, which is held rigid.

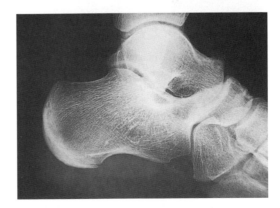

Figure L.89 Same patient as in Fig. L.88. An X-ray confirms the presence of a bony bar between the navicular and the calcaneum.

weakness aggravated by obesity, while a more specific cause is *rupture of the tibialis posterior tendon* (see Pain in the ankle and hindfoot, p. 413).

A *pes cavus deformity* is usually associated with clawing of the toes in addition to the high arch. The majority are 'idiopathic', but ensure that there is no

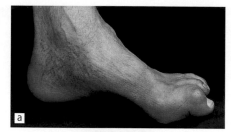

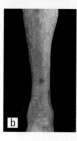

Figure L.90 Hereditary motor sensory peripheral neuropathy (Charcot–Marie–Tooth syndrome). The foot is cavus, the toes are clawed (a), and there is marked wasting of the distal calf (b).

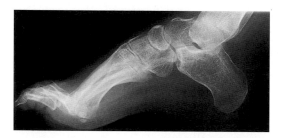

Figure L.91 A severe pes cavus deformity secondary to a neurological imbalance, in this case due to poliomyelitis.

underlying neurological or muscular deficit causing a muscle imbalance that particularly affects the intrinsic muscles. Charcot–Marie–Tooth (peroneal muscular atrophy (Fig. L.90), Friedreich's ataxia and spastic hemiplegia are some examples. Pes cavus was a common deformity in polio (Fig. L.91). In general, pes cavus is a much more troublesome entity than pes planus, since weight-bearing tends to be concentrated along the lateral border of the foot and on the metatarsal heads. In contrast, in the flat foot weight is spread over a wide area. Interestingly, even when there is an underlying pathological reason for a pes

Table L.15 Summary of paralytic causes of foot deformities*

Upper motor neurone lesions
1 Cerebral
- Cerebral palsy
- Meningitis
- Cerebrovascular accident
2 Spinal
- Trauma
- Haemorrhage
- Thrombosis
- Spinal dysraphism
- Diastematomyelia

Lower motor neurone lesions
- Amyotrophic lateral sclerosis
- Cauda equina lesions (e.g. tumours, diastematomyelia)
- Poliomyelitis
- Peroneal muscular atrophy (Charcot–Marie–Tooth, which is now classified as an inherited mixed sensorimotor neuropathy)
- Progressive muscular atrophy (motor neurone disease)

Cerebellar lesions
- Friedreich's ataxia

Primary muscle disease
- Duchenne's disease (pseudo-hypertrophic muscular paralysis)

Acquired muscle conditions
- Ischaemic contracture secondary to compartment syndrome

*In all foot deformities, examine the spine and the neurology.

cavus, the deformity is rarely seen in children under the age of 6 years.

Deformities of the toes

A *claw toe deformity* is due to flexion of the interphalangeal joints and hyperextension at the metatarsophalangeal joint. It is often associated with a pes cavus deformity. Initially, the toe deformities are mobile and can be passively corrected, but they gradually become fixed and eventually the metatarsophalangeal joints may sublux or even dislocate. The condition is usually bilateral. While most cases are idiopathic, it can result from a peripheral neuropathy; in particular, peroneal muscular atrophy should be excluded. Claw toes are also commonly found in *rheumatoid arthritis* secondary to subluxation and dislocation of the metatarsophalangeal joints. Symptoms are secondary to pressure on the prominent metatarsal heads and also over the dorsum of the toes. Callosities are usually present at both sites. In severe cases walking may be difficult.

A *hammer toe deformity* occurs when the proximal interphalangeal joint is fixed in acute flexion while the metatarsophalangeal and distal interphalangeal joints are fixed in extension. The second toe is the most commonly affected. Symptoms are due to painful callosities forming under the metatarsal head and over the dorsum of the toe. In a *mallet toe deformity* there is fixed flexion of the distal interphalangeal joint so that the tip of the toe or the toe nail is impacted down into the sole of the shoe, resulting in a painful callosity. An *overlapping little toe* is a common anomaly in which the little toe sits on the dorsum of the fourth toe. In a *cock-up toe deformity*, the metatarsophalangeal joint is dislocated, with the result that the little toe contracts proximally and sits on the dorsum of the metatarsal head. Both little toe deformities can cause problems with shoe fitting.

Fred Heatley

LYMPHADENOPATHY

Although there are a multitude of causes of lymphadenopathy (Table L.16), it is usually possible to narrow the differential diagnosis considerably by careful review of the patient's history and clinical examination. The differential diagnosis is very dependent on the patient's age and geographical location. Small soft lymphadenopathy is commonly found in healthy children and young adults, particularly in the axillary and inguinal regions. A young adult with significant cervical lymphadenopathy in the UK is likely to have Epstein–Barr (EBV) infection, whereas in Africa the commonest cause is often tuberculosis. Local lymphadenopathy may be secondary to local infection or malignancy, whereas generalized enlargement is indicative of a systemic disorder. Painful, tender nodes in association with a fever and rash indicate a systemic infection, usually of viral aetiology. Firm, painless nodes found in a patient with weight loss or night sweats is likely to be due to malignant disease. Occasionally, it is difficult to identify the cause of enlarged lymph nodes and it is then essential to systematically consider all possibilities listed in Table L.16.

Table L.16 Causes of lymphadenopathy

Infectious diseases

Viral: Epstein–Barr virus, cytomegalovirus, HIV, coxsackie, hepatitis viruses, rubella, measles, herpes simplex, varicella-zoster virus
Bacterial: Local infections (*Staphylococcus*, *Streptococcus*), brucellosis, TB, atypical mycobacteria, syphilis, cat-scratch disease, plague, leprosy, bejel, pinta, yaws, bartonella, tularaemia
Protozoan: Toxoplasmosis, trypanosomiasis, leishmaniasis, filiariasis
Fungal: Blastomycosis, histoplasmosis, paracoccidiomycosis
Chlamydial: Lymphogranuloma venereum, trachoma
Rickettsial: Scrub typhus

Malignant diseases

Secondary deposits from a local malignancy
Hodgkin's disease
Non-Hodgkin's lymphomas: B-cell, T-cell, mycosis fungoides, angioimmunoblastic lymphadenopathy
Acute or chronic lymphatic leukaemia
Myeloproliferative disorders, macroglobulinaemia, amyloidosis

Immunological diseases

Systemic lupus erythematosus
Rheumatoid arthritis, juvenile rheumatoid arthritis
Mixed connective tissue disease
Drug reactions: phenytoin, hydralazine, gold, allopurinol
Serum sickness

Miscellaneous

Sarcoid
Lipid storage diseases
Hyperthyroidism
Familial Mediterranean fever

Infections

Local infections usually result only in regional lymph node enlargement, which may be painful. A viral sore throat may cause swelling of the tonsils and tonsillar lymph nodes. Unilateral cervical, axillary or inguinal lymphadenopathy may be due to bacterial or fungal infection in the field of lymphatic drainage.

EBV infection (*glandular fever*) is a common cause in young adults with generalized lymphadenopathy particularly involving the cervical region. It is clinically very similar to acute cytomegalovirus (CMV) and human immunodeficiency virus (HIV) infection. This latter virus may later cause a persistent painless generalized lymphadenopathy for a period of many months. *Acute brucellosis* or *toxoplasmosis* may also produce a similar syndrome, although usually without a sore throat.

Tuberculosis usually causes enlargement of a single set of nodes, although generalized enlargement is occasionally observed. *Primary syphilis* may initially result in swelling of the inguinal lymph nodes draining the chancre, but generalized lymphadenopathy may be observed in *secondary syphilis* when the primary lesion has healed. *Cat-scratch fever*, which is often seen in children, presents with an inflamed papule at the site of injury, and this may be followed by local lymphadenopathy for several months.

Tropical infections such as filiriasis, African trypanosomiasis and tulareamia may be associated with lymphangitis in association with the primary infection and local lymphadenopathy to which may become generalized later.

Malignant disease

Malignant disease may spread from a primary site along the draining lymphatics to invade the regional lymph nodes; it is unusual for generalized lymphadenopathy to be secondary to disseminated carcinoma, although it is occasionally observed (e.g. melanoma). *Virchow's node* is found in the anterior left supraclavicular region, and is also known as *Troisier's ganglion*. Causes include carcinoma of the breast or bronchus, gastrointestinal malignancy and lymphomas.

Symmetrical generalized painless lymphadenopathy is a common presenting feature of malignancies of the *lymphopoietic system* – for example, Hodgkin's disease in a young person or chronic lymphatic leukaemia or non-Hodgkin's lymphoma in an older adult. *Macroglobulinaemia*, or occasionally *myeloma*, is characterized by painless generalized lymphadenopathy. Such syndromes may be associated with systemic or 'B' symptoms – that is, >10 per cent weight loss, fever >38°C or night sweats. These indicate generalized disease, and in an individual presenting with only a single group of enlarged nodes they are suggestive of more extensive disease. Other malignant disorders of the lymphoreticular system, particularly of T-cell origin, have characteristic features. *Adult T-cell leukaemia/lymphoma* may present with fever, rash and hypercalcaemia as well as extensive hilar lymphadenopathy. *Mycosis fungoides* is recognizable by the cutaneous deposits which, although initially localized as lymphomatous lesions, spread as the

disease progresses to involve nodes, resulting in generalized node enlargement. *Acute lymphatic leukaemia* – especially in children – may present with diffuse lymphadenopathy. *Myeloproliferative disorders* such as chronic myeloid leukaemia, polycythaemia rubra vera and myelofibrosis are occasionally associated with lymphadenopathy.

Other conditions

Lymphadenopathy can occur in *collagenoses* (e.g. SLE and rheumatoid arthritis). *Sarcoid*, in addition to causing bilateral hilar lymphadenopathy, may result in generalized superficial lymphadenopathy. *Drugs* (e.g. phenytoin) may rarely cause lymph node hypertrophy. The unusual condition of angio-immunoblastic lymphadenopathy is often a highly malignant lymphoma, but occasionally it may be secondary to drug therapy (e.g. penicillins and sulphonamides).

Splenomegaly may be a feature of any cause of lymphadenopathy. In acute infections it is usually small and soft, whereas in long-standing infections or malignancies it is often firm on palpation.

Investigations

These should be directed initially at the diagnosis of the most likely conditions, as judged by the history and examination. A full blood count will indicate the presence of a leukaemic process, or atypical lymphocytes will reflect an acute viral infection (e.g. EBV or HIV). A chest X-ray may reveal hilar lymphadenopathy or pulmonary pathology (e.g. tuberculosis). A serological search for infections (e.g. EBV and CMV) may indicate active infection if a high titre of a specific IgM is present. Although a bone-marrow aspirate will reveal the presence of leukaemia, a trephine biopsy is much more reliable for diagnosing an infiltrate (e.g. carcinoma or lymphoma).

An abdominal and chest CT scan is a sensitive investigation for identifying pelvic, para-aortic, coeliac, mesenteric, hilar or paratracheal node enlargement. If the initial blood tests do not provide an early diagnosis, it is essential to perform a lymph node biopsy. If the initial histology reveals reactive change only, or the presence of granulomas, it is often prudent to perform further biopsies if there is a strong clinical indication that the patient may have a malignant condition.

Melvin Lobo

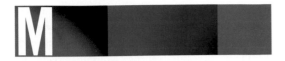

MACULES

A macule is a flat, circumscribed patch of altered skin colour of any size. (In the past, the term was often restricted to small lesions <2 cm across, larger lesions being termed patches.) Macules must be distinguished from papules, the latter being palpable. Macules may be red (e.g. rubella), dark red (e.g. purpura), brown (e.g. freckle) or white (e.g. vitiligo) (see Table M.1). (See also ERYTHEMA, p. 178.)

Table M.1 Macules

Red macules
1 Exanthems
  ■ Measles
  ■ Rubella
2 Typhoid
3 Drug reaction
4 Macular syphilide
5 Tuberculoid leprosy

Purpuric macules
1 Inflammatory skin diseases
  ■ Contact dermatitis
  ■ Drug reactions
  ■ Erythema multiforme
  ■ Vasculitis
2 Pigmented purpuric eruptions
  ■ Schamberg's purpura
  ■ Majocchi's purpura
3 Septicaemia
4 Scurvy

Brown macules
1 Freckles
  ■ Sun-induced
  ■ Xeroderma pigmentosum
  ■ *Peutz–Jegher's* syndrome
  ■ Hutchinson's freckle

2 Flat mole (junctional naevus)
3 Café-au-lait spots
  ■ Neurofibromatosis
  ■ Albright's syndrome
4 Mongolian spot
5 Chloasma
6 Berloque dermatitis
7 Post-inflammatory hyperpigmentation

White macules
1 Post-inflammatory
  ■ Depigmentation
  ■ Pityriasis alba
2 Vitiligo
3 Pityriasis versicolor
4 Naevus anaemicus

Red macules

Redness that is due to hyperaemia and blanches with pressure is known as 'erythema'. A widespread red macular rash occurs at some stage in many infections:

■ In *measles*, the rash begins behind the ears and on the forehead in an ill, coughing, febrile child, with conjunctivitis and lymphadenopathy. The rash spreads over the face, neck and extremities, and comprises small pink macules which become confluent, and subsequently turn brown and desquamate. Vesicles on the buccal mucosae (Koplik's spots) are seen just before the rash appears. The pink macules of *rubella* (*German measles*) also begin behind the ears and spread onto the face, head, neck, and trunk. Occipital lymphadenopathy is common, but fever and malaise are mild. In adults there may be an associated arthropathy.

■ In *typhoid*, 'rose spots' (0.5 cm red maculopapules) appear in crops on the abdomen, chest and back. Successive crops may come and go for 2–3 weeks.

■ The macular *syphilide* is one of the most characteristic lesions of secondary syphilis (Fig. M.1). The eruption, named 'syphilitic roseola', begins as a macular mottling resembling measles, but rather more dusky and distributed over the chest, abdomen and – of great diagnostic importance – on the palms and soles. Eroded red patches are commonly present on the buccal mucosa. Malaise and lymphadenopathy are common and serology will be positive. A primary chancre will often still be present. Generally, about a fortnight after its appearance the rash begins to fade, giving place to a papular or follicular eruption on the trunk, limbs, face and neck. Vesicles are never seen, and characteristically the rash does not itch. It should be distinguished from pityriasis versicolor, in which the scaly patches can be demonstrated by scratching and the

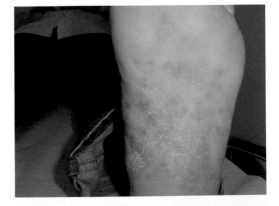

Figure M.1 Rash of secondary syphilis affecting the soles of the feet.

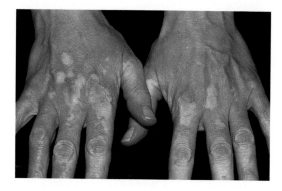

Figure M.2 Tuberculoid leprosy.

fungus can be demonstrated microscopically; from drug reactions by their more vivid redness and the presence of itching and burning; from seborrhoeic dermatitis by its scaliness and pinkish-yellow colour; from measles by the coryza, cough and the different distribution; and from pityriasis rosea by the history of the herald patch, the distribution sparing the face and extremities and the characteristic oval lesions, each with their collarette of scaling.

■ In the earlier stages of *tuberculoid leprosy*, red macular areas may appear. These are often isolated and have hyperpigmented borders, and as they expand to their maximum size of 2–10 cm in diameter, the centre of lesions becomes depigmented and anaesthetic (Fig. M.2). In dark skins the red macules are difficult to discern until the central depigmentation makes them obvious.

■ In *drug reactions*, itching and burning are pronounced and lesions may later become elevated (e.g. maculopapular ampicillin rash), purpuric or even bullous.

Purpuric macules

Purpuric macules are caused by the escape of red blood cells into the skin, and characteristically fail to blanch on pressure. Tiny lesions 1–5 mm are true purpura, larger extravasations are *ecchymoses*, and associated subcutaneous collections are *haematomas*. Purpura appear suddenly, are painless, and change hue from red, to brown, to green and yellow before fading. Where purpura is due to vasculitis, the lesions are generally palpable. Perifollicular purpuric macules may be seen in *scurvy* (ascorbic acid deficiency).

Brown macules

Freckles (ephelides) are small (<0.5 cm), brown, roundish macules in areas of the skin exposed to the sun. They appear in childhood, especially in red-haired, fair-skinned individuals, and are associated with vulnerability to sunburn. They are particularly florid in the rare genetic syndrome *xeroderma pigmentosum*, a condition associated with deficient repair of sun-damaged nuclear protein. By their early teens, affected children are disfigured by atrophy, telangiectasia and multiple cutaneous malignancies, which ultimately prove fatal.

In the *Peutz–Jegher's syndrome*, freckles in great profusion on and around the lips (Fig. M.3) are associated with polyposis of the small bowel, which may be complicated by recurrent intussusception and melaena. The freckles are smaller than usual and may extend inside the mouth and onto the sides and backs of fingers. *Hutchinson's freckle is* a giant freckle that usually occurs on an elderly, sun-exposed skin. Pigmentation is variegate, and malignant pigment cell tumours often eventually arise within their boundaries.

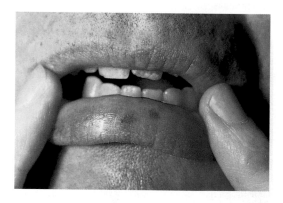

Figure M.3 Lips demonstrating freckles due to Peutz–Jegher's syndrome.

Flat moles (junctional naevi) are either present at birth or develop during the first two decades of life. They have distinct borders and are not uniformly pigmented. They undergo gradual spontaneous involution. Rarely, a more rapid involution of moles – both flat and papular – may be accompanied by a stark, chalk-white halo of depigmentation – a halo naevus (Sutton's naevus). This is a dramatic, but benign, condition.

Café-au-lait spots are well named; they are creamy brown in colour, with smooth borders, and range from 1 to 15 cm in diameter (Fig. M.4). More than six lesions on a child's skin are said to be highly suggestive of the autosomal dominant *von Recklinghausen's neurofibromatosis* (Fig. M.5). The later appearance of axillary freckling is an even stronger diagnostic pointer to the later appearance of multiple pendulous cutaneous nerve sheath tumours. Large brown macules with irregular borders on a child's trunk can also be associated with bone cysts and precocious puberty in girls with *Albright's syndrome.*

The *mongolian spot is* well known to midwives as a marker of Asiatic or Negroid parentage. Large brown or slate-grey macules are seen over the sacrum at birth and gradually fade over the first year of life; the colour is due to melanocytes in the dermis.

Macular facial pigmentation is a feature of *chloasma* (see SKIN, PIGMENTATION OF, p. 648).

White macules

Post-inflammatory depigmentation may occur following inflammatory dermatoses, such as psoriasis or pityriasis rosea. Perhaps more commonly, many skin diseases fail to tan on a sunny holiday. This is particularly seen over the cheeks and outer arms of children with the eczematous condition *pityriasis alba.*

Vitiligo usually begins in the second decade of life as symmetrical chalk-white patches of complete depigmentation around eyes, mouth, genitals and axillae. White locks of hair may occur, but ocular pigmentation is never affected. In dark races the lesions are only too obvious, but in untanned, pale individuals the use of an ultraviolet light may be necessary to demonstrate the full extent of the disease.

Pityriasis versicolor is becoming a more common cause for medical consultation. The original fawny-pink, slightly scaling, round patches on the chest and back may not be noticed until, following sun exposure, partial depigmentation of affected areas occurs. The diagnosis can nearly always be made clinically by noting the slight superficial scale and looking at the margin for typical tiny annular lesions. Microscopic examination of scrapings reveals the possible yeast. The most difficult differential diagnosis is post-inflammatory depigmentation following guttate psoriasis, but here the small round white macules are scattered uniformly over the body and limbs rather than concentrated in the mantle area.

Ash leaf-shaped hypopigmented macules are seen in *tuberose sclerosis*, and may be more readily seen under ultraviolet light.

Naevus anaemicus is present from birth, and may be found at any site as a group of islands of blanched skin. The pigment mechanisms are intact, but there is permanent vasoconstriction due to a congenital neurovascular abnormality.

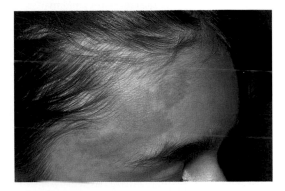

Figure M.4 Café-au-lait macule.

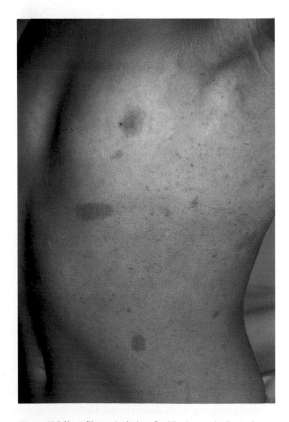

Figure M.5 Neurofibromatosis (von Recklinghausen's disease).

Barry Monk

MANIA

See EUPHORIA (p. 183).

MARASMUS

Severe protein–energy malnutrition in children usually leads to marasmus, which is a body weight less than 60 per cent of the mean for age. Children are often withdrawn and apathetic, their facial appearance is pinched and grey, and they have a curiously senile (wizened) expression. The eyes and the fontanelles are sunken, the skin is tightly stretched over the bones of the skull, whereas on the limbs and body generally the skin is thin and inelastic through dehydration and loss of subcutaneous fat so that it hangs in festoons on the stick-like arms and legs (skin fold thickness and mid-arm circumferences are markedly reduced). The thorax is particularly wasted, and the ribs are unduly prominent. The bony fingers are often stuffed into the mouth as if to obtain nourishment. Oedema is not present. There may be a skin rash with hyperkaratosis, angular stomatitis, sparse depigmented hair, diarrhoea, hypothermia, bradycardia and hypotension, and low levels of electrolytes in the blood. These children are at great risk of intercurrent illness such as gastroenteritis, measles or tuberculosis or by incorrect feeding of carbohydrate rather than protein. Kwashiorkor, a particular manifestation of protein–energy malnutrition, occurs in some developing countries where infants are weaned late from the breast and the child's diet is high in starch. Vitamin and mineral deficiencies also complicate the condition, making treatment far more difficult than in uncomplicated marasmus.

Among the very many conditions which may produce this condition are included: starvation (either from neglect, extreme poverty or the breakdown of normal civilized behaviour, as usually occurs in modern warfare); persistent vomiting (e.g. hiatus hernia) or diarrhoea; chronic infections (the urinary tract, tuberculosis, congenital syphilis, HIV and parasitic infestations); malabsorption – of fat in coeliac disease and cystic fibrosis, of sugar in carbohydrate intolerance, or of protein in protein-losing enteropathy;

Hirschsprung's disease; a group of conditions associated with polyuria, that is to say diabetes mellitus, diabetes insipidus, hypercalcaemia, renal acidosis and renal failure; and, rarely in children, thyrotoxicosis, Addison's disease and malignant disease. Severe cyanotic congenital heart disease which is not corrected may be associated with a marked failure to thrive.

Starvation includes a variety of causes. Because of social and political circumstances, the child may simply not receive enough calories. Because of ignorance, feeding may be imperfect both as regards quantity and quality (see Kwashiorkor, below). Because of structural imperfections (e.g. cleft lip, cleft palate) or feebleness from prematurity, the infant may be unable to suck. Because of an oesophageal stricture dysphagia may prevent adequate intake of food, and persistent vomiting will have a similar disastrous effect.

Chronic infections include serious involvement of the upper renal tract, in which circumstances-associated renal failure, for example in advanced bilateral congenital hydronephrosis, may be an aggravating factor. Congenital syphilis was once a potent cause of marasmus, although its classic features of snuffles, skin lesions, Parrot's nodes, condylomas and enlargement of the liver and spleen are now rarely seen. Chronic infections associated with the acquired immune deficiency syndrome (HIV/AIDS) are the contemporary equivalent. Advanced miliary tuberculosis is now fortunately rare in the UK, as is neglected tuberculous disease of bone with its associated discharging sinuses leading to secondarily infected abscess cavities.

Malabsorption is a potent cause of weight loss in children. Cystic fibrosis and coeliac disease are associated with gross steatorrhoea. Disaccharidase deficiency may result in the infant being unable to split disaccharides into absorbable monosaccharides. Lactase deficiency is the most common example, but the enzymes responsible for splitting sucrose and maltose also may be affected. Not only is the child prevented from absorbing sugar, but this also remains in the small intestine to aggravate the condition by causing diarrhoea by an osmotic effect. Protein-losing enteropathy due to a variety of small intestinal diseases, including Crohn's disease, may result in protein loss into the bowel lumen.

Diabetes mellitus may have a relatively acute onset in children, with thirst, polyuria and severe loss of weight.

Kwashiorkor is a condition seen chiefly in Central Africa in children who are reared in traditional polygamous societies. It has also been widely described in other tropical and subtropical parts of the world, and even in Europe. It is a state produced by gross protein deficiency, and is usually due to late weaning of children from the breast, and a high starch diet. The majority of sufferers are infants under the age of 2 years who are placed on a diet mainly of cereals, with little (if any) animal protein because of shortage of suitable foods or deeply ingrained superstitions. In addition to the failure of growth, there is oedema of the legs, a distended abdomen, hyperpigmentation, and very typical depigmentation of the skin and hair, which produces a reddish hue in African babies.

Dipak Kanabar

MELAENA

Melaena is the term applied to the black bowel motion resulting from haemorrhage which has occurred in the gastrointestinal (GI) tract at a high enough level for chemical alteration to take place (usually the upper GI tract, but it could also be as far down as the caecum). Melaena may also occur after swallowing blood derived from haemoptysis or epistaxis. Melaena stools are black, tarry, with a sticky consistency, rendering it difficult to flush down the toilet. It has been shown by feeding healthy volunteer medical students with increasing aliquots of their own blood, that between 50 and 80 ml of blood is sufficient to cause a melaena stool.

Black or dark stools, simulating melaena, may occur after taking iron preparations by mouth (the iron being converted to the sulphide form), bismuth preparations, liquorice or following the ingestion of charcoal biscuits, black cherries, bilberries or red wine in large quantities, or by the excretion of large amounts of bile pigments. The characteristic thick sticky nature of melaena stools is generally easily differentiated from other causes of black stools, but the diagnosis can be confirmed by laboratory investigation of the stool for the presence of blood.

Melaena is most commonly due to bleeding from the stomach or duodenum, or more rarely from the oesophagus. In such situations it is generally associated with haematemesis, before the melaena is apparent. If melaena occurs alone from these sources, it generally indicates that the rate of bleeding is relatively slow. Melaena is as serious as haematemesis as an indication of upper gastric haemorrhage; patients with melaena should be investigated and managed as urgently as those with haematemesis. It is possible to judge the severity of a gastrointestinal bleed from the patient's description of the stools.

A detailed account of symptoms such as faintness, sweating and collapse, together with the general assessment of the patient's haemodynamic state, allows the clinician to assess the severity of the gastrointestinal bleed leading to the development of melaena. Upper gastrointestinal endoscopy may be required, and blood transfusion may be necessary.

The great majority of patients with melaena will have bled from lesions situated in, or proximal to, the duodenum. The most common cause (perhaps more than 85% of patients) is from duodenal or gastric ulceration, acute gastric erosions and peptic oesophagitis or hiatus hernia. Bleeding from haemorrhagic erosions associated with the use of non-steroidal antiinflammatory drugs (NSAIDs) is an increasingly common cause of melaena, especially in elderly patients.

Lesions distal to the duodenum generally give rise to dark or bright red blood in the stools rather than melaena. However, melaena may occur in the relatively uncommon group of causes of the small intestinal bleeding, which include mesenteric thrombosis or embolism, leiomyoma, leiomyosarcoma, or haemangioma of the upper small intestine, Ehlers–Danlos syndrome, peptic ulcer in a Meckel's diverticulum, Crohn's disease of the small intestine, haemorrhage in typhoid fever from an ulcerated Peyer's patch in the ileum, parasitic disease (e.g. hookworm), angiodysplasia of the small intestine, blood dyscrasias resulting in oozing from the intestinal mucosa, or the use of anticoagulant therapy. Rarely, melaena may be associated with small intestinal ulceration in coeliac disease or secondary to drug-induced damage to the small intestine, a rare but increasing occurrence.

Danielle Harari

MEMORY, DISORDERS OF

Disorders of memory (see also CONFUSION, p. 113) are extremely important in clinical practice. There are

Table M.2 Causes of memory loss

Common	Less common
Head injury	Herpes simplex encephalitis
Cerebrovascular disease	Vertebrobasilar disease (transient global amnesia)
Multi-infarct dementia	Tumours of IIIrd ventricle or hypothalamus
Single infarct in region of posterior cerebral artery	Depression (pseudodementia)
Subarachnoid haemorrhage	Fugue states and psychogenic amnesias
Alzheimer's-type dementia (and other causes	Malingering
of organic confusion states; see p. 314)	
Thiamine deficiency (Werknicke–Korsakoff	**Rare**
syndrome) due to alcoholism, malabsorption,	Bilateral temporal lobectomy for intractible epilepsy
carcinoma of the stomach	Intractible epilepsy
Hyperemesis gravidarum	Carbon monoxide poisoning
Electroconvulsive therapy	Personality disorder
	Pseudologia fantastica
	Ganser state

numerous tests used to assess memory. One of the easiest to use is the Mini Mental State Exam (MMSE) which tests orientation, registration, attention and calculation, recall, language, construction and spatial orientation (areas of higher cortical function). The MMSE has been used widely, but not in all cultures, and depends on education level. The causes of memory loss are given in Table M.2.

Functional memory disturbance/pseudodementia

Pseudodementia is the term used to describe non-organic causes of memory impairment. A depressed person may perform as poorly as a demented person on tests of memory, simply because he or she is retarded and lacks the motivation to take an interest in their surroundings. Similarly, a patient who is psychotic may interpret their recall of events by delusional beliefs. Memory lapses are also common in states of fatigue. In *hysterical fugue states* there is a narrowing of consciousness, a move away from normal surroundings and subsequently complete amnesia for these events. The behaviour of the person may appear quite appropriate during the episode, which can last from hours to weeks. Such dissociative states may be attempts by people of certain personalities to cope with real or imagined stress. The *Ganser state* first described in prisoners awaiting sentence should also be considered an hysterical dissociative state. Two of the main features of the condition are clouding of consciousness and approximate answers (two plus two equals five). Subjects are subsequently amnesic for their abnormal behaviour.

Organic memory impairment

The commonest cause of organic memory impairment is Alzheimer's disease in 60 per cent, followed by 30 per cent due to multiple cerebrovascular accident (CVA). In the West, tertiary syphilis is no longer encountered, but it is an important cause in the developing world. Rare causes of memory impairment need also to be considered. Specific lesions to specific organs can cause specific types of impairment. It has long been known that damage to the temporal lobes and to structures in the limbic system – and in particular to the hippocampus, amygdala, fornix, mammillary bodies and the dorsal medial nucleus of the thalamus – may result in profound amnesia. Bilateral focal lesions affecting these structures – for example, temporal lobe damage following herpes simplex encephalitis or lesions in the mammillary body caused by a thiamine deficiency – may cause severe and specific types of memory impairment. Organic memory disturbance may also be a feature of diffuse cerebral disorder that perhaps involves quite different brain mechanisms. In some situations frontal lobe dysfunction may contribute to memory impairment. Pathological processes that cause bilateral damage to these diencephalic and limbic structures such as head trauma, hypoxia, infarction in the territory of the posterior cerebral arteries and herpes simplex encephalitis can cause memory impairment.

Alzheimer's disease (Alzheimer, 1907) describes a progressive decline in high critical function which eventually leads inexorably to a mute bed-ridden state over 3–10 years. Initially, the patient is able to function at home, but progressive memory loss and increasing behavioural disturbance leads to an inability to do complex followed by simple tasks, which in turn leads to increased care needs by the family and others. Patients die from complications such as pneumonia. There is no cure, although some drugs are available to help alleviate suffering in the mild to moderate stages. *Multi-infarct disease* (MID) is increasingly recognized due to the increasing incidence of cardiovascular disease and successful ageing. It occurs in patients with increased cholesterol, diabetes, hypertension and those with stroke disease.

The main cause of dementia is thromboembolic disease leading to occlusion of the arteries that supply the brain, leading in turn to memory impairment. It manifests as a stepwise decline in cognitive function, and there is no specific treatment. Strategies to reduce the risk factors and control conditions mentioned above are worthwhile.

Lewy body dementia is increasingly recognized as a cause of dementia due to excess deposition of Lewy bodies in the brain's subcortical structures. This leads to presenting symptoms differing from Alzheimer's disease or MID. Typically, patients have psychomotor disturbance, prominent visual hallucinations, fluctuating levels of consciousness (day to day) and an exaggerated sensitivity to major tranquilizers. The disease is incurable and progressive.

Rarer forms encountered include the Wemicke–Korsakoff syndrome, caused by thiamine deficiency in chronic alcoholism, and less frequently due to carcinoma of the stomach, hyperemesis during pregnancy, malabsorption or dietary deficiency. A similar clinical picture can present with tumours of the third ventricle and hypothalamus, carbon monoxide poisoning, tuberculous meningitis or subarachnoid haemorrhage. The acute effects of thiamine depletion include clouding of consciousness, ataxia and nystagmus (Wernicke's encephalopathy), whilst loss of short-term memory is the principal lasting feature. Patients characteristically retain their long-term memory and can accurately recall events before the onset of the illness. They also have an intact immediate memory (digit span), but will be completely unable to store this information for more 1 or 2 seconds. With profound loss of recent memory, patients *confabulate* – which is a way of covering up an exposed memory gap. Sometimes, confabulation will become fantastic in nature as the patient invents situations in their life. Memory loss

in Wemick–Korsakoff syndrome is generally permanent when the cause is alcohol abuse. *Transient global amnesia* describes a memory impairment which starts abruptly and improves over several hours. It generally occurs in middle-aged patients, and is thought to be due to bilateral temporal lobe ischaemia caused by vertebrobasilar disease. During an attack, the patient is unable to form new memories, and their behaviour may be outwardly normal. After recovery the subject is left with a permanent amnesia for the period of the attack. *Closed-brain injury*, which is chiefly a result of road traffic accidents but may also be due to falls, assaults and sports injuries, is a major cause of organic memory impairment. This may be due to focal or diffuse cerebral damage caused by intracranial haematoma, brain swelling, infection, subarachnoid haemorrhage and hydrocephalus, or to extracranial factors such as hypoxia and hypotension. *Post-traumatic amnesia* refers to the period that elapses between injury and the restoration of normal memory. The duration of post-traumatic amnesia is one indicator of the severity of head injury. Typically, patients have impairment in immediate and recent memory following head injury, and have difficulty in performing digit span as well as tests for words and sentences. Most recovery takes place within 1 year of injury.

Mark Kinirons

MENORRHAGIA

Menorrhagia refers to excessive menstrual flow, or undue prolongation of the time during which it takes place. The patient is free from bleeding during the intermenstrual periods, the term 'metrorrhagia' or 'irregular uterine bleeding' being reserved for bleeding which occurs between the periods (see p. 434). The latter may be also associated with heavy periods. Pure menorrhagia is an important symptom of many well-defined conditions which do not, as a rule, give rise to irregular bleeding. Both of these terms must be limited carefully to patients who menstruate, and must not be used for bleeding after the menopause.

Menorrhagia is a very subjective symptom, and menstrual loss consists not only of blood but also tissue and other secretions. Objectively, menorrhagia is taken to be more than 80 ml blood loss per month that will result in iron-deficiency anaemia. The diagnosis of menorrhagia may be difficult because of the absence of anaemia or other signs of severe menstrual blood loss. The diagnosis has to be accepted when the patient complains of having to use more than 18 pads per menstrual period, or when she loses clots or has flooding. It is the second most common cause for hospital referrals, and up to one-third of women may consult their primary care physician about this symptom. It is estimated that in the UK, one in 10 women may have lost their uterus by the age of 43 years as a result of this problem.

Excess of menstrual loss in women without abnormal physical signs is believed to be endocrine in origin, and is called 'dysfunctional menorrhagia'. Acute endometritis of gonococcal or pyogenic origin tends to cure itself owing to the shedding of the endometrium during menstruation. Tuberculous endometritis, a rare cause of infertility in the UK, is due to spread from the Fallopian tubes, and is therefore associated with menorrhagia due to the tuberculous salpingo-oophoritis. If a tuberculous infection is suspected, the uterine curettings should be examined for the typical tubercles and the organism isolated by culture. Causes of menorrhagia are listed in Table M.3.

Dysfunctional menorrhagia

Menorrhagia of puberty is mainly due to hypofunction of the anterior pituitary body, with consequent failure of ovulation and therefore no corpus luteum. The ovaries contain unruptured Graafian follicles; there is increased oestrogen production, and a lack of the luteal hormone progesterone. These cases often right themselves in time as the pituitary gradually assumes its normal cyclic activities. These anovulatory cycles are usually painless.

Menorrhagia of mature women without obvious lesions of the generative or other systems is thought to be due to an imbalance between the secretion by the ovary of oestrogen and progesterone, with an increase in oestrogen and a complete lack (or a deficiency) of progesterone. When there is a complete absence of progesterone in the second half of the menstrual cycle, the cycle is referred to as being 'anovular', drawing attention to a failure of ovulation and formation of a corpus luteum. Sometimes, the ovaries become cystic and the endometrium undergoes polypoidal thickening with a characteristic microscopic appearance known as 'Swiss cheese' endometrium or 'cystic glandular hyperplasia'. In the past, this condition has been known as metropathia haemorrhagica. Bouts of amenorrhoea of some weeks' duration are followed by prolonged irregular bleeding, a symptom-complex which does not properly come under the heading 'menorrhagia'.

Menorrhagia in relation to the menopause and in the years preceding is the result of increasing failure of the ovarian functions and consequent upset in balance between the secretion of oestrogen and progesterone.

Polymenorrhoea is the name given to a form of irregular and excessive menstruation in which the cycle is shortened from the usual 28 days to 21 days, or even

Table M.3 Causes of menorrhagia

Dysfunctional menorrhagia	In the generative system	Circulatory and other systems	In the nervous system
At puberty	Fibromyomas	Uncompensated valvular disease of	Excessive coitus
At maturity without obvious lesions	Salpingo-oophoritis (chronic)	the heart	Prevention of conception
In relation to the menopause,	Endometriosis	Cirrhosis of the liver	*A single excessive period*
and in the years preceding	Adenomyoma	Emphysema of the lungs	Fright
Hyperthyroidism	Tuberculous endometritis	Chronic alcoholism	Violent emotion
Hypothyroidism	IUCD		Sudden changes of
		The blood itself	temperature
	Acute infectious diseases	Deficient coagulability	Cold bath
	Influenza	Scurvy	Dancing
	Typhoid	Purpura	Hunting
	Cholera	Haemophilia	Gymnastics
	Scarlatina	Leukaemia	Bicycling, etc.
	Variola		
	Malaria	*High blood pressure*	
	Diphtheria	Arteriosclerosis	
	Measles		

less. This is due to a disturbed balance of internal secretions, causing ovulation to occur too early in the cycle; in some cases, two corpora lutea have been found at the same stage of development, and fibroids are present in many cases.

Pelvic pathology

Menorrhagia can be associated with fibroids (benign leiomyomas), adenomyosis, pelvic infection, endometrial polyps, endometriosis and the presence of an intrauterine contraceptive device (IUCD). Of all the causes of pure menorrhagia, leiomyoma (fibroids) (Fig. M.6) of the uterus stands out as the only important growth associated with this symptom, and a simple bimanual examination (as a rule) suffices to show that such a tumour exists. The size and shape of the uterus is dependent on the number and size of the fibroids, as there may be more than one tumour in the uterus; its shape may be exceedingly irregular. The uterus feels firm and in most cases is mobile. The only difficulty in diagnosis, as a rule, lies in distinguishing a leiomyoma of the uterus from an ovarian cyst. Sometimes this is difficult, for it is not always possible to say that a given tumour is actually the enlarged uterus. Ultrasound scanning is helpful in the diagnosis of fibroids because it is possible by using this method to determine if a pelvic swelling is both uterine and solid. Fibroids may be submucous, intramural, subserosal or pedunculated. Distortion of the uterine cavity with an increase in the surface area from which menstruation occurs will lead to menorrhagia.

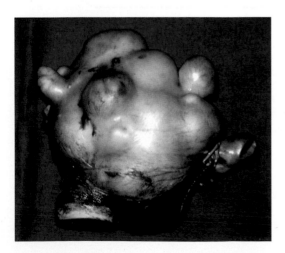

Figure M.6 Hysterectomy specimen of fibroids.

Chronic salpingo-oophoritis (in the form of a pyosalpinx, a hydrosalpinx, a tubo-ovarian abscess or chronic interstitial salpingitis) and ovarian endometriosis both give rise to menorrhagia due to pelvic congestion, but dysmenorrhoea, pelvic pain, dyspareunia and backache are usually more prominent symptoms. In either case, a firm tender swelling in the pouch of Douglas is felt on bimanual palpation. It is unusual to encounter menorrhagia under these conditions without bleeding at other times of the cycle.

Adenomyosis is a condition which can present with menorrhagia and pain at the time of menstruation, and on examination the uterus may be tender. The diagnosis can only be confirmed histologically as endometrial tissue is found in the myometrium. The condition is more common in parous women, and in essence there has been bleeding in the myometrium which gives rise to the pain and tenderness.

There is almost always some increase in menstrual blood loss with the use of IUCDs (copper devices), and in some cases the loss amounts to menorrhagia. This results from the inflammatory reaction that the coil sets up in the myometrium to prevent implantation of the fertilized egg.

Clotting defects

There are certain haemorrhagic disorders that can cause excessive menstrual loss; these include thrombocytopenic purpura, von Willebrand's disease and Christmas disease. These women may suffer excessive menstrual loss and may require surgical intervention. In thrombocytopenia, the blood loss relates to the platelet level, and in some cases splenectomy for the underlying pathology has improved the menstrual symptoms.

Anticoagulation in women who are receiving long-term anticoagulants after prosthetic heart valve implantation, previous pulmonary embolism or, in some cases, with antiphospholipid syndrome, may develop significant period problems depending on the INR level.

Severe menorrhagia may complicate thrombocytopenia, but as soon as it is cured, the period blood loss becomes normal.

Medical disorders

The function of the thyroid and adrenal glands can influence menstrual loss, though the mechanism is unknown. Menorrhagia tends to be more common in hypothyroidism than thyrotoxicosis, and is not uncommon with Cushing's disease.

Antony Hollingworth

METRORRHAGIA (IRREGULAR UTERINE BLEEDING)

Metrorrhagia means loss of blood vaginally between the menstrual periods, and the term should be applied strictly only to irregular haemorrhages during reproductive age range – that is, from puberty to the menopause. It may be used for losses of actual blood or for blood-stained discharges in which mucus is mixed with blood. There has been a tendency of late to refer only to 'menorrhagia', or to use the term 'dysfunctional uterine bleeding'. Metrorrhagia as a term is not commonly used in clinical practice. However, it is a term that includes all types of irregular vaginal bleeding, whether it occurs during menstrual life, before puberty, after the menopause, or during pregnancy. For the purposes of discussion, irregular vaginal bleeding will be considered here under three headings:

- Irregular bleeding during menstrual life.
- Irregular bleeding before puberty and after the menopause.
- Irregular bleeding during pregnancy.

It is important to emphasize that if a woman has had regular periods and then starts to bleed irregularly for no apparent reason, one must exclude pregnancy and where that pregnancy is located. It must be determined if she might have an ectopic pregnancy, as this is still a major cause of maternal death in the UK.

Irregular bleeding during menstrual life

Causes of irregular bleeding are listed in Table M.4.

Malignancy

Carcinoma of the cervix

Cervical cancer (Fig. M.7) is an uncommon disease with an incidence that is reducing as a result of the cervical screening programme. It is estimated that a GP in the UK will see one case of cervical cancer every 7–9 years. The cervix is replaced with a friable mass, which causes irregular bleeding as well as post-coital bleeding. The lesion can be diagnosed macroscopically (Fig. M.8); however, many of these women will be seen in the colposcopy clinic so that a directed biopsy can be undertaken.

Carcinoma of the uterine body

Endometrial carcinoma does occur during the reproductive age group, but it is much more common in post-menopausal women. It is the second most common genital tract tumour, and presents with irregular bleeding. Risk factors include obesity (raised body

Table M.4 Causes of irregular bleeding during menstrual life

Generative system	*Endocrine*
Malignant growths:	Dysfunctional uterine bleeding
Carcinoma of cervix	Metropathia haemorrhagica
Carcinoma of body of uterus	Irregular shedding of the endometrium
Sarcoma	Oestrogen withdrawal bleeding
Chorionic carcinoma	Break-through bleeding from contraceptive pill
Carcinoma of Fallopian tube	Granulosa-cell tumour
Carcinoma of the ovary	
Benign growths:	
Submucous fibroid	
Fibroid polyp	
Mucous polyp	
Endometrial polyp	
Inflammatory lesions:	
Erosion of cervix	
Endometriosis	
Tuberculosis of uterus	

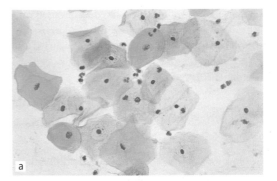

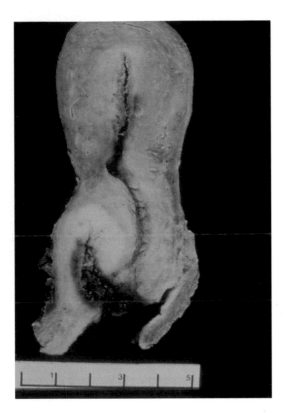

Figure M.7 Cervical cancer. Operative specimen of uterus and upper vagina in sagittal section.

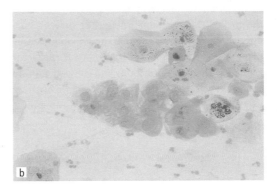

Figure M.8 (a) Normal cervical smear. (b) Severe dyskaryosis.

mass index), nulliparity and a history of polycystic ovarian disease. It is unusual to diagnose this condition before the age of 40 years; hence the Royal College of Gynaecology (RCOG) recommendations which suggest that women with menstrual irregularities before the age of 40 years should receive treatment for 3 months. If the irregularity persists, then a hysteroscopy and endometrial sampling should be undertaken. If the woman is over the age of 40 years, then this would be a first-line investigation.

Sarcoma of the uterus

This is a very uncommon tumour which occurs in fibroids. It may present with irregular bleeding, but many of these women will be post-menopausal and present with a rapidly expanding pelvic mass. The risk of a fibroid becoming malignant is estimated at about 1 in 1000. This tumour may occur in an existing fibroid or appear *de novo*. The difficulty with this condition is the highly aggressive nature of the disease, which as a rule does not respond well to radiotherapy or chemotherapy.

Chorionic carcinoma

Fortunately, this condition is rare, and follows hydatidiform mole in about 5 per cent of recorded cases. It always follows pregnancy, never having been seen in the uterus where pregnancy could be excluded, although the pregnancy may have occurred some years earlier. It is associated with profuse bleeding and the rapid development of a foetid discharge due to decomposition of blood and necrosing tissues *in utero*. Secondary deposits of chorionic carcinoma appear as small plum-coloured ulcerating nodules in the vagina, and secondaries in the lungs cause haemoptysis. The patient rapidly becomes ill with pyrexia and profound anaemia. A raised level of human chorionic gonadotrophin (HCG) is found in the urine. The diagnosis depends upon the finding of masses of trophoblastic cells in uterine curettings, without any evidence of villous formation.

Other malignancies

Carcinoma of the Fallopian tube is a rare tumour which tends to present in the post-menopausal woman, but may present with irregular bleeding. Ovarian cancer is unlikely to cause bleeding unless it has invaded the uterus. Clear cell carcinoma of the vagina is also rare, and has been reported in teenage girls exposed to stilboestrol *in utero*.

Benign lesions

Fibroids

Leiomyomas may cause a mixture of menorrhagia and metrorrhagia. If irregular bleeding tends to occur, then they are submucous (Fig. M.9). They may be in the process of extrusion when they may become infected and sloughing occurs. The reason for this is that in these conditions the tumours are partly strangulated by uterine contractions and consequently are congested with venous blood. This results in bleeding which is unpredictable in both timing and amount.

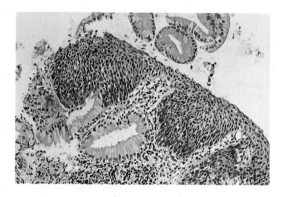

Figure M.9 Histology of fibroid.

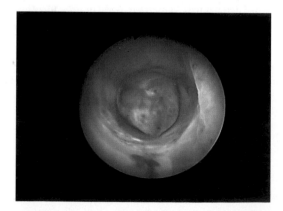

Figure M.10 Benign-looking endometrial polyp as seen through the hysteroscope.

Polyps

Polyps (Fig. M.10) can occur within the cervix and endometrium. Cervical polyps are usually identified at the time of taking a routine cervical smear test, but if the tip becomes inflamed then it can give rise to vaginal bleeding or post-coital bleeding. Polyps within the endometrial cavity – whether fibroid or mucous – are common causes of intermenstrual bleeding, and are usually quite definitive growths. The mucous polyp is soft, strawberry-red in colour, pedunculated, and contains cystic spaces filled with glairy mucus. It rarely gives rise to a malignant growth. The fibroid polyp is hard, and shows the glistening whorled appearance so well known in fibromyomas when sectioned. These growths are liable to infection and sloughing, and are then apt to be mistaken for carcinoma or sarcoma macroscopically.

Inflammatory lesions

Endometriosis

This condition is defined as the finding of tissue outside the uterus that is histologically similar to that of endometrium, and is not strictly an inflammatory lesion. However, it is one of the most common benign gynaecological conditions and may present with a myriad of symptoms, including irregular vaginal bleeding, pain and dyspareunia.

Ectropion of the cervix

This is a physiological condition in which there is eversion of the columnar epithelium from the endocervical canal towards the vagina. The columnar epithelium appears reddened because it is one cell thick and consequently translucent, allowing the blood supply below to be seen. The term 'erosion' should be avoided as it suggests something pathological. The epithelium can become inflamed and give rise to discharge and contact bleeding, though intermenstrual bleeding is unusual.

The columnar epithelium may undergo metaplastic change to squamous epithelium, and the area concerned is known as the 'transformation zone'. It is in this area that precancerous changes may occur. Precancerous changes within the cervix are asymptomatic and usually only diagnosed by cytology (see Fig. M.8).

Tuberculosis

Tuberculosis may affect the genital tract and give rise to irregular bleeding and infertility. It is an uncommon problem within the UK, but is much more common in the developing world. Histology of the endometrial curettings may provide the diagnosis, though a strong suspicion of TB suggests the involvement of a physician.

Dysfunctional uterine bleeding

Although modern techniques of ovarian steroid estimation in serum allow serial measurements to be made of hormone levels throughout the menstrual cycle, no clear pattern has emerged to explain the mechanism underlying dysfunctional uterine bleeding. Dysfunctional bleeding may occur at any age between puberty and the menopause, but 50 per cent of cases occur between the ages of 40 and 50 years, about 10 per cent at puberty, and the remainder between these ages. The bleeding is more commonly menorrhagia, although the interval between bleedings may be shortened. This is particularly the case in this type of bleeding occurring at the time of puberty and the menopause. The bleeding may be profuse or only slightly in excess of normal. In other cases, intermenstrual bleeding occurs which continues for days or weeks; this is usually preceded by amenorrhoea for some weeks. In a large proportion of these cases ovulation fails to occur – that is, the cycle is anovulatory. The histology of any curettings may prove to be essentially normal.

Endometrial hyperplasia can occur as a result of excess oestrogen production. This is likely to occur in women who are obese, due to excess aromatization of androgens to oestrogens within the adipose tissue. It can also occur in women with unruptured follicles, as in polycystic ovarian syndrome (PCOS). This may lead to irregular shedding of the endometrium. Endometrial hyperplasia is classified as:

- Simple hyperplasia, with a 1 per cent risk of becoming malignant.
- Complex hyperplasia, with a 3 per cent risk of malignancy.
- Complex hyperplasia with atypia, which has a 22 per cent risk of malignancy.

These conditions are histological diagnoses, and how the woman is treated will depend on her age and thoughts about fertility.

Contraceptive use

There are three main areas, which can give rise to metrorrhagia:

- Progesterone contraception, whether as the progesterone-only pill, the mirena IUCD or Depoprovera will usually result in the woman being amenorrhoeic. There are a number of women who develop irregular bleeding that may be completely unpredictable.
- The copper-containing IUCDs can give rise to menorrhagia, and in some cases the low-grade inflammatory response of the endometrium to the coil can result in irregular shedding. The treatment would be to remove the coil in the first instance.
- The combined oral contraceptive pill usually gives good cycle control, but breakthrough bleeding can occur due to gastrointestinal upset, absorption and metabolism problems due to other medications (e.g. antibiotics and anti-epileptic drugs), a diet which affects the enterohepatic circulation, and a dosage which is too low for the individual.

Bleeding associated with ovulation

It is not uncommon for women to bleed very slightly about midway between the periods at the time of ovulation. When this is accompanied by lower abdominal pain (Mittelschmerz) the diagnosis is easy.

Bleeding due to granulosa-cell tumour

When irregular bleeding occurs in the presence of an ovarian swelling, the possibility of a granulosa-cell tumour arises. Removal of the tumour and histology reveal its nature. The presence of an intrauterine lesion and a non-secreting ovarian tumour must not be overlooked.

Irregular bleeding before puberty and after the menopause

The causes of irregular bleeding before puberty and after the menopause are listed in Table M.5. The bleeding which occurs from the vagina occasionally in newborn infants is usually due to a high concentration of oestrogen in the fetal circulation. It is usually trivial, but a fatal case has been reported. Bleeding later in childhood may be due to sexual precocity when secondary sexual characteristics will be in evidence; alternatively, it may be due to a new growth

Table M.5 Causes of irregular bleeding

Before puberty and after menopause	During pregnancy
Uterine bleeding in the newborn	Threatened, inevitable or incomplete abortion
Malignant growth of the uterus	Carneous mole
Polyps	Hydatidiform mole
Senile endometritis	Antepartum haemorrhage
Senile atrophic vaginitis	Secondary postpartum haemorrhage
Pyometra	Subinvolution
Granulosa-cell tumour of ovary	Chorionic carcinoma
Oestrogen withdrawal bleeding	Extra-uterine gestation
	Malignant growth of cervix or vagina
	Erosion
	Polyps

such as an embryonal rhabdomyosarcoma (sarcoma botryoides). Vaginoscopy under anaesthesia (and biopsy if a lesion is found) is essential.

After the menopause, the differentiation of malignant growths, polyps and senile endometritis can only be established by uterine curettage. Carcinoma of the body of the uterus (endometrial adenocarcinoma) is the most common malignant growth after the menopause. In any doubtful case, routine dilatation and curettage of the uterus must never be omitted. Senile (atrophic) vaginitis must not be overlooked as a possible cause; the vaginal walls at the fornices become inflamed and may bleed if the surfaces rub together. These surfaces may be partly adherent, and the separation brought about by the examining finger may cause bleeding. Pyometra, or distension of the uterus with pus, may cause haemorrhage, with a foul discharge; although it is almost always due to malignant growth, it may be only the result of infection. The only growth of the ovary that produces uterine haemorrhage is the granulosa-cell tumour. This may occur at almost any age (see PELVIS, SWELLING IN, p. 566).

In women with post-menopausal bleeding, ultrasound scanning to measure the endometrial thickness may be a useful way to triage these patients. If the endometrial thickness is 5 mm or less, then no further action is needed unless the bleeding continues. Otherwise, hysteroscopy and endometrial sampling is performed.

Irregular bleeding during pregnancy

In relation to a recent pregnancy, haemorrhage may result from simple subinvolution, from retained products of conception, or from chorionic carcinoma. The differentiation of these conditions can be established only by exploration of the uterine cavity with, if necessary, the assistance of histology. Such conditions may be termed 'secondary postpartum haemorrhage' in cases occurring within a few days of delivery.

Haemorrhage from the pregnant uterus almost always means separation of the placenta or of the embryo from its attachments, but malignant growth of the cervix, ectropions and polyps may have to be considered. Haemorrhage from a pregnant uterus is never due to malignant growth of the body of the organ, because pregnancy is impossible with this lesion. There are, however, two great difficulties in connection with pregnancy haemorrhages; these are to differentiate:

■ the uterine haemorrhage which occurs with extra-uterine (ectopic) gestation from that due to threatened miscarriage; and

■ the bleeding of placenta praevia from that due to the separation of a normally situated placenta.

In the first case, an ectopic pregnancy usually presents within the first 6–8 weeks of the last normal period. The external haemorrhage occurs when the extra-uterine gestation is separated from its tubal or other attachments and is converted into a tubal mole, when it becomes extruded from the fimbriated extremity of the tube, or when the tube ruptures. These events can cause acute pain in the lower part of the abdomen, faintness, and possibly collapse from internal haemorrhage. On examination, the uterus may not appear enlarged, but there may be fullness and marked tenderness in the adnexa. In the case of ectopic gestation the abdominal pain can be severe and is often referred to the shoulder. It is much more severe than that experienced in an intra-uterine miscarriage, and it almost always precedes the onset of vaginal bleeding. On the other hand, the vaginal blood loss in an inevitable miscarriage is much more than that in ectopic gestation, which is usually scanty. However, these signs are not invariable.

Haemorrhage due to threatened miscarriage cannot be diagnosed unless the presence of an intra-uterine pregnancy can be established and ultrasound scanning has altered the management of these patients. The presence of a live fetus can be demonstrated by the beating of the heart with the aid of real-time ultrasound, and means that the outlook for continuation of the pregnancy is good. The presence of an empty uterus and positive pregnancy test with an adnexal mass and fluid in the pouch of Douglas suggests an ectopic pregnancy until proven otherwise. In the case of a positive pregnancy test using methods employing the detection of low levels of β-HCG and a negative ultrasound scan for intra-uterine pregnancy, laparoscopy would be advisable to exclude the diagnosis. The diagnosis of inevitable miscarriage depends upon finding some part of the uterine contents presenting through the dilating cervix. Incomplete abortion is diagnosed by the continuation of bleeding, or seeing that not all the products of conception have been passed. Retained products are then confirmed on ultrasound scanning.

The management of this condition has changed over the past few years, with an increasing number of women undergoing a natural miscarriage with no curettage. Curettage is reserved for women with excessive or prolonged bleeding.

A hydatidiform mole (Fig. M.11) should be suspected when a rapid increase in uterus size occurs during the early months of pregnancy, associated with uterine bleeding and excessive symptoms of pregnancy. Most patients have a uterus which is larger than would be expected for the dates, but in one-third of cases it is smaller. Sometimes, vesicles are passed and the diagnosis is clear. If not, the finding of a high level of HCG in the blood or urine and the characteristic 'snow-storm' appearance on ultrasound scanning makes the diagnosis certain. In a normal pregnancy, up to 100 000 IU of HCG are passed in the urine each day. Five times this amount is passed in the presence of a hydatidiform mole, and these patients should be registered with one of the three centres in the UK

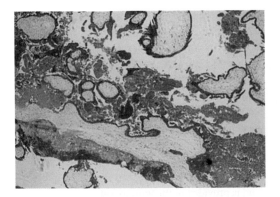

Figure M.11 Hydatidiform mole.

(Charing Cross, Sheffield and Dundee). The centres will monitor the patient for the requisite amount of time, which is dependent on how quickly the HCG returns to normal.

Bleeding due to placenta praevia generally does not occur until 30 weeks of pregnancy. Antepartum haemorrhage is likely to be due to placenta praevia if the fetal presenting part is high above the pelvic brim, or there is a malpresentation such as a breech or a transverse lie. If the fetal head is engaged in the pelvis, antepartum haemorrhage cannot be due to placenta praevia and must therefore be due to accidental haemorrhage, provided that incidental causes such as carcinoma or polyp on the cervix can be excluded. The diagnosis of antepartum haemorrhage has been made much easier with the aid of ultrasound scanning, because the placental echo can be seen clearly and the relationship of the edge of the placenta to the internal os can be accurately determined. It is not uncommon for a low-lying placenta found in the mid-trimester to be seen, on serial scanning, to move wholly into the upper uterine segment as term approaches, due to the development of the lower segment during the third trimester.

In all of these women consideration must be given to the administration of Anti-D if they are Rhesus-negative.

Antony Hollingworth

MICTURITION, FREQUENCY OF

The normal bladder has a capacity of 500 ml, and will store urine until a socially convenient time without urgency, nor incontinence. Urinary frequency should be less than seven times in any 24-hour period, though is of course dependent upon fluid intake. In cold weather most of us notice an increase in urinary frequency. In hot weather, urinary frequency is reduced due to insensible losses reducing urine output. Urinary frequency should be evaluated by asking the patient to fill in a frequency/volume voided chart such that a true indication as to normal intake and output can be discovered. Normal daily fluid intake is somewhere between 1500 and 2000 ml. Additional fluid is provided in the food we eat.

Urinary frequency forms part of the symptom complex of the 'overactive bladder syndrome'. The symptom complex includes daytime frequency, nocturia, urgency and urge incontinence. There are many causes of urinary frequency, some of which are listed in Table M.6.

The majority of pathological conditions within the bladder will be associated with pain or inflammatory symptoms. However, before a diagnosis of overactive bladder can be made, a process of appropriate investigation must exclude the more sinister conditions. The frequency chart (Fig. M.12) will demonstrate the relationship between fluid intake and output. Many patients can significantly reduce nocturia by reducing fluid intake after 7 or 8 p.m.

Daytime frequency, which is not due to a pathological process, can be improved by changes in the volume and timing of fluid intake, and by bladder retraining. The normal volume of urine voided is 200–330 ml in young adults, but tends to reduce with ageing. Many older people do not hold more than 150 ml at any time. Thus, before frequency can be attributed to pathology (unless there are other symptoms), these factors must be taken into consideration.

Nocturia is the awaking to pass urine at night. Normal homeostasis ensures that we do not awake at night to pass urine, the effect of antidiuretic hormone (ADH) on renal homeostasis being in part responsible for the reduction of urine production at night. Normal individuals will awake to pass urine on occasion after drinking larger quantities of fluid prior to going to sleep. As we age, however, more urine is produced at night and thus there is a likelihood that we will awake at night to void as we reach our sixties and seventies. Other causes of nocturia include:

- A reduced bladder capacity, for the reasons listed above.
- Peripheral oedema – particularly dependent oedema in old age, or in association with immobility.
- Congestive cardiac failure.
- Diabetes mellitus and insipidus.

These conditions should be treated according to their need.

Julian Shah

MICTURITION, HESITANCY

There is normally little delay before the start of micturition in normal individuals. In potentially socially embarrassing situations such as in the urinals at motorway service stations there may be a delay in the

Table M.6 Causes of urinary frequency

	Frequency	Nocturia	Urgency	Pain	Incontinence
Urinary tract infection	+	+	+	+	±
Urethral syndrome	+	±	±	±	−
Radiation cystitis	+	+	±	±	−
Prostatic tumours which encroach upon the bladder	+	+	±	±	−
Interstitial cystitis	+	+	±	+	−
Small functional bladder capacity	+	+	±	±	−
Tumour in the bladder	+	+	±	±	−
Bladder stone	+	+	+	+	−
Schistomiasis	+	+	+	+	−
Cyclophosphamide cystitis	+	+	+	+	−
Chronic retention with overflow	+	+	−	−	−
Bladder instability	+	+	+	−	+
Bladder hyperreflexia due to neurological disease	+	+	+	−	+

Frequency Chart

Name: .... Hospital Number: ....

Start date: ....

For three consecutive days please record as accurately as possible the number of times you pass urine in the 'Out' column and also write the volume of fluid you drink and the times that you drink.

Time	Day 1		Day 2		Day 3	
Start	In	Out	In	Out	In	Out
6AM						
7AM						
8AM						
9AM						
10AM						
11AM						
Noon						
1PM						
2PM						
3PM						
4PM						
5PM						
6PM						
7PM						
8PM						
9PM						
10PM						
11PM						
12AM						
1AM						
2AM						
3AM						
4AM						
5AM						

Comments:

Figure M.12 Urinary frequency chart.

start of urine flow when trying to void. This delay may be increased substantially in nervous individuals (those with the 'bashful bladder syndrome').

If there is significant (non-physiological) delay in the start of urine flow, this is known as urinary hesitancy, and it is one of the classical symptoms of bladder out-flow obstruction, which is due to prostatic enlarge-ment. Part of this delay is due to the additional time it takes for the bladder pressure to reach the point at which the outflow resistance is overcome. Hesitancy will also occur due to detrusor hypocontractility or acontractility, which may be due to long-standing obstruction, and has given rise to detrusor dysfunction. These conditions may also be the result of neurological disorders, which have affected the spinal reflex arc or cauda equina.

There is a defined condition – which has been mentioned – of the 'anxious' or 'bashful bladder' or the 'executive bladder' that are associated with hesitancy and the other urinary symptoms that suggest bladder outflow obstruction. Urodynamic testing should be used whenever there is a doubt as to the diagnosis, or where surgery is proposed for a condition in which the diagnosis is not clear.

Julian Shah

MONOPLEGIA, UPPER LIMB

Monoplegia or monoparesis is defined as loss of motor power involving a single limb. In theory, a monoplegia or monoparesis can result from damage anywhere in the motor pathway between the motor cortex and the muscles of the affected limb. When the degree of weakness is only slight, and associated signs such as increased reflexes are absent, accurate diagnosis may be difficult. For example, localized damage to the hand area of the cortex resulting from a stroke can produce weakness of the hand without any obvious reflex change, mimicking a localized nerve or root lesion. To reach a diagnosis in such a case requires a careful history and a detailed examination of motor function, with special efforts being made to delineate the extent and pattern of motor weakness.

A patient may complain of weakness in a limb, when in reality the problem is the result of pain, incoordination, loss of sensation, or akinesia and rigidity, as in Parkinson's disease. The patient with apraxia of a limb often regards it as weak.

Upper motor neurone

A spastic upper limb monoplegia most commonly results from a lesion affecting the motor cortex or the descending corticospinal fibres in the internal capsule. Cerebral infarction, cerebral haemorrhage or tumour are the most likely causes. Muscle atrophy is not a feature, and the appearance of the arm is usually normal.

In an acute lesion muscle tone may be reduced but, given time, spasticity develops and the arm adopts a fixed posture, adducted at the shoulder and flexed at the elbow and wrist. Hand movements are usually more severely affected than shoulder movements. Tendon reflexes are brisk and contractures may develop. Even when symptoms are apparently confined to the arm, there may be some degree of facial weakness, and the plantar response in the ipsilateral foot may be extensor.

In the patient with a progressive upper motor neurone pattern of weakness, the likeliest cause is an intracerebral tumour. A similar pattern of weakness may occasionally be seen in multiple sclerosis, or rarely in spinal cord tumours. A spastic upper limb monoplegia may be mistaken for the rigid akinetic arm of a patient with Parkinson's disease. In such cases the arm moves slowly and is thought by the patient to be weak, yet testing usually reveals no significant loss of power. Similarly, the tendon reflexes in Parkinson's disease are usually unaffected. Finally, it should be possible to differentiate the rigidity of Parkinson's disease from the spasticity of an upper motor neurone lesion.

Hysterical upper limb monoplegia is rare. In such cases the arm appears normal and muscle tone is not increased. The tendon reflexes remain normal and the plantar responses are flexor. There is often apparent dense sensory loss in the affected arm, usually with a sharp line of demarcation at the level of the shoulder. The most difficult cases are those in which there is some genuine weakness with superadded functional overlay.

Lower motor neurone

A flaccid upper limb monoplegia may result from damage to any part of the lower motor neurone between the anterior horn cell and the muscle. Damage to the lower motor neurone typically is associated with muscle weakness, muscle wasting, decrease in the tendon reflexes and fasciculations. Characteristic changes may be found on electromyographic examination.

Anterior horn cell disorders

Localized loss of anterior horn cells may produce a flaccid weakness of one or other arm. This may be seen as a common after-effect of poliomyelitis, and the affected limb is often markedly under-developed. In motor neurone disease, localized loss of anterior horn cells may produce progressive lower motor neurone weakness in the arm, and this may begin in any of the upper limb muscles. A common pattern is for the weakness to begin in the intrinsic hand muscles, with associated muscle wasting. Prominent fasciculations are common in this disorder. Where there is associated damage to the corticospinal tracts, as in amyotrophic lateral sclerosis, the tendon reflexes are brisk despite obvious muscle wasting and fasciculation. This combination of signs is diagnostic.

Localized lesions in the cervical cord may damage the anterior horn cells and produce a lower motor neurone pattern of weakness. This may be seen in syringomyelia and in spinal cord tumours. These may be diagnosed by the associated signs of sensory loss and corticospinal tract signs in the legs. Ischaemic lesions of the cervical cord may produce discrete loss of anterior horn cells, with localized areas of muscle wasting and weakness. This may be one of the mechanisms whereby the lower motor neurone pattern of weakness develops in cervical spondylosis.

Spinal motor root disorders

Localized damage to the spinal roots in the cervical region is common as a result of degenerative cervical spine changes (cervical spondylosis). The C5 and C6 segments are most commonly affected, with muscle wasting and weakness being most prominent in the biceps and shoulder girdle muscles. The biceps and brachioradialis reflexes are depressed, and there is often inversion of these reflexes; that is to say, when the biceps tendon is stretched there is no contraction of the biceps muscle but there is a contraction of the finger flexors, resulting in finger flexion. Extensive cervical spondylosis sometimes produces quite marked wasting and weakness of many of the upper limb muscles. The cause may be recognized by the associated sensory changes and by the presence of pain. Such cases are usually seen in those who have undertaken heavy manual work, and gross changes are usually confined to those over the age of 50 or 60 years. Other causes of damage to spinal motor roots are cervical disc prolapse, trauma to the cervical spine, extramedullary spinal tumours and spinal arachnoiditis.

Herpes zoster is occasionally accompanied by paralysis of one or more muscles within the affected segments. In neuralgic amyotrophy there is localized muscle weakness and wasting occurring a few weeks after the development of severe pain in the affected limb. There is some debate as to the localization of damage to the lower motor neurone in neuralgic amyotrophy; in some cases the damage may be in the ventral roots, in some in the brachial plexus, and in some in peripheral nerves.

The brachial plexus

Brachial plexus damage on one side may usually be recognized by the distribution of muscle weakness and by the associated reflex and sensory changes.

Damage may occur as a result of an injury at birth. Downward traction on the arm in a breech presentation may rupture the upper end of the plexus (C5–C6), with consequent paralysis and atrophy of the spinati, deltoid, brachialis, biceps and brachioradialis. The arm hangs by the side, internally rotated at the shoulder, with the elbow straight and the fingers flexed, the palm of the hand pointed backwards. This is known as Duchenne–Erb paralysis. A similar condition resulting from a fall on the tip of the shoulder is referred to as Erb's paralysis. In both cases the motor disturbances are similar to those produced by a lesion of the 5th and 6th segments of the cervical cord, but there are none of the sensory and pyramidal signs which necessarily occur below the level of the lesion in the latter. A second form of obstetric palsy, described as Klumpke's paralysis, results from injury to the lower cord of the plexus (C8–T1), by traction on the arm in a vertex or shoulder presentation. Atrophic palsy occurs in the intrinsic muscles of the hand and in the flexors of the wrist and fingers. Horner's syndrome may be present if the roots themselves have been torn. Rarer causes of trauma to the brachial plexus are gunshot wounds or stab wounds. In modern times, perhaps the most common traumatic lesion to the brachial plexus is that occurring as a result of a motorcycle accident. In such cases the damage may not only be to the nerves in the brachial plexus but also to the ventral roots themselves, which may become completely avulsed from the spinal cord.

Upward spread of an apical bronchial carcinoma may result in erosion into the brachial plexus, most commonly affecting the lower part (Pancoast's syndrome). Metastatic carcinoma of the breast may produce a similar clinical picture, and this is often difficult to differentiate from post-radiation scarring occurring in a female who has been treated by radiotherapy to the axilla.

The cervical rib

The brachial plexus and subclavian vessels cross the uppermost rib as they pass into the axilla. This may be a normal first rib, an ill-formed rudimentary first rib, or a cervical rib. The last may be a well-developed ossified structure or a fibrous band, but in either case it joins the first thoracic rib lateral to the insertion of the scalenus anterior, at the point where the brachial plexus and vessels pass into the axilla. Such a rib or band tends to angulate the nerves and vessels and to produce friction during respiration and in movements of the shoulder and upper limb, and this in its turn may give rise to pain and paraesthesiae in the ring and little fingers, and atrophic palsy of the small muscles of the hand (see below). However, cervical ribs often give rise to no symptoms at all, and though they are present from birth, symptoms – if they do arise – are uncommon before middle life. They tend to be aggravated by carrying heavy weights and by wearing a heavy overcoat. Friction on the plexus causes atrophy and weakness of the interossei, the thenar and hypothenar muscles, and the long flexors of the fingers and wrist. Fasciculation may be seen in the affected muscles, and slight sensory loss is sometimes found in the medial two fingers and the ulnar border of the hand and forearm. To this essentially neurological picture may be added symptoms and signs of vascular origin: Raynaud's phenomenon, persistent cyanosis of the hand, diminution or even loss of the radial pulse. The subclavian artery is subjected to friction and to costoclavicular compression, and this may lead to thrombosis or even to the formation of an aneurysm at the site of compression. If thrombosis occurs, ischaemia gives rise to pallor of the hand, paraesthesiae in all the fingers, claudication of the forearm and hand and, in elderly subjects, to necrosis of the fingertips.

Costoclavicular compression can occur even in the absence of cervical rib. The motor features are similar to those of a cervical rib, but of milder degree, and vascular symptoms tend to predominate. There is aching pain in the shoulder, paraesthesiae in all the fingers, and a feeling of weakness in the limb. These symptoms are intensified by abduction of the arm, by using the hand above the level of the shoulder, as in doing the hair or painting a ceiling, and by recumbency, so that paraesthesiae is worse at night. These symptoms may come on for the first time in middle age after a period of prolonged and unwanted physical work, and more commonly in females than males. A troublesome form occurs in the late stages of pregnancy, usually disappearing after parturition and recurring in subsequent pregnancies; it is related to the postural readjustments which take place in pregnancy. Care must be taken not to confuse these symptoms with those due to compression of the median nerve in the carpal tunnel, for in the latter there are also complaints of paraesthesiae in the hand on waking in the morning, with or without wasting of the thenar eminence. In the carpal tunnel syndrome, however, the paraesthesiae rarely involve the ulnar part of the hand alone.

Peripheral nerve damage

Peripheral nerve damage in the upper limb usually produces localized muscle weakness in the territory supplied by the relevant nerve. Extensive damage most commonly results from lesions in the nerves of the brachial plexus (see above). The term 'mononeuritis multiplex' implies multiple peripheral nerve lesions. It may occur in diabetes, but is more commonly seen in connective-tissue disorders such as polyarteritis nodosa.

Localized weakness in peripheral nerve lesions

The circumflex (axillary) nerve is liable to injury by fractures of the neck of the humerus, by dislocation of the shoulder, by the use of an unpadded crutch, and by penetrating injuries of the axilla and shoulder. The deltoid is paralysed and there is an area of sensory loss over the proximal half of the lateral aspect of the arm. Paralysis of the radial nerve occurs in fractures of the shaft of the humerus, pressure from callus, gunshot wounds of the axilla and arm and, not infrequently, from sitting with an arm suspended over the back of a chair. With lesions in the neighbourhood of the shaft of the humerus, the triceps escapes, but there is paralysis of the brachioradialis and of the extensors of the wrist and fingers, with consequent wrist-drop and paralysis of finger extension. There is a somewhat variable loss of cutaneous sensation over the radial border of the forearm and the radial half of the dorsum of the hand which may be confined to a small patch over the fast dorsal interosseous space.

Inability to extend the wrist impairs the mechanical efficiency of the flexors of the fingers, so that the grasp is weakened – a circumstance which may lead to an erroneous diagnosis of a coincident lesion of the median nerve. Wrist-drop is a familiar feature of certain general affections – lead poisoning, leprosy, alcoholic neuritis – but in these conditions the weakness is not wholly confined to the radial distribution.

The posterior interosseous nerve is a branch of the radial nerve in the upper forearm, and may suffer entrapment or may become the site of a neurofibroma. There is eventually paralysis of the finger extensors, the thumb extensor and abductor of the wrist. The radial extensor is spared so that there is only partial weakness of wrist extension and no wrist-drop. There is no sensory loss. Spontaneous recovery is unlikely, and early exploration is indicated.

Paralysis of the median nerve is usually due to penetrating injuries of the arm or forearm. If the lesion is above the elbow, atrophic palsy involves the pronator teres, flexor carpi radialis, palmaris longus, flexor digitorum sublimis, flexor pollicis longus, pronator quadratus, the inner half of flexor digitorum profundus, the muscles of the thenar eminence and the lateral two lumbricals. Sensory loss and absence of sweating are limited to the median distribution in the hand.

The anterior interosseous nerve is a branch of the median nerve and supplies, essentially, the flexor profundus of the thumb and index finger so that the patient is unable to make a pincer movement. There is no sensory loss. Lesions usually result from entrapment. Spontaneous recovery may occur, but if there has been none after 2–3 months then exploration is indicated.

Compression of the median nerve in the carpal tunnel may cause wasting of the muscles of the thenar eminence, with paralysis of abduction and opposition of the thumb, and cutaneous sensory loss over the thumb, index, middle and radial half of the ring finger. The full-blown picture is rare, but milder degrees of compression occur and can be responsible for acroparaesthesiae in the hand, even when signs are slight or absent.

The carpal tunnel syndrome occurs mostly in women, and usually for no apparent reason. In men there is likely to be a discoverable cause such as arthritis of the wrist, ganglion at the wrist joint, acromegaly or myxoedema. These causes are not, of course, confined to men, and in women pregnancy is another possible precipitating factor.

The earliest symptom is usually intermittent tingling of the fingers of one hand, often waking the patient from sleep. This tingling may spare the little finger, and is often most prominent in the ring and middle fingers. If the tingling is severe it is likely to be accompanied by pain in the palm of the hand, sometimes at the elbow or even in the shoulder.

As the condition progresses the patient may find that in the morning the fingers feel swollen and numb. Later, symptoms may occur during the day and may be brought on by use of the hands. Finally, abnormal signs may appear. These consist of weakness and wasting of the abductor pollicis brevis and sensory impairment within the distribution of the median nerve in the hand, both of which may be quite mild in degree. The condition is relieved by division of the flexor retinaculum at the wrist.

The ulnar nerve is frequently injured by penetrating wounds of the forearm, and is particularly liable to compression where it lies behind the medial epicondyle of the humerus. This occurs particularly if the groove in which it lies is shallow, in which case it is subject to recurrent injury, as in clerks, telegraphists, and others whose occupation entails resting the elbows on a hard table. Cubitus valgus – whether congenital or as a result of a fracture in the region of the elbow – predisposes to this traumatic neuritis. Pain is rare, but paraesthesiae and wasting of the interossei, the hypothenar muscles, and the medial two lumbricals cause discomfort and disability. Sensory loss of ulnar distribution and palpable thickening of the nerve at the elbow afford confirmatory evidence as to the nature of the condition. An occupational palsy of the muscles supplied by the deep branch of the ulnar nerve is seen in long-distance cyclists, who lean heavily on the handle-bars, and also in individuals using files, with the instrument held in one hand, and downward pressure exerted by the hypothenar eminence of the other on the end of the file. Weakness and wasting are confined to the interossei and there is no sensory loss. Ulnar paralysis can occur in leprosy and may be the sole manifestation.

James Kelly

MOUTH, PIGMENTATION OF

The oral mucous membrane contains melanocytes in the basal layer, as a result of neuroectodermal migration in the fetus, which are similar to those present in the skin. Therefore, any condition which causes abnormal pigmentation in the skin can produce similar changes in the oral cavity, although the effects are usually not as marked. The following are important causes of oral pigmentation.

Melanotic naevae

These occur less often than in the skin, with the hard palate and the buccal mucosa being the most commonly involved site. As in the skin, they represent a collection of the normal melanocytes, but instead of being evenly distributed in the basal layer the cells are aggregated together. Depending on their position in relation to the basement membrane, they give rise to junctional naevae, compound naevae, intramucosal naevae and blue naevae. The lesions are generally small, well-circumscribed, macular or slightly raised. The majority are pigmented with varying shades of brown, blue or black. The lesions are twice as common in females as in males, and tend to occur in middle age.

Malignant melanoma

This is a rare tumour of the oral mucous membrane with a slight male predominance, again occurring in middle age (Figs M.13 and M.14). It is mostly found in the upper jaw, especially the palate, followed by the gingival mucosa. It is more common in the Japanese, Indian and African races, and one-third of cases are preceded by a history of oral pigmentation. As in the skin, any oral pigmented lesion which increases in size or changes its surface characteristics or colour and starts to bleed should be suspected as being a malignant melanoma. Growth of the lesion is

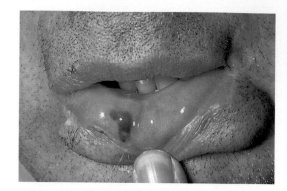

Figure M.14 Malignant melanoma of the lip.

followed by destruction of the underlying bone and loosening of the teeth, with rapid spread to the regional lymph nodes. If malignant change is suspected, then a wide excision of the lesion should be carried out. Rarely, the mouth may be involved, with secondary deposits from a cutaneous melanoma.

Melanotic neuroectodermal tumour of infancy

This pigmented lesion is invariably noted within the first 6 months of life, the majority occurring in the anterior maxilla. The tumour grows rapidly in size, with underlying bone destruction and displacement of the developing teeth. The correct diagnosis is essential as the tumour is benign and responds well to simple enucleation.

Peutz–Jegher's syndrome

This inherited condition is characterized by intestinal polyposis and melanotic spots of the face and mouth (Fig. M.3), with occasionally the hands and feet also being affected. Although it is an inherited condition, a family history will not always be found. There are multiple freckles on the face, especially around the mouth (circum-oral pigmentation), the eyes and the nose. The polyps in the intestine rarely become malignant, as they are hamartomas in origin.

Addison's disease

This condition is caused by bilateral destruction of the suprarenal glands, the most common cause previously being infection with tuberculosis (Fig. F.6). Today, this condition is usually caused by autoimmune destruction or an opportunist infection in immunodeficient

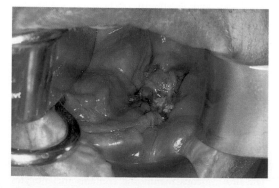

Figure M.13 Malignant melanoma of the alveolus.

patients, and more recently this has been demonstrated in patients suffering from AIDS. The skin becomes pigmented early on in the disease, especially the exposed areas, while the oral cavity shows patchy melanotic pigmentation, which varies in colour from light brown to black. If this disease is suspected, then the diagnosis will be verified by measuring the blood pressure (which is low), the blood urea (which is raised), and serum sodium (which is lowered). The diagnosis is confirmed by the Synacthen test (the measurement of plasma cortisol in response to an injection of synthetic ACTH).

Pigmentation can also occur with tumours secreting ACTH, the most common being bronchiogenic carcinoma, and with Nelson's syndrome.

Racial

This is the most common cause of oral pigmentation, which is most prevalent in the African and Indian races (Fig. M.15). However, 5 per cent of Caucasian people also show pigmentation of the oral mucosa. The pigment is evenly distributed in the palate, buccal and gingival mucosa. The colour of the pigment is not necessarily related to the colour of the skin.

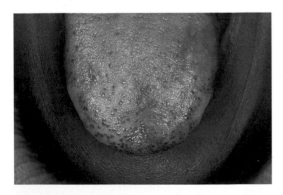

Figure M.15 Racial pigmentation of the tongue.

Amalgam tattoo

This is a common cause of oral pigmentation, and arises by small amounts of amalgam filling material gaining access to the mucosa via a small abrasion during restorative dental procedures or tooth extraction. This produces small regular or irregular areas of pigmentation in the mucosa, which rarely require treatment.

Kaposi's sarcoma

The epidemic form of this vascular tumour is a well-recognized complication of HIV infection. Oral lesions are common, typically affecting the palate or gums. The recognition of oral lesions is important, as there is a strong association with concurrent pulmonary or gastrointestinal disease, which frequently require treatment with chemotherapy.

Lichen planus

The inflammatory process in this condition may cause some degeneration of the basal layer of the mucous membrane, and the pigment released is ingested by macrophages, causing diffuse pigmentation.

Chemicals/drugs

The metals lead, bismuth and mercury – following industrial exposure or their previous use as therapeutic agents – can cause blue, brown or black lines characteristically adjacent to the gingival margin. It is felt that these metals formed sulphides following reactions with the dental plaque, and were deposited in the gingival mucosa. The drugs in current use which have been reported as causing oral pigmentation are the phenothiazines, antimalarials and the oral contraceptive.

Black hairy tongue

This curious phenomena of unknown origin is characterized by overgrowth of the filiform papillae of the tongue which become stained due to proliferation of chromogenic micro-organisms (Fig. M.16). Heavy smoking and the persistent use of antiseptic mouthwashes have been implicated, but in the majority of

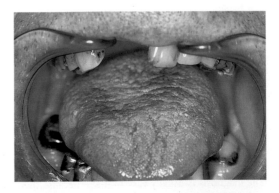

Figure M.16 Black hairy tongue.

cases the cause is unknown. The tongue may be gently cleaned with a soft toothbrush to reduce the amount of staining. Otherwise, reassurance is all that is required.

Oral pigmentation has also been found in thyrotoxicosis, malabsorbtion, cachectic states, disorders of iron metabolism and neurofibromatosis.

Peter Blenkinsopp

MOUTH, ULCERS

The classification of mouth ulcers is outlined in Table M.7.

Table M.7 Classification of mouth ulcers

1 Traumatic
2 Aphthous
3 Ulceration associated with other mucous membranes (Behçet's syndrome, Reiter's disease)
4 Ulceration associated with skin disease
   ■ Lichen planus
   ■ Mucous membrane pemphigoid
   ■ Pemphigus
   ■ Bullous erythema multiforme
5 Blood dyscrasias
   ■ Agranulocytosis
   ■ Leukaemia
6 Ulceration associated with gastrointestinal diseases
   ■ Coeliac disease
   ■ Ulcerative colitis
   ■ Crohn's disease
7 Ulceration associated with connective tissue disorders
   ■ Lupus erythematosus
8 Infection
   ■ Bacterial
       ◆ Acute ulcerative gingivitis
       ◆ Syphilis
       ◆ Tuberculosis
   ■ Fungal
       ◆ *Candida*
   ■ Viral
       ◆ Herpes simplex
       ◆ Herpes zoster
       ◆ Epstein–Barr herpes (infectious mononucleosis)
       ◆ Coxsackie (herpangia, hand, foot and mouth disease)
9 Tumours
   ■ Squamous cell carcinoma

Traumatic

The diagnosis is usually easy to make because there is a definite history of trauma associated with

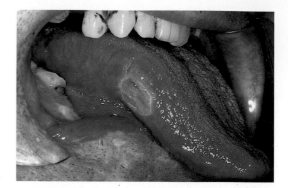

Figure M.17 Traumatic ulcer of the tongue caused by irritation from a carious tooth.

mastication, ill-fitting dentures or other minor injury to the oral cavity. The ulcers are usually shallow and painful, and heal quickly once the noxious stimulant is removed. Secondary bacterial infection can occasionally occur, causing an abscess or cellulitis (Fig. M.17).

Aphthous ulceration

This is the commonest form of oral ulceration, and three types are recognized, depending on the size and number of ulcers (Fig. M.18). The term *minor aphthous ulcer* is given to ulcers less than 5 mm in diameter, which occur intermittently as single ulcers or in crops. The ulcers take from 1 week to 10 days to heal, and in some patients new ulcers may develop before the original ones have healed, so that they are never without ulceration. This type of ulceration tends to commence in childhood and early life, and the attacks diminish as the patient becomes older. They are characteristically found on the buccal mucosa, in the sulcus between the jaws and the cheeks, the ventral

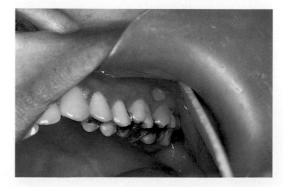

Figure M.18 Minor aphthous ulcer of the left maxillary alveolus.

aspect of the tongue and the floor of the mouth. This condition is often described as recurrent aphthous stomatitis (RAS). The ulcers are round, and have an erythematous periphery with a pale central crater.

Major aphthous ulcers are larger and more persistent and, in addition to the previous sites, may affect the tongue and the palate. They may be up to 1 cm in size and, because of their duration, give concern that the ulcer could be neoplastic. *Herpetiform ulcers* are the third variant, and here the patient suffers from crops of very numerous small ulcers, which are painful and tend to coalesce into one large irregular area on an erythematous background. Anything from 10 to 100 ulcers may be present at one time.

The cause of aphthous ulceration is unknown, although an autoimmune theory has been advanced. Some 10 per cent of patients will have an underlying haematological deficiency, especially of vitamin B_{12}, folate or iron; an additional 3 per cent will be suffering from coeliac disease, and a few may have Crohn's disease. In some female patients the ulcers are related to the menstrual cycle and will respond to hormone therapy. There is also an association with stress and the cessation of smoking. Aphthous ulceration is thought to be a feature of AIDS, but in the majority of cases the cause remains unknown.

Aphthous ulceration is treated by the use of topical steroids and mouthwashes; on occasion, systemic steroids may be required.

Ulceration associated with other mucous membranes

Behçet's syndrome

This syndrome consists of recurrent aphthous ulceration with also genital and ocular involvement in the form of posterior uveitis. The latter may subsequently cause impairment of vision. The disease characteristically affects young men, and there may be associated disease of the skin, joints and nervous system. The cause is unknown, but viral or autoimmune theories have been put forward. The management of the oral ulceration is the same as for recurrent aphthous ulceration.

Reiter's syndrome

The oral manifestations of this complaint are white circinate lines on an area of erythematous mucosa. These lesions are accompanied by urethritis, arthritis and conjunctivitis. The aetiology is again unknown, but may follow infection with *Mycoplasma* or *Shigella*. Some 10 per cent of patients will show small, non-specific ulcers similar to aphthous ulceration.

Mouth ulceration associated with skin disease

Lichen planus

Lichen planus is a common condition affecting both the skin and the mouth, although it can affect either in isolation (Fig. M.19). There are several types of oral lichen planus, with the erosive type being characterized by large, irregular areas of mucosal ulceration; the base of the ulcer is often slightly raised, with a covering of white to yellow slough.

Examination of the mouth elsewhere often demonstrates white lacey striations or a desquamative gingivitis. The aetiology of lichen planus is obscure, but it may be mediated by an immunological process with a lymphocytic infiltration, predominantly T cells, beneath the epithelium. Lichen planus can also be a reaction to liver disease, drugs (e.g. methyldopa, gold salts or antimalarials), or in the graft-versus-host reaction (bone marrow transplantation).

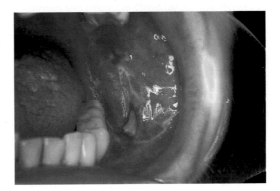

Figure M.19 Erosive lichen planus affecting the cheek.

Pemphigus and pemphigoid

Pemphigus and pemphigoid both may produce oral lesions, which commence as bullae when the epithelium separates from the basal layer in pemphigus, and when the epithelium and basal layers separate from the underlying mesoderm in pemphigoid (Fig. M.20). As a result, the bullae in pemphigus are far more fragile and rupture quickly, whereas the bullae in pemphigoid are more resilient.

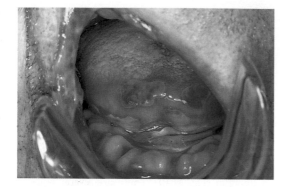

Figure M.20 Ulceration in mucous membrane pemphigoid.

In pemphigus there are circulating autoantibodies against the intercellular attachments of the squamous epithelium, and the level is an indication of the severity of the disease. Immunofluorescence shows deposits of IgG and C3 binding to desmosomes, which is the area of contact between epithelial cells. In pemphigoid, circulating autoantibodies are not detectable, but immunofluorescence studies show IgG and C3 at the basement membrane or dermoepidermal junction.

Pemphigus is a serious vesiculobullous mucocutaneous condition which mostly affects woman in the 40- to 50-year age group. If untreated, the condition may be fatal. The mouth may often be affected first with small bullae or widespread ulceration and loss of the oral epithelium. As the bullae are intra-epithelial, they rupture easily leaving what appears to be a thin layer of tissue paper over an underlying erosion. The diagnosis is made by biopsy (preferably of an intact bulla) and immunofluorescence studies. Treatment is by the use of systemic steroids, with replacement of fluid and protein in the acute phase.

Mucous membrane pemphigoid is a disease of the elderly, and affects females more than males. It affects the oral mucous membrane, and predominantly the conjunctiva of the eyes are involved. Ano-genital lesions may also occur and minor involvement of the skin may also be noted. Because the bullae are more rigid, they tend not to enlarge and rupture late. Once ruptured, they leave areas of irregular ulceration, which is accompanied by considerable scarring. The oesophagus and nasopharynx may also be involved, but the most significant aspect of the disease is conjunctival fibrosis leading to visual disturbance.

Examination of the mouth will demonstrate several intact or ruptured bullae during the active phase of the disease, and the gingivae may be severely affected with a desquamative gingivitis. Treatment is with topical steroids, although occasionally systematic steroids may be necessary.

Bullous erythema multiforme

Bullous erythema multiforme, or Stevens–Johnson syndrome, is the more severe form of erythema multiforme, invariably involving the oral cavity, and this can be the predominant feature of the attack. The appearance is dramatic because of the severe oral ulceration and the blood-stained and crusted lips. It tends to affect children and young adults, and is probably immunologically mediated, via exposure to micro-organisms (e.g. herpes simplex and *Mycoplasma*), or from drugs, typically the sulphonamides, non-steroidal anti-inflammatory agents, phenytoin and penicillin.

Examination of the skin will demonstrate either extensive erythema or a macular rash with target lesions exhibiting central bullae formation or ulceration. There is a conjunctivitis, leading to corneal ulceration. In the mouth, diffuse inflammation leads to vesicle formation followed by widespread erosions and haemorrhage. Epistaxis commonly occurs. Treatment of the minor case is with topical steroids, but the more severe attack may require systemic therapy. Tetracycline antibiotics should be given if infection with *Mycoplasma* is suspected.

Angina bullosa haemorrhagica

This condition of unknown origin is characterized by the spontaneous formation of blood-filled blisters within the mouth, which can develop very rapidly. They may occur while eating, and generally involve the soft palate. The individual is often alarmed by this condition and may develop a sensation of choking.

These blisters normally rupture within 24 hours, leaving an ulcer which heals spontaneously. Although similarities exist between this condition and mucous membrane pemphigoid, immunofluorescence tests are negative. Blood coagulation studies are normal.

Blood dyscrasias

Blood dyscrasias are discussed elsewhere (see GUMS, BLEEDING, p. 245), but ulceration of the gingivae is also common, caused by acute local bacterial infection secondary to the abnormal white cell function.

It should be remembered that the ulceration may also be due to acute bacterial ulcerative gingivitis or acute viral herpetic gingivostomatitis which has arisen because of a blood dyscrasia as the primary cause.

Ulceration associated with gastrointestinal diseases

Whilst coeliac disease, ulcerative colitis and Crohn's disease can be associated with recurrent aphthous ulceration, these conditions may also show distinctive oral signs (Fig. M.21). Crohn's disease characteristically produces a 'cobble-stone' thickening of the buccal mucosa with hyperplastic folds and fissuring. Painful ulcers, which are slow to heal, may also be present. Inflammatory bowel disease may also produce the condition of pyostomatitis vegetans, which is characterized by soft hyperplastic mucosal folds between which fissures and ulcers may form.

The ulceration associated with coeliac disease and gluten hypersensitivity is known as *dermatitis herpetiformas*. The skin is affected by an itchy rash, while in the mouth erythematous areas may appear or extensive erosions. Linear IgA disease may also cause oral ulceration.

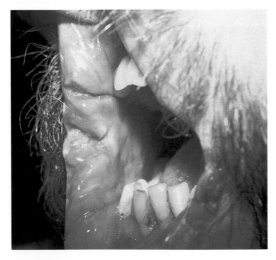

Figure M.21 Oral mucous membrane showing typical 'cobblestone' appearance in a patient with Crohn's disease.

Ulceration associated with connective tissue disorders

Approximately 20 per cent of patients with discoid and systemic lupus erythematosus (SLE) will show oral ulceration. There may be areas of erythema with erosions and, in some areas, these may resemble lichen planus due to minor striae formation. Frank ulceration may also be present.

The differential diagnosis may be difficult to make, but here the lesions often occur on the hard palate, which is rare in lichen planus. The diagnosis is made by biopsy and immunofluorescence studies. Antinuclear antibodies should be sought in the serum, and a history of arthritis and skin rashes should be elicited, particularly an erythematous rash of the face in the butterfly distribution.

Infection

Bacterial infections

Acute ulcerative gingivitis

Bacterial infection of the oral mucous membrane is rare in normal circumstances, the most important example being acute ulcerative gingivitis, which is associated with large numbers of Vincent's organisms (*Treponema vicentii* and *Fusiformis fusiformis*).

There is haemorrhage, inflammation and the formation of painful, shallow ulcers at the crest of the gingival margin. This eventually leads to destruction and flattening of the interdental papillae. Infection is associated with pre-existing periodontal disease and also any condition reducing host immunity. Patients with leukaemia, AIDS, or those receiving chemotherapy are, therefore, all susceptible and infection may follow an episode of acute herpetic stomatitis.

Acute ulcerative gingivitis in the severely debilitated patient may progress to the destructive condition of cancrum oris. This is rare in the developed world, apart from those patients who are immunosuppressed, but still occurs in the Third World as a result of malnutrition and severe viral infections (e.g. herpes and measles). Small areas of gangrene appear in the lips, cheeks or other oral structures, which rapidly progress to larger areas of slough and extensive loss of facial tissue.

Syphilis

The oral cavity may be involved rarely, during the primary stage, to produce a chancre on the lips or the tip of the tongue. Secondary lesions known as the 'mucous patch' are now seldom seen, because of modern effective treatment. Here, there is an erosion in the mucous membrane of a few centimetres with a yellowish slough surrounded by erythema. When these areas coalesce they give an irregular-shaped ulcer known as the 'snail track' ulcer.

The tertiary stage of syphilis, now rarely seen, produces the gumma, which is a deeply punched-out ulcer caused by central necrosis. These may typically affect the tongue or the palate and, in the latter, perforation will produce a central oronasal fistula.

Tuberculosis

With the successful treatment of tuberculosis, oral lesions are rare but, when they do occur, they are usually found in the tongue and lips. The ulcer typically shows undermined edges and a granulating floor. The mode of infection is thought to be expectoration of tubercle bacilli from a primary focus in the lungs, which then become implanted in the oral cavity.

Fungal infections

Candida (thrush)

This infection is caused by the yeast-like fungus, *Candida albicans*, which invades the epithelium, causing erythema of the epithelium and a yellow soft plaque that can be easily removed (Fig. M.22). This leaves an area of haemorrhagic mucosa or ulceration.

A high proportion of patients suffering with HIV infection will commonly develop an infection with *Candida*. This is known as erythematous and pseudomembranous candidosis, which are descriptive terms to describe the appearance of this infection.

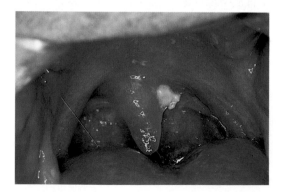

Figure M.22 Mouth demonstrating oral candidiasis.

Viral infections

The majority of acute infections of the oral mucosa are viral in origin. They tend to affect the younger age groups, and are normally associated with constitutional symptoms of fever, malaise and enlarged and tender cervical lymph nodes.

Herpes simplex

The primary infection invariably involves the mouth, with many small vesicles, approximately 2 mm in diameter, of regular shape and size (Fig. M.23). The mouth is generally inflamed, and in areas the ulcers coalesce to produce irregular raw erosions and a yellow slough.

The gingival mucosa is red and swollen and may bleed, even in the absence of ulceration. Herpetic stomatitis may be an opportunist infection and can be severe in immunocompromised patients and patients with AIDS. The lesion of reactivation is known as 'secondary herpes'. This reactivation can be brought on by exposure to sunlight, menstruation, trauma and stress, and particularly immunosuppression. The virus, which has been quiescent in the trigeminal ganglion, becomes active once more, to produce a cold sore or herpes labialis at the mucocutaneous junction of the lip or the nostril. The ulceration occurs in the distribution of the infected nerve. Treatment is by the use of acyclovir.

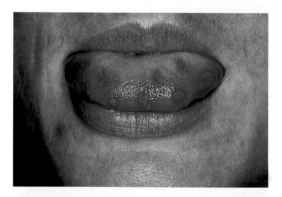

Figure M.23 Primary herpes infection of the oral cavity.

Herpes zoster

Herpes zoster causes chickenpox in the patient who has not been exposed to the virus, and mouth ulcers are common in this condition. The virus again remains quiescent in the trigeminal ganglion, and on reactivation causes painful ulceration within the exact anatomical distribution of the nerve. The ulceration may be preceded by pain or a disturbance in sensation in the same area.

This condition is known as herpes-zoster or shingles, and on occasions can be an indication of a more serious underlying disease. The picture once more is of erythema, small regular ulcers and pain within the distribution of the nerve affected. If the ophthalmic branch is involved then care needs to be given to the cornea. The infection may be complicated by postherpetic neuralgia. Treatment again is with the antiviral agent acyclovir.

Epstein–Barr virus

Infectious mononucleosis is caused by the Epstein–Barr virus (EBV). There may be characteristic petechiae of the soft palate and pharynx, which are often considered diagnostic.

The patient has a sore throat, the fauces and palate become inflamed and oedematous, and the lymph nodes are enlarged. Occasionally, there is extensive ulceration of the fauces. The diagnosis is achieved by the identification of atypical mononuclear cells in the peripheral blood, the Paul–Bunnell test and by EBV serology. Ampicillin should not be given for the sore throat as this exacerbates the condition.

Coxsackie virus

Mouth ulcers may arise from infection with the Coxsackie A virus, which causes a febrile illness, lymphadenopathy and ulcers and intense erythema of the soft palate.

Epidemics – particularly among children with the Coxsackie A virus – give rise to hand, foot and mouth disease. This is a highly infectious condition, characterized by small vesicles, leading to ulcers on the hands, the feet and in the mouth. These infections generally are trivial conditions and are self-limiting.

Tumours

Squamous cell carcinoma is the most common malignant tumour of the oral cavity, and is associated with excessive smoking and alcohol consumption. In the Indian subcontinent it is associated with the chewing of a betel nut quid with added tobacco and other chemicals (Fig. M.24).

The clinical picture of oral carcinoma is very varied, but in the advanced case it is obvious. There is a friable mass arising in the mucous membrane with a rough, irregular surface, which bleeds easily. There is usually deep, irregular central ulceration with an

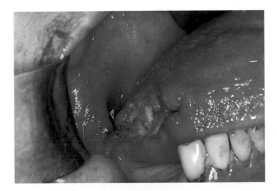

Figure M.24 Ulceration in squamous cell carcinoma of the tongue.

infected slough at its base. Radiographs may show associated bone erosion.

The early lesion may be more difficult to diagnose, showing only an area of erythema or hyperkeratosis, slight roughening of the mucosa and shallow ulceration.

Unfortunately, many oral carcinomas are still diagnosed late. Any ulcer that does not heal within 3 weeks, or does not obviously fall into one of the other categories, should be submitted for a biopsy.

Other tumours of the oral cavity, both benign and malignant, can undergo ulceration due to trauma or ischaemic necrosis; for descriptions, see JAW, SWELLING OF (p. 338).

Peter Blenkinsopp

MUSCULAR ATROPHY

Muscular atrophy occurs for a number of reasons. Patients present complaining of various symptoms such as wasting muscles or, most commonly, weakness of specific muscles leading to inability to perform certain tasks.

Damage to the lower motor neurone

Lesions of the lower motor neurone are responsible for the majority of cases of muscular atrophy encountered in clinical practice. The muscles are weak, flaccid and wasted. Fasciculation is seen. Electromyography shows fibrillation potentials on mechanical stimulation by the exploring needle, and spontaneous fibrillation and fasciculation potentials at rest. The tendon reflexes are depressed or abolished in the affected part unless, as in motor neurone disease, there is a coincident pyramidal lesion, in which case they usually remain brisk as long as there is any power of contraction left in the muscles concerned. It is convenient to classify the causes of this form of atrophy according to whether the lesion is in the anterior horn cells, the motor roots or the peripheral nerves.

Disuse

Disuse of a limb gives rise to extreme degrees of wasting. The best example is provided by the results of prolonged immobilization for fractures of the long bones. It also occurs in muscles acting upon a painful or ankylosed joint, and in rheumatoid arthritis. Voluntary disuse, as practised by some eastern cults, can lead to extreme 'withering' of the entire limb – for example, when penance demands that the arm be held above the head in perpetuity.

Vascular disease

Arterial occlusion is variable in its effects. In tourniquet paralysis, surgical ligation of a major vessel, thrombosis or embolism of the great vessels, the degree of wasting depends on the efficiency of the collateral circulation. In many instances the muscles become fibrosed and hard rather than wasted and flabby. In other cases, there is a true atrophy of muscles due to ischaemia of the motor nerves, as in some cases of Buerger's disease and in polyarteritis nodosa. A special variety of ischaemic palsy, known as Volkmann's contracture, is the result of fractures in the region of the elbow. Oedema and haemorrhage into the soft tissues interfere with the circulation distal to the elbow and cause fibrosis of the flexors of the wrist and fingers, and of the intrinsic muscles of the hand. The affected muscles are hard in consistency, and wasting is comparatively slight owing to replacement with fibrous tissue.

General bodily wasting

Muscular atrophy is often seen in general wasting of the tissues due to chronic or subacute disease such as tuberculosis, malignant disease, neglected or undiagnosed diabetes mellitus, hyperthyroidism, malaria, hookworm infestation, conditions associated with chronic diarrhoea and anorexia nervosa. It is also seen in old age.

Anterior horn cells

Acute poliomyelitis used to be the most common cause of anterior horn cell damage, but the incidence of this has been dramatically reduced. The muscular atrophy seen in late cases of polio is often very striking, and is localized to particular groups of muscles. Localized damage to anterior horn cells may occur at the site of trauma from fracture-dislocation of the spine or as a result of backward protrusion of an intervertebral disc in the cervical or thoracic regions. Spinal tumours may produce a similar effect. In these instances, atrophy is confined to the muscles that are innervated by the affected portion of the cord. Other intraspinal lesions that may produce muscular atrophy are syringomyelia, haematomyelia and intramedullary tumours such as ependymomas and astrocytomas; such cases usually have associated sensory loss and other signs of spinal cord damage. *Motor neurone disease* is a common cause of muscle atrophy in adults. It is prominent in the progressive muscular atrophy form of the disease, and is also seen in the so-called 'amyotrophic lateral sclerosis' form. Fasciculations are prominent in affected muscles in this condition. In the bulbar form, wasting of the tongue may be obvious. The rare syphilitic amyotrophy may mimic motor neurone disease, but the tendon reflexes are depressed and serological tests will confirm the diagnosis. Infarction of a localized area of spinal cord consequent upon thromboembolism of a branch of the anterior spinal artery may cause localized damage to anterior horn cells with segmental muscle wasting. This may occur in atheromatous disease, meningovascular syphilis or in association with arteriovenous malformations or tumours of the spinal cord.

Motor roots

Damage to a single motor root seldom causes much atrophy since most muscles are supplied by several roots. An exception is the first thoracic root, which supplies the intrinsic muscles of the hand (Fig. M.25). Damage to multiple spinal roots may be seen in spinal lesions below the level of the first lumbar vertebra, producing damage to the cauda equina. Apart from muscle weakness and wasting, there will often be associated sensory loss and sphincteric disturbance; pain is often a prominent symptom. Common causes of cauda equina damage include lumbar spondylosis, lumbar canal stenosis, primary

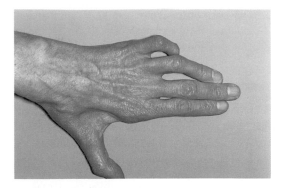

Figure M.25 Atrophy of all the small muscles of the hand due to an old brachial plexus injury involving the first thoracic root.

and secondary spinal tumours, and prolapsed lumbar intervertebral discs. More localized damage to spinal roots may be seen in spondylosis, and muscle atrophy in the upper limbs may be a feature of cervical spondylosis.

The peripheral nerves

Proximal damage to the peripheral nerves may occur at their origin in the brachial or lumbosacral plexus. Malignant infiltration of the brachial plexus typically affects the lower part of the plexus, thereby affecting the nerve supply to the intrinsic hand muscles. Malignant infiltration of the lumbosacral plexus may occur,

but is less common. Pain is a prominent feature. Traumatic avulsion of the plexus in the upper limb is all too common as a consequence of motorcycle injuries and in some instances the avulsion occurs not at the level of the plexus but at the level of the motor roots.

Traumatic damage to the lumbosacral plexus is less common. Localized injuries to the plexus or peripheral nerves may occur as a result of stab wounds, gunshot wounds, and fractures and dislocations in the vicinity of motor nerves.

Compression on motor nerves may produce local damage (so-called 'entrapment neuropathies'). Common sites of damage are the radial nerve in the upper arm, the lower cord of the brachial plexus between the first rib causing thoracic outlet syndrome and a cervical rib, the ulnar nerve at the level of the elbow, the median nerve at the level of the carpal tunnel, and the lateral popliteal nerve at the level of the neck of the fibula. The causes of peripheral neuropathies are listed in Table M.8.

Rates of progression vary considerably, but the common features are those of diffuse involvement of multiple peripheral nerves. In general, the distal parts of the limbs are affected first, with muscle weakness and wasting being most obvious in the lower part of the legs and hands (Fig. M.26). Signs are usually symmetrical, although some types of peripheral neuropathy tend to involve motor fibres more than sensory fibres. However, there is usually an associated distal

Table M.8 Causes of peripheral neuropathy

Inherited neuropathies	Chronic acquired neuropathies	Mononeuropathies
Mixed sensorimotor neuropathies:	Carcinoma	Pressure
1 Idiopathic	Paraproteinaemia	Trauma
2 Metabolic	Uraemic	Idiopathic
Sensory neuropathies	Beri-beri	Serum/post-vaccinal
	Diabetic	Herpes zoster
Acute acquired neuropathies	Hypothyroid	Neoplastic
Guillain–Barré syndrome	Connective tissue	Leprosy
Porphyria	Amyloid	Radiation
Toxic		Diphtheritic
Diphtheritic	*Relapsing neuropathies*	
	Idiopathic	*Mononeuritis multiplex*
Subacute acquired neuropathies	Porphyria	Arteritis
Deficiency states		Diabetes
Heavy metals		
Drug intoxication		
Uraemic		
Diabetic		
Arteritic		

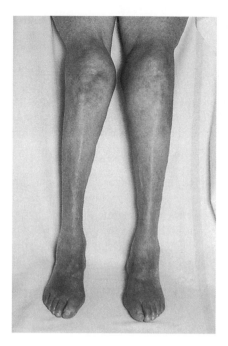

Figure M.26 Distal muscle atrophy due to peripheral neuropathy.

Table M.9 A classification of myopathies

1 *Inflammatory disease of muscle*
Polymyositis
Dermatomyositis

2 *Infective myopathies*
Trichinosis
Toxoplasmosis
Virus infections (e.g. Coxsackie B virus)

3 *Muscular dystrophies*
Duchenne
Becker
Fascioscapulohumeral
Limb girdle
Oculopharyngeal dystrophy
Myotonic dystrophy

4 *Metabolic myopathies*
Glycogen storage myopathies
Carnitine deficiency (and other defects of
fatty acid metabolism)

5 *Endocrine myopathies*
Adrenal dysfunction
Thyroid dysfunction

6 *Spinal muscular atrophies*
Although such conditions are not strictly disorders
of muscle, they are included because of the frequent difficulty
in differentiating them from the true myopathies

sensory loss which is typically in 'glove and stocking' distribution. Tendon reflexes are almost invariably depressed or absent.

Muscle disorders

Muscular atrophy, although not usually a prominent feature in muscle disease, may be seen in any form of myopathy. (For a classification of myopathies, see Table M.9.) Congenital absence of a muscle may occur, and the most common deficiency is the sternocostal portion of pectoralis major. Rupture of a muscle or its tendon may lead to localized atrophy.

Mark Kinirons

MUSCULAR HYPERTROPHY

There is considerable variation in the size of individual skeletal muscles, and the assessment of hypertrophy or enlargement may in some instances be very difficult. For example, the normal calf muscles in a leg that has gross wasting of the quadriceps may appear hypertrophied simply because of the relative disproportion.

Exercising muscles can cause them to hypertrophy: this occurs as a result of an increase in muscle fibre size secondary to an increase in the number of myofibrils per fibre. Such physiological hypertrophy may be generalized as in bodybuilders, or it may be localized as in those who repeatedly use a particular limb, for example tennis players.

The syndrome of hemi-hypertrophy is associated with diffuse enlargement of all the tissues of one half of the body, occasionally affecting only the face or one limb. In this condition, the aetiology of which is unknown, the muscles, subcutaneous tissues and bones all appear to enlarge.

A classification of pathological muscle hypertrophy is provided in Table M.10.

Multiple muscle enlargement

Enlargement of muscles is commonly seen in Duchenne and Becker dystrophy, and occasionally in limb-girdle dystrophy. The most commonly enlarged

Table M.10 Hypertrophy of muscles

Multiple muscle enlargement	Localized muscle enlargement
Duchenne dystrophy	Muscle/tendon rupture
Becker dystrophy	Muscle haemorrhage
Limb-girdle dystrophy	Muscle tumour
Spinal muscular atrophy	Myositis ossificans
Hypothyroidism	Granuloma
Myotonia congenital	Pyogenic abscess
DeLange syndrome	Fibrositis
Cysticercosis	
Malignant hyperpyrexia	
Hypertrophy musculorum vera	

muscle is the gastrocnemius, although hypertrophy of the infraspinatus, deltoid, triceps, quadriceps or gluteus muscles may be encountered. The term 'pseudo-hypertrophy' has been used in reference to Duchenne dystrophy, since in the later stages of the disease the muscle becomes weak but remains enlarged because of replacement of fibres by fat and connective tissues. Often, the pseudohypertrophic muscles will have a rather characteristic firm or doughy feeling.

Rapid enlargement of muscles has been described in spinal muscular atrophy, polymyositis, cysticercosis and in certain families with malignant hyperpyrexia.

Diffuse hypertrophy of muscles may occur in myotonia congenita, and this probably represents work hypertrophy associated with continuous muscle contraction. This produces the so-called 'infant Hercules' appearance. In hypothyroidism, hypertrophy of muscles is more common in children than in adults. The calves, thighs, hands, neck, tongue and face may all enlarge and feel firm or indurated. Often, the patient will complain of pain and stiffness, and this may be accompanied by proximal muscle weakness. In the DeLange syndrome, hypertrophy of muscles is associated with congenital athetosis and mental retardation.

Localized muscle enlargement

This is most commonly seen in the biceps muscle as a result of rupture of the muscle fibres or tearing of the long head. It may also be seen as a result of a muscle haemorrhage, muscle tumour such as rhabdomyosarcoma, angioma, desmoid or metastatic lesion, or as a result of an infective process such as granulomatous disease or pyogenic abscess. Localized enlargement

may occur as a result of trauma leading to myositis ossificans.

Mark Kinirons

MUSCULAR PAIN

Pain in muscles is one of the most common of all complaints, and may occur either as an ache or as a stiffness or cramp. These two types of muscle pain are usually distinguishable, and their causes are different.

Aching pains

Aches and pains in muscles may be transient, recurrent or persistent. They may be classified as follows.

Normal reactions

Fatigue, anxiety, and particularly depression, may be associated with muscle aches and pains. Few healthy people go through an average day, whatever their occupation or activity, without occasional feelings of muscular discomfort. These are usually suppressed or ignored, but in abnormal emotional states they may assume unnatural proportions and become significant and sometimes distressing symptoms. Muscle aches become more common as individuals become increasingly aware of ageing. These aches may be aggravated by postural strain, often resulting from the adoption of fixed positions over prolonged periods.

Injuries

After unduly heavy exertion, muscles may become painful for hours or even days, presumably as a result of small local injuries, tears or haemorrhages, in the muscles themselves or at muscle insertions. Injured fibres, particularly at the points of attachment to bone, may be acutely painful and tender (e.g. tennis or golfer's elbow), and ligaments may be completely torn across, even in the absence of extreme exertion. The largest tendon in the body – the tendo-Achillis – is particularly liable to rupture in those engaged in sporting activities such as squash or cricket. Too-rapid leaping out of bed has been known to rupture both tendons. The supraspinatus muscle and tendon and the quadriceps are perhaps the most frequently injured; a rupture of the long head of biceps, the rhomboids, major or minor, pectoralis major, rectus abdominus, trapezius, levator scapuli, latissimus dorsi or almost any other muscle or tendon may occur and may mislead the unwary diagnostician. It is important that muscle pain in the chest or abdomen should not be mistaken for pain arising from visceral sources. An unusual cause of muscle pain that may be overlooked is spontaneous haemorrhage of the type that may occur in haemophiliacs or in those receiving anticoagulant therapy.

Referred pain

Pains apparently arising in muscles are often referred from inflammatory or degenerative disease in nearby joints. Pains in thigh muscles, for instance, may result from hip joint disease, and muscle pains in the shoulder girdle, chest or abdomen, from degenerative changes in the cervical, dorsal or lumbar spine. Disease or injury of ligaments may be referred to muscles; injections of hypertonic saline into interspinous ligaments, for instance, may cause pains in muscles several inches away. The cause of the extremely common so-called 'fibrositis' or fibromyalgia in muscles in the scapular and shoulder regions is still inadequately explained, but undoubtedly the pain is often referred from adjacent spinal joints and ligaments, allegedly triggered in many cases by cold or damp. These 'fibrositic' pains may sometimes be the first signs of an arthropathy such as rheumatoid arthritis, rarely a disseminated connective-tissue disorder such as systemic lupus erythematosus or polyarteritis nodosa, or more commonly in elderly subjects, polymyalgia rheumatica (see p. 182, p. 454 and p. 458).

Pains of vascular origin

The classical example of ischaemic muscle pain is the intermittent claudication experienced on exertion by victims of occlusive arterial disease in the lower limbs. Inflammatory arterial diseases, for example, polymyalgia rheumatica, giant-cell arteritis and polyarteritis nodosa, may also produce tenderness in muscle, but not pain. Whenever pain is a presenting symptom, consideration of the blood supply is vital in assessment.

Muscle disorders

Several inflammatory disorders of muscle are commonly associated with muscle pain and tenderness, and should be considered in any patient who complains of myalgia. In polymyositis and dermatomyositis, over 50 per cent of sufferers will describe pain as well as muscle weakness. The pain is usually a deep aching within the muscles, and it is often aggravated by activity. The muscles may be swollen as well as tender. Similar symptoms are seen in a variety of other connective-tissue diseases when there is an associated inflammatory myopathy, for example rheumatoid arthritis, Sjögren's syndrome, SLE, polyarteritis nodosa, scleroderma and mixed connective-tissue disease.

Several epidemics of influenza due to type A or B virus have been described in which there was a rather acute onset of severe myalgia lasting for 1 or 2 weeks, with creatine kinase often elevated many times above normal. In epidemic pleurodynia, or Bornholm disease, the acute onset of chest and abdominal pain, chiefly at the costal margins and in the subcostal region, is usually the first symptom. Affected muscles are tender to pressure, and pain is induced by muscle contraction. The acute pain and fever last for several days, and after initial recovery one or more relapses are not uncommon. Care must be taken not to confuse one of these relatively benign and reversible syndromes with polymyositis of acute onset.

An unusual type of muscle disease may result from eating undercooked pork infected with the larvae of *Trichinella spiralis*. Muscle pain and stiffness occur particularly in the masseter. There may be associated malaise, fever, periorbital oedema, skin rash and petechial haemorrhages.

Polymyalgia rheumatica should always be considered in older patients in their sixties and seventies who are complaining of aching muscles and stiffness in the shoulder and hip girdle muscles. The ache tends to be worse at night, and morning stiffness is a prominent feature.

Neuropathic disorders

Pains in the muscles may be marked in the early stages of poliomyelitis, and are common in the Guillain–Barré syndrome. In acute brachial neuritis or neuralgic amyotrophy, severe aching pain in one or both shoulders or arms may precede the development of localized muscle weakness. In diabetic proximal neuropathy, pain often accompanies atrophy of the quadriceps or sometimes other muscles. Other neuropathies associated with severe pain include those seen with alcoholism, arsenical poisoning, polyarteritis and porphyria.

Endocrine causes

In hypothyroidism, acromegaly and hyperparathyroidism, the muscles may ache. Most endocrine disorders, however, are more commonly associated with weakness than with pain.

Drugs

Severe muscle pains may follow the intramuscular injection of suxamethonium, a muscle relaxant used in anaesthesia; these pains can occur 1–5 days after anaesthesia, and are worse if there is an earlier resumption of physical activity. A number of drugs may cause an acute or subacute necrotizing myopathy which may be associated with myoglobinuria, sometimes leading to acute renal failure (Table M.11).

Table M.11 Drugs capable of causing painful myopathy

Suxamethonium
Clofibrate
Epsilon-amino-caproic acid
Heroin
Amphetamine
Vincristine
Alcohol
Guanoclor
Lithium
Emetine
Cimetidine
Isoetharine
Phencyclidine
Statins

Psychogenic

Aching pain in muscles is a common symptom in depression and anxiety, and may also be seen in hysteria or in patients who are frankly malingering.

Muscle stiffness or cramps

Ordinary muscle cramps or painful involuntary contractions of muscle are experienced in almost everyone at some time in their lives, and in most instances the diagnosis presents no difficulty. Benign muscle cramps most commonly occur after unaccustomed exercise and are usually self-limiting. In some patients, however, these cramps can be persistent and quite incapacitating.

Pathological cramps can be produced by an abnormality anywhere along the final common pathway including the anterior horn cell, peripheral nerve, neuromuscular junction and muscle membrane.

Exertional cramps may be seen in a variety of disorders, including cauda equina ischaemia from lumbar canal stenosis, and inborn errors of muscle metabolism such as McArdle's disease or the lipid storage myopathies. In myophosphorylase deficiency and phosphofructokinase deficiency, a true contracture occurs with exercise which may be accompanied by myoglobinuria.

Several of the cramping disorders are characterized by myotonia where the patient observes a delayed relaxation after even a single voluntary contraction.

Muscle cramps and spasms may occur either spontaneously or after exercise in a variety of biochemical disturbances. They are most characteristically seen in tetany, which may occur with hypocalcaemia, alkalosis or hypomagnesaemia.

Several disorders are characterized by an almost continuous state of muscle activity: these include tetanus, strychnine poisoning and the bite of the American black widow spider. A number of rare neuromuscular disorders are associated with persistent contraction of muscles at rest. These include the symptoms of myokymia, continuous muscle fibre activity and the so-called 'stiff-man' syndrome.

A separate and important group of muscle cramp syndromes are the so-called 'professional' cramps or repetitive strain injury (RSI). The most common of these is 'writer's cramp', though similar localized muscle cramps have been described in typists, telephone operators, painters, tailors, seamstresses, pianists, flautists, violinists, cellists, harpists, drummers, piano players, blacksmiths, filemakers and watchmakers! There is considerable debate as to whether these are occupational neuroses or localized dystonias.

Mark Kinirons

MUSCULAR TONE

The tone of a muscle can be regarded as its resistance to passive stretching. This can only be assessed when the muscle is moved; it cannot be judged on the basis of palpation. Postural tone is that state of partial contraction of certain muscles which is needed to maintain the posture of the body.

At the moment a muscle is stretched, receptors in the muscle concerned – particularly in the muscle spindles – transmit afferent stimuli, and reflex partial contraction of the muscle results. The responses to momentary stretching are responsible for the tendon jerks; the responses to more prolonged stretching elicit more complex responses such as tonic contraction.

Forceful continued contraction of a group of muscles – for example, clenching one hand – temporarily causes an increased flow of afferent impulses in the sensory fibres from the spindles. This is associated with exaggeration of the tendon reflexes resulting from increased alpha neuronal discharge. This is known as 'reinforcement', which can be helpful in eliciting depressed reflexes.

Muscle tone is normally regulated by reticulospinal fibres which accompany the pyramidal tract through the spinal cord, and which have an inhibitory effect upon the stretch reflex. This inhibition balances the facilitatory impulses conveyed by the pontine reticulo-spinal and lateral vestibulospinal pathways. These in turn are influenced by multisynaptic reflex arcs traversing the cerebellum, basal ganglia and brainstem.

Alterations in muscle tone

Rigidity

In this form of increased muscle tone, the muscles are continuously or intermittently tense. The increased resistance to passive movement has an even or uniform quality throughout the range of movement of the limb, like that noted when bending a lead pipe. Rigidity is present in all muscle groups, both flexor and extensor, but it tends to be more prominent in those which maintain a flexed posture.

A particular type of rigidity, often encountered in Parkinson's disease, has distinctive characteristics and is described as 'cogwheel'. When the hypertonic muscle is stretched, a ratchet-like resistance is felt.

Rigidity is a prominent feature of many extrapyramidal diseases such as Parkinson's disease, Wilson's disease, dystonia musculorum deformans, multiple system atrophy and basal ganglia calcification.

A special type of variable resistance to passive movement is that in which the patient seems unable to relax. This is sometimes called 'gegenhalten', and is seen in diseases of the frontal lobes. A similar difficulty may be observed in children.

The pathophysiology of rigidity is not fully understood, though it is generally agreed that it results from lesions of the nigro-striatal system. It can often be relieved by dopamine, dopamine agonists, or by stereotactic lesions in the ventrolateral thalamus.

Spasticity

This is a form of increased tone resulting from lesions of the pyramidal pathways and the closely associated reticulo-spinal pathways. The stretch reflexes are released from descending inhibitory influences, and there is increased excitability of fusimotor neurones and alpha motor neurones. The resistance to passive stretch of muscles affected by spasticity often has a distinctive quality. It may be particularly severe initially and then tend to give way – hence the descriptive term, 'clasp-knife rigidity'. The hyperactivity of the tendon reflexes is often accompanied by clonus in which sustained stretch of a muscle evokes repetitive contraction and relaxation.

Decerebrate rigidity

A lesion at the mid-brain, at or about the level of the superior colliculus, releases the brainstem, cerebellum and spinal cord from cerebral control. This results in strong continuous contraction in extensor groups of muscles. In such cases all four limbs are rigidly extended, the back is arched, and there may be neck retraction.

Although the experimental production of decerebrate rigidity by Sherrington appeared to have a specific anatomical substrate, this does not hold quite true in man; for example, unilateral decerebrate rigidity is not uncommonly seen in the early stages of acute cerebral infarction in the territory of the middle cerebral artery.

Hypotonia

Hypotonia, or flaccidity, implies a reduction in tone. It may be seen in cerebral or spinal shock resulting from acute damage to the brain or spinal cord. It is a common manifestation of cerebellar disease, and in this situation is thought to result from diminished gamma efferent activity. It also occurs whenever a lesion interrupts the afferent or efferent pathway of the spinal reflex arc. It is thus seen in damage to the anterior horn cells, spinal roots and peripheral nerves, but it is not a particular feature of muscle disease.

Minor degrees of loss of tone may be difficult to differentiate from normal inherent muscle tone. Gross flaccidity is usually obvious. In the upper limbs, lesser degrees of hypotonia can be elicited by asking the patient to hold the arms out horizontally. Tapping the forearms when hypotonia is present will be associated with slow recoil and a wide arm swing.

Mark Kinirons

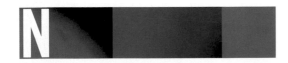

NAILS, AFFECTIONS OF

The nails are absent or hypoplastic from birth in cases of *ectodermal dysplasia*; this may be a familial trait, and a search should be made for associated abnormalities of the hair, teeth, or – most importantly – the sweat glands. In another genetic disorder, *epidermolysis bullosa*, repeated blistering of the finger tips may lead to scarring and loss of the nails. Other genetic syndromes involving the nails include Darier's disease and pachyonychia congenital. Spoon-shaped nails, *koilonychia*, may also be congenital, but in acquired koilonychias there is likely to be a background of chronic iron deficiency. The nails may be shed spontaneously, usually after some major febrile illness; more commonly there is a temporary disruption to nail growth, producing a transverse depression running across each nail (*Beau's lines*) (Fig. N.1) which gradually grow out. Other manifestations of systemic disease including clubbing of the fingers (see FINGERS, CLUBBED, p. 217), whitening of the nails (*leuconychia*) in chronic hepatic disease, and red half-moons are said to be a feature of some cases of cardiac failure. By contrast, white dots and patches within the nailplate, *leuconychia striata* and *leuconychia punctata*, are of no pathological significance. In the *yellow nail syndrome* (Fig. N.2) the nails take on a yellowed, or greeny-yellow colour, grow excessively slowly, and are excessively curved; lymphoedema is often found in association, as are various pulmonary abnormalities including bronchiectasis, and benign pleural effusions. Splinter haemorrhages under the nailplate used to be regarded as a marker of infective endocarditis, but are a non-specific sign, often provoked by trauma. Nailfold infarcts may be a feature of many vasculitic disorders.

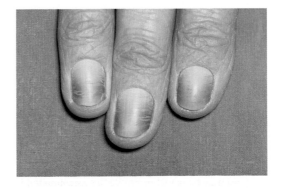

Figure N.1 Beau's lines.

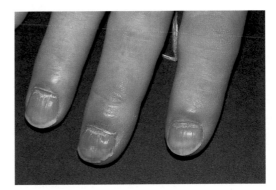

Figure N.2 Yellow nail syndrome.

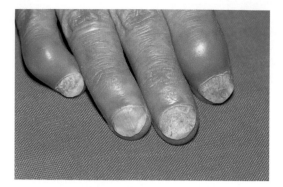

Figure N.3 Psoriatic arthropathy.

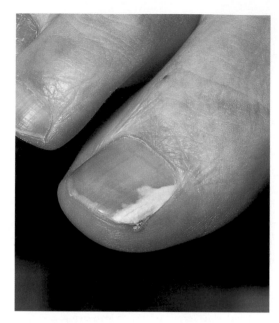

Figure N.4 Tinea of nail (early).

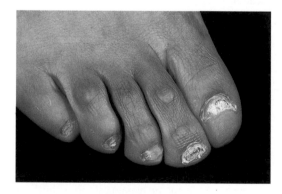

Figure N.5 Tinea of nail (Trichophyton rubrum).

Nail changes are a feature of many inflammatory skin disorders. In psoriasis, the nails are affected in up to 50 per cent of cases (Fig. N.3); changes include pitting of the surface of the nail, *onycholysis* (separation of the distal nailplate producing the appearance of whitening of the distal nail), discoloration of the nail, or a general thickening and friability of the nail. None of these features is totally specific for psoriasis. Thus, onycholysis may be seen in cases of thyrotoxicosis, or alone as an idiopathic phenomenon. Pitting may be an occasional feature of alopecia areata. In dermatitis of the fingers there is quite commonly a rather non-specific ridging of the nailplate, whilst in lichen planus, inflammation around the nailfold may eventuate in scarring destruction of the nail (*pterygium*).

Thickening and crumbling of the nails may be a feature of dermatophyte fungus infection, and this is more common on the toenails than the fingernails. *Trichophyton rubrum* or *Trichophyton mentagrophytes* are the most common causative species (Figs N.4 and N.5). The changes may be indistinguishable from psoriasis, and so it is always wise to confirm the diagnosis by fungal culture before embarking on treatment. However, in their earliest stages, fungal infection may merely present with a localized whitening of the nailplate (*superficial white mycosis*).

In chronic paronychia, which is due to combined candidal and bacterial infection, pockets form under the posterior nailfolds, which will admit the tip of a probe up to 3 mm. Very occasionally, pus may be expressed from these pockets, from which cultures of the yeast may be made. In profile the raised nailfolds over the pockets have a characteristic bolster-like

appearance. The changes in the nailplate are secondary. This disease occurs in those who are obliged to keep their hands wet for long periods, notably bar staff, fishmongers and those with 'wet' occupations. It is much more common in women than in men.

Longitudinal ridging more often has no apparent cause. Brittleness (*onychorrhexis*) or softness of the nails with splitting or terracing of the free edge is more common in women than in men. The cause is unknown, but repeated wetting and drying may be a factor of importance. It has been thought to be aggravated by the use of nail varnish and varnish removers, but many cases occur in women who do not use nail polish. Hypertrophy of the nails (*onychauxis*) occurs more often on the toes and may lead to onychogryphosis (Fig. N.6).

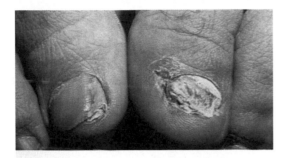

Figure N.6 Onychogryphosis.

Onychia, or inflammation of the nail, is usually septic in origin, but may be the result of trauma or contact with irritants at work. It usually terminates in shedding of the affected nail. *Paronychia*, or whitlow, is usually obvious (Fig. N.7), but a primary chancre of the finger may sometimes imitate it.

Trauma is responsible for many nail deformities. Single injuries produce haematomas which may lead to temporary nail loss or to permanent splits if the nail matrix is injured. Occasionally, an unrecognized injury which leads to a haematoma may lead to the mistaken impression of a *subungual malignant melanoma*. Periungual warts may distort nail growth, as may an adjacent *myxoid cyst*.

Barry Monk

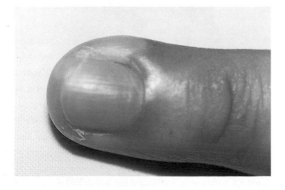

Figure N.7 Acute paronychia.

NAPKIN (PERINEAL) ERUPTIONS

Eruptions in children

Napkin dermatitis, at least in transient form, occurs in all babies at some stage. It is usually responsive to emollients and home remedies. Most examples are caused by irritation of the skin due to prolonged contact with urine or faeces, and are favoured by infrequent nappy changes, particularly when occlusive plastic pants are worn. The convexities are affected by shiny red plaques, sometimes eroded, which spare the flexural creases. If the flexures are the main site of inflammation, secondary *candidiasis* should be suspected and a search made at the edge for typical 'satellite pustulation'. *Infantile seborrhoeic dermatitis* is an acute, self-limiting red scaly eruption in which the napkin area is usually severely affected. The condition begins with cradle cap and spreads to the face, chest, back and limb flexures as well as the napkin area. Despite the widespread eruption, infants show little sign of discomfort. This is in marked contrast to those infants with *atopic dermatitis*, who may also have a napkin eruption, but who are distressed by itch, and sleep poorly.

Irritable children with erosions and papules around their napkin areas should be carefully examined for scabies. Other common sites for burrows are anterior axillary folds, wrists, finger webs, ankles, palms and soles. Nursing mothers may have burrows around their nipples as well as the usual sites. *Molluscum contagiosum* causes persistent irritating papules around the ano-genital area in both children and adults. Patients are frequently atopic, and individual lesions may heal spontaneously, sometimes with considerable purulent reaction or a stark halo of eczema.

Earlier editions of this book dwelt on the details of the nappy rash seen as a manifestation of *congenital syphilis*. Affected infants are irritable, feed poorly and have a purulent, often bloody, nasal discharge. Perianal and peri-oral erosions and rhagades are prominent and highly infectious. At 2 months of age the napkin area as well as the palms and soles may be affected by a new pinkish rash resembling the rash of secondary syphilis in adults.

In the extremely rare *acro-dermatitis enteropathica*, zinc absorption is deficient. Affected infants have diarrhoea and characteristic peri-orificial erosions, which may spread on to the limbs, sometimes in a livedoid pattern. Similar lesions can occur in zinc-deficient premature babies. If a napkin eruption becomes purpuric, *Letterer–Siwe disease* (histiocytosis) should be suspected. Other flexures, the gums and external auditory meatuses should be inspected for lesions.

White patches in the perineum can be due to *vitiligo*, which may begin in childhood and has a predilection for genital skin.

Lichen sclerosus of the vulva (white spot disease) is rare in infancy, but young children are affected. The physical signs of a porcelain-white, scarred, purpuric vulva may lead to suspicions of molestation.

Hyperpigmentation is most commonly due to the *mongolian spot*, a reliable marker of Negroid or Asiatic parentage, which causes considerable and extensive bluish pigmentation of the sacral napkin area and is due to dermal dendritic pigment cells.

Eruptions in adults

In adults, the perineum may be involved in numerous dermatoses with scaly eruptions (e.g. tinea, erythrasma, candidiasis or psoriasis). The area can be infested in pediculosis pubis, as well as scabies. *Molluscum contagiosum* can cause irritating papular lesions. Venereal warts are increasing in frequency, and can be a marker of other sexually transmitted infections or cervical intraepithelial neoplasia in women. *Syphilitic chancre* occurs more commonly within the anal canal or vagina, but rarely syphilitic *condyloma acuminata* may be seen on the perineum. In *pruritus ani*, lichenification from scratching and rubbing will be seen. There may be a complicating contact dermatitis due to one of the topical remedies employed (e.g. local anaesthetics, local antibiotics or lanolin).

Dipak Kanabar

NASAL DEFORMITY

Nasal deformity can be congenital or developmental, but is most often acquired. Abnormalities of either the bony or cartilaginous nasal skeleton contribute to the deformity.

Minor degrees of septal deformity are extremely common, and are thought to be the result of undetected minor injuries during birth or early childhood. These may compromise nasal airflow but rarely cause significant external nasal deformity. However, in some, deformity may develop during adolescence. Some postulate that this is caused by unequal growth of the nasal skeleton as a result of previous trauma.

The most common cause of an acquired deformity is a simple, displaced, fracture of the nasal bones. More severe blunt injuries to the nose are often associated with fractures and severe distortion and deviation of the nasal septum. In this situation there is a visible displacement of the nasal tip. From a practical standpoint, nasal fracture should be diagnosed clinically rather than radiologically, as non-displaced fractures are irrelevant and plain X-rays can be extremely unreliable and difficult to interpret.

Saddle nose deformities are usually acquired as a result of destruction of the septal cartilage (Fig. N.8). Septal abscesses or haematoma, arteritides (e.g. Wegener's disease, relapsing polychondritis) or, nowadays rarely, congenital syphilis may cause this appearance. It is also a recognized complication of excessive resection of septal cartilage during surgery.

It must be recognized that *perception of appearance* is very subjective, and can even be influenced by fashion. Humps, bulbous, broad, raised or drooping nasal

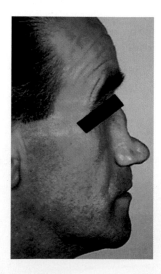

Figure N.8 Saddle nose. The cause of this was an SMR operation for a septal haematoma.

tips are inherent in some. These features may detract from the patient's potential appearance and can have a profound effect on personality. Rhinoplasty can go some way to correcting or changing these deformities in selected cases and significantly improve the patient's quality of life (Fig. N.9). Unfortunately, there are a few patients for whom surgery can never provide a satisfactory solution, and they require psychiatric help.

Michael Gleeson

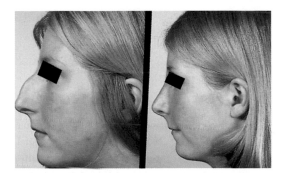

Figure N.9 Left: Congenital bony cartilaginous hump. Right: Corrected by rhinoplasty.

NASAL DISCHARGE

The causes of nasal discharge are listed in Table N.1.

Table N.1 Conditions causing nasal discharge

Congenital	Trauma
Choanal atresia	Foreign body
	Rhinolith
Infective	CSF rhinorrhoea
Acute rhinitis	Atopy or hypersensitivity
Rhinosinusitis	Allergic rhinitis
Caseous rhinitis	Vasomotor rhinitis
Atrophic rhinitis	
Chronic infective granulomas	**Neoplastic**
■ Syphilis	Carcinoma
■ Tuberculosis	Lymphoma
■ Leprosy	
■ Rhinoscleroma	**Miscellaneous**
	Wegener's granulomatosis
	Old age

Congenital causes

Choanal atresia, by blocking the posterior choana, prevents the normal nasal mucus stream from reaching the pharynx. A mucoid anterior nasal discharge results and intermittent infections ensure that the discharge is mucopurulent at times.

Infective causes

Acute viral infection, the common cold, and the prodromal stages of many infectious fevers, give rise to a clear mucoid discharge. The discharge becomes increasingly purulent as secondary bacterial infection follows. Persistent purulent discharge, either unilateral or bilateral, is seen in sinusitis. Careful inspection of the nasal passages may reveal the origin of the discharge and indicate the sinus or sinuses involved. The maxillary sinuses open into the middle meatus, as do the anterior ethmoid sinuses. The posterior ethmoid and sphenoid sinuses drain more posteriorly. About 10 per cent of maxillary sinus infections have a dental cause, for example, peri-apical infection. If pus aspirated from the maxillary sinus is foetid, a dental cause should be suspected. Sometimes, the pus becomes inspissated, giving rise to the so-called 'caseous sinusitis' or 'rhinitis'. This is particularly common with fungal infection. The material is whitish, cheesy and foul-smelling. Even worse are the crusts and dry discharge of an atrophic rhinitis. In these patients the nasal fossae are unduly wide and the mucosa thin and devoid of mucus cells. The especially disgusting odour is called 'ozaena'.

Pathogenic fungi and yeasts are a common cause of nasal infection and discharge in tropical countries but, of course, nowadays these infections are occasionally seen in this country in immigrants and travellers returning from exotic places.

To summarize the nasal symptoms of the main fungal diseases:

- *Rhinosporidiosis* predominantly affects the nasal mucosa, where the characteristic lesion is a bleeding polyp containing the sporangium from which spores spread via the lymphatics (Fig. N.10). This condition chiefly affects the peoples of Sri Lanka, Bangladesh and India.
- *Phycomycoses* cause serious disease, often starting with granulomatous lesions in the nose and considerable mucoid discharge. This fungus is also found in the tropics.

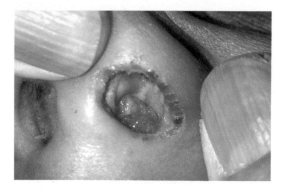

Figure N.10 The typical appearance of rhinosporidiosis, seen here in a young girl from Bangladesh.

- *Aspergillus* infection is sometimes contracted from captive birds. It is characterized by a watery, mouldy smelling discharge and a greyish membrane on the mucosa.
- *Actinomycosis* rarely affects the sinuses and nose. There is a woody mass and multiple sinuses from which the pus exudes.
- *Candida albicans* is found commonly in the mouth and occasionally in the nose of the young and those in a poor state of general health. It forms white patches that can be removed without bleeding. Many patients start with nasal discharge and bleeding. The diagnosis is made by identifying the fungus in scrapings, or by biopsy.
- *Secondary syphilis* affects the nose, causing a simple catarrhal rhinitis. Other accompanying lesions usually suggest the diagnosis. *Tertiary syphilitic gummas* were, at one time, relatively common and frequently affected the nose with destruction of bone and cartilage. Secondary infection causes offensive discharge and there is bleeding, often with the later development of an atrophic rhinitis.
- *Lupus vulgaris* is the most common tuberculous infection of the nose. There is nasal discharge, and the typical lesion – a reddish, firm nodule – is found at the anterior end of the nasal septum. The septum may perforate.
- *Leprosy* affects the nose as almost the earliest sign of the disease. Nodular thickening of the mucosa with inflammation and obstruction are associated with discharge. Later, perforation of the septum and destruction of tissue allows for secondary infection and very offensive discharge.
- *Rhinoscleroma* is a progressive granuloma beginning in the nose in an atrophic form with ozaena. Nodules form

later, and there is considerable scarring. The diagnosis is made by biopsy.
- *AIDS* is associated with a watery nasal discharge that is frequently found concomitantly in this disease.

Foreign bodies

A unilateral nasal discharge in an infant or child is pathognomonic of a foreign body, often a piece of foam rubber or paper inserted into the nasal fossa. Small hard objects may remain in the nose for some time before symptoms develop. Long-standing foreign bodies calcify to form rhinoliths. These are associated with chronic discharge and halitosis.

Trauma

A clear watery discharge following a head injury suggests a fracture of the anterior cranial fossa or cribriform plate and a cerebrospinal fluid (CSF) leak. Such a discharge will increase on leaning the head forward, or on compression of the jugular veins. The presence of sugar in this fluid confirms that it is CSF. This can be further confirmed by serological tests for β-transferrin.

Atopy

Copious clear mucoid nasal discharge, almost as freely flowing as water, is present in allergic rhinitis, and may be associated with violent attacks of sneezing, lacrimation and conjunctival injection. The diagnosis is confirmed by the history and by RAST and PRIST tests. Nasal allergy is liable to be confused with less non-specific vasomotor rhinitis, which is also very common. Numerous provocative factors are present in this troublesome condition, including changes of environmental temperature and humidity, mechanical irritation from dusts and vapours, psychological factors, pregnancy and drug reactions. Patients with vasomotor instability not infrequently carry boxes of paper tissues. The diagnosis is made after excluding nasal allergy.

Neoplastic

Malignant nasal disease (squamous cell carcinoma, adenocarcinoma, olfactory neuroblastoma) is usually heralded by progressive unilateral obstruction, followed shortly by nasal discharge. This is often clear to start with, but later becomes blood-stained, offensive and thick. The growth may be in the nasal fossa, one or other of sinuses or the nasopharynx. This sequence of events should prompt the clinician to obtain a CT scan of the patient and to examine the nose under anaesthetic so that a biopsy can be obtained.

The so called 'midline granuloma', is in fact a T-cell lymphoma that presents as a slowly progressing ulceration of the face, starting in the region of the nose and pre-maxilla. The localized destruction of tissue produces a blood-stained nasal discharge.

Miscellaneous

Wegener's granulomatosis commonly involves the nose, and usually presents with symptoms referable to the paranasal sinuses. It also affects the kidneys, lungs and lower respiratory tract. Patients present with malaise, severe facial pain, nasal obstruction and discharge spotted with blood.

Senile rhinorrhoea is thought to be a form of vasomotor rhinitis. It is a common and sometimes distressing condition for the elderly to bear, and is not easy to treat. There are no physical signs apart from a watery nasal drip.

Michael Gleeson

NASAL OBSTRUCTION

Nasal obstruction – the inability to breathe through one or both nostrils – is a very common complaint, and the reason for referral to an ENT outpatient clinic. The causes of nasal obstruction and discharge are listed in Table N.2.

Choanal atresia may be membranous or bony, unilateral or bilateral. Nasal respiration is innate and therefore, in bilateral cases, the obstruction must be bypassed immediately after birth, by placement of an oropharyngeal airway. Surgical correction of the abnormality is undertaken in the first few days of life. Unilateral choanal atresia is sometimes not discovered until later. Babies breathe continuously

Table N.2 Causes of nasal obstruction and discharge

Congenital	Neoplastic
Choanal atresia	*Epithelial*
■ Bilateral	■ Papilloma
■ Unilateral	■ Inverted papilloma
	(Ringertz tumour)
Acquired	■ Schneiderian polyp
Physical obstruction	■ Squamous cell carcinoma
■ Adenoids	■ Transitional cell carcinoma
■ Deviated nasal septum	
■ Concha bullosa	*Non-epidermoid*
	■ Adenocarcinoma
Trauma	■ Adenocystic carcinoma
■ Haematoma and abscess of	
septum	*Neuro-ectodermal*
	■ Olfactory neuroblastoma
Inflammation	
■ Viral, bacterial, fungal rhinitis	*Vascular*
■ Allergic rhinitis	■ Angiofibroma
■ Nasal polyps	
■ Rhinitis medicamentosa	*Connective tissue tumours*
	■ Fibroma
Autonomic imbalance	■ Fibrous dysplasia
■ Vasomotor rhinitis	■ Fibrosarcoma
	■ Chondrosarcoma
	Miscellaneous
	■ Lymphoma
	■ Plasmocytoma

while feeding; hence, those with unilateral choanal atresia are unable to do so when the patent nostril is blocked by their mother's breast. Consequently, they suckle better from one breast rather than the other.

Deviations of the nasal septum are extremely common, and present in up to 30 per cent of normal individuals. It has been speculated that these deviations are caused by birth trauma, but there is little evidence to support this contention. The majority of deviations are acquired by trauma after birth as a result of sports injuries, falls or physical conflicts. Some of these deviations are severe enough to cause either unilateral or bilateral obstruction. In some, the sinus outflow tracts are impaired and recurrent sinus infection ensues. For these patients, septoplasty is a simple and effective remedy. Septoplasty alone is unlikely to restore a normal nasal contour or profile in those who have acquired their deviations traumatically. For these, a septorhinoplasty (see NASAL DEFORMITY, p. 464) will be more appropriate. Septal deviation can be seen with a nasal speculum. It will often be found that the inferior turbinate in the concavity of the deviation will have hypertrophied, thus increasing the obstruction. It is important to remember that the spur of the deflected septum may obscure other pathology behind.

Adenoid enlargement is probably the most common cause of nasal obstruction in childhood. These lymphoid masses usually regress in the first decade of life. In a few children hypertrophy can cause near-complete obstruction and result in loud snoring and obstructive sleep apnoea. Adenoidectomy is curative.

In recent years, it has been realized that pneumatization of anterior end of the middle turbinate can be a cause of nasal obstruction and recurrent sinus infections. This condition, termed 'concha bullosa', is easily eradicated by a small endoscopic procedure.

A *subperichondrial haematoma of the nasal septum* may develop spontaneously, but is more commonly caused by blunt trauma or inadequate packing after nasal surgery. It may be either unilateral or bilateral, and presents as a tender soft tissue swelling within the nose. The haematoma should be evacuated by removal of a patch of mucosa, as the pressure may cause cartilage necrosis and later a saddle nose deformity. Infection sometimes intervenes to produce a septal abscess; this is an extremely painful condition, and is almost always followed by significant cosmetic deformity.

Swelling of the mucosa, sufficient to block the airway, may be caused by acute or chronic infection (*rhinitis*). The common cold is the most simple and frequent example of this. Chronic rhinitis is most often associated with sinusitis, which needs to be addressed in order to relieve the obstructive symptoms.

In certain parts of the world, specific *bacterial infections* (rhinosporidiosis, rhinoscleroma) are a relatively common cause of protracted nasal obstruction. These conditions require long-term antimicrobial therapy and, in the case of rhinosporidiosis, surgical resection of the obstructive growth (Fig. N.11).

Allergic rhinitis is the most common manifestation of Type I allergy, affecting up to 20 per cent of the population in Western countries. Both acute and chronic forms are recognized. In the acute form – hayfever – the patient complains of bouts of sneezing associated with watery rhinorrhea, nasal obstruction and sometimes conjunctival irritation. In the chronic form, nasal obstruction is the most prominent

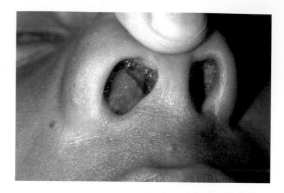

Figure N.11 A typical case of rhinosporidiosis that had developed in a young child living in Bangladesh. The growth was extremely friable and bled furiously when excised.

symptom, while discharge and sneezing are sometimes absent. Possible treatment includes allergen avoidance, specific immunotherapy, mast cell degranulation inhibitors, and antihistamine or steroid preparations.

Polyps appear as bilateral, glassy swellings which progressively fill the nose and are associated with chronic sinusitis, anosmia and chronic nasal discharge. The aetiology of nasal polyps is unknown, but they are not (as previously thought) due to atopy. In some patients, a dramatic response to systemic steroids may be maintained by the regular use of topical steroid drops. In others, the response is less satisfactory or more short-lived, and for these patients surgical removal of the polyps is required. However, polyps tend to recur and it is not unusual for patients to have multiple surgical procedures throughout their lives. Nasal polyposis in a few patients is associated with hypersensitivity to salicylates, and their management may be improved with a special diet.

Rhinitis medicamentosa is an uncommon condition caused by the abuse of nasal vasoconstrictor medication. Some of these patients use ten or more bottles of nasoconstrictor drops per day (Fig. N.12). Nasal obstruction is the predominant symptom, and is extremely resistant to therapy. Topical steroid nasal drops can be effective, but care must be taken as they are absorbed extremely well by the chronically inflamed mucosa, and significant adrenal suppression can result.

Vasomotor rhinitis or autonomic imbalance is a diagnosis of exclusion made when no other cause for nasal obstruction can be incriminated. The nasal

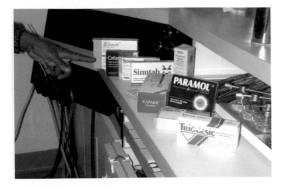

Figure N.12 The contents of a patient's handbag who had severe rhinitis medicamentosa. The patient consumed up to 10 bottles of decongestant nose sprays each day, together with the oral preparations shown.

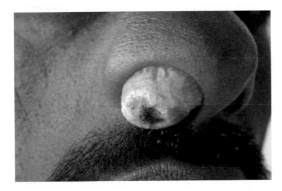

Figure N.13 Nasal obstruction caused by a large Ringertz tumour (inverted papilloma).

vasculature undergoes cyclical and alternate changes (physiological nasal cycle). In this way, the mucosa of one or other nostril is congested while the other is relatively constricted. Vasomotor rhinitis is thought to be the derangement or exaggeration of this physiological process.

Nasal tumours, especially malignant neoplasms, are extremely rare. However, progressive unilateral nasal obstruction should always alert one to the possibility of a sinonasal tumour, particularly when associated with intermittent epistaxis and pain (Fig. N.13). Tumours may develop in all age groups. A list of the neoplasms found in the nose is provided in Table N.2. The diagnosis is made on the basis of clinical examination and biopsy.

Michael Gleeson

NASAL REGURGITATION

Most people have experienced the regurgitation of food or drink through their nose at some time or other in their life. It is most unpleasant, and is usually caused by a lapse of concentration when swallowing. Progressive and persistent nasal regurgitation may be caused by a number of conditions that are classified in Table N.3.

Chronic pathological nasal regurgitation occurs when either the soft palate is too short, too rigid,

Table N.3 Causes of nasal regurgitation

Structural abnormalities of the palate
Congenital
- Cleft palate

Trauma
- Surgical
  - Oro-antral fistula after dental extraction
  - Palatal fenestration following surgery for malignancy of maxillary antrum
- Non-surgical
  - Attempted suicide

Inflammatory
- Destruction or perforation of palate due to syphilis, tuberculosis or leprosy
- Mucomycosis

Malignant disease

Fixation of the soft palate
Post-surgical deformity

Paralysis of the soft palate
Damage to the nucleus of the 10th nerve
- Postero-inferior cerebellar artery thrombosis
- Tumours of the medulla
- Bulbar palsy
- Poliomyelitis
- Landry's ascending paralysis

Posterior fossa lesions
- Tumours
- Syphilitic meningitis
- Glomus jugulare tumour
- Hydrocephalus

Extracranial lesions
- Malignant disease

Miscellaneous
- Post-diphtheritic paralysis
- Myopathies
- Myasthenia gravis

paralysed, or when there is a defect in the hard palate, alveolus or buccal sulcus.

Abnormalities of the soft palate preclude complete closure of the post-nasal space during swallowing. A cleft palate is the most common structural cause, and is almost always diagnosed directly after birth. Surgical correction is not always entirely successful, and minor degrees of regurgitation may persist. Subtle abnormalities of the soft palate may not be diagnosed for some time, for example, submucosal clefts. Removal of the adenoids in all of these patients can exacerbate regurgitation. Less common causes include post-tonsillectomy scarring and over-enthusiastic uvulopalatopharyngoplasty.

Oro-antral fistulae arise following difficult dental extractions when the floor of the maxillary anthrum is damaged or fractured. The majority close spontaneously, but occasionally some persist and require a secondary surgical closure. Other reasons for structural defects of the palate are listed in Table N.3.

The motor nerve supply of the palate is through the pharyngeal plexus, of which the major contribution is from the vagus. The sensory supply is shared by the Vth and IXth nerves. Interruption or interference with any of these nerves may result in regurgitation. Damage to the vagus and glossopharyngeal nerves may be caused by lesions within the posterior fossa, jugular foramen or parapharyngeal space. Lesions responsible for damage to the maxillary division of the Vth nerve are usually found in the floor of the cavernous sinus or pterygopalatine fossa.

Paralysis of the palate, when bilateral, may be difficult to notice at rest, but it remains immobile on phonation and is even more obvious if the patient is made to gag. In addition, the patient is unable to blow up a balloon. When the paralysis is unilateral the normal side is drawn up like a curtain and the uvula is displaced to the normal side.

Michael Gleeson

NAUSEA

The term 'nausea' reflects a constellation of unpleasant symptoms including bloating, post-prandial fullness, early satiety and a sensation of an impending need to vomit. Nausea may be an acute or chronic phenomenon that develops from a stimulus anywhere in the gastrointestinal tract or systemically. The majority of cases are trivial, the cause evident, and their resolution spontaneous.

In order to search more widely for a cause of nausea, it is important to consider the potential physiological mechanisms underlying this symptom, namely luminal (noxious stimulus), gut wall (mucosa, muscle and nerve endings) local feedback pathways (splanchnic nerves) and higher centres.

Nausea is a symptom that easily can be rationally ascribed to a cause in the upper gastrointestinal tract, in particular to pathology of the stomach. It is a noxious symptom, and noxious causes ought to be considered first: dietary (fatty or spicy/hot foods); toxins (alcohol; medications of any type, although especially NSAIDs, metronidazole, erythromycin, cholestyramine); peptic ulcer disease (gastritis, duodenitis, reflux oesophagitis or peptic ulceration; *Helicobacter pylori*); infections, whether bacterial (food poisoning: *Staphylococcus aureus*, *Bacillus cereus*; giardiasis), viral (Norwalk virus, cytomegalovirus, Epstein–Barr virus, HIV) or fungal (oesophageal candida); or cancer (adenocarcinoma, gastric mucosa-associated lymphoid tissue lymphoma, small-bowel lymphoma).

Nausea is a primary symptom of gastrointestinal motility disorders. The best known of these is diabetic gastroparesis, but other systemic conditions involving the gut wall (scleroderma, amyloid, Chagas' disease), muscle (dystrophies) or nerves (HIV, autoimmune diseases) may present with nausea. Although surgery is usually associated with acute ileus, blind-loop or sump syndromes and their potential for associated bacterial overgrowth may underlie chronic nausea. A history of previous surgery (Billroth II gastrectomy; biliary surgery or gastro-jejunostomy) is of significance.

The gut has a limited repertoire of symptoms through which it can highlight pathology. A degree of malabsorption due to pancreatic exocrine insufficiency or coeliac disease/tropical sprue and the rare Whipple's disease may result in nausea. The presence of inflammation in the bowel wall (Crohn's disease, ulcerative colitis, ischaemic colitis, diverticulitis) can cause nausea on account of irritation of the visceral peritoneum. Similarly, the presence of peritoneal deposits of tumour, endometriosis or the accumulation of ascites may also give rise to nausea.

Altered gut blood flow, whether portal hypertension (cirrhosis, mesenteric vein occlusion, hepatic vein occlusion) or small/medium vessel disease (auto-immune disease, atherosclerosis, Henoch–Schönlein purpura), or right ventricular heart failure can present with nausea. Mesenteric ischaemia is an important differential diagnosis for acute-onset nausea, particularly in the setting of atrial fibrillation or recent heart surgery. Similarly, acute nausea with fruitless vomiting is a key symptom of gastric volvulus. Compression of the duodenum between the superior mesenteric artery and the aorta is thought to be associated with subacute obstructive symptoms.

Metabolic disorders, whether endocrine (hypoadrenalism, hypothyroidism, phaeochromocytoma, pregnancy), renal (acute/chronic renal impairment), hepatic (acute/chronic impairment) or manifesting as electrolyte imbalances of other causes (e.g. hypercalcaemia) commonly result in the onset of nausea.

Migraine is associated with recurrent nausea and headache. Other intra-cranial causes of nausea (hydrocephalus, tumour, infarct, middle-ear disease), although uncommon, must be considered in the absence of any other credible cause.

As the potential causes for nausea are myriad, a *detailed history* is vital to provide the starting point for further investigation. The history must detail setting (acute/chronic, during travel, exposure to toxins, relation to meals, recent foreign travel, others with similar symptoms, possibility of pregnancy), the presence of other gut symptoms (lower/upper bowel) or of systemic features (flu-like illness, rash, joint pains, headache, general well-being). Past medical history (surgery, peptic ulcer disease, diabetes mellitus, previous malignancy) and medication history (NSAIDs, iron, azathioprine, sulphonamides, steroids, bisphosphonates, choles-tyramine, statins, potassium/vitamin supplements, chemotherapy, metronidazole, erythromycin, digoxin, hormones/hormonal antagonists) are very important. A family history may provide some clue as to cause (coeliac disease, inflammatory bowel disease, muscular dystrophies).

The *physical examination* too must be thorough. In the absence of focal gastrointestinal signs, evidence for systemic (metabolic, autoimmune) or vascular (atrial fibrillation) disease must be sought, and raised intra-cranial pressure excluded.

The broad nature of the conditions that give rise to nausea preclude a limited list of investigations. In the absence of further focal symptoms or signs, general tests such as urea/electrolytes, liver blood tests, serum calcium/phosphate, full blood count and ESR may provide some leads. Gastroscopy with biopsy will identify the presence of peptic ulcer disease, cancer, infiltrative conditions, viral inclusions and gastric stasis. An ultrasound of the abdomen and pelvis will identify focal pathology in the absence of focal signs.

John Meenan

NECK, ENGORGED VEINS IN

For practical purposes, the jugular venous pressure may be regarded as raised if jugular pulsation is visible, or the internal jugular vein is seen to be distended, with the patient sitting erect (Fig. N.14). This is more reproducible than the older criterion of 4 cm above the sternal angle with the patient lying at 45°, and a grossly elevated venous pressure is less likely to be missed. The first major distinction is between non-pulsatile and pulsatile elevation of the venous pressure.

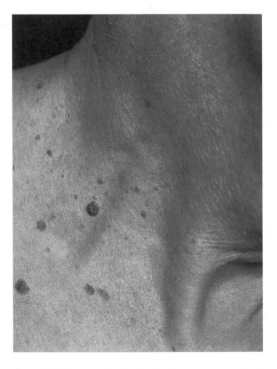

Figure N.14 Engorged veins due to raised jugular pressure due to heart failure.

Non-pulsatile elevation of the jugular venous pressure

This is due to obstruction of the jugular or brachiocephalic vein or, most commonly, of the superior vena cava. The causes of this are listed below:

- Common causes:
  - ◆ Thrombosis following implantation of pacemaker/defibrillator.
  - ◆ Bronchial neoplasm.
  - ◆ Mediastinal tumour (e.g. lymphoma, thymoma).
- Less common causes:
  - ◆ Fibrosing mediastinitis.
  - ◆ Right atrial or pericardial tumours.
  - ◆ Late complication of Mustard's operation for transposition of the great arteries.

The diagnosis of venous obstruction can be confirmed by venography; the cause of the obstruction may be more difficult to diagnose, and needs further investigation with chest radiography supplemented by CT/MRI scanning.

Pulsatile elevation of the jugular venous pressure

This condition is much more common, the causes including:

- Common causes:
  - ◆ Congestive cardiac failure.
  - ◆ Over-transfusion.
  - ◆ Cor pulmonale/right heart failure.
  - ◆ Tricuspid regurgitation.
- Less common causes:
  - ◆ Pericardial effusion.
  - ◆ Massive pulmonary embolism.
  - ◆ Constrictive pericarditis.
  - ◆ Tricuspid stenosis.
- Rare causes:
  - ◆ Restrictive cardiomyopathy.
  - ◆ Carcinoid syndrome.
  - ◆ Right atrial tumours.

An analysis of the venous waveform helps to identify the cause of the elevation (Table N.4). A 'normal' jugular pulse has three 'humps' (the a, c and v waves) and two 'dips' (x and y descents). The a wave is transmitted atrial systole, the c wave occurs early in systole as the tricuspid valve closes and braces back towards

the atrium, and the v wave is produced by the filling of the atrium from the venae cavae followed by the emptying of the atrium after tricuspid valve opening (Fig. N.15). The relationship of this pattern to those

Table N.4 Abnormalities of the jugular venous pulse

Cause	Most prominent feature
Congestive failure	Raised mean pressure with early diastolic descent
Tricuspid regurgitation	Systolic v waves
Right atrial hypertrophy	Presystolic a waves
Complete heart block, ventricular tachycardia, pacemaker, etc.	Cannon waves (sporadic or regular sharp v waves)
Constrictive pericarditis	Very high pressure, sharp early diastolic descent
Tricuspid stenosis	High pressure, slow diastolic descent

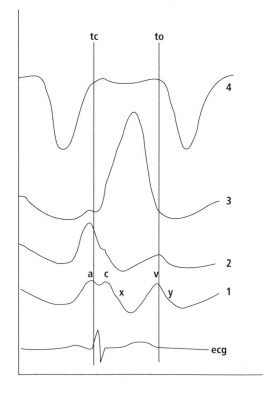

Figure N.15 Diagram showing the relationship of different jugular waveforms to the cardiac cycle. ecg = electrocardiogram; tc = tricuspid valve closes; to = tricuspid valve opens. 1, Normal trace to show a, c, v waves and x and y descents. 2, Exaggerated a wave due to right atrial hypertrophy. 3, Tricuspid regurgitation wave (note different timing from normal v wave). 4, Prominent y descent in severe cardiac failure, pericardial effusion or constrictive pericarditis.

found in disease is not always straightforward. Where an increased load on the right heart develops gradually – as in pulmonary/tricuspid stenosis or some forms of pulmonary hypertension – the right atrium has time to hypertrophy and there may be a prominent a wave. If the tricuspid valve becomes incompetent, the jugular pulse shows a systolic pulsation in time with the arterial pulse. This is traditionally called a v wave, though its timing and cause are both different from the 'normal' v wave. The v waves of tricuspid regurgitation are often striking in appearance and readily palpable.

Cannon waves are also prominent systolic waves appearing in the venous pulse, but these are due to contraction of the atrium against a closed tricuspid valve. Classical cannon waves are seen in patients with complete heart block and atrioventricular dissociation, when the atria and ventricles contract at their own independent frequencies. When atrial and ventricular contractions coincide, the cannon waves are seen as striking, sharp pulsations in the jugular pulse. Cannon waves may also occur in patients in junctional rhythm and in those with a permanent ventricular pacemaker who have preserved retrograde atrioventricular conduction; in such cases retrograde atrial activation and cannon waves may occur in a series of consecutive beats. The murmur of tricuspid regurgitation is, of course, absent.

When the mean jugular venous pressure is considerably raised, the sudden fall in pressure (and consequent collapse of the vein) as the tricuspid valve opens at the beginning of ventricular diastole (y descent) is usually the most prominent feature of the venous pulse. In patients with tricuspid stenosis this fall in pressure occurs more slowly as the right ventricle fills via the stenotic valve. In patients with constrictive pericarditis, the y descent is usually prominent, but a proportion of patients show a more pronounced dip in early systole (x descent), possibly because ventricular contraction causes a transiently negative intrapericardial pressure. This may also be seen in pericardial tamponade, although many cases simply show a prominent y descent. Patients with constrictive pericarditis or pericardial tamponade may also show a paradoxical elevation of venous pressure on inspiration (Kussmaul's sign). The probable mechanism is due to a corresponding increase in right ventricular filling pressure in a

patient unable to increase the right ventricular stroke volume.

Melvin Lobo

NECK, PAIN AND/OR STIFFNESS

These two symptoms usually co-exist, or else stiffness will be 'residual' to a previous painful episode, for example a cervical disc prolapse. The exception is the congenital causes, which are usually painless and present with stiffness accompanied by deformity.

The causes of neck stiffness and/or pain are listed in Table N.5.

Congenital causes

Congenital torticollis or *wryneck* (see SPINE, DEFORMITY OF, p. 661) is due to a contracture of the sternocleidomastoid muscle on one side, and is generally considered to be the result of an injury during obstetric delivery, possibly ischaemic in nature. The muscle stands out as a tight band in the neck, and its contracture leads to a characteristic deformity. The head is pulled down towards the affected side, and the face and chin are tilted towards the opposite shoulder. The movements of the head are necessarily restricted owing to the shortening of the muscle, which in longstanding cases leads to a marked asymmetry of the face. The consequences are not limited to the head and neck, for the spine shares in the general obliquity and shows marked lateral curvature in old cases. This condition must not be confused with a secondary torticollis, which is an acquired condition and may indicate underlying disease, for example vertebral injury, pyogenic infection, intraspinal tumour, intracranial tumour of the posterior fossa, or unusual bone pathology (e.g. an osteoid osteoma).

In the *Klippel–Feil syndrome* there is a congenital fusion of one or more cervical vertebrae resulting in a short, thick, stiff neck, the head being set low on the shoulders. Other co-existing abnormalities are common: undescended scapulae (Sprengel's deformity), platybasia, etc. (see UPPER LIMB, PAIN IN, p. 738, Fig. U.2).

Table N.5 Causes of neck stiffness and/or pain

Congenital
- Congenital (infantile) torticollis of 'wryneck'
- Congenital deformities (e.g. Klippel–Feil syndrome)

Acquired: acute
Traumatic
- Fractures, dislocation and subluxations of the cervical spine
- Soft tissue injuries to muscles and ligaments including whiplash injury

Infective: local
- Acute pyogenic infection
- Abscess in the neck
- Reflex spasm due to adenitis from otitis media, tonsillitis, etc.

Infective: systemic
- Meningitis
- Typhus
- Brain abscess
- Poliomyelitis
- Psittacosis
- Arborvirus infections (e.g. sandfly fever)
- Leptospirosis
- Tetanus, etc.

Malignant
- Metastatic neoplasms (N.B. primary neoplasms are exceptionally rare)
- Multiple myeloma

Degenerative
- Acute cervical disc prolapse
- Acute painful episode in cervical spondylosis

Miscellaneous
- Exposure to cold
- Positional
- Intracerebral and subarachnoid haemorrhage
- Cerebral tumour
- Hysteria (remember, this is diagnosed by 'excluding' other causes).

Acquired: chronic
Post-traumatic
- Untreated acute traumatic lesions
- Contractures following burns, nerve injuries etc.

Infective
- Tuberculosis

Degenerative
- Cervical spondylosis
- Ossification of the posterior longitudinal ligament

Arthritic
- Chronic juvenile arthritis (Still's disease)
- Rheumatoid arthritis
- Ankylosing spondylitis
- Other spondylarthropathies

Acquired acute causes

Traumatic

Exposure to cold – for example a cold draught from air conditioning or sleeping in a cramped position – may give rise to a *transient stiff neck*, which is associated with no other symptoms. The patient wakes up in the morning with a stiff neck, and the diagnosis is made by exclusion. The symptoms settle rapidly.

Fractures and *dislocations* may be rapidly fatal, particularly when they affect the upper cervical spine. A classic example is a fracture through the pedicles of C2, often referred to as the 'hangman injury'. Road traffic accidents are the most common cause. A second group of patients present with associated cord or nerve root compression, and consequently there is a clear pointer to the underlying injury. Beware however, the third group in which there may be major instability but no abnormal neurology and apparently normal plain X-rays. These injuries are easy to miss, but the patient is of course still at major risk of developing a paralysis should they suffer a simple fall. They are by no means all high-velocity injuries, but they may occur following relatively simple falls and landing on the forehead – for example, falling downstairs, skiing, playing sports, etc. A common sign in this third group is that the patient supports the head with his/her hands. When taking lateral flexion/extension views, these movements should be made by the physician, and not left to a radiographer. The cervicothoracic junctional zone is difficult to visualize in broad-shouldered men. Imaging with CT and MRI scans are very helpful in making a precise diagnosis.

Whiplash injuries have not only become a common cause of cervical pain but are also a major source of medico-legal compensation. The majority are due to a rear impact collision to a car, causing a hyperextension injury of the neck. The precise soft-tissue pathology is a matter of dispute, but the disc, the anterior longitudinal ligament and the facet joints have all been implicated. Neck pain and headaches are the most common symptoms, and often appear disproportionately great in comparison to the physical signs. Most patients recover within 2–3 months. Some take one to two years to resolve, while a few are left with a permanent disability.

Acute local infection

Acute pyogenic infection of the cervical spine is uncommon, but is increasing in incidence secondary to infection around intravenous cannulae. It is usually staphylococcal in nature. In the early stages, it is extremely easy to overlook and, as with other infections in the spine, it may present as a pyrexia of unknown origin.

Inflammation around the cervical lymph nodes commonly causes reflex muscle spasm. The primary infection may be obvious – for example, a boil or carbuncle – but do not overlook carious teeth or infected tonsils.

Acute systemic infection

Many acute infections are accompanied by a stiff neck (meningism), particularly in children; pneumonia, once a common cause in childhood, is now much less so. Fever is almost always present. Meningitis from any cause, bacterial or viral, almost always causes some neck rigidity. Neck stiffness may be an early prodromal sign in paralytic or non-paralytic poliomyelitis, and changes in the cerebrospinal fluid (CSF) are found. *Phelbotomus* (sandfly) fever – an arbovirus infection – presents as fever, malaise, myalgia and sometimes headache, in some cases with findings of an aseptic meningitis. Stiffness of the neck may be an early sign of tetanus, but other signs such as trismus (inability to open mouth due to tonic contraction of the jaw muscles) rapidly appear (see TRISMUS (LOCK JAW), p. 731).

Malignant causes

By far the most common group of tumours affecting the cervical spine are metastatic deposits. In order of frequency these are carcinoma of the breast, prostate, lung, kidney and thyroid, but rarely of the bladder and gastrointestinal tract. By the time the patient is symptomatic, destructive or sclerotic X-ray changes are usually obvious, although sometimes it is easy to overlook the destruction of a pedicle (see SPINE, TENDERNESS IN, p. 665; Figs S.52 and S.53). By contrast, X-rays in multiple myeloma may show nothing more than osteopenia until a vertebral body collapses (Fig. N.16). Benign tumours of the cervical spine are uncommon, but are a differential diagnosis of a cervical disc presenting with radiculopathy or myelopathy. An example is a neurofibroma producing nerve root compression at an exit foramen.

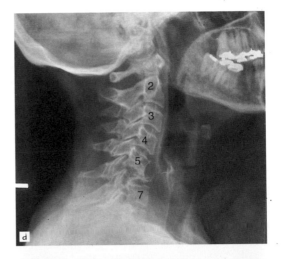

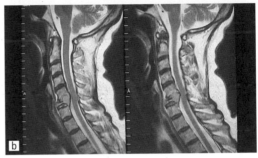

Figure N.16 Myelomatous destruction of C6. (a) Lateral X-ray. (b) MRI scan.

Degenerative causes

An acute cervical disc is often precipitated by a local strain, especially sudden unguarded flexion and rotation. In essence, there are three clinical pictures:

- Symptoms and signs confined to the cervical spine.
- Pressure on a nerve root with radicular symptoms radiating into an arm.
- A central prolapse with pressure on the cord producing myelopathy (for further details, see UPPER LIMB, PAIN REFERRED INTO THE ARM, p. 733).

Miscellaneous causes

Cerebral or subarachnoid haemorrhage

Conscious patients who have intracranial bleeding usually complain of headache and stiffness of the neck. Indeed, after subarachnoid haemorrhage the main physical sign is marked neck rigidity and pain on trying to move the head. A brain tumour may cause a stiff neck due to meningeal irritation from bleeding into the subarachnoid space, by direct meningeal involvement, or by causing cerebellar herniation through the foramen magnum.

Hysteria

A theatrical and over-dramatic symptom of neck stiffness is accompanied by other features of hysteria, but not by any objective physical signs of organic disease.

Acquired chronic causes

Degenerative

Cervical spondylosis is the most common disorder of the cervical spine. The symptoms come on gradually over many years, and are typically episodic, acute exacerbations interspersed with long periods in which underlying stiffness only causes minor inconvenience. As with an acute disc, symptoms essentially fall into three patterns:

■ Neck pain with radiation up into the occiput, out over the shoulder or down the thorax over the scapula.
■ Radicular pain secondary to osteophytic impingement and narrowing of an exit foramen.
■ Myelopathy due to central impingement on the cord, often from multi-level disease.

This third group, which particularly affects the elderly, is often of insidious onset, and neurological features – particularly unsteadiness of gait – are all too easy to attribute to 'old age'. Radiological changes in the neck are the norm in those aged over 60, so care must be taken in relating radiology to symptoms. If neurological compression – either of a nerve root or the cord – is suspected, a MRI scan is the investigation of choice.

Ossification of the posterior longitudinal ligament is a rare disease, with the majority of cases having been reported from Japan. In addition to neck pain and stiffness, nerve root compression is common, and myelopathy may result from central compression as the ossification increases.

Rheumatoid arthritis involves the cervical spine in as many as 30 per cent of cases. Rheumatoid erosion leads to instability, which can be a cause of sudden death. The myelopathy is not easy to diagnose as the

neurological deficiency in the limbs is often masked by the peripheral joint disease. There are three categories: (i) basilar invagination with the odontoid (dens) migrating through the foramen magnum affecting the brainstem and upper cervical cord: (ii) atlanto-axial instability usually with anterior displacement of C1 on C2 (Fig. N.17b); and (iii) subaxial instability which can affect any part of the remainder of the cervical spine. Beware, therefore, of the long-standing chronic rheumatoid patient (Figs N.17 and N.18) who presents with increasing pain in the cervical spine, a progression of their pain up over the

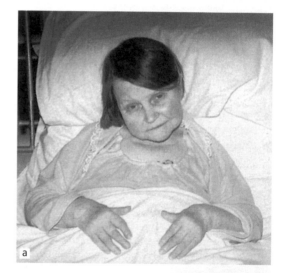

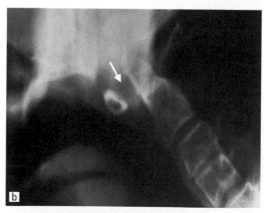

Figure N.17 (a) Rheumatoid arthritis of the spine: atlanto-axial instability and migration of the odontoid. (b) The point of the arrow marks the site where the tip of the odontoid should lie. It has moved proximally and posteriorly secondary to rupture of the transverse ligament of the atlas.

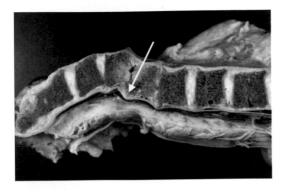

Figure N.18 Rheumatoid arthritis: post-mortem specimen. C4 has subluxed anteriorly on C5, the sharp posterior proximal border of the body of which has compressed the cervical cord (arrow).

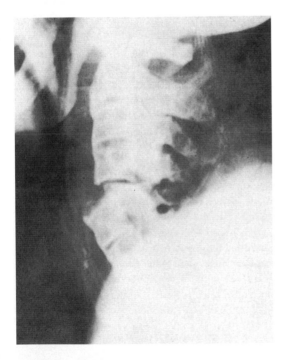

Figure N.19 Ankylosing spondylitis: fracture dislocation of the cervical spine with severe posterior displacement of the head and proximal spine at the C4/C5 level following a fall.

occiput indicative of compression of the posterior primary rami; and symptoms such as tinnitus, vertigo, visual disturbances or dysphagia and L'Hermitte's syndrome with flashing electrical shock-like pains involving all or part of the body and being indicative of cord compression.

Ankylosing spondylitis can extend up to involve the cervical spine (see BACK, PAIN IN, p. 58). Even when it becomes 'burnt out', the spine remains at increased risk of injury due to the loss of its flexibility. Do not therefore dismiss the recurrence of cervical spine pain in an old ankylosing spondylitic patient as being due to a recurrence of the disease, for there may well be an un-united fracture which has occurred secondary to a relatively minor injury (Fig. N.19).

Cervical vertebral tuberculosis

The greatest care must be taken not to overlook tuberculous disease of the cervical vertebrae as a cause of reflex muscular rigidity of the neck. Pain and rigidity are among the earliest signs; the pain is increased by the least movement, and the child – for it is generally a child that is affected – takes the greatest precaution to avoid any movement, even holding the head between the two hands. The position of the head varies; it is most often held very stiff and straight, the natural backward curve of the neck being lost. In the late stages there may be an angular or lateral curve.

Fred Heatley

NECK, SWELLING OF

See also THYROID ENLARGEMENT (p. 714).

Anatomy

The neck on either side is divided into anterior and posterior triangles by the sternocleidomastoid muscle arising from the sternum, sternoclavicular junction and medial third of the clavicle below and being inserted into the mastoid process of the temporal bone above. At the upper end of the anterior triangle the digastric muscle defines the lower borders of a subsidiary space known as the 'digastric triangle', and at the lower end of the posterior triangle the posterior belly of the omohyoid muscle defines the upper border of a subsidiary space known as the 'supraclavicular fossa'.

The sternocleidomastoid muscles are enclosed within the deep cervical fascia, which splits to embrace them. If even a part of a mass in the neck overlaps either border of the sternocleidomastoid muscle, then, by putting one or other of these muscles into contraction, the relationship of the mass to the sternocleidomastoid muscle and so to the deep fascia can readily be determined. This method is applicable to practically all masses in the neck, except for the majority of those situated in the midline. The right sternocleidomastoid muscle is put into contraction by rotating the head to the left while resistance is applied to the chin, and vice versa; both sternocleidomastoids are made to contract when the forehead is pressed forwards against resistance.

Lumps in the neck arising from structures superficial to the deep cervical fascia are not specific to the neck. Thus, sebaceous cysts, lipomas, carbuncles, etc. are common, particularly in or deep to the skin at the back of the neck. It is the masses deep to the deep cervical fascia which have particular relevance in regard to the neck and it is the differential diagnosis of these that must be considered.

It is conventional to divide swellings in the neck into midline swellings and lateral swellings, although this is a little misleading as nearly all so-called 'midline swellings' can deviate slightly to one side or the other. They can, however, be divided appropriately into masses arising from unpaired midline structures and masses arising from paired lateral structures.

Masses arising from unpaired midline structures

Thyroglossal cyst

The thyroid gland is developed from an epithelial-lined duct which grows downwards from the region of the foramen caecum of the tongue, passing close in front of and then behind the hyoid bone, and so towards the site of the adult thyroid isthmus from which the lateral lobes expand. A cyst may form in any part of this track by failure of obliteration of the duct, but the most common site is at the lower border of the hyoid bone, anterior to the thyrohyoid membrane. These cysts usually appear at about puberty and enlarge to a variable size slightly to one or other side of the midline. They are fluctuant, globular masses which, if superficial, may transilluminate. If the jaw is held open and the tongue steadily protruded, the swelling will rise in the neck, demonstrating its attachment to the base of the tongue (Fig. N.20). These cysts

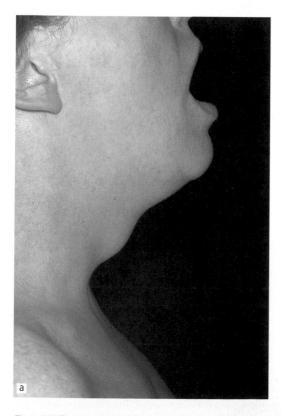
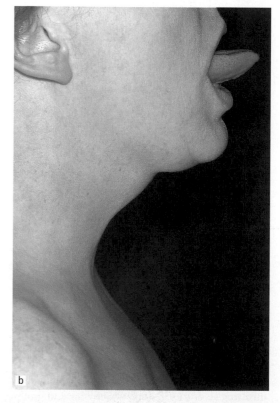

Figure N.20 Thyroglossal cyst showing: (a) elevation with (b) protrusion of the tongue.

occasionally become infected and may rupture, leading to a fistula.

Swellings arising from the isthmus of the thyroid gland

All of those pathological conditions described (see p. 715) and which give rise to swellings of the thyroid gland can arise in the isthmus. It should be repeated again that practically all thyroid swellings move up and down on deglutition owing to their intimate relationship to the larynx and upper part of the trachea, the movements of which they follow during this act.

Rare cases of swelling arising in midline structures

These include:

- Subhyoid bursa – a cystic swelling which arises behind the hyoid bone and is indistinguishable clinically from a thyroglossal cyst.
- Perichondritis of the thyroid cartilage.
- An advanced carcinoma of the larynx, trachea or oesophagus penetrating the walls of these viscera and protruding to one or other side.
- The so-called 'Delphic lymph node', which lies in the midline on the thyrohyoid membrane; this may enlarge in carcinoma of the thyroid gland and may be the first evidence of this disease.

Masses arising from paired lateral structures

Lymph nodes

See LYMPHADENOPATHY (p. 423).
The most common swellings in the neck are undoubtedly due to pathological processes arising in the lymph nodes, usually secondary to some acute or chronic inflammatory or a neoplastic process in one of the organs which they drain, but sometimes (as in the lymphomas) appearing to arise primarily within these nodes.

The distribution of the lymph nodes in the neck is variable, but the general disposition is as follows. In the upper part of the neck there is a horizontally disposed system consisting of the submental, suprahyoid, submaxillary and upper deep cervical groups. The names of these groups indicate sufficiently their situation, except for the upper deep cervical group, which is situated in relation to the internal jugular vein where it is crossed by the posterior belly of the digastric muscle. One important node of this group – the jugulo-digastric node – is particularly significant in relation to pathological conditions of the tongue and tonsil. As a general rule, the anterior nodes drain anteriorly placed structures in the head, while the posterior nodes drain more posteriorly situated organs. Thus, the tip of the tongue drains to the submental nodes, while the posterior aspect of the scalp drains to the occipital nodes.

In addition to the horizontal system, there is a vertical system ranged along the internal jugular vein. At the upper end there is the upper deep cervical group, which is common to both systems, and at the lower end the lower deep cervical group with subsidiary groups in between. The lower deep cervical group of lymph nodes is in relation to the internal jugular vein where it is crossed by the posterior belly of the omohyoid, and one large node of this group – the jugulo-omohyoid node – is again of significance in relation to pathological processes in the tongue, receiving lymphatics from this organ without the interposition of any intervening lymphatic nodes. In this way, a carcinoma of the side of the tongue can give rise to secondary deposits in the supraclavicular fossa, where this node is situated, without the enlargement of any of the systems in the upper part of the neck. The Delphic node on the thyrohyoid membrane, which has already been referred to, should also be mentioned at this point. For a description of the differential diagnosis of the various types of enlarged lymph nodes, see page 423.

Thyroid swellings

These are the second most common cause of swellings situated laterally in the neck (see p. 714). Nearly all these swellings move up and down with deglutition, by which property they may be recognized. There are, however, some exceptions to this rule. If the mass is very large and fills one or both anterior triangles and perhaps also the midline, there may not be room for the thyroid to move on deglutition. Again, in certain types of carcinoma with infiltration of the pretracheal muscles the growth may not move on deglutition. This is because the larynx, which causes the thyroid to move, cannot itself do so as there is no elasticity left in the infiltrated pretracheal muscles. Indeed, it is this tethering of the larynx by infiltration of the surrounding structures which leads to dysphagia in carcinoma of the thyroid, as can readily be appreciated by anyone who attempts to swallow while holding down their thyroid cartilage by placing a finger on its upper border. Sometimes, in a nodular goitre the excursion of the mass on swallowing or on coughing may be so considerable that it rises up from 'plunging down' into the superior mediastinum or retroclavicular spaces during these movements. This so-called 'plunging goitre' is only a type of retrosternal or retroclavicular goitre with an abnormally free range of movement. Its very mobility argues that it will probably be a simple matter to deal with surgically.

More rare cases of swelling laterally placed in the neck

These may be listed as:

- Branchial cyst
- Sternomastoid tumour
- Cervical rib
- Cystic hygroma
- Aneurysm
- Carotid body tumour
- Submandibular salivary swellings (sialectasia or tumour)
- Actinomycosis
- Cold abscess from spinal TB
- Pharyngeal pouch
- Laryngocele

Branchial cyst

This is a congenital condition believed to arise in the remains of the second branchial cleft and to give rise to a cystic swelling in the lateral part of the neck. Another theory is that it represents cystic degeneration within a lymph node. The condition may arise at any age, but usually occurs in young people and is rare after the age of 40 (Fig. N.21). The swelling, which varies in size, usually protrudes into the anterior triangle from the deep surface of the upper part of the sternocleidomastoid muscle. It is usually rather soft and fluctuates readily, but it is generally too deeply

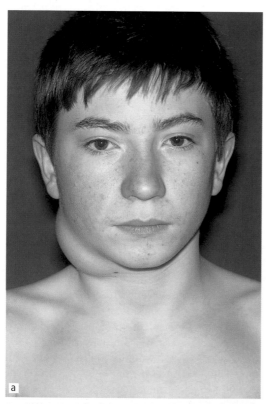
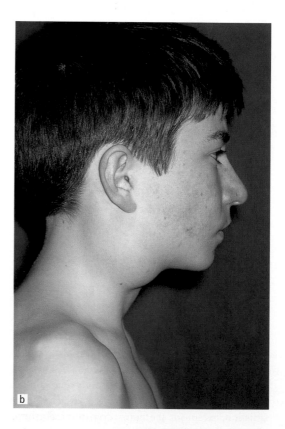

Figure N.21 Branchial cyst. (a) Anterior view; (b) lateral aspect.

situated to demonstrate translucency or transillumination. Occasionally, these cysts become infected, when the differential diagnosis from breaking-down tuberculous nodes may be difficult.

However, the diagnosis can usually be determined by aspiration, which will yield either tuberculous pus in the latter case or, on the other hand, turbid yellow fluid containing numerous cholesterol crystals on microscopic examination which is typical of a branchial cyst.

Although not strictly a swelling in the neck, it should be mentioned here that the unobliterated second branchial cleft, instead of forming a cyst, may communicate with the exterior, usually just medial to the sternal head of the sternocleidomastoid muscle below and into the pharynx in the supratonsillar fossa above, forming a *branchial fistula.*

Sternomastoid tumour

As a result of birth or intra-uterine injury, some fibres of the sternocleidomastoid muscle may be torn and a haematoma appears in this muscle, leading to torticollis (wryneck).

Cervical rib

This is another congenital abnormality which may give rise to a swelling in the supraclavicular fossa. The swelling may be due to the rib itself, or there may be a pulsatile swelling due to a 'post-stenotic' dilatation of the subclavian artery.

Cystic hygroma

This rare congenital abnormality is a lymphangiomatous condition that usually arises in the supraclavicular fossa of infants. It forms a soft, fluctuating, extremely translucent and painless swelling which may grow rapidly. These masses are liable to attacks of infection.

Aneurysm and arteriovenous fistula

The large vessels of the neck are liable to the same pathological changes as vessels elsewhere. Aneurysms may occur in the cervical part of the subclavian artery, or the carotid arteries. A penetrating injury of the neck, as by a metallic fragment, may damage both the carotid artery and the internal jugular vein, leading to an arteriovenous fistula.

Carotid body tumour

This is a rare lesion arising in the chromaffin tissue situated at the bifurcation of the common carotid artery. It appears at any time after infancy as a very firm 'potato-like' tumour in close association with the carotid sheath so that pulsation is usually, but not invariably, transmitted to it (Fig. N.22). Its steady growth over a period of years serves to distinguish it from tuberculous cervical adenitis, with which it may readily be confused. Carotid angiography demonstrates the diagnostic splaying apart of the internal and external carotid arteries at their origins by the tumour mass at the bifurcation.

Swellings of the submandibular salivary gland

These arise in the digastric triangle (see SALIVARY GLANDS, SWELLING OF, p. 627). *Ludwig's angina* is an acute inflammatory process of the cellular tissue around the submandibular gland, usually arising from the floor of the mouth or the teeth. The physical signs extend into the floor of the mouth, and give rise to considerable oedema which, without treatment, may spread to the glottis and demand tracheotomy.

Actinomycosis

This is a chronic inflammatory swelling of the cellular tissue about the angle of the mandible. The diffuse induration with the eventual development of multiple sinuses and the accompanying trismus should make the diagnosis obvious.

Late in the disease, 'sulphur granules' containing the streptothrix may be discharged, but the diagnosis should not await bacteriological confirmation, which may be equivocal in the early stages.

Cold abscess from spinal TB

In certain cases of tuberculosis of the cervical spine, the abscess may track from the retropharyngeal region laterally, and present as a fluctuant mass in the upper part of the posterior triangle and deep to the insertion of the sternocleidomastoid muscle. The accompanying stiffness of the neck, together with the general evidence of a chronic infection, should alert the examiner to this possibility. If untreated, the abscess breaks down, discharges, and forms multiple sinuses in the apex of the posterior triangle. An X-ray examination will reveal typical destruction of the involved vertebra or vertebrae and adjacent disc.

Pharyngeal pouch

At the back of the inferior constrictor muscle of the pharynx there is a triangular area (Killian's dehiscence),

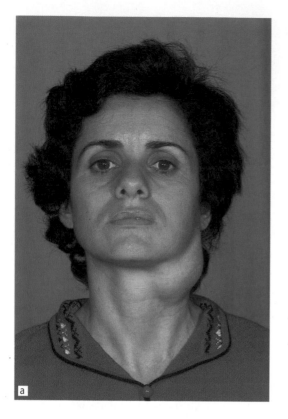

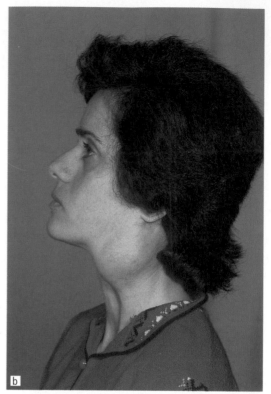

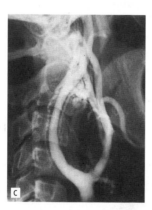

Figure N.22 Carotid body tumour. (a) Anterior view; (b) lateral aspect; (c) carotid angiogram of a carotid body tumour to demonstrate the typical splaying apart of the external and internal carotid arteries. [Prof. Gerald Westbury.]

located between the upper border of the transversely running fibres of the cricopharyngeus below and the lower border of the obliquely running fibres of the thyropharyngeus above, where the wall is deficient in muscle. A pouch of mucosa, covered only by the fascia propria of the pharynx, may protrude through this defect. This pouch gradually enlarges, usually towards the left side of the neck, and tends to fill up when food or fluid is swallowed. At first, this is just a nuisance and gives rise to an uncomfortable feeling on swallowing together with a rapidly developing swelling which may be emptied by pressing on the mass. This may be accompanied by regurgitation of fluid, often foul-smelling, into the pharynx and mouth. Later, the mass becomes sufficiently large to press upon the oesophagus, against which it lies, to produce severe dysphagia with inanition.

Food is apt to stagnate within the pouch, leading to diverticulitis which may spread and give rise to pharyngitis or oesophagitis, so adding to the burden of dysphagia. This condition may appear at any age, but usually arises during the third and fourth decades of life. It is readily demonstrated by a barium swallow X-ray (Fig. N.23). Treatment, after attention to the nutritional needs of the patient, is by surgical excision.

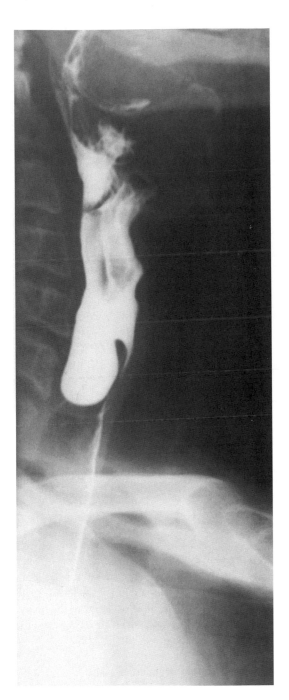

Figure N.23 Pharyngeal pouch demonstrated by a barium swallow, lateral view.

Laryngocele

This is a narrow-necked, air-containing diverticulum consequent on herniation of the laryngeal mucosa through a defect of the thyrohyoid membrane, where

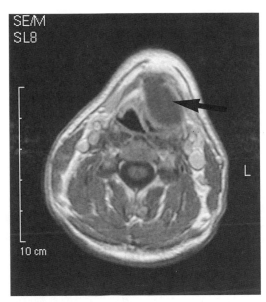

Figure N.24 Computed tomogram of the neck, showing a left-sided laryngocele (arrowed).

this is pierced by the superior laryngeal vessels and the deep branch of the superior laryngeal nerve. Occasionally it is bilateral.

It appears as a swelling in the anterior triangle of the neck just above the lamina of the thyroid cartilage when the patient blows his/her nose – it may then remain distended for some days. It is likely to be found in professional trumpet players and glass-blowers.

A lateral X-ray of the neck reveals the air-filled mass, also visible on CT (Fig. N.24).

Harold Ellis

NIPPLE, ABNORMALITIES OF

Deformities of the nipple may be classified as follows:

- Congenital
  - Congenital absence
  - Supernumery (Fig. N.25)
  - Congenital inversion
  - Bifid nipple
- Acquired
  - Acquired inversion
  - Plasma cell mastitis

◆ Mammillary duct fistula
◆ Duct ectasia
◆ Tumour
  ■ Retro-areolar carcinoma
  ■ Paget's disease

Congenital abnormalities

Rarely, there can be complete absence of the development of the breast and the nipple. This may be associated with failure of development of the pectoral muscles, when the condition is known as Poland's syndrome. Supernumery nipple areolar complexes are quite common, running down the milk line from the subclavicular area across the lateral part of the abdomen, ending in the region of the anterior superior iliac spine. Congenital inversions of the nipples are common, and must be distinguished from the acquired inversion of the nipple associated with either carcinoma of the breast or duct ectasia. A bifid nipple is a rare, but well-recognized, entity.

Acquired inversion of the nipple may be a consequence of duct ectasia/plasma cell mastitis syndrome (see BREAST LUMP, p. 79). In this condition, inversion of the nipple is usually bilateral, central and slit-like. Apart from this, acquired inversion of the nipple is usually of sinister significance and may represent a retro-areolar carcinoma, or even the first sign of a cancer in one of the outer quadrants of the breast.

Paget's disease of the nipple is a relatively rare presenting sign of carcinoma of the breast, and may be an eczematous condition affecting the nipple and areola. This is usually associated with an intraduct element of carcinoma invading along the terminal portions of the lactiferous ducts to infiltrate the dermis of the nipple and areola. If this eczematous condition is unilateral and not associated with patches of eczema elsewhere on the body, then it should be treated seriously by an immediate biopsy. The histological appearance is characteristic, with foamy cells with large atypical nuclei seen scattered throughout the dermis and subdermal layers.

Mammillary duct fistula is a sequel of periductal mastitis, and presents as a discharging sinus at the areolar margin. For a description of this complex of diseases, see BREAST LUMP (p. 79).

Michael Baum

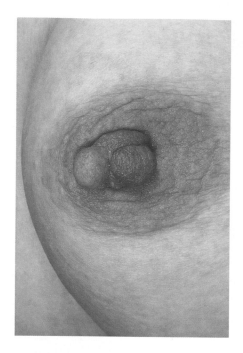

Figure N.25 Bifid nipple.

NIPPLE, DISCHARGE FROM

Discharge from the nipple may be divided into three classes.

Normal discharges

A discharge of milk from the breast during pregnancy is not uncommon, especially in multiparae. Both then and during lactation it is usually of small amount, except when the child is put to the breast, but occasionally the flow at other times may be sufficient to be distressing.

Normal discharges at abnormal times

A secretion similar to colostrum sometimes occurs from the breasts of both sexes in the newly born, and again at puberty. This is due to endocrine stimulation, but it may predispose to a true infective mastitis when the breast, already tender and swollen, becomes hot and red, and the discharge may change from being clear to purulent.

Occasionally, the normal secretion of milk during lactation is prolonged for many months or years after the stimulus of suckling has been removed. This is probably due to some endocrine abnormality. Apart from being a serious nuisance, and sometimes also a source of anxiety to the patient, it has no sinister significance. It usually resolves spontaneously and unpredictably after a varying period, with or without the aid of endocrine therapy. Women with prolactin-secreting tumours of the anterior pituitary may present with galactorrhoea and amenorrhoea.

Abnormal discharges

Serous fluid

A discharge of serous fluid from the nipple is a common accompaniment of duct ectasia, epithelial hyperplasia or duct papilloma.

Pigmented fluids

Green fluid

When the colour is due to melanin or pigments other than derivatives of haemoglobin, its admixture with yellow serum gives to the resultant discharges a green colour of varying shades. If the discharge is very dark, dilution with water will disclose the green colour. In cases of real difficulty, the discharge may be submitted to spectroscopic or chemical assay for haemoglobin. Such discharges have precisely the same significance as the non-pigmented serous discharges discussed above.

Haemorrhagic

Blood-stained discharges can usually be recognized on sight; the colour is red to black, and again if there is real doubt the final arbiters are the microscope and the chemical test. Blood-stained discharges are indicative of duct papilloma, epithelial proliferation, and intraduct carcinoma, in that order of frequency.

The nipple should be examined through a magnifying glass, and a bead of blood or a speck of clot may reveal from which of the 20 or so ducts the bleeding is arising. Such evidence is important in determining from which section of the breast the bleeding is

originating. Having examined the nipple thus, it should be wiped clean and (with the breast rendered moderately tense by an assistant if available) the tip of the finger pressed on to the breast at successive sites, working spirally from the nipple. Particular attention should be paid to the subareolar region, where the source of the bleeding lies in the majority of cases. By this means it will be found possible to cause blood to issue from the nipple on pressure over quite a restricted area, whereas pressure elsewhere has no effect. If the affected duct has been previously identified, the significant area will be found to be in the segment of the breast drained by that duct, and the pathological region is confirmed. The segment of the breast affected should be removed by local operation, and the pathological condition causing the bleeding determined by naked-eye inspection and histological study. Further treatment depends upon the nature of the lesion so determined. Solitary papillomas adjacent to the nipple are the commonest cause of this symptom, but if they are removed in this way the bleeding seldom recurs.

Should it be impossible to localize the origin of the bleeding – and with care and practice this is most unusual – the diagnosis depends on an assessment of probabilities. The younger the patient, the more likely is the cause to be benign; the older the patient, the more likely to be malignant. Mammography is valuable in demonstrating or excluding an occult neoplasm as the source of the haemorrhage. Where the discharge of pigmented fluids from multiple ducts associated with duct ectasia is profuse and embarrassing, total excision of the subareolar duct system (Hadfield's operation) will effect a cure.

Grumous material

The discharge of 'cheese-like' material or material having the consistency of toothpaste or putty, grey or green in colour, indicates the condition known as 'comedo mastitis'. This is another variant of the duct ectasia/periductal mastitis complex (see p. 79).

Pus

Pus, or pus mixed with milk, generally indicates acute suppurative mastitis; the other signs of inflammation or abscess are well marked as a rule, so that there is no difficulty in arriving at a diagnosis. A tuberculous lesion also causes a discharge of pus, and it may simulate carcinoma. The discharge may contain demonstrable tubercle bacilli, but specific bacteriological culture – together with a radiograph of the chest – will very likely be required before a positive answer on the nature of the infection can be given.

Michael Baum

NODULES

Nodules are larger than papules (>5 mm in diameter), but are distinguished by depth rather than by diameter. They may be free in the dermis or fixed to overlying skin or underlying subcutaneous tissue. Nodules must be distinguished from cysts, which have a fluid or semi-fluid content. The causes of nodular skin lesions are many (see Table N.6), but persistent non-tender nodules should always be biopsied.

Neoplasms

Nodules are a stage in the development of tumours, both benign and malignant. Most nodular skin neoplasms are aetiologically related to ultraviolet light

Table N.6 Causes of nodular skin lesions

Neoplasms	Acne
Basal cell carcinoma	Nodular prurigo
Squamous cell carcinoma	
Kerato-acanthoma	**Metabolic**
Malignant melanoma	Xanthoma
Lymphoma	Gouty tophus
Kaposi's sarcoma	Lipoid proteinosis
Dermatofibroma	Pretibial myxoedema
Pyogenic granuloma	
Keloid	**Infections**
	Mycobacteria
Vasculitis	Fungi
Erythema nodosum	Leprosy
Nodular vasculitis	*Treponema*
Wegener's granulomatosis	Oncocerciasis
Polyarteritis nodosa	Infestation (including post-scabetic
Temporal arteritis	nodules)
Chronic inflammation	**Miscellaneous**
Sarcoid	Heberden's nodes
Rheumatoid nodules	Chondrodermatitis nodularis
Bromoderma	chronica helicis

(sunlight) exposure, and are thus most common on exposed areas of skin, in fair-skinned subjects, and especially in those who already show evidence of other ultraviolet-induced changes in the skin. The most common tumour is a *basal cell carcinoma*. Although these are also known as *rodent ulcers*, ulceration is not invariably a feature, and is often a relatively late stage. Lesions begin as a small, rounded, pearly, translucent papule, showing telangiectasia. The head and neck are the most common sites, and the incidence rises with increasing age; lesions occurring below the age of 40 years are uncommon, though not unknown. Nodulocystic lesions grow as solid tumours composed of lobulated masses of cells in which cystic degeneration may occur. Enlarging lesions eventually ulcerate centrally, where a haemorrhagic crust forms. The *morphoeic variant* of rodent ulcer may erode widely, with a poorly defined infiltrating margin, and may thus be difficult to eradicate surgically.

A *squamous cell carcinoma* is a harder, fleshy nodule, often with overlying crust, generally arising on the face, including lips and ears, or the dorsa of the hands (curiously an uncommon site for basal cell lesions). They tend to grow in a more aggressive fashion, to become secondarily infected (often with an unpleasant odour), and to metastasize to draining lymph nodes. They are especially common in patients who are immunosuppressed (e.g. following transplant surgery). Occasionally, squamous cell carcinoma arises in an old scar or sinus, or on the margin of a chronic leg ulcer; in such a case it is easy to overlook the true diagnosis unless one is especially vigilant.

A *kerato-acanthoma* is a rather remarkable lesion which shows some histological similarity to a squamous cell carcinoma, but has a very different natural history. This lesion presents acutely as a neat, dome-shaped nodule which grows alarmingly in weeks on the exposed skin of the face and limbs. A juicy hyperkeratotic central plug forms which may discharge later, giving the lesion the appearance of a giant molluscum contagiosum. Keratoacanthoma is a benign tumour which eventually involutes spontaneously after some 3 months, leaving no trace save for a small irregular depressed scar.

Nodular *malignant melanomas* are usually ominously obvious, though the amelanotic variant is often first diagnosed by the histopathologist (Figs N.26 and N.27). Early changes in moles which can point to malignant change include haemorrhage, loss of plaques and nodules, particularly on the lower limbs. A more aggressive form occurs widely on the body in HIV-positive individuals (and is now an accepted AIDS-defining diagnosis).

Secondary deposits of an internal malignancy may present in the skin as hard dermal nodules (Fig. N.28); the diagnosis may be confirmed histologically, but it is usually a late presentation, so that even if the primary tumour can be identified, cure is rarely possible.

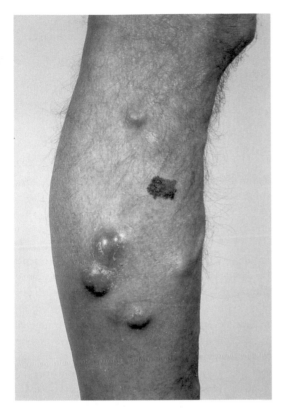

Figure N.26 Malignant melanoma with cutaneous secondaries.

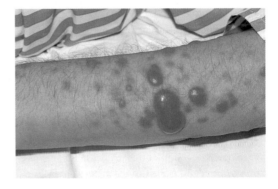

Figure N.28 Leukaemia with secondary deposits in skin.

The most common benign nodular neoplasm is a *dermatofibroma* (histiocytoma), which develops as a firm red/brown nodule in the upper dermis fixed to overlying skin usually on the legs (Fig. N.29). Histology shows a dense proliferation of fibrocytes, which may represent a tissue reaction to a preceding insect bite.

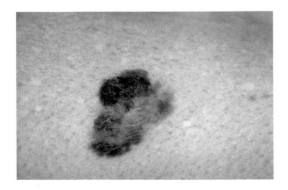

Figure N.27 Primary malignant melanoma.

hairs growing from the mole, pigment spilling into surrounding skin, ulceration and inflammation. *Lymphomatous infiltrates* in the skin are often nodular, and the later stages of *cutaneous cell lymphoma* (mycosis fungoides) are nodular and tumorous. *Kaposi's sarcoma* comprises slow-growing, port-wine-coloured

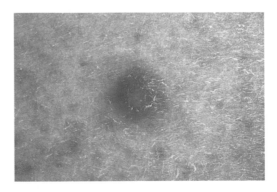

Figure N.29 Histiocytoma (dermatofibroma).

A *pyogenic granuloma* is a firm, small, cherry-red pedunculated nodule of hypertrophic granulation tissue, which bleeds easily on slight trauma and occurs most frequently on the lips and extremities. Its rapid growth and characteristic collarette are helpful diagnostic pointers, but histological confirmation is essential.

Vasculitis

Skin nodules can be caused by swollen, inflamed, dermal blood vessels, and are seen particularly on the legs. Small vessels are involved in *erythema nodosum*, larger in *nodular vasculitis* and *Wegener's granulomatosis*, and arteries in *polyarteritis nodosa* and *temporal arteritis*.

Erythema nodosum occurs most often in females in their second and third decades of life as crops of painful, tender, red nodules. These occur on the shins, are 1–8 cm in diameter, and heal over several weeks without breaking the surface, and going through the colour changes of a bruise. A cause for this reaction can be found in half of the affected individuals. Examples include sarcoidosis, inflammatory bowel disease, infections (*Streptococcus*, tuberculosis, leprosy and deep fungus) and drugs (sulphonamides and thiazides).

Nodular vasculitis is also more common in women, but occurs later in life, in their third and fourth decades. The calves are the usual site of well-demarcated, bluish, fixed, subcutaneous nodules. Underlying tuberculosis must be excluded, but often a cause is not determined. *Polyarteritis nodosa* affects adult men, with nodules usually occurring along the course of arteries. There is severe illness with fever, arthralgia, hypertension, peripheral neuropathy and eosinophilia. Nodular lesions may be seen along retinal arteries. The prognosis is related to the degree of renal vascular involvement. In *giant-cell arteritis*, exquisitely tender, nodular swellings occur most commonly along the course of the temporal artery. Sometimes, extensive ischaemic scalp ulceration is seen. Early recognition and treatment is important, as irreversible retinal artery thrombosis – and consequent blindness – can occur.

Chronic inflammation

Non-infectious granulomatous nodules are seen in sarcoidosis, rheumatoid arthritis, bromoderma and

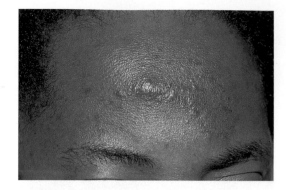

Figure N.30 Sarcoid.

around ruptured pilosebaceous glands in acne. *Sarcoidosis* usually begins in early adult life, most commonly in women, and with marked racial variation in prevalence. Skin presentations are varied, but include dermal nodules, papules and infiltration of scars. Erythema nodosum is a common presentation of acute sarcoid (Fig. N.30). The nodules of *rheumatoid arthritis* occur over the bony prominences at points of pressure, such as on the hands (Fig. N.31) and especially just below the elbow. They are painful, very rarely ulcerate, and vary in size from a pin-head to 2 cm in diameter. When present, they indicate seropositivity (Rose–Waaler or latex). Reaction to ingested bromides and iodides (bromoderma, iododerma) can rarely produce dramatic purplish, nodular and vegetative lesions on the face of infants or extremities of adults. The lesions may persist for long periods until recognized; they are now a rarity with the decline in use of these agents. Firm, suppurating nodules are seen in *nodulo-cystic acne vulgaris*, due to granulomatous reactions around ruptured, swollen sebaceous glands. Similar lesions in the axillae, groins and peri-anal skin are seen in *hidradenitis suppurativa*, but these abscesses are based on apocrine glands. Young adults are chiefly affected, and the nodules are accompanied by draining sinuses.

Metabolic

The deposition of *metabolic products* in the dermis may cause nodular swelling. These begin as papules, and include xanthoma, pretibial myxoedema, gouty tophi and lipoid proteinosis. Xanthomas are reddish-brown nodules of varying size, and are usually found

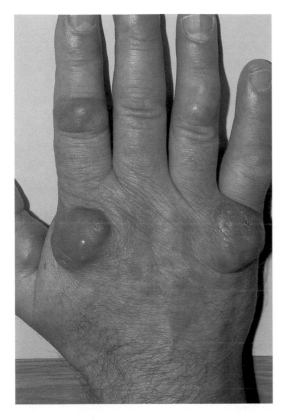

Figure N.31 Rheumatoid nodules.

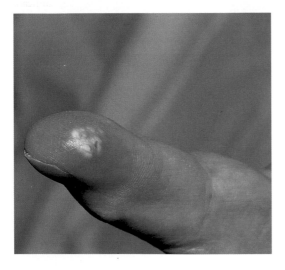

Figure N.32 Tophi in a case of gout.

on the elbows and knees and dorsa of hands and feet. They indicate an underlying disturbance of carbohydrate/lipid metabolism, usually primary but sometimes secondary (e.g. uncontrolled diabetes).

Gouty tophi are hard, yellow-white waxy nodules, on the helix or antihelix of the ear, palms or soles, tarsal plates of eyelids and tendons of hands or feet (Fig. N.32). Sometimes, tophi ulcerate and discharge a 'cheesy' material containing crystals of sodium biurate.

Lipoid proteinosis is a very rare inherited tendency to infiltrate the skin and mucosa with a hyaline material (mucopolysaccharide). Affected patients have a hoarse voice and characteristic beading along eyelid margins.

In *pretibial myxoedema*, firm red nodules or plaques arise on the lower legs, over the front of the shin, and on the dorsa of the feet. The hair and follicle orifices are grossly hypertrophied, giving a peau d'orange appearance.

Infections

Nodules due to infection are less common in Western countries, except for the ubiquitous furuncle or boil. Boils appear chiefly on the face, neck and buttocks, and are painful red nodules, often with a yellow pustule at the apex. The cause is a follicular infection with *Staphylococcus aureus*, and lesions may be recurrent for many weeks or months. They are more frequent in diabetic and debilitated people.

Any organism which induces a chronic granulomatous tissue reaction seems particularly prone to produce skin nodules (see Table N.6).

Mycobacteria

Lupus vulgaris is now extremely uncommon. Small, softish, reddish-brown or yellowish nodules appear on the face or mucous membrane in childhood. When examined compressed under a glass slide (diascopy), the nodules have a typical 'apple jelly' appearance. The nodules progress and slowly coalesce over very many years to form annular scaling plaques with central atrophy and fibrosis. More common now are nodules caused by infections with atypical mycobacteria, for example *fish-tank granuloma* (Fig. N.33). Usually, a finger is abraded against an infected fish-tank, and soft subcutaneous nodulo-cystic lesions develop. These are followed by a succession of nodules appearing along a lymphatic chain (sporotricoid spread). In *swimming-pool granuloma*, lesions are smaller papulo-nodules on the elbows, knees or any skin area traumatized against an infected pool wall – sporotricoid spread does not occur.

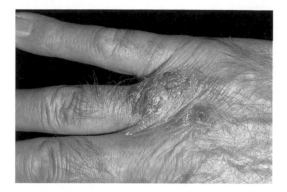

Figure N.33 Fish-tank granuloma (*Mycobacterium marinum*).

Fungi

In the UK, fungi and other infections in the immuno-suppressed – and particularly those with HIV disease – should be thought of as the cause of nodules. *Actinomycosis* causes abscesses around carious teeth, tonsils or gastrointestinal tract. The pus contains 'sulphur' granules of the penicillin-sensitive 'ray fungus', *Actinomyces israeli*. *Cryptococcosis* (torulosis) occurs in all parts of the world, usually involving the central nervous system, where meningitis, abscess or brain tumour may be suggested. Sometimes, transient skin nodules occur. *Sporotrichosis* begins with a skin nodule at the site of injury of hand or forearm, in contact with infected wood, soil or plant. There may be a considerable local inflammation before the characteristic succession of nodules appears up the draining lymphatic chain. Occasionally, a superficial dermatophyte infection elicits so violent a reaction that a boggy nodulopustule, rather like a carbuncle, develops. This is called a *kerion*, and it usually occurs in a hairy area (e.g. scalp or beard).

Leprosy

During the later stages of *lepromatous leprosy*, dull, red-brown nodules or plaques may be seen in symmetrical distribution on the limbs, face and ears. There may be hypopigmented anaesthetic macules elsewhere on the body, impaired eyebrow growth, and the diagnosis is made by finding acid-fast organisms in tissue smears.

Treponema

Late *syphilis* can produce nodular skin lesions. For example, nodulo-ulcerative tertiary syphilis is characterized by groups of crusted, copper-coloured nodules which spread peripherally and heal centrally in bizarrely shaped patterns. Sometimes, these ulcerate and are seen on the face, trunk or limbs. The solitary syphilitic gumma begins as a dermal or subcutaneous bluish-red nodule. Later, this sloughs to produce a punched-out ulcer with a rubbery necrotic base, and may cause gross tissue destruction. In secondary *yaws*, exuberant moist red nodules, rich in *Treponema pertenue*, may occur widely – particularly in the groins and at the angles of the mouth (their resemblance to raspberries gives rise to the alternative name, 'framboesia'). Juxta-articular nodules can occur in the tertiary stage of yaws.

Other infections

Leishmaniasis (Baghdad boil) is common in young adults and children in the Middle East, but can also be seen in European holidaymakers on their return from the south shore of the Mediterranean and the Middle East. Pruritic papules slowly develop into ulcerating nodules on exposed sites following the bite of an infected phlebotomus fly. Giemsa staining of material readily reveals the intracellular parasite. *Onchocerciasis* (see p. 556) gives rise to pruritus and indolent non-tender nodules varying in size from 0.5 to 5 cm on the head, shoulders and trunk. These nodules contain the adult worm. In *loaiasis*, or Calabar swelling, transient hot, skin-coloured nodules occur on the face and extremities. Tick bites can be the cause of remarkably persistent dermal nodules.

Miscellaneous

Heberden's nodes, which are small bony swellings on the terminal interphalangeal joints, are more common in women, and are a sign of osteoarthritis. *Chondrodermatitis nodularis chronica helicis* is the descriptive title given to a not uncommon exquisitely painful nodule, which occurs in the upper third of the helix of the ear. The lesions are probably due to pressure, like a corn, causing underlying perichondritis with fibrinoid degeneration of the cartilage.

Barry Monk

NYSTAGMUS

Nystagmus refers to an involuntary rhythmic to-and-fro oscillatory movement of the eyes due to a disorder of the mechanisms responsible for maintaining steady gaze. Nystagmus may result from dysfunction of the visual system, vestibular apparatus, vestibular nerves, brainstem or cerebellum. There are three mechanisms for maintaining steady gaze:

- When the eyes are in the primary position, the *fixation system* is responsible.
- When the eyes are turned to an eccentric gaze position (e.g. looking to the left), the neural integrator or *eccentric gaze-holding mechanism* maintains gaze.
- When the head is being rotated or looking at a moving object, the vestibulo-ocular system is involved.

A problem with any of these systems will cause the eyes repeatedly to drift away from the desired position, leading each time to a corrective phase (a *saccade*) that leads to nystagmus.

Fixation system

Fixation involves the ability to detect an eye drift and then to initiate an appropriate corrective movement of the eye to keep the desired object on the macula. This requires intact visual input via the optic pathways, as well as a complex network involving the parieto-occipital eye fields and the brainstem.

The neural integrator

The neural integrator is responsible for sustaining eyes at a desired eccentric position in the orbit, against the mechanical opposing forces of the orbital tissues. To maintain eccentric gaze requires tonic contraction of the extraocular muscles. This ability is impaired by central disorders of the cerebellum or brainstem, or drug intoxication – for example with anticonvulsants. The important brainstem nuclei that constitute this system include the nucleus prepositus hypoglossi, medial vestibular nucleus for horizontal gaze, the interstitial nucleus of Cajal for vertical gaze, and the vestibulocerebellum. The cerebellar component of the gaze-holding system tends to move the eyes towards the active side of the cerebellum, so that if there is damage to one side the eyes tend to drift away from the lesioned side. This explains why the fast phase of nystagmus due to cerebellar damage is towards the side of the lesion, and tends to be maximal in this direction.

The vestibulo-ocular system

The vestibulo-ocular reflex produces eye movements to compensate for head movements, thus allowing clear vision when the person is moving. Each peripheral vestibular apparatus horizontal semi-circular canal has a tonic input to the brainstem tending to push the eyes over toward the opposite side. When one side is damaged, the contralateral vestibular apparatus is unopposed and drives the eyes towards the lesioned side, creating the abnormal drift (slow phase) towards the lesion, with corrective jerks (fast phase) away from the lesion. Eye movements away from the lesion will be weakened because of the tonic drift towards the lesion, so when the eyes are moved in the direction of the fast phase the nystagmus becomes more prominent (Alexander's law).

Describing nystagmus

There are two main types of nystagmus, *jerk* and *pendular*, both of which can be either horizontal or vertical. Jerk nystagmus consists of a slow phase drifting away from the fixation target, followed by a fast saccade back towards the target. The direction of the nystagmus is conventionally defined by the fast phase. In pendular nystagmus, both phases of the nystagmus are of the same velocity. Pendular nystagmus is always due to central (brainstem or cerebellar) dysfunction. Nystagmus can be horizontal, vertical or torsional (where the eyes rotate).

Opsoclonus–myoclonus is a dramatic form of abnormal eye movements that may be confused with nystagmus. It is characterized by spontaneous, chaotic, multi-directional saccades. It is often associated with myoclonic limb jerking (see MYOCLONUS, p. 110).

Examination of the patient with nystagmus

To examine for nystagmus, the eyes should be examined at rest, fixating on a target straight ahead (the primary position) to see if there is any nystagmus in this position. The patient should then be asked to follow an object – for example the examiner's index finger – to the extremes of lateral, upward and downward gaze. Note should be made of whether pursuit movements are smooth or jerky. Any nystagmus should be carefully noted in terms of whether it is jerk or pendular, its direction, and in which gaze positions it occurs. The patient should be asked to look in each direction of gaze to assess saccades. Note should be made of any deviation of eye positions at rest (strabismus). The head impulse should be tested: the patient fixates ahead and the head is rotated rapidly to one side. Intact peripheral vestibular function should mean that the eyes continue to point forwards due to brainstem input resulting from the sudden movement of fluid in the lateral semicircular canals. A full neurological examination should be performed, including visual acuities, fundoscopy (during which very small amplitude oscillations can be seen), cerebellar and pyramidal functions. Nystagmus may occur in normal subjects at extremes of gaze or with repeated testing, but usually dampens after a few seconds. Conventionally, three beats is deemed within physiological limits. Signs of congenital disorder (e.g. ocular albinism) should be sought.

Clinical types of nystagmus

Nystagmus in childhood

Congenital nystagmus

Typically, this condition arises in the first 3 months of life. There may be a clear pattern of inheritance. The nystagmus is horizontal, in all gaze positions (including the primary position), of jerk or pendular type, and is worsened by attempted fixation. About one in six patients will also have eye deviation (strabismus). It may be associated with visual impairment, sometimes with ocular albinism. Brainstem disease can also cause this presentation, so full investigation may be necessary. Latent nystagmus is only manifest when one eye is covered.

Acquired childhood nystagmus

Any condition reducing visual acuity in early childhood may cause nystagmus. If acuity is lost before 2 years of age, nystagmus is invariable; if lost between 2 and 6 years it may develop; if visual loss is after 6 years, nystagmus will not usually occur as a result of the visual loss. There are many possible causes, including retinal disorders (e.g. rod or cone dystrophy) or visual pathway damage (e.g. optic chiasm tumour, hereditary optic nerve atrophy, ocular albinism). Extensive investigation may be required, including retinal electrophysiology. Optic nerve glioma is a rare cause of highly asymmetric or uniocular nystagmus. Spasmus nutans refers to a syndrome of nystagmus,

head nodding and abnormal head posture. This usually develops at between 4 and 12 months of age, and resolves spontaneously by age 3 years.

Acquired horizontal jerk nystagmus

This occurs when attempting to maintain an eccentric gaze position, and is the most common type of nystagmus seen clinically. The important distinction is between a peripheral cause due to vestibular dysfunction, and a central cause due to disease of the brainstem or its connections (the neural integrator). This is important, because if a central cause is suspected then urgent neuroimaging must be performed to determine the cause. There are several ways to distinguish between these possibilities:

- The nystagmus of peripheral vestibular dysfunction is suppressed (to some extent) by visual fixation.
- In vestibular dysfunction, the fast phase is always directed away from the damaged ear, and this remains true in both directions of horizontal gaze (i.e. it is unidirectional); the nystagmus is maximal looking away from the lesion.
- In peripheral vestibular damage the head impulse test will be impaired.
- In peripheral vestibular disturbance there is often a torsional component.
- In peripheral vestibular nystagmus the patient is usually unable to walk due to severe vertigo and disequilibrium, and will often have nausea, vomiting, sweating or diarrhoea (vegetative symptoms). In the nystagmus due to central disease (causing weakness of the gaze holding system), the eyes tend to drift back to the central position, causing the fast phase to change depending on the gaze direction, generally being in the direction of gaze (i.e. it is bidirectional); the nystagmus is maximal towards the lesion.

Peripheral acquired horizontal jerk nystagmus

The common peripheral causes of acquired horizontal jerk nystagmus are vestibular neuronitis (labyrinthitis) and benign positional paroxysmal vertigo (BPPV). Most patients with vestibular neuronitis (perhaps better termed acute peripheral vestibulopathy, a label which does not imply a definite aetiology) will be prostrated with vomiting, nausea and dizziness without hearing loss, facial weakness or other brainstem dysfunction. The symptoms resolve within a week or so but may recur. Vestibular sedatives (e.g. cinnarizine) may be helpful in reducing symptom severity. BPPV is a symptom complex implying benign end-organ disease. The patient reports brief (<40 seconds) vertigo on sudden movements of the head, classically on turning over in bed or lying down. Symptoms ameliorate to some degree when the head is still. There may be a history of viral illness (e.g. upper respiratory tract infection) associated with severe vertigo, or of head trauma. Symptoms can be reproduced by laying the patient supine with their head hanging back over the end of the examination couch (the Hallpike manoeuvre). Treatment with Cawthorne–Cooksey exercises (vestibular rehabilitation) may be helpful.

Drugs may damage the vestibular nerve or end organ; the main cause is from the aminoglycosides, including streptomycin and gentamicin.

Menière's disease is characterized by recurrent episodes of severe vertigo, vomiting, and tinnitus on a background of fluctuating, but progressive, hearing loss.

Central causes of acquired horizontal jerk nystagmus

These typically lead to less severe vertigo and vegetative symptoms than peripheral causes. Any cause of brainstem or cerebellar disease may be responsible. The acute onset of symptoms may be due to trauma or brainstem or cerebellar infarction; subacute onset may be due to demyelination (multiple sclerosis); slower onset may be due to tumour (either intrinsic, e.g. brainstem glioma or extrinsic, e.g. cerebellopontine angle tumour). Patients with a cerebellopontine angle lesion may have nystagmus with the characteristics of both peripheral and central nystagmus. Drugs are an important cause of central horizontal jerk nystagmus, for example anticonvulsants (phenytoin) or alcohol.

In normal subjects, caloric stimulation induces vestibular nystagmus. Cold water produces horizontal jerk nystagmus to the opposite side; warm water to the same side (mnemonic COWS – Cold: Other; Warm: Same).

Special types of nystagmus

Downbeat nystagmus

This is jerk nystagmus where the fast phase is downwards, usually present in the primary position. The best way to elicit this clinically is in eccentric down and lateral gaze positions, which typically increase the oscillations. It is an important clinical sign as it has some localizing value. Downbeat nystagmus classically occurs in structural craniocervical junction disease, for example Arnold–Chiari malformation or Paget's disease. It may also result from cerebellar degenerations (spinocerebellar ataxias or paraneoplastic cerebellar degeneration); brainstem disease (e.g. multiple sclerosis, glioma or infarction); drugs (lithium, alcohol); brainstem encephalitis; magnesium depletion; or Wernicke's encephalopathy.

Upbeat nystagmus

Jerk nystagmus with a fast phase upwards, usually present in the primary position, suggests structural disease of the cerebellar vermis or brainstem (e.g. posterior fossa tumour).

See-saw nystagmus

This is a striking disorder where one eye elevates and intorts, whilst the other eye drops and extorts. It occurs with abnormalities at the junction of the mesencephalon and diencephalons (e.g. a tumour).

Convergence–retraction nystagmus

This is characterized by rhythmical convergence or retraction movements of the eyes when the patient tries to look up. It is a component of Parinaud's syndrome, together with light–near dissociation, lid retraction, vertical gaze paresis and impaired accommodation. This syndrome is due to pathology in the dorsal midbrain at the level of the superior colliculus. A pineal gland tumour (pinealoma) is a classic cause.

Periodic alternating nystagmus

This is spontaneous horizontal jerk nystagmus that reverses every 90–120 seconds, with 1- to 10-second pause between reversals. Its localizing significance is similar to down-beating nystagmus. It may respond to baclofen.

Voluntary nystagmus

A few people can perform very high-frequency horizontal saccades that resemble pendular nystagmus. The eyelids often flutter at the same time, and the movements usually fatigue after more than a few minutes.

David Werring

O

OBSESSIONS

The term 'obsession' has a specific meaning in medical writing that is very different from the tabloid journalist, who tells us about the man 'obsessed with Madonna'. It does not refer to a preoccupation *per se*. Rather, an obsession is defined as a repetitive, intrusive, unwelcome thought, image or impulse that is recognized as one's own thought (rather than an inserted foreign thought), but also recognized as absurd. The typical themes are sex, violence and contamination. Obsessions are usually resisted, but at the cost of some anxiety. It will be noted that obsessions are intrapsychic phenomena as opposed to the more visible behavioural compulsions, such as checking, cleaning or counting, that often accompany them. Obsessional slowness may arise due to lengthy obsessional ruminations or due to prolonged rituals of bathing, eating and dressing. Such individuals may take hours to leave their house each morning.

The most common cause of obsessions is depressive illness. A rarer cause is primary obsessive–compulsive disorder (OCD). In practice, it is fairly straightforward to separate these two possible underlying diagnoses: primary OCD typically has its onset in the mid teens, while depression more often arises in people over the age of 30. If depression is the problem, then the obsessions resolve as the depression is treated. Primary OCD requires rather different management with high-dose serotonin-specific antidepressants for the obsessions, and behaviour therapy (exposure with response prevention) for the compulsions or rituals. Obsessive–compulsive symptoms are prominent in Gilles de la Tourette syndrome, and there is growing interest in the neurology of OCD. There is also an interesting debate about the extent to which anorexia nervosa can be conceptualized as a variant of OCD.

Finally, one other usage of the term 'obsessional' must be mentioned. Psychiatrists talk about obsessional personality traits and obsessional (or anankastic) personality disorder. Here, they are referring to traits such as meticulousness, pedantry, punctuality, perfectionism and rigidity. These can all be adaptive and valuable in certain walks of life, such as academic work, but sometimes are so marked as to make the individual difficult to live with. Once harm to self or others occurs, then the personality may be considered disordered.

Andrew Hodgkiss

OEDEMA, DEPENDENT

The fact that oedema typically 'pits' on pressure is because the fluid can be easily displaced from one part of the subcutaneous tissue to another. It is this free mobility of the fluid within the tissues that is responsible for the fact that, whenever there is a significant expansion of the extracellular fluid volume, the excess fluid accumulates under the influence of gravity in the dependent parts of the body. The term 'dependent oedema' has, therefore, no specific diagnostic significance, and its only value is as a reminder to beginners to look for oedema in those parts of the body which are dependent at that time. Thus, a decrease in ankle oedema after a night's rest is not necessarily a sign of improvement; in such circumstances, the oedema may well have moved and be found in the back and sides of the calves and thighs. This behaviour of the oedema fluid accounts for an occasional curious finding such as rings of oedema around the olecranon processes; this can be due to the patient spending much of their time in bed leaning forward with their elbows on a bed table in front of them.

The causes of oedema, nearly always dependent, are discussed under OEDEMA, GENERALIZED, below.

Boris Lams

OEDEMA, GENERALIZED

Generalized oedema is due to an increase in the volume of extracellular fluid. This is brought about by excessive renal tubular reabsorption of sodium and water; the mechanism of this reabsorption is complex, and the renin–angiotensin–aldosterone system is only one of the factors involved. The accumulation of fluid in the extravascular space which causes oedema is determined by the relationship between the hydrostatic and oncotic pressures in the capillaries and the interstitial tissue. Thus, a rise in capillary hydrostatic pressure due, for example, to venous obstruction and a fall in capillary oncotic pressure, as a result of hypoalbuminaemia, increases the net movement of fluid from the capillaries to the tissues. When sufficient fluid has been transferred in this way – at least 5 litres in adults – clinically detectable oedema results. Another factor concerned in the transfer of fluid across capillary walls is their permeability; in practice, an increase in this is more important in the production of localized rather than generalized oedema. Impairment of the lymphatic drainage of tissues is also a cause of localized oedema (see LEG, OEDEMA OF, p. 368). In any patient with generalized oedema, fluid may also accumulate in serous cavities in the form of ascites and pleural or pericardial effusion.

Gravity determines the fact that, in any situation in which sodium and water retention occurs, the oedema fluid tends to accumulate in the dependent parts of the body (see OEDEMA, DEPENDENT, p. 494). This tendency is so marked that, even in normal subjects, a little ankle oedema is common following prolonged periods of immobility in the seated position. It is particularly common during long journeys by air and, sometimes, by train or coach; it is probable that this is mainly due to a reduction in lymphatic drainage which is critically dependent on muscular activity. Also, in about 90 per cent of pregnant women, slight oedema is present at term and is, in fact, associated with a more favourable outcome to the pregnancy than when no oedema is present. The pathological situations in which generalized oedema most commonly occurs are heart failure and renal, hepatic and, less often, gastrointestinal disease. These, and other less common causes of oedema, are discussed below.

Heart failure

The oedema of heart failure is typically dependent, affecting particularly the ankles and, in recumbent patients, the sacral region. Despite this clear evidence of a hydrostatic component in determining the site of the oedema, the rise in central venous pressure in heart failure is a minor factor in the production of the oedema, compared with the reduction in renal blood flow and glomerular filtration rate and the increase in tubular reabsorption of sodium and water. These mechanisms operate whatever the cause of the heart failure but, in cor pulmonale, an additional factor may be a movement of fluid from the cells to the interstitial tissue; this is believed to occur in order to provide more buffers for the associated respiratory acidosis. The oedema is usually symmetrical but, sometimes, it is more marked in the left leg than the right; this is thought to be due to pressure on the left common iliac vein by the right common iliac artery as it crosses it. It is heart failure which is the mechanism of the oedema of so-called 'wet beri-beri', due to a dietary deficiency of thiamine, and also of the oedema seen commonly in severe anaemia from any cause.

Renal disease

Slight transient generalized oedema is a characteristic feature of acute post-streptococcal glomerulonephritis, but this is not due to the proteinuria, which is of no more than moderate severity. It is in the nephrotic syndrome that hypoalbuminaemia, due to heavy proteinuria, is severe enough to lower the intracapillary oncotic pressure to a level at which oedema occurs. In this condition the urinary protein loss is usually more than 3 g per 24 hours, and the serum albumin below 30 g per litre. It is probable that the hypovolaemia resulting from massive loss of fluid from the capillaries stimulates the renin–angiotensin–aldosterone system, and this leads to renal retention of sodium and water. The oedema is usually dependent but, in children, it may be as prominent in the trunk and face as in the legs; the external genitalia are commonly very swollen. Spontaneous disappearance of the oedema is not necessarily a good sign as, with advancing renal failure, the fall in glomerular filtration rate may markedly reduce the amount of protein lost.

There are numerous conditions which can cause the nephrotic syndrome. In children, by far the commonest cause is *minimal change nephropathy*, in which, as the name implies, the glomeruli are nearly normal on light microscopy but show characteristic changes on electron microscopy; clinically, the most typical feature is the complete remission produced by steroid therapy. In adults, *membranous* and *proliferative nephropathy* are at least as common as the minimal change lesion, and these three conditions together represent about three-quarters of all cases of the nephrotic syndrome. Less common causes include *focal glomerulosclerosis*, a condition of unknown aetiology with patchy glomerular scarring without previous inflammatory changes, *systemic lupus erythematosus*, *amyloidosis* and *diabetic nephropathy*. Oedema is quite common in diabetics, even in the absence of heavy proteinuria, perhaps due to microvascular disease. There is also a recognized association of the nephrotic syndrome with *malaria* due to *Plasmodium malariae* and with *malignant disease*, especially adenocarcinoma and lymphoma. The high venous pressure of *constrictive pericarditis* is also known occasionally to cause the nephrotic syndrome, which has also been seen in *cyanotic congenital heart disease*. Renal vein thrombosis *per se*, however, is no longer thought to be a cause but rather a complication of the nephrotic syndrome. A number of *drugs and other substances* are known to cause a membranous glomerular lesion and proteinuria heavy enough to cause oedema; these include mercurials, gold, penicillamine and captopril. A specific allergy is probably responsible for the nephrotic syndrome associated with certain foods, pollens, penicillin, bee stings and poison ivy.

Liver disease

Fluid retention is common in hepatic failure in which it is due to impaired protein synthesis and consequent hypoalbuminaemia. The changes in renal function are similar to those in the nephrotic syndrome. Both oedema and ascites can occur, often together, but one can be present without the other. Any form of cirrhosis may be the underlying disorder, but *cryptogenic* and *alcoholic cirrhosis* and *chronic active hepatitis* are those most likely to be associated with oedema.

Protein-losing enteropathy

Protein may be lost from the body, not only in the urine but also via the gastrointestinal tract. Marked hypoalbuminaemia can develop, causing oedema and, sometimes, ascites and pleural effusion. This situation arises particularly with *intestinal lymphoma* and *giant hypertrophic gastritis* (*Menetrier's disease*), but has been seen in many other disorders such as *coeliac disease, ulcerative colitis, Crohn's disease, tumours of the stomach* and *colon and intestinal allergies*.

Other causes of oedema

Oedema, more or less generalized, is a recognized feature of a number of other conditions, all rather rare in

the UK. *Malnutrition*, of course, is far from rare in developing countries where it is an all too common cause of oedema. It is usually due to dietary deficiency of protein, causing hypoalbuminaemia, and is a constant feature of kwashiorkor. A condition affecting emotionally labile women of reproductive age is known, non-committally, as *idiopathic oedema*. The distribution of the oedema is curious, affecting particularly the face, hands, breasts, thighs, buttocks and abdominal wall and, hardly ever, the ankles. The aetiology is unknown, but in some cases it may follow the use of diuretics in an attempt to lose weight; in that case it would be described as 'rebound' oedema. Oedema of the face, hands and ankles sometimes occurs at *high altitudes*. It may or may not be accompanied by the more severe manifestations of acute mountain sickness, such as pulmonary oedema, and is relieved by a spontaneous diuresis on return to a lower altitude. Very rarely, oedema may occur in diabetics on first being given *insulin*; this resolves completely in a week or so.

Boris Lams

OLIGOMENORRHOEA

Oligomenorrhoea is a term that defines menstrual periods occurring repeatedly at intervals between 6 weeks and 6 months. It is an arbitrary definition, and may be misleading. It is considered that the normal menstrual cycle has an upper limit of 35 days. The proliferative phase – that is, the time during which the follicle develops – is variable, whilst the secretory phase – that time from ovulation to menstruation – is usually 14 days. Cycles of 6 weeks' duration seem to show no difference from normal length cycles from the point of follicular and hormone development.

A number of conditions can cause oligomenorrhoea, and these range from normal to the same causes as amenorrhoea (see p. 22). Polycystic ovarian syndrome (Fig. O.1) accounts for about 90 per cent of cases of oligomenorrhoea, compared with only 33 per cent of amenorrhoea. Usually, the periods are also light and the condition is often associated with anovulation. A prolonged proliferative phase is associated with ovulatory oligomenorrhoea. It often occurs in adolescent girls or at the time of menarche and in older

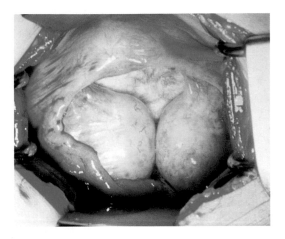

Figure O.1 Polycystic ovaries; appearance at laparotomy.

women in the perimenopausal phase. Prolonged corpus luteum activity may also lead to oligomenorrhoea and a prolonged cycle, but is usually associated with prolonged menstruation.

Clinically, oligomenorrhoea should be considered in the same way as amenorrhoea for investigations and further management.

Antony Hollingworth

OLIGURIA

The volume of urine which constitutes clinically significant oliguria varies with the pre-existing state of the kidneys. With a urine volume of less than 400 ml per 24 hours, even a normal kidney is unable to concentrate the glomerular filtrate sufficiently to prevent a rise in plasma urea and creatinine. Much larger volumes may be needed to maintain homeostasis if renal function has been impaired for any reason. Oliguria is present in most, but by no means all, cases of acute renal failure of which the causes (see Table O.1) are conventionally classified as pre-renal, renal and post-renal. Although these categories are not entirely mutually exclusive, it is important to identify – in any individual patient – the dominant factor causing renal failure, because the management is very different for these three groups. It is also important to decide whether the condition from which the patient is suffering is acute renal failure with previously normal

kidneys, or an acute exacerbation of chronic renal disease. The latter is more likely if the patient is very anaemic, shows evidence of long-standing hypertension, has biochemical or radiographic evidence of osteodystrophy or, most significantly, the kidneys can be shown – by plain X-rays of the abdomen or ultrasound scanning – to be shrunken.

Table O.1 Causes of oliguria

- Renal circulatory insufficiency
- Primary renal disease
  - Acute tubular necrosis
  - Acute cortical necrosis
  - Drugs and poisons
  - Acute interstitial nephritis
  - Acute glomerulonephritis
  - Vascular lesions (e.g. accelerated hypertension)
  - Other causes (e.g. hepatorenal syndrome, mismatched blood transfusion)
- Obstructive
  - Calculi
  - Pelvic tumours
  - Retroperitoneal fibrosis

Renal circulatory insufficiency (pre-renal uraemia)

This situation arises whenever the renal blood flow falls steeply. It is most commonly due to a fall in cardiac output secondary to a reduction in circulating blood volume. The implication of a diagnosis of pre-renal uraemia is that normal renal function will be restored as soon as the circulatory abnormality has been corrected. The cause of the circulatory failure is usually obvious. External loss of fluid is a common cause; severe diarrhoea and vomiting, haemorrhage, burns and previous polyuria in diabetes mellitus or Addison's disease are all well-known causes of, usually transient, oliguria. Other mechanisms operate in so-called 'cardiogenic' shock following myocardial infarction, acute pancreatitis and septicaemia, often due to Gram-negative organisms. All of these conditions can also cause acute tubular necrosis, a poorly defined pathological entity but a diagnosis which is made when renal function does not improve rapidly following restoration of normal renal perfusion. It is clearly important not to delay the recognition that this change for the worse has taken place, and a useful indication may be provided by estimation of the urinary sodium concentration. With oliguria due to renal circulatory insufficiency this is typically low (around 20 mmol/l), whereas in acute tubular necrosis with oliguria it will be about three times that level.

Renal causes of oliguria

Acute tubular necrosis

As mentioned previously, acute tubular necrosis is an imprecise term, and will be used here to designate only those cases of acute, usually oliguric, renal failure due to those circulatory disorders described above under pre-renal uraemia. Other specific disorders causing a similar clinical syndrome will be discussed separately. In practice, the diagnosis will usually be made in patients under observation and treatment for the causative condition. The symptoms are those of uraemia (i.e. anorexia, nausea and vomiting), perhaps muscle cramps and a 'flapping' tremor. Bleeding into the skin and gastrointestinal tract and fits can occur. Hypertension is unusual, and suggests a different cause for the renal failure. The plasma creatinine will rise progressively unless effective treatment is started, and dangerous hyperkalaemia – especially when there has been much tissue destruction – is common. Improvement can usually be expected in 6 weeks or less and, if this does not occur, renal biopsy may reveal that the damage is severe, perhaps in the form of acute cortical necrosis. In such a case the recovery is very slow, and may be incomplete.

Acute cortical necrosis

This condition may follow insults similar to those which cause acute tubular necrosis. It is a recognized feature of severe obstetric emergencies such as antepartum haemorrhage, eclampsia and septic abortion. Irreversible renal damage occurs, but the changes may be patchy and, therefore, compatible with some recovery. Radiography may show shrunken kidneys with cortical calcification as early as 2 months after the onset.

Acute renal failure due to drugs and poisons

Many drugs are known to damage the kidneys and cause acute renal failure. Some do so by causing acute interstitial nephritis (see below). Others, such as the aminoglycoside antibiotics, amphotericin, colistin, polymyxin B and radiographic contrast media, do so by other mechanisms. Heavy metals, organic solvents (particularly carbon tetrachloride), paraquat, snake bite and mushroom poisoning can also cause acute renal failure.

Acute interstitial nephritis

This is a common cause of acute oliguric renal failure, and is most often due to drugs. Those most commonly implicated include the NSAIDs, the penicillin and cephalosporin groups of antibiotics and diuretics, although many other drugs are known on occasion to cause this syndrome. The same type of renal damage is occasionally caused by bacterial and viral infections.

Acute glomerulonephritis

Some reduction in urine volume is common in most cases of acute nephritis, and severe oliguric renal failure is a common feature, particularly in adults, of the more rapidly progressive forms of glomerulonephritis (see HAEMATURIA, p. 261).

Vascular lesions

Renal infarction, if extensive, may cause acute renal failure; *renal vein thrombosis* is much less likely to do so except in infants. The fibrinous necrosis of *accelerated (malignant) hypertension* as well as the similar vascular damage seen occasionally in *systemic sclerosis*, together with intravascular coagulation occurring in the *haemolytic–uraemic syndrome* of children, *thrombotic thrombocytopenic purpura* and the rare *idiopathic postpartum renal failure* are all rare causes of oliguria and renal failure.

Other causes of acute oliguric renal failure

Renal failure may complicate hepatic failure from any cause; the term *hepatorenal syndrome* is applied, particularly, to the acute renal failure which may follow surgery in patients with obstructive jaundice. Muscle damage is an important contributory cause of renal failure following trauma, and *rhabdomyolysis* in the absence of trauma can also cause renal damage. This can be due to acute myositis, either idiopathic or in association with viral infections, prolonged convulsions or marathon running, malignant hyperpyrexia following general anaesthesia, carbon monoxide poisoning and a number of other conditions. It is probably the myoglobinuria which is responsible for the renal damage, though the mechanism by which this occurs is unclear. Similar damage can occur as a result of intra-vascular haemolysis, as in *malignant malaria* or follow-ing a *mismatched blood transfusion*. In *myelomatosis*, acute renal failure may occur probably due to hyper-calcaemia as well as the specific renal lesion of that condition. Finally, obstruction of the renal tubules by crystals of *urate*, during treatment of leukaemia and similar conditions or following starvation, is a rare but important and preventable cause of acute olig-uric renal failure.

Post-renal (obstructive) causes of oliguria

Unlike primary renal disease, obstructive lesions below the renal papillae more commonly cause total anuria than oliguria, and this is sometimes a helpful differen-tial diagnostic feature. Also the rate of deterioration – both clinical and biochemical – is slower with obstructive than with renal lesions. Conventionally, the term 'anuria' is applied to obstruction in the ureters or above; obstruction to outflow from the bladder is termed urinary retention (see URINE, RETENTION OF, p. 765). It goes without saying, therefore, that obstructive anuria can occur only if the outflow from both kidneys or from the only functioning kidney is obstructed. In a patient with acute renal failure and anuria, or severe oliguria, it is clearly important to dis-tinguish between an obstructive cause which can usu-ally be quickly dealt with surgically, and a primary renal cause in which other treatment is required. The situation is not always clear-cut. For example, chronic calculous disease may cause severe renal damage and chronic renal failure without much in the way of symptoms as well as acute anuria from obstruction; alternatively, chronic ureteric obstruction by spread from a uterine carcinoma might be complicated by pyonephrosis and Gram-negative septicaemia causing acute tubular necrosis.

Calculous disease is the most common cause of obstructive anuria. It is rare for this to occur as a result of simultaneous obstruction of both ureters by calculi; it is more common to find that one kidney has been severely damaged by chronic disease and that there is a calculus in the other ureter. Exceptionally, the blockage of one ureter may cause reflex anuria in the other kid-ney. The patient will usually complain of pain in the acutely obstructed kidney with renal colic; they may also feel a constant desire to micturate, despite the empty bladder. If the patient has total anuria, it is necessary to confirm the diagnosis and to localize the obstruction. Radiographic examination of the kidneys and ureters is essential, perhaps by using tomography to demonstrate a small or poorly radio-opaque calcu-lus. At cystoscopy the ureteric orifice on the affected side may be congested and show ecchymoses; ureteric catheterization may localize the calculus precisely.

Other causes of anuria from ureteric obstruction include *vesical carcinoma*; in such cases it is likely that the diagnosis will already have been made and chronic partial bilateral ureteric obstruction will have caused hydroureter and hydronephrosis with severe renal damage. A similar situation can arise in *carcin-oma of the uterine cervix*, but occasionally anuria may be the presenting feature. Other *pelvic* or *abdominal tumours* can also cause bilateral ureteric obstruction, and *ligation of both ureters* is an occasional complica-tion of extensive pelvic surgery for malignant disease. *Retroperitoneal fibrosis* is a rare cause of bilateral ureteric obstruction; in most cases no cause can be found, but there is a recognized association with retroperitoneal lymphoma, abdominal aortic aneurysm and exposure to methysergide, used in the prophylaxis of migraine; the ureters are seen to be displaced medi-ally on urography.

Sulphonamide crystalluria with blockage of both ureters is now very rare, although the need for a high fluid intake in patients receiving these drugs remains.

Boris Lams

OPTIC FUNDUS, ABNORMALITIES IN

The features visible on examination of the normal fundus are the optic disc, the retinal vessels, the mac-ula and the retinal periphery. The neurosensory retina comprises (from vitreous to choroid) the nerve fibre layer, ganglion cell layer, photoreceptors (rods and cones), inner nuclear and plexiform layers, outer nuclear and plexiform layers; it is transparent. Behind this lies the retinal pigment epithelium and then the choroid, both of which contribute to the normal red reflex. The outermost eye layer is the sclera. When the retinal pigment is deficient, the choroidal vessels are more easily seen; when both are thinned, the white sclera is visible. This is most obvious in coloboma of the choroid, a congenital defect (see below).

Physiological variations in the normal fundus

A physiological cup (Fig. O.2) varies in size, but usually occupies the centre of the optic disc. The retinal vessels dip over the edge, usually more steeply on the nasal than the temporal side. At the base of the cup is the lamina cribrosa, which is mottled by the scleral openings through which the retinal nerve fibres pass.

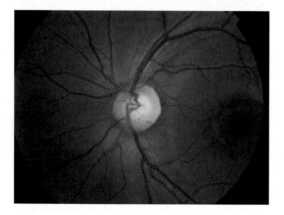

Figure O.2 Physiological cupping of the disc.

The physiological cup may be absent altogether, or when present may be filled with embryonic connective tissue which blurs the details. The vessels may sometimes bifurcate whilst still in the substance of the optic nerve, and separate branches are seen to enter and leave the disc instead of the single artery

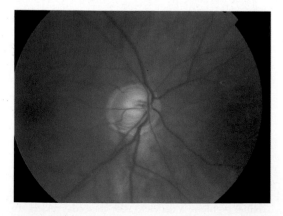

Figure O.3 Glaucomatous cupping of the disc.

and vein. A physiological cup is distinguished from the pathological cup caused by glaucoma (Fig. O.3) by the fact that it occupies only the centre and is usually not more than 60 per cent of the area of the disc.

Congenital crescents

Congenital crescents are common and are usually situated at the lower part of the disc, in contrast to myopic crescents (Fig. O.4), which are more usually seen on the temporal side (see below). The myopic crescent is usually on the temporal side of the disc, and may vary in size and extent from a thin crescent to a large atrophic area surrounding the whole disc. Usually, the size of the crescent varies with the amount of the myopia, and increases with age. Considerable difficulty may be experienced in viewing a highly myopic fundus even through a dilated pupil, though the patient's own spectacles *in situ* reduce magnification and provide a better view. When the condition is marked and associated with distortion of the disc itself, it is referred to as disc *coloboma*; astigmatism or hypermetropia is then often marked and the vision reduced, even with correction of the refractive error.

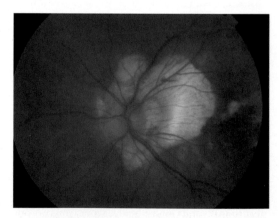

Figure O.4 Myopic crescent and retinal atrophy.

Pigmentation

The disc margin is variably pigmented, from a small crescent to a complete ring. The pigment has no pathological significance. The degree of pigmentation of the fundus varies considerably, generally corresponding to the complexion of the patient. When there is little or no retinal epithelial pigment the choroidal vessels are plainly seen (albinoid fundus); when retinal pigmentation is intense, the appearance of tigroid fundus is presented. The retina may also show small congenital oval or round greyish-black pigment spots.

Myelinated nerve fibres

This normal variant can be recognized by the brilliant white colour of the myelinated nerve fibres, the feathered, striated appearance, and the embedding of the retinal vessels among the nerve fibres (Fig. O.5).

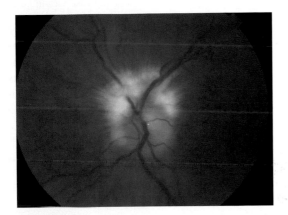

Figure 0.5 Myelinated nerve fibres in the retina.

Drusen (colloid bodies)

These are seen as multiple oval or round, yellowish spots, especially around the optic disc. They are common in later life and usually do not affect vision. They may be confused with papilloedema. Calcified drusen can be detected on CT or ultrasound scanning.

Pseudo-papilloedema

In marked hypermetropia the disc may be small, crowded and elevated, with no physiological cup and an ill-defined margin; the vessels may be tortuous (though not dilated), and unless the error or refraction is observed the condition may be mistaken for papilloedema. In true disc swelling the vascular changes are usually prominent, with capillary dilatation, exudates and haemorrhages. If spontaneous venous pulsation of the central retinal vein is seen, raised intracranial pressure (ICP) is virtually excluded – though the absence of pulsation is common in normal individuals and is *not* a helpful indicator of raised ICP. Flourescein angiography may be helpful in distinguishing pseudopapilloedema from true swelling.

Coloboma of the choroid

This is a congenital defect that may be recognized by its situation, which is usually below the disc, as an oval area of exposed sclera that may extend from the periphery and include the optic disc, with overlying healthy retinal vessels on its surface (Fig. O.6). It may be associated with other congenital abnormalities such as coloboma of the iris or lens.

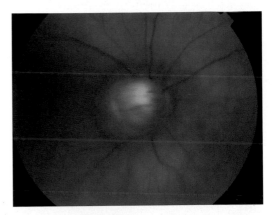

Figure 0.6 Coloboma of the choroid.

Abnormalities of the optic disc

Optic disc swelling (papilloedema)

Although the terms 'optic disc swelling' and 'papilloedema' are often used interchangeably, papilloedema is conventionally applied specifically to disc swelling (usually bilateral) due to raised ICP. The underlying cause of any optic disc swelling is stasis of retrograde axonal transport along the optic nerve. This may be due to a variety of different pathologies. Raised ICP increases pressure in the anterior optic nerve sheath, impairing axonal function at the lamina cribrosa, whilst in anterior ischaemic optic neuropathy an impaired blood supply to the nerve head disrupts axonal transport. In optic neuritis, inflammatory cell accumulation around vessels, with interstitial oedema, compresses axons at the optic nerve head.

Swelling of the disc causes loss of the normal physiological cup and blurring of the disc margin. The retinal veins are often dilated, and there may be flame-shaped haemorrhages on the disc surface. The main causes of optic disc swelling are listed in Table O.2. In the differential diagnosis of optic disc swelling it is helpful to distinguish between disc swelling due to raised ICP and

Table O.2 Differential diagnosis of optic disc swelling

Raised intracranial pressure (usually bilateral)
- Tumour
- Abscess
- Haematoma
- Cerebral venous sinus thrombosis
- Meningitis (granulomatous, carcinomatous, haemorrhagic)
- Subarachnoid haemorrhage
- CSF secreting tumour (choroid plexus tumour) – rare
- Malignant hypertension

Local pathology (usually unilateral – unless the disease affects both optic nerves at the same time)
- Anterior optic neuritis
- Anterior ischaemic optic neuropathy
- Optic nerve compression by tumour, e.g. glioma, lymphoma
- Optic nerve infiltration (e.g. granulomatous disease; TB, sarcoid)
- Central retinal vein occlusion

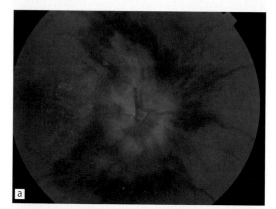

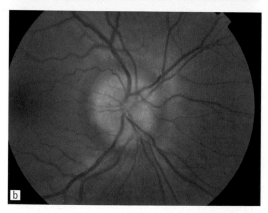

Figure O.7 (a) Acute papilloedema; (b) chronic papilloedema.

that due to local disease affecting the optic nerve. A raised ICP usually causes bilateral, symmetrical optic disc swelling, with acuity and colour vision usually preserved (Fig. O.7). Local pathology of the optic nerve

usually causes unilateral disc swelling with early loss of acuity and colour vision, for example in anterior optic neuritis or ischaemic optic neuropathy.

Papilloedema due to raised ICP has a characteristic natural history: early (blurred margins, loss of venous pulsation); acute (secondary haemorrhages, hard exudates, cotton wool spots); chronic (swelling with mild venous congestion); vintage (early disc pallor); and finally atrophic (established optic atrophy). When the atrophy follows papilloedema (Fig. O.8) there may be glial sheathing of the vessels at the disc (secondary optic atrophy), oedema residues may fill the physiological cup, the colour is then greyish-white, the retinal vessels are thin and tortuous, and the edge of the disc is irregular.

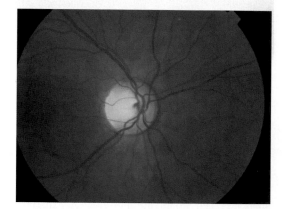

Figure O.8 Primary optic atrophy.

Optic disc cupping

Excavation of the optic disc (cupping), occurs in chronic glaucoma (see Fig. O.3). There is enlargement of the cup associated with thinning of the normally pink neuroretinal rim with associated peripheral visual field loss. The cupping is particularly evident in the vertical meridian. The cupping of the optic disc in cases of glaucoma may be distinguished from the physiological cup by the fact that it extends beyond the physiological norm – that is, more than 60 per cent of the size of the disc in the vertical meridian. The retinal vessels bend sharply over the edge, and may disappear from view behind the overhanging margin of the disc, reappearing on the base of the cup. The lamina cribrosa is clearly seen and the disc becomes white and atrophic.

Optic atrophy

Pallor of the disc (Fig. O.9) signifies atrophy of the disc (i.e. reduction in the number of nerve fibres which arise in the retina and converge to form the optic disc). The causes are listed in Table O.3.

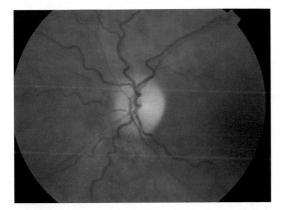

Figure 0.9 Atrophic papilloedema.

Table 0.3 Differential diagnosis of optic atrophy

Congenital
- Leber's optic atrophy
- Autosomal dominant optic atrophy
- Retinal degenerations (e.g. retinitis pigmentosa)
- Spinocerebellar ataxias (SCA) Types 1–4
- Freidreich's ataxia

Acquired
- Optic neuritis – typical demyelinating (±multiple sclerosis), atypical
- Pressure on optic nerve – glaucoma, tumour (pituitary or anterior visual pathways), Paget's disease, aneurysm
- Infection (chorioretinitis, e.g. treponemal infection, tuberculosis)
- Deficiency (vitamin B_1/B_{12})
- Toxic/drugs (ethambutol, lead, quinine, chloroquine, methanol)
- Long-standing raised ICP with papilloedema (any cause)
- Vascular – central retinal artery or vein occlusion

Peripapillary atrophy

Atrophy of the tissues around the disc occurs with age. In younger patients, it is most frequently seen with myopia (i.e. myopic crescent) (see Fig. O.4). This is usually found on the temporal side of the disc, and may vary in size and extent from a thin crescent to a large atrophic area around the whole disc.

Retinal vascular abnormalities

Central retinal vein occlusion

This condition makes the disc extremely swollen and oedematous, with dramatic blurring of the edge (Fig. O.10). There may be macular oedema. The retinal veins are dilated and tortuous, and the whole fundus may be covered with flame-shaped and blotchy haemorrhages. The oedema of the retina may be entirely obscure retinal venous segments. Cotton wool spots may be seen. The causes and associations are listed in Table O.4.

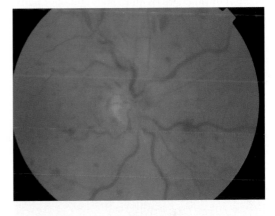

Figure 0.10 Central retinal vein occlusion.

Table 0.4 Causes and associations of central retinal vein occlusion

Systemic arterial vascular disease
- Hypertension
- Diabetes
- Ischaemic heart disease

Haematological disorders (hyperviscosity)
- Polycythaemia
- Lymphoma
- Leukaemia
- Paraproteinaemia
- Multiple myeloma
- Cryoglobulinaemia

Thrombophilic tendency
- Protein C, S or antithrombin III deficiency
- Antiphospholipid/anticardiolipin antibodies
- Oral contraceptive use

Vasculitis
- Lupus
- Sarcoidosis
- Syphilis

Distal to the occlusion there are numerous scattered haemorrhages, dilated tortuous veins and retinal oedema. Central retinal vein occlusion is associated with severe visual loss with little prospect of recovery, while branch retinal vein occlusion has a much more favourable prognosis.

Central retinal artery occlusion

This condition occurs more commonly in the middle-aged or elderly. Visual loss occurs following loss of blood supply to the inner layer of the retina (Fig. O.11). The central retinal artery is the first intra-orbital branch of the ophthalmic artery, which enters the optic nerve behind the globe to supply the retina. Short posterior ciliary arteries arise more distally from the ophthalmic artery and supply the choroid.

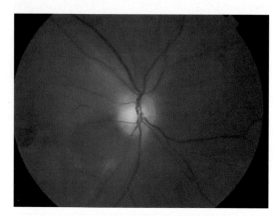

Figure O.11 Occlusion of the central retinal artery.

Cardiac embolism must always be considered, especially in young patients who may have valvular disease, right-to-left shunting from patent foramen ovale, or endocarditis. The emboli are usually cholesterol, but they may be bacterial or talc in some patients (e.g. intravenous drug users). In older patients, carotid atherosclerosis and thromboembolism, and giant cell arteritis, are important causes of retinal artery occlusion. The main causes of central retinal artery occlusion are listed in Table O.5.

The infarcted retina is pale due to secondary oedema. The central macula (fovea) is spared because it has additional supply from the choroidal capillary circulation, and appears as a bright 'cherry-red' spot. The differential diagnosis of a cherry-red spot includes a number of lipid storage diseases (see Table O.6), which

Table O.5. Causes and associations of central retinal artery occlusion

Systemic arterial disease
- Hypertension
- Diabetes

Cardiac disease
- Valve disease, including endocarditis
- Patent foramen ovale

Carotid disease
- Atherosclerotic carotid stenosis

Coagulopathies
- Sickle cell disease
- Antiphospholipid antibodies
- Polycythaemia
- Oral contraceptive

Vasculitis
- Giant cell arteritis
- Polyarteritis nodosa
- Behçet's disease
- Syphilis

Migranous retinal infarction

Table O.6 Differential diagnosis of a cherry-red spot

- Tay–Sachs disease
- Sandhoff disease
- Niemann–Pick disease
- Generalized gangliosidosis
- Sialidosis types I and II

are characterized by more widespread neurological dysfunction.

No visual recovery is likely following central retinal artery occlusion. The pallor of the inner retina slowly clears, and secondary atrophy of the optic disc later develops. If giant cell arteritis is suspected (history of preceding amaurosis, age >60 years, constitutional symptoms, high ESR), then urgent treatment with high-dose corticosteroids may save vision in the other eye.

Investigation will depend on age and clinical presentation, but may include carotid or cardiac imaging to seek sources of emboli.

Renal retinopathy

Renal retinopathy is characterized by the presence of flame-shaped haemorrhages in the nerve-fibre layer of the retina. There are also two types of white patches: in the early stages of the disease, ill-defined 'cotton wool spots' are scattered irregularly throughout the macular region; in later stages, smaller linear patches of white exudate may be seen radiating from the macula.

Hypertensive retinopathy

The arteries are narrow, show a heightened light reflex (silver or copper wiring), and compress the veins at the crossings (arteriovenous nipping), which may show local deflections at these points. In more severe hypertension there is retinal ischaemia and loss of the integrity of the small vessels; this results in the appearance of retinal exudates (due to oedema) and 'cotton wool spots', which can be confused with diabetic retinopathy (see below). Cotton wool spots are white, fluffy lesions that result from occlusion of pre-capillary arterioles supplying the retinal nerve fibre layer, with subsequent swelling of nerve fibres (Fig. O.12). They are also called 'soft exudates' or 'nerve-fibre layer infarctions'. Fluorescein angiography shows no capillary perfusion in a cotton wool spot. Other causes of cotton wool spots are listed in Table O.7. Disc swelling is also evident in malignant hypertension. Hard exudates (intra-retinal lipid

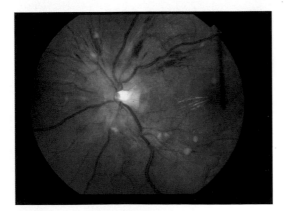

Figure O.12 Hypertensive retinopathy.

Table O.7 Differential diagnosis of cotton wool spots

- Pre-proliferative diabetic retinopathy
- Hypertension
- Retinal vein or branch retinal artery occlusion
- HIV retinopathy
- Autoimmune disorders (e.g. SLE)
- Scleroderma
- Haematological disorders

exudates) result from the leakage of lipid through damaged capillaries, and may be visible as well-defined yellow deposits within the retina, sometimes in a circinate pattern. Hyperlipidaemia may correlate with the development of hard exudates.

Diabetic retinopathy

This frequent complication of long-standing diabetes mellitus is a common cause of blindness in adults in the Western world. The complex damage to the retinal microcirculation causes a number of characteristic features, including microaneurysms, dot and blot haemorrhages, neovascularization, cotton wool spots and hard exudates (Fig. O.13). Microaneurysms (focal dilatations) of abnormal retinal capillaries are seen as small red dots. Visual loss may occur due to leakage of lipids and water from abnormal capillaries into the retina. Deep retinal haemorrhages occur when vessel walls or aneurysms rupture ('dot' or 'blot' haemorrhages). More superficial haemorrhages may be flame-shaped and indistinguishable from those of hypertensive retinopathy. Retinal ischaemia due to widespread capillary occlusion or hypoperfusion results in the production of vasoproliferative substances and to neovascularization. Neovascularization can involve the retina, optic disc or the iris, the latter being an ominous sign of severe proliferative disease that may be complicated by intractable glaucoma. The new retinal vessels bleed easily, causing vitreous haemorrhage (Fig. O.14) and may give rise to fibrous proliferation, which may cause traction retinal detachment. Nerve-fibre layer infarcts (cotton wool spots) and hard exudates are also features of diabetic

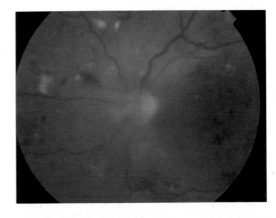

Figure O.13 Diabetic retinopathy.

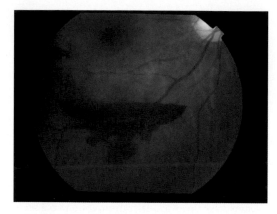

Figure O.14 Vitreous haemorrhage in diabetes.

retinopathy, particularly in patients who are also hypertensive.

Retinal vasculitis

There are many systemic associations with retinal vasculitis, which is characterized by perivascular sheathing by inflammatory cells. The important causes are listed in Table O.8.

Table O.8 Causes of retinal vasculitis

Idiopathic
Infectious
- Herpes (zoster or simplex)
- Cytomegalovirus
- Human immunodeficiency virus (HIV)
- Syphilis
- Tuberculosis
- Toxoplasmosis

Collagen vascular diseases
- Systemic lupus erythematosus
- Polyarteritis nodosa
- Wegener's granulomatosis
- Giant cell arteritis
- Scleroderma

Other systemic diseases
- Sarcoidosis
- Behçet's disease
- Multiple sclerosis
- Malignancy
- Crohn's disease
- Churg–Strauss syndrome
- Whipple's disease
- Miscellaneous
- Eales' disease

Macular diseases

Age-related macular degeneration

This is the most common cause of blindness in Western countries. It is due to age-related changes in the retinal pigment epithelium (the most metabolically active part of the retina), and small choroidal vessels. The fundus changes include atrophy and clumping of the pigment and atrophy and sclerosis of the choroidal blood vessels. Drusen (hyaline deposits) between the retinal pigment epithelium and choroid also appear (Fig. O.15). In some patients, sudden visual loss results in haemorrhage in subretinal neovascularization. Occasionally, laser treatment may halt the progress of subretinal neovascularization, but otherwise no treatment is available for this condition. Patients often benefit however from low visual aids.

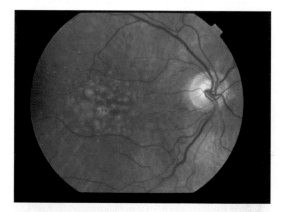

Figure O.15 Age-related macular degeneration.

Macular oedema

Macular oedema may be caused by many disease processes, all of which have in common a breakdown of the blood retinal barrier with an increase in extracellular fluid within the retina. The retinal capillary endothelium and the retinal pigment epithelium form this barrier, and diseases affecting either may cause oedema with accompanying visual loss. The main causes are retinal vascular disease (e.g. retinal vein occlusion and diabetic retinopathy).

Peripheral retinal abnormalities

Retinal detachment

The retina may become detached from the underlying retinal pigment epithelium by a variety of mechanisms.

Most commonly, fluid vitreous tracks through a break or tear in the retina, progressively lifting the retina around the break. The area of detachment slowly spreads until the whole retina is detached (Fig. O.16). Unless the retinal break is sealed surgically, vision will be lost. Retinal breaks are most common in myopic patients and may follow trauma. The second mechanism is when traction forces from the vitreous pull the retina off. This may occur under conditions where there is fibrous proliferation within the eye, for example in advanced diabetic retinopathy or following penetrating injuries of the eye. Finally, the retina may detach because it is pushed off either by a tumour of the underlying choroid or by subretinal exudate which may complicate inflammatory choroidal disease or vascular anomalies. The detached retina has a grey appearance, and the retinal vessels are tortuous and thin and appear dark in colour.

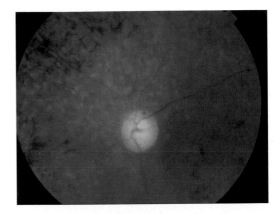

Figure O.17 Retinitis pigmentosa.

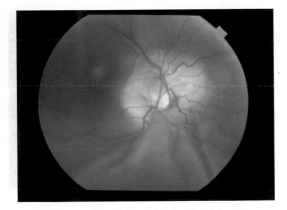

Figure O.16 Retinal detachment.

Retinitis pigmentosa

This is a group of hereditary diseases affecting the photoreceptors and retinal pigment epithelium. Night blindness and constriction of the visual fields (tunnel vision) are variably progressive, with eventual blindness. The earliest fundus changes occur in the equatorial zone with areas of hyperpigmentation (typically in a bone spicule pattern), which spread to involve the whole fundus. Waxy pallor of the disc and gross attenuation of the retinal arterioles are also features (Fig. O.17).

Choroiditis

Active choroiditis manifests itself as a greyish-white, ill-defined, slightly raised area. Overlying vitreous

opacities are commonly associated with such areas of active choroiditis. When healed, the patch appears white because there is atrophy of the choroid and overlying retinal pigment epithelium. Such scars are generally surrounded by clumps of dense pigment (Fig. O.18).

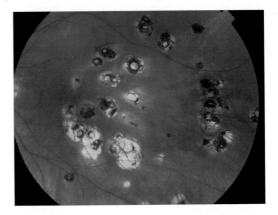

Figure O.18 Scars from old choroiditis.

Eales's disease

This rare disorder manifests itself as recurrent intraocular haemorrhages in young adults, and is generally attributed to retinal phlebitis. Sudden obscuration of vision results from haemorrhage into the vitreous. Recurrence is the rule, and proliferative retinopathy may ensue with fibrovascular membrane formation and traction retinal detachment.

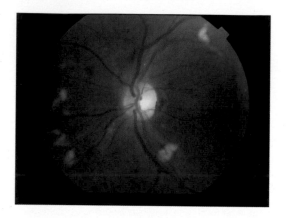

Figure O.19 AIDS-related retinal disease.

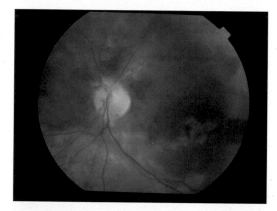

Figure O.20 Cytomegalovirus (CMV) retinitis.

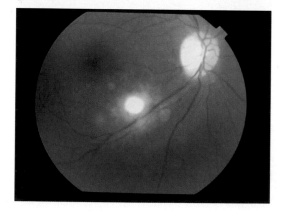

Figure O.21 Retinitis due to toxoplasmosis.

HIV retinopathy

Untreated advanced HIV disease is associated with a retinopathy characterized by multiple cotton wool spots, usually without accompanying haemorrhages (Fig. O.19). It is asymptomatic, and usually clears with effective antiretroviral therapy. It may occasionally be difficult to distinguish this from early cytomegalovirus (CMV) retinitis, which typically occurs in patients with CD4 + lymphocyte counts below 50 per mm^3. CMV retinitis causes irreversible retinal damage, and is characterized by large perivascular exudates and haemorrhages (Fig. O.20). Retinitis due to toxoplasmosis has also been described (Fig. O.21).

David Werring

ORTHOPNOEA

See also DYSPNOEA (p. 159)

A patient is said to have orthopnoea if they experience breathlessness, especially when lying down. Most patients suffering breathlessness at rest are more comfortable in the sitting position, but a clear history of intense breathlessness in the recumbent position is particularly characteristic of left ventricular failure, mitral stenosis and other conditions which cause pulmonary venous hypertension. The paroxysmal nocturnal dyspnoea of patients with left ventricular failure is at least partly related to posture in bed. Orthopnoea, and episodic breathlessness at night, is also a common feature of asthma.

Boris Lams

OTORRHOEA

Otorrhoea (aural discharge) may arise from the external auditory meatus, middle ear or, occasionally, intracranial or adjacent structures. It is an unpleasant and worrying symptom for the patient. At the outset it is important to note the character of the discharge, whether it is watery or mucoid, continuous or intermittent, its colour, quantity and whether it is inoffensive or offensive. Some discharges are very subtle, and all require a very thorough inspection of the ear with a microscope and microsuction. The causes of discharge are listed in Table O.9.

Table O.9 Causes of otorrhoea

External auditory canal
- Wax
- Otitis externa
  - ◆ Atopic or eczematous
  - ◆ Infective
    - Bacterial
    - Fungal
    - Viral
- Neoplasia
- Trauma
- Salivary fistula
- Branchial anomaly

Middle ear
- Acute otitis media
- Chronic otitis media
- Neoplasia
- CSF

External auditory meatus

Wax (cerumen) is so variable in colour and consistency that it can be mistaken for something else. Most often just present in small flakes or boluses, it can change as a result of infection or water contamination into a light yellow, semi-liquid discharge. Wax is nature's disinfectant. It provides the first barrier against infection, and dissolves squamous epithelium shed from the tympanic membrane. Wax is transported laterally by an inherent pattern of epithelial movement and, in normal circumstances, should not need to be removed. In some situations it may become impacted in the deep meatus or contaminated with water; in these circumstances microsuction or syringing is appropriate. *Keratosis obturans* is a condition where wax and desquamated squamous epithelium forms an adherent mass in the bony meatus, sometimes even causing bony erosion. This condition may be associated with bronchiectasis and sinusitis as part of the *immotile cilia syndrome*.

Otitis externa

This is a very common disease, and is sometimes part of a generalized dermatitis, for example, eczema or psoriasis. Some patients may precipitate the condition by the use of hairsprays, perfumes and even eardrops to which they are allergic. Indeed, even some wax solvents can cause enough irritation to create the condition.

The most common cause of otitis externa, however, is a breakdown in the migratory mechanism of the skin of the deep meatus referred to above. Elsewhere in the body where skin divides, movement, clothes, friction and washing all serve to dispose of the dead skin. The external meatus is not exposed to any of these factors, and so a different mechanism exists to dispose of the dead epithelium. The viable epithelium in the area has the property of migrating dead epithelium from the deep meatus to the wax glands in the outer part of the ear canal. If, for any reason, this migratory process breaks down, then dead epithelium collects in the deep meatus. The entrapped skin acts as an excellent culture medium for bacteria, particularly if it is wet. Secondary bacterial infection takes place rapidly, giving rise to symptoms of pain and discharge. Treatment consists of thorough aural toilet and antibiotic drops. It may take some time for the mechanisms within the external ear to return to normal. Throughout this time, the patient should be careful not to itch or scratch the ear, and to avoid further water contamination.

Fungal otitis externa will not respond to the usual antibiotic eardrops, and may even be caused by their over-use. It has a distinct appearance, and so can be recognized immediately without recourse to fungal cultures. In these patients the ear canal is filled with moist, whitish debris that looks and suctions like damp blotting paper. In *Aspergillus niger* infection, black spots are seen amidst the fungal debris. The other common causative fungus is *Candida albicans*.

Viral otitis externa exists in two forms, each of which can cause a type of otitis externa. Reactivation of *herpes zoster* causes excruciatingly severe pain, and may sometimes be accompanied by facial paralysis (*Ramsay–Hunt syndrome*) (Fig. O.22). The other type is *meningitis bullosa haemorrhagica*, which is often seen in conjunction with the flu virus. Blood blisters form on the drum and lead to a serosanguinous discharge and bouts of very severe pain. Both of these conditions cause pain that is significantly more severe than the clinician would expect from the physical signs alone.

In many cases it is not possible, because of oedema, to see the tympanic membrane. It is most important to differentiate between simple otitis externa and otitis externa secondary to otitis media as soon as possible. One useful differentiating feature is that the pain of external otitis is precipitated or exacerbated by movement of the pinna, while in otitis media it is

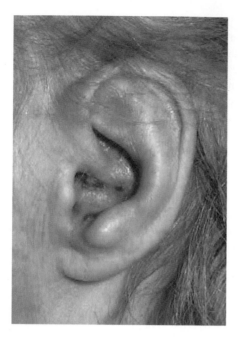

Figure O.22 Typical appearance of vesicles and crusted lesions in the concha of an elderly patient who presented with an acute facial palsy caused by Ramsay–Hunt syndrome.

pressure above and behind the ear that is painful. If in addition to the characteristic pain, the patient has good hearing and a positive Rinne test, even though the meatus may be almost completely occluded, the condition is most unlikely to be otitis media.

Malignant otitis externa is a poor term as it wrongly implies a neoplastic process. Unfortunately, this term has become enshrined in otological practice and is unlikely to be changed. It refers to a *Pseudomonas* or fungal infection of the tissues immediately beneath the skull base. This infection gains access by a breach of the skin in the external auditory canal at the junction of the bony and cartilaginous parts. Malignant otitis externa is a very severe and sometimes fatal infection which tends to develop in those who are either elderly or immunocompromised for any reason – for example, diabetics, chemotherapy and AIDS. Scant discharge precedes the spreading infection that presents with consummate, unremitting pain together with progressive cranial nerve palsies. In late cases gross destruction of the skull base takes place.

More correctly, malignant otitis externa should refer to patients with *carcinoma of the external auditory canal*. This too is extremely painful, is almost

always misdiagnosed, and is under-estimated for months until the discharge becomes blood-stained and facial palsy supervenes. Fortunately, it is a very uncommon form of squamous cell carcinoma as it has a poor prognosis (Fig. O.23).

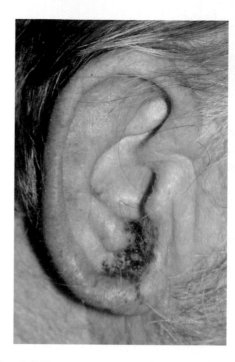

Figure O.23 Blood-stained discharge coming from a squamous cell carcinoma of the external auditory canal.

Rarely, a *salivary fistula* involves the cartilaginous meatus and may follow injury that involves the ear, the temporomandibular joint and the parotid gland. Discharge can also be caused by a first branchial arch sinus that classically communicates with the bony cartilaginous junction and may pass through the parotid and intermingle with branches of the facial nerve (Fig. O.24).

Middle ear cleft

Acute otitis media gives rise to discharge once the tympanic membrane has ruptured. Until then, the patient suffers from pain, increasing deafness and malaise. The pain subsides as soon as the pus is released. Initially, the discharge is blood-stained, but it soon becomes frankly mucopurulent and often profuse, pouring down the cheek and soiling the patient's pillow. This continues for some days until the infection comes

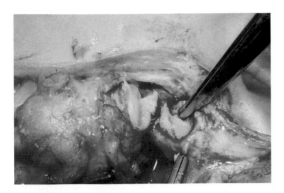

Figure 0.24 First branchial fistula being removed at surgery. It was filled with thick, cream-coloured material that had discharged into the floor of the ear canal (opened) and onto the skin through a small punctum that has also been excised in continuity.

under control, either as a result of antibiotic therapy or natural immunity. If the eardrum is inspected carefully, the perforation can be seen through which a pulsating discharge escapes. The pus is usually inoffensive. Acute otitis media is caused by either viral or bacterial infection. The organisms most commonly implicated are *Streptococcus*, *Pneumococcus* and *Haemophilus*.

Chronic suppurative otitis media (CSOM) is classified as either *tubo-tympanic* or attico-antral. The hallmark of tubo-tympanic otitis media is a central perforation, a defect in the pars tensa of the drum. Few ears with persistent perforations are entirely dry. Most are moist with episodes of increased and sometimes profuse discharge during acute exacerbations. In some cases it may be possible to close the perforation by surgical means, thereby eradicating the discharge. In others this is not possible, and the discharge must be kept to a minimum by strict water precautions and intermittent courses of antibiotics. Continuous infection in the middle ear cleft stimulates hyperplasia of the mucosal lining which ultimately prolapses through the perforation as a polyp.

The fundamental lesion of attico-antral chronic otitis media disease is an attic retraction pocket, with or without cholesteatoma, or ingrowth of skin from a marginal perforation. In some cases – particularly children – polyps develop adjacent to the attic defect. The precise cause of these pathological processes is not known. Cholesteatoma, a nidus or collection of moist and often infected epithelium, releases enzymes that help to destroy bone and erode the temporal bone. As a result, the cholesteatoma can extend into the mastoid, disrupt the ossicular chain, and destroy the bony labyrinth and facial nerve. Given time, the cholesteatoma eventually abuts the dura of the middle and posterior cranial fossas from where infection can spread intracranially and either meningitis or brain abscess will develop. This disease can be extremely serious, and the cholesteatoma should be eradicated by mastoid surgery.

Primary malignant neoplasia of the middle ear is extremely rare, but usually presents with a blood-stained, muco-purulent discharge arising from granular tissue that has destroyed the tympanic membrane. The diagnosis can only be made by biopsy. Malignant tumours arising in the middle ear cleft include squamous cell carcinoma, metastatic tumours and eosinophilic granuloma (histiocytosis X).

Cerebrospinal fluid (CSF) can escape from the ear and appear as a watery discharge. Although spontaneous CSF leaks are possible, they would have to develop in a patient with a perforated eardrum in order to drain from the ear rather than the Eustachian tube. Most patients with CSF otorrhoea have a clear history of severe trauma, sufficient to have fractured the temporal bone.

Michael Gleeson

OVER-ACTIVITY

The causes of over-activity may be classified as follows:

- Common causes
  - ◆ Mania
  - ◆ Organic brain disease (see CONFUSION, p. 114)
  - ◆ Delirium
  - ◆ Agitated depression
  - ◆ Anxiety neurosis
  - ◆ Schizophrenia
  - ◆ Hyperthyroidism
  - ◆ Hyperparathyroidism
  - ◆ Drugs
  - ◆ Caffeine intoxication
  - ◆ Withdrawal from: sedatives, hypnotics, anxiolytics, alcohol
  - ◆ Abuse of: hallucinogens (LSD), amphetamine, cocaine, phencyclidine
  - ◆ Akathisia and restless leg syndrome
  - ◆ Attention-deficit hyperactivity disorder in children

- Less common causes
  - Post head injury (in children)
  - Anorexia nervosa
  - Temporal lobe epilepsy (post-ictal confusional state)
  - Neurosyphilis

Disorders of movement may frequently provide valuable clues about a diagnosis, especially when a patient is confused, mute or otherwise unable to give a clear account of symptoms. Disorders of movement include *overactivity*, *underactivity* (p. 734) and abnormal *involuntary movements*. Over-activity describes behaviour where there is an increase in physical activity, over-talkativeness and sometimes aggressiveness. The subject may make exaggerated gestures and facial expressions, and at interview will have difficulty in sitting still; they feel impelled to move about the room, their attention being easily distracted by external stimuli. This type of over-activity typically occurs in *mania*, when it is associated with elevated or irritable mood, pressure of speech and flight of ideas, grandiose plans and, in severe forms, grandiose or paranoid delusions. Sleep is disturbed and patients may remain awake and active all night with apparently undiminished energy levels next morning. Libido and appetite may both be increased. Such a typical presentation of a manic illness presents few diagnostic problems, especially if there is a history of previous mood swings or a family history of affective disorder. Restless over-activity may also be drug-induced or a feature of organic brain disease. Both *acute* and *chronic organic confusional states* (see CONFUSION, p. 113) may present with irritability, restlessness and excitement, and this can be particularly marked in states of *drug intoxication* and withdrawal from *alcohol* and *sedatives*. In the early stages of *Alzheimer's-type dementia*, a state may develop resembling mania, and the diagnosis should be made from the history of increasing memory impairment. *Neurosyphilis* could also present in this way, and associated signs such as Argyll Robertson pupils, peripheral neuropathy and evidence of dementia combined with serological tests will confirm the diagnosis. Patients with *temporal lobe epilepsy* may rarely develop *post-ictal confusional states* with over-activity, irritability or senseless aggression. These episodes are usually brief and in the context of a known history of epilepsy. *Akathisia* is a particular form of restlessness found frequently in Parkinson's disease and as a side effect of antipsychotic medication. Subjects are unable to remain still through a subjective sense of unease and restlessness. They have an urge to get up to move their feet and legs, or rock the body. Restless legs may keep them awake at night and be troublesome to a partner.

Overactivity may be a main presenting feature of *agitated depression* when the subject's complaint of worry is reflected in their appearance, thought content and behaviour. The person will appear restless, tense and fidgety, constantly seeking reassurance, because of feelings of guilt about the past and uncertainty about the future. Agitation may also be a principal feature of an *anxiety neurosis*, and in patients with *schizophrenia*. In all of these psychiatric conditions, and in physical illnesses including *hyperthyroidism* and *hypoparathyroidism*, agitation may be associated with signs of increased autonomic activity including sweating, tachycardia, palpitations, shallow breathing and gastrointestinal disturbance.

Over-activity without significant mood disturbance can be a feature of *anorexia nervosa*. These patients will exercise relentlessly and methodically in order to keep their weight low. The exercise may take the form of housework or regular training in a gym, or various sports.

Hyperkinesis is the commonest and most disruptive sequela of *head injury* in children. Features include restlessness and impulsive disobedience at home and at school, sometimes with explosive outbursts of anger. A similar pattern of hyperactivity and resistance to discipline has been observed in children with epilepsy and after *encephalitis lethargica*, although fortunately epidemic encephalitis has now largely disappeared. Both organic and psychogenic factors are involved, and the pre-traumatic personality of the child and the family setting may be as important as the severity or nature of head injury. The *attention deficit hyperactivity disorder* in children is viewed as a developmental abnormality presenting around the time the child enters school or earlier, with inappropriate degrees of inattention, impulsiveness and hyperactivity. The disorder is manifest in all situations including home, school and in play activity. There may be inappropriate running about in the classroom, fidgetiness, and over-talkativeness. These children tend to be academic under-achievers with low self-esteem, low mood and temper outbursts. There is an increased likelihood of 'soft' neurological signs, including poor coordination. Enuresis and encopresis are more common. Children may show features of conduct disorder and impairment of social and school functioning persisting throughout childhood.

Andrew Hodgkiss

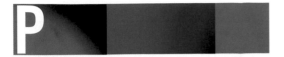

PAIN, PSYCHOGENIC

Pain is the most common complaint brought to a doctor, and is probably the most complex of subjective experiences. All pain has sensory, emotional and cognitive dimensions which require management. For example, there is a large literature to show that patients who are well-informed about surgical procedures preoperatively suffer less pain and anxiety postoperatively and require less analgesia. Thus, the 'psychological aspects' of all acute and chronic pains need to be managed. However, it is the large numbers of patients with chronic, medically unexplained pain that will be focused upon here.

A large proportion of chronic pain remains medically unexplained. Half of all diagnostic laparoscopies for chronic pelvic pain appear normal. Many patients disabled by headache, facial pain and back pain have repeatedly normal investigation results. Are these chronic pains of psychological origin?

Two routes of psychogenesis of pain have been described throughout the twentieth century: (i) an hysterical mechanism (conversion of a psychological conflict into a meaning-laden somatic symptom); and (ii) pain as a 'depressive equivalent'. These two rather different psychogeneses have tended to be lumped together under the term 'psychogenic pain' or pain disorder. A good example of an hysterical mechanism would be the chronic pelvic pain of the female patient sexually abused in childhood. The pain can be interpreted as a result of the repressed memories of this trauma. Pain as a depressive equivalent rests on the idea that some patients suffer in a non-localized way and report low mood to doctors, while others, lacking words for emotional states (alexithymic patients), localize their suffering within the space of their bodies and report bodily pain instead. These patients often have positive family histories of depressive illness.

Today, the treatment of patients with pain disorder is well established, particularly in the USA and France. Patients there are offered pain management programmes with multidisciplinary components including psychologists and occupational therapists. A cognitive–behavioural approach is usually adopted, with pain behaviour being left unrewarded and habits of thought when in pain examined and corrected. Opiate dependence, which often comes to complicate the chronic pain, is tackled. In addition, antidepressant medication – particularly the tricyclics – is valuable. Despite the hysterical mechanism underlying a proportion of these pains, it was Freud's experience – and that of others since – that psychoanalytic treatment is less successful with pain than with other hysterical somatic symptoms.

It is best to reserve the use of the term 'psychogenic pain' for those patients where positive evidence of psychogenesis is evident. The remainder are best left in the category of 'medically unexplained symptoms'. There is growing interest and understanding about how this large number of patients should be managed.

A number of psychiatric disorders can present with pains – for example, muscular tension pains in anxiety disorders (especially non-cardiac chest pain), a gripping abdominal pain in depression, or hallucinatory pain in schizophrenia. Pain is a popular symptom choice for those with factitious disorders and malingering.

Finally, it is important to distinguish psychogenic pain from neuropathic pain. Confusion often arises clinically because both respond to tricyclic antidepressants. However, neuropathic pain is medically explicable and has a characteristic distribution and nature – for example, the burning sensation in the soles of the feet in the sensory peripheral neuropathy associated with alcohol misuse.

Andrew Hodgkiss

PALLOR

Pallor is a very subjective sign indicating a reduction in skin or mucous membrane colouring. It usually refers to a generalized reduction rather than localized depigmentation, as in vitiligo.

Pallor may be a congenital characteristic resulting in an individual always looking pale, even when healthy.

Anaemia, for any reason, is the most common cause of pallor. Pallor of the conjunctivae or mucous membranes is a very unreliable indication of a reduced haemoglobin, except when there is severe anaemia. Pallor may be accentuated in hypopituitarism when, in addition to the anaemia, there is a reduction in skin pigmentation.

A reduction in blood flow to the skin will result in acute pallor. This can arise either due to hypotension as in shock or due to hypothermia.

Any increase in the thickness of the skin – particularly the epidermis – will tend to obscure the haemoglobin in the capillaries, resulting in pallor. Skin thickness is increased in acromegaly and myxoedema.

Melvin Lobo

PANIC

Panic is an extreme form of anxiety characterized by: (i) severe, acute, brief attacks; and (ii) the feeling of loss of personal control. The symptoms are predominantly the somatic (especially cardiovascular) features of anxiety and hyperventilation, so that a primarily physical presentation is common. The emotions experienced are stark and distressing: terror, fear of dying, going mad or losing control. Attacks may be triggered by specific stimuli or be unpredictable, and life frequently becomes dominated by the apprehension of the acute distress and helplessness engendered. Panic attacks are common, occurring at some time in 10 per cent of the adult population, and to a persistently disabling degree in one in five of those affected. The causes of panic are listed in Table P.1.

There are a number of *physical conditions* which enter the differential diagnosis. Hyperthyroidism and phaeochromocytoma can mimic closely, whilst – particularly in a diabetic or partial gastrectomy patient – the possibility of hypoglycaemia should be excluded. Other episodic medical conditions that can be confused with somatic presentations of panic attacks are migraine, Ménière's disease, temporal lobe epilepsy and carcinoid syndrome. Not uncommonly, patients with these conditions develop genuine panic attacks as an emotional reaction to the uncertainty they experience. They may begin to report symptom differences between attacks which can confound the physician, unless he or she is aware of the possibility of a superimposed panic disorder. In addition to the symptom content, the brief duration of panic attacks

Table P.1 Causes of panic

Commonest
Normal
Stress-related
Anxiety
Panic disorder

Less common
Drugs
- Stimulants
- Hallucinogens
Drug withdrawal
Physical disorders
- Hyperthyroidism
- Hypoglycaemia
- Phaeochromocytoma
- Carcinoid syndrome
- Asthma
- Ménière's disease
- Temporal lobe epilepsy
- Migraine
Psychiatric disorders
- Phobia
- Depression
- Chronic hyperventilation syndrome
- Post-traumatic stress disorder

Rare
As for anxiety (see p. 35)

(usually lasting for a few minutes) is a pointer in distinguishing panic from most physical disorders.

Panic attacks are frequently predominant features in the setting of other *psychological conditions*. In phobias, panic is often experienced when exposed to the phobic stimulus, but anticipating or even thinking about exposure may trigger panic. Panic attacks occur, and may occasionally be the presenting complaint in depressive illness, or develop subsequently during recovery. Episodes occurring regularly early in the day are a clue, but usually there are readily identifiable features of depressive change evident in the history and mental state. Hyperventilation may be involved in the development of panic attacks, and may also be exacerbated by them.

Panic attacks are induced by stimulants, both illicit drugs (e.g. amphetamine and cocaine) and the socially acceptable caffeine – a note of coffee consumption is worth taking. Drug withdrawal also precipitates episodes, perhaps most commonly implicated are the benzodiazepines and alcohol.

Finally, the relationship between *anxiety* and panic is disputed. It is evident that patients who suffer from generalized 'free-floating' anxiety are likely to experience panic attacks of varying degree and frequency, while patients having panic attacks become appreciably anxious about these alarming experiences, and commonly develop a secondary chronic anxiety state or agoraphobia. The controversy stems from the American view that panic disorder is a separate diagnostic entity, based essentially on the discovery that tricyclic antidepressant drugs have a specific anti-panic action in patients without clinically apparent depression. Whilst British psychiatry has not yet cleaved panic from anxiety, panic attacks have now become regarded as a distinct focus for research and, if putative differences in inheritance, pathophysiology, natural history and treatment responses are confirmed, the status of panic is likely to change from a subcategory of anxiety to independence as an emotional disorder.

Andrew Hodgkiss

Table P.2 Characteristics of papules

White	Black/blue
Milia	Malignant melanoma
Keratosis pilaris	Blue naevus
Phrynoderma	
Molluscum contagiosum	**Yellow**
Syringomas	Xanthelasmas
Lipoid proteinosis	Naevoxanthoendothelioma
	Pseudoxanthoma elasticum
Brown	Sebaceous adenoma
Acrochrodia (skin tags)	Fordyce's disease
Viral warts	
Seborrhoeic warts	**Red**
Plane warts	Guttate psoriasis
Venereal viral warts	Pityriasis lichenoides chronica
Lichen amyloidosis	Pityriasis lichenoides acuta
Darier's disease	Pityriasis rosea
Acanthosis nigricans	Acne vulgaris
Dermatosis papulosa nigra	Dermatitis
Tuberous sclerosis	Eczema
	Lichen simplex chronicus
Violaceous	Papular syphilide
Lichen planus	Campbell de Morgan spots
Kaposi's sarcoma	Angiokeratoma of Fordyce

PAPULES

Papules are solid, circumscribed elevations of the skin up to the size of a split pea (5 mm). Similar lesions, if larger, are nodules or tumours. Papules are usually round or oval in shape, but they may be irregular, whilst in lichen planus they are polygonal. Their colour can vary from white, red, brown, yellow to violaceous. Their profile may be domed, pointed or flat-topped, and their surface smooth, warty or scaly. Papules may be transitional lesions, becoming vesicles or growing into nodules and tumours, or breaking down into ulcers (Table P.2).

White or pearly papules

Milia are tiny firm papules filled with white solid material, most often found on the face and, once present, persist until incised. They may also follow blister formation (e.g. porphyria cutanea tarda and epidermolysis bullosa). They consist of keratin.

Keratosis pilaris is a common condition of children and young adults, and consists of rough, firm, white papules, approximately 1 mm in diameter. It is found over the lateral upper arm and the anterior thighs above the knees; the buttocks are occasionally involved. The papules give the skin a nutmeg grater-like feeling, and are occasionally surrounded by an inflammatory halo. They are caused by keratin plugs in the ostia of hair follicles. The development of keratosis pilaris is determined by a dominant gene, and the condition is closely related to ichthyosis and atopic dermatitis. Rarely, it is a manifestation of vitamin A deficiency (*phrynoderma*).

Molluscum contagiosum is a common viral infection (Fig. P.1), occurring especially in children and young adults. It is readily transmitted from person to person, and in addition individual lesions may be auto-inoculated. Typical lesions present as pearly white or skin-coloured papules, 2–10 mm in diameter. They have a smooth shiny surface with central umbilication, from which a cheesy material may be expressed, and the typical inclusion bodies may be demonstrated under the microscope. In children, especially atopics, lesions may be widespread on the face and limbs; in adults they are more common around the genitals. After a period of some months, the body mounts an immune reaction, the lesions become acutely inflamed, and then resolve spontaneously, sometimes leaving a minute scar.

Syringomas are common benign lesions, frequently multiple, arising from the sweat duct apparatus. They

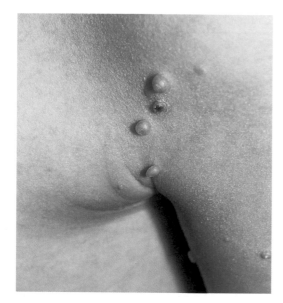

Figure P.1 Molluscum contagiosum.

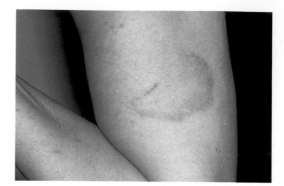

Figure P.2 Granuloma annulare.

are generally multiple, and usually occur on the upper cheeks just below the eyes as smooth white oval papules 2–4 mm in length. Lesions accumulate over the years, and must be differentiated from *xanthelasmata*, which are yellower and larger and fewer in number and may be associated with hyperlipidaemia. In the rare disorder *lipoid proteinosis*, pearly translucent white papules occur widely on mucous membranes and skin, particularly the eyelid margins.

Skin-coloured papules

Viral warts are a common cause of skin-coloured papules, and occur particularly over the dorsa of fingers and on the soles. Flat *plane warts* can also occur on the backs of hands and may form subtle tan papules over the chin and cheeks, especially in young women.

In older subjects, viral warts are uncommon, and small multiple keratotic papules on the backs of the hands or scalp are more likely to be *solar (actinic) keratoses*. These lesions are important, because malignant transformation may occur.

Clustered subcutaneous papules formed into an annular configuration are suggestive of *granuloma annulare*. They are seen most commonly on the fingers, backs of hands, elbows or ankles, and resolve spontaneously over a number of years (Fig. P.2).

Brown papules

Basal cell papillomas (seborrhoeic warts) – the most common benign tumour of the elderly – may grow to form large brown plaques, but they begin as light brown tiny verrucous papules scattered widely on the chest and back.

Venereal viral warts are usually small, brown, flat-topped and smooth with an angular outline. This is in contrast to *condylomata acuminata* seen in secondary syphilis, where extensive crops of soft, skin-coloured or pink pedunculated papules or nodules, covered with tiny moist papillary projections, occur on the genitalia, scrotum and peri-anal region (and also between the toes and at the angles of the mouth). The serology will be positive.

An *acrochrodion* (skin tag) is a tiny brown pedunculated soft papule with a narrow neck found in the flexures of patients from middle age onwards. Lesions may be numerous around the neck, axillae and groins. They are more profuse in the obese, and are particularly marked in *acanthosis nigricans*. In *Darier's disease* the papules are brownish, perifollicular, and covered by a brown-grey crust. The papules may be grouped or accumulate into sheets, and the sites of predilection are the seborrhoeic areas of scalp, behind the ears, nasolabial folds, midback and interscapular regions. They may be crusty on the scalp, and vegetating in the intertrigenous areas. Palmar pits and notching of the nails are associated features which may assist in the clinical diagnosis; if in doubt, the histology is characteristic. The disease often flares during the summer months, and is dominantly inherited.

Dermatosis papulosa nigra is the rather grand and cumbersome title of tiny common jet black papules over the cheeks of black subjects. In *lichen amyloidosis* multiple, closely spaced, uniform, rounded, hard papules, that may be red, brown or skin-coloured, occur over the anterior shins, or rarely more widely. The lesions are intensely pruritic, resistant to treatment, and not associated with systemic amyloidosis. Even more rare are the brown/skin-coloured papules crowded around the nose seen in *tuberose sclerosis*, the so-called *adenoma sebaceum of Pringle* (Fig. P.3). Other cutaneous manifestations are shagreen patches, ashy leaf hypopigmented macules and periungual fibromas. There may be associated neurological, cardiac and renal problems.

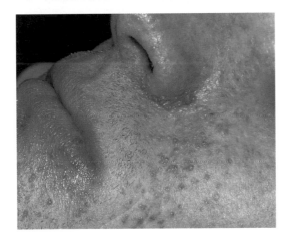

Figure P.3 Adenoma sebaceum in tuberose sclerosis.

Violaceous papules

Flat-topped shiny polygonal papules are the hallmark of *lichen planus*. The colour is characteristically lilac-pink. The papules are smooth and not crusted, and may be crossed by tiny white lines known as 'Wickham's striae'. They are intensively irritating and may appear in areas of skin damage, known as the Koebner (isomorphic) phenomenon. The eruption is usually symmetrical, particularly on the flexural aspects of wrists and forearms, anterior and inner aspects of calves and ankles, and over the upper abdomen and lumbar region. In Caucasians, a delicate white lace-like pattern is common on the buccal mucosa, and this is an important diagnostic sign. Similar lesions may be present on other mucous membranes (medial aspect of labia majora, glans penis). Lesions may be simulated by a lichenoid drug eruption; mepacrine,

oral hypoglycaemics, beta-blockers and gold have all been implicated. Lichen planus resolves spontaneously after a year or two, leaving macular post-inflammatory pigmentation at the previously affected sites.

Black papules

A solitary uniform sharply marginated blue-black papule is highly suggestive of a *blue naevus*. The lesions remain unchanged over many years, and malignant transformation is vanishingly rare. The sudden appearance of multiple uniform black papules may indicate satellite spread of a *malignant melanoma*. In *multiple idiopathic haemorrhagic sarcoma of Kaposi*, dark purplish papules appear usually over the feet and ankles of elderly patients of Jewish or Italian lineage. Gradually, the lesions become elevated to form multiple papules and later soft nodules, plaques and angiomatous tumours. They may ulcerate, bleed and crust. A more generalized, aggressive and metastasizing form of the disease is endemic in East Africa and is seen in association with HIV infection.

Yellow papules

Xanthelasmas are found on the upper cheeks and eyelids in middle-aged men and women. Investigation should exclude hyperlipidaemia, coronary artery disease, diabetes, myxoedema or primary biliary cirrhosis. The sudden appearance of numerous yellow papules over the buttocks and elsewhere indicates *eruptive xanthoma*, a condition in which abnormalities of lipid metabolism are invariable. *Naevoxanthoendothelioma* (juvenile xanthogranuloma) occur as rounded yellow firm papules or nodules over extensor surfaces within a few weeks of birth. They involute spontaneously in 1–3 years and are not associated with underlying lipid abnormalities. The skin of the neck and axillae may be covered in sheets of yellowish papules in *pseudoxanthoma elasticum*. This is inherited as an autosomal recessive condition and is a generalized defect of support tissue. There may be associated tears in Bruch's membrane in the eye and aneurysms of small and large arteries.

Tiny yellow papules on the face and forehead of older people can be caused by *sebaceous hyperplasia*; the lesions are usually flat-topped, with an erythematous halo and a tiny central depression. They must be differentiated from molluscum contagiosum, which

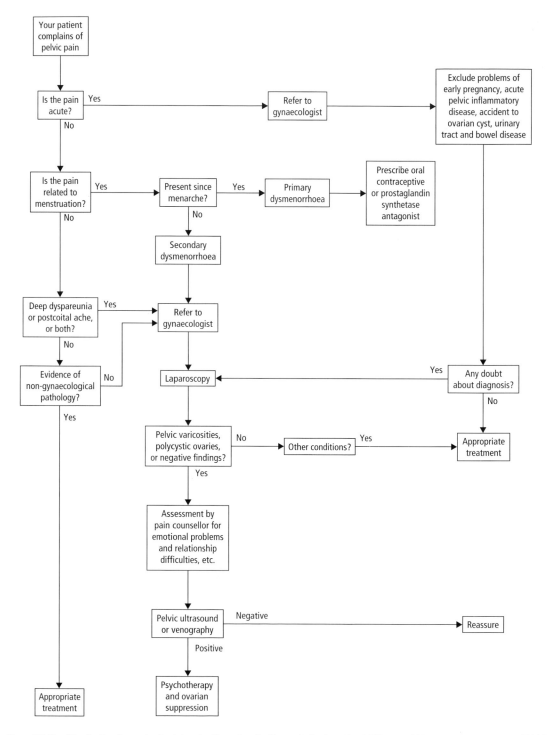

Figure P.5 Algorithm for the diagnosis of pelvic pain. [Reproduced with permission from Beard RW, *et al.* (1986) Pelvic pain in women. *British Medical Journal* **293**, 1161.]

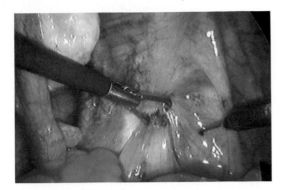

Figure P.6 Rectovaginal endometriosis; appearance at laparoscopy.

and pelvic clearance. Whilst there is a place for this with endometriosis and chronic PID, if there is no obvious pathology then it will not result in cure for all women.

- *Adhesions.* These may be found in up to 20 per cent of patients with chronic pain, though they may not be the cause of the pain.
- *Residual ovary syndrome* in women who have had a hysterectomy associated with pain and dyspareunia and a fixed tender ovary at the vaginal vault. Treatment may be by suppression of the ovary, or its removal.
- *Endometriosis.* In this condition there is abnormal implantation of endometrium outside the uterine cavity (Fig. P.6). This may cause dysmenorrhoea, dyspareunia, menstrual upset, pelvic pain and infertility. Diagnosis is usually by laparoscopy. *Adenomyosis* is a variant of this condition, when endometrium invades the myometrium, and this causes pain with the period and a very tender uterus. The surgical option is dependent on symptoms.
- *Chronic PID.* This is a consequence of acute infection, and leads to damage and consequent pain and menstrual upset.
- *Irritable bowel syndrome.* This condition is often confused with a gynaecological cause of lower abdominal pain.
- *Pelvic congestion.* The pain is dull and aching, with occasional sharp exacerbations. There may be local tenderness. The women are usually in their reproductive years, and may be nulliparous. Diagnosis can be made by venography, laparoscopy or ultrasound, and treatment is medically with progestogens or surgically with a pelvic clearance followed by hormone replacement therapy (HRT).

Antony Hollingworth

PELVIS, SWELLING IN

Swellings that arise from the pelvis can be considered under their anatomical origins. A number of structures may appear to be pelvic, when their original site of origin is really abdominal. Ultrasound scanning has improved the detection of lesions that are not necessarily palpable without a vaginal or rectal examination. The background to the swellings can be simply described by the five 'F's – namely fat, fluid, faeces, flatus and fat. Careful history taking, clinical examination and appropriate imaging should be able to establish the diagnosis. Anatomically, pelvic swellings will arise from a variety of sources, as follows.

Bladder

Pelvic swelling related to the bladder is most likely to result from:

- Simple distension or retention.
- Transitional cell carcinoma (see HAEMATURIA, p. 261).

The most common difficulty in the diagnosis of pelvic swellings is to differentiate between the distended bladder, pregnant uterus, ovarian cyst and uterine fibromyoma, and the most common mistakes are made between these swellings. The distended bladder is the easiest to ascertain, the passage of a catheter settling the question. Nonetheless, neglect of this simple procedure has led to the abdomen being opened.

Vagina

Pelvic swelling related to the vagina is most likely to result from:

- Haematocolpos.
- Hydrocolpos.

Distension of the vagina by menstrual fluid is not likely to be mistaken for anything else, if only on account of the absolute closure of the atretic membrane which gives rise to it. This condition is often referred to as 'imperforate hymen'. This is not correct, because the atresia is at a higher level in the vagina than the hymen, which is always perforate.

Haematocolpos is practically the only central tumour occurring between the rectum and the bladder reaching from the hymen to the pelvic brim. It presents in girls about the age of 16 or 17 years who frequently present with acute retention of urine due to the fact that the swelling fills the pelvis, such that the distended bladder in front is forced upwards into the abdomen. Primary amenorrhoea is present, although monthly symptoms without loss of blood may have taken place. Two swellings are described: (i) the tender distended bladder in the lower abdomen, reaching as high as the umbilicus; and (ii) the distended vagina filled with menstrual fluid in the pelvis. The uterus can usually be felt like a cork movable upon its upper extremity. The lower pole of the haematocolpos presents a blue-coloured swelling at the vulva. A similar swelling may be found on rare occasions in newborn girl babies: the vagina is filled with a milky fluid (hydrocolpos).

Uterus

Pelvic swelling related to the uterus is most likely to be either of the following:

- Pregnancy-related, either normal or abnormal, with or without associated tumours of the uterus or ovary.
- Non-pregnancy-related, the most common of which includes fibroids (leiomyoma) (Fig. P.7), haematometra and pyometra (blood or pus in the uterine cavity), endometrial carcinoma and, more rarely, uterine sarcoma or choriocarcinoma.

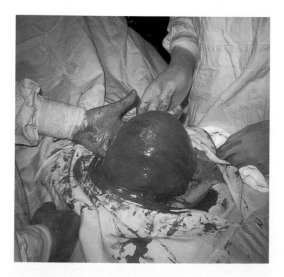

Figure P.7 Fibroid uterus.

Patient history is of great value to differentiate these cases, with amenorrhoea being the usual story with pregnancy, and menorrhagia and pressure effects being common with fibroids. Bleeding can occur in early pregnancy at the time when the periods would be due, or as a result of threatened miscarriage. Fibroids may cause menorrhagia depending on their location within the uterus. As regards the other pathologies, they tend to be linked with age. *Haematometra* may be related to cervical stenosis following treatment to the cervix for precancer, whilst *pyometra* may be seen in post-menopausal women and suggest malignancy. *Endometrial carcinoma* may present with menstrual upset, but most present in the post-menopausal age group with bleeding or discharge.

Palpation may be difficult to differentiate, as during the early months of pregnancy the uterus may fluctuate like a cyst. A softened fibroid may act in the same manner, whilst a tense ovarian cyst may feel so hard as to be mistaken for a fibroid. While the presence of the sound of the fetal heart is characteristic of pregnancy, its absence cannot be taken as evidence of a fibroid or of an ovarian tumour. If the pedicle of a tumour can be felt definitely attached to one uterine cornua, it is strong presumptive evidence of an ovarian tumour. When small tumours are in question, the first point to arise is whether the tumour can be separated from the uterus bimanually. If so, it is unlikely to be a fibromyoma of the uterus, nor a normal uterine pregnancy. This point can only be made out by careful bimanual examination, and requires considerable skill in some cases. A pedunculated fibroid is, of course, extrauterine and may have the same anatomical arrangement to the uterus as an ovarian tumour. If it is a fibroid that has undergone cystic change, the physical signs are identical to those of an ovarian cyst, and only a laparotomy will reveal the true state of affairs.

Early pregnancy in a retroverted uterus should not give rise to diagnostic difficulties if it is remembered that the soft, cystic fundus is felt through the posterior fornix, that the cervix looks down the vagina or forwards to the symphysis, and that the posterior mass is continuous with the cervix. If the retroverted uterus is associated with bladder distension, the picture is usually clear enough. The history of urinary retention followed by constant dribbling of urine (distension with overflow), amenorrhoea, other signs of pregnancy, the presence of two tumours – one in front, tense, tender and elastic, the other behind, soft and cystic – and, finally, the passage of a catheter will settle the question. The diagnosis of solid ovarian tumours is not always possible as the pedicle is often short and the tumour is then so close to the uterus that the two cannot be separated. They are therefore likely to be mistaken for fibroids of the uterus.

In the case of definite uterine tumours, the diagnosis of malignant growths is not often difficult because they cause irregular bleeding in addition to uterine enlargement. However, the diagnosis should always be confirmed by microscopic examination of curetted fragments. Fibroids are only likely to be mistaken for malignant growths when they produce constant bleeding as a result of extrusion, infection and sloughing. Rapid growth of a fibroid is more likely to be the result of degenerative changes, such as formation of cysts or necrobiosis, than to the developing of a sarcoma or other malignant growth along with it. The growth of a fibroid after the menopause, however, should make one consider sarcomatous change in it.

Ovary

Pelvic swelling related to the ovary is most likely to be one of the following:

- Benign, including cysts (Fig. P.8) and fibromas.
- Malignant – the primary origin in the form of epithelial tumours (85%), sex cord tumours (6%), germ cell tumours (2%) and uncommonly sarcomas or lymphomas. Secondary tumours (6%) originate from the gut, breast, lung and thyroid.

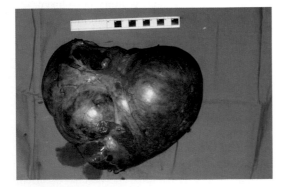

Figure P.8 Ovarian cyst after surgery.

Large tumours arising in the pelvis are not often difficult to differentiate one from another, bearing in mind those ovarian tumours; uterine fibroids and pregnancy are the most commonly occurring conditions. It cannot be repeated too often that amenorrhoea stands for pregnancy, and occasionally for ovarian tumours when bilateral; whilst menorrhagia goes with uterine fibroids except in the case of subperitoneal tumours. Exceptions to these general statements are uncommon, and mistakes in diagnosis will occur, but seldom if these concepts are borne in mind. Ascites must be differentiated from ovarian cysts. In general, ascites give dullness in the flanks on percussion, with resonance over an area somewhere about the umbilicus, whilst ovarian cysts give dullness over the front of the abdomen, with resonance in the flanks. When ascites exist along with ovarian tumours, the free fluid may be so large in amount that the tumour cannot be felt; as a rule, however, it can be touched on dipping through the fluid and the omentum may be ballotable as an omental cake. Ascites with an ovarian tumour does not necessarily mean malignancy. Some fluid may also accompany fibroma of the ovary, or a simple ovarian cyst with a twisted pedicle. Ovarian fibromas may be accompanied by a large amount of ascites and bilateral pleural effusions (Meigs' syndrome). Some of the ascites may be sent for cytology.

When pregnancy is associated with a tumour, the diagnosis may be difficult. This does not lie in the recognition of the pregnancy; amenorrhoea, breast changes, fetal movements and the fetal heart will usually make that clear enough. It lies in deciding the nature, or even the presence of a tumour along with the pregnant uterus. In the early months, when the presence of two tumours can be demonstrated, the diagnosis is easier, but in the later months the great size of the abdomen, and the way in which the swellings merge into one another, may obscure the picture. The relationship to the uterus, whether a part of it, or attached to it by a pedicle; the feel of the tumour, whether solid or cystic, soft or hard; and the previous history, will assist in making out the nature of the growth. Fibroids are likely to soften and degenerate during pregnancy, so that they are liable to be mistaken for ovarian cysts.

In the case of ovarian tumours, it is often impossible to be sure of the exact nature of the growth until this has been decided microscopically after removal. Because of this doubt, there should be no undue delay in the removal of an ovarian tumour larger than the size of an orange, or one that is growing. Small follicular cysts may be left as they are harmless and eventually disappear. Fixation of the growth in the pelvis, obvious ascites, unilateral oedema of the leg, emaciation of the patient, abdominal pain and rapid growth in size of the abdomen all point to malignancy.

As a rule of thumb, a cyst less than 5 cm in diameter may resolve without any action except for repeat scanning after two to three normal periods. If the cyst is larger than 5 cm, it will probably need to be formally removed. Very large cysts tend to be either benign or borderline malignant (Figs P.9 and P.10). The largest cyst ever removed in the UK weighed 63 kg, whilst the world's largest was removed in 1905 in the US and weighed approximately 145 kg. The ovary should not be palpable in a post-menopausal woman, and any ovarian cyst in these women should be considered malignant until proved otherwise.

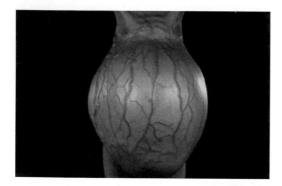

Figure P.9 Clinical picture of patient with ovarian cyst, full frontal.

Fallopian tubes

Pelvic swellings should be one of the following:

- Pregnancy-related, tubal gestation or progressive extra-uterine pregnancy.
- Inflammatory – salpingitis, which may lead to a hydrosalpinx or pyosalpinx.
- Malignant, carcinoma of the Fallopian tube being very uncommon.

With small tumours confined to the pelvis, or rising only a little above the brim, diagnosis is often difficult. In practice, however, extra-uterine gestation and its resulting blood-tumour stand out pre-eminently as a swelling, which must be recognized at once if treatment is to be successful. Before rupture or abortion has occurred, a tubal gestation is essentially a

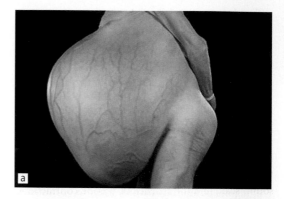

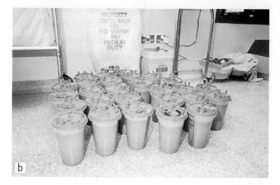

Figure P.10 Same patient as Fig. P.9. (a) Clinical picture of patient, lateral aspect. (b) Contents drained from the cyst.

small tumour in one posterolateral corner of the pelvis, attached to the uterus, indefinite in consistency, remarkably tender, and perhaps – though not always – associated with amenorrhoea of short duration and acute attacks of pain in the pelvis. Definite signs of pregnancy may be entirely wanting, but a pregnancy test will be positive. It may be mistaken for a chronic salpingo-oophoritis, a small cystic ovary, a small pedunculated fibroid or a small ovarian dermoid. The differential diagnosis may be difficult, but attacks of pain unassociated with menstruation are not likely to occur in any of the above conditions; the pains are usually the result of over-distension and stretching of the tube from haemorrhage into its wall or lumen around the fertilized ovum. Unless the swelling is tender (often very tender), it is not likely to be due to a tubal pregnancy. When tubal abortion has occurred, or tubal rupture, the signs of internal bleeding accompanied by sudden pain and collapse, with haemorrhage from the uterus or the passage of a decidual cast, usually create an unmistakable picture. Intraperitoneal haemorrhage is more commonly severe and copious with tubal rupture than with tubal abortion. If the patient recovers from the initial bleeding, the clinical picture may be that of a retro-uterine or peritubal haematocele. The uterus is pushed forwards and upwards against the symphysis pubis, and the mass of blood clot can be felt posteriorly bulging the posterior fornix and also the anterior wall of the rectum. It is very tender. Tubal miscarriage is most likely to be mistaken for an ordinary intra-uterine miscarriage; however, the presence of a tender mass on one side of the uterus, with a closed cervix and a negative ultrasound scan, and the absence of uterine contractions or extrusion of any products of conception, should make the case clear. Pain is much more severe, but external bleeding is much less in extra-uterine pregnancy. The essential point in diagnosing an ectopic pregnancy is to approach every woman of childbearing age who complains of irregular bleeding and abdominal pain with the possibility in mind. No two cases are alike, and there are more exceptions to the rule in the symptomatology of this condition than in any other. It must be emphasized that whilst maternal death is not common in the UK, ectopic pregnancy remains a major cause of it.

Progressive extra-uterine gestation is a rare occurrence, and is the result of continued growth of an embryo after a partial separation from the tube as a result of rupture, or extrusion from the fimbriated end (abortion). The continued enlargement of a mass beside the uterus, with amenorrhoea and progressive signs of pregnancy, are the most characteristic points. Abdominal pain in late pregnancy is a characteristic feature. The uterus may be felt in the pelvis separate from the fetal sac. The diagnosis, however, is difficult, because there is always some effused blood, which obscures the outlines of the uterus, and makes it appear to be a part of the pelvic mass. The fetus is often situated high above the pelvis and it tends to lie transversely facing downward. A radiograph reveals the fetus adopting a position that is characteristically odd, with the spine hyperextended or acutely flexed and the head and limbs at unusual angles to the trunk. If, on a lateral view, radiography shows fetal parts overlapping the maternal spine the pregnancy must be extra-uterine. Ultrasonography will establish the absence of an intra-uterine gestation and also the size of the uterus, which never exceeds that of a 5 months' gestation, even in the presence of a full-term extra-uterine pregnancy, and the cervix does not soften to the same degree. In those cases where the fetus lies in the front of the false sac it will feel very superficial owing the absence of uterine wall in front of it, and between it and the examining hand. However, the fetus is often difficult to palpate, due perhaps to the placenta in front, which may give rise to a loud vascular souffle just medial to the anterior superior iliac spine on the side from which it derives its main blood supply (via the ovarian vessels).

The swellings due to salpingo-oophoritis are usually easy to distinguish. They form fixed tender masses in the pelvis, seldom of any definite shape, but occasionally presenting the characteristic retort shape (with its narrow end near the uterus) which the tube assumes when distended with fluid. The history is usually that of an acute illness at some time, with pain in the pelvis, rise of temperature and peritoneal irritation. It is preceded, as a rule, by uterine discharge and menorrhagia. This inflammatory disturbance in married women is associated with long periods of infertility, owing to the sealing up of the tubes. In the chronic state, the patient complains of pelvic pain, congestive dysmenorrhoea, dyspareunia, vaginal discharge, menorrhagia and infertility. The signs of suppuration, pyrexia, leucocytosis, wasting and daily sweating are usually absent, and the pus in the tubes is sterile.

A large pelvic abscess may accompany salpingo-oophoritis, or it may occur alone without infection of the tubes, as is seen occasionally in puerperal septic infections. When it does occur, it is of course peritoneal; it fixes the uterus in a central position, bulges into the posterior fornix and rectum, tends to rupture into the rectum, before which occurrence there is a copious discharge of mucus per anum, is acute in onset, and accompanied by signs of local peritonitis. A swinging temperature, leucocytosis, sweats and the symptoms of fever are present, all of which suddenly improve when the abscess discharges itself. It is likely to be confounded with pelvic cellulitis, in which the uterus is fixed in a laterally displaced position. This swelling bulges one lateral fornix and extends right out to the lateral pelvic wall, tends to burrow along the round ligament to the groin, and may point there like a psoas abscess, is slow in onset, chronic and not accompanied by signs of local peritonitis. It always follows labour, or abortion, whereas pelvic abscess of peritoneal origin may occur with salpingo-oophoritis or appendicitis, quite apart from pregnancy. Pelvic cellulitis never bears any relationship to salpingo-oophoritis. It may take many weeks to resolve, which it usually does without pointing.

Pelvic peritoneum, retroperitoneal swellings and connective tissue

Encysted peritoneal fluid, hydatid cysts and retroperitoneal lipomas are generally diagnosed as ovarian cysts, and their true nature is only discovered at operation. There are no definite signs by which these conditions may be diagnosed, and as they all require operative treatment, postoperative diagnosis meets their requirements. Encysted peritoneal fluid due to tuberculosis may be suspected if tuberculous lesions are present elsewhere in the body. They lack the definite outline of an ovarian cyst and are often semi-resonant on percussion.

Urachal cysts occur in front of the uterus and in close relation to the bladder; however, in spite of this they are usually mistaken for ovarian cysts. It is to be remembered that ovarian cysts are only likely to locate in front of the uterus when they are large, although small-sized dermoid cysts of the ovary occasionally do so. Urachal cysts are embryological remnants and rarely attain a large size.

The omentum should also be included in this group, which can form a 'cake' as a result of secondary spread from an ovarian tumour. Usually, they tend to be abdominal but can become involved with the tumour pelvically.

Bowel

Appendicitis with pregnancy occurs occasionally, and may be mistaken for such a condition as torsion of an ovarian pedicle. The swelling due to appendix inflammation is, however, in close relation to the anterior superior spine of the ilium, and apparently adherent to the iliac fossa. The lump is ill-defined, and rarely fluctuates unless there is a large abscess. The acute onset may be similar to that of torsion of an ovarian pedicle. There is usually a definite fluctuating tumour when an ovarian cyst is present, and some interval between it and the iliac crest can usually be felt. Bowel cancer is more common than the common gynaecological tumours, as is diverticulitis; these patients tend to display altered bowel problems.

Bone

Tumours of the pelvic bones are rare, but they may be cartilaginous or sarcomatous in origin. They may be mistaken for fixed tissues which arise secondary to chronic pelvic infection, leading to a frozen pelvis. They will be found to be continuous with the bones forming the pelvis, and when growing from the sacrum may have the rectum in front of them; all other pelvic tumours have the rectum behind them. In most cases of this nature the uterus and adnexae can be palpated bimanually, and shown to be free from disease and unconnected with the mass. When complicated by the presence of a pregnant uterus, their true nature may be difficult to determine unless examination reveals that they are absolutely fixed and are continuous with the bones of the pelvis.

Other structures

Many of these lesions are not primarily pelvic, but they are included in the list because they are liable to be mistaken for pelvic tumours. Thus, renal, splenic or pancreatic tumours may reach the pelvic brim, but the history ought to show that they have grown down from above, not up from below. Renal swellings may be associated with urinary changes, or an absence of urinary secretion on the affected side as detected by cystoscopy or intravenous pyelogram. Malformations of the genital tract are associated with developmental abnormalities of the renal tract. It is not uncommon to find a solitary pelvic kidney in patients with a congenital absence of the vagina and uterus. Splenic enlargements may be associated with blood changes. Pancreatic cysts are the least likely to be mistaken for pelvic swellings, but they have been difficult to distinguish from ovarian tumours with long pedicles.

Antony Hollingworth

PENILE SORES

Sores on the penis may be present on the thin mucous covering of the glans or prepuce, or on the cutaneous surface of the body of the penis; they are more common in the former situation.

Ulceration in the neighbourhood of the glans penis may be due to:

- Balanitis
- Herpes genitalis
- Soft sore
- Granuloma venereum (inguinale)
- Lymphogranuloma inguinale (venereum)
- Chancre
- Epithelioma
- Papilloma

Balanitis

If inflammatory processes have been allowed to continue beneath the prepuce, ulceration and excoriation of the mucous membrane covering the glans penis or lining the prepuce will occur, accompanied by a stinking, purulent discharge. Multiple shallow ulcers are formed, rapidly coalescing and causing considerable discomfort. The prepuce often becomes swollen and oedematous, preventing retraction, so that a condition of phimosis occurs. Alternatively, if retraction has taken place, the analogous state of paraphimosis will occur, almost strangulating the end of the penis and even causing it to become gangrenous. Care must be exercised in diagnosing a simple balanitis from one accompanying acute gonorrhoeal urethritis or an underlying syphilitic or soft chancre. The so-called balanitis circinata is part of Reiter's syndrome, occurring in association with urethritis, arthritis, conjunctivitis (often slight and transient) and buccal ulceration. In Behçet's syndrome, ulcerative penile and scrotal lesions may also occur in association with buccal ulcers. With an acute urethritis there will be a history of infection and pain along the course of the urethra during micturition; the intracellular gonococcus may be identified in a Gram-stained smear of the discharge.

If a chancre exists under the swollen phimosed prepuce, there is often a tender spot about the corona or at the fraenum. With a soft sore, consecutive sores may appear about the orifice of the prepuce, while the inguinal nodes are much more likely to be inflamed or to suppurate than with simple balanitis. A syphilitic chancre obscured by a phimosis can usually be felt distinctly under the skin, and causes a comparatively small amount of discharge, while the inguinal nodes become enlarged but do not suppurate. The interval of about 4 weeks from the time of the possible source of infection until the appearance of the sore will suggest, and the finding of spirochaetes (*Treponema pallidum*) in the fluid expressed from the ulcer will prove, the diagnosis. In later cases, enlargement of the inguinal nodes, secondary cutaneous rash, sore throat and positive serological reactions will be present.

A form of balanitis, which is frequently very obstinate to treatment, may occur in patients with diabetes mellitus. The main causative organism is *Candida albicans*. Phimosis appearing in an adult male is often due to unsuspected diabetes; the urine should always be tested for sugar.

Herpes genitalis

Herpes may attack the genital organs as part of a herpes zoster which is unilateral. This is a rarity compared with herpes simplex, which is now regarded as an important sexually transmitted disease. Recent studies have implicated *herpes simplex virus* Type 2 in the aetiology of uterine cervical cancer. The disease begins as a patch of erythema on the inner surface of the prepuce or on the glans penis, followed by vesicles and pustules; the latter become rubbed by the clothes, and form small ulcers. Herpes of the genital organs tends to recur, so that a previous history of a similar attack is often forthcoming. If seen during the vesicular stage no difficulty will be met with in the diagnosis; however, if suppuration has followed it must be diagnosed from a venereal sore. Soft chancres are usually deeper, with marked edges; their bases are sloughing, and they are usually accompanied by a bubo (enlarged inguinal lymph node, which may suppurate), which is exceptional with herpes. A syphilitic chancre is usually single, indurated and raised, and is accompanied by the typical multiple, discrete nodes in the inguinal region. It should be remembered that syphilis may become inoculated upon a herpetic patch or that herpes may appear in an area already infected with syphilis.

Soft sores or chancroids

Soft sores or chancroids of the penis occur almost invariably from infection during sexual connection. The incubation period is short, a vesicle occurs in 2 days, and this breaks down rapidly to form a rounded or oval ulcer with undermined edges and a yellowish, sloughing base. The ulcers appear usually on the mucous surface of the glans, fraenum or corona, and are multiple, with direct inoculation occurring from each ulcer to the contiguous part. They may cause rapid destruction of tissue, perforating the fraenum or spreading over the surface of the glans. The soft sore must be differentiated from others occurring on the gland, and above all from a syphilitic chancre, and serum from the edge of the lesion should be examined for *Haemophilus ducreyi* (Ducrey's bacillus) as well as by dark-ground illumination for *Treponema pallidum*. At the same time, it must be remembered that besides the infection with chancroid, a simultaneous infection with syphilis may have taken place, so that a soft sore may ultimately become indurated and assume the character of a primary syphilitic lesion. The chancroids are multiple, are accompanied by a good deal of thin, purulent discharge, and by a painful swelling of the inguinal nodes, usually of one side, which have a marked tendency to suppurate. On the other hand, a syphilitic chancre is single, is raised and indurated, has little discharge, and is accompanied by enlarged but firm and indolent nodes in both inguinal regions; the incubation period of a syphilitic chancre is from 21 to 28 days. The multiple ulcerations caused by herpes are more superficial.

Granuloma inguinale

Granuloma inguinale (granuloma venereum) is a chronic granulomatous ulceration which may affect the perineum and the inguinal regions, as well as the penis. The condition occurs in tropical countries and is mildly contagious. The lesion on the penis starts as a papule which appears after a few days' or weeks' incubation period, and breaks down to form a superficial ulcer. Examination of the discharge shows intracellular capsulated Gram-negative rods known as Donovan bodies (*Donvania granulomatis*). Lymph nodes are not involved.

Lymphogranuloma venereum

Lymphogranuloma venereum (lymphogranuloma inguinale) is also more common in the tropics, and is a chronic condition characterized by a small initial lesion on the penis with marked glandular enlargement in the groins and severe constitutional disturbances. The nodes tend to break down and form sinuses. The lesion on the penis appears, after an incubation period of about a week, as a vesicle, papule or ulcer, and this tends to disappear by the time that the lymphatic nodes are enlarged. It is due to a filter-passing organism, *Chlamydia trachomatis*, which can be diagnosed by complement fixation reactions, demonstration of specific skin reactivity (Frei's test) and, if necessary, a biopsy of the primary lesion or lymph node. It must be distinguished from chancroid and from granuloma venereum. Rectal stricture and effusions into joints are other lesions caused by this disease.

Chancre

Chancre – the initial lesion of syphilis – generally appears on the penis, and is most common in the neighbourhood of the fraenum or coronary sulcus. A chancre appears about 25 days after infection as a reddened patch, which becomes raised above the surface of the mucous membrane, with distinctly indurated margins. The central part breaks down into an ulcer (Fig. P.11), discharging a thin, purulent fluid, and at the same time the inguinal nodes of both sides become palpable, slightly enlarged but discrete, and with no tendency to suppurate. The chancre increases only slowly in size, or may occasionally become smaller without any treatment. After a further lapse of from 4 to 6 weeks, if the condition remains untreated, the typical secondary symptoms make their appearance – namely, a roseolar rash on the chest, abdomen, face and thighs, general adenitis, and mucous patches about the faucial pillars and tonsils, accompanied by low pyrexia. The diagnosis of the primary lesion of syphilis frequently presents no difficulties, the indurated character of the sore, the date of its appearance after infection, and the presence of firm, indurated nodes in the inguinal region being distinctive. If the character of

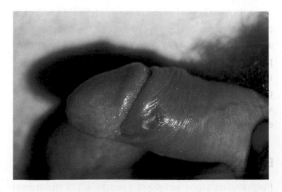

Figure P.11 Primary chancre of the penis.

the sore is not distinctive it is necessary to differentiate it from other lesions of the penis. A careful search must be made using dark-ground illumination for *Treponema pallidum* in serum expressed from the sore; negative serological reactions in the early stage of the disease are not reliable. If the sore is syphilitic, the secondary manifestations of the disease will follow, provided that the doubtful ulcer is not treated as a chancre.

A chancre may be simulated by an inflamed soft sore; soft sores are, however, frequently multiple, appear within a few days of infection, and are accompanied by painful enlargement of the inguinal lymphatic nodes, which are particularly prone to suppurate. It must not be forgotten that a double infection may have occurred, so that a soft sore may show little inclination to heal or, by becoming indurated, may present the features of a chancre after about 3 weeks, followed later by the symptoms of constitutional syphilis.

Epithelioma of the penis (see below) in the early stage may be confused with syphilitic chancre. In epithelioma, there is no history of infection; it occurs usually in elderly uncircumcised patients, and there is frequently a greater destruction of tissue than in syphilis. The inguinal nodes are not enlarged until the sore has been present for some weeks, and there are no secondary lesions such as the faucial ulceration and cutaneous rash. Diagnosis is confirmed by histological examination of a biopsy specimen.

Perhaps the greatest difficulty in the diagnosis of a chancre is experienced when it is hidden beneath an inflamed and phimosed prepuce. There is a purulent and foul discharge from beneath the oedematous and swollen prepuce; the inguinal nodes are enlarged from the associated sepsis. If a chancre is present, it can frequently be felt as an indurated area under the prepuce, but if it has been present for some time the secondary lesions of syphilis may be identified. If any doubt exists as to whether an indurated subpreputial area is an early epithelioma or a syphilitic sore, the prepuce should be split up along the dorsal aspect under anaesthesia, the ulceration inspected, a small piece submitted to microscopical examination if necessary, or some serum expressed from the ulcer and examined on a dark stage for *Treponema pallidum*.

Epithelioma

Epithelioma (squamous cell carcinoma) is the most common form of malignant growth of the penis

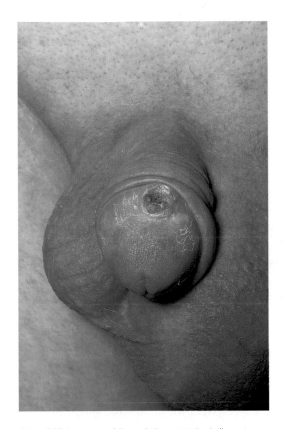

Figure P.12 Carcinoma of the penis (prepuce retracted).

(Fig. P.12). It arises most frequently from the inner aspect of the prepuce, or from the mucous membrane of the glans, as a small, raised ulcer with friable, irregular edges. It is rarely present before the age of 40 years, and frequently occurs on the site of previous ulceration or long-standing irritation. It is unknown where circumcision has been performed in infancy, although later circumcision does not confer this near-total immunity. An epitheliomatous ulcer increases in size gradually in spite of various forms of treatment, and with it is frequently associated enlargement of the inguinal lymph nodes. At first, the nodes may be enlarged from septic infection, but later from malignant infiltration. An epitheliomatous ulcer may in some cases be confused with a chancre; however, the friable, irregular edges of the former, the liability to bleed, and the gradual progressive increase in size in spite of treatment, in an elderly patient, together with the extensive induration of the base, should give rise to grave suspicion of malignant disease. Microscopical examination of a biopsy from the edge of the ulcer will provide direct evidence of epithelioma.

Carcinoma of the penis may also occur in a *papillary form*, which grows to produce a large 'cauliflower' excrescence. In this form, any enlargement of the inguinal nodes is more likely to be due to infection than to metastasis.

Papillomas

Papillomas (venereal warts or condylomata acuminata) occur on the glans and contiguous surface of the prepuce, and are most frequently found on the corona. They are simple papillomas, usually multiple, and are distinguished from epithelioma by the absence of induration in the base.

Gummatous ulceration

Today, gummatous ulceration of the penis occurs with great rarity, resulting from the disintegration of a small gumma of the glans or prepuce, frequently in the position of an old scar. A gumma begins as a small, elevated nodule which, if left untreated, softens and discharges its contents, leaving an ulcer bounded by thin edges and with a yellowish, sloughy base.

Tuberculous ulceration

Tuberculous ulceration of the penis is rare, and is generally associated with advanced tuberculous infiltration elsewhere. Tuberculous ulcers are usually shallow, with thin overhanging edges, painful and multiple. The diagnosis is clinched by discovering tubercle bacilli in films made from the discharge.

Injury

Injury is an uncommon cause of a penile sore.

Harold Ellis

PENIS, PAIN IN

Pain in the penis is a symptom which occurs not only in association with lesions of the penis or urethra, but also as a referred pain from disease of the prostate, bladder or kidney. Penile pain may be present either during or immediately after micturition, or it may be entirely independent of the act. If pain is felt only during micturition there is probably some inflammatory lesion of the urethra or prostate; however, if it occurs immediately after the flow of urine it suggests the presence of a lesion in the urinary bladder, whilst pain present quite apart from micturition may be due to various diseases of the penis, bladder, ureter or kidney.

The term 'pain' is also a relative quantity, varying with the nervous susceptibility of the patient. What is pain in one patient may be merely discomfort in another; thus, the patient's description may have to be discounted to a certain extent by the clinician.

Penile pain experienced during micturition

- Diseases of the urethra
  - Acute inflammation, gonorrhoeal or other
  - The passage or impaction of a calculus
  - Stricture of the urethra
  - Injury of the urethra
  - Foreign body in the urethra
- Diseases of the prostate
  - Acute prostatitis
  - Prostatic abscess
  - Prostatic carcinoma
- Diseases of the bladder
  - Acute cystitis
  - Vesicle calculus
  - Papilloma
  - Pedunculated carcinoma

Diseases of the urethra

The most common cause of pain in the penis during micturition is acute inflammation of the urethra, often gonorrhoeal. However, such pain may also result from other organisms, and is particularly common following catheterization. Non-specific urethritis – a common sexually transmitted infection – is diagnosed when gonorrhoea and other bacterial infections have been excluded. Frequently this is due to *Chlamydia trachomatis* or *Trichomonas vaginalis* (see URETHRAL DISCHARGE, p. 762). In the earliest stages of an acute urethritis, before any marked urethral discharge is apparent, there is usually a sense of smarting or tingling in the terminal urethra, and this becomes more marked as the discharge increases, when it is of a burning or scalding character. The pain during micturition within a few days of sexual connection is frequently the earliest symptom of urethral infection;

a purulent discharge from the urethra is usually present when the patient comes under observation.

The passage of a calculus through the urethra causes a sharp, cutting pain along the urethra, the cause of which is apparent when the calculus is voided. A stone may, however, pass into the urethra during micturition and become arrested at some narrowed portion of the canal, usually at the membranous portion or at the distal end. At this point a sudden sharp pain is felt in the urethra, and at the same time the flow of urine is partially or completely stopped before the bladder has been emptied. Further efforts to expel urine result only in a forceless stream. The whole length of the urethra should be examined by passing the finger along its course, when a stone may be actually felt; alternatively, the calculus may be seen through an endoscope or identified on a plain radiograph.

Occasionally, a calculus may remain in the urethra, becoming gradually enlarged in size and causing pain on micturition. These calculi usually lie in the dilated posterior urethra behind a stricture in the bulb.

Urethral stricture occasionally causes pain during micturition, especially if the calibre is small, and if there is septic infection or ulceration of the urethral mucosa behind the stricture, though as a rule a stricture causes little pain. A gradually increasing difficulty in micturition, a feeble stream and dribbling of urine from the meatus after the stream has terminated are common symptoms. The diagnosis will be confirmed by the obstruction offered to the passage of a full-sized bougie or, better, by direct observation of the urethra through a urethroscope.

Injury of the urethra may cause pain during micturition. The urethra may be injured by a fall on the perineum, by a kick or blow, or by the faulty or careless passage of instruments; it may also be injured or lacerated in association with a fracture of the pelvis. The urethra may be merely bruised, lacerated on one aspect, or completely ruptured. If it is lacerated by direct injury, blood usually appears at the external urinary meatus, together with a contusion in the perineum or along the course of the urethra. Any attempt at micturition causes pain in the penis, while urine may or may not be expelled from the meatus, depending upon the extent of the injury, or it may be extravasated into the perineal or scrotal tissues (Fig. P.13). As a rule, there will be no difficulty in the diagnosis.

A *foreign body* in the urethra may cause considerable pain. In some cases the history will be clear; for

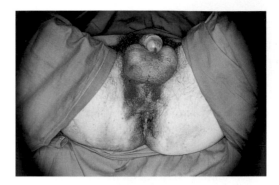

Figure P.13 Traumatic rupture of the bulb of the urethra showing blood at the meatus and perineal haematoma limited posteriorly by the attachment of Colle's fascia to the perineal membrane.

instance, the end of a catheter or bougie may have broken off within the urethra. However, in other cases – and especially in weak-minded individuals – no history of the insertion of a foreign body into the urethra will be forthcoming. Urethroscopy will show the foreign body; various articles have been found in the urethra, such as a wax taper, a seed of barley with its barb, a hairpin, a small shell, a nail and a windscreen wiper rubber.

Diseases of the prostate

Acute prostatitis and *prostatic abscess* both give rise to pain during micturition in addition to increased frequency and difficulty during the act. Both are usually sequelae of an acute urethritis, and whereas an acute prostatitis is accompanied by a temperature raised to 38°C (100–101°F), a prostatic abscess causes the usual rise and fall common to septic processes. The diagnosis of the two conditions is made by careful rectal examination, the acutely inflamed gland presenting a much enlarged, smooth-surfaced prominence in the rectum. By contrast, if an abscess is present a softer, acutely tender area in the inflamed gland can usually be detected.

Adenomatous enlargement of the prostate does not give rise to any penile pain during micturition; however, pain in the penis is present during micturition occasionally in cases of prostatic carcinoma, owing to direct infiltration of the urethral mucous membrane. Prostatic carcinoma is by no means uncommon (indeed, it is the fourth most common cause of death from cancer in the UK), and whilst in terms of its general symptoms it resembles prostatic adenoma, a marked difference is found on digital examination of the gland per rectum. The carcinomatous gland, once clinically obvious, presents rounded areas of densely infiltrated tissue, in contradistinction to the elastic, uniform feel of the adenomatous variety. The whole gland becomes fixed and immovable, and in advanced stages distinct infiltration of the lateral pelvic lymphatics and soft tissues may be felt extending laterally from the affected organ. It is often tender on palpation.

Care must be taken not to mistake the hard nodules felt in a prostate containing calculi for carcinoma. With calculous disease, the gland is not fixed and is only slightly enlarged. Radiography will distinguish the two conditions (see Fig. K.10), but they may co-exist.

Diseases of the bladder

Diseases of the bladder may cause penile pain during micturition under certain circumstances, although it is much more common to find that pain in vesical disease follows the completion of micturition. In acute cystitis, penile pain is present throughout micturition, due to the intense congestion of the vesical mucous membrane of the trigone and around the internal urethral orifice. The other symptoms of acute cystitis, namely surprapubic pain, pyrexia, increased frequency of micturition and the presence of pus and blood in the urine, suggest the diagnosis.

Pain during micturition in other vesical lesions is caused whenever there is sudden obstruction to the normal flow of urine by the impaction of something against the internal urethral orifice. This may occur with a small calculus or with a pedunculated tumour (whether simple or malignant) when, during micturition, the flow is arrested suddenly. This is accompanied by a shooting pain in the urethra, and after an interval of a few seconds the stream may be re-established. With vesical calculus the urine may be normal or may contain pus and blood if the bladder has become infected; there is penile pain after micturition, and the stone will be seen both on plain X-ray of the pelvis and with cystoscopy. With a simple villous papilloma there is no pain unless part of the fimbriated portion of the tumour engages in the urethral orifice during micturition; however, there are usually recurrent attacks of profuse haematuria. With a carcinoma, there is increased frequency of micturition, with pain following the act, and more frequent

haematuria. Upon rectal examination, the base of the bladder may be felt to be infiltrated, but by far the most valuable means of diagnosis between the three conditions is by cystoscopy, when a calculus or villous tumour is seen readily, whereas a pedunculated carcinoma appears as a dark red tumour covered with stunted processes.

Penile pain following micturition

This symptom is common to many lesions of the urinary bladder, more especially those in which there is ulceration or infiltration of the basal areas. The particular pain felt by the patient is described as a sharp pricking or tingling at the terminal part of the penis on the cessation of micturition, lasting some minutes, and causing a desire to squeeze the glans. It was thought to be diagnostic of vesical calculus, but this is far from being the case, for it may be due to almost any affection of the trigone.

The common causes of pain in the penis following upon micturition are:

- Vesical
  - ◆ Calculus
  - ◆ Tuberculosis
  - ◆ Tumour (carcinoma, papilloma)
  - ◆ Acute cystitis
  - ◆ Billharzia (schistosomiasis)
- Ureteric
  - ◆ Calculus in lower end
  - ◆ Tuberculous ureteritis
- Prostatic
  - ◆ Acute inflammation
  - ◆ Abscess
- Vesicular
  - ◆ Acute seminal vesiculitis
- Rectal
  - ◆ Carcinoma
- Anal
  - ◆ Fissure or ulcer
  - ◆ Inflamed haemorrhoids

Diseases of the bladder

A *calculus* in the bladder, unless it is trapped in the pouch behind an enlarged prostate or in a diverticulum, causes pain in the glans penis after micturition. It may exist without causing cystitis, although commonly there is some degree of pyuria when the case is first seen. There is increased frequency of micturition during active exercise or during the jolting of travelling, but not during complete rest unless cystitis is marked.

The terminal drops of urine during micturition are often tinged with blood, and on some occasions there may have been a sudden stoppage of the stream during micturition. In some cases there is a history of acutely painful colic due to the descent of a stone from the kidney without the subsequent passage of a calculus in the urine. Patients subjected to vesical stone have usually reached the later part of life in the UK, although bladder stones in children are still common in the tropics.

The great majority of vesical calculi are radio-opaque and can be seen on a plain X-ray of the pelvis. At cystoscopy, stones can be seen, their approximate size determined, and any other conditions of the bladder accompanying or simulating calculus may be diagnosed with certainty.

Vesical tuberculosis is usually secondary to tuberculous disease in some other part of the genitourinary tract, particularly the kidney. It causes marked penile pain after micturition, together with pyuria and a tinge of blood in the terminal drops of urine. The frequency of micturition is increased during both day and night, and is uninfluenced by rest, thus differing from the increased frequency of calculous disease. Vesical tuberculosis occurs in young adults, and is usually associated with renal tuberculosis in which symptoms referable to the bladder are commonly present before the bladder is attacked by disease. In a young patient in whom increased frequency of micturition, pyuria and penile pain are present, a search should be made for any tuberculous focus, especially in the kidneys by excretion urography, and in the epididymes, prostate or seminal vesicles, or for marked thickening of the terminal ureter as felt per rectum.

Routine laboratory examination of the urine reveals an acid urine, with pus cells but no growth on routine culture – the so-called 'sterile acid pyuria'. The deposit from three early morning specimens should be examined for acid-fast bacilli, and if this is negative, the search should be continued by culture, which requires up to 6 weeks in special nutrient-reinforced media. A cystoscopic examination may be necessary to determine the extent of the disease.

Vesical tumours: carcinoma of the bladder occurs in either a papillary or a solid form. Papillary

carcinoma is at first non-infiltrating, while the solid nodular and ulcerative types and adenocarcinoma are infiltrating. They begin most commonly in the base of the bladder; the submucous coat and the muscular wall become infiltrated by malignant cells so that contraction of the bladder during micturition causes pain which is referred to the terminal portion of the urethra. All forms occur in elderly patients, mostly men, and give rise to increased frequency of micturition during both day and night, and to haematuria. They also often give rise to renal pain when the infiltration has extended to the ureteric orifice in the bladder.

The incidental cystogram of intravenous urography (Figs P.14 and P.15) may sometimes afford visual proof of the deformity that the new growth is producing, or of a filling defect in the otherwise regular contour of the bladder.

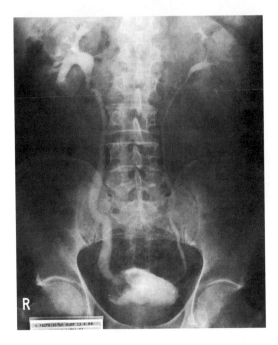

Figure P.14 Intravenous urogram taken 20 minutes after injection. There is a filling defect on the right side of the bladder due to a large benign papilliferous tumour. Both kidneys are normal.

Under anaesthesia, the base of the bladder may be felt per rectum to be thickened, or lymphatic infiltration may be felt in the lateral pelvic space, and a cystoscopic examination, together with biopsy, will usually clarify the diagnosis.

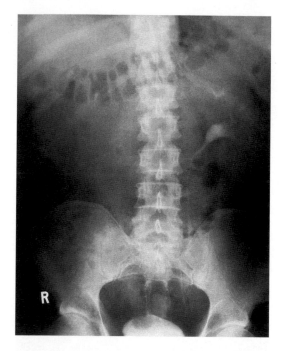

Figure P.15 Intravenous urogram. There is a filling defect on the right side of the bladder caused by infiltrating carcinoma. The right ureteric orifice has been obstructed, and there is no function of the right kidney.

Whereas solid infiltrating growths of the bladder give rise to penile pain after micturition as a result of direct infiltration of the vesical walls, the pedunculated papillary carcinoma and the simple villous papilloma may occasionally give rise to sharp penile pain during micturition from blocking of the internal urethral orifice by a process of growth. The occurrence of this, together with attacks of profuse haematuria, is suggestive of a pedunculated growth. On cystoscopic examination the carcinomatous pedunculated tumour is seen to be covered by blunt, stunted processes, whereas the innocent villous papilloma presents much more delicate fimbriae.

Acute cystitis causes tingling pain in the penis after micturition from the inflammatory infiltration of the trigonal area. The mode of onset, the character of the pain and other symptoms of cystitis will point to the cause of the pain.

Bilharzia (*schistosomiasis*), due to infection with the trematode *Schistosoma haematobium*, gives rise to clinical symptoms that are very similar to those of vesical tuberculosis. The history of residence in an infected district (e.g. Egypt or East Africa), microscopical examination of the urine for parasitic ova, and the typical cystoscopic appearance of the bladder establish the diagnosis.

Radiographs may show calcification of the bladder or ureters, and pyelography often demonstrates stricture formation and gross dilatation of the ureters.

Ureteric lesions

Ureteric lesions infrequently produce pain in the glans penis after micturition, and may cause considerable difficulty in the diagnosis from vesical disease.

When a calculus becomes impacted in the narrowed terminal or intramural portion of the ureter, symptoms are produced almost exactly similar to those of vesical calculus or tuberculosis, namely increased frequency of micturition, referred pain in the glans penis after micturition, and a small amount of pus and blood in the urine. Intimate knowledge of the history of the illness will often be of value in these cases; the first attack of pain is usually described as being sudden, and felt in the renal angle posteriorly, passing forwards above the iliac crest and spine and finally becoming localized at the situation of the external abdominal ring. The calculus may become impacted in the terminal 2.5 cm of the ureter when, in addition to this pain, there will be increased frequency of micturition and penile pain, and possible haematuria. With ureteric calculus there is usually aching pain in the kidney of the affected side from the dilatation of its pelvis. The diagnosis of these cases is not difficult if a careful inquiry is made into the history and symptoms, and so long as it is remembered that increased frequency of micturition and penile pain may be caused by ureteric impaction of a calculus. A good radiographic examination of the pelvic area areas may show the shadow of a stone. Indeed, some 90 per cent of these calculi are radio-opaque but, when small, may mimic phleboliths or be obscured by gas shadows or underlying bony structures. A cystoscopic examination also affords valuable information, not only in excluding vesical lesions, but by giving a distinct indication of ureteric calculus by the marked congestion and dilatation of the blood vessels in the immediate vicinity of the ureteric orifice. An intravenous pyelogram may demonstrate obstruction of the ureter and confirm that the calculus lies in its lumen. A catheter passed into the ureter may meet with obstruction in its passage; a radiograph of the pelvis with an opaque catheter passed into the ureter will show the shadow to be in the immediate line of the ureter.

Ureteritis descending from infection of the renal pelvis may give rise to slight penile pain and to increased frequency of micturition, and thus simulate vesical disease before the bladder is actually infected. This is seen most commonly in the tuberculosis form, but is present in a less marked degree with infection by other organisms, of which the most common are *Escherichia coli* and *Streptococcus faecalis*.

In renal tuberculosis, the penile pain and increased frequency of micturition are more marked, the kidney may be felt enlarged and tender, and tubercle bacilli will be found in the urine. Apart from this, typical changes in the ureteric orifice are seen on cystoscopic examination, the orifice being pulled up or retracted or horseshoe-shaped, and usually occupying a position slightly above and outside the situation of the normal orifice, due to the actual shortening of the ureter by infiltration of the submucous coats. The rigid 'golf-hole' ureteric orifice is a late manifestation caused by contraction of scar tissue around it and in the ureter above it.

Diseases of the prostate

These often cause pain in the penis immediately following micturition. This is seen most commonly with acute inflammation or abscess in the gland as a sequela of acute gonorrhoea or septic urethritis. In either case there is penile pain, sometimes associated with erection, but little difficulty will be experienced in the diagnosis on due consideration of the symptoms and upon rectal examination.

Diseases of the seminal vesicles

These are seldom present without accompanying disease of the prostate or bladder. Acute vesiculitis may follow urethritis and give rise to pain after micturition, but in most cases it will be associated with prostatitis. Similarly, tuberculous nodules in the vesicle will be associated with foci in the epididymis, prostate or bladder.

Diseases of the rectum and anus

These may occasionally give rise to penile pain following micturition, apart from any infection of the bladder or prostate. Thus, an infiltrating carcinoma in the anal canal, a rectal fissure or an inflamed haemorrhoid may occasionally cause pain in the penis, but in each the local symptoms of the trouble will be the more marked, and little difficulty will be found in the diagnosis if a local examination is made with care.

Pain in the penis apart from micturition

Under the above divisions, the symptom of penile pain has been considered in relation to the act of micturition, and it remains to consider some conditions giving rise to pain in the penis apart from urination. These include certain lesions of the penis and urethra, and also the pains referred from disease elsewhere. Although a local lesion may cause little more than discomfort in many patients, in some it is described as pain, the degree of which depends upon the nervous susceptibility of the individual. Thus, penile pain may be present with acute urethritis, with balanitis in association with phimosis or with paraphimosis. In some instances herpes of the prepuce of penile skin causes distinct pain. Any infiltration of the cavernous tissue of the penis causes pain during erection of the organ; thus, during an attack of acute urethritis the symptom known as chordee arises from this cause. It may occur in a chronic form in Peyronie's disease (chronic indurative cavernositis), a condition of unknown aetiology but similar to – and sometimes associated with – Dupuytren's contracture and retroperitoneal fibrosis. In this condition, erection is not only painful but may be accompanied by lateral deviation of the organ. Another condition causing the same trouble arises from the organization of a haematoma in the cavernous tissues of the penis following upon a local injury, due either to external violence or arising during forcible attempts at coitus. A similar condition may arise spontaneously in blood diseases, especially lymphatic or myelocytic leukaemia.

Epithelioma of the penis on rare occasions gives rise to pain in the organ.

Pain may be felt in the penis in some cases of renal colic, in which case it is classed as a referred pain. Thus, in the acute colic accompanying the passage of a calculus, blood clot or debris of caseous material, aching pain may be felt in the penis quite apart from the increased desire to pass urine. Penile pain is, however, only a minor detail in the presence of the severe pain in the loin, and along the course of the ureter, and is often only lightly alluded to or revealed on direct questioning of the patient.

Finally, pain in the penis may be based on an anxiety state or some other mental cause rather than organic disease.

Harold Ellis

PERINEUM, PAIN IN

Pain in the perineum is a symptom often mentioned by patients in giving their history of some affection of the genitourinary apparatus or of other organs, but usually only as a dull aching, of which little notice is taken, as it is generally of minor degree in comparison with other more striking symptoms. The complaint of perineal pain *per se* does not convey much information to the clinician, and it is practically never present as the only symptom in a case. It may be a manifestation of an anxiety state.

Aching in the perineum is frequently present in diseases of the following organs:

- Prostate
  - ◆ Chronic prostatitis
  - ◆ Abscess
  - ◆ Calculus
  - ◆ Adenomatous enlargement
  - ◆ Carcinoma
- Seminal vesicles
  - ◆ Acute inflammation
  - ◆ Tuberculosis
- Testis
  - ◆ Congenital misplacement in perineum
- Urinary bladder
  - ◆ Cystitis
  - ◆ Tuberculosis
  - ◆ Calculus
  - ◆ Carcinoma
- Urethra
  - ◆ Injury
  - ◆ Gonorrhoea
  - ◆ Stricture with extravasation or urethral abscess
  - ◆ Fistula
  - ◆ Calculus impacted in bulbo-prostatic portion
- Anal area
  - ◆ Haemorrhoids

- ◆ Fissure
- ◆ Carcinoma
- Vagina
  - ◆ Acute inflammation
  - ◆ Inflammation or abscess of Bartholin's glands
  - ◆ Cystocele
  - ◆ Epithelioma
- Cutaneous diseases
  - ◆ Intertrigo
  - ◆ Diabetic inflammation
  - ◆ Condylomas

From the foregoing list it will be seen that aching in the perineum occurs with numerous different lesions, but other symptoms discussed elsewhere are in almost every case more marked. In prostatic disease it is an indication of inflammation rather than of enlargement. In clinical practice, it is most commonly found to be due to chronic prostatitis. Examination of the secretion expressed after prostatic massage will show the presence of many pus cells.

Harold Ellis

PERINEUM, ULCERATION IN

Ulceration may be present in the perineum as the result of:

- Cutaneous inflammation or injury
- Urethral suppurations or fistulas
- Prostatic suppuration
- Anal fistula
- Syphilis
- Granuloma venereum (inguinale)
- Lymphogranuloma inguinale (venereum)
- Epithelioma and other cutaneous cancers

Cutaneous inflammation or injury

An ulcer in the perineum may result from direct injury to the area, or from infection of the sebaceous or hair follicles. An ulcer from these causes may be placed at the centre or to one side of the perineum, is movable on the deeper parts, and shows no track into which a probe can be passed. In women, ulceration of the perineal area may be associated with gonorrhoeal or septic vaginal discharge. It may also arise from severe scratching caused by the irritation of such skin infections as tinea cruris or pruritus ani.

Urethral suppurations or fistulas

During the progress of an acute urethritis a glandular follicle may become infected. The suppurative process leading from this in the bulbous urethra may extend towards the perineum and open externally, leaving a small fistula which may or may not discharge urine during the act of micturition. In a similar manner, urinary fistulas may result from inflammatory processes behind a urethral stricture, and in an old-standing case it is not uncommon to find a urinary calculus in the dilated portion of the urethra behind the stricture. Where the urethral suppuration is acute and an abscess bursts in the perineum, the diagnosis will be obvious, and the ordinary treatment for an abscess, in addition to that of the acute urethritis, will usually suffice to cure the condition. If the perineal wound discharges urine this occurs usually only during the act of micturition, as there is no interference with the vesical sphincter. A stricture of the urethra, not necessarily of sufficient degree to cause severe interference with micturition, will generally be seen on endoscopic examination, the sloughy granulations behind it denoting the position of the urethral opening of the fistula.

Diseases of the prostate

An abscess or tuberculous focus in the prostate may occasionally discharge in the perineum, and remain as a sinus. An abscess in the prostate arises practically always from some infection in the posterior urethra, from venereal causes, or after septic instrumentation. It is accompanied by urethral discharge, or there is a history of a recent infection, whilst per rectum the prostate may be felt to be inflamed, or scarred from the shrinkage of the abscess cavity.

Anal fistula

An ulcer on the perineum may be present as the result of an anal fistula – commonly from perianal suppuration and occasionally as a tuberculous infection. The history of pain on defecation followed by the rupture of an abscess and the history of passage of flatus or faecal matter from the fistula are usually present, or a probe may be passed into the fistula and felt by a finger passed into the rectum. Perianal and perirectal abscesses, fissures and fistulas may occur in Crohn's disease, especially when the colon is involved, and less commonly in ulcerative colitis.

Syphilis

Syphilis may cause ulceration on the perineum either as a chancre or as mucous tubercles. A chancre at this site is rare. It forms a small ulcer with slightly indurated borders, indolent in character, and accompanied by slight enlargement of the inguinal lymph nodes. A chancre of the skin may not possess the usual features of a genital chancre, and is not usually diagnosed with certainty until the secondary lesions of syphilis become apparent; but an ulcer with raised, infiltrated edges, which shows no tendency to heal under aseptic precautions, should always give rise to a suspicion of syphilis. *Treponema pallidum* should be looked for, under dark-ground illumination, and serological tests for syphilis performed.

Condylomas may be present about the perineum in association with active syphilis. They may extend from the anal or vulval orifice, and form oval or rounded, flat-topped, sessile masses, covered by macerated greyish epithelium, or they may be ulcerated on the surface. The accompanying signs of syphilis will indicate the diagnosis.

Soft sores may occur in the perineum as well as on the scrotum or the vulva; they are generally venereal, but are not in themselves syphilitic; they are generally multiple, are apt to be foul, and cultures from them yield Ducrey's bacillus (*Haemophilus ducreyi*).

Ulceration of granuloma inguinale

Ulceration of granuloma inguinale sometimes attacks the perineum, and fistulas there can be caused by lymphogranuloma venereum (see PENILE SORES, p. 530).

Epitheliomatous ulceration

Epitheliomatous ulceration of the perineum is seen as a direct spread of a growth of the anus or vulval area, when the diagnosis presents no difficulty. An epithelioma may develop in the scar of some former cutaneous affection, particularly in long-standing fistula-in-ano, in which case an ulceration may exist showing the usual characteristics of a cutaneous epithelioma. The inguinal nodes may be enlarged early from the inflammatory process, or later by invasion with malignant disease. Other cutaneous cancers, malignant melanoma and basal cell carcinoma, may also occur in this situation. In case of doubt, a biopsy specimen is taken for microscopical examination.

Harold Ellis

PERISTALSIS, VISIBLE

(See also BORBORYGMI, p. 77).

Usually, visible peristalsis is pathological. However, in a number of conditions the normal movements of the bowel may be visible; these circumstances are divarication of the abdominal recti muscles, an incisional or massive umbilical hernia containing bowel, and extreme thinness of the abdominal parietes – the result of emaciation or, rarely, congenital absence of the recti. It is not uncommon to see visible peristalsis within the sac of a very large ventral or inguinoscrotal hernia (Fig. P.16). In all these circumstances the diagnosis can be made at inspection, and the patient is otherwise symptomless. In all other situations, visible peristalsis is pathological and may be of two types, gastric and intestinal.

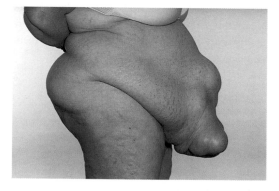

Figure P.16 Visible peristalsis was obvious in this large, thin-walled but unobstructed umbilical hernia.

Gastric peristalsis

Gastric peristalsis takes the form of a comparatively large swelling in the upper abdomen showing slow waves of peristalsis which progress from under the

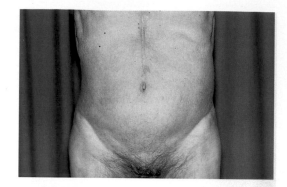

Figure P.17 Gross gastric dilatation due to a stenosing duodenal ulcer. The stomach was visible, gave a loud succussion splash, and showed typical gastric peristalsis, passing from left to right. The mid-line upper abdominal scar was from a previous repair of a perforation of the ulcer.

region of the left ribs, slowing downwards and to the right. This swelling indicates obstruction to the gastric outlet. There may be other signs of gastric dilatation and distension, particularly a loud succussion splash (Fig. P.17). Typically, there is a history of the vomiting of large amounts of liquid in a projectile manner, and which may contain fragments of food ingested 24 hours or more previously. The diagnosis can be confirmed by the passage of a nasogastric tube, which will yield a pint or more of fluid several hours after the last food or drink has been taken. The aspirate has a typical stale, unpleasant smell, and may contain recognizable particles of food eaten even several days before. A barium X-ray examination will clinch the diagnosis by demonstrating the gastric retention and dilatation. An X-ray taken 6–8 hours after the ingestion of the barium is particularly valuable as this will confirm the extent of gastric holdup (Fig. P.18). In doubtful cases of visible gastric peristalsis, the sign may be accentuated by asking the patient to swallow several glasses of soda-water. In the normal subject no peristalsis is seen, but in cases of pyloric obstruction, previously invisible peristalsis may now become obvious.

In congenital hypertrophic pyloric stenosis of infancy, not only can gastric peristalsis be seen after a drink from a bottle but the hypertrophied pylorus can often also be felt. This interesting and eminently treatable condition does not become apparent immediately, but some four weeks after birth.

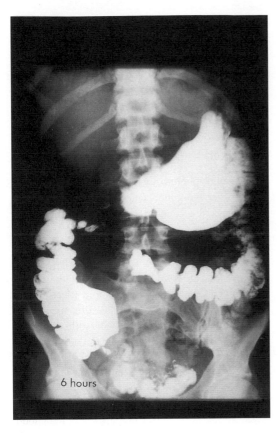

Figure P.18 At 6 hours after ingestion of barium, this patient with gross pyloric stenosis from a duodenal ulcer, and with obvious visible gastric peristalsis, still has considerable residue in the stomach. The barium which has escaped through the stenosis has already reached the splenic flexure of the colon.

Visible intestinal peristalsis

Visible intestinal peristalsis is a feature of advanced intestinal obstruction, with the limitations discussed above. As a pathological entity it will not occur alone, but is accompanied by colicky abdominal pain, abdominal distension, vomiting and absolute constipation. The discussion of the differential diagnosis of the different causes of the symptoms will be found elsewhere. If the small intestine alone is involved, the waves are multiple and run more or less transversely across the abdomen – the ladder pattern. When the colon is obstructed, peristalsis takes the form of vertical waves, especially in one or both flanks, but this is much more rarely seen.

Plain radiographs of the abdomen taken in the erect and supine positions are invaluable; the first

demonstrate multiple fluid levels, the second the distribution of gas shadows within the dilated loops of bowel which will often enable the clinician to determine whether small or large bowel is obstructed.

Harold Ellis

PHOBIAS

A phobia is a persistent, irrational, morbid fear of a specific object, situation or activity that induces a compelling desire to avoid that stimulus. This reaction is acknowledged as inappropriate or disproportionate, but nevertheless the individual is unable to desist from avoidance behaviour because of the anxiety that develops when exposure occurs or is anticipated. The causes of phobias are listed in Table P.3.

Most people probably harbour mild phobic responses to such common stimuli as harmless insects

Table P.3 Causes of phobias

Commonest
- Primary phobia
- Anxiety

Less common
- Drugs
  - Alcohol abuse
  - Hallucinogens
  - Sympathomimetics
  - Stimulants
- Drug withdrawal
- Psychiatric disorders
  - Depression
  - Panic
  - Schizophrenia
  - Paranoid disorder
  - Obsessive–compulsive disorder
  - Post-traumatic stress disorder
  - Personality disorder
    - Avoidant
    - Schizoid

Rare
- Neurological disorders
  - Brain tumour
- Cerebrovascular disease
- Multiple sclerosis
- Epilepsy
- Head injury

and snakes, spiders, dogs, small furry animals, lifts, heights, air travel, darkness, tunnels, blood, vomiting, dentists – and even doctors! All are catalogued by classically derived prefixes which can be employed to impress. Typically, these exaggerated fears can be overcome if necessary, place no limitations upon lifestyle, and are often regarded as socially acceptable reactions, so treatment is rarely sought or required. Clinically appreciable phobias are reported in about 8 per cent of the adult population, about 1 in 40 cases being severely disabling.

Simple phobias

Simple phobias (monophobias) become a medical problem when either they are intense and distressing or else impair social functioning – common examples include the pregnant women who cannot permit venepuncture, the businessman who cannot fly when his job demands it, or the child who will not leave home because of the neighbour's dog. In children, this type of development is usually brief and over-come with reassurance, but in adults specialist assistance and behaviour therapy are more likely to be required. Secondary simple phobias are uncommon. In schizophrenia, a phobia can represent the response to an unrevealed delusion and remit when the delusion subsides, while in obsessional neurosis phobias frequently develop in the context of cleaning rituals with the patient avoiding objects or situations through which contamination is feared.

Illness phobias

These differ in that the phobia consists of endless ruminations about the possibility of suffering from a disease, rather than primary avoidance. The patient will seek reassurance from the doctor that they do not have the disease, which contrasts importantly with hypochondriacal delusions where the patient is already convinced the disease is present. Common illness phobias concern cancer, heart disease and ven-ereal disease, but any disorder can become implicated – and particularly when attracting media attention. Hence, topical illness phobias include AIDS, radi-ation and food additives. Illness phobias are more common in patients with appreciable obsessional or hypochondriacal traits in their personality, and often signify an underlying stress. The presentation is dis-tinguishable from obsessional ruminations in that

the patient feels no tension to resist their thoughts, and from hypochrondriasis in that there is a single concern with reassurance often effective. Illness phobias can be the presenting feature of a primary depressive ill-ness when they respond to antidepressant treatment; but if unrecognized, phobias may progress to frank hypochondriacal delusions in depressed patients.

Agoraphobia

While simple phobias are the most common form of the disorder, agoraphobia tends to be the most incap-acitating, and accounts for over half of the phobic presentations to specialists. The essential features of agoraphobia are a marked fear of being alone, accom-panied by apprehension of becoming helpless in, or unable to escape from, a public place. Life becomes increasingly constricted as fears about streets, travel-ling, shopping, crowds and enclosed or open spaces take root: typically, the patient will battle unsuccess-fully and present when virtually restricted to their home or dependent upon others for accomplishing routine daily activities. This condition is twice as com-mon in women than men, usually develops in early adult life, and is associated with personality traits of passivity, dependence and anxiousness. A precipitant which may threaten the individual's security is often evident. Commonly, this may be a social change such as marriage, divorce, bereavement or childbirth, but less commonly it is an incapacitating, unpredictably episodic illness such as asthma, epilepsy or Menière's disease. Sometimes, the condition may be precipi-tated by a more persistent physical change, for example, following a head injury or other brain disease, ampu-tation, transplantation or other forms of major sur-gery. Once established for about a year, agoraphobia usually persists with remissions and relapses linked to life stresses.

Agoraphobia is almost always accompanied by other neurotic features – panic attacks, free-floating anxiety, depression, hyperventilation, obsessions and depersonalization are all frequently reported. As with simple phobias, schizophrenia or obsessional neurosis may occasionally be underlying, but the commonest cause of secondary agoraphobia is depressive illness.

Sometimes it can be impossible to decide clinically whether the patient has depression with secondary agoraphobia or agoraphobia with secondary depres-sion, although evidence of agoraphobic changes over months or years would point to the latter. In circumstances of uncertainty it is worthwhile prescribing an antidepressant drug, as secondary agoraphobia will remit.

Finally, it is advisable to inquire about health and education problems in the children of agoraphobic women. Children may not be going to school either because their mother would be stranded at school or, more seriously, requires them as a crutch at home. Sometimes school phobia or other emotional problems emerge, and occasionally the child can form the initial presentation.

Social phobias

These are especially common in adolescents. The patient avoids social situations because of the intense fear of behaving in an embarrassing or humiliating manner, and the feeling of being under scrutiny by an audience who are able to detect minor signs of their anxiety. Common social phobias are speaking, eating, drinking, writing or blushing in public, and using public lavatories. Usually, the patient has a single phobia linked to a specific situation, but occasionally all forms of social contact are avoided and the patient leads the life of a recluse.

Many social phobics treat their fear and anxiety by using alcohol or tranquillizers, and consequently some present with alcohol or drug dependence. Other phobias can co-exist, although agoraphobia tends to develop later in life: incidental agoraphobics also fear groups of people, but their phobia centres upon the mass of people, while social phobics are apprehensive of the individuals within the crowd. Again, schizophrenia and obsessional neurosis may underlie a social phobia, although in depressive illness unresisted social withdrawal is more common and motivated by anhedonia rather than fear. In more profound social phobia the possibility of a developing schizophrenic illness should be kept in mind, particularly if the patient is less concerned about their impoverished lifestyle than would be anticipated. For some patients with avoidant personality disorder, social phobias establish a persistent, unwelcome impairment of life, with work and relationships grossly affected. Such patients are rare, however, and the majority of social phobics have an excellent outlook, often with a minimum of advice and assistance.

Andrew Hodgkiss

PHOTOPHOBIA

Photophobia is an intolerance of light. The causes can be grouped into ocular and non-ocular. Ocular causes may be due to lack of retinal pigment, ocular inflammation or other ocular damage. Reduced retinal pigment occurs in cone dystrophies, albinism, which may be associated with Chediak–Higashi syndrome together with immune deficiency, easy bruising and bleeding, and recurrent infections. Causes of ocular inflammation include uveitis and keratitis. Some patients complain of photophobia in an eye with a mydriatic pupil because of the increased light through the wider aperture. Other ocular causes of photophobia include corneal abrasion, congestive glaucoma, retinal detachment, and refractive surgery. The diagnosis can be made by detailed ophthalmological assessment.

Migraine is commonly associated with photophobia, and can usually be diagnosed by the accompanying features; these include lateralized, throbbing headache with phonophobia (intolerance of sounds), desire to lie still, nausea and sometimes vomiting. Photophobia is an important component of the syndrome of *meningeal irritation*, together with neck stiffness and positive *Kernig* and *Brudzinski* signs. Kernig's sign is limitation or pain on extending the knee with the leg flexed at the hip; Brudzinski's sign is flexion of the hips when the head is pushed forward on to the chest. Meningeal irritation may be due to meningitis (acute or chronic), encephalitis or subarachnoid haemorrhage. The diagnosis should be suggested by the associated neurological symptoms and signs.

David Werring

PICA

Pica is a pattern of eating non-nutritive substances (e.g. dirt or paper), lasting for at least 1 month. It is seen more in young children than adults, with 10–32 per cent of children aged 1 to 6 years old exhibiting these behaviors. Clay, dirt, ice, sand, animal faeces, paint and hairballs are just a few examples of what children and adults with pica have been known to eat.

Pica is seen in children with emotional deprivation, neglect or even child abuse, especially between the ages of 2 and 5 years; it is interpreted as the child's symbolic response to a lack of maternal affection and care. It may lead to poisoning if noxious substances are eaten accidentally, or to obstruction of the stomach if multiple foreign bodies are eaten (e.g. pebbles). If the swallowed material is fibrous, it may bind together to form a *bezoar*, which forms a cast of the stomach with consequent obstruction. A variant of pica is *trichotillomania* where hair is pulled out and eaten with the formation of a trichobezoar.

There is no single test that confirms pica. However, since pica is associated with abnormal nutrient or raised toxic metal levels, and in some cases malnutrition, several tests may be performed. Serum levels of lead, iron and zinc should be taken. Haemoglobin should also be checked to test for anaemia. Lead levels should always be checked in children, who may have eaten paint or objects covered in lead paint dust. The presence of infection may be detected, if contaminated soil or animal waste is being ingested.

Identified nutritional deficiencies and other problems, such as lead toxicity, should be addressed medically. Treatment emphasizes psychosocial, environmental and family guidance approaches. Other successful treatments have been mild aversion therapy followed by positive reinforcement. Medications may be helpful in reducing the abnormal eating behavior, if pica occurs in the course of a developmental disorder, such as mental retardation, or pervasive developmental disorder.

Dipak Kanabar

PILIMICTION

Pilimiction – that is, the passage of hairs in the urine – is a rare condition which almost invariably signifies that the patient has a pelvic dermoid cyst that has become inflamed, thereafter opening into the bladder and discharging its contents via the urinary passages. This condition has been observed in men, but it occurs more often in women. Subacute or acute cystitis accompanies the event with vesical pain, frequency of micturition and pyuria. The obvious fallacy in diagnosis arises from the possibility of contamination in the urine of hairs which were not, as supposed, passed per urethram.

Harold Ellis

PLEURAL EFFUSION

Pleural effusion – the presence of fluid lying between the visceral and parietal pleura – is common, and may be associated with a large number of conditions. Pulmonary embolic disease, cardiac failure, malignant pleural infiltration and pneumonia are the four most important conditions which are responsible for more than 90 per cent of pleural effusions seen in clinical practice.

Physiology of the pleura

In health, the two pleural surfaces are in close contact but separated by a thin layer of fluid. Estimates of the volume vary, but quoted figures range from 1 to 20 ml with an electrolyte content similar to serum and a low protein concentration. The fluid is formed by transudation from the parietal pleura and is absorbed by the visceral pleura. It is in a dynamic state, with some two-thirds of the fluid being absorbed and replaced every hour.

The pleura transmits the forces generated by the respiratory muscles to the lungs, and there is a negative pressure within the pleural space of about $-5\,mmHg$. Capillary fluid and gas would enter the pleural space were it not for a number of balancing factors, including a hydrostatic pressure difference between the parietal capillaries and the capillaries of the visceral pleura which are supplied by the low-pressure pulmonary arterial system. Plasma oncotic pressure is the same in both sets of capillaries (about $35\,mmHg$), while pleural osmotic pressure is only about $6\,mmHg$ due to its low protein content.

Thus, fluid is driven in sequence from the parietal pleural capillaries to the pleural space and then on to the visceral pleural capillaries and lymphatics resulting in a continuous transfer of low protein fluid.

In the case of gas entering the pleural space, there is a driving force of about $40\,mmHg$ (atmospheric pressure − pleural pressure + pleural capillary blood gas tension) which assists gas absorption, as occurs in closed pneumothoraces.

Clinical features

Symptoms associated with the accumulation of fluid in the pleural space depend upon the cause, volume and rate of formation of fluid. Small effusions are often symptomless, and even quite large effusions can cause little disability, provided that the fluid has accumulated slowly. Effusions caused by inflammatory disease often present with pleuritic pain which may be relieved as the fluid accumulates. Large effusions eventually cause symptoms including dry cough, shortness of breath, initially on exercise and later at rest, together with dull, aching discomfort over the affected side of the chest.

The clinical findings are influenced by the size and site of the effusion. Most effusions occupy the dependent part of the pleural space, and so when the patient is sitting the characteristic findings of stony dullness to percussion and distant or absent breath sounds are most prominent at the lung bases. Bronchial breath sounds or aegophony may be heard directly above an effusion. Large effusions displace the mediastinum towards the unaffected side unless the underlying lung is fibrosed from previous inflammation (tuberculosis) or collapsed due to a proximal bronchial lesion. Very large effusions may displace the mediastinal contents to produce an area of dullness at the opposite base close to the midline (Grocco's sign).

Radiological features

Effusions may be small, moderate, large, encysted, mediastinal or subpleural. Small effusions may be difficult to detect clinically, but can be seen radiographically as non-specific blunting of the costophrenic angles. Moderate-sized free effusions cast a characteristic homogeneous shadow over the lower lung fields, obscuring the diaphragm and cardiac silhouette. At the upper border of the effusion there is decreased density of the radiographic opacification with a superior concave curvature which appears to reach its highest level in the axilla when seen on posteroanterior films or posteriorly on lateral films. In fact, the level of the effusion is horizontal and the radiographic appearances are artifactual due to the increased distance traversed by the radiation. Massive effusions cause complete opacification of the hemithorax, often with very marked displacement of the mediastinal structures to the opposite side. Sometimes, the fluid collects in the pleural cavity under the lung adjacent to the diaphragm – the so-called diaphragmatic or subpulmonary pleural effusion. The upper margin of the fluid shadow runs parallel to, and may be mistaken for, an elevated diaphragm. On the left side the apparent separation of the transradiant gastric 'air bubble' from the transradiant lung tissue may draw attention to the effusion. If the presence of fluid is in doubt, a lateral decubitus film may help to differentiate between effusion or pleural thickening when, in the former, the fluid is seen to shift to the lateral chest wall or mediastinum. Interlobar pleural effusions are quite commonly seen as an extension of an effusion and result in a characteristic ovoid homogeneous shadowing with well-demarcated margins lying in one of the interlobar fissures. Interlobar effusions may mimic tumours and occur particularly in cardiac failure, when clearance following diuretic treatment gives rise to the term 'vanishing pulmonary tumour'.

Encysted effusions can give rise to diagnostic difficulties, especially if they lie posteriorly and cause homogeneous shadowing suggesting consolidation when seen on posteroanterior films. The nature of the abnormality becomes apparent in a lateral view when opacification is seen to lie posteriorly.

Aetiology

The majority of pleural effusions are related to increased pleural capillary permeability and occur in response to inflammation (both infective and other), ischaemia (pulmonary infarction) and pleural neoplasia. The clinical findings may provide some diagnostic clues, as may radiology which will also localize the position of the fluid and reveal its extent. In most cases the fluid must be examined cytologically and biochemically, and also cultured for organisms.

The appearance of the freshly aspirated fluid can be informative. It is usually straw-coloured or cloudy, but can be frankly purulent (empyema), blood-stained (haemothorax) or opalescent (chylothorax). Blood-stained effusions are relatively common and, setting aside trauma to the chest or accidental haemorrhage resulting from a traumatic pleural tap, is most commonly seen in malignancy or pulmonary infarction. A pleural fluid red blood cell (RBC) count of $<10\,000$ per ml is not diagnostic, but $>100\,000$ RBC per ml is significant.

The pleural fluid formed through normal capillary membranes is a transudate with a low protein content, whereas fluid formed through abnormally permeable capillary walls contains a higher concentration of protein. The distinction between a transudate and exudates may be obvious on clinical grounds, for instance when there is cardiac, renal or hepatic failure. By convention, a transudate has a specific gravity <1.016 or a protein content <30 g/l. However, up to 30 per cent of transudates are shown to have a specific gravity in excess of 1.016, and 10 per cent have a protein content >30 g/l. An improved discrimination between transudate and exudate can be achieved by considering the pleural fluid lactate dehydrogenase (LDH) level, where activity in excess of 200 IU or a pleural fluid/serum LDH ratio >0.6 is characteristic of an exudate.

The pleural fluid cytological findings in benign effusions are variable. Mesothelial cells and macrophages are found in most transudates. Mesothelial cells predominate in exudates, especially when due to pulmonary infarction. Neutrophil polymorphonuclear leucocytes are frequently present in sterile and infected effusions associated with pulmonary inflammation. The exception to this pattern is tuberculosis, where an initial neutrophil excess is quickly replaced by lymphocytes which may account for between 80–100 per cent of all the cells present in the effusion. Lymphocytic pleural effusions are not specific to tuberculosis and occur in sarcoidosis or some forms of malignancy (e.g. lymphoma).

A high pleural fluid eosinophil count is seldom associated with allergy, but is seen in occasional pulmonary infarcts, malignancy or simply when there has been bleeding into the pleural space.

Malignant cells are present in about two-thirds of cases where there is malignant invasion of the pleura. The appearances are often diagnostic of the cell type and, when due to metastases, often can reveal the site from where the primary tumour has arisen. Other useful characteristics of the fluid include measurements of pH and blood glucose. A low pH (pH <7.3) is occasionally seen in tuberculosis or in parapneumonic effusions prior to the onset of frank empyema. A pH greater than 7.4 is most frequently found in malignancy. The presence of a low pleural fluid glucose (<1–7 mmol/l or 13 mg/100 ml) and normal serum glucose suggests rheumatoid pleural disease, although rarer cases of tuberculosis, malignancy and empyema may also be found to have a low pleural fluid glucose.

Boris Lams

PLEURAL RUB

The diagnostic sign of pleurisy is a rub of a creaking superficial nature usually located close to the site of pain.

The pleura is a double serous membrane separating the lung from the chest wall and mediastinum. The pleural surface consists of a uniform layer of mesothelial cells supported on a connective tissue framework which is well supplied with capillary and lymph vessels. The parietal pleura is innervated with pain-sensitive nerve fibres supplied by the intercostal and phrenic nerves, and is exquisitely sensitive to painful stimuli.

In health, the visceral and parietal pleural surfaces are smooth, glistening and separated by a small amount of fluid, allowing low friction movement of the lungs with respiration.

In contrast, if the pleural surfaces become thickened or roughened by inflammation or neoplastic infiltration, movement with breathing will cause increased friction, which may be heard with a stethoscope. Patients commonly complain of thoracic pain on breathing or coughing. On auscultation, sounds of varying intensity may be heard during inspiration and expiration, often described as having a 'leathery' or 'creaking' quality that may be exaggerated when the stethoscope is applied firmly to the chest wall. Pain associated with a pleural rub may vary in degree from lancinating discomfort during slight inspiratory effort to a less sharp 'catch' of pain at the end of maximum inspiration. Pleural pain is often reduced by breath-holding or by exerting firm pressure over the affected thoracic segment. Except when it involves the diaphragm, the affected pleura typically underlies the area in which pain is perceived. The central portion of the diaphragm is innervated from the third and fourth cervical posterior nerve roots running via the phrenic nerve. Pain caused by diaphragmatic pleural irritation is often referred to the neck and shoulders.

A pleural rub may last for as little as a few hours in short-lived inflammatory conditions such as pneumonia, but to months or even years in patients with more chronic causes of pleurisy. Typically, as the pleurisy settles the pain and physical signs (including the rub) become less obvious, although in some patients the rub may persist after the pain has gone and occasionally a loud rub may persist indefinitely.

Most pleuritic conditions giving rise to pain and auscultatory rub are inflammatory in origin. Infection associated with community-acquired pneumonias – especially pneumococcal, mycoplasma and other 'atypical' infections – may present with severe pleurisy and a pleural rub accompanied by signs of pneumonic consolidation. Pulmonary infarction secondary to pulmonary embolism is another frequent cause, and is especially common following major surgery, in patients with underlying abdominal malignancy when thromboembolism may be the first sign of gastric or pancreatic carcinoma, or in females taking oestrogen preparations. Tumours invading the chest wall typically cause a continuous persistent pain, but may occasionally present with pleurisy and a pleural rub. Rather less frequently, a pleural rub may occur in association with asbestos-induced pleural disease, or connective-tissue diseases such as systemic lupus erythematosus, or rheumatoid arthritis. Recurrent pleurisy at the same site should suggest bronchiectasis, and at different sites, bronchopulmonary aspergillosis. If pleurisy progresses to a pleural effusion, the sharp pain and pleural rub largely disappear to be replaced by a dull and more constant ache and heaviness.

The pain of pleurisy may be mimicked by a number of *chest wall conditions*, such as rib fractures, intercostal muscle pain due to tearing or strain, Tietze's syndrome, and neurogenic causes such as intercostal nerve root compression and herpes zoster. Pain due to intercostal muscle strain and tears can be quite sharp, may be caused by coughing, and can result in shallow breathing. However, local tenderness over the affected site is common and typically no pleural rub is heard.

Epidemic myalgia (pleurodynia, Bornholm disease, devil's grip, epidemic dry pleurisy) is an acute febrile viral illness that affects skeletal muscle and is characterized by an abrupt onset of intense pain in the lower chest or upper abdomen. In about 25 per cent of patients, headache, malaise, anorexia, sore throat and deep myalgia precede the onset by 1 or 2 days. The afflicted patient complains of a fever of 38–40°C and multiple paroxysms of excruciating pain lasting from a few minutes to several hours. The illness is often biphasic, with an initial bout of pain and fever settling, only to recur after a day or two. The acute illness usually settles within a week, but rarely patients have several recurrences over a period of several weeks. The illness may be accompanied by myocarditis or pericarditis.

Epidemic myalgia is caused by enteroviruses, usually Coxsackie B3 or B5 but also Coxsackie A or echoviruses. The incubation period is short (about 3–5 days) and, as with other enteroviral infections, the majority of illnesses occur in the summer and autumn. A specific diagnosis can be made by isolating virus from the throat and faeces during the acute illness, or demonstrating a rising titre of serotype-specific neutralizing antibodies in acute and convalescent sera. The level of creatine phosphokinase in the serum may also be elevated, reflecting injury to striated muscle.

Confusion with acute *myocardial infarction* is inevitable in those patients presenting with abnormal electrocardiograms and raised creatine phosphokinase. The condition may also be confused with pre-eruptive *herpes zoster*, although in the latter condition pain is more constant and no pleural rub is detected.

Recurrent polyserositis (familial Mediterranean fever) is an autosomal recessive, recurrent inflammatory disease of unknown cause, characterized by recurrent inflammation of serous membranes. Attacks occur at irregular intervals from several days to several years with pleurisy, abdominal and joint pain, and other systemic symptoms which typically settle spontaneously within 12–48 hours. This condition usually manifests in children and is recognized in many parts of the world, but is largely restricted to ethnic groups originating in the eastern Mediterranean area.

Investigation of patients presenting with pleurisy and a pleural rub will almost inevitably include a chest radiograph, which is frequently useful in showing a primacy lung condition. If the chest X-ray is normal, or if it only shows a small pleural reaction, it may be important to consider the possibility of a pulmonary embolism, and further examination of the legs – together with scanning – may help in coming to a therapeutic decision. If pulmonary embolism is considered unlikely, and there is an absence of any other features, it is reasonable to make a provisional diagnosis of viral pleurisy, and to treat the patient with adequate analgesia.

Boris Lams

PNEUMATURIA

The passage of gas per urethram, either with or independently of urine, is a rare but striking peculiarity, particularly when it occurs in males. It may be due to one or other of two distinct groups of causes, namely:

- Communications between the rectum, caecum, vermiform appendix or other part of the alimentary canal and the bladder, ureter or renal pelvis, either directly or via an intermediate gas-containing abscess cavity.
- Infection of the bladder or other part of the urinary tract by gas-producing micro-organisms.

When the cause lies among the first of these groups, the patient is apt to pass faecal material as well as gas. It should be added, however, that the passage of gas without faeces per urethram by no means excludes a fistulous communication between some part of the alimentary canal and the urinary tract; the fistula may be of such a character that while gas can traverse it, faeces cannot. It may also happen that a lesion such as appendicitis or, most commonly, acute sigmoid diverticulitis has led to the formation of a local abscess which, owing to infection by *Escherichia coli*, contains gas. This abscess may open into the bladder and cause the discharge of pus and gas, but no faeces, per urethram. The same applies to similar abscesses which, though not arising primarily in connection with the bowel, nevertheless contain gas from infection by *E. coli* and *Aspergillus aerogenes*, which produce gas when they grow in urine, as may various *yeasts* in patients with glycosuria.

If no sign of a fistulous communication between any part of the bowel or a gas-containing abscess cavity with the urinary tract can be distinguished on cytoscopic examination, it may be presumed with confidence that the pneumaturia is due to infection. Such patients are usually elderly female diabetics with considerable glycosuria. The infecting organisms are usually *E. coli*, *A. aerogenes*, yeasts, or combinations of these.

The urine in such a case contains pus, sugar and albumin. It may be acid, and not foul-smelling or ammoniacal; however, it may sometimes be so foul and faeculent as to arouse unwarranted suspicion of a communication between the colon and the bladder. A cystoscopic examination will serve to exclude a fistulous opening into the bladder, but it may be much more difficult to exclude a similar communication with the higher parts of the urinary tract, especially the renal pelvis. Such a condition is very rare, so that urinary infection is the more probable unless there is a known or recognizable cause for communication

between the bowel and the renal pelvis, such as a carcinoma.

Harold Ellis

POLYDIPSIA

Polydipsia is defined as excessive or abnormal thirst. The primary stimulus to the sensation of thirst is dehydration, which gives rise to an increase in the plasma osmolality of the blood passing through the thirst centre in the hypothalamus. An increase in plasma osmolality can also be achieved by increasing the solute load, for example by drinking salt water. The sensation of thirst must be distinguished from a dry mouth caused by Sjögren's syndrome, or mouth breathing or by drugs (in particular antidepressant and anti-psychotic medications with pronounced anti-muscarinic activity). Apparent thirst may also be due to a psychiatric disorder, when it is called 'psychogenic polydipsia'.

True polydipsia due to dehydration may be associated with disorders, which cause polyuria (see below), including diabetes mellitus, cranial diabetes insipidus, nephrogenic diabetes insipidus and diuretic therapy. Other causes of dehydration not associated with polyuria include inadequate fluid intake, excessive loss of fluid from the skin (fever, thyrotoxicosis, burns injuries), from the stomach (repeated vomiting), from the bowel (diarrhoea), and into serous-lined cavities, as in acute peritonitis.

Melvin Lobo

POLYURIA

The term 'polyuria' signifies a larger than normal daily volume of urine. There is considerable variation from subject to subject in the amount of urine passed, but a urinary output of more than 2–5 litres per 24 hours is nearly always abnormal. Polyuria must not be confused with frequency of micturition due, for example, to prostatic hypertrophy or cystitis. Also, although polyuria will almost always lead to a complaint of nocturia, many individuals complaining of the latter have no increase in the total output of urine but show a reversal of the normal diurnal variation in urine flow. This is the case in most cases of sodium and water retention, as in cardiac failure or the nephrotic syndrome, in suprarenal disorders, and in chronic renal failure. Polyuria may be due either to an increased solute load with obligatory water loss or to a primary water diuresis, and will be discussed under these headings. The main causes are summarized in Table P.4.

Table P.4 Causes of polyuria

Due to increased solute load
Diabetes mellitus
Diuretic therapy
Chronic renal failure
Following relief of obstruction
During recovery from acute tubular necrosis
Resolving haematoma

Due to water diuresis
Psychogenic polydipsia
Cranial diabetes insipidus
Nephrogenic diabetes insipidus
- X-linked
- Potassium depletion
- Hypercalcaemia
- Drugs
- Sickle-cell anaemia
- Early chronic pyelonephritis

Other causes
Following fevers
After attacks of migraine, etc.
Paroxysmal tachycardia

Polyuria due to increased solute load

Any osmotically active solute will produce a diuresis if present in excess in the distal tubular fluid. For example, the massive protein breakdown occurring in a large *haematoma* may be associated with a diuresis, urea itself being the active solute. It is also the mechanism of *diuretic therapy* in which the solute concerned is sodium. *Diabetes mellitus* is much the most common pathological condition in which this type of polyuria occurs. The daily urine volume is often 4 litres or more, and polyuria and excessive thirst are the most common symptoms. In children who were previously dry at night, enuresis may be an early symptom of diabetes. The diagnosis is usually straightforward. In *chronic renal failure* the total

solute load may be normal, but the reduction in the number of nephrons results in a greater than normal load per nephron and consequent polyuria which is usually only of moderate severity. The polyuria which may follow the relief of chronic *urinary tract obstruction* is also partly due to this mechanism, but some defect of concentrating power may also be present. Diuresis is also common during recovery from *acute tubular necrosis*; this is partly due to the elimination of water and electrolytes retained during the phase of oliguria, and partly to incomplete recovery of tubular function.

Polyuria due to water diuresis

The simplest cause of this is an increased water intake, which may reach pathological dimensions in the condition known as *psychogenic polydipsia* or *compulsive water-drinking*. This is an hysterical manifestation and simulates diabetes insipidus. The differentiation is discussed below but, clinically, marked fluctuations in urine output would strongly suggest psychogenic polydipsia. Patients with Sjögren's syndrome may try to relieve the dryness of their mouths by drinking large volumes of water, with a consequent modest polyuria.

The urine is normally concentrated in the distal tubules and collecting ducts. Antidiuretic hormone (ADH) is secreted by the posterior pituitary in response to a rise in plasma osmolality; its action is to increase the permeability of the tubular epithelium to water. The effect of this is to increase the transport of water from the tubular lumen into the hypertonic renal medulla through which these tubules pass. Thus, a pathological water diuresis may be due either to failure of secretion of ADH or to failure of the renal tubules to respond to its action.

Cranial (neurogenic) diabetes insipidus is often caused by an identifiable lesion of the hypothalamus or pituitary (or both), but in about one-third of cases no such cause can be found. Tumours in that region are a common cause and include craniopharyngioma, pinealoma, glioma and metastases from distant primary growths. Diabetes insipidus may also follow trauma to the skull (including operative), infections such as exanthemas in childhood, or infiltration with granulomatous lesions such as sarcoidosis or histiocytosis X. In such cases other evidence of hypothalamic pituitary disease may well be present.

Occasionally, diabetes insipidus is complicated by a destructive lesion of the 'thirst' centre in the hypothalamus so that polydipsia does not accompany the polyuria; water loss is severe, and hypernatraemia with brain damage may result. There is a very rare familial form of cranial diabetes insipidus, inherited as an autosomal dominant trait; even rarer is the DIDMOAD syndrome (Diabetes Insipidus, Diabetes Mellitus, Optic Atrophy, Deafness), with autosomal recessive inheritance.

Failure of the renal tubules to respond to the action of ADH is termed *nephrogenic diabetes insipidus*. A familial form is seen in males only, inherited as a sex-linked recessive (X-linked). It may also be a part of other renal tubular defects such as the Fanconi syndrome with cystinosis and proximal renal tubular acidosis (Type 2); it can also occur in renal amyloidosis, myelomatosis and hyperglobulinaemia.

The differentiation of the two types of diabetes insipidus from each other and from psychogenic polydipsia may be difficult. This is because a prolonged water diuresis from any cause may lead to partial resistance to the action of ADH. Thus, deprivation of water in psychogenic polydipsia may not cause immediate cessation of the polyuria, although there will usually be a considerable reduction. In diabetes insipidus, whether nephrogenic or of cranial origin, the polyuria will continue despite water deprivation, and the patient becomes very thirsty and ill; the test is not without its dangers in this situation. Further information may be obtained from the administration of desmopressin, an ADH analogue. This will clearly have no effect in nephrogenic diabetes insipidus, but will reduce the urine output in cranial diabetes insipidus and in psychogenic polydipsia. Once again, the result may not be clear-cut, and the effect of desmopressin may not be apparent for several days. There is a danger that, in psychogenic polydipsia, the continued ingestion of large amounts of water after the administration of ADH may cause water intoxication.

Several other conditions cause nephrogenic diabetes insipidus. Polyuria is a common feature of the renal lesion of *potassium depletion*; this condition might be suspected if muscular weakness is a prominent complaint, or the deep reflexes are absent. Potassium depletion may be due to chronic diarrhoea, diuretic therapy, primary aldosteronism, excessive doses of corticosteroids and alkalosis from any cause; it is particularly seen in the type of Cushing's syndrome produced by an ACTH-secreting bronchial carcinoma. The polyuria fails to respond to desmopressin, but is reversible if the potassium balance can be restored to normal.

Hypercalcaemia also can cause a water diuresis, and might be suggested by associated abdominal pain and vomiting. Thus, polyuria may be a feature of primary hyperparathyroidism, vitamin D intoxication, sarcoidosis, multiple bony metastases or primary tumours secreting parathyroid hormone related protein. The renal lesion is reversible unless severe nephrocalcinosis has developed or renal calculi have produced irreversible damage. As in hypokalaemia, there is no response to ADH. A reversible nephrogenic diabetes insipidus can also be produced by a number of drugs including lithium carbonate, demeclocycline, amphotericin B, glibenclamide and gentamicin.

Other conditions in which failure of urinary concentration occurs are *sickle-cell anaemia* and chronic *pyelonephritis* at an early stage. The polyuria due to the latter must not be confused with the osmotic diuresis of chronic renal failure discussed above.

Transient polyuria

Polyuria lasting for only a few hours can occur in various circumstances. It is rarely of any great significance, and indeed is often physiological. The diuresis which follows excessive water drinking needs no comment. The same applies to polyuria in the course of *diuretic therapy*, although the diuretic effect of such substances as tea or coffee may occasionally provoke a complaint from a patient who has not realized the association. Cold weather may also induce polyuria as a result of reduced fluid loss from the skin; travellers returning from a long stay in the tropics and accustomed to a large fluid intake may occasionally complain of polyuria on return to a colder country. It is this contrast with previous oliguria that partly explains the polyuria following *fevers*; there may also be a temporary impairment of ADH secretion.

Polyuria can also occur following various stressful situations, and has been described after attacks of *migraine*, *asthma* and *angina*. A more striking polyuria may occur during and after attacks of *paroxysmal tachycardia*. Any arrhythmia – either supraventricular or ventricular – which lasts for more than half an hour may produce this effect. This is probably due to the release of atrial natriuretic peptide.

Boris Lams

POPLITEAL SWELLING

Popliteal swellings may be divided into:

- Fluid swellings
  - ◆ Bursae
  - ◆ Morrant Baker's cyst
  - ◆ Varicose veins
  - ◆ Abscess
  - ◆ Aneurysm
- Solid swellings not connected with bone
  - ◆ Enlarged lymph nodes
  - ◆ Innocent tumours
  - ◆ Malignant tumours
- Solid swellings connected with bone
  - ◆ Exostosis
  - ◆ Sarcoma
  - ◆ Separation of the epiphysis

Fluid swellings

Bursae

There are numerous bursae associated with muscles and tendons around the knee. Communications between two bursae and between a bursa and the knee joint are common.

The semi-membranous bursa on the posterior aspect of the knee is the most often enlarged of the bursae. When the leg is extended, the bursa stands out as a tense fluctuating swelling on the inner side of the popliteal space; on flexion, it disappears completely. It may be found enlarged in young athletes, but causes no symptoms whatever. On account of its fairly frequent communication with the knee joint, it may be distended when that joint is the seat of an effusion, acting, as it were, as an overflow tank. Where the joint condition is an acute one, the bursa may be very tender. In rheumatoid arthritis it is common for fluid to pass from the joint into the bursa, but not in the reverse direction – thus, a ball-valve mechanism appears to be in operation.

The bursae under either of the two heads of the gastrocnemius muscle or those connected with the insertion of the semi-tendinosus may be enlarged similarly, but these are more rare.

Morrant Baker's cyst

This is a herniation of the synovial membrane which only occurs in connection with chronic inflammatory changes in the joint, most commonly in rheumatoid arthritis. However, the semi-membranous bursa is usually also affected and is also distended. The extension from the joint tends to spread along fascial planes and may point at varying distances from its origin. The 'cysts' may be multiple. Such extensions of the knee joint may sometimes rupture and cause an inflammatory reaction in the calf muscles, and this may be mistaken for a deep venous thrombosis. In diagnosis, CT or MRI may be of value.

Varicose veins

Varicosities of the short (small) saphenous vein are often present in the popliteal space; the diagnosis presents no difficulties, as the veins in the lower part of the leg will also be varicose. However, they become much more obvious when the patient stands.

Whilst the above-described are the most common causes of popliteal swelling, the following conditions are much more rarely encountered.

Acute abscess

This is recognized by the signs of acute inflammation; the skin is red and oedematous, the pulse and temperature are raised, and the swelling is very painful. The knee is kept flexed in order to minimize the tension of the part. The abscess may be caused by suppurating lymph nodes or by suppurative periostitis or necrosis of the lower end of the femur. In the former case, the abscess will be superficial, whilst in the latter case it is deep to the popliteal vessels.

Aneurysm of the popliteal artery

This gives rise to an expansile pulsating tumour, the pulsation being synchronous with the heart beat. Pressure on the femoral artery above will cause a diminution in size of the swelling and cessation of pulsation. The pulse at the ankle on the affected side may be smaller than that on the opposite, and delayed. If a stethoscope is placed over the swelling a distinct bruit can be heard.

The major complaint of the patient will probably be of pain, which may be referred down the leg if either popliteal nerve is pressed on, or in the site of the swelling if the bone is eroded. Varicose veins are almost always present on account of pressure on the popliteal vein. Owing to its pulsatile character, an aneurysm is not often mistaken for anything else, but every swelling that pulsates is not an aneurysm. A soft vascular sarcoma growing from the end of the femur may be pulsatile, and over it a bruit may be heard, but the tumour is not as compressible as an aneurysm is and the effects on the distal pulse are less marked. A radiograph (or better, a CT scan) will usually settle the question at once. Distinction must also be drawn between a tumour that pulsates and a tumour to which pulsation is communicated. For instance, an abscess or a solid swelling lying over the popliteal artery may appear to pulsate, but the movement is heaving in character and not expansile. In the rare event of an aneurysm having become filled with clot it might be taken for a solid tumour growing either from the soft parts or from the bone. Finally, the aneurysm may present on the medial side of the lower end of the thigh, anterior to the tendon of the sartorius.

Solid swellings not connected with bone

Enlarged nodes

It is not common to find the popliteal nodes enlarged from any cause. It is possible that they may become infected with pyogenic organisms from a sore on the back of the leg.

Tumours

Tumours are rare; they may be either innocent (e.g. *lipoma* and *neurofibroma*) or *sarcomatous*, starting in the connective tissue of the popliteal space, or attached to one of the muscles. The innocent tumours are of long history and are well defined; the malignant lesions are rapidly growing and infiltrating.

A lipomatous mass, either in the popliteal fossa or on the medial aspect of the knee, is not infrequently present in osteoarthritis of this joint, and is part of the general fatty infiltration which gives rise inside the joint to the *lipoma arborescens* of the synovial membrane.

Solid swellings connected with bone

In all cases of bony tumour a radiograph should always be obtained.

Benign tumours

Exostoses may be found, generally in children and young adults, growing from the region of the epiphysial cartilage of the femur. Others may occur in other parts of the skeleton, and sometimes several members of the family are similarly affected. The swelling is of slow growth, well-defined and rarely causes any problems. It is most often found at the inner side of the popliteal space. Exostoses may be confused with *ossification of the insertion of a tendon* or muscle, the adductor longus muscle being the most commonly affected (rider's bone).

Osteoclastoma is prone to occur in the upper end of the tibia or lower end of the femur, and may cause an asymmetrical expansion of the cortex presenting in the popliteal fossa. Usually, expansion of the bone can be detected on other aspects, and if the condition is advanced the shell may be so thin in some places that 'eggshell crackling' can be elicited. The radiographic appearances are typical – expansion and thinning of the cortex, an absence of new bone formation, and trabeculation.

Malignant tumours

These include osteosarcoma, fibrosarcoma arising from the fibrous periosteum and metastases from neoplasm elsewhere. Here, as in giant-cell tumour, enlargement of the bone is not usually confined to the popliteal space. The differential diagnosis from inflammatory lesions can be very difficult, even with radiography, and is often impossible without. The type of osteosarcoma which shows a palisade of bony spicules perpendicular to the line of the cortex is easily diagnosed by radiography, but it must be remembered that a sarcoma may present itself with an obvious clinical swelling but with little or no radiographic changes. This usually – but not always – denotes a *fibrosarcoma of the periosteum*, particularly if a thin line of periosteal new bone is laid down. Occasionally, a small central area of erosion with a clinical swelling may indicate the presence of a bone sarcoma of the osteolytic type. Although there may be marked swelling, there is usually less effusion into the joint than is the case if the lesion is inflammatory. Computed tomography is useful in providing accurate anatomical delineation of the tumour mass. Serological tests for syphilis and a biopsy of the diseased part should be performed in all doubtful bone lesions. A *gumma* is indicated by dense sclerosis around the lesion, clear-cut central softening without erosion, and regular bone formation.

Separation of the epiphysis

In the somewhat rare accident of separation of the lower epiphysis of the femur, the lower fragment becomes displaced backwards, forms a prominence in the popliteal space, and presses on the vessels – sometimes to a dangerous extent. It is unlikely that such a condition would present itself as a doubtful popliteal swelling for diagnosis.

Harold Ellis

POSTURE, ABNORMAL

The term 'posture' refers to the position either of one particular part of the body such as an arm or leg, or to the position of the body as a whole. Abnormalities of posture may thus be limited to either individual parts of the body or to the appearance of the whole body. In general, posture cannot be considered in isolation as part of a differential diagnosis. Posture is altered in many conditions (muscles, skeletal, neurological, psychological, etc.).

In the conscious patient, disorders of the basal ganglia produce some of the most characteristic abnormalities of posture. Dystonia may affect the body as a whole in the generalized dystonic disorders such as dystonia musculorum deformans. Focal dystonias may produce a local abnormality such as spasmodic torticollis or writer's cramp. Parkinson's disease is associated with a very characteristic flexed posture in the late stages. In athetosis and chorea, postural abnormalities may be seen in addition to the involuntary movements.

Kyphosis for example is increasingly common with advancing age. It can be taken to be due to a degenerative arthritis or osteoporosis. Rarely, such a posture is hysterical.

Mark Kinirons

PREMENSTRUAL SYNDROME

Premenstrual syndrome (PMS) can be defined as cyclical recurrence of psychological, behavioural and physical symptoms during the luteal phase of the menstrual cycle. This is essentially the two weeks prior to menstruation, and the symptoms resolve by the end of menstruation, after which the woman should be free of symptoms between the end of menstruation and ovulation. Psychological and somatic disturbances are part of the normal physiology of the menstrual cycle, but when exaggerated they may lead to severe psychological disturbance and behavioural abnormalities. The symptoms include bloating, cramping, pain and tenderness in the breasts, temporary gain in weight and some swelling of the hands and feet. They also include emotional tension, bad-temper, nervousness, irritability, and headache, lack of concentration, depression and insomnia, sufficient to interfere with the normal enjoyment of life. The majority of women (95%) will have some symptoms, only a small percentage (5%) is totally symptom-free. In a small group of women (5%), the symptoms of PMS have a major impact on their lives and have led to suicide, acts of aggression, and even cited as defence in murder trials.

The aetiology remains obscure, and consequently presents therapeutic difficulties when dealing with this problem. The underlying cause may be a combination of imbalances/abnormalities of the ovarian steroid production and central nervous transmitters. It has been shown that women with PMS have lowered levels of whole blood serotonin concentrations and platelet serotonin. Several serotonin re-uptake inhibitors (SSRIs) have now been shown to improve PMS symptoms. Elimination of the cyclical ovarian function results in the complete suppression of symptoms. Despite cyclical ovarian steroid function being the trigger for PMS, there is no definitive test to distinguish it from other disorders. The nature of the symptoms are less important than the timing, and keeping a diary of symptoms may be useful to distinguish primary PMS from secondary. The latter are a group of patients who have true PMS with underlying psychopathology.

Treatment depends on the severity of symptoms, and may range from a mixture of counselling, education and reassurance in patients with mild problems. Essential fatty acids and pyridoxine have been used in the past. SSRIs may be used to good effect in moderate cases. In more severe cases, ovulation suppression can be used, and this can start with continuous combined oral contraceptive (OCP) usage, provided that there is no contraindication to OCP use, or continuous progestogens. Danazol and GnRH analogues can be used. If these treatments are successful, then total abdominal hysterectomy and bilateral salpingo-oophorectomy may be indicated, but these patients would need subsequent HRT in the form of continuous oestrogen only.

Antony Hollingworth

PRIAPISM

'Priapism' (see also PENIS, PAIN IN, p. 532) signifies erection of the penis which is persistent, of troublesome degree, and not necessarily accompanied by sexual desire. Though generally spoken of in connection with the male sex, a precisely similar affection may occur in the female clitoris. The symptom is not often by itself of diagnostic importance. Although it may be due to a considerable number of different conditions, the ultimate cause is usually thrombosis in the vascular spaces of the cavernous tissue, which are found to contain thick black grumous blood.

The important causes are:

- After injury to the upper dorsal region of the spinal cord. The damage may have produced fracture-dislocation of the spine with paraplegia, in which case the diagnosis will be obvious. Short of this, however, a minor degree of injury, with contusion and small haemorrhages into the substance of the cord, may be followed by painful priapism, persisting sometimes for weeks before recovery occurs. Cerebrospinal syphilis or tumour may also rarely be responsible.
- In leukaemia. Apart from obvious changes in the penis (e.g. cavernous haemorrhage), priapism has been noted in both myelocytic and lymphatic leukaemia even before the other symptoms and signs have led to a haematological diagnosis. The cause of the priapism in leukaemia is obscure, but the diagnosis is suggested by the concomitant splenomegaly and/or lymphadenopathy, and is confirmed by the haematological findings.
- Sickle-cell anaemia.
- New growths of the urethra, either primary or secondary to carcinoma of the bladder or testis.
- Trauma with haematoma formation.

Chronic intermittent priapism is the term used to describe frequently repeated erections which are of long duration but lack the persistence of true priapism. The attacks occur in the night, and may or may not be associated with sexual desire. They are due to nerve irritation arising from lesions of the central nervous system or from local lesions in the posterior urethra, prostate or seminal vesicles. In elderly men they are frequently associated with enlargement of the prostate. Seldom will priapism be the only symptom in that case; the diagnosis will be made from the history and from the other symptoms and signs.

Harold Ellis

PRURITUS ANI

Pruritus ani – the sensation of itching around the anal verge – is a common symptom. In more than half the patients, no obvious cause can be found (idiopathic pruritus), but in every case the following checklist should be considered:

- The pruritus may be the result of a general disease associated with itching (see PRURITUS, GENERALIZED, p. 555). Examples are lymphoma, advanced renal failure, severe jaundice and diabetes mellitus. The latter is often associated with *Candida albicans* infection (thrush), and this may occur, of course, in the non-diabetic patient. Moreover, *Candida* is often a secondary invader on any moist and excoriated skin and so may well not be the primary cause of the condition.
- The localized itching may be due to a skin disease which happens particularly to affect the perianal region. Examples include: scabies, where characteristic lesions may be seen elsewhere in the body, notably between the fingers and on the anterior aspects of the wrists; pediculosis pubis, where the parasites may be noted in the anal region, as well as in their usual site in the pubic hairs; and fungal infection. The latter is particularly to be thought of where the skin lesion has a well-defined border at its lateral extent. Other lesions may be found between the toes and in the groin, and proof may be obtained by examination of scrapings from the affected skin. Erythrasma, due to infection with *Corynebacterium minutissimum*, may be diagnosed by demonstrating coral pink luminescence when viewed with a Wood's lamp.
- Any condition within the anus or rectum which produces moisture and sogginess of the anal skin is liable to cause

pruritus ani. These lesions include prolapsing piles, prolapse of the rectum, anal fissure, anal fistula, anal papillomata or condylomata, carcinoma or benign tumours of the rectum, colitis or colonic Crohn's disease (Fig. P.19). Anal incontinence due to sphincteric injury may result in constant soiling of the perianal skin. Careful inspection of the anal verge, digital examination of the anal canal, proctoscopy and sigmoidoscopy, where necessary, will rapidly expose the underlying cause of this condition.

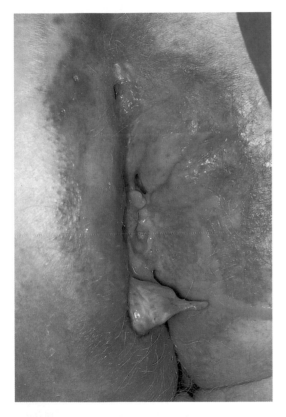

Figure P.19 Severe pruritus extending forward to the vulva in a young girl with extensive Crohn's disease of the colon and distal rectum.

Excessive sweating, especially in hot weather and in hairy men, may be associated with pruritus ani, especially in subjects who wear thick and rough undergarments.

Pruritus ani is unusual in children and, when it occurs, a well-recognized cause is infestation with threadworms (*Enterobius vermicularis* or *Oxyuris vermicularis*). Characteristically, the worms migrate to the anal verge (especially at night), and scratching results in auto-infection. The parasite is white, about

6 mm long, and the thickness of cotton thread. The parasites may be noted at the anal verge or seen at proctoscopy. If the diagnosis is suspected but no parasites immediately seen, a wash-out of the rectum with normal saline should be inspected against a black background, when the white parasites can be detected. It should be noted that threadworm infection may also occur in adults.

Idiopathic pruritus is diagnosed when no obvious cause can be found. A number of theories have been suggested, including: allergy; that the original cause has now disappeared but the pruritus has persisted because of continued scratching of the anal region by the patient; irritation of the perianal skin by faecal contamination even when no gross soiling is evident; or some psychogenic cause.

Harold Ellis

PRURITUS, GENERALIZED

Pruritus, or itching, is that sensation of the skin which excites the urge to rub or scratch. It is sensed by undifferentiated endings of unmyelinated C-fibres at the dermo-epidermal junction; the fibres pass centrally with pain fibres, and itching appears to be caused by stimuli too weak to cause pain. Itching is most pronounced in those areas served by the greatest number of pain-conducting fibres, for example around the lips and nose, and in the anogenital area. For the same reason, itching is more easily provoked in the flexures than on extensor surfaces, and this may be a factor in the localization of atopic lichenification. Response to itch stimuli, like pain, is immensely variable between individuals. The threshold for pruritus can be lowered by warming the skin, by stimulants such as dexedrine and caffeine, and by emotional tension. It is probable that rubbing a particular area may 'facilitate' the itch pathway, which would explain why itching may be worsened by scratching (Fig. P.20): the so-called 'itch–scratch cycle' as seen in pruritus ani and lichen simplex chronicus. The causes of pruritus are listed in Table P.5.

Some dermatoses are tremendously pruritic, and the debilitating nature of a chronic, nagging pruritus, depriving the patient of sleep, may easily be underestimated by physicians. The degree of pruritus is

Table P.5 Causes of pruritus

Itchy dermatoses
Infestations (scabies, lice, insect bites)
Dermatitis – all causes
Lichen planus
Prickly heat
Urticaria, including cholinergic urticaria and dermographism
Dermatitis herpetiformis
Pemphigoid gestationis
Cutaneous T-cell lymphoma
Onchocerciasis

Generalized pruritus
Senile asteatosis
Liver: obstructive hepatopathy (including primary biliary cirrhosis)
Kidney: chronic renal failure
Blood: polycythaemia, anaemia, iron deficiency
Endocrine: hyperthyroidism, myxoedema
Malignancy: lymphoma; liver secondaries; T-cell leukaemia
Pregnancy: last trimester (especially in atopics)
Hydroxyethyl starch (plasma expanders)
Psychological: delusional state of parasitosis
Drugs, gold salts, detergents, de-greasing agents

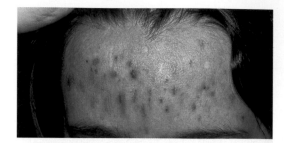

Figure P.20 Excoriations.

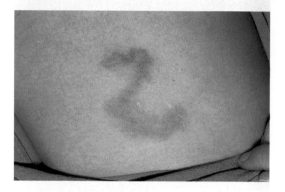

Figure P.21 Cutaneous larva migrans.

seldom of great diagnostic help, largely because of variability of individual response, the possible exceptions being *cutaneous syphilis* which never itches, and the intense nocturnal itching of scabies. In general, the most itchy dermatoses – apart from the infestations – are *dermatitis* of all causes particularly atopic dermatitis, *lichen planus, urticaria, dermatitis herpetiformis* and *pemphigoid gestationis*.

Faced with a scratching patient, it is important not to overlook an *infestation* (e.g. scabies or pediculosis) (Fig. P.21). One condition often forgotten by Western physicians is *onchocerciasis* (estimated by WHO recently to affect 20 000 000 people worldwide), where pruritus may be intense, and localized to the legs and buttocks or involve the whole body. Onchocerciasis occurs in a broad belt worldwide from 19° North to 15° South, as well as scattered foci in Mexico, Central and South America, the Yemen and parts of Saudi Arabia. Onchocercoma nodules containing the adult worm may be found around the pelvic girdle or on the head and neck, and the diagnosis will be confirmed by finding microfilariae from skin snips.

The term *generalized pruritus* is usually reserved for those patients in whom no cutaneous lesions are present except those due to scratching. In the elderly, the most common cause is a subclinical dryness of skin, *senile asteatosis*, due to inadequate secretion of

sebum and sweat. A subtle scaling may be seen, and perhaps an eczema craquele on the anterior shins or forearms (Figs P.22 and P.23). The rather evanescent but intensely itchy rash of cholinergic urticaria can also be easily missed. Likewise, patients who have received infusions of plasma expanders based on hydroxyethyl starch may experience an intense and persistent itch out of all proportion to the rather minimal rash. If no primary dermatosis can be identified, the following possibilities should be considered:

- *Liver disease.* Pruritus is severe in obstructive jaundice, but in hepatitis and primary biliary cirrhosis can begin before icterus is obvious.
- *Renal disease.* The skin in advanced uraemia may be intensely pruritic, and in patients receiving dialysis sudden shifts in electrolytes may cause pruritus, as may secondary hyperparathyroidism.
- *Blood disease.* Pruritus is common in polycythaemia rubra vera and also in iron deficiency, even without anaemia.
- *Endocrine disease.* Generalized itching is occasionally a presenting feature of hyperthyroidism, and can accompany

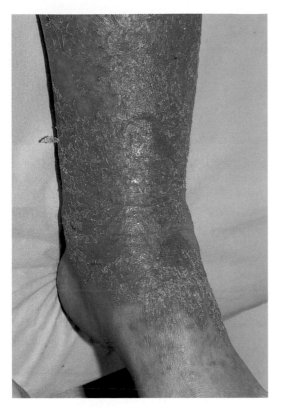

Figure P.22 Acute eczema.

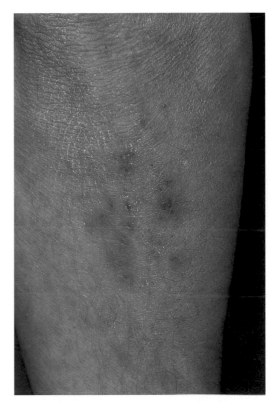

Figure P.23 Excoriated eczema.

the dry skin of myxoedema. Diabetes mellitus is said to cause generalized pruritus, but this is more often found to relate to localized infection with *Candida* (e.g. candidal vulvo-vaginitis).

- *Malignancy.* Generalized pruritus, sometimes with prurigo nodules, can be the presenting feature of underlying cancers, especially lymphomas. T-cell leukaemia – particularly the Sézary syndrome – produces a notoriously itchy erythroderma.
- *Pregnancy.* Itching is common during the last trimester of pregnancy, and a proportion of patients, probably atopics, will produce prurigo nodules on the arms and legs. The itch disappears after parturition.
- *Psychological.* Scratching may be associated with delusions, particularly that parasites are crawling over the skin – a symptom which may indicate serious underlying mental disturbance. Cocaine is also said to be capable of producing an intense itching sensation which has been likened to ants crawling on the skin (formication).

Barry Monk

PRURITUS VULVAE

Pruritus vulvae is a term used to denote vulval irritation without an obvious cause being found. In reality, gynaecologists use the term to describe the sensation of itching around the vulval area, which causes the woman to scratch herself. It is a condition which is much more common after the age of 40 years.

As with conditions affecting the skin, it may be due to local dermatoses, or it may reflect a systemic condition. This symptom may also be due to a local vaginal infection.

General causes of pruritus vulvae

General conditions for pruritus vulvae include:

- Skin diseases including eczema, psoriasis and contact dermatitis to local deodorant use, washing products or man-made fibres. Intertrigo can occur whenever the skin is moist and susceptible to inflammation and secondary infection. This may be a particular problem in over-weight women – especially if diabetic, in which case they may have a greater chance of developing *Candida* infection.

- Drug reactions.
- Psychogenic problems.
- Medical conditions which include:
  - ◆ Diabetes
  - ◆ Hypothyroidism
  - ◆ Liver disease
  - ◆ Chronic renal failure
  - ◆ Crohn's disease
  - ◆ Haematological disorders, including polycythaemia, leukaemia and Hodgkin's disease.

In some women with this symptom it may be useful to check the serum iron levels. These may be low, but not necessarily anaemic; the iron stores are low, but treatment with oral iron to supplement the diet can improve symptoms.

Local causes of pruritus vulvae

These include:

- Atrophic vulvitis in post-menopausal women
- Vulval dystrophies
- Tumours
- Infections
  - ◆ *Candida*
  - ◆ Herpes
  - ◆ Warts
  - ◆ Threadworm, lice and scabies
  - ◆ Other sexually transmitted diseases

Infection of the vagina and vulva with *Candida albicans* (thrush) is a common problem, which may be associated with combined oral contraceptive use, antibiotics, diabetes and pregnancy. The itching is intense and is associated with a typical curdy, white discharge that causes local inflammatory change resulting in a very reddened vagina. It can be treated with local preparations of antifungal agents; fluconazole can be given systemically if local treatment is unsuccessful. Vaginal discharge from any cause may be responsible for pruritus, as may infection from the urinary tract. The mucoid discharge from an ectropion, however, does not usually cause pruritus, and infection with *Trichomonas vaginalis* is more inclined

to give rise to vulval soreness. Pubic lice and scabies can cause considerable distress from itching, but can be treated with topical agents.

Vulval dystrophies are a common cause of pruritus vulvae. They include lichen sclerosus (Fig. P.24), squamous cell hyperplasia plus the other skin conditions mentioned earlier. The most common of these is lichen sclerosus; this has typical features of loss of the architecture of the vulva with fusion of the labia majora and minora, while the skin appears thickened and white, but can be thin and reddened as a result of scratching. The appearance of the skin can resemble cigarette paper. Treatment of this condition is with high-dose steroid cream (dermovate), initially to control the symptoms, then to change to a less potent formulation, and eventually to wean the patient off the steroid treatment. However, if the condition flares up, the same regimen can be repeated. There is a small risk that this may predispose the woman to invasive cancer of the vulva (approximately 4% of cases). It must be emphasized that carcinoma of the vulva is an extremely uncommon condition in the UK.

Hyperplastic dystrophy may have atypical cells in the epidermis, and such a finding is regarded as being pre-malignant. Vulval intra-epithelial neoplasia (precancerous changes) and Paget's disease are also found

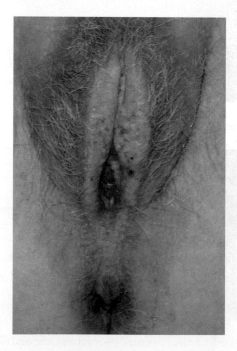

Figure P.24 Lichen sclerosus.

on the vulva. These both cause pruritus and require biopsy for diagnosis. Conservative measures using steroid creams are adopted for dystrophies without cell atypia, but excision of the affected area must be undertaken when atypia denotes pre-malignancy.

Antony Hollingworth

PTOSIS

Ptosis is the term applied to drooping of the upper eyelid with inability to elevate it to the full extent (Fig. P.25). The most common form is a congenital defect, and if the pupil is in consequence covered, then urgent surgical correction is indicated to prevent amblyopia. The acquired form is usually caused by paralysis of the IIIrd nerve, when it may also be associated with paralysis of other ocular muscles, either external or internal.

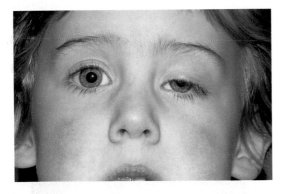

Figure P.25 Ptosis of left upper lid.

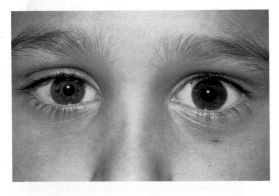

Figure P.26 Horner's syndrome: ptosis and constricted pupil on the right side.

In paralysis of the cervical sympathetic nerve, slight ptosis may be associated with diminution in the size of the pupil on the affected side, retraction of the eyeball or 'enophthalmos' and absence of sweating – Horner's syndrome (Fig. P.26). Ptosis occurs in myasthenia gravis, and is diagnosed using the Tensilon test.

Ptosis, associated with oedema and infiltration of the lids, is also found in inflammatory disorders of the conjunctiva and upper lids. Gross oedema may occur in angioneurotic oedema. It also follows direct injury of the elevating muscle or its nerve supply following lid laceration or blunt trauma.

Congenital ptosis is often bilateral, and associated with smoothness of the upper lids and an absence of all the usual cutaneous folds. The levator palpebrae may be absent or ill-developed, and efforts to open the eye are made by the occipito-frontalis muscle.

In the congenital condition called 'jaw-winking', movements of the jaw – especially lateral movements – cause the ptotic lid to rise. The patient is thus seen to 'wink' whilst eating or chewing. The cause appears to be a misdirection of nerve fibres resulting in a faulty innervation of the levator muscle.

The causes of ptosis are listed in Table P.6.

Table P.6 Causes of ptosis

Congenital
Paresis or maldevelopment of levator muscle, jaw-winking syndrome, blepharophimosis syndrome

Acquired
■ Traumatic
   ◆ Eyelid laceration, post-surgical (following enucleation or orbital surgery)
■ Neurogenic
   ◆ IIIrd nerve palsy (due to trauma, ischaemia, inflammation, neoplasm or aneurysm), Horner's syndrome, multiple sclerosis, neurosyphilis
■ Myogenic
   ◆ Dystrophia myotonica, myasthenia gravis, primary muscular atrophy, chronic progressive external ophthalmoplegia, senility, iatrogenic, chronic ocular inflammation
■ Mechanical
   ◆ Lid tumours, cicatricial, inflammation

Reginald Daniel

PTYALISM

Pytalism means excessive secretion of saliva. It is not always easy to determine if there really is excess, or if the patient is merely allowing the normal volume of saliva to dribble from the mouth. Thus, the difficulty may be solely that of swallowing the normal secretion, as in bulbar paralysis. There may be both excess of secretion and difficulty in swallowing, as in mercurial stomatitis. In other instances there is too much secretion but no difficulty in swallowing, as in functional or hysterical ptyalorrhoea. The first step towards ascertaining the cause is to inquire as to any medicine or *drug* the patient may be taking orally or applying externally.

Mercury was the most important of these when it was used as a drug in the treatment of syphilis; its effects were worst when the mouth was not kept clean. Iodides, bromide and arsenic were also often responsible in the past.

If the salivation is not attributable to any drug, it may be the result of one of the many forms of *general stomatitis*. The nature of a severe stomatitis will be ascertained by local examination; by bacteriological examination of swabbings from the mouth; by serological tests for syphilis; or by microscopical examination of a fragment of the affected tissues. Tuberculous stomatitis is one of the rarer but severe forms; it may be primary, but is more often associated with pulmonary tuberculosis.

If drugs and general stomatitis can be excluded, a local examination may still serve to detect a cause acting by reflex irritation of the Vth cranial (trigeminal) nerve, especially:

- a jagged carious tooth;
- a stump left beneath a dental plate;
- a broken or ill-fitting dental plate;
- a foreign body impacted in the gum; and/or
- an ulcerating tumour of the oral cavity.

If appropriate examination serves to exclude these causes, the salivation – apparently rather than actually increased – may be found to result from *mechanical difficulties in swallowing* (see DYSPHAGIA, p. 157). The excessive salivation seen in many cases of advanced carcinoma of the oesophagus results from the oesophago-salivary reflex; a constant excess flow of saliva is secreted in an attempt to 'swallow' the obstructing bolus of tumour in the gullet.

In the absence of an obvious local structural lesion, apparent salivation may be due to inability to swallow, as in cases of:

- Parkinsonism
- Bulbar paralysis
- Pseudo-bulbar paralysis
- Bilateral facial paralysis
- Myasthenia gravis
- Hypoglossal nerve paralysis

The differential diagnosis of these conditions is discussed elsewhere. It is only in bulbar and pseudo-bulbar paralysis that the dribbling of much saliva is a prominent symptom. Pseudo-bulbar paralysis, being of cortical and not of medullary nuclear origin, does not exhibit wasting of the tongue.

Slovenliness and lack of cerebral control are responsible for the slobbering and salivation of some elderly or mentally handicapped patients.

Harold Ellis

PUBERTY, DELAYED

Delayed puberty is rather more common in boys than in girls, and may be defined as the total absence of sexual development in a boy over the age of 15 years, or in a girl who is aged more than 14 years. Constitutional delayed puberty accounts for half of the male cases, but is much less likely to be the cause in a girl, in whom well over 80 per cent will have some pathological condition. For practical purposes, the first sign of puberty in a girl is the appearance of pubic hair or a breast bud, whereas in a boy enlargement of the testes is the earliest sign, before rugosity of the scrotum or pubic hair growth. Pre-pubertal testes are less than 2 cm in length. A length of more than 2.5 cm indicates that pubertal testicular stimulation is taking place. Alternatively, the size of the testes may be compared with a Prader orchidometer. A volume of more than 4 ml indicates pubertal change.

It is important to distinguish children who are undergoing a constitutional delay in onset of puberty from those who have pathological disorders that require treatment. Delayed puberty will fall into one of three categories: (i) constitutional delayed puberty; (ii) hypogonadotrophic hypogonadism or hypothalamic–pituitary abnormalities; and (iii) primary gonadal failure or hypergonadotrophic hypogonadism. The causes of delayed puberty are listed in Table P.7.

Constitutional delayed puberty

Constitutional delayed puberty accounts for 50 per cent of cases in boys, but only 16 per cent in girls. There is often a family history, and there may be an indication of a recent slowing of growth. This may, in fact, be the normal pre-pubertal deceleration of growth. Bone age is correlated better with the time of onset of puberty than with chronological age. As the bone age advances,

serum gonadotrophin levels increase. As long as the penis is not very small and there is no anosmia, it is reasonable to review these patients every 6 months, especially if the testosterone response to human chorionic gonadotrophin (HCG) is appropriate for the bone age. If the boy is becoming embarrassed by his lack of sexual development, and if his height is adequate, one may consider low doses of androgen. Similarly, oestrogens may be used in girls. Generally speaking, however, these individuals usually develop perfectly normally, albeit in their late teens or even in their early twenties.

Hypothalmic and pituitary causes

Altogether, abnormalities of the hypothalamus and pituitary account for approximately one-third of cases

Table P.7 Causes of delayed puberty

Constitutional	■ Destructive lesions
	◆ Castration
Hypothalamic syndromes	◆ Mumps (damage occurs very rarely in children)
■ Lack of gonadotrophin-releasing hormone (Kallmann's syndrome)	◆ Tuberculosis
■ Laurence–Moon–Biedl syndrome	◆ X-irradiation
■ Prader–Willi syndrome	◆ Cytotoxic therapy
■ Lyndi's syndrome	
	Adrenal disease
Destructive lesions of hypothalamus and/or pituitary	■ X-linked congenital adrenal hypoplasia
■ Craniopharyngioma	■ Cushing's syndrome
■ Germinoma	
■ Chromophobe adenoma	**Thyroid disease**
■ Prolactinoma	■ Hypothyroidism
■ Optic chiasma glioma (neurofibromatosis)	■ Hyperthyroidism
■ Meningioma	
■ Langerhans cell histocytosis	**Chronic disease** (functional gonadotrophin deficiencies)
■ Hydrocephalus	■ Anorexia nervosa
■ Trauma	■ Malnutrition
■ Vascular lesions	■ Tuberculosis
■ Granulomas	■ Severe uncontrolled diabetes
■ Infections (tuberculosis)	■ Chronic renal failure
■ Cranial irradiation	■ Cyanotic congenital heart disease
	■ Cystic fibrosis
Isolated pituitary deficiencies	■ Gluten enteropathy and other malabsorption syndromes
■ Growth hormone	■ Connective-tissue diseases
■ Luteinizing hormone (fertile eunuch syndrome)	■ Haemoglobinopathies
	■ Acquired immune deficiency syndrome
Gonadal abnormalities	
■ Anorchism	**Rigorous physical training**
■ Ovarian dysgenesis	
◆ Turner's syndrome	**Drugs**
◆ Pure dysgenesis	■ Girls
■ Noonan's syndrome (boys and girls)	◆ Androgens
■ Klinefelter's syndrome (rarely causes delayed puberty)	◆ Anabolic steroids
■ Autoimmune ovarian failure	■ Both sexes
■ Resistant ovary syndrome	◆ Excess thyroid hormones
■ Hormonal	
◆ Masculinizing tumour of ovary	

of delayed puberty in both girls and boys. The cause may be a space-occupying lesion, trauma, or the result of infection or granulomatous infiltration involving the hypothalamus or the pituitary, or both. The hormone defects in these cases tend to be multiple, so that in addition to delayed puberty due to lack of gonadotrophins there may be short stature due to growth hormone deficiency, lethargy and weakness due to lack of adrenocorticotrophic hormone (ACTH), cold insensitivity due to low thyroid-stimulating hormone (TSH) levels, or polydipsia and polyuria due to deficiency of vasopressin (diabetes insipidus). However, patients with solitary growth hormone deficiency (see p. 676) may present not only with short stature (and often obesity) but also with delayed puberty, though sexual development usually occurs normally later on. Chromophobe adenomas and prolactinomas may cause hypogonadism due to the secretion of high levels of prolactin. High prolactin levels may also be produced by lesions that interfere with the production of prolactin-inhibiting factor (dopamine), or its delivery to the pituitary.

A hypothalamic lack of gonadotrophin-releasing hormone (GnRH) accounts for about 7 per cent of all cases of delayed puberty. This may be due to a midline developmental defect, since in some of these cases anosmia due to hypoplasia of the olfactory bulbs is present (Kallmann's syndrome, male:female ratio, 4:1) and there may be cleft palate, hare lip and other congenital abnormalities. These patients tend to be tall because of their hypogonadism.

Male patients have been reported with isolated luteinizing hormone (LH) deficiency. They are tall, with eunuchoidal skeletal proportions (the arm span is more than 5 cm >body height, and the lower body segment [heel to pubis] is more than 5 cm >upper body segment [pubis to crown]), and are sexually immature. Full maturation can be achieved by injections of HCG.

In some cases of the Laurence–Moon–Biedl syndrome (see p. 676), a hypothalamic deficiency of GnRH has been shown. This also occurs in the Prader–Willi syndrome (see p. 678), and in the Lyndi's syndrome of male hypogonadism and congenital ichthyosis.

Gonadal abnormalities

A primary gonadal abnormality is responsible for over 30 per cent of cases of delayed puberty in girls,

but in little over 5 per cent of boys. The most common cause in girls is *Turner's syndrome* (see p. 672), in which ovarian dysgenesis is classically associated with the karyotype 45,XO. Unlike most other patients with hypogonadism, the girl is short and there are usually several physical abnormalities, such as a webbed neck, a low hairline posterolaterally, an increased carrying angle of the elbows, short fourth and/or fifth metatarsals and metacarpals, a shield-shaped chest with widely spaced nipples, pigmented naevi, renal anomalies, coarctation of the aorta, atrial and ventricular defects and aortic stenosis. In about one-quarter of patients, not all the cell lines carry the karyotype 45,XO. These are mosaics, and cells may be XO,XX, XO,XXY or XO,XX,XXX. Patients with mosaicism tend to be taller than those with XO Turner's syndrome, and the physical features outlined above may be less apparent. The serum gonadotrophins, LH and follicle-stimulating hormone (FSH), will be elevated. Buccal smear examinations will usually show absent Barr bodies, indicating the presence of one X chromosome, but if there is any doubt then a full karyotyping should be carried out, as there could be mosaicism.

In a small number of cases of ovarian dysgenesis there are none of the features of Turner's syndrome, the stature is normal, and the appearance female, though hypogonadism is present ('pure dysgenesis'). Half of the patients have a normal female karyotype, 46,XX; in the other half the karyotype is male, 46,XY. Serum gonadotrophin levels are high. It is advisable in these patients to perform a laparoscopy in order to confirm dysgenesis of the ovaries.

Noonan's syndrome (see p. 672), which superficially resembles Turner's syndrome, may occur in both sexes and may present with delayed puberty.

In the *resistant ovary syndrome* the ovaries fail to respond to gonadotrophins, probably owing to lack of receptors, and an adolescent girl may present with lack of pubertal development.

In a small proportion of girls suffering from autoimmune disease (of the adrenals, thyroid and parathyroid especially), delayed puberty may be due to autoimmune ovarian failure; antibodies against the ovaries can be demonstrated in the serum.

In boys, *anorechism* will cause delayed puberty, but will usually have been investigated long before the expected age of puberty because of the absence of testes in the scrotum. High levels of LH and FSH in the blood will confirm the diagnosis.

In both sexes surgical removal of the gonads (castration), for whatever reason, will lead to delayed puberty. *Mumps* usually only damages the post-pubertal gonad, while *tuberculosis* has become rare in the developed world. *Irradiation* for the treatment of lymphomas is becoming a more common cause of hypogonadism, particularly in girls. The Leydig cells of the testis seem to be more resistant. Cytotoxic *chemotherapy* may cause gonadal damage.

A *masculinizing tumour of the ovary* will cause delayed puberty in a girl because of the suppression of gonadotrophins by the excess androgens. Secondary sexual hair and even hirsutism will be present, and there may be clitoromegaly.

Suprarenal disease

In girls, *congenital suprarenal hyperplasia* (see p. 563) or *Cushing's syndrome* (see p. 794) may lead to failure of breast development and to primary amenorrhoea because of the production of excess amounts of androgen. Pubic and axillary hair will almost always be present, for the same reason. A boy with either of the above two conditions may be thought to be well developed, but examination of his testes will show them to be small because of suppression of pituitary gonadotrophins by the excess androgens. In *Cushing's syndrome* in both sexes the hyperproduction of cortisol also may have an effect in reducing gonadotrophin secretion.

Thyroid disease

Where *hypothyroidism* is associated with delayed puberty in a girl it is usually due to autoimmune ovarian failure. Hypothyroidism is, in fact, more often associated with precocious puberty (see below). *Hyperthyroidism* in a child of either sex may lead to delayed puberty due to suppression of gonadotrophin release.

Chronic disease

Chronic debilitating diseases of any type, particularly those causing poor nutrition, may cause delayed puberty by interfering with the hypothalamic control of pituitary gonadotrophins. *Anorexia nervosa*, which occurs in about 1 per cent of all teenage girls in Western society, may be missed as a diagnosis, but a careful history may reveal abnormal eating habits and

fads and evidence of vomiting or purgation. Fine 'lanugo' hair may be seen over the body (see p. 38).

Malnutrition such as marasmus and kwashiorkor will be obvious causes of delayed puberty in underdeveloped countries. *Tuberculosis, chronic renal failure, cyanotic congenital heart disease, connective-tissue disease* and severe *uncontrolled diabetes* should present no problems in diagnosis. Patients with *cystic fibrosis*, in addition to having chronic respiratory infections, may also have evidence of gastrointestinal malabsorption due to pancreatic enzyme deficiencies. *Gluten enteropathy*, which occurs in approximately 1 in 2000 children, may be more difficult to recognize as a cause of delayed puberty. Bowel symptoms may be very subtle, but the diagnosis should be suspected in a short child who has a protubertant abdomen and scanty subcutaneous fat elsewhere. Low red cell folate and antigliadin and anti-endomysial antibodies are useful screening tests, but the definitive investigation is a small-bowel biopsy. In gluten enteropathy the villi are flattened.

Rigorous physical exercise in boys and girls can delay the onset of puberty. This is particularly prominent in young female athletes (e.g. ballet dancers and gymnasts), though it also happens in boys. There is evidence that the luteinizing hormone-releasing hormone (LHRH) pulse generator may be inhibited by endogenous endorphins. With the delay in menarche in females, long-term osteopoenia may result from chronic low oestrogen.

Drugs

In girls, the administration of either *androgens* or *anabolic steroids* will lead to suppression of sexual development due to inhibition of gonadotrophin release. Pubic and axillary hair will, however, usually be present. In both boys and girls, the ingestion of excess *thyroid hormones* in the treatment of hypothyroidism or thyroid cancer may lead to delayed puberty owing to the inhibition of gonadotrophin release.

Sharon O'Byrne

PUBERTY, PRECOCIOUS

Before puberty, blood levels of luteinizing hormone (LH) and follicle-stimulating hormone (FSH) are low and are poorly responsive to administered gonadotrophin-releasing hormone. At the time of puberty, gonadotrophin secretion begins to increase and gonadal stimulation occurs, with a consequent rise of testosterone in boys and of oestradiol in girls. In both sexes, puberty is preceded by an increase in

the production of the suprarenal androgens dehydroepiandrosterone and androstenedione. The causes of precocious puberty are listed in Table P.8.

In 95 per cent of girls the first sign of puberty, which is either breast bud or pubic hair development, appears between the ages of 8.5 and 13 years. Puberty is precocious if either of these two events occurs before the age of 8 in a girl. Menarche occurs in 95 per cent of girls between the ages of 11 and 13 years.

In 95 per cent of boys the testes begin to enlarge between the ages of 9.5 and 13.5 years (mean 11.6 years), and reach adult size between the ages of 13 and 17 (mean 14.9 years). Pubic hair growth develops after testicular enlargement has begun, so it is rare before the age of 9.5 years. Testicular growth is

Table P.8 Causes of precocious puberty

True (LHRH-dependent)
Constitutional
Cerebral
- Trauma
- Cranial irradiation
- Granulomata
- Brain abscess
- Hypothyroidism
- Hydrocephalus
- Encephalitis
- Meningitis
- Tuberose sclerosis
- Neurofibromatosis
- Cerebral tumour
- Pineal tumour
- Craniopharyngioma
- Hamartoma
- McCune–Albright syndrome (polyostotic fibrous dysplasia with cutaneous pigmentation)
- Russell–Silver syndrome

False (LHRH-independent)
Gonadotrophin-producing tumours
- Hepatoma
- Hepatoblastoma
- Teratoma
- Chorionepithelioma

Suprarenal
- Congenital adrenal hyperplasia
- Tumours
- Cushing's syndrome

Testicular
- Leydig cell tumour
- Leydig cell hyperplasia

Ovarian
- Granulosa cell tumour
- Androblastoma
- Lipoid cell tumour
- Chorionepithelioma
- Benign ovarian cyst

Drugs
- Androgens
- Anabolic steroids
- Oestrogens

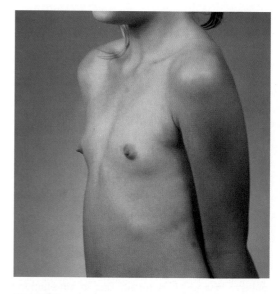

Figure P.27

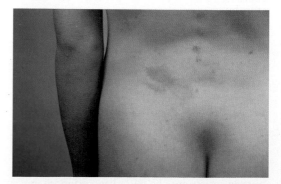

Figure P.28

stimulated by the action of FSH on germinal epithelium and of LH on Leydig cells. The testosterone produced by the Leydig cells is responsible for the growth of the penis. Puberty is precocious in a boy if any of the abovementioned changes takes place before the 9th birthday.

Precocious puberty can be either a true puberty or a false pseudo-puberty. In true puberty, the changes proceed in the normal physiological manner, albeit at an early age. In false puberty, on the other hand, changes such as secondary sexual hair growth and enlargement of the phallus occur because of abnormal androgen production, and gonadal function is in fact inhibited. A rare intermediate variety may be produced by non-pituitary, gonadotrophin-secreting tumours.

Constitutional precocious puberty

This is the most common cause of precocious puberty, especially in girls, where it accounts for 80 per cent of cases. Early puberty in boys is five times less common than in girls, and in boys a pathological cause (especially neurological) is found in 50 per cent. A family history of precocious puberty may be found, though the majority of cases are sporadic. Ovarian cysts may be detected in girls on ultrasound examination. They should not be confused with granulosa cell tumours.

Other variants of premature puberty may be present. *Premature adrenarche* is characterized by the early growth of pubic hair and a slightly advanced bone age. There are no other signs of premature sexual development, and full puberty develops at the normal age. *Premature thelarche* refers to the early development of breast tissue, often in the second year of life. It usually regresses spontaneously within 2 years but may lead on to a full early puberty.

The important implication for a child who enters early puberty is that, because bone maturation is advanced, final adult stature may be below that predicted for an offspring of that family.

Cerebral

Hypothyroidism is included under cerebral causes of precocious puberty because it seems likely that the mechanism is via the stimulation by thyrotrophin-releasing hormone (TRH) of gonadotrophins in addition to TSH and prolactin.

A wide variety of other cerebral conditions can give rise to precocious puberty if the area posterior to the median eminence, including the mamillary bodies and the posterior part of the floor of the IIIrd ventricle are involved.

The *McCune–Albright syndrome* is only tentatively included under cerebral causes of precocious puberty because it has been postulated that there may be inappropriate secretion of hypothalamic releasing hormones in this condition. The syndrome is rare and is much more common in girls than in boys. Precocious puberty is usual, but other endocrine abnormalities such as thyrotoxicosis, hyperparathyroidism and Cushing's syndrome may occur. One of the characteristic features is polyostotic fibrous dysplasia, which may be unilateral. There are pigmented areas on the skin roughly corresponding to the underlying bony lesions.

Patients with the Russell–Silver syndrome (see p. 677) may develop early puberty. The cause is unknown.

True precocious puberty can develop in children who are adopted from under-developed countries. This is thought to be secondary to correction of malnutrition generally after 3 years of age. The correction of a virilizing condition can be followed by true precocious puberty due to activation of the hypothalamic–pituitary–gonadotrophin–gonadal axis. This occurs in boys and girls with congenital adrenal hyperplasia who have received treatment with glucocorticoids after the ages of 4–8 years.

Gonadotrophin-producing tumours are exceedingly rare, and produce testicular enlargement in boys and vaginal bleeding in girls as the first sign. They are usually malignant.

Suprarenal causes of false puberty

The secretion of excess androgens by the suprarenal causes false puberty. The growth of secondary sexual hair is stimulated and the phallus enlarges. Gonadotrophins, however, are suppressed so the testes remain small in a boy, and periods do not develop in a girl. Suprarenal tumours and Cushing's syndrome can be distinguished from congenital adrenal hyperplasia by the presence of raised plasma 17-hydroxyprogesterone and urinary excretion of pregnanetriol in the latter when it is due to a 21-hydroxylase defect, and by normal suppressibility of urinary 17-oxosteroids.

Testicular causes of false puberty

Testicular Leydig cell tumours causing false puberty are exceedingly rare. Occasional cases of Leydig cell hyperplasia have been described. The tumours are usually palpable, but occasionally may be small. However, a useful clue to the presence of a testicular tumour is that the contralateral testis is even smaller because gonadotrophins are suppressed. In most cases the condition is fully established by the age of 6 years.

Precocity is marked: the physique is muscular, body hair growth is considerable, the voice is strikingly gruff and manly, and the penis and prostate are enlarged. In half the cases there may be grossly overt psychosexual behaviour. Because the tumour is secreting testosterone, high levels of 17-oxosteroids are not always found in the urine, but raised plasma testosterone is diagnostic.

Ovarian causes of false puberty

Ovarian tumours account for only a few per cent of cases of precocious puberty in girls. They usually present at about the age of 4 years with irregular vaginal bleeding, breast development and pubic and axillary hair growth. There may be abdominal pain and the tumour may be palpable. The usual type of tumour producing endocrine effects is a granulosa cell tumour. This is usually benign, but about one-fifth are malignant.

Androgen-producing tumours of the ovary (andro-blastomas) cause heterosexual precocious puberty with the development of secondary sexual hair, hirsutism and virilization.

Drugs

The accidental or deliberate ingestion of oestrogens (commonly mother's contraceptive pills) by girls may lead to vaginal withdrawal bleeding and to some breast development. Androgens and anabolic steroids may cause secondary sexual hair growth and phallic enlargement.

Sharon O'Byrne

PUBIC HAIR, LOSS OF

The amount of pubic hair varies from individual to individual and is less in some races than others, for example in orientals compared with Caucasians. In the female, secretion of the adrenal androgens, androstenedione and dehydroepiandrosterone, is responsible for the development of pubic hair, via their peripheral conversion into testosterone. In the male, the secretion of testosterone by the testis and its conversion to dihydrotestosterone brings about pubic hair growth. Bearing these facts in mind, it can be seen that any disease process which affects the adrenal gland in a female, or testicular function in a male, may lead to loss of pubic hair. The causes of loss of pubic hair are listed in Table P.9. Thus, hypothalamic or pituitary disease may cause loss of adrenocortico-trophic hormone (ACTH) or of the gonadotrophins, luteinizing hormone being the one responsible for testosterone production by the testis. Primary disease of the adrenals such as Addison's disease will cause loss of pubic hair in females, whereas in males destruction by disease or removal of the testes will lead to pubic hair loss. The testes can be damaged by mumps or orchitis in adult life, by trauma, or by cyto-toxic drugs. The testes may be removed surgically or their function inhibited medically in the treatment of prostatic carcinoma. In this condition the loss of pubic hair may also be caused by the administration of oestrogens. Oestrogens may sometimes be secreted in a male by a Leydig secreting tumour of the testis. Other conditions which can lead to a rise in the ratio of oestrogen to androgen in the male include cirrhosis of the liver and haemochromatosis.

Table P.9 Causes of pubic hair loss

Males	*Females*
Hypothalamic disease	Hypothalamic disease
Pituitary disease	Pituitary disease
Testicular disease, damage or removal	Addison's disease
Oestrogen therapy	Hypothyroidism
Cirrhosis of the liver	Hypoparathyroidism
Haemochromatosis	Alopecia universalis
Hypothyroidism	
Thyrotoxicosis	
Hypoparathyroidism	
Alopecia universalis	

In addition to adrenal and testicular androgens, other hormones affect the growth of pubic hair. The low calcium levels of hypoparathyroidism may lead to coarse and scanty pubic hair, while there is loss of genital hair in hypothyroidism and, in some cases of thyrotoxicosis, loss of pubic hair has been described. Finally, pubic hair may disappear completely in the condition of alopecia universalis.

Sharon O'Byrne

PULSE, CHARACTER OF

An essential part of the cardiovascular system examination is assessment of the pulse character, rate and rhythm at a major artery, usually radial or carotid. The character of the pulse is understood to be the shape which would be inscribed by an instrument recording the movement of the artery. The most important deviation from the normal character is in the rate of rise of the pulse. This, together with variations in the amplitude – often referred to as the 'volume' of the pulse – produces patterns which are characteristic of various cardiac lesions – usually of the valves. These observations are best described in simple, unambiguous terms; for example the pulse volume should be referred to as 'small', 'normal' or 'large' and not as 'good' or 'poor'.

The most common abnormality in the character of the pulse is a rapid rate of rise. The most typical form of this is the pulse of aortic regurgitation. This pulse is of large volume and is described as *collapsing*, although it also used to be known as a *water-hammer* pulse. It is best examined by feeling with the palmar surfaces rather than the tips of the fingers, with the hand placed over the wrist and then elevating the patient's arm rather sharply above shoulder level. A collapsing pulse is also found in patients with a large persistent ductus arteriosus or arteriovenous fistula. Other rarer congenital causes include pulmonary atresia with a large ventricular septal defect and persistent truncus arteriosus. A large-volume pulse which is not necessarily collapsing in nature can arise due to high-output cardiac states (thyrotoxicosis, Paget's disease and severe anaemia), bradycardia and arteriosclerotic arteries in older patients.

Normal- or small-volume pulses with a rapid rate of rise are felt in such conditions as gross mitral regurgitation, hypertrophic obstructive cardiomyopathy and fixed subvalvar aortic stenosis. This type of pulse is sometimes described as *jerky*.

A *slow-rising* pulse is seen with significant aortic valve stenosis. The volume of the pulse is usually small, and this type of pulse is more easily missed than is the collapsing pulse. Sometimes a notch is felt low down on the upstroke of the pulse so that there appears to be a very small impulse followed by a much larger one. If this is the case, the pulse is described as *anacrotic* (an abbreviation of anadicrotic meaning 'twice-beating on the upstroke'). This pulse can often be felt in the radial and brachial arteries, but it is much more easily detected in the carotids where it is often accompanied by a systolic thrill – the palpable counterpart of the murmur transmitted to the neck. A variation of this pulse is when the notch is very much higher on the upstroke, producing the impression of two more nearly equal impulses. This is the *bisferiens* pulse, and it is felt when aortic stenosis is accompanied by aortic regurgitation of at least moderate severity. This type of pulse is rather uncommon, and must not be confused with one in which a small notch is felt at the very apex of the pulse; this is sometimes felt in aortic regurgitation, especially if the palpating finger is applied more firmly than usual. A very well-marked bisferiens pulse is very occasionally visible in the carotid arteries.

Melvin Lobo

PULSE RATE, ABNORMAL

A normal pulse rate varies from about 60 to 100 beats per minute: bradycardia is defined as a rate of less than 60, and tachycardia as a rate of greater than 100 beats per minute. This does not imply that rates outside this range are necessarily abnormal; for example, a rate of 40 or so is quite common in athletes in training, and a rate of over 100 would not necessarily be remarkable in an exceedingly anxious patient.

Bradycardia

Bradycardia may be due either to a slow rate of discharge of the sino-atrial node or to various disorders of impulse formation or conduction. It should not be diagnosed solely from the rate as felt at the radial pulse as, in various conditions such as atrial fibrillation or extrasystoles, only a proportion of the beats may reach the wrist; the true heart rate can then be determined only by auscultation. The causes are summarized in Table P.10.

Table P.10 Causes of bradycardia

Sinus bradycardia
- Athletics
- Reflex
- Obstructive jaundice
- Myxoedema
- Anorexia nervosa
- Hypothermia
- Aortic stenosis
- Drugs (e.g. beta-blocking agents)

Sick sinus syndrome

Junctional rhythm

Conduction defects
- 2:1 atrioventricular block (or higher degrees of partial a-v block)
- Complete heart block

Sinus bradycardia is not uncommon in otherwise normal individuals, especially during sleep when rates as low as 30 to 40 per minute have been recorded during continuous monitoring. The pulse rate may also be slow during convalescence after influenza and other fevers. In acute nephritis, bradycardia is probably a reflex result of the acute hypertension. A similar mechanism operates in cases of phaeochromocytoma releasing predominantly noradrenaline; the paroxysms of hypertension are associated with striking bradycardia, unlike the type of attack due to release of adrenaline. Bradycardia is also a well-recognized, but far from constant, finding in obstructive jaundice and when the intracranial pressure is raised for any reason; in the latter case the slow rate may be due to direct stimulation of the vagal centre. Myxoedema is another cause of bradycardia which may be profound in myxoedema coma. The pulse is also often very slow in anorexia nervosa. The only valve lesion to be associated with a slow pulse is aortic stenosis; in some severe cases a rate as low as 50 may be found, even in the presence of left ventricular failure. As in myxoedema, the reduced metabolic rate of hypothermia, either accidental or induced, is associated with bradycardia; even in atrial fibrillation, a common

complication of hypothermia, the ventricular rate is quite slow. As a transient phenomenon, bradycardia occurs in carotid sinus syncope and in vasovagal attacks in general. Drugs which commonly cause bradycardia include beta-blockers, non-dihydropyridine calcium-channel blockers and anti-arrhythmic medications such as amiodarone. Bradycardia may also be found after large doses of cholinergic drugs (e.g. carbachol) and anticholinesterases (e.g. neostigmine). Sinus bradycardia may also be seen in digoxin intoxication.

The *sick sinus syndrome* is caused by impairment of sino-atrial node function. It is thus characterized by sinus bradycardia (Fig. P.29), sinus arrest, which may cause Stokes–Adams attacks, and sino-atrial block. The latter, like sinus bradycardia, may occur normally during sleep, and is a result of failure of transmission of a sinus impulse to the atria; a whole electrocardiographic complex is thus deleted. With 2:1 sino-atrial block the electrocardiogram resembles sinus bradycardia, but exercise or atropine will cause the rate suddenly to double. A well-known association of the sick sinus syndrome is the occurrence of paroxysms of atrial fibrillation, often with a slow ventricular rate, and atrial flutter – the so-called bradycardia–tachycardia syndrome.

Junctional rhythm, originating in the atrioventricular node or the main bundle of His, is a common arrhythmia. It is most often due to digoxin, but may occur after myocardial infarction or in healthy individuals; the rate is usually around 60. The atria and ventricles contract simultaneously so that, clinically, the diagnostic feature is a cannon wave in the jugular venous pulse with each beat. In the electrocardiogram the P wave is inverted in leads II, III and aVF, and may be just before, incorporated in or just after the QRS complex (Fig. P.30). Junctional rhythm is rarely of any serious significance.

Disorders of the atrioventricular conducting system are an important cause of bradycardia. In first-degree heart block, with prolongation of the P-R interval as the only abnormality, the heart rate is

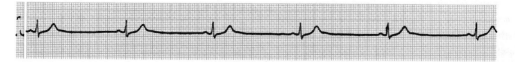

Figure P.29 Electrocardiogram (lead II), showing profound sinus bradycardia at a rate of 31 per minute, in a man, aged 61 years, complaining of recurrent syncope. A 2:1 sino-atrial block was suspected, but the rate increased gradually during exercise and after atropine administration.

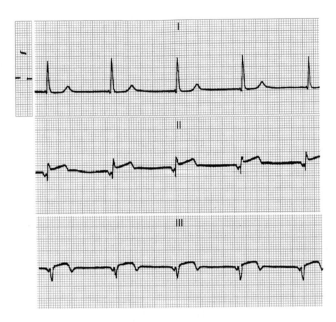

Figure P.30 Electrocardiogram of a woman, aged 66 years, at 24 hours after inferior myocardial infarction. Apart from the changes of recent infarction, the P wave is inverted in leads II and III and closely precedes the QRS complex. Junctional rhythm at a rate of 60 per minute.

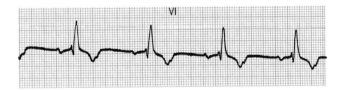

Figure P.31 Electrocardiogram of a woman, aged 58 years, admitted following a Stokes–Adams attack. The record shows a 2:1 atrioventricular block with right bundle-branch block; the unconducted P waves deform the upstroke of the T waves of the preceding QRS complex.

normal. The pulse is slow and regular, however, if second-degree heart block has progressed to 2:1 block. This is the case whether the conduction defect has progressed via Wenckebach periods (Mobitz Type I) or is the more serious Mobitz Type II block. Clinically, these two types can be differentiated by the response to exercise or atropine. In Type I block, conduction improves and a normal heart rate results (see Fig. P.44); an increase in the severity of the block is the rule following these manoeuvres in Type II block. A 2:1 block is most often diagnosed from the electrocardiogram (Fig. P.31).

In *complete heart block*, atrioventricular dissociation is present and the ventricular rate is that of a pacemaker somewhere in the conducting system distal to the block. The site of this pacemaker can be determined approximately from the surface electrocardiogram. If the QRS complexes are of normal configuration, the pacemaker must be above the bifurcation of the main bundle; a pacemaker in one or other bundle branch produces complexes with the pattern of bundle-branch block. Precise localization of the site of the block is possible by intracardiac electrocardiography. The most common cause of heart block is fibrosis of the atrioventricular bundle and its branches; the cause of this fibrosis is not known, and the remaining myocardium is usually healthy. Ischaemia – particularly myocardial infarction – is a less common cause, as are digoxin intoxication and cardiomyopathy of almost any type; cardiac amyloidosis is particularly likely to be associated with conduction defects. Even less common causes include myocarditis, particularly diphtheritic and, in South America, trypanosomiasis (Chagas' disease); calcification of the atrioventricular rings in and around the aortic valve may encroach on the bundle and cause heart block. Congenital heart block is a rare condition; the ventricular rate is usually rather faster than in the acquired variety.

The most common symptom of heart block is the Stokes–Adams attack, particularly if the degree of block is changing. Established complete heart block may also cause some reduction in exercise tolerance with fatigue, dyspnoea and even heart failure. The diagnosis of Stokes–Adams attacks is discussed under FAINTS (see p. 213). Clinical diagnosis of complete heart block is almost always possible. Apart from marked bradycardia with a ventricular rate around 30 or 40 or less, the diagnostic signs include 'a' waves in the jugular venous pulse at a faster rate than the arterial pulse with, in addition, cannon waves occurring whenever atrial and ventricular systole happen to coincide. On auscultation, the first heart sound varies markedly in intensity, the louder sounds occurring when ventricular systole follows closely upon atrial systole, so that the atrioventricular valve cusps are wide apart when the ventricles contract (Fig. P.32) (see also HEART SOUNDS, p. 285). Occasionally, it may be possible to hear separate atrial sounds. Importantly, when complete heart block is complicated by atrial fibrillation, none of these signs – which result from a coordinated atrial contraction – is present. An ejection systolic murmur is commonly present due to the large stroke volume, which is also the reason for the wide pulse pressure; these two signs are present in bradycardia from any cause. In the electrocardiogram P waves and QRS complexes can be identified with no mathematical relationship between the atrial and ventricular rates.

Tachycardia

Tachycardia may be due to an increased frequency of discharge of the sino-atrial node (sinus tachycardia) or to an arrhythmia. (For a discussion of arrhythmias causing an irregular pulse, see PULSE, RHYTHM OF, p. 573). In this section only those arrhythmias producing a rapid regular pulse will be discussed in any detail. The common causes of tachycardia are summarized in Table P.11.

Sinus tachycardia is present in most febrile conditions due to a direct effect of the pyrexia on the sino-atrial node. In tetanus, the rapid pulse is probably due to involvement of the autonomic nervous system by the toxin. In a few infections, such as typhoid, the rise in pulse rate may be rather less than expected from the degree of fever; this relative bradycardia may be of

Table P.11 Causes of tachycardia

Sinus tachycardia
- Anxiety
- Febrile conditions
- Hyperthyroidism
- Drugs (e.g. sympathomimetic agents)
- Reflex (e.g. heart failure, hypertension)

Supraventricular tachycardia
- a-v re-entrant tachycardia
- Atrial and junctional tachycardia
- Atrial flutter
- Atrial fibrillation

Ventricular tachycardia

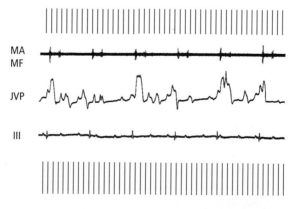

Figure P.32 Phonocardiogram, jugular venous pulse and lead III of the electrocardiogram of a man, aged 47 years, with long-standing complete heart block. In the first and last beats the P waves closely precede the QRS complexes, and the first heart sound is loud. In the third beat, the P wave coincides with the QRS complex and a tall cannon wave is present in the venous pulse. Smaller cannon waves are seen from time to time, and 'a' waves can also be identified occurring 0.14 s after each P wave. Time markers are 0.2 s.

some slight diagnostic significance. The sino-atrial node is affected directly in a number of other situations in which tachycardia is prominent. These include: hyperthyroidism in which there is also the reflex effect of the high cardiac output discussed below; phaeochromocytoma secreting predominantly adrenaline; and anxiety states and other conditions (e.g. severe pain) in which there is a raised level of circulating catecholamines. Da Costa's syndrome, known also as cardiac neurosis and effort syndrome, is an important cause of moderate tachycardia which persists sometimes for many years. Various drugs, including atropine and sympathomimetic agents such as ephedrine and isoprenaline, also produce tachycardia which is also a characteristic feature of poisoning by tricyclic antidepressant drugs.

Sinus tachycardia can also be caused by reflex mechanisms. In conditions causing a rise in right atrial pressure the sinus rate is increased via the Bainbridge reflex. Hypotension from any cause or, more precisely, a fall in pulse pressure, also causes tachycardia via baroceptors in the aortic arch and carotid sinus. This is the mechanism, for example, of the tachycardia during the straining period of a Valsalva manoeuvre. In high-output states the tachycardia is probably secondary to the tendency of the right atrial pressure to rise as a result of the increased venous return; therefore, the pulse rate is rapid in hyperthyroidism, severe anaemia, pregnancy, beri-beri, widespread Paget's disease and arteriovenous fistula. If such a fistula is accessible, the effect of the high cardiac output can be convincingly demonstrated by the abrupt fall in pulse rate which results from digital occlusion of the fistula. In cardiac failure the tendency to a reduction in pulse pressure, acting on the aortic and carotid baroceptors, combines with the rise in right atrial pressure to produce considerable tachycardia in most, though not all, cases. Tachycardia is also a feature of severe myocardial disease even in the absence of frank failure; thus, it is found in most cases of myocarditis and in some cases of ischaemic heart disease. Hypotension due to extracardiac factors is also a cause of tachycardia which is seen in shock and as a result of the administration of vasodilating agents.

Disproportionate tachycardia on exertion, with a normal resting pulse rate, is seen in patients less severely affected by the conditions discussed above, and is also a measure of an individual's lack of training. Physical fitness can be roughly quantified by the amount of work that can be done at any given heart rate.

Lesions of the vagus nerve may occasionally cause tachycardia which has been described with subtentorial tumours and in various types of peripheral neuropathy including alcoholic and diphtheritic. There is also a rare primary disorder of the sino-atrial node (sinus node re-entry) in which tachycardia is a feature.

There are several varieties of *supraventricular tachycardia*. The most common is *a-v re-entrant tachycardia*, which occurs when there is a conducting pathway between the atria and ventricles in addition to the atrioventricular node. This is either in – but functionally separate from – the node, or is anatomically separate, as in the pre-excitation syndromes. Differences in the conductivity and refractoriness of these two pathways can result in a circus movement, with an impulse re-entering the atria from the ventricles via one pathway and then being transmitted again to the ventricles via the other. There is usually no other evidence of heart disease, and paroxysms of tachycardia occur throughout life. The attacks begin abruptly, and patients may describe symptoms of palpitation and lightheadedness. The associated anxiety may cause hyperventilation and paraesthesiae in the fingers, or even frank tetany may occur. In such cases it is clearly important to distinguish cause from effect in the manifestations. The attack may last for minutes, hours or (rarely) for days, and ends as abruptly as it began. Prolonged attacks, lasting for a week or more at a very fast rate, can cause cardiac failure even in otherwise normal individuals, but this resolves rapidly and completely once the attack is over. In older patients more serious symptoms may occur; in particular, ischaemic pain is common even though the associated coronary artery disease may be quite mild. Paroxysms of a-v re-entrant tachycardia are common in the *pre-excitation syndromes*, of which the Wolff–Parkinson–White syndrome is the most common. In this syndrome, the P-R interval is pathologically short and the initial part of the QRS rises or falls slowly to form the so-called 'delta' wave (Fig. P.33). In paroxysms of tachycardia in such cases the QRS assumes a normal configuration. This condition is often benign, but paroxysms of atrial fibrillation with a very rapid ventricular rate can occur and sudden death, due probably to ventricular fibrillation, has been reported.

Atrial and *junctional tachycardia* due to enhanced automaticity of a focus in the atria or atria-ventricular junction are much less common than a-v re-entrant

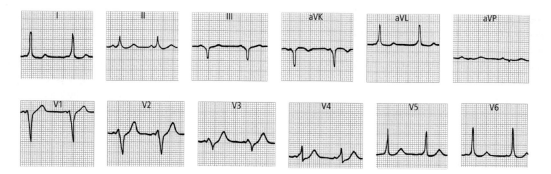

Figure P.33 Wolff–Parkinson–White syndrome showing short P-R interval and broad QRS complexes. The slowly rising initial part of the QRS complex (the delta wave) is well shown in leads aVL and V6.

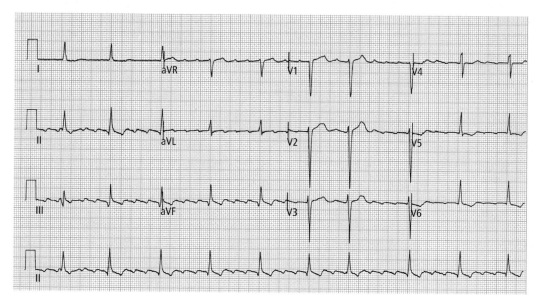

Figure P.34 Atrial flutter with variable atrioventricular block. The baseline demonstrates rapid, regular flutter waves with characteristic 'saw-tooth' appearance.

tachycardia. They may occur in paroxysms, but are more often sustained for long periods. There is often some degree of atrioventricular block which never occurs in a-v re-entrant tachycardia, and there is usually associated heart disease such as ischaemia or cardiomyopathy; digoxin toxicity may also cause such arrhythmias.

Faster atrial rates than those found in the tachycardias already considered produce *atrial flutter*. Here, the atrial rate is often around 300 per minute; this is faster than the AV node can conduct, and some degree of atrioventricular block is almost inevitable. A 2:1 ratio is most common, producing a regular ventricular rhythm at about 150 per minute. This particular rate is rather characteristic of atrial flutter as it is

faster than most sinus tachycardias and slower than many other supraventricular tachycardias. The diagnosis can be made with near-certainty by studying the effect of pressure on the carotid sinus. In atrial flutter, the degree of atrioventricular block is increased with, characteristically, an abrupt halving of the pulse rate. In sinus tachycardia, carotid sinus pressure produces a more gradual slowing, and in other supraventricular tachycardias the attack is either terminated or continues unabated. In atrial flutter the electrocardiogram shows rapid regular flutter waves with QRS complexes at one-half or one-quarter of the atrial rate. The atrial rate is so rapid that, in most leads, the flutter waves produce a continuous 'saw-tooth' appearance of the baseline (Fig. P.34). The absence of any isoelectric segments in the baseline has been suggested as a diagnostic criterion of flutter. There is, however, no real justification for this view, and many authorities prefer to use the term 'flutter' for all supraventricular arrhythmias with an atrial rate of 250–350 per minute. The causes of atrial flutter are similar to those of atrial fibrillation (see p. 576), except that it is not so common in mitral valve disease or hyperthyroidism.

Atrial fibrillation presents with an irregular tachycardia, and is discussed at length in the section on PULSE, RHYTHM OF (below).

The electrocardiographic diagnosis of a supraventricular tachycardia depends on finding a regular tachycardia with P waves which are abnormal both in their timing in relationship to the QRS and in their shape (Fig. P.35). The QRS complexes are usually normal, although they may be widened and deformed as a result of aberrant ventricular conduction and resemble bundle-branch block.

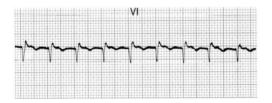

Figure P.35 Supraventricular tachycardia at 160 per minute, probably junctional as P waves cannot be certainly identified, in a patient 1 week after an inferior myocardial infarction.

Ventricular tachycardia is a much more serious arrhythmia than its supraventricular counterparts. Although it can occur in patients with otherwise normal hearts, there is usually serious underlying heart disease. Much the commonest cause is ischaemic heart disease, and this is particularly common after myocardial infarction when it can cause serious deterioration in the patient's condition and may be a forerunner of ventricular fibrillation. Ventricular

tachycardia also occurs in a group of syndromes characterized by a prolonged Q-T interval in the electrocardiogram and, sometimes, congenital deafness. In ventricular tachycardia the rate is very variable (most commonly around 180 per minute, though it may be as low as 100 or less), in which case some prefer to use the term 'idioventricular rhythm' rather than 'tachycardia'. The electrocardiogram shows broad, often notched, QRS complexes with no preceding P waves; a variation in which the QRS axis changes gradually and repeatedly so that the complexes appear to twist around the baseline is known as 'torsades de pointes'. In the usual type it may sometimes be possible to identify P waves separately at a slower rate; in this case, the diagnosis of ventricular tachycardia is certain (Fig. P.36). Otherwise, there can be confusion with supraventricular tachycardia with aberrant ventricular conduction. This is a difficult diagnostic problem as the certain identification of P waves in such a record may be impossible.

See also PULSE, RHYTHM OF (below).

Melvin Lobo

PULSE, RHYTHM OF

An absolutely regular pulse is rare. Even in normal sinus rhythm slight fluctuations in rate can be detected by measuring successive R-R intervals in the electrocardiogram. This can hardly be detected by palpation of the pulse, however, and this section will deal with irregularities that are apparent clinically. When examining the pulse, it is necessary first to determine whether it is regular or irregular and, if the latter, whether any pattern can be detected within the irregularity. Complete clinical analysis of an irregular pulse includes inspection of the jugular venous pulse and auscultation at the apex beat in addition to feeling the arterial pulse. The venous pulse provides evidence of

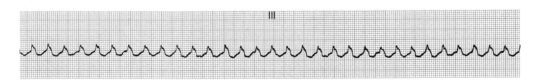

Figure P.36 Ventricular tachycardia at 190 per minute in a patient a few hours after a myocardial infarction. Low-amplitude deflections which are probably P waves at a slower rate can be seen between some of the ventricular complexes; this confirms the ventricular origin of the arrhythmia.

the presence and frequency of atrial contractions; auscultation allows the detection of ventricular contractions too feeble to produce a pulse at the wrist. Many arrhythmias can be diagnosed clinically, but electrocardiographic confirmation is essential.

There are two main mechanisms that can produce an irregular pulse. The first is a disorder of impulse formation in which, most commonly, an abnormal (ectopic) pacemaker drives the ventricles either directly or via the atrioventricular bundle. The other mechanism is a disorder of conduction in which a block develops somewhere along the long pathway from the sino-atrial node to the ventricular myocardium; if this block is intermittent, an irregular pulse is likely to result. The common causes of an irregular pulse are summarized in Table P.12. For a more detailed discussion of the genesis of arrhythmias, see PULSE RATE, ABNORMAL (p. 567).

Disorders of impulse formation

The rate of discharge of the sino-atrial node can vary, more or less rhythmically, in many normal subjects;

Table P.12 Causes of an irregular pulse

Disorders of impulse formation
Sinus arrhythmia
Ectopic beats (supraventricular or ventricular)
- Escape beats
- Extrasystoles
- Parasystole
Atrial fibrillation
Atrial flutter with varying atrioventricular block

Disorders of conduction
Sino-atrial block
Partial atrioventricular block
- Mobitz Type I (Wenckebach)
- Mobitz Type II

Apparent irregularity in normal rhythm
Pulsus alternans
Pulsus paradoxus

---

this condition, termed *sinus arrhythmia*, is quite benign and hardly justifies classification as a 'disorder'. The fluctuations in rate are most commonly in phase with respiration, the rate increasing during inspiration and slowing during expiration. This is very common in children and is due to reflex variations in vagal tone (Fig. P.37). The absence of respiratory sinus arrhythmia is sometimes of some slight diagnostic significance in a child, as this is a feature of a large atrial septal defect. There are also two, much rarer, types of non-respiratory sinus arrhythmia. In one, the cycles of tachycardia and bradycardia are much longer and are quite unrelated to respiration; the P waves of the electrocardiogram are normal and constant in configuration. In the other type, the P waves vary slightly in shape and the irregularity is believed to be due to changes in the site of the pacemaker within the sino-atrial node itself. The irregularity in respiratory sinus arrhythmia is exaggerated by deep breathing and, in all types, is abolished or markedly reduced by exercise or other causes of tachycardia.

Ectopic beats are a very common cause of an irregular pulse. They are due to the discharge of an abnormal pacemaker in the atria, atrioventricular junction (AV node and main bundle of His) or ventricles. Apart from their site of origin, they can be classified as escape beats, extrasystoles and parasystoles. *Escape beats* should be regarded as a protective mechanism against asystole. They arise either from the atrioventricular junction or from the ventricles and occur whenever, for any reason, there is a prolonged pause in the activity of the sino-atrial node. Thus, they may be seen in sinus bradycardia and during the slow phase of sinus arrhythmia. They are difficult to recognize clinically, but can be identified in the electrocardiogram by the abnormally long pause preceding an ectopic beat identified, as described below, as junctional or ventricular in origin.

Extrasystoles most frequently arise from the ventricles, but atrial and junctional extrasystoles are also common. If a ventricular extrasystole occurs early in

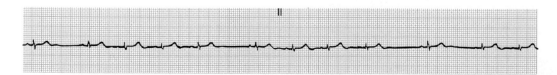

Figure P.37 Electrocardiogram showing gross respiratory sinus arrhythmia. The cycle lengths vary from 0.7 to 1.24 seconds.

diastole, ventricular filling will be incomplete and the contraction may fail to open the aortic valve; even if it does so, the pulse may be so feeble that it does not reach the wrist. Thus, in the radial pulse a 'dropped beat' will be noticed; on auscultation the extrasystole will be heard either as the first sound only or as both sounds. Ventricular extrasystoles occurring later in diastole are more likely to produce a palpable impulse at the radial pulse. Often an extrasystole follows each sinus beat to produce pulsus bigeminus or coupled beats, or every second sinus beat to produce trigeminus. The patient with extrasystoles may have noticed no abnormality, or they may describe symptoms of palpitations.

In the electrocardiogram ventricular extrasystoles are identified by the bizarre configuration of the QRS complex and by the absence of a P wave (Fig. P.38). The pause following the extrasystole is usually fully compensatory, that is the sum of the R-R intervals preceding and following the ectopic beat equals two complete cycles. Rarely, if the sinus rate is slow, interpolated ventricular extrasystoles occur – the only true 'extra' systole. Occasional ventricular extrasystoles are usually benign and do not necessarily indicate organic heart disease; they are more common following overindulgence in tea, coffee, alcohol or tobacco. Frequent ventricular extrasystoles occurring at rest are of more importance and probably indicate heart disease of some kind; however, their exact significance is uncertain and, provided that the standard investigations (including an exercise electrocardiogram) are normal, a good prognosis can be given. They are certainly of more serious significance following myocardial infarction, when, if they are multifocal, or appear in salvoes, or are so premature as to deform the T wave of the preceding complex (R-on-T), they may presage ventricular tachycardia or fibrillation.

Atrial and junctional (supraventricular) extrasystoles produce very much the same symptoms and signs as ventricular. The electrocardiogram shows abnormal P waves indicating the site of the ectopic focus; with junctional extrasystoles the P wave is typically inverted in leads II, III and aVF. The form of the QRS complex is usually normal as the impulse reaches the ventricles via the normal conducting pathways. Occasionally, however, if the supraventricular extrasystole is very premature, one or other branch of the bundle may still be partially refractory so that intraventricular conduction proceeds abnormally and the configuration of the QRS is bizarre, simulating bundle-branch block. This phenomenon is known as 'aberrant ventricular conduction', and can only be decisively distinguished from a ventricular extrasystole by the finding of an ectopic P wave preceding the QRS (Fig. P.39). The pause following a supraventricular extrasystole is usually less than fully compensatory. Supraventricular extrasystoles are nearly always benign, but if they are frequent – for example in a patient with mitral stenosis – they may indicate that atrial fibrillation is impending.

With extrasystoles in general, the interval between a sinus beat and an extrasystole – the coupling interval – is remarkably constant, implying that the discharge of the ectopic focus is in some way dependent on the preceding sinus beat. This is not the case in the phenomenon known as *parasystole*. In this situation an ectopic focus, most often in the ventricles but occasionally in the atria or atrioventricular junction, discharges at its own intrinsic rate regardless of the rate of the sino-atrial node or other dominant pacemaker. The ectopic focus is 'protected' from discharge by the normal sinus beats so that, whenever the ectopic discharge finds the ventricles in a non-refractory state, an ectopic beat appears. The diagnosis is made from the electrocardiogram by finding ectopic beats with varying coupling intervals and a succession of interectopic intervals all of which are multiples of a single shorter interval – the intrinsic cycle length of the ectopic focus (Fig. P.40).

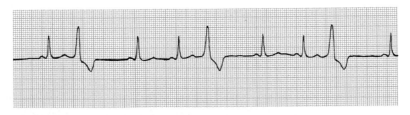

Figure P.38 Electrocardiogram showing ventricular extrasystoles producing pulsus bigeminus (second complex) and trigeminus (fifth and eighth complexes).

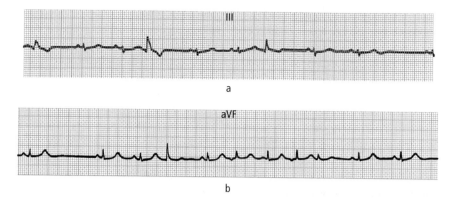

Figure P.39 Electrocardiogram showing frequent supraventricular extrasystoles conducted normally or with ventricular aberration. (a) The first, fourth and seventh complexes are supraventricular in origin, despite their abnormal configuration, as shown by the preceding P waves which deform the T waves of the previous complexes. The long pause at the end of the strip is preceded by an ectopic P wave which is completely blocked. (b) The sixth and eighth complexes are supraventricular extrasystoles conducted normally, the fourth and ninth complexes show ventricular aberration.

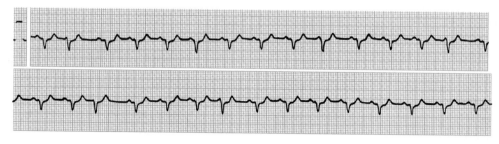

Figure P.40 Two strips of continuous record showing junctional parasystole with retrograde block. The sinus P waves continue uninterruptedly with a cycle length of 0.7 second. The second, 10th and 14th complexes in the upper strip and the third and seventh in the lower are junctional in origin. The inter-ectopic intervals are 5.76 seconds ($= 2 \times 2.88$) and 2.88 seconds.

The clinical diagnosis of extrasystoles is usually easy but, if they occur frequently, they may be difficult to distinguish from atrial fibrillation. Exercise will usually abolish extrasystoles and, if anything, cause greater irregularity in atrial fibrillation. The jugular venous pulse may also be helpful as cannon waves are a constant finding in junctional extrasystoles and may occur in other varieties also, if atrial and ventricular systole happen to coincide. A cannon wave implies an effective atrial contraction and therefore rules out atrial fibrillation.

Progressively more rapid rates of discharge of an ectopic atrial focus lead to atrial tachycardia and atrial flutter, which can be regarded as a series of atrial ectopic beats. In these conditions the ventricular rhythm is usually regular, but when the rate of discharge of the ectopic focus exceeds about 400 per minute, coordinated atrial depolarization and contraction are impossible and

atrial fibrillation results. The supraventricular impulses impinge more or less at random on the atrioventricular node, finding it and the remainder of the conducting tissue more or less refractory at any given time so that the ventricular response is totally irregular.

Atrial fibrillation is an extremely common finding in almost any type of heart disease. Probably the most common cause is rheumatic heart disease, especially mitral valve disease; it is much less common, except as a terminal event, in isolated aortic valve disease. It is also a well-known complication in hyperthyroidism, especially in the toxic nodular goitre of older subjects. It is not very common in uncomplicated angina, but it occurs quite frequently after myocardial infarction and when cardiac failure develops. In hypertensive heart disease, as well, it is rather unusual except late in the course of the disease. Other conditions characterized by chronic atrial fibrillation (as distinct from the transient type to be discussed below) are constrictive pericarditis, invasion of the pericardium by bronchial carcinoma or other mediastinal tumours, tumours of the heart itself, many varieties of cardiomyopathy and atrial septal defect, but not other types of congenital heart disease. Idiopathic or 'lone' atrial fibrillation, with no other evidence of heart disease, is well recognized and not uncommon. Infections – particularly respiratory – can precipitate atrial fibrillation, especially in patients predisposed by rheumatic heart disease. Once the infection is over, sinus rhythm may be restored, either spontaneously or by DC cardioversion. Return to sinus rhythm is also possible if atrial fibrillation has been caused by myocardial infarction, and is almost the rule in thyrotoxic atrial fibrillation once the patient is euthyroid. Other causes of transient atrial fibrillation include pulmonary embolism (although it is rather unusual in chronic cor pulmonale), sick sinus syndrome, alcohol abuse, thoracotomy for any purpose, electric shock and hypothermia, either accidental or induced. It can rarely be caused by drugs such as digoxin and anaesthetic agents.

The development of atrial fibrillation will usually cause the patient to complain of palpitation, and cardiac failure may be precipitated in those with severe heart disease. This is particularly the case in mitral stenosis in which the rapid ventricular rate, by restricting the time available for ventricular filling, causes a steep rise in left atrial pressure and may precipitate pulmonary oedema (Fig. P.41). Once the ventricular rate has been brought under control with anti-arrythmic therapy, most patients with atrial

fibrillation have few, if any, symptoms attributable to the arrhythmia. The pulse is totally irregular and rapid in uncontrolled atrial fibrillation. The true ventricular rate can be determined only by auscultation as many of the impulses fail to reach the radial pulse. The difference between the rates as determined at the radial pulse and by auscultation – the 'pulse deficit' – is some measure of the lack of control. Once the ventricular rate is under control there is no pulse deficit, and the irregularity of the pulse, though still present, may be less easy to detect. The other diagnostic feature is the absence of evidence of atrial systole; no 'a' waves are seen in the jugular venous pulse and the pre-systolic murmur of mitral stenosis disappears, as does an atrial gallop rhythm if one has been heard previously. The electrocardiogram shows three diagnostic features: a totally irregular ventricular rhythm; absence of P waves; and their replacement by 'f' waves, fairly large in amplitude if the atrial fibrillation is of recent onset and becoming smaller as the months and years go by (Fig. P.42).

Atrial flutter, although usually associated with a regular ventricular rhythm, may produce an irregular pulse if the degree of atrioventricular block is variable. Clinically, this is very difficult to distinguish from atrial fibrillation and, indeed, at fast atrial rates the two conditions merge in so-called 'flutter-fibrillation'. This unsatisfactory term should be avoided if possible; if each of the varying R-R intervals is a multiple of the interval between two 'f' waves, flutter should be diagnosed. For further discussion on atrial flutter, see PULSE RATE, ABNORMAL (p. 572).

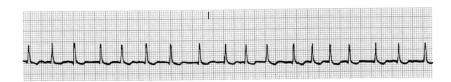

Figure P.41 Atrial fibrillation with a ventricular rate of 140 per minute. Recorded from a man, aged 51 years, with mitral stenosis who was in pulmonary oedema at the time. He became virtually symptom-free when the ventricular rate was controlled with digoxin.

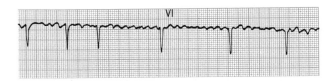

Figure P.42 Electrocardiogram showing atrial fibrillation with a ventricular rate of 60 per minute. The f waves are well shown, as is usually the case in lead VI.

Disorders of conduction

Failure of transmission of the impulse from the sino-atrial node to the ventricles causes 'dropped beats'. The ventricular rhythm will be regular only if every other beat is dropped (as in 2:1 atrioventricular block) or if the beat is complete and a lower pacemaker is driving the ventricles. Any other pattern of failure of conduction will cause an irregular pulse.

Sino-atrial block is a rather rare conduction defect in which the impulse fails to pass from the sino-atrial node to the atrial myocardium. Although sino-atrial block can be classified into first, second or third degree, only second degree can be diagnosed reliably from the ECG (Fig. P.43). The patients may be symptom-free, but Stokes–Adams attacks can occur. The condition can occur in the absence of other evidence of heart disease, especially during sleep, but it is quite often associated with ischaemic heart disease or, as a transient phenomenon, with acute rheumatic carditis. It is one of the typical features of the sick sinus syndrome and can also occasionally be produced by digoxin.

Partial atrioventricular block can also produce an irregular pulse. In Mobitz Type 1 (Wenckebach) second-degree block, conduction in the atrioventricular bundle becomes progressively more impaired from beat to beat, as shown by an increasing P-R interval in the electrocardiogram, until conduction fails completely and a ventricular beat is missed (Fig. P.44) Thus, in the radial pulse, every third, fourth or fifth beat may be dropped; there is also a slight progressive increase in ventricular rate during the runs of conducted beats, but this cannot be detected by palpation alone. This type of atrioventricular block is relatively benign and may be a transient occurrence in myocardial infarction or digoxin intoxication. Normal conduction is almost always restored by exercise, atropine or any other measure which increases the atrial rate (see Fig. P.44). Mobitz Type II second-degree

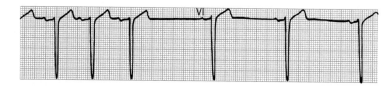

Figure P.43 Electrocardiogram showing the sudden development of 2:1 sino-atrial block (from a woman, aged 59 years, with severe hypertensive and ischaemic heart disease) between complexes 3–4, 4–5 and 5–6. P waves and QRS complexes are dropped for one cycle.

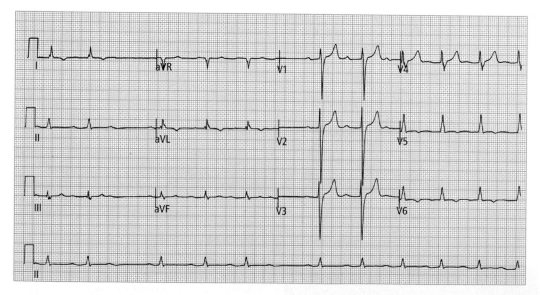

Figure P.44 Electrocardiogram showing Type I (Wenckebach) partial atrioventricular block. The P-R intervals progressively lengthen until conduction fails and a QRS complex is deleted (between 2nd and 3rd and between 5th and 6th QRS complexes on rhythm strip).

block is a much more serious condition. In its mildest form beats may be dropped intermittently, as in Type I, but without any previous lengthening of the P-R interval; later 2:1 or 3:1 block with a slow regular ventricular rhythm is common. Increasing the atrial rate, by any means, increases the severity of the block (see also PULSE RATE, ABNORMAL, p. 567).

Two mechanical causes of a palpably irregular pulse should be mentioned. *Pulsus alternans* is characterized by a regular rhythm with alternation in amplitude of the equally spaced beats. It may be easily palpable but, more often, is detected by sphygmomanometry. As the cuff pressure is lowered, half of the beats are heard at the higher systolic pressure and, as the pressure of the smaller amplitude beats is reached, the rate seems suddenly to double. A run of pulsus alternans is often initiated by an extrasystole, but it must not be confused with pulsus bigeminus. Nor should it be confused with electrical alternans in which the QRS complexes alternate in amplitude; the two conditions may co-exist, however. Though rather rare, pulsus alternans is an important sign of left ventricular failure.

Pulsus paradoxus is a feature of constrictive pericarditis, high pressure pericardial effusion and other less common conditions in which the primary abnormality is failure of the ventricles to fill adequately (restrictive cardiomyopathy). It is also important evidence of the severity of an attack of asthma. The normal tendency of the pulse-pressure to fall slightly during inspiration is much exaggerated so that, in a gross example, the arterial pulse may become impalpable during inspiration. At first, the impression is of a grossly irregular pulse but there is little difficulty in relating the changes to the phases of respiration; the diagnosis is confirmed by finding other evidence of pericardial constriction. This includes a rise in the already elevated venous pressure on inspiration instead of the usual fall, known also as Kussmaul's sign. The arterial changes are an exaggeration of, not opposite to, the normal; the term 'paradoxical' was applied because the heart's action appeared to have ceased during inspiration and yet, paradoxically, heart sounds could still be heard normally at this time.

Melvin Lobo

PULSES, UNEQUAL

See also GANGRENE, Diseases of blood vessels (p. 235).

A thorough physical examination should include palpation of all the easily accessible arterial pulses. The pulses on the two sides should be compared and, in the arms, inequalities should be confirmed by sphygmomanometry. It must be remembered that, in normal subjects, the blood pressure in the right arm may be slightly higher than that in the left; this difference is, however, rarely palpable. It is always worth recording the arteries in which the pulse has been felt, if only for future reference; the significance of an absent pulse is much greater if it is known to have been present on a previous occasion.

The pulse in one or other radial artery may be reduced or absent as a result of a minor *congenital abnormality* in the course or calibre of the vessel. Other congenital conditions in which the radial pulses may be unequal include a few cases of *coarctation of the aorta*. In 2 per cent of cases the lesion is proximal to the left subclavian artery so that the pulses in the left arm are weaker than those in the right; in addition, stenosis of the origin of a subclavian artery is a rare complication of coarctation. *Supravalvar aortic stenosis* is another, very rare, cause of unequal pulses; in this condition the blood pressure in the right arm is often a good deal higher than that in the left, and the difference may be palpable. There is no convincing explanation for this finding.

Inequality of pulses previously known to be equal is a most important sign. In the legs, *atherosclerosis* of the larger arteries is the commonest cause, and the level of occlusion should be sought by comparing the pulses in the femoral, popliteal, posterior tibial and dorsalis pedis arteries. Another cause of unequal pulses, usually in the legs, is *Buerger's disease*, also known as *thromboangiitis obliterans*. Atherosclerosis is less common in the vessels of the upper limbs, but can certainly involve the branches of the aortic arch and cause inequality of the brachial and radial pulses. Giant-cell *arteritis* and other inflammatory diseases of arteries occasionally cause occlusion of major limb vessels.

Arterial embolism is an important cause of unequal pulses in the upper or lower limbs. The three most common sources of such an embolism are: the left atrium in atrial fibrillation, particularly in association with mitral valve disease; vegetations in infective endocarditis of the mitral or aortic valve; and mural thrombus laid down on the endocardial surface of a myocardial infarct. Less common causes of systemic embolism are left atrial myxoma, left ventricular endocardial thrombus in a ventricular aneurysm or in dilated cardiomyopathy, thrombus detached from an atherosclerotic plaque in the aorta, and a so-called 'paradoxical embolus' passing from veins in the legs via a patent foramen ovale to the systemic circulation. This last phenomenon occurs only if the pressures on the right side of the heart have been raised, often by a previous pulmonary embolism.

Arterial thrombosis of major vessels is a less common but well-recognized cause of unequal pulses. It may arise as a complication of severe septicaemia, particularly pneumococcal or meningococcal. In addition, underlying malignancy, hyperviscosity syndromes and the thrombophilias are all predisposing factors for arterial (and venous) thrombosis which may manifest with acute limb ischaemia giving rise to unequal pulses. *Pseudoxanthoma elasticum* is a rare cause of occlusive arteriopathy involving mainly the coronary and peripheral circulations leading to unequal lower limb pulses.

Frequent palpation of the arterial pulses is most important when *dissecting aneurysm* of the aorta is suspected. As the dissection proceeds along the length of the aorta, the branches may be occluded one by one over a period of a few hours; the process may be capricious, branches past which the dissection has spread unexpectedly remaining patent. If re-entry occurs, the pulse may return in arteries previously occluded.

Takayasu's disease, or the 'pulseless disease', is a rare form of arteritis involving the branches of the aortic arch. Apart from inequality in the pulses in the arms or, perhaps more commonly, obliteration of the pulses in both arms, signs and symptoms of cerebral ischaemia are common. Takayasu's disease is one of the causes of so-called 'reversed coarctation', a not very satisfactory term implying diminished (or absent) pulses in the arms with normal femoral pulses. This situation can also occur as a result of *aortic aneurysm*, particularly of the arch, in which unequal pulses in the arms may be of diagnostic importance.

Occlusion of a subclavian artery by external pressure, such as by a *cervical rib* or a *tumour* in that region, must be remembered. With cervical rib particularly, pain, paraesthesiae and weakness and wasting of the small muscles of the hand, due to compression of the first thoracic root, are common associated features.

Iatrogenic causes of unequal pulses include intra-arterial cannulation and drug administration, previous *subclavian pulmonary anastomosis* for cyanotic congenital heart disease, and brachial *embolectomy*.

Melvin Lobo

PUPILS, ABNORMALITIES OF

Abnormalities of the pupil are a vital aid to neurological and ophthalmological diagnosis. Careful examination of the shape, size and reactions of the pupils provides important information about the integrity of the autonomic (parasympathetic and sympathetic) pathways, the anterior visual pathways, and the brainstem. No special equipment is needed to examine the pupils – simply a bright torch, a dark environment, and a few minutes to allow accurate observations to be made. It is important to have an understanding of normal pupil function.

Anatomy

Normal pupil function depends on the integrity of the pupillary light reflex pathway. This pathway comprises afferent and efferent limbs. The afferent limb consists of retinal receptors; ganglion cell axons in the optic nerve; the optic chiasma, optic tract (excluding the lateral geniculate body); and the pretectal nucleus of the midbrain. From the pretectal nucleus interneurons stimulate the pupilloconstrictor motor (Edinger–Westphal) nuclei on both sides of the midbrain. The efferent limb begins with parasympathetic fibres that pass in the IIIrd (oculomotor) nerve to the ciliary ganglion and then the short ciliary nerves. This system is affected by the amount of light falling on the retina, the degree of retinal light adaptation, the accommodation effort of the eyes, input from frontal and occipital cortex, and from the reticular formation. A lesion in one afferent limb diminishes the input to the ipsilateral pretectal nucleus, which is relayed to *both* Edinger–Westphal nuclei. Thus, a lesion in one afferent limb (e.g. the optic nerve) decreases pupil constriction in both eyes when the affected side is stimulated compared to when the normal side limb is stimulated. The ipsilateral response is termed the 'direct pupillary reaction'; the contralateral response is termed the 'consensual pupillary reaction'. An afferent lesion can be detected clinically during the swinging light test as a relative afferent pupillary defect (RAPD). A bright light is shone into the affected eye and maintained until the pupillary constriction is static, then rapidly into the unaffected eye, with a similar reaction. When the light is swung again rapidly from the normal to the affected eye, there is a paradoxical dilatation of the pupil (Marcus–Gunn phenomenon). In clinical practice, a RAPD is diagnostic of an incomplete optic nerve lesion. Pupil sizes are always equal as long as the output signals (efferent limb) are equal, so an isolated afferent pathway lesion does not give papillary size inequality (anisocoria).

Regulation of pupil size

The size of the pupil is determined by the balance between two opposing iris muscles: the circular sphincter (pupilloconstrictor) muscle (under parasympathetic control) and the longitudinal radial pupillodilator muscle (under sympathetic control). As described above, the two-neuron parasympathetic pathway begins in the Edinger–Westphal (pupillomotor constrictor) subnucleus of the oculomotor complex, travelling to the ciliary ganglion where it synapses with the post-ganglionic short ciliary nerves innervating the iris pupilloconstrictor muscle. The sympathetic pathway consists of a three-neuron chain, originating in the posterolateral hypothalamus. The first neuron traverses the lateral brainstem, descending to the spinal cord segments C8–T2. The second neuron ascends across the lung apex and then the neck to synapse in the superior cervical ganglion. The third (post-ganglionic) neuron follows alongside the internal carotid artery into the skull (carotid canal) and exits the superior orbital fissure with the ophthalmic division of the trigeminal (Vth) nerve. The sympathetic pathway continues to the nasociliary branch to the pupillodilator iris muscle.

Differences in pupil size are common; about 20 per cent of the normal population have a physiological anisocoria.

Abnormalities of pupil shape

The normal pupil is circular or slightly oval, with its longer axis horizontal. An irregularly shaped pupil is due to local damage to the iris. The circular shape of the pupil is also lost in coloboma. Common causes

include adhesions between the iris and the lens due to previous iritis, trauma or surgery. If an iris anomaly or iris damage is suspected from the patient's history or examination (iris atrophy, distorted pupillary margin, heterochromia), the patient is most appropriately referred to an ophthalmologist. Anisocoria in eyes with normal iris muscles can be presumed to have pathological damage to the nerves innervating the iris muscles – that is, anisocoria of neurological origin. This is subdivided into two groups: (i) anisocoria that is greater in darkness (when the abnormal pupil is smallest because of abnormal dilation); and (ii) anisocoria that is greater in light (when the abnormal pupil is the largest because of abnormal constriction).

Abnormalities of pupil size

Enlargement of the pupil is termed mydriasis; constriction of the pupil is termed meiosis.

Abnormally small pupil (anisocoria greater in darkness)

Physiological anisocoria

Anisocoria, usually of less than 1 mm, occurs in about 20 per cent of the general population, and may be of no pathological significance. The anisocoria may alternate between sides. More pronounced difference in the size of the pupils is likely to be symptomatic of an organic lesion.

Horner's syndrome

This is a defect in the sympathetic innervation of the eye (Fig. P.26). The full syndrome consists of ptosis, meiosis and anhidrosis. The upper lid ptosis is mild, and lower lid ptosis creates the false impression of enophthalmos. The anisocoria is of the order of 1 mm, and is less in bright light, greater in darkness. The most specific clinical sign of Horner's syndrome is dilation lag of the meiotic pupil compared to the normal pupil when viewed over 15–20 seconds in darkness. The pupillary light reflex and the accommodation reflex are preserved.

Aberrant regeneration

After the oculomotor nerve suffers a traumatic or compressive injury, the regenerating axons may grow along an aberrant course. Axons originally destined to supply extra-ocular muscles may instead sprout to innervate the iris sphincter. Therefore, whenever the patient uses the extra-ocular muscle concerned, the pupil constricts – a type of synkinesis. Any of the oculomotor nerve branches that innervate extra-ocular muscles can aberrantly innervate the iris sphincter.

Old Adie's (tonic) pupil

A tonic pupil (see below) that has been denervated for years eventually becomes smaller than the normal pupil, and does not dilate properly. This reason for this is not known.

Pontine stroke

In pontine stroke there is bilateral pupillary constriction. Opiate drugs can cause a similar papillary appearance.

Abnormally large pupil (anisocoria greater in bright light)

Adie's (tonic) pupil

This is due to injury of the ciliary ganglion, short ciliary nerves, and post-ganglionic parasympathetic denervation of the iris sphincter and ciliary muscles. Because the iris sphincter constricts the pupil and the ciliary muscle regulates accommodation (near vision), the affected pupil is large and reacts poorly to light and accommodation so that the patient develops difficulty with close work. After several weeks, the injured post-ganglionic parasympathetic fibres (short ciliary nerves) begin to sprout collaterals and regenerate. Because there are many more accommodation fibres than pupilloconstrictor fibres, these predominate. Some accommodation fibres are imperfectly directed to the sphincter muscle, resulting in segmental areas of palsy and constriction of the iris sphincter with *vermiform movements* and a slow (tonic) contraction of the sphincter whenever the patient attempts to accommodate. The iris remains poorly responsive to light, so there is light–near dissociation. Over months and years, the pupil becomes smaller.

Oculomotor (IIIrd) nerve palsy

The oculomotor nerve supplies the iris sphincter and ciliary muscles, levator palpebrae, superior rectus, inferior rectus, medial rectus, and inferior oblique extraocular muscles. The clinical features of oculomotor palsy are therefore ptosis, pupil dilatation (mydriasis) and ophthalmoplegia. The patient will be able to abduct the affected eye if the VIth (abducens) nerve is intact, but will have impaired movement in all other directions. The unopposed lateral rectus action will cause the eye to be deviated outward (exotropia) at rest. The upper lid ptosis can be mild or complete. A compressive lesion ('surgical third nerve palsy') is likely to affect the fibres to the sphincter muscle since these traverse the outer aspect of the oculomotor nerve. The pupil is larger than the normal pupil and reacts poorly to light and accommodation. The most common cause of a pupil-involving IIIrd nerve palsy is a posterior communicating artery aneurysm, in which the pupil is involved in about 80–90 per cent of cases. In the comatose patient whose assessment of lid and eye movement function is difficult, pupillary enlargement may be the most important sign of tentorial herniation ('coning'). If the pupillary size and responses are spared ('non-surgical third nerve palsy'), then a process affecting the inner oculomotor fibres is more likely. The most common cause of a pupil-sparing IIIrd nerve palsy is a 'microvascular' lesion, often in the context of diabetes. Other causes include mononeuritis due to vasculitis, granuloma (e.g. sarcoidosis) or treponemal infection. It should be remembered, however, that up to 40 per cent of microvascular oculomotor palsies may show pupillary involvement. A fixed dilated pupil that remains an isolated abnormality for more than one week in a neurologically intact patient is probably not an acute oculomotor nerve palsy.

Pharmacological mydriasis

Topical agents that can pharmacologically dilate the pupil fall into two classes: (i) sympathomimetics, which stimulate the pupillodilator; or (ii) anticholinergics, which inhibit the pupilloconstrictor. Topical agents include phenylephrine, cocaine, hydroxyamphetamine, guanethidine, atropine, scopolamine, cyclopentolate and tropicamide. Inadvertent exposure to mydriatic agents may occur from eye drops used for red eyes, scopolamine skin patches used for motion sickness, anticholinergic agents used for asthma, or certain plants. Occasionally, mydriatics may be instilled deliberately by patients, particularly those in medical or allied professions, in order to mimic true pathology.

An isolated fixed, dilated pupil

This clinical finding deserves special mention as it sometimes causes unnecessary emergency assessment of a patient. Confirmation that the dilated pupil is an isolated clinical finding is important – there are truly no other signs of focal neurological deficit, ipsilateral ptosis or ophthalmoplegia. If the patient complains of diplopia, then it should be assumed that there is weakness of one or more extra-ocular muscles. An early oculomotor palsy may have very subtle ocular motility abnormalities. If no ophthalmoplegia is present, the two most common causes of an isolated, fixed dilated pupil are tonic pupil or pharmacologically induced mydriasis. Rare causes include a fascicular or very early compressive IIIrd nerve palsy. If there is better accommodation than light response (light–near dissociation), the likely diagnosis is an Adie (tonic) pupil. If the dilated pupil is unreactive to light or accommodation, an acute tonic pupil is still possible, but pharmacological mydriasis must be considered. Pilocarpine (1%) will usually constrict a tonic pupil or oculomotor palsy, but not a pharmacologically manipulated pupil.

Transient pupillary abnormalities

The pupil varies in size depending on age. In infancy it is small, but it becomes larger during young adult and middle life, and then small again in old age. As a general rule the pupil is smaller in hypermetropic (long-sighted) and larger in myopic (short-sighted) eyes.

Ophthalmoplegic migraine occurs in children and adolescents, and typical migraine is followed by a unilateral oculomotor nerve palsy. Ophthalmoplegia and pupillary involvement are usual, and the deficit takes 1–4 weeks to resolve. The diagnosis is based on a characteristic history and negative evaluation for other possible causes of an oculomotor palsy.

Benign episodic unilateral mydriasis has been noted in young women with migraines, and lasts for an average of 12 hours; it recurs with a frequency of two to three attacks per month.

Tadpole-shaped pupils due to intermittent segmental spasm of the dilator muscle last for a few minutes, and recur several times daily or weekly. The episodic distortion eventually resolves spontaneously. Conditions associated with tadpole pupils are Horner's syndrome, tonic pupil and migraines.

Hippus is a benign cause of spontaneous papillary movement; both pupils are seen to constrict and dilate simultaneously, without any obvious stimulus being applied. This is simply an exaggeration of physiological variation in pupil size due to fluctuations in the different inputs to the pupillomotor pathways.

David Werring

PURPURA

See also BLEEDING (p. 64); BRUISES (p. 84).

The presence of purpura usually indicates thrombocytopenia (Table P.13), although there are additionally, non-thrombocytopenic causes (Table P.14). In any patient with purpura due to a reduced platelet count it is important to ascertain the cause and severity because purpura usually indicates a severe haemorrhagic potential. Whereas purpura on the skin is not life-threatening, thrombocytopenia can result in rapidly fatal intracranial or massive gastrointestinal haemorrhage. Purpura usually indicates a platelet count less than $30 \times 10^9/l$.

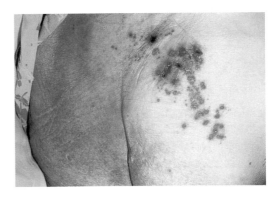

Figure P.45 Purpura due to vasculitis.

Platelet functional disorders (e.g. thrombasthenia or platelet storage pool disorder) do not usually result in purpura unless there is a secondary provocative stimulus (e.g. protracted coughing). The presence of purpura in an individual with a normal platelet count is indicative of a vasculitis (Fig. P.45). Whereas thrombocytopenia results in flat purpura lesions, those due to a vasculitis are often slightly raised and on some occasions may be up to 1 cm in diameter.

Melvin Lobo

Table P.13 Causes of thrombocytopenia

Impaired production of platelets	**Drugs causing immune destruction**

Impaired production of platelets

Congenital megakaryocytic abnormalities
- Wiscott–Aldrich
- May–Hegglin anomaly
- Thrombocytopenia with absent radii (TAR)

Marrow hypoplasia

Aplastic anaemia

Megaloblastosis
- Vitamin B_{12}/folate deficiency
- Folate antagonists

Toxins
- Chemotherapy
- Drugs
  - Phenylbutazone
  - Sulphonamides
  - Choramphenicol
  - Procainamide
  - Thiazides
  - Oestrogens
  - Ethanol
- Ionizing radiation

Infiltration by:
- Leukaemia
- Lymphoma
- Myeloma
- Carcinoma
- Paroxysmal nocturnal haemoglobinuria
- Myelodysplasia

Increased utilization/destruction of platelets

Immune-mediated
- Acute idiopathic thrombocytopenic purpura
- Chronic idiopathic thrombocytopenic purpura

Secondary to immune abnormalities
- Systemic lupus erythematosus
- Chronic lymphatic leukaemia
- Hodgkin's disease
- Non-Hodgkin's lymphoma
- Hyperthyroidism

Drugs causing immune destruction
- Quinine
- Gold
- Penicillins
- Para-amino salicylic acid
- Rifampicin
- Methyldopa
- Heparin

Neonatal thrombocytopenia
- Maternal auto-antibody
- Maternal iso-antibody
- Post-transfusional purpura

Disseminated intravascular coagulation

Pregnancy-associated conditions
- Eclampsia
- Abruptio placentae
- Retained dead foetus

Septicaemia

Hypothermia

Asphyxia

Cardiopulmonary arrest

Local thrombosis
- Massive thromboembolism
- Giant haemangiomas
- Thrombotic thrombocytopenic purpura (Moschcowitz syndrome)

Haemolytic uraemic syndrome

Virus
- Rubella
- Cytomegalovirus
- Ebstein–Barr virus
- HIV
- Herpes

Other infections
- Toxoplasmosis
- Syphilis

Abnormality of distribution of platelets

Splenomegaly

Massive transfusion

Table P.14 Non-thrombocytopenic causes of purpura

Vasculitis

Henoch–Schönlein purpura

Systemic lupus erythematosus

Drugs

Mechanical

Coughing

Orthostatic

Senile

Steroid-induced

Scurvy

Factitious purpurae

PUSTULES

A pustule is an elevation of the skin containing pus, differing from a vesicle or bulla only in its contents.

Pustules may develop from vesicles that have become purulent, or from papules. They may develop so rapidly that their origin cannot be observed. They vary in colour from bright yellow to cream, orange, grey or green. Examination with a hand lens may show them to arise in hair follicles, but they may occur on normal skin or around sweat pores (Table P.15). Establishing the diagnosis of a pustular lesion or rash

Table P.15 Pustules

Pustules of infectious origin

Staphylococcal
- Folliculitis, boils, carbuncle, ecthyma, hordeolum (stye), sycosis barbae

Candidiasis
Dermatophyte
Gonococcal septicaemia
Gram-negative folliculitis
Anthrax
Glanders
Smallpox
Chickenpox
Pustular syphilide
Jacuzzi folliculitis (Pseudomonas)

Sterile pustules

Pustular psoriasis
- Localized, generalized

Facial
- Acne, rosacea, peri-oral dermatitis, itchy

Widespread
- Miliaria, drug-induced, Behçet's disease, subcorneal pustular dermatitis, dermatitis herpetiformis

---

may be assisted by determining whether or not the pus is sterile on bacteriological examination.

Pustules of infectious origin

The most common bacterial cause of a pustule is infection with *Staphylococcus*. Systemic factors (e.g. diabetes) may predispose, as may the effect on the skin of heat and humidity, friction, or the use of topical corticosteroids on the skin. Recurrent infection may result from chronic staphylococcal carriage in the anterior nares, or the perineum.

Folliculitis is a superficial infection of the hair follicles; it presents with multiple symptomless superficial pustules which, when examined with a hand lens, can be seen to be arising from a hair follicle. A *boil* (furuncle) is a deeper staphylococcal follicular pustule or abscess. The neck, buttocks and face are the commonest sites for boil formation. There is often considerable acute inflammation surrounding boils, and the lesions can be hot and very tender. The central painful papule undergoes rapid necrosis, a yellow pustule is formed, which becomes boggy, fluctuates and ultimately ruptures and discharges pus. In many cases a hard 'core' of necrotic material is extruded before healing takes place. Occasionally, the contents

of the boil are absorbed before rupture occurs and the lesion regresses; this is termed a 'blind-boil'. After poulticing a boil a ring of small satellite boils may form around the original lesion. Boils beginning in the hair follicles of the eyelid are known as *styes* (hordeolum).

A *carbuncle* resembles a boil, but the infection spreads to the deeper tissues, and when rupture occurs there may be several openings onto the skin. Boils may follow one another in series for many months, when the condition is known as *chronic furunculosis*. *Sycosis barbae* is staphylococcal folliculitis of the hairy areas of the face, including the eyebrows. It differs in no way from the other forms of staphylococcal folliculitis; it may be localized to small areas or it may affect the whole of the face and neck. The pustules are grouped on a bright erythematous base, and in the centre of each pustule there is a hair which pulls out easily. It must be distinguished from the more common seborrhoeic sycosis in which the predominating lesions are red papules with little or no pustule formation. In all forms of staphylococcal folliculitis the diagnosis is fairly simple. Only rarely do other organisms (e.g. *Streptococcus* or Gram-negative organisms) produce similar lesions.

An *ecthyma* begins as a burning painful vesicopustule on an erythematous base, either singly or as sparse lesions scattered over buttocks and lower legs. Later, deep-crusted ulcers form which heal slowly with considerable scarring. Patients are usually young women, debilitated by anaemia or systemic illness or suffering from HIV disease. Streptococci or staphylococci may be cultured.

Boils in the axillae and groins can be the presentation of *hidradenitis suppurativa*, an intractable purulent condition affecting the apocrine sweat glands.

Recurrent purulent skin infections in a child, especially with crops of pustules in the webs of fingers and on wrists, is sometimes a feature of neglected *scabies*. Pustules are also a feature of secondarily infected dermatitis, and can be particularly widespread in *atopic dermatitis*.

Satellite vesicopustules at the edge of a moist eroded patch are highly suggestive of *candidiasis* (thrush). This particularly favours damp, intertriginous areas, such as the submammary, perineal and perioral folds of skin. Scrapings from lesions warmed with 10 per cent potassium hydroxide show small oval budding thin-walled spores on microscopy; culture shows *Candida albicans*.

Some *dermatophyte* species appear to proliferate deep in hair follicles, especially *Trichophyton mentagrophytes*. Inappropriate treatment of superficial fungal infections with topical corticosteroids often leads to an apparent initial improvement of the condition, but fungal growth persists deep in the hair follicles and a curious resistant pustular eruption may result – the so-called *tinea incognito*. Scalp ringworm in cases where there is a vigorous inflammatory reaction may present with a discharging pustular mass (*kerion*). Fungal elements will be seen on microscopy.

Characteristic discrete inflammatory pustules (which may become haemorrhagic) accompany the fever, arthritis and tenosynovitis of *gonococcal septicaemia*. Recognition of this skin lesion can lead to making this important diagnosis at an earlier stage, particularly in women who may have little in the way of genital symptoms.

Anthrax infection of the skin in its localized variety takes the form of a carbuncle-like inflammatory lesion caused by *Bacillus anthracis*. It is contracted from the hides or hairs of cattle or goats, or rarely from shaving brushes. It attacks an exposed area of skin, and the incubation period is 1–3 days. The first sign is a small, itching red macule, not unlike a flea bite. In 2 days a papule forms which rapidly becomes a pustule; this soon ruptures and sometimes blood as well as pus is extruded. There results a gangrenous ulcer which, in a simple case, heals in a few weeks. However, in severe cases there may be grave constitutional symptoms with septicaemia and rapid death, and sometimes there are multiple skin lesions. It must be distinguished from a carbuncle and extragenital syphilitic chancre. Scrapings from the lesion contain the causal organism in large numbers. Anthrax is mostly an occupational disease in handlers of hides or wool, but is endemic in some parts of the world.

Glanders is a disease of horses, mules and donkeys which very rarely affects humans, and then only those in contact with these animals. The main lesion is an ulcerating pustule. It is not unlike a carbuncle in its early stages, and occurs on exposed areas of skin. The general symptoms are those of septicaemia, and there is always a purulent nasal discharge. The presence of *Pseudomonas mallei* in this or material from the

ulcers or pustules is diagnostic. The disease is almost invariably fatal.

The pustule was an important manifestation of *smallpox*. After an incubation period of 5–12 days the disease began with fever, headache, backache and vomiting. On the third and fourth days, there was macular erythema and after a few hours shotty papules developed. These became vesicles, and by the fifth day pustulated. The rash was most profuse on the head and limbs and there was only one crop of lesions which matured in 'majestic' concert. The vesicles were tough, firm and often multilocular, and showed definite umbilication. By the time the pustules formed the umbilication was less well marked. In severe cases there was confluence of the pustules, particularly on the face. The mucous membranes were often also involved. As a rule, the temperature fell slightly with the eruption, but rose again on the eighth or the ninth day when the pustules ruptured. In the final stage the pustules dried up to form brown crusts. Pitting or scarring was the rule. Previous vaccination modified the course of the disease considerably, and there was a type of the disease known as *alastrim* (variola minor).

Chickenpox can be distinguished by the usually milder nature of disease, which is vesicular rather than pustular, and its profusion on the trunk rather than the extremities. In chickenpox the eruption comes out in successive crops and the vesicles are unilocular, fragile and do not exhibit umbilication. In spite of these differences, mild smallpox and severe chickenpox were difficult to differentiate.

Other viral diseases causing pustules are *vaccinia*, *cowpox* and *orf*. In the so-called *pustular syphilides* there are no true pustules, their resemblance to pustules being only superficial; on incision, they will be found to be solid and contain no pus. The histology is diagnostic, and the serology will be positive.

Perhaps the most modern form of folliculitis is a new epidemic of *Pseudomonas folliculitis* that has been described in those indulging in jacuzzi bathing. The organism is inoculated on to the skin by the high-pressure water jets.

Sterile pustules

Pustules do not always indicate cutaneous infection, and can arise during inflammatory dermatoses. These are often referred to as 'sterile' pustules, as routine bacteriological examination of the pus always yields negative results. The classical example is *pustular psoriasis of palms and soles* (acrodermatitis perstans), where bright yellow sterile pustules arise within well-demarcated areas on palms and soles (Fig. P.46). As they age, the pustules change to dark-brown macules and eventually peel off. The condition is most common in middle-aged women, and is notoriously resistant to conventional treatment. Only 25 per cent of such patients have evidence of psoriasis elsewhere on the body. On very rare occasions psoriasis may produce widespread sheets of sterile yellow pustules, associated with considerable toxicity and fever – a phenomenon known as generalized pustular psoriasis of von Zumbusch. The incidence of this rare and dangerous complication of psoriasis rose dramatically following the introduction of potent topical steroids; it has become uncommon again, now that steroids are used more cautiously and appropriately in treatment.

Sterile pustules on the face are seen in *acne, rosacea* and *perioral dermatitis*. In *acne* these are associated with evidence of comedones, acne papules and perhaps acne cysts (Fig. P.47). The distribution is more peripheral on the face than in *rosacea*, where pustules surround the 'muzzle' area, and are associated with vascular changes (erythema, flushing, telangiectasia), as well as papules and sometimes hypertrophied and patulous pilosebaceous pores on the nose (rhinophyma). *Perioral dermatitis* is a modern condition which was unknown before the introduction of fluorinated topical corticosteroids; the pustules are tiny and surmount painful small red papules, which abound around the mouth. A further diagnostic feature is a background of perioral erythema with a halo of pallor around the lip margins.

Unilateral pustules near the lips may have developed from *herpes simplex* vesicles, and tend to be greyish in colour. The grouped distribution and a history of

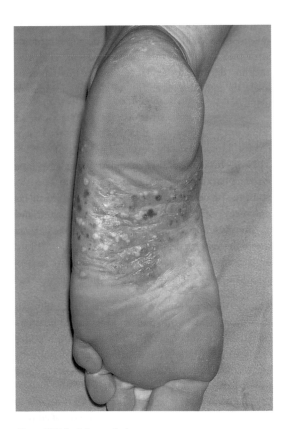

Figure P.46 Pustular psoriasis.

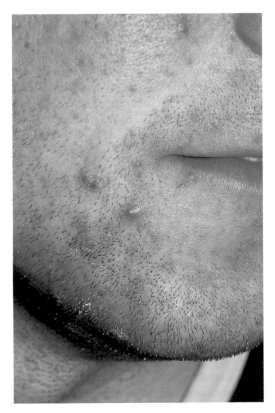

Figure P.47 Acne vulgaris.

and, to a lesser extent, from time to time. The more common conditions to consider are listed in Table P.16. Inevitably, such a list is bound to be incomplete and cannot be comprehensive. Space does not permit a full description of each of the diseases mentioned, but the following are some of the salient points.

Specific fevers

Today, *infectious mononucleosis* is one of the most common causes of prolonged fever in children and young adults, and diagnosis is often difficult. Paul–Bunnell or 'Monospot' tests are useful in diagnosis after the first

Table P.16 Causes of prolonged pyrexia

Specific fevers
- Viral:
  - Infectious mononucleosis
- *Salmonella*:
  - *S. typhi*
  - *S. paratyphi*
- Rickettsia:
  - Epidemic and scrub typhus
  - Rocky Mountain spotted fever
  - Q fever
  - Trench fever
- Legionella:
  - Legionnaire's disease
- *Chlamydia*:
  - Psittacosis
- Fungus:
  - Coccidioidomycosis
  - Histoplasmosis
- Spirochaete:
  - Syphilis
  - Leptospirosis
  - Lyme disease
- Brucella:
  - Abortus and melitensis fever
- Tuberculosis
- Listeriosis
- Streptobacillary rat-bite fever
- Tularaemia

Bacteraemia
- Staphylococcal
- Streptococcal
- Meningococcal
- Gonococcal
- Coliforms
- Infective endocarditis

Localized infection
- Prostatic abscess
- Ischiorectal abscess
- Pyosalpinx
- Suppurating ovarian cyst
- Parametritic abscess
- Empyema of the maxillary antrum, frontal sinus or ethmoidal air cells
- Osteomyelitis
- Infected lymph nodes in neck, axilla, groin
- Mammary or submammary abscess

- Empyema thoracis
- Lung abscess
- Hepatic abscess
- Renal abscess
- Splenic abscess
- Empyema of gallbladder
- Suppurative cholangitis
- Suppurative pyelophlebitis
- Subdiaphragmatic abscess
- Bronchiectasis
- Appendix abscess
- Perinephric abscess
- Diverticulitis
- Lumbar and iliac retroperitoneal abscess
- Psoas abscess
- Actinomycosis of jaw, cheek, neck, lung, liver, spine or caecum

Infective and inflammatory conditions
- Pyelonephritis and other urinary infections
- Papillary necrosis
- Chronic cystitis
- Chronic cholecystitis
- Phlebitis
- Thyroiditis
- Pneumonia and pneumonitis
- Bronchopneumonia
- Parametritis
- Vesiculitis
- Dysenteric colitis, bacillary or amoebic
- Ulcerative colitis
- Crohn's disease (regional enteritis)
- Pancreatitis
- Familial Mediterranean fever
- Sarcoidosis

Non-purulent hepatic affections
- Cirrhosis
- Secondary carcinoma
- Hepatitis, subacute and chronic

Connective-tissue disorders
- Rheumatoid arthritis
- Rheumatic fever
- Systemic lupus erythematosus
- Polyarteritis nodosa and other arteritides
- Polymyositis and dermatomyositis
- Giant-cell arthritis
- Still's disease (childhood and adult)

Blood diseases
- Aplastic anaemia
- Agranulocytosis
- Lymphatic, myeloid or monocytic leukaemia, acute or chronic
- Haemolytic anaemias

Diseases of the tropics and subtropics
- Trypanosomiasis
- Malaria
- Kala-azar
- Plague
- Relapsing fever
- Filariasis
- Leprosy
- Schistosomiasis

Meningeal and cerebral haemorrhage

Skin conditions
- Pemphigus
- Severe or exfoliative dermatitis
- Bullous pemphigoid

Malignancy
- Lymphoma (e.g. Hodgkin's disease, lymphosarcoma)
- Sarcoma
- Carcinoma

Allergic (antigen–antibody reactive) conditions
- Henoch–Schönlein syndrome
- Allergic skin rashes
- Post-cardiac injury syndrome

Factitious pyrexia produced by malingerers

Drug reactions
- Sulphonamides
- Antibiotics
- Arsenicals
- Iodides
- Barbiturates, etc.

2 weeks or so. These are tests for heterophile antibodies; several specific antibodies against components of the Epstein–Barr virus (EBV) have also been identified.

Infectious mononucleosis should be seriously considered in any prolonged, low-grade fever with malaise and loss of weight in children and young adults, as lymphadenopathy, splenomegaly and typical blood counts are not invariably present in all cases, or may have been present earlier and have disappeared. Some authors consider infectious mononucleosis to be a clinical syndrome rather than a single entity, as the same picture can be due to EBV, cytomegalovirus (CMV) or toxoplasma. However, as only EBV gives a positive Paul–Bunnell test, full serological tests should be carried out in all cases.

Typhoid fever suggests itself when a patient, who was previously in good health, suffers from a progressive fever of considerable and increasing degree with a pulse rate that is relatively slow in relation to the temperature. The illness starts with headache and malaise, but without any conspicuously abnormal signs. During the first week, the temperature rises each night to a slightly higher level than that of the previous night, until a maximum is attained and maintained during the second week. After this time there is a progressive diminution during the third week until normal temperature is reached again. Diarrhoea may occur with foul-smelling stools of pea-soup consistency, but constipation is more usual. Abdominal pain is usually confined to the right lower quadrant. The headache, which is in most cases a conspicuous feature, persists for about a week, at which time it almost invariably ceases, thus contrasting with the headache of tuberculous meningitis. Blood cultures are positive during the first 10 days and in acute relapse; similar cultures later prove negative, although urine and faecal cultures may by then be positive. The spleen becomes palpable early in the disease and remains so until defervescence; it enlarges again in a relapse. Typical typhoid rose spots appear – chiefly on the abdomen, less often on the chest or back, and seldom on the limbs – from the seventh day onwards, and in successive crops. They are about 2–3 mm in diameter, rose red in colour, fade on pressure, and are without a central punctum. The majority of patients, but not all, develop a rise in agglutinins against the O antigens of the typhoid bacillus during the course of the disease. Another help in diagnosis is the absence of leucocytosis, and in the differential leucocyte count the lymphocytes are relatively

increased, the polymorphonuclear cells being absolutely reduced. The leucocyte count may, however, be influenced by complications. Rigors are exceptional, a fact which sometimes helps in diagnosis from conditions such as septicaemia and malaria. Some difficulty arises in the diagnosis of those cases in which there has been previous immunization of the patient by antityphoid inoculations; the fever is then of shorter duration and the illness relatively mild.

The *Ricketisial disorders* are numerous, ranging from epidemic typhus to trench fever. Different Rickettsiae are transmitted by lice, fleas, ticks and mites via man, wild rodents, domestic animals and cattle. In the history of mankind they rank high as a cause of epidemic disease causing great suffering and death, but they do not usually persist beyond 20 days and rarely cause prolonged fever.

Legionnaire's disease usually resolves or proves fatal within 3 weeks, but the pneumonia caused may extend to lobes of both lungs and prolong the febrile disorder. The causative organism resembles a Rickettsia in some cultural characteristics, but it is larger in size and does not react with the standard Rickettsial antigens in complement fixation tests. Diagnosis via the Legionella direct antigen test (DAT) performed on urine is now possible.

Psittacosis or *ornithosis* is transmitted to man from parrots and the parrot family, pigeons and a number of other birds, including ducks, turkeys and chickens. It is due to a Gram-negative obligate intracellular parasite, *Chlamydia psittaci*, formerly classified as a virus. The illness may be transmitted from the patient to others by contact. Clinically, the illness is similar to typhoid fever, with liability to serious pulmonary complications. The fever lasts for about 3 weeks, and tends to end abruptly followed by a slow convalescence, but it may last for as long as 3 months. When the disease is contracted from parrots or parakeets it tends to be more severe and prolonged. The diagnosis is suggested in a patient with an illness that bears a general resemblance to typhoid fever, but whose blood does not give the agglutination test, and especially if there has been contact with a recently imported parrot, budgerigar or pigeon. The organism may be isolated from the blood or sputum. A rising titre of complement-fixing antibody in the patient's blood is useful in diagnosis.

Secondary syphilis may be a febrile illness. The diagnosis becomes obvious when the rash is associated with a fading primary sore, typical snail-track ulcers of tonsils, fauces and pharynx, and generalized enlargement of most of the palpable lymph nodes. Spirochaetes may be isolated from the skin lesions.

Lyme disease is caused by a tick-borne spirochaete, *Borrelia burgdorferi*. Cases have been reported from most parts of the USA, Scandinavia and Europe. The early disease is characterized by the annular skin lesion, erythema chronicum migrans (ECM). At this stage there may be fever, lymphadenopathy, myalgia and arthralgia. A history of tick-bite is often obtained. After several weeks of this flu-like illness, neurological, cardiac and joint changes can develop. with the latter often becoming permanent. The diagnosis can be confirmed serologically and by culture of the organisms or their demonstration in skin biopsies of ECM.

Abortus fever is a not uncommon cause of prolonged unexplained pyrexia, lasting usually for several months and occasionally for a year. It is due to infection by *Brucella abortus*. This organism causes fatal abortion in cows, and apart from the geographical circumstances the fever is identical to Mediterranean fever in which the disease is communicated by goat's milk. Infection may arise from the ingestion of milk or the handling of infected animals or excreta.

This infection may underlie obscure, long-continued febrile illness either in children or in adults. There are no characteristic symptoms, although arthritis is a frequent accompaniment. Diagnosis is usually by agglutination tests, and rarely by blood cultures. Rarely, the organism causes endocarditis, which is sometimes fatal. Cultures taken from bone marrow or liver may be positive when blood cultures are negative. Brucellar infections are particularly persistent, probably due to the intracellular location of the organism in the reticuloendothelial tissues.

Melitensis, *Mediterranean* or *Malta fever* is one of the most prolonged of the fevers due to a known specific organism, in this case *Brucella melitensis*. In the undulant form of the disease, successive exacerbations of pyrexia may prolong the illness into the sixteenth, eighteenth or twentieth week, or longer (Fig. P.48). The condition may simulate typhoid fever, including the enlargement of the spleen and the paucity of abnormal physical signs, but there are no rose spots or other eruption. The diagnosis may be suggested by geographical factors; for example, recent residence in some parts of the Mediterranean coast or islands, or Spain, Portugal, the Canary Islands or parts of South America – and especially if the patient has been drinking goat's milk,

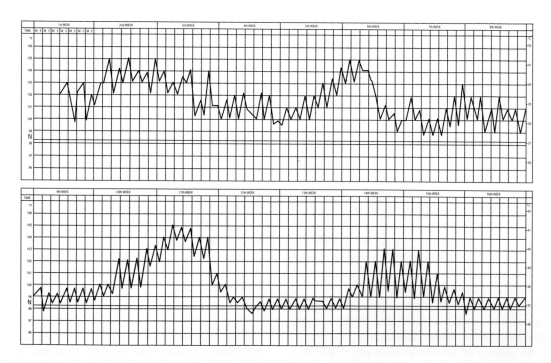

Figure P.48 Temperature chart of a case of Mediterranean fever of undulant type (*Brucella melitensis*).

by which the infection is transmitted. The diagnosis is established by serum-agglutination tests, which may be positive from the fifth day onwards, the patient's diluted blood serum agglutinating cultures of *Br. melitensis*. Blood cultures should be carried out. *Brucella suis* infections, contracted from pigs, are also diagnosed by agglutination tests and blood cultures.

Tuberculosis lesions often occur without pyrexia. On the other hand, the occurrence of some degree of fever without any apparent cause may be the sole evidence of such disease, especially the miliary form. Pulmonary tuberculosis is almost invariably pyrexial, but in an earlier stage there are often long periods of apyrexia even when the tuberculous process is active, with brief febrile spells. Tuberculous disease of the joints may be apyrexial unless secondarily infected. Glandular tuberculosis is less likely to be pyrexial when the nodes involved are cervical or bronchial than when the mesenteric and other abdominal nodes are caseous and softening ('tabes mesenterica'), when there may be – and usually is prolonged pyrexia. The diagnosis may be easy if there is ascites in a child or if there are palpable abdominal masses, but it may be difficult in the absence of lumps and ascites in a condition of ill health with pyrexia and with vague abdominal pains which may be mistaken for some other non-tuberculous abdominal disease. The patient is usually young, and in European countries may be an immigrant. The presence of enlarged cervical lymph nodes supports this diagnosis.

Listeriosis is an infectious disease of animals and man world-wide. Its distribution is due to a Gram-positive bacillus, *Listeria monocytogenes*. Clinically the condition may present as a meningitis, or resemble infectious mononucleosis with pharyngitis and diffuse lymphadenopathy, influenza or miliary tuberculosis. Untreated severe cases with meningitis often prove fatal. It may occur in infancy or in pregnancy. Diagnosis rests on isolating the micro-organisms, which resemble diphtheroid bacilli in culture, and on rising agglutination titres in the serum.

Streptobacillary rat-bite fever is caused by bites from rats and, sometimes, mice, cats, dogs and weasels. The causative organism is *Streptobacillus moniliformis* or *Spirillum minus*, and the condition is characterized by acute febrile attacks at fairly regular intervals of a few days. These persist for from two to ten months.

Tularaemia is uncommon in England, but cases have occurred amongst those handling live rabbits, for example in bacteriological laboratories. It is a specific infectious disease due to *Pasteurella* (*Francisella*) *tularensis*, and is transmitted from rodents by ticks or deer flies, by the handling or ingestion of infected animal tissues, or by inhalation of infected aerosols. It is not transmitted directly from human to human. A sore on a finger is commonly the start, the sore becoming a small ulcer in a day or two, with associated enlargement of the epitrochlear and axillary lymph nodes; a chill or rigor is usual, and pyrexia continues for 2–3 weeks with marked prostration followed by slow convalescence. There may be erythematous blotches on the skin, or even purpura. Swallowing a very large number of bacilli may cause a typhoid-like disorder with high fever, abdominal pain and toxicity. Lung involvement may occur, in addition to enlargement of the cervical glands. Rigors seen initially in severely ill patients may be followed by pyrexia persisting for several weeks. The diagnosis can be confirmed by a skin test which becomes positive in the first week, or the organism can be recovered from a mucocutaneous ulcer or regional lymph node, and occasionally from sputum on appropriate culture. Specific agglutinins appear in the serum within 8–10 weeks of onset of the illness, which is severe and prolonged, though the prognosis is good.

Bacteraemia

Disseminated infection may occur in association with a local lesion and metastasize to new areas. This may occur with many organisms. As an example, in *meningococcal infection* meningitis is not always present. In the early stages patients are acutely ill, with fever, chills, arthralgia and myalgia, particularly severe in the legs and back. They are very prostrated, hypotensive, and 70 per cent develop a characteristic petechial rash (Fig. P.49). Meningococci are cultured from the blood and sometimes from scrapings from the skin lesions, and from the cerebrospinal fluid in cases with meningitis. A rare form of chronic meningococcaemia has been identified which lasts for weeks or months, and is characterized by fever, rash and arthritis or arthralgia.

Infective endocarditis

The comparatively rare acute or malignant endocarditis is due to infection by one of the pyogenic bacteria, such as haemolytic *Streptococcus*, *Pneumococcus*,

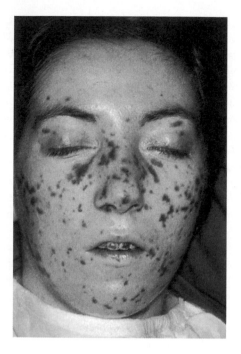

Figure P.49 Meningococcal septicaemia which presented as sub-arachnoid haemorrhage and purpuric rash.

Gonococcus and *Staphylococcus.* Many other organisms may cause endocarditis: *Corynebacterium diphtheriae*, *Brucella* and numerous others have been reported as causative agents. Pseudomonal endocarditis may follow open-heart surgery. The type formerly termed the 'subacute' variety occurs in a subject with chronic valvular disease of congenital or rheumatic origin when the organism is usually *Streptococcus viridans*. Patients present with cardiac symptoms, anaemia, cerebral vascular lesions or, most commonly, with pyrexia of unknown origin, a feature which arouses suspicion when progressive anaemia of normocytic and orthochromic type develops. The white cell count is variable, and a polymorphonuclear leucocytosis up to about 9000–12 000 per mm^3 is common. Other diagnostic features are an enlarged spleen, clubbing of the fingers in half of the subacute cases (but rarely in the malignant type), petechial haemorrhages under the nails and in the retina and conjunctiva, and Osler's nodes. Emboli may occur in any organ or tissue. Red blood cells in the urine are invariably found to a greater or lesser degree.

Blood cultures should be performed immediately, as treatment must not be delayed. If over middle age,

a patient who is not immediately treated may be cured of the infection but die of cardiac failure due to the damage to the heart.

Localized infection

Many cases of continued fever are due to localized infection (e.g. abscess formation). The elicitation of local signs, in addition to pyrexia and other evidence of generalized systemic illness, will provide the diagnosis, though it may be long delayed.

A rectal or vaginal examination should serve to detect *prostatic abscess, periproctal abscess, ischiorectal abscess, pyosalpinx, suppurating ovarian cyst* or *parametric abscess*, all of which are likely to cause local pain in the perineum, anal region, sacral region, back or lower abdomen.

In its acute form, *empyema of the maxillary antrum* causes pain and tenderness over the affected maxilla with oedematous swelling of that side of the face, but in chronic cases the symptoms may be much less definite. The diagnosis may be suggested by facial pain, local swelling and perhaps an intermittent purulent discharge from one nostril. Radiographs and antral aspiration will confirm the diagnosis.

Empyema of a frontal sinus may be acute or chronic, causing pyrexia in either case. The diagnosis may be suggested by the complaint of local headache above the eyes, generally on one or other side of the midline rather than central, and especially if the headache is associated with local tenderness to percussion. Identification becomes easy if the abscess points above the inner canthus of the orbit near the root of the nose, though doubt may persist for a long time. Difficulty in diagnosis applies still more to *empyema of the ethmoidal* or *sphenoidal sinuses* in which few objective signs are to be expected. The patient may complain of severe frontal headaches which are often worse in the morning but pass off later in the day. A purulent nasal discharge may also be present, whilst the pyrexia may be only slight, but generally persistent.

Suppurating lymph nodes will be diagnosed from the character of the tender swellings that precede the skin-reddening and the actual formation of an abscess. The site is likely to be the neck, axilla or groin, and there will usually be an indication of the source of the problem in the form of a septic focus in the skin corresponding to the lymph drainage of the node concerned – impetigo, a septic cut, a wound or a whitlow.

One source of trouble that may be overlooked is *pediculosis* of the scalp; this should be suspected if there is irritation of the back of the neck at the roots of the hair in association with enlargement of the occipital as well as of the cervical lymph nodes.

Mammary and *submammary abscess* may be of the chronic type, and cause pyrexia without much pain. *Empyema thoracis* is generally easy to diagnose. The abnormal physical signs at the base of one lung suggest the presence of fluid, whilst pus may be found on needle aspiration. The condition may be simulated by subdiaphragmatic abscess, but X-ray examination or ultrasonography will usually help in distinguishing between the two. In some cases both conditions are present. Difficulty in diagnosis may on occasion be considerable when the empyema is interlobar, or between the pericardium and the pleura, or between the diaphragm and the lower lobe.

Lung abscess may be either single or multiple, and may be part of a blood-borne or local infection or be associated with a bronchial neoplasm (Fig. P.50). In the latter situation, much of the fever and acute systemic upset is due to infection rather than to the primary neoplasma. Imaging will help in the differential diagnosis.

Hepatic abscess, especially amoebic, may be a sub-acute or chronic rather than an acute condition, with

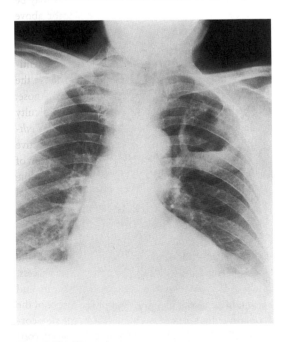

Figure P.50 Left lung abscess.

fluctuating pyrexia persisting for months. The diagnosis may be suggested by complaint of pain or tenderness over the lower part of the right chest in front or behind, by dullness at the base of the right lung, or by friction sounds over the liver. A history of amoebic dysentery is not always forthcoming. Pain is in some instances referred to the right shoulder. When pyrexia and rigors are the only objective features, malaria is simulated, but a high polymorphonuclear leucocytosis is against this diagnosis. Elevation of alkaline phosphatase may be the only clue in some cases. The diagnosis of hepatic abscess is clinched by ultrasound-guided needle aspiration which reveals pus, or fluid resembling 'anchovy sauce' in amoebic abscess. On rare occasions this may be coughed up as the result of ulceration through the diaphragm and pleura into a bronchus.

In *empyema of the gall bladder*, jaundice is generally absent. The pyrexia may be considerable and prolonged, and rigors are to be expected. The diagnosis depends largely upon the patient's complaint of pain in the right hypochondrium, associated either with an enlarged gall bladder or with acute pain and tenderness on palpation of the gall bladder region below the tip of the right ninth rib cartilage.

Suppurative cholangitis is the result of extension of pyogenic infection up the hepatic ducts into the biliary canals within the liver. It generally is associated with obstruction in the bile duct by stone or growth. By the time the infection has extended to become suppurative cholangitis, the patient will have become increasingly ill. The supervention of cholangitis may be indicated by progressive, soft, uniform and tender enlargement of the liver, associated as a rule with jaundice. Recurrent rigors are almost invariable.

Suppurative pylephlebitis arises from infection somewhere in the periphery of the portal area – for example, previous appendicitis. The condition is often fatal. The liver becomes studded with multiple small abscesses around the intrahepatic subdivisions of the portal vein. The liver becomes progressively, smoothly and uniformly enlarged, and generally tender; jaundice is present in less than half the cases. The high degree of pyrexia, the rigors, the asthenia and wasting all indicate that the patient has developed some form of septic extension of the original disease. There is a high degree of leucocytosis.

Subdiaphragmatic abscess is often difficult to diagnose. There may be no abnormal physical signs, but more usually infection of the pleura through the diaphragm leads to an impaired percussion note at the base of one lung, accompanied by pleuritic friction and rales. Diagnosis is aided by the use of ultrasonography or computed tomography, followed by needle aspiration.

Bronchiectasis may be responsible for prolonged periods of pyrexia with afebrile intervals of varying length. The pyrexial bouts are due either to invasion of the pus-containing cavities by fresh organisms or to recrudescence of infection already present, possibly brought about by impaired bronchial drainage. The abnormal physical signs in the lungs, the abundant foul sputum and the clubbed fingers indicate the diagnosis. Not infrequently there is considerable inflammation in the lung tissues around the area of bronchiectasis – the so-called 'peribronchiectatic pneumonitis'. This condition should be suspected in any patient where consolidation, often with pleurisy, recurs repeatedly in one area of the lung.

An *appendix abscess* may be easy to diagnose on palpating the tender swelling in the right iliac fossa. In other locations, the abscess may be difficult to diagnose; a rectal examination leads to the detection of the abscess when it descends into the pelvis. Pyrexia ceases as a rule when the pus obtains free drainage, so that it is exceptional for appendix abscess to be the cause of prolonged pyrexia.

Perinephric abscess may cause pyrexia of considerable degree, possibly lasting for several weeks. Pain in the loin is almost always present, eventually with tenderness to palpation in both the loin and the lumbar region, but it is often absent in the early stages, and may not appear until the patient has been febrile for some weeks. There may be no defined swelling but only a sense of resistance evident when, with the patient recumbent, the examiner places one hand behind each loin with the fingertips external to the erector spinae muscles, and then makes as if to raise the patient from the bed though without actually lifting. The fingers on the affected side will not feel the hollow of the loin as clearly as will those on the sound side. The signs may be yet more striking if the patient lies prone. If they are well enough to sit up in bed with the back bared, the observer may then look down the patient's spine from above. It may often be apparent that the loin on the sound side is slightly concave, whilst that of the perinephric abscess side is either flat or slightly convex. Only in pronounced cases does the loin show a distinct convexity. Peri-nephric abscess is generally the result of pyogenic infection, within the kidney; alternatively, it may be due to pus tracking up behind the colon from appendicitis, or it may be a delayed result of a loin injury, a haematoma due to the injury becoming infected and slowly forming a perinephric abscess weeks or months after the trauma. In many cases the history is obtainable of a suppurative process a short time previously. Pre-existing neutropenia, or corticosteroid therapy will in these cases – as in all infective processes – predispose to abscess formation.

Diverticular abscess may be subacute and yet cause prolonged pyrexia. It is generally situated in the left lower part of the abdomen, producing a tender swelling that may simulate carcinoma. It is preceded by chronic bowel symptoms, constipation and colic. Bleeding may occur, sometimes profusely. It is a disease of the second half of life.

Psoas abscess results from tuberculous spinal disease; the condition may be apyrexial but, like any other form of tuberculosis, it may cause protracted irregular pyrexia. Pain localized to some part of the back and stiffness of the corresponding part of the spine in a child are suggestive features. Radiographs must be taken. On the other hand, the diagnosis may remain unsuspected until a tender swelling appears above or below one groin as the abscess tracks down from the spine along the course of the psoas muscle, ultimately causing fluctuation from above to below the inguinal ligament.

Actinomycosis is diagnosed by the discovery of the organism. It may be in the discharge from a sinus communicating with the focus infected, generally the cheek, jaw, neck, lung, liver, caecum or spine. It may, however, occur anywhere in the skin or viscera, and the disease is likely to be missed if specific bacterial investigation is not undertaken. An actinomycotic ischiorectal abscess, for instance, may be regarded as of merely pyogenic origin. There is diffuse infiltration of deep as well as superficial parts, a liability to discharge through one or more sinuses, and a suggestive purplish red colour of the skin adherent to the lesion. The course is chronic and often apyrexial, but frequently there are periods of pyrexia.

Infective and inflammatory conditions

Coliform infection of the urinary tract may be chronic and apyrexial, but is liable to exacerbations with prolonged pyrexia, aching or pain in one or both loins, frequency of micturition, and pain during micturition. It may exist, however, especially in children, with so few symptoms of urinary disease that its responsibility for continued pyrexia may be missed.

Chronic or recurring pyelonephritis is more common in women than men, but it may be associated with an enlarged prostate or urethral stricture. The patient is ill, with rigors and high, long-continued pyrexia; the urine is purulent and yields a positive culture of the causative organism or organisms. In papillary necrosis the renal calices become clubbed and pyuria is common, even when urine cultures are sterile. Prolonged fever is not uncommon. It may be due to prolonged taking of compound analgesic tablets or diabetes mellitus.

Gallstones may be silent, causing no symptoms, or they may be associated with irregular and sometimes prolonged pyrexia and with bouts of pyrexia in attacks of biliary colic.

Phlebitis in a superficial vein is indicated by tenderness, with or without redness and swelling along the course of the vein; pyrexia of variable degree and duration accompanies the disorder in the earlier stages, but usually subsides in a few days. The diagnosis is much more difficult when the inflamed vein is deeply situated. Intra-abdominal phlebitis may be responsible for both continued pyrexia and vague, but possibly severe, abdominal pain in certain cases for which no explanation is forthcoming. *Thrombophlebitis migrans* occurs uncommonly. Venous thrombosis in the pelvis, not necessarily associated with obvious femoral or popliteal thrombosis, may account for pyrexia after childbirth.

Thyroiditis, an inflammatory but non-infective condition, may cause the complaint of sore throat, the thyroid itself being painful and tender.

Parametritis is diagnosed by pelvic examination. It is likely to be the after-effect of recent labour, and is often associated with continued pyrexia, pain in the pelvis and lower part of the back. Abscess formation may occur. Elderly women are apt to develop a purulent form of endometritis, sometimes pyrexial, with pelvic pain, bearing-down pain, pain in the back, and a foul vaginal discharge which is often blood-stained, the condition simulating advanced carcinoma of the body of the uterus.

Vesiculitis, though perhaps of local origin, is generally due to a gonococcal infection of the seminal vesicles. The complaint is mainly of hot burning pain in the rectum, aggravated by defecation; proctitis, or carcinoma of the rectum or acute prostatitis, are simulated. Diagnosis is established by rectal examination, the finger locating a tender swelling in the vesicles.

Colitis, whether infective or ulcerative, will be suggested by a history of diarrhoea, with the passage of blood and mucus associated with more or less pain along the course of the colon, particularly the descending colon; carcinoma or diverticulitis may be simulated. The diagnosis is confirmed by endoscopy, barium enema and/or bacteriological studies.

Crohn's disease (regional enteritis) should be suspected when there is a history of chronic intermittent diarrhoea, fever, loss of weight and abdominal pains or distension. Barium studies are necessary. Intermittent small-bowel obstruction is common. *Pancreatitis*, when subacute or chronic, may be very difficult to diagnose. It is sometimes (but not always) pyrexial, and it may simulate other abdominal lesions such as gallstones. Glycosuria in association with pyrexia and a dull aching pain in the abdomen across the site of the pancreas may be suggestive, but the symptoms are generally too vague to be characteristic. There is often a curious dull-brown pigmentation of the skin. Chronic pancreatitis should be suspected in a patient with recurrent abdominal pain, particularly if the pain or tenderness extends to the left of the midline, if gallstones are present, and if there have been bouts of over-consumption of alcohol. Radiographs may show pancreatic calcifications. Repeated serum amylase estimations taken within 12 hours of an acute episode are elevated in most cases, but as more acinar and ductal cells are destroyed these become less evident. Following acute pancreatitis, suppurative pancreatitis may occur in the second or third week with a return of fever.

Familial Mediterranean fever (paroxysmal polyserositis, periodic fever) is an inherited disease of unknown aetiology that is characterized by acute episodes of self-limited fever with signs of inflammation of the peritoneum, pleura and joints. The febrile episodes recur irregularly and unpredictably. The disease occurs most commonly in patients of Mediterranean or Middle East origin, particularly in Sephardic (but not Ashkenazic) Jews, Armenians, Turks, Arabs, Greeks and, less commonly, in Italians and others. In the acute form, attacks of fever may reach 40°C (104°F), but symptoms of peritonitis or 'pleurisy'

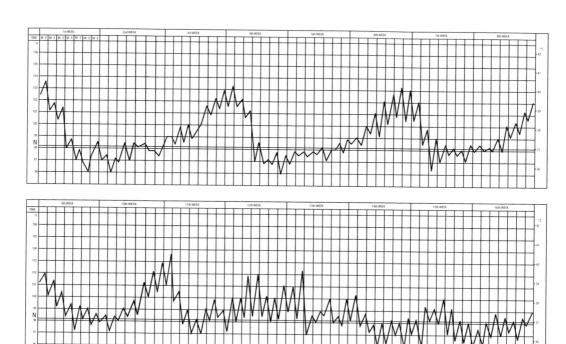

Figure P.55 Morning and evening temperature charts in a case of Hodgkin's disease, illustrating the Pel–Ebstein type of recurrent or periodic pyrexia that may occur in this disease.

Drug reactions

In any persistent unexplained fever where drug treatment is being given, the possibility of the therapy being the cause should be considered. Fever occurring in the treatment of pulmonary tuberculosis, for example, may be due to isoniazid, aminosalicylate or streptomycin, or to all three drugs. Antibiotics, sulphonamides, arsenicals, iodides, barbiturates and many others may be responsible. When in doubt, the motto should be, if possible, 'Stop treatment'.

Boris Lams

PYURIA

Pyuria means no more than the presence of pus in the urine. It will be present when there are infective processes affecting the urinary tract, in some chronic non-infective conditions such as bladder carcinoma-in-situ and interstitial cystitis, and occasionally following the rupture of an abscess outside the urinary tract into the system. The quantity of pus may vary;

when present in large quantities, it forms a thick, grey or yellow sediment. The sediment of urate crystals is usually pink or red in colour, and this clears when the sample is warmed to body temperature. The sediment of phosphate is cleared by the addition of acetic acid. Pus in the urine will be unchanged by both these tests.

When the urine is alkaline, pus cells tend to aggregate either into a dense viscid deposit or into large clumps, the deposit or clumps separating to leave a slightly turbid supernatant. On microscopy, pus cells are seen as rounded multi-nucleated bodies about twice the size of a red cell. As pus cells are, in fact, protein, dipstick testing is almost invariably positive for this substance. This test will also be positive if there are abnormally large numbers of epithelial cells in the sample so that microscopy of a urine sample is the only reliable simple test for the presence of pus.

The site of the pus-producing lesion cannot be determined simply by examination of the urine. The general and specific history of the individual case are essential although, in general, vesical lesions are often consequent upon renal lesions, particularly when these are infective. For example, when a pyelitis arises as a result of haematogeneous spread, the initial symptom may be frequently due to cystitis. In time, the hyperpyrexia, rigors and sweating attacks of pyelitis become manifest, together with severe loin pain on the affected side. A pyonephrosis need not necessarily present with pyuria if outflow from the kidney is blocked for one reason or another, such as a stone.

Special investigations

Imaging

If the patient is investigated during an acute illness associated with pyuria, imaging investigations of the urinary tract may provide specific answers with regard to the site of the pus. The kidney which is the seat of acute pyelitis will appear larger on *ultrasound examination*, and the fluid in the collecting system will appear less transonic than normal urine, implying turbidity.

Urography during an acute episode of pyelitis may show spasm of the collecting systems on the affected side, or dilatation if there is sufficient oedema of the pelvi-ureteric junction to obstruct the outflow of urine. Complete cessation of renal function is occasionally observed in acute interstitial bacterial nephritis.

Cystoscopy

Instrumentation of the lower urinary tract has little to commend it during an acute illness as the risk of septicaemia is considerable. However, following appropriate antibiotic therapy and the resolution of gross infection, cystoscopy under further intravenous antibiotic cover may provide useful information.

It is most likely that the bladder will be the source of pyuria if it shows the obvious features of a cystitis, but if the viscus is normal on cystoscopy, inspection of the two ureteric orifices may yield valuable information:

- A ureterocele is seen as a bulge above and lateral to the ureteric orifice, disappearing as the pressure inside the bladder increases with filling.
- A refluxing ureter is wider than it should be, and is often placed far lateral. The ureteric efflux may be thick and turbid, and exuding like toothpaste from the orifice if the urine production from that side is diminished.
- The ureteric orifice may be oedematous if pyelitis has extended along the whole length of the ureter as secondary ureteritis.

- The ureteric orifice in chronic tuberculosis is characteristically 'golf-hole' in appearance.
- Tiny nodules resembling sand granules are seen around the orifice in schistosomiasis.
- The areas above and lateral to the orifices are those characteristically affected by early carcinoma-in-situ, looking very much like inflammatory patches.
- Interstitial cystitis (Hunner's ulcer), presents as a red vertical line on the posterior wall of the bladder. This line extends into a split as the bladder is distended and rivulets of blood are seen on the back wall of the bladder, falling down as a curtain into the area behind the trigone.

A classified list of the causes of pyuria is provided in Table P.17.

Urinary tract pyuria

The kidneys

Recurrent attacks of pyelitis are commonest in childhood, during pregnancy and after childbirth. In childhood, pyelitis secondary to reflux often remains undetected and therefore untreated; chronic pyelonephritis in later life is a serious complication.

The kidneys may be infected:

- *Through the blood stream* – it is surprising that they are not infected more frequently, remembering the enormous renal blood flow.
- *By direct spread from the bladder* – which can occur if there is vesico-ureteric reflux.
- *By infections ascending through peri-ureteric lymphatics* – from an infected bladder or from a para-vesical structure.
- *By direct spread from the bladder* – along submucosal planes.

Outflow tract obstruction will predispose to ascending infection, particularly if the bladder has to contract violently in order to expel urine. This explains the occasional association of pyelitis with prostatic hypertrophy, and almost certainly accounts for the increase of incidence of pyelitis in pregnancy. It is unusual for both kidneys to be affected simultaneously, but it is certainly true to say that once a kidney is damaged it is more likely to be a seat of infection on subsequent occasions.

Congenital abnormalities in themselves will not predispose towards sepsis, but if there is interference with free drainage in a horseshoe kidney (Fig. P.56),

Table P.17 Causes of pyuria

Pyuria from diseases of the urinary organs

- Renal
  - Pyelitis
  - Pyelonephritis
  - Renal abscess
  - Renal papillary necrosis
  - Pyonephrosis
  - Tuberculosis
  - Calculus
  - Medullary sponge kidney
- Ureteric
  - Calculus
  - Megaureter
  - Ureteric foreign body
  - Vesicoureteric reflux
- Vesical
  - Cystitis
  - Tuberculosis
  - Calculus or foreign body
  - Ulcer – simple, epitheliomatous
  - Tumour – sloughing papillary or solid carcinoma
  - Diverticula
  - *Bilharzia haematobia*
  - Trichomoniasis
  - Carcinoma-in-situ
  - Interstitial cystitis
- Urethral
  - Urethritis
    - specific
    - gonococcal
    - chlamydial
    - trichomonal
    - monilial
    - non-specific
  - Stricture
  - Calculus or foreign body
- Prostatic
  - Prostatis, acute or chronic
  - Prostatic abscess
  - Calculus
  - Prostatic carcinoma
- Vesicular
  - Seminal vesiculitis, acute or chronic vesicular abscess

Pyuria from diseases outside the urinary organs

- Leucorrhoea
- Balanitis with phimosis
- From the extension of inflammatory processes to the bladder, or the rupture into the bladder or urethra of an abscess such as:
  - Prostatic abscess
  - Appendicular abscess
  - Iliac or pelvic abscess
  - Abscess due to colonic diverticulitis
  - Psoas abscess
  - Pyosalpinx
  - Carcinoma of the uterus, rectum, caecum, sigmoid or pelvic colon
  - Ulceration of the small intestine, tuberculous or dysenteric

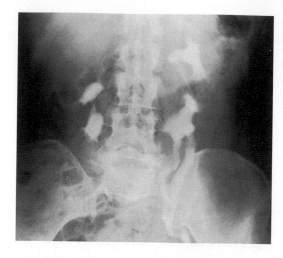

Figure P.56 Horseshoe kidney. The classical malrotation is shown. The picture is complicated by a duplex left kidney with distal obstruction of both ureters.

an ectopic kidney or a kidney with a degree of pelvi-ureteric junction obstruction, it may be the seat of infection more frequently than a normal system. A duplex kidney may become infected in one or other of its moieties.

Vesicoureteric reflux arises when the intramural course of the ureter is short and the normally acute 'ureterovesical angle' is lost. The normal 'hydraulic valve' which prevents reflux is not therefore present and there is no obstruction to the retrograde passage of urine. At the same time, acute cystitis may in itself alter the efficiency of this ureterovesical angle so that reflux can occur secondary to the primary cystitis.

Cystoscopy of a patient with reflux often shows a small saccule or shallow diverticulum above and lateral to the ureteric orifice. It seems more likely that this is part of the original maldevelopment than a traction diverticulum.

Megaureter in children is a condition in which the whole of the ureter may be dilated, although the condition more commonly affects the distal ureter only. A megaureter may be obstructed or non-obstructed, and may reflux or may not. Paradoxically, an obstructed megaureter may also reflux, with relative obstruction to the passage of urine from upper tract to bladder but a facilitated passage from lower tract to upper.

Megaureter is physiological during pregnancy, either as a result of direct obstruction from the gravid uterus or secondary to the progestogen effect of a maintained pregnancy. Whatever the aetiology of megaureter, the resulting stasis predisposes to sepsis, stone formation, squamous metaplasia, and so on. Reflux may occur in severe cases of outflow tract obstruction where the intravesical pressure rises to a level that overcomes the resistance of the most normal ureteric orifice.

Reflux is demonstrated by a micturating cystogram, and also by ultrasound assessment. Reflux is sometimes severe enough to cause gross distention of the upper urinary tract especially when there is congenital outflow obstruction, as in urethral valves.

The congenital megaureter megacystis syndrome arises because of incorrect development of the urinary tract, and the ureteric orifices are widely patent (Fig. P.57). A similar picture may be seen in severe chronic retention when dilatation of the bladder and ureters has occurred beyond the point of recovery when the obstruction is relieved.

Pyelitis

Haematogeneous pyelitis arising as an entity separate from other urinary tract pathology is not unusual

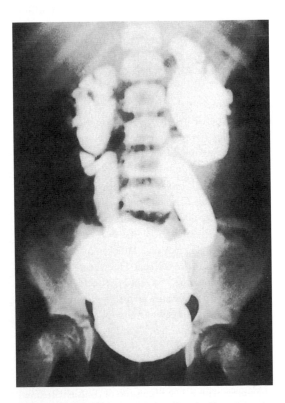

Figure P.57 Bilateral vesicoureteric reflux in the megaureter megacystis syndrome.

following acute febrile illness or secondary to suppuration elsewhere in the body. The organisms responsible are usually *Escherichia coli*, *Proteus* and *Klebsiella*; *Pseudomonas* is common as a hospital-based infection, as is the increasingly common multiple-resistant *Staphylococcus aureus*.

The symptoms of *acute pyelitis* are severe. There is loin pain, symptoms of an associated acute cystitis, hyperpyrexia, tachycardia, rigors and sweating. The urine is turbid, opalescent, may be bright red from haematuria and positive for protein, while microscopy reveals large numbers of free bacteria with pus cells and red cells. The patient may be oliguric because of fluid loss.

While examination reveals a high white cell count and ESR, urography may show reduced function on the affected side; calculi will almost always show up as radio-opaque bodies overlying the urinary tract.

Chronic pyelitis is dangerous because there may be few symptoms early in the course of the disease. A slight stinging during micturition and vague pain in the renal areas may be ignored, and general malaise, lassitude secondary to anaemia, a low-grade persisting pyrexia and hypertension are often presenting features. The urine classically has a specific gravity of 1.010, the blood urea and plasma creatinine are raised, and creatinine clearance is diminished. Excretion urography may be impractical because of poor renal function, but delayed films will show irregularity and blunting of the calyces, cortical atrophy and a reduction in renal size. The physical signs of hypertension may be manifest.

Renal abscess

Renal abscesses follow acute haematogeneous infections and are initially situated in the peripheral area of the cortex. There are general symptoms and signs of a systemic abscess, with acute tenderness in the loin, developing into a mass with an overlying hyperaemic skin. It is rare for renal abscesses to discharge spontaneously through the skin as they are usually seen and treated well before this happens. Occasionally, they may discharge into nearby viscera, the ascending or descending colon and the second and third parts of the duodenum, depending on the side affected. It is uncommon for a left-sided abscess to involve the tail of the pancreas. An abscess may occasionally follow a renal infarct.

Renal papillary necrosis

Renal papillary necrosis is common in diabetics. It is now rarely seen following phenacetin abuse as the substance was withdrawn following the discovery of the association between its abuse and renal failure. The renal papillae undergo avascular necrosis and separate from the kidney. They may be passed as sloughs, in which case the patient may present with ureteric colic, or retained within the pelvicalyceal system, where they calcify. An acute bacterial infection often supervenes and presentation with an acute pyelitis or cystitis is not unusual.

Urography shows several changes depending on the severity of the process. In the early stage, a line of contrast can be seen crossing the base of each papilla; as the papilla sloughs it may be seen as a filling defect within a dilated calyx. Later still, a triangular zone of calcification lying within the pelvicalyceal system is readily apparent. Bilateral renal papillary necrosis can lead to progressive renal failure and death from uraemia.

Pyonephrosis

In pyonephrosis, the urine within an obstructed pelvicalyceal system becomes infected, usually secondary to congenital pelvi-ureteric junction or impaction of a stone at the junction. Obstruction of a ureteric orifice by stone or tumour, or ureteric involvement from a primary bladder or primary uterine carcinoma, are less common causes of pyonephrosis. The symptoms are not as severe as those of an acute pyelitis and are more gradual in their onset. Examination almost invariably shows tenderness in the affected loin, together with a palpable renal mass.

Radiological examination often reveals the presence of a stone, while renal function is rarely preserved. The quickest way of proving the diagnosis is by establishing a nephrostomy under local anaesthesia and ultrasound control; this will not only allow aspiration of pus for diagnostic and therapeutic purposes but will also provide drainage of the system. Nephrectomy is usually required together with appropriate management of the precipitating cause.

Renal tuberculosis

This disease – once commonplace – is now relatively rare in the Western world, and there must always be the danger that the diagnosis will be missed unless it is remembered that all cases of persistent sterile and acid pyuria must be considered as tuberculosis until disproved by the examination of no fewer than three early morning urine samples. Even this number may be insufficient to exclude the diagnosis with certainty, and as many as 12 samples could be reasonably cultured for tubercle bacilli if the clinical suspicion of the disease is relatively high. Culture, on specially reinforced media, must be continued for 6 weeks.

The miliary form of tuberculosis which was once seen in childhood is now extremely rare; it is not associated with urinary symptoms. Renal tuberculosis, however, is still very much a reality, the kidney at first being attacked by a tuberculous infection on a microscopic basis. The resultant small tuberculous nodules eventually coalesce to form an area of caseation, which then bursts into the renal pelvis by direct ulceration into a calyx. The transitional cell lining of the pelvis and ureter are subsequently infected with tubercle bacilli, becoming thickened by submucosal infiltration and by oedema.

The symptoms prior to discharge into the urinary tract may be very slight. Aching in the loin may be the only symptom, and albuminuria the only finding once the septic focus has discharged. The symptoms mimic a low-grade pyelitis and cystitis; there is increased aching in the renal area, whilst the frequency of micturition, discomfort while passing urine and polyuria also occur.

The urine is pale, acid, of low specific gravity and turbid; tubercle bacilli may sometimes be found after appropriate staining of a centrifuged sample.

Cystoscopy may show areas of oedema within the bladder, and sometimes small tubercles are visible. The ureteric orifice is usually oedematous and pouting into the bladder. The 'golf-ball' change is seen in long-standing disease when fibrosis has caused contraction of the orifice. Digital examination per rectum or per vagina may reveal thickening of the bladder wall, and pencil-like thickened ureters are occasionally felt as they hook their way into the bladder base.

Urography may show reduced function on one side, together with cavities, ureteric dilatation, and a thick-walled bladder. The caseating areas occasionally undergo calcification, these areas being poorly defined, in contrast to the clear-cut margins of a renal calculus. Calcific caseous debris is sometimes seen passing along the ureter, with a dilated column of contrast proximal. Renal tuberculosis should be considered strictly in relation to the rest of the genitourinary system; the male frequently has lesions in the bladder, epididymis, prostate and vesicles, while the female may have tuberculosis secondarily in the Fallopian tubes. Evidence of former disease in the spine, joints, chest or mesenteric lymph nodes may also be noted.

Renal calculus

The symptoms of stones will depend on their site, size and pathological effects (see Fig. H.2). Renal stones may be asymptomatic. A stone floating free within the renal pelvis may cause intermittent obstruction and loin pain; a stone in the ureter presents as acute ureteric colic. Macroscopic haematuria is rare, but microscopic bleeding is almost invariable. Secondary infection is most likely to occur if calculi impact at a narrow area – a calycine neck, the pelvi-ureteric junction, the ureter as it crosses the iliac vessels or at the ureterovesical junction. Some 90 per cent of renal calculi are radio-opaque (Figs P.58 and P.59); all stones are shown on ultrasound of the kidneys or on CT scanning.

Medullary sponge kidney

This is a congenital abnormality which probably represents a minor form of polycystic kidneys. The condition is not always bilateral, and is often associated with the unusual physical sign of body hemihypertrophy. Unless the family history is known, the condition usually presents as renal angle pain, pyuria, supervening upper tract sepsis and ureteric colic. The stones may erode into the pelvicalycine system and from there make their way along the ureter. The radiological changes are pathognomonic of the condition, showing the typical 'bouquet of flowers'.

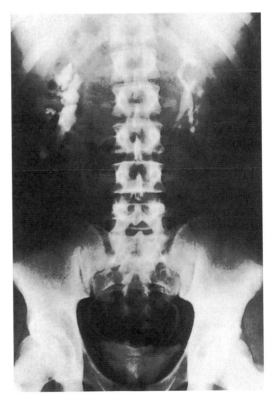

Figure P.59 Excretion pyelogram in the same case as Fig. P.56, showing caliceal saccules which contain the stones. From a boy aged 16 years.

Ureteric disease

Ureteric calculus

Most ureteric calculi will pass of their own accord once they have passed the pelvi-ureteric junction.

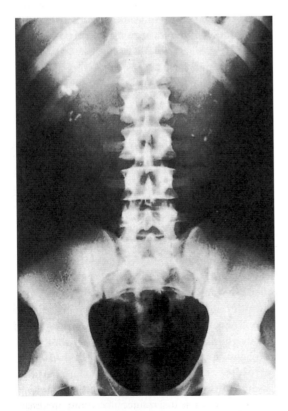

Figure P.58 Multiple small bilateral renal calculi in a case of medullary sponge kidney.

This is the rule in 95 per cent of cases if the stone is less than 1 cm in diameter. The smaller and smoother the stone, the more likely it is to pass. It is probable that acute ureteric colic is the most severe pain known to man (or woman), the severe pain starting on the affected side radiating upwards to the renal area and downwards towards the bladder and into the testicles or labia. It is surprising how many ureteric stones are, in fact, asymptomatic and present as an incidental finding. Complete blockage of a ureter by a calculus is unusual but, if it happens, it can result in a non-functioning and atrophic kidney. The lower down the ureter the stone impacts, the more lower urinary tract symptoms will be manifest; a stone impacting very near to the bladder can exactly mimic an acute cystitis, with supervening pyelitis, except that there is no pyrexia unless the obstructed and retained urine becomes infected. Calculi are well demonstrated by urinary tract ultrasound; most stones show on plain X-rays; ultrasound will also give an accurate picture of the degree of upper tract dilatation.

Ureteric foreign bodies

It might seem inappropriate to discuss foreign bodies within the ureter, but with the increasing frequency of endoscopic stone surgery, iatrogenic foreign bodies are now introduced with increasing regularity. One of the disadvantages of over-vigorous ultrasound stone destruction is fragmentation of the metal probe-tip; these metal fragments may embed in the mucosa of the ureter and predispose to pyuria.

It should be noted that non-absorbable suture materials should never be used to close surgical incisions in the ureter as they form an excellent nidus for calculus formation.

Vesical diseases

Pyuria will be present in any lesion of the bladder which is associated with inflammation. This applies to acute and chronic bacterial infections, parasitic infections, the presence of stone, primary and secondary malignant disease, squamous metaplasia, leucoplakia and interstitial cystitis.

Cystitis

Cystitis may be acute or chronic and, while both forms are usually associated with infection by a micro-organism, a true infective cause is not essential as any

process which produces congestion of the bladder will give rise to cystitis.

In *acute cystitis* the mucosa of the bladder is oedematous and congested, leading to epithelial desquamation, pyuria, haemorrhage, the development of small abscesses within the mucosa and occasionally to areas of ulceration. The changes are sometimes sufficiently severe to cause sloughing of the whole of the mucosa of the bladder, with profuse haemorrhage.

The symptoms of acute cystitis are well known: there is frequency, urgency, dysuria, perineal pain and pain in the suprapubic area, haematuria and pyuria. The diagnosis of an acute bacterial cystitis depends on the positive culture of an infective organism. While the precipitating cause may be evident in some cases, such as lower tract instrumentation, over-vigorous intercourse or acquired urethritis, many cases cannot be attributed to a specific event. An attack of acute abacterial cystitis may exactly mimic a true cystitis; the inflammatory agent in these cases must be a chemical irritant which is irrigated into the bladder by the turbulent urine flow associated with distal urethral stenosis in women. A causative organism can never be found, but red cells and pus cells are frequently present on urine testing. The condition is most frequently seen in young women after they become sexually active, but is also common in peri-menopausal women. The name 'honeymoon cystitis' is often given to the condition, but it seems rather inappropriate nowadays. Because of the common incidence of the condition at the extremes of reproductive life it seems reasonable to postulate distal urethral stenosis as a very real aetiological factor, the stenosis arising because of the hormone imbalances which occur at these two stages of a woman's development.

Chronic cystitis may follow an improperly or inadequately treated acute episode. While the symptoms are less severe, increased frequency or micturition, pyuria and a persisting alkaline urine are noted. It is often seen with some form of urinary obstruction or retention and is sometimes found in cases of urinary incontinence, of whatever cause. The main differential diagnosis is from pyelitis, which can also cause increased frequency of micturition with pyuria, but the urine is usually acid, pale, generally turbid and has little inclination to form a deposit. An important second diagnosis is to consider tuberculous cystitis.

At cystoscopy, the bladder wall is red, smooth and oedematous; in pyelitis, the cystoscopic appearance of the bladder is normal apart from possible modifications in the appearances of the ureteric orifices, the efflux of which is often cloudy as it contains more particulate matter.

Tuberculosis

This is part of a tuberculous infective process affecting the whole of the urinary system, together with the reproductive system of both sexes. Frequency is the predominant presenting symptom, by day and by night, associated with a minor discomfort usually felt at the end of the urethra. A few drops of terminal haematuria are often observed. Pyuria is constant. Vesical calculus and vesical carcinoma, particularly carcinoma-in-situ, present in a similar fashion. Bladder calculi are usually found in older patients with symptoms of outflow tract obstruction or a history of previous lower urinary tract instrumentation and catheterization. Calculi in the bladder often give pain only on movement; haematuria in calculous disease is observed throughout the stream and is often a more regular occurrence than with carcinoma.

The symptoms of bacterial cystitis may supervene in both calculus and carcinoma, accompanied by frequency, urgency and painful micturition by day and night. Vesical carcinoma may be felt per rectum, especially when the patient is thin and the tumour is extensive. The early stages of tuberculous cystitis are characterized cystoscopically by the appearance of greyish tubercles in the submucosal coat of the bladder, particularly around the ureteric orifice. At this stage frequency of micturition may be the only symptom, but as the disease progresses the tubercles enlarge, coalesce and eventually ulcerate, by which time pus and blood will both be present in the urine; tubercle bacilli should show up on special staining. The bladder becomes extremely small, with micturition occurring every 15 minutes or so throughout the 24 hours.

As a general diagnostic rule, any patient with increased frequency of micturition and a sterile acid urine should be considered as suffering from tuberculosis until disproved. As noted previously, as many as 12 negative early-morning sample cultures may be required before the clinical suspicion of tuberculosis can be dismissed. Culture, on special media, must be continued for 6 weeks. Tuberculosis within the bladder is often associated with tuberculosis in the Fallopian tubes, vas deferens, epididymis, prostate and seminal vesicles.

Tuberculosis in the bladder usually arises secondarily from an infection in the upper tract. A caseous lesion, however small, in the kidney ruptures and discharges its contents into the renal pelvis so that the urothelium of the pelvis, the ureter and the bladder become affected in turn. The primary site may similarly be within the epididymis, infection ascending through the vas deferens to affect the bladder, seminal vesicles and prostate. Prostatic tuberculosis is rare but may involve the bladder by direct ulceration. As with simple infective pyelitis, renal tuberculosis may present with lower urinary tract symptoms; the amount of blood present in the urine is usually less than if the bladder is chiefly involved and blood will, of course, be noted and found throughout the urinary stream. In renal tuberculosis there may be tenderness in the loin, while the kidney may be more readily palpable than usual and the distal end of the lower ureter can sometimes be felt on rectal or vaginal examination.

It is not, however, critical to establish whether the kidneys or the bladder are the primary sites of the disease, and in many cases it is impossible to do this. Intravenous urography may provide useful information with regard to the state of the upper tract. Cystoscopy in renal tuberculosis may show pathological changes surrounding one ureter but not the other. The affected ureter is primarily oedematous, and the wall is thickened and patulous. Later on, the orifice becomes rigid and patent, representing the 'golf-hole', and is drawn up towards the affected kidney by fibrotic shortening of the ureter. The final stage of vesical tuberculosis is a small thick-walled bladder (the 'golf-ball' bladder).

Vesical calculus

Calculus in the bladder often presents as simple bacterial cystitis, and under these circumstances there is little that will distinguish cystitis from many other forms except, perhaps, that the urine may be loaded with crystals. An increase in the amount of blood after exercise is noted frequently, while pyuria is usually constant. Haematuria may occur after exercise, as it does in joggers.

The constant symptoms of vesical calculus are frequency and discomfort during the daytime, especially when erect and moving, penile pain after micturition and haematuria. Except for those patients who have had indwelling catheters or complex lower urinary tract surgery, vesical calculus is almost always secondary to sepsis and stasis from outflow obstruction. Management must aim not only to remove the calculus but also to eliminate the source of obstruction. A suspected calculus will almost always show on plain pelvic X-ray or ultrasound. It may not always be possible to determine whether a stone lies within a diverticulum, except by cystoscopy.

Stones which form in the upper tract and pass into the bladder without producing the symptoms of ureteric colic are almost always small enough to pass per urethra, unless the bladder outlet is obstructed. Radiolucent stones within the bladder (e.g. uric acid stones) are unusual as they accumulate calcium once within the viscus and take on a laminated appearance. If a pure uric acid stone is present within the bladder, it will not show on plain X-ray but will probably be detected as a filling defect at urography.

Ulceration of the bladder

This occurs secondary to chronic cystitis, following traumatic cystoscopy, secondary to a long-standing stone and as a consequence of radiotherapy for pelvic malignancy. Hunner's ulcer (interstitial cystitis) is a disease which is peculiar to women, causing severe frequency, pain on micturition, urgency with incontinence, and occasional haematuria. The diagnosis is established cystoscopically when a vertical ulcer is usually observed on the posterior bladder wall. The ulcer splits as the bladder is distended, resulting in a curtain of blood rivulets falling down the posterior wall. Biopsy of the area, usually taken to exclude malignancy, shows chronic inflammatory changes with a heavy mast-cell infiltrate. Calcium encrustation occurs, so that pyuria and calcific debris are often seen. The bladder capacity in this condition is relatively small, and therapy often consists of forcible distention.

Tuberculous ulceration, malignant ulceration and ulceration secondary to radiotherapy have similar presenting symptoms of frequency, haematuria, urgency and additional pain at the termination of micturition. The cystoscopic appearances of these different ulcers are not always easy to distinguish, and multiple biopsies are often necessary in order to establish the diagnosis with certainty.

Malignant ulceration of the bladder

Malignant ulceration of the bladder and papillary transitional cell carcinoma of the bladder are common conditions, giving rise to irregular haemorrhage, which is often profuse and almost always painless. Well-differentiated tumours tend to protrude into the bladder lumen, supported by a pedicle of rather narrow size, which accounts for the fact that the surface is often necrotic and ulcerated, giving rise to pyuria in conjunction with haematuria. The pathognomonic symptom is painless haematuria, but increased frequency can occur if the tumour(s) is sufficiently large to disturb bladder capacity. Pain is unusual unless secondary infection has occurred. Tumours are often multiple because of the 'field change' that occurs within the whole of the transitional cell lining of the urinary tract – the urothelium.

When tumours are less well differentiated and situated near the ureteric orifices, there may be ureteric obstruction and loin pain secondary to distention of the affected upper tract. Diagnosis can almost always be established preoperatively by a combination of urography and ultrasound examination of the urinary tract. Endoscopic examination of the bladder is conclusive, and with the advent of continuous-irrigation instruments the presence of a bleeding lesion offers no handicap to the endoscopist.

When the tumours are large, clumps of the frond-like lesions may separate and be present in the urine. Cytological examination of voided samples is relatively unsatisfactory if the tumour is well differentiated as the cells are barely different from normal bladder epithelial cells. As soon as relative de-differentiation occurs, cytological examination of the urine is a useful diagnostic and monitoring tool.

It is probably true to say that the more poorly differentiated a transitional cell carcinoma, the more solid-looking it becomes. The solid carcinomas are nodular, sessile, often solitary, and involve the trigone rather than affecting the lateral walls. Ureteric obstruction is a frequent complication, and early invasion of the muscle wall occurs. The presence of a mass on bimanual palpation reveals that the tumour is probably beyond the scope of endoscopic resection, while fixity to the pelvis implies inoperability.

Diverticulum of the bladder

A bladder diverticulum may give rise to intermittent or persistent and excessive pyuria together with increased frequency, pain and difficulty with micturition. The last symptom relates to the outflow tract obstruction. A common symptom is that bladder emptying is often followed quickly by the need to empty the bladder again; as the bladder 'empties' it expels as much urine into the diverticulum as it does through the urethra, so that when the sphincter apparatus has closed, urine flows back into the bladder cavity from the distended diverticulum.

The diagnosis is established by urography or ultrasound, but the size of the orifice into the bladder is rarely established without endoscopic examination. A cystogram gives a reasonable idea of the size of the diverticulum, but an exaggerated impression may be obtained because of the magnification seen on this kind of X-ray, and the relatively forceful distention which occurs during the examination.

Schistosomiasis

This causes pus in the urine when the small submucosal nodules – the 'sandy' patches – ulcerate into the bladder. Ova are often observed in the urine, together with pus and blood, but microscopic examination of a biopsy is pathognomonic. Complement fixation testing is specific. In advanced cases, calcification, appearing as a ring in the bladder wall, may show on plain X-ray while urography shows upper tract dilatation, due to the presence of ureterovesical stricture. Complication of the disease process by carcinoma is all too common, and is to some extent related to the duration of the disease; the consequent bladder carcinoma frequently affects young people.

Trichomoniasis

This condition is relatively rare in males, but may be acquired from an infected partner. The pyuria is relatively symptom-free, but trichomonas are found on staining the urine, or motile organisms are seen in centrifuged urine deposits. They can also be found in urethral discharge, semen, or fluid massaged from the prostate.

Urethral causes

Urethral pyuria will be caused by any condition which causes a purulent urethritis. A profuse discharge, together with a history of recent unprotected sexual contact, are enough to provide the diagnosis, but urethritis may be secondary to cystitis as well as the converse. The symptoms of urethritis are discharge, urethral pain and occasional initial haematuria; if there is also increased frequency, suprapubic pain and bleeding throughout the stream, cystitis is also probably present. The pyuria of urethritis is usually confined to the initial sample of urine; in cystitis, the mid-stream sample will also be contaminated. Urethral calculi, foreign bodies and self-inflicted urethral trauma will also cause purulent urethritis.

Prostatic causes

Acute prostatitis presents with increased frequency, perineal and suprapubic pain, discomfort on micturition, pyuria, and even acute retention. Prostatitis may arise by haematogeneous spread, or it may complicate cystitis or urethritis. A rectal examination reveals a large prostate which is exquisitely tender, to the degree that touching the oedematous gland causes acute reflex contraction of the external sphincter and straightening of the hips.

Prostatic abscess usually follows an acute urethritis which has affected the posterior urethra and caused an acute prostatitis. It may be secondary to a sexually transmitted infection, such as gonorrhoea or chlamydia, and may also follow instrumentation of the urethra. The prostate is intrinsically infected subclinically, and endoscopy can trigger this infection – however carefully performed. Acute prostatitis may result in the formation of an abscess, almost always unilateral, which may discharge spontaneously into the urethra, bladder or rectum unless de-roofed by transurethal resection. Acute prostatitis presents with increased frequency of micturition, perineal and hypogastric pain, fever, rigors and difficulty with micturition. The abscess can be felt as a soft area within the tender and oedematous prostate.

Prostatic calculi are frequent, but prostatic abscesses complicating calculi are relatively unusual, as are abscesses related to genitourinary tuberculosis. Involvement of the prostate is a very late manifestation of this disease, presenting as increased frequency, perineal pain, difficulty with micturition and a sudden episode of initial haematuria.

Pyuria is invariable following prostatic surgery, whether covered by prophylactic antibiotics or not. The healing cavity of a prostatectomy, carried out transurethrally or retropubically, can take as long as 8 weeks to epithelialize, and pyuria during the whole of this period is common.

Vesicular causes

Seminal vesiculitis often accompanies acute prostatitis, and often causes persistent symptoms following gonococcal or non-specific urethritis. It is a very rare complication of prostatectomy, but an abscess may develop if the openings of the vesicles are involved in the cicatrization process postoperatively. Tuberculous vesiculitis also occurs.

The symptoms of vesiculitis are pain in the bladder area, in the perineum, and in the low back. Pyuria may be scant, but if the channels between the vesicles and urethra are free it may be profuse. Haematospermia is not infrequent, while ascending inflammation of the vas and acute epididymitis are also often associated. The inflamed vesicle can be felt above the prostate on rectal examination. Whilst massage can produce a bead of pus at the urethral meatus, it is difficult to distinguish this sign from the similar phenomenon encountered in acute prostatitis.

Pyuria caused by diseases outside the urinary system

The most common cause of pyuria is the incorrect collection of a sample, in that the urinary meatus, in the male or female, is improperly cleaned prior to collection. If the sample has been collected appropriately, pyuria can occur by secondary inflammatory changes within the bladder, prostate or urethra, from septic foci or malignant processes outside. In the male, retained secretions behind a phimosis can result in pyuria; an excess of physiological discharge in the female may have the same effect. If there is persistent doubt with regard to the presence of pyuria in a woman, suprapubic fine-needle aspiration of a bladder which is well distended with urine is a relatively safe method of establishing the diagnosis with certainty.

The presence and spread of inflammatory processes outside the urinary tract into the urinary passages will cause pyuria, as will the rupture of an extravesical abscess. When the symptoms suggest urinary problems (e.g. increased frequency, urgency, pain on micturition, haematuria), and are followed by the sudden appearance of a quantity of pus in the urine, there is a strong possibility of the rupture of an extra-urinary abscess into the bladder or urethra or (very rarely) into the ureter, provided that the sudden emptying of a renal abscess or pyonephrosis can be eliminated. This spontaneous discharge is often associated with a relief of the primary symptom. The history will often provide some indication of the primary diagnosis, of which the most frequent are

prostatic abscess, appendix abscess, pyosalpinx, psoas, iliac and pelvic abscess and an abscess around a carcinoma or diverticulitis of the colon, the last of these being the most common of all.

Pyuria in acute appendicitis

If the appendix is in its usual position the bladder is rarely affected, but if the appendix passes downwards across the pelvic brim it is not unusual to find that the patient complains of frequency and pain on micturition when appendicitis occurs. If the appendix is severely inflamed it may adhere to the bladder, and both pus and blood may be present in the urine. If cytoscopy is carried out, a localized area of congestion will be seen on the right lateral wall. Very occasionally, a small abscess may develop in the adhesions between the appendix and the bladder, and if this abscess discharges into the bladder pyuria results and an enterovesical fistula is established. Diagnosis in the case of a dependent appendix is difficult; the pain is much lower in the pelvis than is usual with appendicitis, while the lower urinary tract symptoms point to a bladder disorder. The onset of the condition is gradual, however, and there is an elevation of temperature and pulse rate with right-sided abdominal rigidity. None of these is present in acute cystitis, and the possibility of an alternative acute intra-abdominal lesion must be considered. A right-sided pelvic abscess arising from a burst appendix may rupture into the bladder. The usual history of acute appendicitis is accompanied by the presence of a mass in the right iliac fossa or the pelvic space, bimanually palpable if in the later. Pyrexia continues and is associated with rigors. If the abscess discharges into the bladder, the fever resolves and a large quantity of pus appears in the urine. Rectal examination reveals not only the tenderness of acute appendicitis but also considerable thickening relating to the thick wall of the abscess cavity.

Pyosalpinx may cause cystitis by direct spread of the inflammatory process to the bladder, and may eventually rupture. There has usually been a history of profuse vaginal discharge associated with constant aching in the pelvic region and in the lower back; there are often frequent attacks of severe pain and malaise at variable intervals, together with an intermittent pyrexia. Periods may be profuse, frequent, and more painful than usual, while vaginal examination reveals fullness or a mass in one or both vaginal fornices.

Psoas and iliac abscesses may rupture into the bladder, and the former has been known to discharge into a ureter. There is a swelling in the iliac fossa and sometimes in the inguinal region, and clinical and radiological evidence of spinal osteomyelitis, together with lateral displacement of the psoas shadow.

Diverticulitis of the pelvic colon often becomes adherent to the bladder, and if peridiverticular abscesses form these may rupture into the bladder, causing pyuria and formation of an enterovesical fistula. Pneumaturia – the passage of flatus per urethram – is pathognomonic, but it is surprising how rarely it occurs; the appearance of solid faecal particles in the urine is more common; when air is passed in the urine the stream hisses or whistles. The main differential diagnosis of pneumaturia is an acute cystitis with a gas-forming organism, particularly in diabetic patients. A colovesical fistula occurs far more frequently following rupture of a peridiverticular abscess than by direct extension of a colonic carcinoma.

Carcinoma of the pelvic structures often involves the bladder by direct extension. This is particularly true of carcinoma of the cervix and of the rectum, but it may also happen from carcinoma of the pelvic colon, sigmoid and caecum. Spread of disease to the bladder occurs relatively late, and the symptoms of the primary condition have usually given a clear indication of the diagnosis before pyuria results. Involvement of the bladder is first shown by frequency, dysuria and urgency, while the presence of blood and pus in the urine are late features, representing ulceration through the whole thickness of the bladder wall. Uterovesical and vesicovaginal fistulae may result from extension of primary tumours from either of these two structures into the bladder; the pathognomonic symptom is continuous incontinence by day and night. It is hardly likely that this incontinence will need to be distinguished from that secondary to an ectopic ureter as this will be evident from birth. Penetration of the bladder by a carcinoma of the rectum or colon will give rise to pneumaturia and the passage of pus, blood and faecal debris in the urinary stream. Occasionally, the urine flow passes in the other direction and the urine output falls while the passage of watery stools, alternating with reasonably well-formed motions, may occur.

Tuberculosis, or *dysenteric ulcers* of the intestines and *caecal actinomycosis* are rare causes of pyuria. In the last of these, the fungus, instead of infiltrating the skin and pointing in the groin externally as it usually does, extends downwards into the pelvis and opens into the bladder or rectum. The diagnosis depends on the discovery of ray fungi in the urine, and it is unlikely that they would be found unless specifically sought. Actinomycosis of the kidney is usually mistaken for tuberculosis until the fungi are discovered by microscopy.

The most common causes of the intermittent appearance of large amounts of pus in the urine are pyonephrosis, diverticulum of the bladder and vesicocolic fistula. The presence of a persistent low-grade pyuria which cannot be explained otherwise may indicate carcinoma-in-situ of the bladder or urinary tract tuberculosis.

Harold Ellis

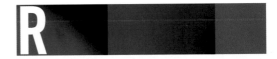

RECTAL BLEEDING

Bleeding from the rectum is one of the most common presenting symptoms in clinical practice, and is also the most commonly mismanaged. A classification of causes is listed in Table R.1.

The majority of patients with rectal bleeding are found to have haemorrhoids (or piles, the terms are interchangeable) as the underlying cause. Haemorrhoids are cushions of erectile tissue containing extensive arteriovenous anastomoses and, when traumatized, arterial bleeding results (Fig. R.1). Usually, the bleeding is of a minor nature; there is light staining of the lavatory paper following defaecation. Rarely, profuse bleeding leading to hypovolaemic shock can occur. The possibility of a neoplasm must always be a consideration, irrespective of the age of the patient. Although the incidence of rectal carcinoma is highest in the sixth and seventh decades of life, it is not uncommon in younger age groups. The presence of malignancy must be considered particularly when there are constitutional symptoms or

Table R.1 Major causes of rectal bleeding

Anal causes	Neoplasia
Haemorrhoids	■ Adenoma
Anal fissure	■ Carcinoma
Anal fistula	■ Malignant melanoma
Perianal haematoma	
Condylomata	**Colonic causes**
Trauma	Diverticular disease
Malignancy	Infective (e.g. dysentery)
■ Squamous carcinoma	Inflammatory
■ Adenocarcinoma	■ Ulcerative colitis
■ Paget's disease	■ Crohn's colitis
■ Malignant melanoma	Angiodysplasia
■ Bowen's disease	Intussusception
■ Basal cell carcinoma	Ischaemia
	Neoplasia
Rectal causes	■ Adenoma
Angiodysplasmia	■ Carcinoma
Ischaemia	
Infective (e.g. tuberculosis)	**General causes**
Inflammatory (e.g. ulcerative colitis)	Clotting deficiencies
Solitary rectal ulcer syndrome	Anticoagulants
Trauma	Uraemia

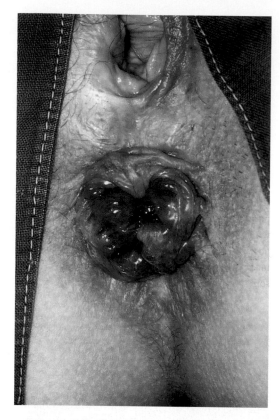

Figure R.1 Third-degree haemorrhoids, or piles. The patient is lying on the operating table in the lithotomy position awaiting haemorrhoidectomy.

there is a history of recent irregularity of bowel function. Profuse mucous discharge in association with bleeding is consistent with a villous adenoma or carcinoma, and a history of bloody diarrhoea is most consistent with a diagnosis of inflammatory bowel disease.

Approximately 80 per cent of rectal neoplasms are within range of digital examination, and a per rectum examination should be conducted in all patients with rectal bleeding. If a lesion is palpated an assessment should be made of its mobility and fixity to surrounding tissues. A highly mobile lesion is indicative of a benign adenoma, whereas any degree of fixity is strongly suggestive of invasion and hence of malignancy. Haemorrhoids, in contrast, are not usually palpable and not tender on palpation in the absence of strangulation. Undue local tenderness suggests the presence of underlying fissure, infection (intersphincteric abscess) or haematoma.

Sigmoidoscopy is an essential step in the exclusion of carcinoma and inflammatory bowel disease, and where there is dispute over the macroscopic appearances then biopsy is mandatory. The presence of oedema, erythema or a shallow discrete ulcer, usually confined to the anterior rectal wall, are features which may be indicative of the solitary rectal ulcer syndrome. This is a benign condition associated with excessive defaecation straining, and can readily be confused with carcinoma on its sigmoidoscopic appearances.

The diagnosis of haemorrhoids largely rests on the appearances at proctoscopy. Most commonly, the right anterior haemorrhoid is noted to be enlarged and congested, and is the putative cause of bleeding since it is rare to see the active bleeding source at the time of the examination.

Patients with a history of blood mixed in with the stool, or where there is a major loss of altered or of venous blood, may require more detailed investigation which will include barium enema and colonoscopy. If angiodysplasia is to be excluded, arteriography may be necessary. Finally, rectal bleeding may be readily confused with bleeding from the upper gastrointestinal tract and small intestine (see MELAENA, p. 429).

For other causes particularly related to disorders in the upper gastrointestinal tract and small intestine, see also MELAENA, p. 429.

Harold Ellis

RECTAL DISCHARGE

The causes of rectal discharge are classified and listed in Table R.2.

Secretion from sweat glands in the perianal area and from the anal glands is a common and normal phenomenon which rarely gives rise to significant problems. Profuse mucous secretion, however, often causes considerable discomfort and pruritus ani as a consequence of inflammation of the perianal skin. Such secretion is commonly observed with *haemorrhoids*, particularly where there is a combination of *prolapse* with a weak internal anal sphincter. More serious *pelvic floor disorders* (e.g. complete prolapse, solitary rectal ulcer syndrome) may be responsible for profuse and sometimes blood-stained mucous secretion which can

Table R.2 Classification of major causes of rectal discharge

Discharge of mucus
Haemorrhoids
Rectal prolapse
Solitary rectal ulcer syndrome
Villous adenoma
Carcinoma rectum
Proctitis

Discharge of pus
Anal fistula
Perianal Crohn's
Anal tuberculosis
Anal neoplasms
Anal fissure
Syphilis
Gonorrhoea
Condyloma accuminata

be incapacitating. *Inflammation* of the rectal mucosa from ulcerative colitis or Crohn's disease of the rectum may similarly produce a mucous discharge which is usually blood-stained and accompanied by diarrhoea.

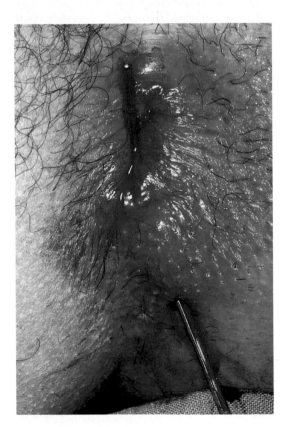

Figure R.2 Fistula-in-ano. The patient is on the operating table in the lithotomy position. Under anaesthetic, a probe has been passed through the external opening of the fistula at the 5 o-clock position, and can be seen to emerge through the internal opening in the midline.

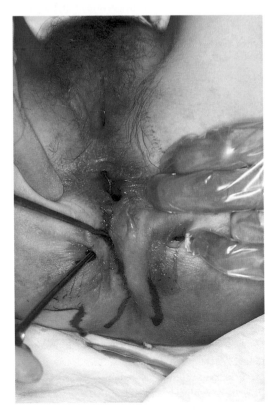

Figure R.3 Multiple fistulae-in-ano in Crohn's disease involving the rectum.

The existence of *neoplasia* should always be suspected, since copious secretion is a particular feature of villous adenomas of the rectum in which the potassium loss may be sufficient to induce hypokalaemia. Carcinoma may also be a cause of mucous secretion, although bleeding is usually a more prominent feature and there may be constitutional symptoms.

A purulent discharge is usually caused by *anal* and *perianal sepsis*. On inspection of the perineum, a small opening discharging pus to the side of the anus is highly suggestive of fistula (Fig. R.2). The diagnosis can be confirmed by palpation and observation at proctoscopy of the internal opening. Ulcerating and purulent perianal lesions should raise the possibility of Crohn's disease (Fig. R.3), anal tuberculosis or sexually transmitted disease (e.g. syphilis, gonorrhoea, HIV infection). Where there is doubt, bacteriological examination of the pus and histological examination of the biopsy from the perianal skin should be performed. Anal neoplasms and condylomata can be responsible for an offensive purulent discharge; the diagnosis is apparent on inspection, but biopsy is always mandatory even if simple condyloma is diagnosed since malignant development can occur with this lesion.

Harold Ellis

RECTAL MASS

Every medical practitioner should be aware of the importance of conducting a digital examination of the anal canal and rectum in all patients with anorectal symptoms, since the majority of rectal neoplasms are well within reach of the examining finger. The relevance of performing a rectal examination as part of a general examination in a patient without rectal symptoms is less clear. Since rectal cancer is a common malignancy in patients aged over 60 years, a strong argument can be made that all patients in this age group should undergo rectal examination as part of any general physical examination. Clearly, if there are urinary symptoms, a digital assessment of the prostate is highly relevant and similarly digital examination of the rectum (and, where relevant, vaginal examination) may be valuable in patients with pelvic or perineal symptoms.

Digital examination of the rectum should be conducted, where possible, with the patient lying in the left lateral position, and should not be attempted until a full inspection of the perineum has been conducted to exclude fissure or other pathology which might give rise to severe pain on palpation. Initially, a digital assessment is made of anal sphincter tone, which may be increased in the presence of fissure and decreased in functional disorders such as anorectal incontinence. Each quadrant of the anus and rectum should be examined sequentially. Within the anus, lesions may extend caudally from the rectum, and vice versa. In the normal state, haemorrhoids are not palpable and no specific structure is palpated until the examining finger reaches the rectum. In women, the cervix frequently projects into the anterior rectal wall and is readily palpable; this is frequently mistaken by an inexperienced clinician for a rectal neoplasm, as may a vaginal tampon! In men, the prostate is easily palpable anteriorly. Laterally, the ischial spines may be palpated, and this may be of value in the location of the pudendal nerves (to provide a pudendal nerve blockade). Posteriorly, the shelf created by the levator ani, and in thin subjects, the bony coccyx may be palpable.

A classification of major causes of rectal masses is provided in Table R.3.

Intrinsic lesions

If a mass is perceived on digital examination, it is not always possible to decide on palpation alone if the lesion is intrinsic or extrinsic. The differentiation may only be possible after sigmoidoscopy and histological examination. The consistency and mobility may closely relate to the diagnosis. Hence, a *benign villous adenoma* (Fig. R.4) will feel soft, fleshy and highly mobile. In contrast, a *carcinoma* (Fig. R.5) may feel hard with obvious fixation of the mucosal lesion to the underlying muscle or perirectal fat. Sometimes, nearby *extrarectal lymph nodes* containing secondary tumour deposits may be palpable.

A circumferential stenosis of the rectum may be seen following *trauma* (e.g. previous surgery) or be a complication of (i) *infection* (e.g. lymphogranuloma); (ii) *inflammation* (e.g. ulcerative colitis); or (iii) *ischaemia*. Digital examination under these circumstances is usually accompanied by marked tenderness and pain. *Anal neoplasms* may extend from the anus and upwards into

Table R.3 Classification of major causes of rectal masses (common causes are indicated by asterisks)

Intrinsic causes	Gynaecological causes
Rectal neoplasia	◆ Carcinoma body uterus*
■ Benign	◆ Carcinoma cervix*
◆ Polyps*	◆ Carcinoma ovary*
◆ Villous adenoma*	◆ Fibroid uterus*
◆ Leiomyoma	◆ Ovarian cyst*
■ Malignant	◆ Pyosalpinx
◆ Carcinoma*	◆ Ectopic gestation
◆ Carcinoid	◆ Endometriosis
◆ Leiomyosarcoma	■ Presacral lesions
◆ Lymphoma	
◆ Melanoma	**Presacral (retrorectal)**
Anal neoplasia	**causes**
■ Benign	■ Congenital
◆ Condylomata*	◆ Epidermoid cyst
◆ Polyps*	◆ Teratoma/carcinoma
■ Malignant	◆ Meningocoele
◆ Adenocarcinoma*	◆ Chordoma
◆ Squamous carcinoma*	■ Causes arising from
◆ Melanoma	bone/cartilage
◆ Bowen's disease	◆ Osteogenic sarcoma
◆ Paget's disease	◆ Ewing's sarcoma
◆ Basal cell carcinoma	◆ Osteochondroma
■ Infection	◆ Myeloma
◆ Lymphogranuloma	Giant-cell tumour
◆ Tuberculosis	■ Neurological causes
	◆ Neurilemmoma
Extrinsic causes	◆ Ependymoma
■ Benign prostatic hypertrophy*	◆ Neuroblastoma
■ Infection	■ Miscellaneous
◆ Pelvic abscess	◆ Lymphoma
◆ Anal fistula with	◆ Lipoma
supralevator extension	◆ Haemangioma
■ Tumour	
◆ Secondary spread to	
pelvis/pouch of Douglas	
◆ Carcinoma prostate*	

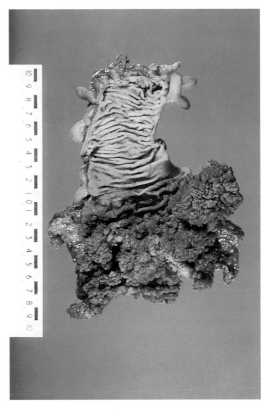

Figure R.4 An extensive villous adenoma of the rectum; operative specimen.

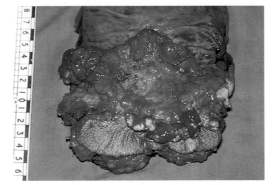

Figure R.5 Adenocarcinoma of the lower rectum invading the anal canal; specimen of abdomino-perineal excision of the rectum.

the rectum, in which case there may be a marked stenosis and the examination will cause pain.

Extrinsic lesions

Rectal examination is a simple clinical means of diagnosing the presence of *pelvic pus* or *pelvic tumour*. A tender mass in the presence of oedematous rectal mucosa suggests a collection of pus, whereas a hard, fixed extrinsic mass in which there is no mobility of the rectal wall or uterus would be strong evidence in favour of pelvic malignancy. Infection may arise secondary to gynaecological or intestinal sepsis, but may be secondary to an anal fistula where pus has tracked superiorly to

create a collection above the levator musculature. Such fistulas are important to recognize since their treatment is complex. *Benign enlargement of the prostate* may give rise to symmetrical hypertrophy of the gland in which the midline sulcus is preserved. *Malignant enlargement* gives rise to a mass which is denser and asymmetrical, and the midline sulcus is invaded.

A mass which is clearly situated posterior to the rectum arises in the potential space ventral to the sacrum and coccyx bounded distally by the levator ani, and proximally by the pelvic peritoneal reflection. The important primary distinction is whether the lesion is solid or cystic; this may require ultrasound examination for confirmation. The majority of solid lesions are *chordomas* and a cystic lesion is usually one of the following: (a) *epidermoid cyst*; (b) *mucus-secreting cyst*; (c) *teratoma*; (d) *teratocarcinoma*; or (e) *meningocele*. Neurogenic and osseous tumours are rare in this region. Clinically, presacral masses usually present with a history of low back pain radiating to the rectum and buttocks. Pressure on the bladder may lead to urinary retention, and constipation is a frequent symptom. On sacral radiographs, presacral lesions may show up as an area of calcification with rarefaction of the sacrum; if there is bony destruction malignancy should always be suspected. A barium enema should always be performed to exclude colonic communication with the mass; and similarly, communication with the subarachnoid space should be excluded by CT or MRI.

Harold Ellis

RECTAL TENESMUS

Rectal tenesmus is a non-specific term employed to describe a state in which there is either difficulty with, or repeated, painful and sometimes *futile* defaecation. A similar condition has been described affecting micturition and is referred to as urinary tenesmus (or strangury). The repeated defaecation is often accompanied by the passage of mucus and/or blood, and this collection of symptoms should be distinguished from the symptom of diarrhoea. In the latter, there is either a complaint of stool of loose consistency or there is increase in frequency but, in contrast to patients with tenesmus, defaecation is usually productive of stool.

As with all rectal symptoms, there may be a sinister underlying cause, and a full clinical assessment – which includes digital examination of the anus/rectum and sigmoidoscopy – is essential.

Inflammatory and infective causes (proctitis)

Proctitis (see RECTAL ULCERATION, p. 619) may be either inflammatory (e.g. ulcerative colitis, Crohn's disease) or infective in origin. The tenesmus may be associated with constitutional symptoms (e.g. malaise, weight loss, anorexia) and with severe diarrhoea. In patients with ulcerative colitis, the bleeding may be substantial, so leading to severe anaemia. The diagnosis is readily made by sigmoidoscopy, biopsy and, where relevant, by stool culture. Less commonly, perianal sepsis (e.g. fistula) can cause tenesmus. The diagnosis is suggested either by the presence of extreme tenderness on digital examination of the anus or by the presence of a sinus/fistula opening in the perianal region.

Neoplastic causes

Benign (e.g. villous adenoma) or malignant lesions of the rectum or anus frequently cause tenesmus. An extensive villous adenoma of the rectum is notorious as a cause of excessive secretion of rectal mucus, which is sufficiently rich in potassium to lead to hypokalaemia. Adenocarcinoma of the rectum may similarly be responsible for the secretion of mucus, but to a lesser degree. Rectal bleeding is a more pronounced feature in the history; the bleeding may be bright or dark red, may be mixed in with the stool, and accompanies defaecation. In the case of advanced malignancy the rectal symptoms may be accompanied by constitutional symptoms, such as weight loss. Squamous carcinoma of the anal margin should be recognizable on simple inspection of the anal verge, and examination of the inguinal region may reveal lymphadenopathy in the presence of metastatic spread to the regional nodes.

Mechanical causes

Tenesmus occasionally results from a poorly understood condition in which the pelvic floor and external anal sphincter musculature fail to relax, or may actively contract during attempted defaecation. Under normal circumstances these muscles relax reflexly to enable easy passage of the faecal bolus through the anal canal. This condition is usually diagnosed only either by conventional electromyography or by defaecography (radiographic imaging of the rectum during defaecation after barium installation), and may be associated with a solitary rectal ulcer as seen on sigmoidoscopy (see RECTAL ULCERATION, p. 619). The cause is usually not known, but occasionally pelvic floor 'spasticity' is identified in patients with multiple sclerosis and the symptom of tenesmus may be the first symptom noted by patients with demyelinating diseases.

Minor anorectal disorders, particularly in an acute presentation (e.g. perianal thrombosis), may cause tenesmus, since the lesion within the anus may cause stimulation of anal sensory receptors at and below the dentate line which gives rise to a false impression that there is faecal matter present within the anus and lower rectum.

Harold Ellis

RECTAL ULCERATION

Normally, a diagnosis of rectal ulceration will be made from the macroscopic appearances of the rectum either at sigmoidoscopy or radiologically at barium enema. Only under certain circumstances (see below) will an ulcer be palpable.

The major causes of rectal ulceration are listed in Table R.4.

Table R.4 Major causes of rectal ulceration

- Inflammatory
  - Ulcerative colitis
  - Crohn's disease
  - Post radiation
- Infective
  - *Shigella*
  - *Salmonella*
  - *Campylobacter*
  - Tuberculosis
  - Gonococcal
  - Amoebiasis
  - Pseudomembranous colitis (*Clostridium difficile*)
  - Lymphogranuloma
  - *Schistosoma*
  - Syphilis
  - Herpes simplex
  - Enterovirus
  - Cytomegalovirus
  - HIV infection
- Solitary rectal ulcer syndrome
- Trauma
- Malignant ulcer
  - Carcinoma
  - Leukaemia
- Ischaemia

The clinical distinction between inflammatory bowel disease and infection can rarely be made on macroscopic appearances alone. Hence, ulcerative colitis or *Shigella* infection may both give rise to: (i) shallow ulceration; (ii) granular appearances; (ii) haemorrhagic friable mucosa; and (iv) oedematous mucosa in the rectum. The presence of pseudopolyps is more closely allied to ulcerative colitis, but these rarely occur in the rectum and are more a feature of colonic disease. Bacterial infections tend to be of more sudden onset and are often associated with severe abdominal pain. Patients with ulcerative colitis develop symptoms usually over a prolonged period, and rarely complain of significant abdominal pain. The presence of multiple, yellowish-white plaques varying in size from a few millimetres to 15–20 mm in diameter may be suggestive of pseudomembranous or antibiotic-associated colitis. The latter condition is now recognized to be a toxin-mediated disease induced by *Clostridium difficile* following exposure to antibiotics. The organism is a component of the normal flora of approximately 30 per cent of healthy adults, but exogenous infection can probably occur as well.

Where ulceration is observed sigmoidoscopically, a portion of mucosa should be biopsied in most instances. Unfortunately, the discrimination between infection and inflammation is not always possible on the microscopic appearances alone, particularly in the early stage of inflammatory disease. The diagnosis in these patients will depend on bacteriology of the stool. If the stool culture is negative for pathogenic flora, the microscopic appearances will be important in the distinction between Crohn's proctitis and ulcerative colitis. The presence of granulomas, fissures, transmural inflammation and an anal lesion would provide strong evidence in favour of Crohn's disease. A non-specific microscopic inflammation may also be a feature of post-irradiation proctitis, and can often only be distinguished by the history alone. The list of infective agents which can give rise to a proctitis is legion; only the more important are listed in Table R.4. If rare organisms are cultured, such as the protozoan cryptosoporidia or viruses (e.g. cytomegalovirus, herpes simplex), the possibility of immune deficiency (e.g. HIV infection, leukaemia) should always be considered.

Ischaemia rarely affects the rectum, but when present it is usually prevalent in older age groups, it is of sudden onset, and is associated with profuse bleeding

Table R.7 Causes of mononeuritis multiplex

Diabetes
Ischaemic neuropathy
Vasculitis
Polyarteritis nodosa
Churg–Strauss syndrome (with asthma/eosinophilia)
Wegener's granulomatosis
Essential mixed cryoglobulinaemia
Rheumatoid arthritis
Lupus
Brachial neuritis
Hepatitis C (with or without cryoglobulinaemia)
HIV
Sarcoidosis
Lyme disease
Sjögren–Sicca syndrome (dorsal root ganglionopathy)
Chronic ataxic neuropathy (idiopathic sensory ganglionopathy)
Migrant polyneuritis of Wartenburg
Coeliac disease

Table R.8 Causes of generalized polyneuropathy

Acute motor paralysis
- Guillain–Barré syndrome
- Diphtheria
- Porphyria

Subacute sensorimotor paralysis
- Vitamin B_{12} deficiency
- Beri-beri
- Alcohol
- Drugs (e.g. isoniazid, chemotherapy (vincristine, cisplatin, etc.), phenytoin, chloramphenicol)
- Heavy metal poisoning (e.g. arsenic, mercury, lead, thallium)

Chronic sensorimotor neuropathies
- Associated with neoplasia: carcinoma, lymphoma, myeloma, paraproteinaemias, others
- Chronic inflammatory demyelinating polyneuropathy (CIDP)
- Amyloid
- Diabetes
- Leprosy

Inherited neuropathies
- Hereditary motor-sensory neuropathy (HSMN) (Charcot–Marie–Tooth)
- Hypertrophic (Dejerine–Sottas disease)
- Hereditary liability to pressure palsies
- Metabolic (Refsum's disease, leukodystrophies, abetalipoproteinaemia)
- Mitochondrial diseases
- Riley–Day syndrome

Spinocerebellar degenerations

of this book. The more important ones are listed in Table R.8. In clinical practice, Guillain–Barré syndrome is the most important cause of an acute sensorimotor polyneuropathy, while diabetes, alcohol and chronic inflammatory demyelinating polyradiculopathy are common causes of a chronic sensorimotor polyneuropathy. Neurophysiological characterization of the neuropathy as predominantly demyelinating (with slowed conduction) or axonal (with reduced sensor and motor action potential amplitudes) can be helpful in narrowing the differential diagnosis. Demyelinating neuropathies include Guillain–Barré syndrome, chronic inflammatory demyelinating polyneuropathy, paraproteinaemic neuropathy and Charcot–Marie–Tooth disease (Type 1).

Disease of the motor or sensory spinal roots

Damage to either the afferent or efferent part of the spinal reflex as a result of root damage is a common cause of loss of a localized tendon reflex. Common causes are cervical and lumbar spondylosis, with or without disc herniation, intraspinal tumours, and brachial or lumbar plexopathy (e.g. from neoplastic infiltration or radiation). Tabes dorsalis produces areflexia due to damage to the posterior nerve roots.

Disease of the spinal cord

Damage within the spinal cord, either within the dorsal root entry zone, between the dorsal root entry zone and the anterior horn cell, or in the anterior horn cell itself,

may produce loss of the tendon reflex. This may occur in intramedullary lesions, such as syringomyelia or intramedullary tumours. A syrinx classically gives dissociated sensory loss (reduced pain and temperature sensation, but preserved joint position and light touch) with reduced reflexes at the involved segmental level, commonly C5–C6. In motor neuron disease there is usually damage to both upper and lower motor neurons, so that the reflexes are pathologically brisk in wasted (denervated) muscles.

David Werring

REGURGITATION

In regurgitation, the patient is aware of food that is passed from the oesophagus into the mouth. There is therefore relaxation of the upper oesophageal sphincter to allow the contents of the oesophagus to enter the mouth. It is important to distinguish between regurgitation, reflux and vomiting. In *vomiting*, the food passes through open lower and upper oesophageal sphincters, and is the consequence of forceful contractions of the abdominal wall and the stomach muscles. *Reflux* is the passage of food from either the duodenum or the stomach into the oesophagus. If the food fails to pass the upper oesophageal sphincter, then the patient is said to be suffering from gastro-oesophageal reflux. If, however, the food passes into the mouth, the term *regurgitation* can be used. Thus, reflux and regurgitation are often used synonymously. While regurgitation can be regarded as a classical symptom of oesophageal disorder, it is not necessarily so, and this is seen to best effect in infants where regurgitation can be a common and normal phenomenon and is related to the passage of gastric contents into the child's mouth.

Patients who complain of regurgitation will often indicate that there is a postural element, with the symptom being most marked by change of position, particularly when bending forward and often on physical exercise. The symptom occurs classically in *achalasia* (or achalasia of the cardia, or cardiospasm). In this motor disorder of the oesophagus there is a reduction in the number of ganglion cells which innervate the oesophageal musculature. This is particularly so in the region of the lower oesophageal sphincter. The patient is usually between 20 and 40 years of age, and classically describes dysphagia, painful swallowing and regurgitation. The regurgitation of food into the mouth at night-time can be associated with inhalation pneumonia and bronchopneumonia. Halitosis may be a symptom. The diagnosis is made manometrically when reduced contractions in the body of the oesophagus will be noted. The resting pressure in the lower oesophageal sphincter is usually elevated and fails to fall, as is normal with swallowing. A poorly contracting, dilated oesophagus will be seen on barium swallow with the non-relaxing lower oesophageal sphincter giving the appearance of a 'beak' on the X-ray. Oesophagoscopy is usually unnecessary, but is useful to exclude the association of a squamous carcinoma of the oesophagus, which is a recognized complication of achalasia.

Gastro-oesophageal reflux is often known as reflux oesophagitis. The two terms are not necessarily synonymous, because reflux into the oesophagus from the stomach is not necessarily associated with inflammation. By definition, in reflux oesophagitis there is the regurgitation of fluid from the stomach into the oesophagus. The cause for the reflux is not always clear.

Reflux is associated with a reduced tone in the lower oesophageal sphincter, which has inappropriate relaxation. In addition to this it has been claimed that the secondary peristaltic clearing mechanisms in the oesophagus are inadequate. In other words, instead of refluxed material being promptly cleared back into the stomach it remains for a longer period than normal in the oesophagus, thereby causing symptoms and possibly inflammation. It is controversial whether in patients with severe reflux there is an element of ineffective clearing of the oesophagus. A reduced lower oesophageal sphincter pressure has been seen following the ingestion of fat and alcohol. Smoking also tends to cause relaxation of the oesophageal sphincter, as do drugs such as morphine, pethidine and diazepam. Carminatives such as coffee will cause a temporary relaxation of the sphincter.

Whether or not a *sliding hiatus hernia* is associated with regurgitation is a much more controversial issue. It is true that regurgitation, gastro-oesophageal reflux and a hiatus hernia may co-exist, but the two conditions can exist independently and many authorities believe that the position of the lower oesophageal sphincter in relation to the diaphragm is irrelevant in the genesis of the symptoms from hiatus hernia. Patients with a sliding hiatus hernia in which the gastro-oesophageal junction lies in the thorax above the diaphragm complain of heartburn, dysphagia and reflux. A small percentage of the patients may actually have a haematemesis. The hiatus hernia may be diagnosed on endoscopy or on a barium swallow and meal.

Evidence of reflux may be obtained by various tests in which the oesophageal pH is measured. There are tests available to measure oesophageal pressures, sphincter function, and the ability of the oesophagus to clear material in its lumen. It must be emphasized, however, that the demonstration of a hiatus hernia is no guarantee that it is the cause of oesophageal reflux or of the symptoms.

A picture very similar to achalasia is produced by *Chagas' disease* due to *Trypanosoma cruzi*, which is encountered in South and Central America. The disease is characterized by a mega-oesophagus, mega-colon and severe cardiac dilatation and dysfunction. It is the cardiac complications of the disease that usually bring the patient to medical attention, but occasionally the oesophageal symptoms may be dominant and they are then identical to that of classic achalasia.

Other motor disorders which may occasionally cause dysphagia include the *collagen vascular disorders* such as *scleroderma*, *diabetes mellitus* and *alcoholic neuropathy*. In these conditions reflux or regurgitation is not a prominent feature, dysphagia or heartburn being more frequently the predominant symptoms.

It is well worth stressing that in many patients who have a complaint of reflux as manifested by heartburn, or occasionally by regurgitation of food into the mouth, no clear aetiological factor can be determined. Tests of oesophageal motor function and 24-hour monitoring of oesophageal pH will very often not demonstrate any evidence of abnormality, despite the patient complaining of quite severe symptoms. These are important considerations in deciding whether or not a patient with the symptoms of regurgitation and who has a hiatus hernia demonstrated should be subjected to surgery.

Mark Kinirons

RUB, PERICARDIAL

A pericardial rub, once identified as such, is pathognomonic of acute pericarditis. A rub has a characteristic 'creaking' or 'leathery' character, but this quality does not certainly differentiate it from a cardiac murmur. A typical rub is virtually continuous throughout the cardiac cycle, but three components have been identified; systolic, early diastolic and, if the patient is in sinus rhythm, late diastolic. If all three components are heard there is little doubt about the diagnosis, but the to-and-fro cadence of the systolic and early diastolic components can sometimes be confused with the murmurs of aortic stenosis and regurgitation. If the rub is heard in systole only – as is often the case when the pericarditis is resolving – it may often be confused with a murmur.

A rub may be heard anywhere over the precordium. It may be markedly influenced by respiration (increasing on lying and reducing on sitting up) and posture, although the changes are not predictable and, to be sure of not missing a rub, it is necessary to auscultate in all phases of deep respiration and with the patient in several postures. Sometimes it may be possible to increase the intensity of a rub by increasing the pressure with which the stethoscope is applied to the chest.

In practice, there is rarely much difficulty in identifying a pericardial rub, but there may occasionally be confusion with the 'scratchy' murmur of Ebstein's anomaly or the late systolic murmur of mitral valve prolapse. When doubt remains, the passage of time will usually resolve the issue as pericardial rubs are evanescent and usually disappear within a few days.

The causes of pericarditis are discussed under CHEST PAIN (p. 101).

Mark Kinirons

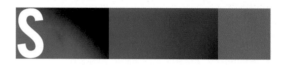

SALIVARY GLANDS, PAIN IN

Pain in one or other of the major salivary glands is associated with enlargement of the affected organ itself (see SALIVARY GLANDS, SWELLING OF, p. 627). For practical purposes, this symptom is confined to the parotid and submandibular salivary glands. Painful enlargement of the sublingual gland is rare; it is occasionally seen as a manifestation of mumps, together with painful enlargement of the other glands, and in the unusual condition of an advanced carcinoma of the gland itself or invasion from adjacent structures. This gland will not be considered further.

The painful salivary swellings may be classified as follows:

- ■ Parotid gland
  - ◆ Mumps (epidemic parotitis)
  - ◆ Acute bacterial suppurative parotitis – postoperative, dehydration, following radiotherapy
  - ◆ Parotitis association with duct obstruction (calculus, trauma)
  - ◆ Carcinoma (primary or spread from another focus)
- ■ Submandibular gland
  - ◆ Mumps (rare)
  - ◆ Inflammation associated with duct obstruction
  - ◆ Carcinoma

Mumps

Mumps (epidemic parotitis) is a viral disease which is transmitted by droplet infection and has an incubation period of 17–21 days. It is the commonest cause of a painful parotid swelling.

Children are most often affected. There is usually prodromal fever with malaise. Only one gland may be involved, or both may be affected simultaneously, or one gland may become enlarged after the other. The swelling progresses for several days with a marked tenderness of the gland and thickening of the overlying skin. There is characteristic uplifting of the lobe of the ear and stiffness of the jaw. Rarely, the submandibular glands may also become swollen, and this may also unusually implicate the sublingual glands.

After 7–10 days, the swelling gradually subsides. There may be an associated acute orchitis, which may be bilateral, and which may proceed to testicular atrophy. A rare complication is pancreatitis.

Acute suppurative parotitis

Acute parotitis as a complication of major surgery is now quite unusual (Fig. S.1); this is because it results from postoperative dehydration in a patient with poor oral hygiene and septic dental stumps. Nowadays, this condition is usually obviated by adequate fluid replacement and by both preoperative and postoperative oral care. Acute parotitis is also occasionally seen as a complication of the severe dehydration in conditions such as typhoid fever and cholera. Radiotherapy to the parotid region may result in damage to the gland, reduction in its secretion and a propensity, therefore, for ascending infection to occur.

On examination, the whole of the gland is enlarged with a tender red swelling of the side of the face. This may progress to overlying cellulitis. Pus can be expressed from the parotid duct on the affected side. Because of the dense overlying fascia, which confines the enlarged gland, pain may be intense. There are the associated features of severe infection with pyrexia and toxaemia.

Parotitis associated with duct obstruction

Obstruction of a salivary duct, from any cause, results in a typical syndrome in which the gland becomes painful and swollen at meal times, due to the increased

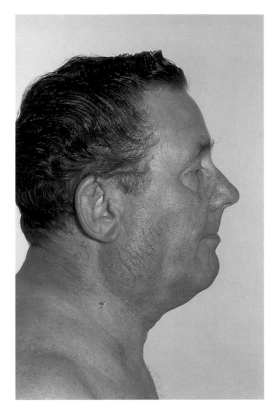

Figure S.1 Acute postoperative right-sided parotitis following gastrectomy for gastric carcinoma.

secretion of saliva being unable to discharge through the duct. Between meals, as the saliva gradually escapes, the swelling and pain subside. Frequently, inflammation of the obstructed gland occurs as a result of ascending infection from mouth organisms. Under these circumstances, there may be the associated features of infection (Fig. S.2) and there may be a discharge of pus from the mouth of the duct.

Although less common than in the submandibular duct, calculi in the parotid duct are not rare. They tend to be smaller and less radio-opaque than in the submandibular duct or gland, so that only larger ones are seen on a plain X-ray of the region. A sialogram may be necessary to identify the stone, which will then be seen as a filling defect.

Other causes of parotid duct stenosis are trauma from the irritation of an adjacent tooth stump or, occasionally, from traumatic division of the duct, for example following a knife laceration of the cheek.

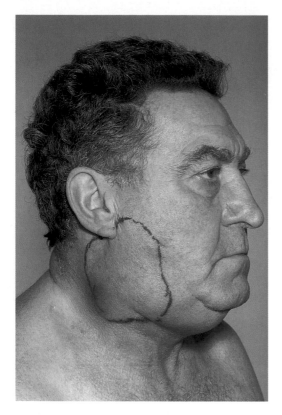

Figure S.2 Parotitis secondary to calculus obstruction. The outline of the gland has been marked with a skin pen. Note that the whole gland is diffusely enlarged, in contrast to a tumour of the gland, which causes localized swelling.

Submandibular calculus

Calculi are the commonest cause of a painful swelling of the submandibular gland, and account for some 95 per cent of all salivary stones. There are several reasons for the comparative frequency of stones in the submandibular gland and its duct. Its secretion contains more mucus than the parotid duct so that it is more viscid. Its duct is longer and slopes upwards from the gland so that there is more tendency for a small concretion to remain within the duct. Furthermore, its orifice, being on the floor of the mouth, is more exposed to trauma than that of the parotid duct. The aetiology of these stones remains the subject of debate. Their size varies from minute to the size and shape of a date stone. Numbers vary; there may be a single stone in the duct or the gland itself may contain numerous stones throughout a dilated duct system (sialectasia).

The classical story of a swelling and pain associated with food is elicited in the history. The gland itself can be felt as a tender enlargement on bimanual palpation with one finger below the angle of the jaw and the other in the sulcus between the tongue and the mandible. Occasionally, a calculus can be seen to extrude through the duct orifice at the side of the base of the fraenulum linguae. At other times it may be palpated along the course of the duct in the floor of the mouth or stones may be felt in the gland itself. Pus may be expressed from the duct orifice by pressure on the gland.

Submandibular calculi are nearly all radio-opaque and can be visualized on a plain X-ray of the floor of the mouth (Fig. S.3).

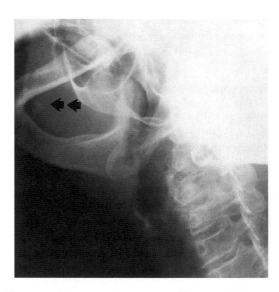

Figure S.3 Radio-opaque submandibular salivary calculus (arrowed).

Carcinoma of the salivary glands

In its late stages, a carcinoma of the salivary gland (commonest in the parotid, less often seen in the submandibular gland and rare in the sublingual gland and the accessory salivary glands) will invade adjacent tissues and produce severe pain. Invasion of a salivary gland from an adjacent tumour, for example a carcinoma of the floor of the mouth, a squamous carcinoma of the overlying skin or a malignant melanoma, will be associated with intense pain.

Harold Ellis

SALIVARY GLANDS, SWELLING OF

The salivary glands are subject to swelling due to inflammation and new growth in the same way as any other organ. In common with other externally secreting glands, they are also subject to swelling resulting from retention of secretion. This most commonly occurs as a result of blockage of a duct by a stone. Parotid swelling with fever, often with lacrimal adenitis and uveitis (Mikulicz's syndrome), may occur in leukaemia, Hodgkin's disease, tuberculosis, systemic lupus erythematosus and sarcoidosis. Confusion in diagnosis may result from the close proximity of the lymph nodes; in the case of the submandibular gland, the lymph nodes may be right in the centre of the salivary tissue. The different salivary glands do not exhibit the same liability to each lesion, the submandibular for instance being the most liable to calculus formation, while inflammatory lesions are only common in the parotid. Mumps is the commonest cause of all parotid swellings; it may occasionally involve glands other than the parotid, but this is a rare exception and usually occurs only after the parotid is first attacked. Here, as in all diagnosis, it is important to decide the exact anatomical site of the lesion before considering its pathology. For example, swelling of the loose tissues over the jaw from alveolar inflammation may mimic parotitis. A useful point in this connection is that a generalized parotid swelling tends to lift the auricle away from the head and inspection of the orifice of Stensen's duct within the mouth will usually reveal some abnormality (Fig. S.4). If lymph nodes are suspected as a site of swellings, the presence of other enlarged nodes and of a primary lesion should be sought.

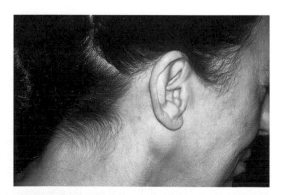

Figure S.4 Mixed parotid tumour (pleomorphic adenoma).

Sialography may prove helpful. Radio-opaque contrast is injected into the appropriate orifice (Wharton's submandibular or Stensen's parotid; the lingual ducts are not suitable for injection). The branching system of ducts is well visualized in the radiograph. Blockage by a stone or by growth, sialectasia (dilatation and beading of the duct system, especially in the parotid gland) or the presence of a fistula is the lesion most likely to be demonstrated in this way. The lesions of the salivary glands are summarized in Table S.1.

Salivary tumours can be classified as:

- Benign
  - Pleomorphic adenoma ('mixed tumour')
  - Adenolymphoma (Warthin's tumour)
- Malignant
  - Primary – carcinoma
  - Secondary
    - Invasion from overlying skin (e.g. malignant melanoma)
    - Secondarily involved lymph nodes.

Some 90 per cent of the *pleomorphic adenomata* (Fig. S.5) occur in the parotid, although occasionally the lesion is found in the submandibular gland and, rarely, in the sublingual and accessory salivary glands. Likewise, 90 per cent are present before the age of 50 years, and the gender distribution is equal.

Characteristically, the tumour arises as a lobulated firm mass, noticed first when about the size of a cherry, and of variable consistency. The lump is painless and is typically situated between the ascending ramus of the mandible and the mastoid process, although no part of the parotid is exempt from this change and these tumours may be found as low as 2.5 cm (1 inch) below the angle of the mandible. A frequent history is that the lump, over a period of years, shows a progressive slow increase in size.

Adenolymphoma accounts for about 10 per cent of parotid tumours, and is very rare elsewhere. It usually occurs in men over the age of 50 years, and may be bilateral. The tumour feels soft and cystic.

Carcinoma again usually affects the parotid, but may occur rarely in the other main, and accessory, salivary glands. Usually the patient is over the age of 50 years. Clinically, the diagnosis is based on rapid growth, pain, involvement of the facial nerve (in the case of the parotid) and of the regional nodes. Eventually, the surrounding tissues are infiltrated and the overlying skin becomes ulcerated.

Table S.1 Lesions of the salivary glands

Salivary gland	Acute unilateral enlargement	Acute bilateral enlargement	Chronic unilateral enlargement	Chronic bilateral enlargement
Parotid	Non-specific infective Parotitis (rarely bilateral)	Mumps. (One side usually appears first, second commonly appears 24–36 hours later, but occasionally up to 4–5 days later)	(1) Progressive growth or inflammation. May involve part of gland only; differentiate from preauricular adenitis by searching area drained, etc. (2) Intermittent – sialectasia (calculus uncommon)	Sarcoidosis
	Both of these show signs of inflammation with much pain. In both, orifice of Stensen's duct is red and pouting.			
Submandibular	As for parotid, but both very rare. N.B. Inflammation of submandibular lymphatic nodes common.		(1) Progressive – growth (rare) (2) Intermittent – stone. Swelling occurs at mealtimes when the flow of saliva is stimulated, but the gland is permanently swollen when condition is of long standing. Stone may be palpable in duct and will show on X-ray. Orifice of duct inflamed.	
Sublingual	Uncommon. Ranula was originally thought to be due to retention of secretion in this gland, but retention in adjacent simple mucous glands is the more probable explanation.			
All glands	Mikulicz's syndrome – characterized by chronic painless swelling of all the salivary glands and the lacrimals. This occurs in Hodgkin's disease, tuberculosis, leukaemia, sarcoidosis and systemic lupus erythematosus.			

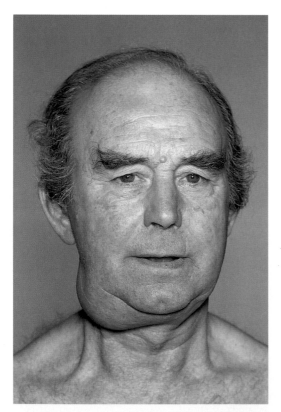

Figure S.5 Pleomorphic adenoma of the right submandibular gland.

Sarcoidosis

In sarcoidosis, asymptomatic enlargement of the parotid, sublingual and submandibular glands occurs in about 6 per cent of cases. Spontaneous resolution often occurs. The glands are not tender. Facial palsy may occur with parotid enlargement. The syndrome of fever, uveitis and lacrimal and salivary gland enlargement is known as 'uveoparotid' fever.

Harold Ellis

SCALP AND BEARD, FUNGUS AFFECTIONS OF

Tinea capitis

Scalp ringworm (tinea capitis) is a fungal infection of the scalp, and predominantly a disease of childhood. It is contracted by direct contact. The infection may be caused by a number of species of fungus; some such as *Trichophyton violaceum* and *Microsporum audouini* are anthropophilic, and may thus be spread from child to child, including through fomites such as school caps or hair brushes. Other species, such as

Microsporum canis, are zoophilic and are usually acquired by contact with animals, especially household pets. *Trichophyton verrucosum*, the causative organism of cattle ringworm, may cause a particularly violent inflammatory infection in children, and should be suspected if there is a history of contact with cows. In some cases of scalp ringworm the inflammatory reaction is so marked as to produce a boggy discharging mass, termed a 'kerion', and is usually associated with local lymphadenopathy.

In cases of scalp ringworm, the hair follicles are first infected, causing small, red, scaly patches in which hairs break off short, rather like down-trodden

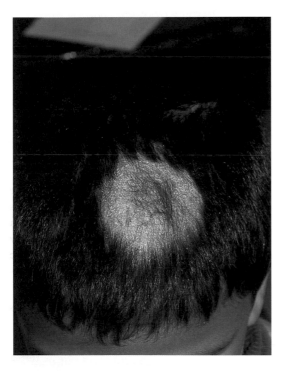

Figure S.6 Tinea capitis (scalp ringworm).

stubble (Fig. S.6). Lesions may remain solitary or be multiple. Itching may or may not be present, and the degree of scaliness varies from a fine branny desquamation to heaped-up masses of soft scale. Diagnosis is confirmed by microscopic examination of a few stumps that have been soaked in 10 per cent potassium hydroxide, but specimens should also be sent for laboratory culture, because identifying the species of fungus is important in determining the likely source. Scalp examination using an ultraviolet lamp (Wood's light) can be most helpful, especially in screening groups of patients, as infections with small-spored fungi cause green fluorescence (Table S.2).

Tinea capitis must be differentiated from *seborrhoeic dermatitis*, where there may be diffuse fine scaling but no broken-off hairs. In scalp *psoriasis* there are well-demarcated areas of scale heaped over red plaques through which the hairs grow undisturbed. In *alopecia areata* there are one or more sharply demarcated bald areas entirely devoid of scaling or inflammation.

Tinea faciei

Ringworm on the face is likewise usually seen in children as the result of exposure to an animal harbouring a zoophilic species of fungus.

Tinea barbae

Ringworm of the beard area is largely a disease of the adult male, and confined almost exclusively to agricultural workers who contract the disease from infected animals. It may take the form of superficial patches with folliculitis, or more usually a deep suppurative type (*kerion*) (Fig. S.7). *Trichophyton verrucosum* (cattle) and *Trichophyton mentagrophytes* (hedgehogs) are responsible for the majority of cases. Anthropophilic

Table S.2 Fungus infections of scalp or beard

		Fluorescence with Wood's light	Clinical features	Usual geographical location
Small-spored	M. audounini	+	Scaling bald patches	Canada, USA, Nigeria
	M. canis	+	Inflammatory scalp ringworm	Worldwide
	T. violaceum	−	Black dot fungi	S. America, E. Europe, Far and Middle East
Large-spored	T. schoenleinii	−	Favus with scutuli	Iran, Iraq, Pakistan, Greenland
	T. tonsurans	−	Scaling bald patches. Occasionally kerion	Worldwide

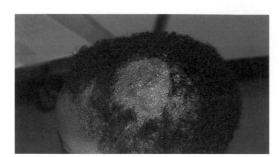

Figure S.7 Kerion (inflammatory ringworm).

species are occasionally causes, and *Microsporum canis* can affect eyebrows and eyelashes.

Barry Monk

SCALY ERUPTIONS

Scales are dried-up thin plates of keratinized epithelial cells which occur as a result of an alteration of the normal keratinization process. Normally, as the epithelial cells become slowly impregnated with keratin, their nuclei are lost; eventually, they desquamate invisibly from the surface and are responsible for the majority of house dust. When the process is abnormally speeded up, keratinized cells may reach the surface of the skin before losing their nuclei and adhere together in abnormal clumps; these appear white or silvery rather than translucent, and are shed as visible scales. This can occur in many chronic inflammatory conditions of the epidermis, particularly psoriasis. When the rate of epithelial turnover is markedly slowed (e.g. in myxoedema, severe malnutrition or ichthyosis), keratinized cells may accumulate abnormally at the skin surface, which again loses its translucency and is shed in large abnormal pieces.

Ichthyosis is an inherited disorder in which there is a generalized scaling of the skin without associated inflammation. *Acquired ichthyosis* should raise the suspicion of an underlying malignancy.

The major causes of scaly skin conditions are listed in Table S.3.

Red scaly lesions

Psoriasis is a common disorder of keratinization, which may start at any age. It presents with sharply

Table S.3 Scaly eruptions

Red scaly rash
Psoriasis
Eczema
■ Discoid, lichen simplex chronicus, atopic eczema, contact dermatitis, seborrhoeic
Dermatophyte infection
Pityriasis rosea
Pityriasis lichenoides chronica
Parapsoriasis
Mycosis fungoides (cutaneous T-cell lymphoma)
Secondary syphilis

Scaly papules
Guttate psoriasis
Pityriasis lichenoides chronica
Darier's disease

Scaling without erythema
Ichthyosis
Tinea versicolor

Erythroderma
Eczema
Psoriasis
Pityriasis rubra pilaris
Drug reaction
Sézary syndrome
Lymphoma

demarcated thickened red plaques, surmounted by an easily detachable silvery scale (Figs S.8 and S.9). When affected areas are rubbed, punctate haemorrhage may be noted on the affected surface. In flexural areas, scaling may be absent, but there is a sharply demarcated glazed erythema. All areas of the body – from the top of the scalp to the soles of the feet – may be affected, but there is a predisposition to extensor surfaces and sites of friction. Lesions may localize in sites of injury to the skin, such as cat scratches or surgical wounds (Koebner phenomenon). The scalp is commonly affected, but hair loss is uncommon. The extent of the eruption may vary from the inconsequential to whole body involvement. When very extensive, systemic disturbance may arise through excessive vasodilatation of the skin. The nails are involved in about 50 per cent of cases, and there may be an associated arthropathy. Psoriatic plaques may go into spontaneous remission, and when they do so, they commonly clear from the centre, leaving an annular patter.

In psoriasis, the lesions are generally multiple, and the presence of a solitary lesion of psoriasis should cause one to question the diagnosis. There may in fact

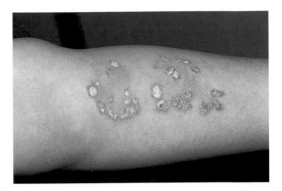

Figure S.8 Psoriasis.

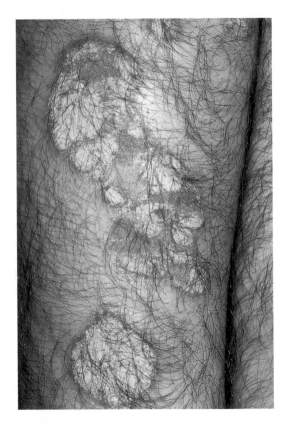

Figure S.9 Psoriasis.

be lesions in occult sites such as the scalp or ears, but if truly solitary the possibility of Bowen's disease or a superficial basal cell carcinoma should be considered. *Keratoderma blenorrhagica* is a cutaneous reaction pattern comprising thickly scaled, red plaques often in bizarre shapes and occurring chiefly on soles,

palms and genitalia. The lesions have a great similarity to psoriasis, but follow urethritis and are accompanied by uveitis, fever, arthralgia and sacroiliitis. This symptom complex is called Reiter's syndrome, and many authorities believe that it occurs only in those with the psoriatic genotype. Another distinctive variant is *guttate psoriasis*, in which a streptococcal infection is followed by the sudden onset of a profuse eruption of tiny psoriatic lesions The condition must be differentiated from *pityriasis lichenoides chronica*, which affects an older age group, does not follow a streptococcal sore throat, and where individual papules are covered by a single translucent 'mica' scale which detaches *en masse*. The lesions are also less numerous and in varying stages of evolution at different sites.

Chronic eczema may also manifest itself with multiple red scaly plaques. In *discoid (nummular) eczema*, there are multiple, intensely itchy coin-shaped lesions scattered randomly over the trunk and limbs. This form of eczema is most commonly seen in middle-aged men, and is commonly provoked by stress. Eczematous lesions are markedly less sharply demarcated than those in psoriasis, and the scales usually finer and more adherent.

Eczema is not, of course, a diagnosis, but rather a pattern of reaction which may arise from a number of causes such as contact allergy, chronic exposure to irritants, photosensitivity, or endogenous factors. The pattern of the eruption may give a clue to the cause; for example, a localized area of eczema under a wristwatch may be caused by nickel sensitivity. In any case of unexplained eczema, investigation by patch testing should be undertaken if possible.

Seborrhoeic dermatitis is a distinctive pattern of endogenous eczema in which rather greasy superficial scales arise on a background of erythema; typically, the eruption is symmetrical, and affects the scalp, eyebrows, nasolabial folds and presternum. *Intertrigo* is a term used to describe any flexural rash, especially of the submammary folds and groins; many cases are due to seborrhoeic dermatitis, sometimes with superimposed candidiasis.

As with psoriasis, the possibility of a solitary scaly patch of eczema should be regarded with some suspicion, as this may in fact be a presentation of Bowen's disease or superficial basal cell carcinoma. However, one exception to this rule is provided by *lichen simplex chronicus*; this is a form of neurodermatitis caused by habitual scratching, and presents with a thickened scaly plaque in which the skin markings are accentuated. The ankle is a common site in males, and the nape of the neck in women.

In *pityriasis rosea*, an acute eruption of unknown cause, the onset is often marked by the development of a solitary scaly oval lesion on the trunk (the herald patch), followed some days later by a widespread eruption of scaly ovoid lesions over the bathing trunk area. The degree of pruritus is very variable, and the rash resolves in 6–8 weeks. Inspection of individual oval lesions reveals the scale to be concentrated in a collarette just inside the edge. If lesions extend to palms and soles and are accompanied by malaise, lymphadenopathy, fever and a sore throat, then *secondary syphilis* should be suspected. The plaques are less pink and more of a ham colour. There is often patchy alopecia, 'snail-track' ulceration of the oral mucosa, the serology will be positive, and a primary chancre may still be present.

Pityriasis versicolor is a common superficial yeast infection which is generally seen in young adults (Fig. S.10). The individual lesions are symmetrically arranged over the neck and upper trunk, and are composed of flat oval macules with a slight scale and minimal inflammatory reaction. Microscopy of the skin scrapings will reveal the causative organisms.

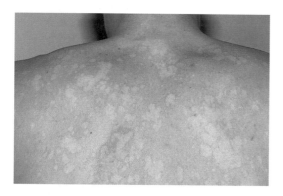

Figure S.10 Pityriasis versicolor.

Dermatophyte infection can cause isolated red scaly plaques, usually with a central clearing and a raised red edge with an advancing scaly border; zoophilic fungi show considerable inflammation and rapidly expanding rings, anthropophilic species being more indolent (Fig. S.11).

Mycosis fungoides (cutaneous T-cell lymphoma) generally presents with a slowly progressing rash which may in places resemble eczema, and in others psoriasis. It is distinguished from both by its characteristically

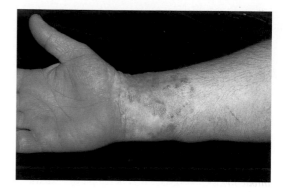

Figure S.11 Tinea incognito (fungal infection spread by use of topical corticosteroids).

bizarre arcuate patterning, sometimes with islands of sparing. There may be rather variable erythema and scaling and a notable lack of response to topical therapy. Over the course of many years the lesions extend, become more indurated, and may ultimately progress to tumours and systemic dissemination. Occasionally, cases present with tumours from the outset (*tumour d'emble*).

Scaly palms

A unilateral scaly palm is the hallmark of *tinea manuum*. The colour is of a dull, lustreless greyish red, and the scaling is fine and concentrated in skin creases. There may be associated fungal onychodystrophy of one or many fingernails, and signs of tinea elsewhere on the body. The condition is often of very long standing. Bilateral scaly symmetrical palms can be inherited as a familial trait in the extremely rare *tylosis palmaris*. The hyperkeratosis is tightly packed and yellowish in colour. Similar yellowish, thick hyperkeratosis of palms is seen in *pityriasis rubra pilaris*, an uncommon condition which may be seen at all ages and accompanied by a widespread psoriasiform rash with follicular accentuation.

Scaly scalp

The scalp is one of the sites of election of *psoriasis*, where well-demarcated plaques of thick scale cause surprisingly little disturbance of hair growth. The shedding of large amounts of silvery scales from these lesions is often a source of great embarrassment for patients. *Seborrhoeic dermatitis* causes a more confluent scaly eruption, and the scales are greasier and more adherent. Corroborative evidence should be sought of seborrhoeic dermatitis in the classic areas elsewhere on the skin. *Tinea capitis* usually causes asymmetrical scaling eruptions of the scalp. The hairs are usually broken off close to the surface, giving a stubbled appearance.

Scaling of whole skin surface

Inflammatory skin conditions can, on occasion, affect the whole skin surface causing an erythroderma; when large amounts of scale are shed, the term *exfoliative erythroderma* is applied. This may develop from extension of a previously diagnosed skin condition (e.g. psoriasis), or present in this manner when the diagnosis may be more difficult to establish. Possible causes include drug allergy (e.g. gold, antimalarials, sulphonamides), severe contact dermatitis, atopic dermatitis, seborrhoeic dermatitis, psoriasis, underlying lymphoma and the Sézary syndrome (the erythrodermic stage of mycosis fungoides). Erythroderma is often associated with significant constitutional upset, with difficulty of thermoregulation and loss of fluid and protein. It has a significant mortality.

Barry Monk

SCIATICA

See LOWER LIMB, PAIN IN (p. 378).

SCOLIOSIS

See SPINE, DEFORMITY OF (p. 659).

SCROTUM, SURFACE AFFECTIONS OF

The skin of the scrotum may be affected as part of a generalized eruption, such as seborrhoeic dermatitis or psoriasis. It may be the only area affected, and skin disorders in this site may be influenced by the local environment – heat, humidity and mobility of the part, local friction, and the thinness of the scrotal skin. In a bed-ridden patient, it may be irritated by urine or faeces, or the drugs they may contain

Table S.4 Surface affections of the scrotum

- Generalized eruptions affecting scrotal skin
  - ◆ Examples: drug eruptions, exanthema, exfoliative dermatitis
- Eruptions confined to the scrotum
  - ◆ Rashes
    - Irritant dermatitis
    - Seborrhoeic dermatitis
    - Tinea cruris
    - Erythrasma
    - Psoriasis
    - Syphilis
  - ◆ Malignancies
    - Bowen's disease,
    - Basal cell carcinoma
    - Extramammary Paget's disease
  - ◆ Ulcers
    - Behçet's syndrome
    - Herpes simplex
  - ◆ Papules/nodules
    - Angiokeratomas of Fordyce
    - Scabies (post scabetic nodules)
    - Hidradenitis suppurativa
  - ◆ Erosions
    - Herpes simplex
    - Fixed drug eruption
  - ◆ Thickening
    - Lichen simplex

(e.g. danthron breakdown products); an analogous situation may arise in infants allowed to stay in soiled nappies (ammoniacal dermatitis). Acute dermatitis and intertrigo are common on scrotal skin (see Table S.4).

Acute dermatitis of the scrotum frequently follows over-treatment; the thin skin is particularly sensitive to medicaments such as those used in the treatment of pediculosis pubis or tinea cruris. Topical steroids penetrate the scrotal skin more readily than other sites, and this may lead to atrophy, and increased sensitivity of the scrotal skin. *Seborrhoeic dermatitis* may affect the scrotum and be confused with candida (Fig. S.12), or

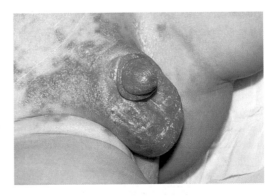

Figure S.12 Candidiasis.

with *tinea*. The latter nearly always affects the neighbouring groin skin, has a well-defined wavy edge, and shows mycelia when the scales are examined under the microscope. Moreover, patches of white macerated or scaly skin produced by the same fungus can often be found elsewhere (e.g. between the toes). It is when a seborrhoeic dermatitis of the scrotum and groin is mistakenly treated for tinea (e.g. with Whitfield's ointment) that a particularly acute and painful dermatitis can occur.

Erythrasma occurs as a discoid plaque of a beefy, brownish-red colour covered with fine scales; unlike tinea, there is no central healing and the plaques are uniform in appearance. They fluoresce pink under Wood's light, and culture reveals the causative *Corynebacterium minutissimi*. Plaques of *psoriasis* can affect the scrotum, especially in flexural psoriasis. Scaling is less prominent at this site, but plaques will have the typical well-defined edge and salmon pink colour. There should be evidence of psoriasis elsewhere on the body (e.g. elbows, knees, sacrum and scalp).

Syphilis gives rise to moist papules or serpiginous, erythematous patches and ulcers; however, in contrast with dermatitis, the whole of the scrotal skin is not affected, itching is absent and the serology will be positive. Hard and soft chancres may affect the scrotum as well as other parts of the genitals; the differential diagnosis is discussed under SCROTUM, ULCERATION OF (below).

Boils, warts, sebaceous cysts and tumours are referred to under TESTICULAR SWELLING (p. 702). Some scrotal neoplasms may cause non-healing erosive and ulcerating lesions; examples include *Bowen's disease*, *basal cell carcinoma* and rarely *extramammary Paget's disease*. Moles and malignant melanomas can also occur on scrotal skin.

Ulceration of the scrotum may be a feature of *Behçet's syndrome*, the features of which are recurrent orogenital ulceration, together with iritis, keratitis, diffuse pustulation, polyarthritis, thrombophlebitis, and sometimes neural infarcts.

Small angiomas are very common on the scrotum in elderly persons, and are known as *angiokeratomas of Fordyce*. Small nodules on the scrotum and penis are characteristic of *scabies*. Discharging nodular lesions on the scrotum, spreading into the groins and often affecting the axillae, are seen in *hidradenitis suppurativa*.

Recurrent erosions in the same site can be caused by both *herpes simplex* and *fixed drug eruptions*. In the former case, multiple vesicles and minimal scarring will be seen. In the latter case, considerable post-inflammatory hyper-pigmentation is the rule, and a carefully taken drug history will usually reveal the culprit (e.g. codeine, laxatives, sulphonamides).

In *lichen simplex chronicus*, the habit of regular rubbing and scratching leads to considerable thickening and lichenification of the skin; this is common in peri-anal skin, but it also occurs on the scrotum.

Barry Monk

SCROTUM, ULCERATION OF

Ulceration of the scrotum occurs in association with:

- Underlying disease of testis
  - ◆ inflammatory
  - ◆ tuberculous
  - ◆ syphilitic
  - ◆ neoplasm
- Fistula
- Syphilis involving the scrotum
- Suppurating cutaneous cysts
- Infected haematocele
- Cutaneous neoplasms
- Behçet's syndrome, herpes simplex, candidiasis.

Underlying disease of the testis

In some cases, extension of disease in the testicle may involve the coverings of the scrotum, and may even perforate them to form a scrotal sore. This sequence occasionally occurs with:

- Testicular abscess
- Tuberculosis of the epididymis
- Gumma of the testis
- Malignant disease of the testis.

A testicular abscess is somewhat uncommon, but may arise from direct extension from the urethra via the vesiculae seminales and vasa deferentia, or by a haematogenous infection during the course of a specific fever, such as scarlet fever, mumps or typhoid fever. With urethral disease, the primary problem may be due to gonorrhoea, or more frequently to a septic urethritis from the introduction of infected instruments. In cases in which the infective process extends from the urethra, the epididymis is affected first, whilst in the metastatic cases the body of the tesis usually shows the first sign of enlargement.

On occasion, following vasectomy for sterilization, the swelling and possible abscess will occur in the upper part of the scrotum at the site of the division. The acute inflammations of the testis occasionally suppurate, when the scrotal tunics become inflamed and adherent, whilst softening occurs later. Unless surgically relieved, the abscess opens through the skin, leaving an ulcer, and a sinus discharging pus. An unusual form of abscess of the testicle is caused by a suppurating dermoid cyst of the testicle, and this may discharge through the scrotal coverings to form an ulcer.

Tuberculosis of the testis rarely occurs as a primary disease but more often as a secondary deposit in association with tuberculosis elsewhere in the genito-urinary tract. Testicular tubercle almost always begins as a nodule in the epididymis, but in the later progress of the disease may extend into the testis proper. If the tuberculous nodule progresses rather than under-goes cure, the scrotal skin becomes adherent, thinned and finally perforated, leaving a shallow ulcer with thin, undermined edges and discharging thin pus. The ulcer in this case is most likely to be on the posterior aspect of the scrotum. Occasionally, the necrotic epi-didymis fungates through the opening in the scro-tum, appearing as a greyish, sloughy projection from the cutaneous opening – the so-called 'hernia testis'.

A gumma of the testis (once common, now very rare), causes a swelling in the body of the testis rather than in the epididymis. A gumma which remains unrecognized or untreated may soften and ulcerate through the scrotal skin in a manner similar to tuber-culous disease, leaving a clearly defined ulcerated area with sharply cut margins and a wash-leather-like, sloughy base. Such ulcers are usually placed on the front of the scrotum. The gummatous granulation tissue may fungate through the scrotal aperture, forming a yellowish necrotic mass.

The diagnosis of these three conditions may pro-duce some difficulty in the earlier stages (see TES-TICULAR SWELLING, p. 702), but in the advanced stage now under consideration, when an open scrotal sore is present, the diagnosis is easier.

The opening of a testicular abscess on the scrotum leaves a small sinus discharging pus and accompanied by a general enlargement of the organ. Preceding the rupture of the abscess there is acute pain in the testicle,

with a rise in temperature, rigors and general signs of suppuration, though these are much diminished as soon as the abscess bursts or is incised. There is often a urethral discharge, but this is frequently much lessened with the onset of acute epididymitis, with distinct thickening of the cord and aching pain in the neigh-bourhood of the external abdominal ring. In metastatic cases the abscess occurs during the progress of an acute fever. The general history is one of acute pain beginning in the testicle, with rapid and extremely tender swelling of the organ, followed by abscess formation.

In tuberculosis of the epididymis the progress is much more gradual. A nodule may have been present in the epididymis for some time, gradually enlarging, but causing very little pain. In some cases a nodule may have been present for months without any apparent change, and then it may enlarge rapidly, involve the scrotal tunics, and discharge its contents. By the time the disease has reached this stage it is probable that evidence of tuberculosis will be found in other organs, particularly the other testicle, prostate, seminal ves-icles or bladder. The affected testicle usually presents several nodules in the epididymis and is tender on pressure, whilst small nodules may also be felt in the vas deferens.

The opening remaining from the discharge of a gummatous orchitis is usually a rounded ulcer with sharply cut edges and yellowish base. The whole testis is enlarged and practically painless. The cord is not thickened, and there is no evidence of disease in the other testicle, prostate or seminal vesicles. There is prob-ably a history of syphilis, and other tertiary syphilitic lesions may be present elsewhere, such as gummatous periostitis.

A hernial protrusion of nectrotic testicular tissue may be present either with tuberculous disease or from a gumma. In tuberculosis, the mass is greyish and necrotic, discharging thin pus, and there will be evi-dence of tuberculous disease in the underlying testis and other genital organs. Very rarely, tubercle bacilli may be found in the discharge. A distinctive feature of the gum-matous hernia testis is found in the appearance of the cutaneous opening; if the fungating mass is pushed aside, the opening in the scrotal skin will be seen to be cleanly cut and to encircle the protruding tissue tightly. The fungating hernia testis of tubercle or syphilis must also be diagnosed from other conditions producing a raised tumour on the scrotum. An epithelioma of the scrotum has raised borders, but the centre is excavated, and there is rarely any enlargement of the testis. A sloughing papilloma of the scrotum may more nearly reproduce the appearance, but the tumour and the skin are freely movable on the underlying testis, while in hernia testis the mass is connected with the testicle, and the tubular structure of the latter is often apparent on picking up a small fragment of the fungating tumour.

Neoplasms of the testis seldom cause ulceration of the scrotum because they have generally been removed surgically before such a late stage is reached. Any variety, however – whether seminoma or teratoma – may cause local recurrence in the scar, with ulceration. The diagnosis depends upon histological examination, either of the tumour previously removed or of a biopsy from the edge of the recurrence. Occasionally, fungation of the tumour is seen through the scar of the biopsy site in the scrotal skin when there has been delay in carrying out definitive treatment, though this state of affairs should never be allowed to happen.

Fistula

Fistulas may occur in the scrotum and cause ulceration. Sinuses occur in association with tuberculosis or syphilitic disease of the testes, but fistulas may follow urine extravasation, or burrowing from rectal suppuration. An abscess may form and open through the scrotal skin from a peri-urethral abscess accompanying an acute urethritis or formed by septic infection behind a urethral stricture. In either case, a small amount of urine may leak through the opening during micturition whilst the history of the urethral discharge, or of difficulty in micturition and other symptoms of stricture, will point to the diagnosis.

Syphilis involving the scrotum

This may be present either as a primary chancre or as a mucous tubercle. A primary chancre in this situation is by no means easy to recognize unless other signs of syphilis are present. However, the presence of a cutaneous sore which does not show much inclination to heal under antiseptic dressings should always give a suspicion of syphilis. There is often only slight induration of the ulcer compared with that of a penile chancre, but the edge is raised and of a rolled appearance. The inguinal lymph nodes are enlarged and discrete, but it is some 5–6 weeks after the commencement of the ulcer that the usual secondary symptoms of syphilis become manifest.

Mucous tubercles of secondary syphilis may be present on the scrotum, usually on the lateral aspect. They may extend directly from the anal area. No difficulty will be met with in the diagnosis, as other signs of syphilis are obvious and the specific serological tests are positive.

Suppurating cutaneous cysts

A sebaceous cyst in the scrotal skin may suppurate and leave an open sore. The areas remaining present raised borders, and are easily mistaken for an early epithelioma. An accurate history of the previous swelling in the skin is of little assistance in these cases, but microscopical examination of a piece removed from the margin of the ulcer will exclude malignancy. A suppurating cyst in the scrotum is less common than epithelioma.

Infected haematocele

A haematocele which becomes infected may form an abscess that bursts through the scrotal coverings. It may have a superficial resemblance to a gumma.

Cutaneous neoplasms

Carcinoma of the scrotum, formerly known as 'chimney-sweep's cancer' or 'tar-worker's cancer', is by no means limited to these occupations, but is certainly more common in men engaged in work in which they are exposed to much irritation from solid particles or from noxious fumes. Hence the disease is, or was, most commonly seen amongst chimney sweeps, employees in gas works, paraffin, tar and chemical works, and coalmines and in spinners in the cotton trade. It often begins as a small subcutaneous nodule, over which the skin is thinned and adherent. The nodule enlarges slowly, and the thinned covering gives way to form an ulcer with thickened irregular edges and a tendency to bleed on slight injury. The ulcerated area extends both radially and into the tissues of the scrotum, later involving the testes. The inguinal nodes become enlarged soon after active ulceration begins, at first from inflammatory causes, but later from malignant infiltration. If left untreated, these nodes will ulcerate, and indeed the common mode of death in this condition is from repeated haemorrhages. In other cases a scrotal epithelioma begins in a wart or papilloma, which may have been present for years with only slight increase in growth (Fig. S.13). These soft papillomas are not unusually the starting point of malignant change, when they become more vascular, while the surface epithelium becomes thinned and easily excoriated. A small amount of foul discharge is present, often encrusted into a scab which, on removal, leaves an ulcer with indurated, everted edges, with the gradual progress of a cutaneous epithelioma. Any ulcer on the scrotum – especially if indurated or readily caused to bleed – must be looked upon with extreme suspicion and immediately subjected to biopsy for microscopic examination. It is not unusual, however, for a large mass of nodes to be found in the groin when the primary lesion is very small and almost imperceptible. The scrotum must be examined very carefully in such cases lest the primary lesion be missed.

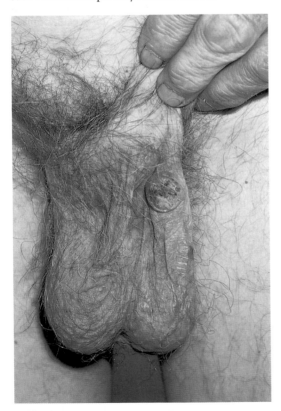

Figure S.13 Epithelioma of the scrotum.

Behçet's syndrome, herpes simplex and candidiasis

Behçet's syndrome causes painful ulcerative lesions of the scrotum as well as the penis, unlike the lesions in the vulva and vagina, which are often painless and therefore often missed. Behçet's may be accompanied by abscess or herpes-like lesions of the scrotum. Herpes simplex – both types I and II – may cause vesicular lesions less commonly, and very rarely candidiasis.

Harold Ellis

SELF-HARM, DELIBERATE

Deliberate self-harm – sometimes termed parasuicide – remains the most common reason for emergency hospital care in young adults, accounting for 10 per cent of all acute admissions, or about 100 000 cases each year in England and Wales.

The initial management is of course the medical and/or surgical evaluation and treatment of the physical presentation. Psychosocial assessment of the behaviour takes place subsequently when the patient is fit to be interviewed, which may not coincide with when physical evidence of toxicity has subsided.

The first psychological task is to confirm whether deliberate self-harm actually took place, and to accomplish this the account of an individual close to the patient is always desirable and may prove essential. The types of self-harm are listed in Table S.5.

Table S.5 Types of self-harm

Commonest
- Deliberate

Less common
- Experimental
- Accidental
- Feigned
- Self-mutilation in the mentally impaired

Feigned self-poisoning is by no means rare, the suspicions being raised by atypical symptoms, responses or behaviour and the absence of confirmatory physical signs or evidence. Such patients may be habitual self-poisoners who eventually only go through the motions, or they may be a self-referral from out of town with a dramatic story and no corroboration available, when the possibility of Munchausen's syndrome should be considered. Gains from simulating self-harm may sometimes emerge later from another source.

Experimental self-poisoning is usually evident from the drugs taken and the account of somebody present at the time. The most common are illicit substances such as opiates, barbiturates, amphetamines, magic mushrooms and solvents, but prescribed drugs – particularly minor tranquillizers, hypnotics, analgesics, anticholinergics and inhalers – are taken for this purpose; proprietary medicines such as Actifed and Benylin may also be abused. It should not be uncritically assumed that the employment of an illicit substance necessarily implies that the purpose of the act was for recreation – the circumstances must also be taken into account.

Accidental self-poisoning can be more difficult to establish, and if doubt persists the patient should be considered to have acted deliberately. This problem occurs most commonly when the patient's judgement was impaired by alcohol, drugs or other physical causes of confusion, with an invariably sketchy recall of events. The most difficult situation is the depressed elderly individual recently prescribed antidepressants, when heavy reliance has to be placed on a relative's observations of changes in behaviour and mental functioning in the days leading up to the overdose. These presentations are not uncommonly caused by good compliance with a large dose of medication leading to anticholinergic-induced confusion. The necessity for an independent account is crucial in cases where accident is asserted by the patient, as this may be a ploy for evading recognition in an acutely suicidal person.

Deliberate self-harm or *self-mutilation in people with more profound degrees of mental impairment* is usually regarded as distinct from parasuicide in that these patients have diminished judgement which raises doubts into their capability to form intent. Self-injurious behaviour should never be assumed to be acceptable or normal in the mentally handicapped, however: its origins may lie in factors as diverse as epilepsy, manic–depressive psychosis, under-stimulation and relationship problems within the family.

Having ascertained that deliberate self-harm has occurred, the next step is to *evaluate the act*. It is important to appreciate that parasuicide is a common end-point of behaviour, and not a medical diagnosis. The circumstances surrounding the act are a pointer to the degree of suicide intent, while the events leading up to taking the decision also help to establish motive(s). It is crucial to understand that the majority of patients who deliberately harm themselves have no wish to kill themselves. Other common motives include ridding oneself of unpleasant feelings, escaping from a stressful situation, obtaining help (the classic 'cry for help'), and as a form of communication with another person. Next, precipitating and vulnerability factors should be inquired about in the patient's social and personal history. Symptoms of mental illness – especially depression – should be sought specifically.

Table S.6 Profile of suicidal risk factors

Circumstances surrounding the act
- Evidence of planning and timing
- Evidence of precautions against discovery
- No communication or seeking help afterwards
- Suicide note, will, gifts, insurance changes

Self-report about the act
- Expectations of fatality
- Concepts of method's lethality and reversibility (more important than quantity taken)
- Intention/motive(s)

Socio-demographical variables
- Male
- Middle-aged or elderly
- Widowed,* divorced,* separated* or single
- Unemployment*
- Social isolation or rejection*
- Financial difficulties*

Physical variables
- Any disabling, painful, chronic or life-threatening illness*
- Epilepsy

Psychological variables
- Family history of suicide
- Previous deliberate self-harm or psychiatric history
- Alcoholism or drug addiction
- Personality disorder
- Schizophrenia (especially during a quiescent phase)
- Depression especially if:
  - suicidal ideation/impulses
  - pessimism
  - self-denigration
  - hypochondriacal or guilt delusions
  - self-neglect
  - sleep disturbance
  - mood is cycling
  - early stages of treatment
- Hopelessness – may be the single most important predictor, irrespective of mood state

*Especially if this represents recent, abrupt change

Recent life events, especially losses and interpersonal difficulties, are particularly important. Other background factors that are associated with increased suicidal risk are presented in Table S.6.

Finally, mental state assessment should seek objective evidence of mental illness as well as considering continuing suicidal risk. How the patient views their action and their future are essential inquiries; hopelessness is consistently reported to be strongly associated with subsequent self-harm and suicide.

This interview is often more difficult than usual situations because it rarely takes place at the patient's request. Resentment at the suggestion of a psychiatric label, embarrassment about the behaviour with fear of the consequences, and an unwillingness to disclose the true motive may all lead to poor compliance, whilst the lingering effects of alcohol or drugs may subtly impair the mental state. Nevertheless, it is important to persevere for three purposes:

1 The identification of a treatable mental disorder.

2 The identification of issues where intervention may help the patient and thus (hopefully) reduce the likelihood of recurrence.

3 The evaluation of suicidal risk.

Much effort has been spent upon refining methods of identifying high-risk groups with the aim of preventing suicide. However, this has proved of little practical value because suicide is a very uncommon early outcome, even among patients who have demonstrated high lethality in their attempt. Default rates in follow-up are around 50 per cent, and treatment interventions have generally proved ineffective in preventing recurrent parasuicide, even when social stresses are alleviated and the patient reports an improved satisfaction with life. The problem may be that not enough is understood yet about this behaviour when the circumstances do not fit the medical model – that is, when it is not a failed attempt at suicide by a person suffering from serious mental illness.

Andrew Hodgkiss

SENSATION, ABNORMALITIES OF

Sensory disturbances are referred to in many sections of this book, but it is convenient here to consider the subject as a whole under the present heading.

Terminology

The inaccurate application of an exact terminology gives rise to so much confusion in the literature that it is often preferable to describe sensory experiences and sensory findings in plain language. 'Paraesthesia' is used for sensations of tingling, pins-and-needles, subjective numbness and feelings of cold and heat, whether they appear spontaneously or as a result of touching or manipulating the part. Since the term covers so many different sensations, it should be avoided when precise descriptive work is required, as for instance in case histories.

Anaesthesia means 'without feeling', but neurologists use it for loss of sensibility to light touch; partial reduction of such sensibility is called 'hypoaesthesia' or 'hypaesthesia'. Analgesia (loss of pain) and hypoalgesia or hypalgesia (reduction of pain sensibility) are useful terms, free from ambiguity. Thermanaesthesia and thermhypaesthesia (loss of, and reduction of, temperature sensibility) are explicit, if inelegant. These cutaneous sensibilities, together with those derived from the special senses, are called 'exteroceptive'. 'Proprioceptive' sensibility is concerned with information received from the labyrinths and from muscle and joint receptors. Vibration sense is difficult to classify and is of no apparent value to humans (but it did warn our ancestors of the herd of animals they couldn't see but their naked feet could feel by vibration), but its loss may help to localize a lesion, especially of the spinal cord.

Hyperaesthesia, hyperalgesia and hyperthermaesthesia refer to increased sensibility to touch, pain and temperature, respectively. Increased sensibility to proprioceptive stimulation has not been described.

Anatomy and physiology

The four common cutaneous sensations – touch, pain, heat and cold – together with the deep sensations of pressure and proprioception – are referred to as the 'somatic sensations'. These are consciously appreciated in all parts of the body, and they have a common pathway within the nervous system. An appropriate stimulus generates an impulse at the periphery which passes into the central nervous system, is relayed by the thalamus, and thence, by a final relay, is passed to the appropriate part of the cerebral cortex. In simple terms, the pathway for somatic sensation is subserved by three orders of neurones: the first-order neurone is concerned with transmitting information from the periphery to the spinal cord; the second-order neurone transmits information from the spinal cord to the thalamus; and the third-order neurone transmits information from the thalamus to the cerebral cortex.

Receptors

Information to the first-order neurones comes from a variety of receptors. Every sensation depends on impulses excited by the adequate stimulation of these receptors, which comprise two main groups – those in skin, and those in the deeper somatic structures. Although individual cutaneous sensory receptors are most sensitive to a particular form of natural stimulation, this specificity is not absolute and other forms of stimulation may also excite the receptors.

Transmission of information from receptors

The stimulation of a sensory ending gives rise to a receptor potential which appears at the specialized end of an afferent nerve fibre. This is not an all-or-none phenomenon, but varies in amplitude and time course, and may be rapidly dissipated even though the stimulus continues, with resulting falling away of the firing frequency in the nerve fibre. Impulses from the receptors travel centrally through the first-order neurones, the cell bodies of which are in the dorsal root ganglia.

The afferent pathways to the spinal cord

The afferent sensory fibres from the various receptors pass up the differing peripheral nerves and enter the spinal cord via the dorsal roots. To understand the variety of peripheral nerve disturbances that may occur requires knowledge of the anatomy of the distribution of peripheral sensory nerves and sensory roots. It should be emphasized that there is considerable overlap in the peripheral nerve distributions and in the dermatome distributions.

There is some evidence to suggest that a number of afferent fibres enter the cord in the ventral roots. The significance of these is uncertain, but their presence may be responsible for the persistence of pain in some patients after dorsal rhizotomy.

Somatic sensory pathways

All of the somatic sensory pathways are crossed and terminate in the opposite sensory cortex in the cerebral hemisphere. Three anatomically separate pathways may be recognized.

Dorsal column medial lemniscus pathway

Input to this pathway within the spinal cord is via large, thickly myelinated fibres which pass through the medial division of the dorsal spinal nerve root to enter the dorsal white column of their own side, dividing into ascending and descending branches. The descending branches establish reflex connections by sending collateral branches into the dorsal grey column; the ascending branches are the first link in the sensory pathway. At their entrance, these ascending fibres are situated immediately medial to the dorsal horn, but during their course up the spinal cord they are steadily pushed to a more medial position because the fibres entering at succeeding rostral levels intrude between the ascending fibres and the dorsal horn. As a consequence of this, the fibres occupying the most medial part of the dorsal column in the upper cervical region will belong to the sacral roots, whilst the fibres from the upper extremity are found most laterally. The fibres terminate at the cervicomedullary junction in the nucleus gracilis and nucleus cuneatus. The fibres terminate synaptically on to the second-order neurones in the gracile and cuneate nuclei and the axons of these neurones curve ventrally and medially, crossing the midline, and then turn upwards to form a prominent bundle of fibres, the medial lemniscus.

The classical view is that the impulses ascending in the fibres of the dorsal columns mediate the sensations of touch, deep pressure, vibratory sense and sense of position of joints, and are particularly important for sensory discrimination. During the past few years, this view has been challenged and, although the matter is far from certain, it appears that the dorsal columns mediate sensory signals necessary for complex tasks.

The segmental somatotopic organization present in the dorsal columns and their nuclei is maintained in the medial lemniscus as it ascends to the thalamus, where the fibres enter the ventroposterior lateral nucleus which contains the cell bodies of the third-order sensory neurones.

Lateral spinothalamic pathway

This transmits impulses which are concerned with the appreciation of heat, cold and pain. It also provides an alternative pathway for touch sensibility – the so-called 'crude' or 'coarse' touch. The first-order neurones have their cell bodies in the dorsal root ganglia, and their fibres are thinner than those of the dorsal column medial lemniscus pathway; some, indeed (the C fibres), have no myelin at all. They enter the spinal cord in the lateral part of the dorsal root and divide into short descending and ascending branches. The ascending branches run for one or two segments in the posterolateral column before synapsing with second-order sensory neurones which lie deep in the dorsal column. The axons then cross the midline, the so-called 'ventral white commissure', and ascend in the ventrolateral white column as the spinothalamic tract. Some of the spinothalamic fibres give off collaterals to certain nuclear regions such as the reticular formation.

In the brainstem the spinothalamic tract lies lateral to the medial lemniscus, which it accompanies to terminate in the thalamus in the ventroposterior lateral nucleus. Important features of the spinothalamic pathway include the following:

- The second-order neurone fibres cross the midline only one or two segments above the level of entry of the dorsal root fibres.
- The site of decussation of the fibres in the cord exposes them to damage by expanding ventral cord lesions.
- Fibres concerned with pain and temperature sensibility are situated dorsally to those involved with touch and pressure.
- The spinothalamic tract is less compactly organized than the medial lemniscus, being intermingled with other ascending pathways giving off collaterals to the brainstem reticular formation.

The trigeminothalamic pathway

This pathway carries information from the distribution of the trigeminal nerve which serves most of the skin of the face, the forehead as far as the vertex, the mucous membranes of the nasal cavities, paranasal sinuses, mouth, tongue and parts of the pharynx, the teeth and gums, and part of the dura mater.

About half of the fibres entering in the trigeminal nerve divide into a branch which terminates in the chief nucleus of the trigeminal nerve, while the other half descends in the spinal tract to end in the spinal nucleus. The chief nucleus, which is in the lateral part of the pons, contains the second-order neurones concerned with tactile and postural sensibility; it gives rise to fibres which cross the midline to ascend near the medial lemniscus. The nucleus of the spinal tract, which extends downwards in the lateral part of the medulla to about the level of C2, contains the second-order neurones concerned with pain and temperature sensibility. Second-order neurones cross to the quintothalamic tract, which ascends close to the spinothalamic tract. Both sets of second-order neurone fibres terminate in the ventroposterior medial nucleus of the thalamus.

The thalamus and thalamocortical projections

The third neuronal link in the ascending somatic sensory fibre system is made up of neurones the nuclei of which are in the thalamus. The axons of these neurones transmit impulses to the cerebral cortex.

The somatosensory cortical areas

From clinical and physiological observations it has been known for many years that, in man, the postcentral gyrus is the main (primary) somatosensory area. Another area beneath the lower end of the postcentral gyrus is known as the secondary somatosensory area. Since the work of Penfield, it has been known that there is a clear somatotopic representation in the sensory cortex. The first sensory area appears principally to reflect activity in the dorsal column medial lemniscus system and also in the associated trigeminal system. The thalamic relay for these impulses passes through the internal capsule.

However inadequate our understanding of the sensory cortex, one thing is clear: provided that the subcortical structures – especially the thalamus – are intact, certain sensations such as pain, touch, pressure and extremes of temperature can reach consciousness.

The accurate localization, however, as well as the patient's ability to make sensory discriminations, depend on the integrity of the sensory cortex. This is a fundamental distinction and will be discussed further when considering individual sensory syndromes.

Patterns of sensory disturbance

Figures S.14 to S.19 illustrate some of the sensory syndromes discussed below.

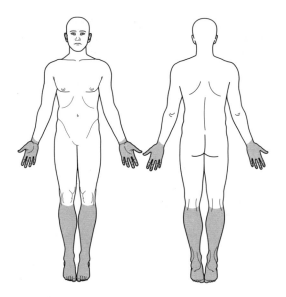

Figure S.14 Peripheral neuritis. 'Glove and stocking anaesthesia'. Cotton-wool and pinprick sensibility impaired or lost over the dotted areas. This is associated with hyperalgesia of the underlying muscles.

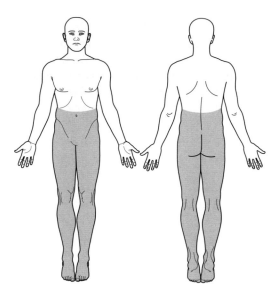

Figure S.16 Dorsal myelitis affecting the cord as high as the 9th dorsal segment. The shaded parts are insensitive to touch, pain and all degrees of temperature.

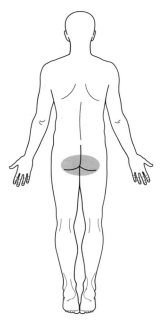

Figure S.15 Comminuted fracture of the sacrum, with injury to the 3rd, 4th and 5th sacral roots. Complete loss of sensibility to touch, pain, heat and cold resulted in the shaded area.

Mononeuropathy

Changes in this instance will vary, depending on whether the nerve involved is predominantly motor,

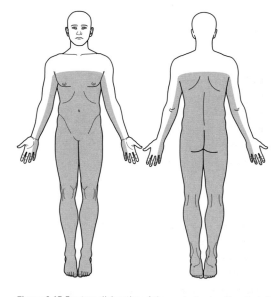

Figure S.17 Fracture-dislocation of the cervical spine. The shaded area represents the loss of sensibility to touch, pain, heat and cold.

sensory or mixed. In sensory nerves the area of touch loss is usually more extensive than the area of pain loss. Because of overlap from adjacent nerves, the area of sensory loss following damage to a cutaneous nerve is always less than its anatomical distribution. Deep pressure and joint position senses remain intact

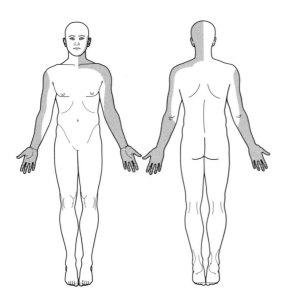

Figure S.18 Syringomyelia. The shaded parts show the areas of dissociated anaesthesia (i.e. of thermo-anaesthesia and analgesia). This was associated with atrophic palsy of the upper extremities.

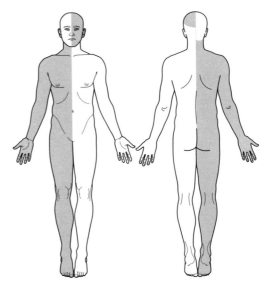

Figure S.19 Thrombosis of the left posterior inferior cerebellar artery. The dotted areas show the regions of dissociated anaesthesia (i.e. loss of sensibility to pain and temperature of all degrees).

because they are mediated by nerve fibres from the subcutaneous structures and joints. Particular types of pathological lesion may differentially affect the fibres in a sensory nerve. Compression typically disturbs large touch and pressure fibres and leaves intact small pain, thermal and autonomic fibres. Lesions of the brachial or lumbosacral plexus may be differentiated from multiple peripheral nerve involvement by the distribution of the sensory and motor loss (see Radiculopathy, below).

Polyneuropathy

In most instances of polyneuropathy the longest and largest fibres tend to be involved. The sensory loss is most severe over the feet and legs and less severe over the hands, and the trunk and face are usually spared except in the most severe cases. Typically, the sensory loss involves all the modalities, although this varies depending on the type of neuropathy. The term 'glove and stocking' sensory loss draws attention to the distal pattern of involvement (see Fig. S.14). However, it is an inaccurate term as the border between normal and abnormal sensation is not sharp, and the sensory loss shades off gradually. In hysteria, the border between normal and abnormal sensation is usually sharp.

Radiculopathy

Irritative symptoms may be present when the dorsal roots are the subject of traction or compression. This shows itself as pain which is often limited to the dermatome belonging to the affected root. In some root disorders pain is absent and paraesthesiae in the dermatome distribution are present. Damage to a dorsal root will result in a loss of sensory modalities of all types within the distribution of the dermatome. Because of overlap between dermatomes, interruption of one single dorsal root will often give no definite sensory loss. When two or more roots have been completely divided, the zone of sensory loss is usually greater for pain than for touch. Surrounding the area of complete loss will be a zone of partial loss.

Spinal cord syndromes

Lesions of the dorsal horn (the tabetic syndrome)

Lesions of the dorsal horn produce syndromes similar to those seen in lesions of the dorsal roots. Depending on the number of segments involved, there will be a segmental sensory loss affecting vibration and position senses in particular. Accompanying this may be pain which often is called 'lightning pain'. This repeated severe pain is described as occurring at right-angles to the skin and penetrating through the affected limb. Most commonly, this syndrome results from neurosyphilis, although it may be seen in diabetes mellitus.

Transverse cord lesions

A complete transverse lesion of the spinal cord will be associated with loss of all forms of sensation below the segmental level which corresponds to the lesion. There may be a narrow band of hyperaesthesia at the upper margin of the level of sensory loss. Loss of pain, temperature and touch sensation is usually evident two or three segments below the level of the lesion, whereas vibratory and position sense is less easy to delimit. A compressive cord lesion is usually associated with descending loss of sensation as the outermost fibres carrying pain and temperature sensation are from the legs. A lesion expanding from the centre of the cord, such as an intramedullary tumour, will tend to involve the innermost fibres carrying pain and temperature sensation, and thus there may be relative sparing of the most superficial fibres from the sacral segments; this may lead to so-called 'sacral sparing'.

Hemisection of the spinal cord (the Brown–Sequard syndrome)

Occasionally in spinal cord disorders pathology is limited to one side of the spinal cord. Loss of pain and temperature sensation is found on the opposite side, and the upper margin of this is usually two or three segments below the level of the lesion. Proprioceptive sensation is affected on the same side as the lesion and an associated motor paralysis occurs on the same side. Touch sensation is not involved, because the fibres are distributed in both posterior columns and the spinothalamic pathway on both sides of the cord. In clinical practice a complete hemisection of the spinal cord is rarely seen, although a partial syndrome occurs in multiple sclerosis.

Central spinal cord lesions (the syringomyelic syndrome)

A central spinal cord lesion characteristically will involve the pain and temperature fibres as they cross in the anterior commissure. Typically, these modalities are affected on one or both sides over a number of dermatomes, with relative preservation of tactile sensation (so-called dissociated sensory loss). Abolition of tendon

reflexes in the affected segment is usually seen. The most common cause of this syndrome is syringomyelia (see Fig. S.18), but intramedullary tumours (e.g. ghomas or ependymomas) may also produce it.

The posterior column syndrome

In lesions preferentially affecting the dorsal columns there is loss of vibration and position sense below the level of the lesion, with preservation of pain, temperature and touch. When such sensory loss affects the legs there is typically a sensory ataxia and a positive Romberg's sign. Sensory loss of this type in the hands produces clumsiness when manipulating small objects, and an inability to recognize shapes such as coins in the pocket. Tingling and pins-and-needles sensations are common, and patients often complain that the hands and feet feel swollen or tight. Causes include vitamin B_{12} deficiency and syphilis.

The anterior cord syndrome

In anterior cord disturbances there is typically damage to the spinothalamic tracts producing pain and temperature loss below the level of the lesion.

Brainstem syndromes

Because of the complex structure of the brainstem, with multiple ascending and descending tracts intermingled with a variety of cranial nerve nuclei, lesions result in far more complex clinical pictures than those which may be seen in spinal cord disorders. A characteristic feature of a medullary or lower pontine lesion is that the sensory disorder is crossed – that is, there is loss of pain and temperature sensation on one side of the face and on the opposite side of the body. This results from involvement of the trigeminal tract or nucleus, resulting in ipsilateral facial sensory loss, and of the lateral spinothalamic tract, resulting in contralateral loss of sensation of the trunk and limbs. Higher in the brainstem, the trigeminothalamic and lateral spinothalamic tracts run together, and a lesion will therefore produce contralateral loss of pain and temperature sense on the whole of the opposite side of the body. In the upper brainstem the spinothalamic tract and the medial lemniscus become confluent, so that a lesion at this level may cause contralateral sensory loss of all types.

In brainstem lesions there is frequently bilateral involvement, and a variety of syndromes have been described involving sensory, motor and cerebellar dysfunction accompanied by cranial nerve palsies. Lesions, particularly vascular lesions, are rarely discrete and it requires a detailed knowledge of the anatomical structure of the brainstem to achieve accurate localization. Another point of practical importance is that partial involvement of the sensory tracts may produce sensory impairment which may mimic lesions in the cord.

Thalamic disorders

Thalamic sensory disorders usually result from discrete cerebral infarcts. A destruction of the entire thalamic area receiving sensory fibre systems would be expected to result in an impairment or loss of somatic sensation in the whole of the opposite half of the body. In documented cases where such a lesion was identified, the perception of pain has often been found to be only slightly affected. Position sense typically is affected more profoundly than any other sensory function. Pure lesions of the ventroposterior lateral nucleus of the thalamus will be associated with contralateral sensory disorders of the limbs and trunk, whereas involvement of the ventroposterior medial nucleus will produce sensory impairment of the contralateral face.

In thalamic disorders there is often accompanying spontaneous pain or discomfort. These thalamic pains are often very intense and occur in paroxysms affecting the opposite side of the body. They typically are more pronounced in the face, hand or lower leg and are uncommon on the trunk. Causes include tumours and vascular lesions.

Cortical disorders

Circumscribed lesions of the postcentral gyros will be followed by localized sensory loss in parts of the opposite half of the body. This is typically a loss of discriminatory sensory function, and includes loss of position sense, impaired ability to localize touch and pain stimuli, elevation of the two-point threshold, and astereognosis. In acute lesions of the parietal cortex there may appear to be impairment of pain sensibility, but this is rarely prominent or persistent.

Occasionally, sensory seizures are seen in lesions of the sensory cortex, although these are rare. Typically, they show themselves as a wave of sensory irritative symptoms spreading over the body in accordance with the somatotopic organization of the sensory cortex.

Simulated sensory loss

A variety of sensory disorders may be simulated. Patients may complain of the sensory loss, but more commonly it is found incidentally during examination. The area of sensory loss is usually sharply demarcated and, in other than medical personnel, does not conform to a recognized anatomical distribution. Characteristically, pain loss is the most striking feature and loss of position sense is uncommon. Bearing in mind the difficulties of the sensory examination it is probably safer to ignore sensory findings that do not fit with any other neurological abnormalities that are present. Often it is possible to make a positive diagnosis of a simulated sensory loss because the individual's knowledge of anatomy is not sufficient to enable them to get it right. For example, anybody who is found to have unilateral loss of vibration sense on the skull can be confidently diagnosed as simulating. It must be added, however, that the positive finding of non-organic sensory loss does not necessarily indicate that the whole of the neurological problem is simulated. Sensory loss that is simulated is often added on to symptoms and signs as part of a functional overlay.

Mark Kinirons

SEXUAL DYSFUNCTION

Most commonly, advice is sought for problems arising in the context of heterosexual relationships. For women, the two main categories of complaint are disorders of arousal and disorders of orgasm during sexual intercourse. For men, complaints can be grouped as *erectile impotence* (when erection cannot be obtained or maintained), *premature ejaculation* and *retarded ejaculation*. There appear to be quite marked differences between men and women in their expectations from sexual intercourse, the majority of men complaining of problems with erection or ejaculation and only a minority seeking help on account of lack of interest or enjoyment of sex. An approach to understanding sexual dysfunction must take account of the social, emotional psychological and physiological effects which may all influence the sexual response, so that when advice is sought for sexual problems from patients with multiple sclerosis, hypertension, epilepsy, colostomy, mastectomy and with many other physical conditions the clinician must consider the effects of the reaction of the patient and their spouse to the disability as well as the direct physiological disturbances and the effects of medication.

Disorders of arousal and orgasm in both men and women are most commonly connected with psychological and emotional factors. Particularly in the young there may be *anxiety* about sexual prowess and performance. Negative feelings about intercourse may arise in people with *obsessional personalities* because of a general fastidiousness and a fear of losing control of feelings and bodily functions. *Fear of pregnancy* is possibly the most widespread and realistic inhibiting factor, while pleasant sexual experience in childhood may lead to difficulties in establishing normal relations in adulthood. It is also normal for many women to achieve orgasm only through sexual activities other than full intercourse. In women, pain during intercourse (dyspareunia) may result from vaginal infection or other pathology in the pelvis. There may also be inadequate lubrication of the vagina, particularly in post-menopausal or lactating women. In some women there is a tendency to develop spasm of the pelvic floor muscles during intercourse, resulting in *vaginismus* which makes intercourse painful or impossible.

Failure to achieve orgasm (anorgasmia) may be the outcome of dyspareunia or occasionally severe physical malformation of the genital tract, but in the majority of cases there appears to be no good physical or psychological reason for the inability to achieve orgasm. Women depend on tactile stimulation for arousal, and anorgasmia may be due simply to poor technique by the partner.

Libido may be severely impaired in *depressive illness*. *Chronic alcoholism* may cause reduced libido in both sexes. Organic causes of impotence include *autonomic neuropathy* (e.g. diabetes mellitus), *spinal cord damage* and sometimes central nervous system impairment as in *tumours* in the region of the third ventricle and *temporal lobe epilepsy*. Endocrine disorders include primary and secondary *hypogonadism*. The only drugs which clearly and directly interfere with vascular mechanisms leading to erection are the *ganglion blockers*. Adrenergic receptor blockers interfere with ejaculation, and drugs may interfere with the male sexual function by effects on the central nervous system, on blood pressure, or endocrine effects. For example, the reduced libido in some patients with temporal lobe epilepsy has been attributed to the effect of anticonvulsant drugs in lowering testosterone levels.

Medical advice may be sought by homosexuals because of sexual and relationship difficulties, and these may be exacerbated by the attitudes of society. A group of sexual disorders which may lead the person into trouble with their partner or with the law are the disorders of sexual preferences (the *paraphilias*) which include abnormalities of the sexual object (*fetishism*, *paedophilia*) and abnormalities of the sexual act (*exhibitionism*, *voyeurism*, *frotteurism* and *sadomasochistic sexual practices*). Fetishism and sadomasochism may be quite common and easily concealed in a stable relationship. Help may be sought only when such practices cause strain in a heterosexual or homosexual partnership. Fetishism occurs almost only in men, and describes the use of objects such as clothing, parts of the body or specific textures such as rubber, leather or plastic to stimulate erection. Sadomasochism related to sexual arousal occurs in both men and women, and has a role more frequently in fantasy than in reality. The sadist inflicts pain, while the masochist adopts a passive role, as in sexual practices involving bondage. Generally these practices do not lead to conflict with society. A medical opinion is most likely to be sought with sexual offenders, the common deviations being *exhibitionism* and *paedophilia*. Exhibitionism or *indecent exposure* is the gaining of sexual stimulation by exposing the genitalia. Unlike other forms of sexual deviation, there is no attempt to establish further contact with the 'victim'. In some instances the exhibitionist may derive satisfaction in a sadomasochistic way by evoking fear in a witness. Some become highly sexually aroused and masturbate during or shortly after the exposure. *Frotteurism* describes the achievement of sexual arousal by rubbing against a stranger, often in crowds.

Paedophilia describes sexual activity with children in preference to adults. Usually a paedophile will be attracted either to boys or to girls, but not to both. It is recognized almost exclusively in men.

Factors sometimes associated with sexual deviations include disturbed rearing and parental disharmony, leading to difficulties in establishing stable adult relationships, and personality disorders, particularly in those who are inadequate or psychopathic. The role of low IQ, alcohol abuse and mental illness (manic–depressive illness and schizophrenia) should also be considered in the clinical assessment of a case.

Problems with gender identity reflected in cross-dressing behaviour (*transvestism* and *trans-sexualism*) may reflect a number of quite distinct sexual problems.

For some men the wearing of female clothes is sexually arousing, and the clothes are objects of fetishism. A homosexual of either sex may cross-dress out of preference, but in the absence of any genuine gender confusion or desire to be of the opposite sex. Finally, there are genuine trans-sexuals of either sex who often since early childhood have been aware that their psychological sex is opposite to their anatomical sex. These trans-sexuals may proceed to successful surgical sexual reassignment.

Mark Kinirons

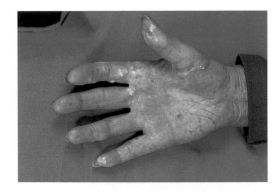

Figure S.20 Calcinosis in CRST syndrome.

SKIN HARDENING

Hardening of the skin is the principal feature of *scleroderma*. This occurs in localized and progressive systemic forms. Localized scleroderma, or *morphoea*, usually begins in patients under the age of 30 years as asymptomatic, round or oval, firm, smooth, reddish plaques many centimetres in diameter. They are commonest on the trunk, and may have a lilac or telangiectatic border. After several years the centre of lesions may become atrophic and hyperpigmented. More rarely, morphoea appears in linear form either in paramedian distribution on the scalp (*coup de sabre*) or along the line of a limb. Sclerosis in linear morphoea is very marked, and there can be associated atrophy of underlying bone or muscle. The linear type shows little tendency to spontaneous resolution. At times the whole of a limb or one side of the head may be affected in a child, resulting in a deforming hemi-atrophy. Even more rarely very large areas of skin may be involved in a *generalized morphoea*.

The progressive type of scleroderma is a systemic disease, probably of autoimmune aetiology. It occurs in two distinct forms. In the calcinosis, Raynaud's phenomenon, sclerodactyly, telangiectases (CRST) syndrome, symptoms of Raynaud's phenomenon are followed by progressive *acrosclerosis* (hardening of the extremities), with an associated loss of mobility; calcinosis of the fingertips may be a prominent feature. In addition, telangiectasia is seen, and the skin on the face – especially around the mouth – becomes tight and fixed. Disorders of oesophageal mobility are common, and pulmonary hypertension is a late, but ominous, feature (Figs S.20 and S.21).

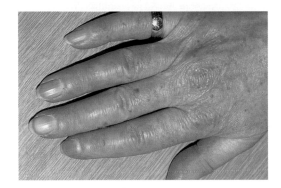

Figure S.21 Acrosclerosis in CRST syndrome.

In the more generalized form of progressive systemic sclerosis, the whole skin becomes thickened and immobile; the lungs, kidneys and heart may also be affected, and there is little tendency to spontaneous improvement. Features mimicking the hardening of the skin in scleroderma may be seen occasionally in the late stages of *porphyria cutanea tarda*, in *carcinoid syndrome*, and in patients affected by occupational exposure to the manufacture of vinyl chloride.

Hard, bead-like infiltration of the skin is seen with *lipoid proteinosis*, and this is particularly noticeable around the eyelid margins. Hardening of the skin of the chest can follow secondary infiltration with *scirrhous carcinoma*. A tender, hard plaque appearing on the head and face at the site of inoculation by 'kissing' bugs can occur with *Chagas' disease* in South America. The skin of the lower legs may become hard in patients with long-standing venous insufficiency (*lipodermatosclerosis*), and a general hardening of the skin may be evident in diabetes of long standing.

Barry Monk

SKIN, PIGMENTATION OF

The main component of normal skin pigment is the amount of melanin produced by the melanocytes situated at the dermo-epidermal junction. A genetic defect in the ability to produce melanin may cause *albinism*, whilst an acquired localized loss of pigment arises from destruction of melanocytes in *vitiligo*. The pigment loss in vitiligo is usually patchy and often symmetrical; autoimmune disorders may be seen in association. In red-haired subjects, the melanocytes do not produce melanin, but a related pigment, phaeomelanin, which although present in abundant quantities does not provide photo-protection, and this accounts for the high incidence of skin cancers in red-haired people.

Excessive pigmentation may arise from localized or generalized abnormal or excessive production of melanin, from deposition of haemosiderin, or from exogenous pigmenting agents.

Generalized hyperpigmentation

Diffuse hyperpigmentation, including pigmentation of the buccal mucosae, gingival margins, palmar creases and nailbeds, is a feature of Addison's disease. In fact, this disorder is remarkably rare in clinical practice, and a more likely cause is the presence of an *ectopic hormone-secreting tumour*; for example, various lung carcinomas secrete peptides, some of which have MSH-like (melanocyte-stimulating hormone) properties. Similarly, ACTH for intramuscular injection is often contaminated with similar peptides and can cause hyperpigmentation. Diffuse pigmentation can be a feature of *malignant cachexia*, the late wasting phase of HIV disease, and can be very marked in those dying with a heavy tumour load of secondary *malignant melanoma*, sometimes accompanied by melanuria. The diffuse hyperpigmentation of *haemochromatosis* (bronze diabetes) is due to an excess of both melanin and iron.

Localized hyperpigmentation

Many skin disorders appear able to cause a non-specific post-inflammatory hyperpigmentation. This is particularly seen following *lichen planus* (Fig. S.22) and in a *fixed drug eruption*, where the condition can

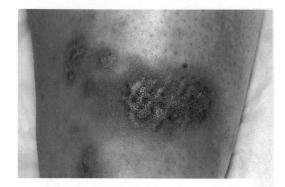

Figure S.22 Hypertrophic lichen planus.

be diagnosed retrospectively from the distribution of the pigmentation. Dark-skinned races seem more susceptible to the phenomenon of post-inflammatory changes in pigment, and in lichen planus in South Asian races, for example, this can be most disfiguring. In some chronic conditions pigmentation forms part of the spectrum of diagnostic physical signs, for example, *atopic dermatitis, morphoea, urticaria pigmentosa* and *acanthosis nigricans*. In a *berloque dermatitis* an acute photo-toxic reaction occurs to perfume or eau de cologne, due to the psoralens which they contain. In its most florid form, the condition can be dramatic and even bullous, but patches of hyperpigmentation on the sides of women's necks are extremely common. A similar hyperpigmentation can follow a photo-toxic reaction to plant chemicals – a *photophytodermatitis* – as seen with plants of the Compositae family.

A common cause of a symmetrical hyperpigmentation on the forehead and cheeks in middle-aged ladies is *chloasma (melasma)*. This condition is of unknown cause, but may be exacerbated by pregnancy or the oral contraceptive pill, and by sunlight. Less common causes of localized hyperpigmentation include lichen amyloid (Fig. S.23) and naevus of Ota (Fig. S.24).

Hyperpigmentation of exposed areas

Ultraviolet (sunlight) exposure will tan the skin in those with appropriate skin types, but tanning may be accentuated by certain *drugs*, including thiazides, sulphonamides, amiodarone, nalidixic acid, tetracyclines and chlorpromazine. A similar phenomenon may arise in metabolic disorders such as *pellagra* and *porphyria cutanea tarda*.

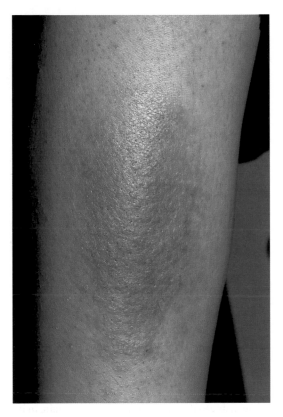

Figure S.23 Lichen amyloid.

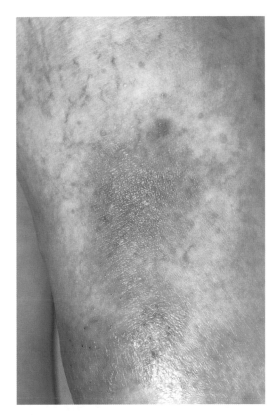

Figure S.25 Haemosiderosis.

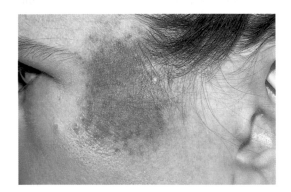

Figure S.24 Naevus of Ota.

Haemosiderin

Haemosiderin is a breakdown product of haemo-globin, and will be precipitated in the skin leaving a persistent, localized orangy-brown discoloration in situations where there has been chronic extravasation of blood, as in *stasis ulceration* of the legs, and in some cutaneous vasculitic disorders (*pigmented purpuric eruption, Majocci–Shamberg disease*) (Fig. S.25).

Other chemicals

Obstructive hepatopathy causes acute or insidious *jaundice* of differing hue, for example the greenish colour of primary biliary cirrhosis. *Carotinaemia* results in a yellowish or orange discoloration of the skin, sparing the sclerae, and follows the ingestion of large quantities of carrots, oranges and other vege-tables. Yellowing of the skin can be caused by drugs, particularly *mepacrine*. In *alcaptonuric ochronosis*, the pigment precursor tyrosine cannot be catabolized, and a bluish-black pigment accumulates, particularly in the cartilaginous tissues of the ears, sclerae, joints and vertebral column. The urine becomes black on standing for 24 hours. Topical use of hydroxyquinone-based chemicals, which are sold in some countries as skin lighteners, can also produce a permanent deep pigmentation due to *ochronosis*. The history in such cases may be misleading, as patients may be too embarrassed to admit use of such products, but the histology is characteristic. A generalized bluish discoloration is seen with *methaemoglobinaemia* which can be drug-induced (e.g. by dapsone). A deeper colour is induced by the deposition of silver in *argyria*; this may arise from chronic occupational exposure or from the medicinal use of silver salts. High-dose, long-term treatment of acne or rosacea with minocycline can result in pigment deposition within acne scars, and sometimes more widely (Fig. S.26). Zidovudine (AZT) can cause linear pigmentation of nails (melanonychia striata) and sometimes diffuse hyperpigmentation.

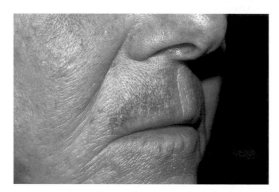

Figure S.26 Minocycline pigmentation.

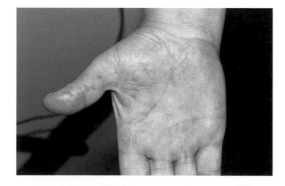

Figure S.27 Accidental tattooing.

Tattooing of the skin is usually obvious, but may produce unusual patterns when it has arisen accidentally from blast injuries (Fig. S.27). Occasionally, bizarre colouring of the skin arises from attempts to fool doctors or alarm relatives (*factitious dermatitis*).

Barry Monk

SKIN TUMOURS

Cutaneous tumours are growths on the skin which are larger than nodules. They may be firm, fleshy, cystic, multi-lobulated or ulcerated, and they may be solitary or multiple. The chief causes are neoplasms, both benign and malignant.

A brief classification of skin tumours is listed in Table S.7.

Table S.7 Skin tumours

Malignant
- Secondary deposits
- Kaposi's sarcoma
- Primary malignant tumours
  - Squamous-cell carcinoma (epithelioma)
  - Malignant melanoma
  - Rodent ulcer (basal cell carcinoma)
  - Mycosis fungoides (cutaneous T-cell lymphoma)
  - Xeroderma pigmentosum

Benign
- Sebaceous cyst
- Lipoma
- Seborrhoeic keratosis (basal cell papilloma)
- Cutaneous horn
- Pyogenic granuloma
- Adnexal tumours (syringoma, hidrocystoma, etc.)

Genetic syndromes with multiple skin tumours
- Gorlin syndrome
- Xeroderma pigmentosum (XP)
- Neurofibromatosis (von Recklinghausen's disease)

Malignant tumours

Secondary deposits

These commonly occur late, as multiple, hard, fleshy nodules of any colour (Fig. S.28). Subcutaneous secondaries can masquerade as benign lesions, and a high level of suspicion should be maintained. Even infectious lesions can be simulated, for example by *lymphangitis carcinomatosa* on the chest of a patient with breast cancer. Certain areas are predisposed to metastases, including the scalp (breast, lung and genitourinary tract carcinoma), the chest wall (breast cancer) and the abdominal wall especially around the umbilicus (carcinoma of the stomach and the colon). The cell type identified on histology may give a clue as to the primary source. The skin is sometimes infiltrated by leukaemia or lymphoma, the patients presenting with multiple randomly scattered erythematous nodules; it is a late, and usually pre-terminal, manifestation. Paget's disease (Fig. S.29) is invariably associated with an underlying malignancy of the breast.

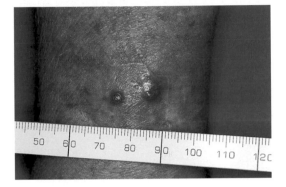

Figure S.28 Secondary deposits.

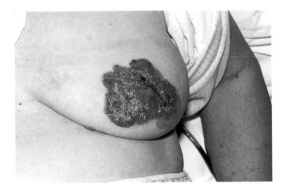

Figure S.29 Paget's disease of the nipple.

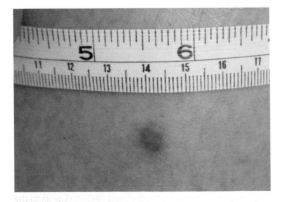

Figure S.30 Papular Kaposi's sarcoma.

Kaposi's sarcoma

This is a malignant proliferation of vascular endothelial cells giving rise to superficial, subcutaneous or deeper vascular tumours (Fig. S.30). The tumours do not metastasize, but are multi-site in origin. They are probably due to infection with human herpes virus-8. Tumours flourish when immunity is depressed, for example in HIV, post-transplant and old age. The classical lesions, which were first described in patients of Jewish or Italian descent living in Vienna in the 1870s, are probably acquired on the genome and expressed in old age. Endemic Kaposi's sarcoma was first recognized in the 1950s as a common tumour in sub-Saharan Africa, in younger patients, and was seen to follow a much more aggressive course.

Individual lesions begin as pink vascular macules, often in multiple sites, and they gradually enlarge and become palpable and darken with time. Draining oedema is often prominent. The vascular lesions can simulate granulomata, histiocytomata or haemangiomata. Internal lesions can occur chiefly in the gastrointestinal tract and lungs. If immunity improves (i.e. with anti-retroviral therapy), the tumours may shrink.

Primary malignant skin tumours

Squamous cell carcinoma (Fig. S.31) is usually single and, as a rule, is fairly slow growing, extending peripherally and infiltrating deeply while ulcerating at its centre. Eventually, the lymphatic nodes draining the affected area become involved and enlarged. The usual sites for squamous cell carcinoma are the lips, especially the lower lip and sun-exposed areas, as well as glans penis and vulva. Solar keratoses, X-ray scars and lupus vulgaris may all undergo malignant squamous change. The main diagnostic features are its origin as a single growth, its craggy hardness, its slow development, and the metastases to neighbouring lymph nodes.

Malignant melanoma (Fig. S.32) can arise anywhere on the skin surface at any age, although it is rare in childhood; it may arise *de novo* or from a pre-existing mole. It is rare in blacks, and increases in frequency with the fairness of the skin and the amount of previous sun exposure. Patients with a history of severe sunburn in childhood, with more than 50 moles on their skin, more than five unusually large moles or a family history of malignant melanoma, are at increased risk. This tumour may occur on the scalp, under a nail, or on anogenital skin.

is highly malignant, but early diagnosis and excision is curative. The prognosis depends on the thickness of the primary lesion at the time of excision.

Rodent ulcer (*basal cell carcinoma*) (Fig. S.33) usually affects the face (see FACE, ULCERATION OF, p. 204). These are the most common primary skin malignancies. They do not metastasize, but local invasive destruction can be extensive if the lesions are neglected.

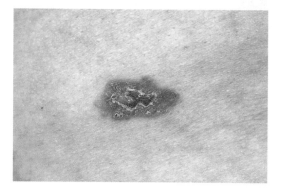

Figure S.33 Basal cell carcinoma (rodent ulcer).

Mycosis fungoides (cutaneous T-cell lymphoma) (Fig. S.34) is a rare, chronic, slowly fatal disease which is characterized in its final stage by tomato-like growths which may ulcerate. For many years a 'pre-mycotic', non-specific, red scaly rash is present, later (sometimes 30 years plus) forming red plaques of differing hue, and finally tumours.

Xeroderma pigmentosum is an extremely rare disorder of nuclear protein repair which is inherited as a recessive trait. It presents in childhood as a proneness to sunburn and early gross sun damage with elastosis, atrophy, telangiectasia and finally multiple skin tumours (squamous cell carcinoma, rodent ulcer, malignant melanoma, kerato-acanthoma).

Benign cutaneous tumours

Sebaceous cysts, which occur most commonly on the back, face, scalp and scrotum, are of variable size, cystic on palpation, and with a minute orifice (punctum) to be found somewhere on their surface. *Lipomas* are usually multiple subcutaneous nodules which may be lobulated, and found on any part of the body. They occur as a familial trait, but can often not be discerned until adulthood. *Seborrhoeic keratosis* (basal-cell papillomas) (Fig. S.35) are extremely common and start as papules in middle age, growing into larger, flat, greasy, warty

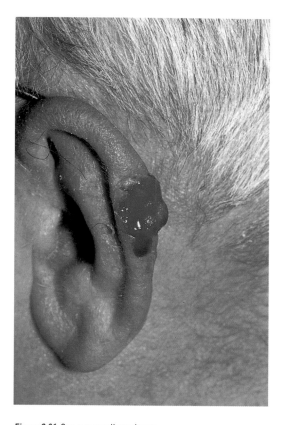

Figure S.31 Squamous cell carcinoma.

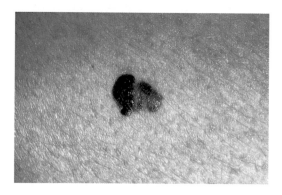

Figure S.32 Malignant melanoma.

Occasionally, melanomas lose the capacity to produce pigment; this is termed *amelanotic melanoma*. The characteristics of malignant melanoma are its rapid development and growth, its deepening colour, its ulceration, areas of depigmentation, bleeding and crust formation, and its rapid metastases. Sometimes multiple metastases occur in the skin itself. The disease

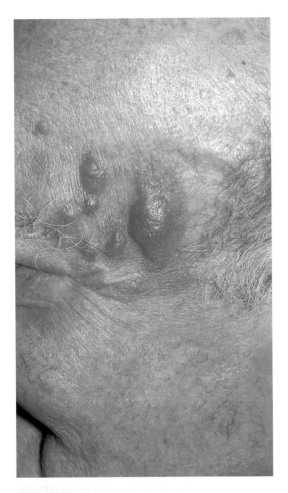

Figure S.34 Mycosis fungoides.

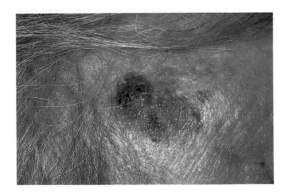

Figure S.35 Seborrhoeic keratosis (basal cell papilloma).

pigmented neoplasms. They are sometimes unkindly called 'senile keratoses'.

A *cutaneous horn* is a peculiar cutaneous neoplasm surmounted by a spectacular horny overgrowth. The nature of the underlying neoplasm can only be safely diagnosed by examining the histopathology, for example actinic keratosis, squamous-cell carcinoma, viral wart, keratoacanthoma and seborrhoeic wart (basal cell papilloma).

A *pyogenic granuloma* (granuloma telangiectaticum) is a fairly common skin lesion. It often develops at the site of a recent injury, and is composed of proliferating capillaries in a loose stroma. This produces a rapidly growing vascular nodule which bleeds easily when traumatized. It is distinctive, being bright red, 0.5–1 cm in diameter, often pedunculated, and surrounded by a collar of thickened epidermis. The most common sites are the fingers, upper chest, lips and toes. It must be differentiated from amelanotic melanoma, and glomus tumour. Kaposi's sarcoma in HIV-infected patients can accurately mimic pyogenic granuloma, and for this reason histological analysis after curettage or excision is advisable.

The superficial dermis contains many specialized tissues, some of ectodermal and some of mesodermal origin, forming the various adnexal structures (e.g. hair, sebaceous glands, sweat glands). Benign, or rarely malignant, neoplasms of all these specialized tissues can occur, for example *leiomyoma*, *hydradenoma*, *neurofibroma*, *sebaceous adenoma*, *tricho-epithelioma* and *glomus tumour*. The diagnosis of these uncommon adnexal lesions requires many years' experience, and is often first made by the pathologist.

Barry Monk

SLEEP, DISORDERS OF

The most common complaint is of insomnia, although some patients will seek advice on account of too much sleep (hypersomnia) or occasionally for abnormal events which occur during sleep (the parasomnias) (Table S.8).

Poor sleep is a very common complaint, more so amongst women than men, and especially in the elderly. Self-reports from patients are frequently inaccurate, because patients typically over-estimate the time taken to get to sleep and under-estimate the total duration of sleep. Patients generally sleep longer than they think. Complaints of poor sleep come from people who are under stress at home or at work, or who have

Table S.8 Disorders of sleep

Insomnia
- Normal variant
- Physical illness (pain, respiratory disease, delirium)
- Mood disorder
  - Depression
  - Anxiety
  - Mania
- Post-traumatic stress disorder
- Drugs
  - Stimulants (including coffee, tea, nicotine, amphetamine)
  - Alcohol
  - Sedative withdrawal

Hypersomnia
- Sleep apnoea/hypopnoea syndrome
- Intracranial space-occupying lesions
- Metabolic disorder
  - Uraemia
  - Hepatic failure
- Narcolepsy
- Kleine–Levin syndrome
- Idiopathic (sleep drunkenness)
- Drugs
  - Benzodiazepines
  - Barbiturates
  - Phenothiazines
  - Tricyclic antidepressants

anxious personalities. Such people tend to be highly aroused and stay awake thinking about stressful situations and planning how to cope. In others, their reports of poor sleep may be due to stimulants such as coffee, tea or smoking cigarettes, and there is a high rate of reported poor sleep in patients with an alcohol problem. The normal requirement for sleep varies widely, and a small number of individuals require only 3–4 hours of sleep each night. During a painful physical illness, or in a person with respiratory difficulties, the causes of disturbed sleep will be obvious. Poor nutritional status and low weight may also be accompanied by diminished sleep.

A change in sleep pattern is extremely common in all forms of mood disturbance. The manic patient may remain cheerful and active throughout the night and show little sign of fatigue, whereas the anxiety-prone patient may have difficulty falling to sleep because of worrying thoughts. In depression there may be initial, middle and late insomnia, early morning wakening being one of the features of endogenous or melancholic depression. Such subjects may wake 2–3 hours

earlier than normal, feeling depressed and dreading the coming day.

Hypersomnia may be the complaint of someone who lacks a day-time schedule and has no motivation to rise. Poor motivation and the effects of medication can account for the apparently increased sleep of some psychiatric patients, especially those with a schizophrenic defect state.

In *narcolepsy*, the person experiences bouts of drowsiness leading to short periods of sleep of a few minutes' duration recurring two or three times a day. The condition may be associated with cataplexy, a sudden loss of muscle tone lasting for a few seconds, often triggered by strong emotions. Other features of the condition include sleep paralysis, in which the subject is momentarily paralysed and unable to move (as happens sometimes with normal people awaking from a bad dream), and hypnagogic hallucinations which may be auditory, visual or tactile. Usually, the diagnosis of narcolepsy is made from the clinical history and electroencephalography findings that on falling asleep the patient goes spontaneously into rapid eye movement (REM) sleep, without passing through a non-REM stage.

One rare form of hypersomnia that usually occurs in young men is the *Kleine–Levin syndrome*. The patient sleeps excessively by day and night but is rousable. Such patients often eat excessively. *Organic lesions of the midbrain or hypothalamus* may also cause increased hunger, weight gain and drowsiness. The abrupt onset of daytime sleepiness or drowsiness should, however, immediately alert the clinician to the possibility of an intracranial space-occupying lesion. When unusual behaviour patterns during sleep develop suddenly in a patient, a drug effect should be rapidly excluded.

Nightmares are a normal phenomenon with no psychiatric significance. Frequent nightmares may occur during anxiety states and depression, in post-traumatic stress disorders, and with alcohol abuse or following a change of hypnotic. *Sleep walking* and *night terrors* may be familial, and can be precipitated by drugs such as antidepressants, anticonvulsants, analgesics, lithium and phenothiazines. These sometimes follow a febrile illness. A child experiencing a night terror which usually occurs within the first 2 hours of sleep may sit up with an expression of fear and remain oblivious to the surroundings for a few minutes before dropping soundly to sleep again. The child will have no memory of the event in the morning. Sometimes, *sleep walking* occurs during a night terror. Usually, patients will sleep walk in a calm, gentle way, but sleep walkers are at high risk of injuring themselves by falling downstairs or through windows. The subject is in a state of automatism and may walk some distance and carry out quite complicated series of actions. Both night terrors and sleep walking are more frequent during times of stress, and families will require reassurance.

In *bruxism*, the grinding of teeth during the night causes dental problems, and can be provoked by psychotropic medication. *Nocturnal enuresis* is a common occurrence, and multifactorial sources of stress should be sought in a family when this develops in a child after a period of established bladder control.

Sleep apnoea/hypopnoea syndrome

The major complaint of patients with the sleep apnoea/hypopnoea syndrome is usually day-time sleepiness which may vary in severity from trivial to dangerous. Indeed, many patients fall asleep during driving, working or in mid-conversation. The patient is usually unaware of the hundreds of brief awakenings per night which result in the day-time sleepiness, although around one-third of patients are aware of awaking occasionally at night with choking episodes. The sleep disruption results from total or partial occlusion of the upper airway at the level of the soft palate or tongue each time a patient goes to sleep. This produces apnoeas or severe hypopnoeas which are only terminated when the patient awakens briefly, perhaps, due to the fall in arterial oxygen levels. The awakening is so brief that the patient is not aware of it, but it is sufficient to increase the tone to the upper airway-opening muscles, and breathing resumes for a few seconds until the patient goes back to sleep and becomes apnoeic or hypopnoeic again. Patients do not find nocturnal sleep satisfying and sometimes awaken with a headache. Their bed partners report very loud snoring punctuated with breathing pauses, and that the patient is a very restless sleeper, often thrashing around the bed.

This condition affects around 1 per cent of adults, with 85 per cent of patients being male and 50 per cent being overweight. Severe long-standing cases, particularly in patients with co-existing lung disease, may be complicated by cyanosis (see CYANOSIS, p. 133) and right heart failure.

Boris Lams

SMELL, ABNORMALITIES OF

Abnormalities of the sense of smell are commonplace, and most people will have experienced this at some time or other. Although some claim increased sensitivity to odours (*hyperosmia*), this is not a pathological condition, merely an expression of normal variation. Similarly, some normal people seem perversely unaware of smells (*hyposmia*), yet are able to perceive other odours. This too is rarely abnormal. Complete loss of the sense of smell (*anosmia*) through one or both nostrils is of importance as it may be treatable and can be a sign of potentially serious disease. Perhaps more disturbing for the patient is distortion of the sense of smell (*dysosmia*), or the perception of non-existent odours (*parosmia*). The common causes of anosmia are listed in Table S.9.

Table S.9 Causes of anosmia

Nasal obstruction
- Rhinitis and rhino-sinusitis
- Deviated nasal septum
- Sino-nasal malignancy

Abnormalities of the olfactory mucosa
- Rhinitis medicamentosa and atrophic rhinitis
- Post-viral neuropathy

Abnormalities of the olfactory nerves and pathways
- Congenital absence
- Trauma
- Neoplasia (olfactory neuroblastoma, meningioma)
- Alzheimer's, Parkinson's disease, Huntington's chorea, temporal lobe epilepsy

Psychological

Reduced or total loss of the sense of smell is a common accompaniment of *rhinitis* and *rhino-sinusitis*. Polyps are usually clearly visible by inspection of the nasal cavities, and occasionally in severe cases protrude from the nose (Figs S.36 and S.37). Sometimes, mucopus can been seen escaping from under the middle turbinate, indicating paranasal sinus infection. However, signs of infection may not be apparent on clinical examination and are only evident after scanning the patient. Treatment of rhinitis or rhino-sinusitis by medical or surgical means may restore the sense of smell for some. Patients who lose their sense of smell after viral infection, but have no obvious residual sepsis,

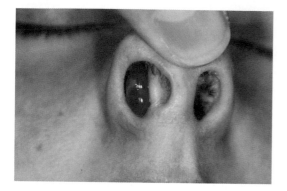

Figure S.36 A simple nasal polyp that was easily seen by elevation of the nasal tip.

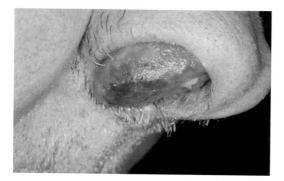

Figure S.37 A large nasal polyp that has prolapsed through the nostril. In severe, bilateral cases the polyps expand and distort the nostrils so much that the patient develops the so-called 'frog face' deformity.

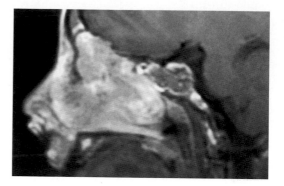

Figure S.38 Magnetic resonance scan of an extensive olfactory neuroblastoma that developed in a 17-year-old girl. Her presenting symptoms were long-standing anosmia and more recent nasal obstruction.

damage to the olfactory nerves. Common causes include head injury, tumours and nasal infection. Olfactory hallucinations represent a common and striking symptom of partial seizures originating in the medial aspect of the temporal lobe (uncinate seizures). These hallucinations tend to be pungent, sometimes likened to burning rubber, or a smell of gas. Olfactory hallucination is not uncommon in psychosis, when unpleasant smells may be attributed either to the patient him/herself, or to others. Patients with rhinoliths sometimes describe an offensive smell that is not always apparent to others.

Michael Gleeson

may also be helped by topical steroid drops, but these fortunate patients are few and far between. Those who lose their sense of smell as a result of an anterior cranial base fracture rarely, if ever, recover it.

Tumours affecting or arising in or around the cribriform plate of the ethmoid produce a slowly progressive deterioration and loss of the sense of smell. *Olfactory neuroblastoma* (aesthesioneuroblastoma), meningioma and juvenile angiofibroma are the most common tumours in this region, and it is prudent to remember that they may develop in relatively young patients. Loss of the sense of smell is an early symptom and sign in these patients and becomes established well before proptosis, nasal obstruction and blood-stained nasal discharge (Fig. S.38).

Parosmia is a perverted sense of smell that is characteristically unpleasant and usually develops after

SNEEZING

Sneezing is usually initiated by irritation of the nasal mucosa, especially that of the anterior part of the nasal septum or the turbinates. The sneeze reflex is protective in nature and essentially similar to the cough reflex. It is a sudden and involuntary expulsion of air through the nose and mouth, and is controlled by a reflex initiated by the Vth and Xth cranial nerves. Sneezing may be caused by local irritation or increased sensitivity of the nasal mucosa. The early stage of the common cold is probably the most common cause of sneezing that subsides once the bacterial secondary infection supervenes with a thicker nasal discharge. Sneezing is common in the prodromal stages of measles and the other infectious fevers, but is not common in more chronic nasal infections.

The inhalation of fine dusts and powders causes sneezing due to local irritation. Riot control gas and war gases irritate the eyes as well as the nasal mucosa; lacrimation, nasal discharge and sneezing may be incapacitating to those exposed. Some individuals are particularly sensitive to changes of temperature and light. Many people sneeze once or twice on their first exposure to bright light. Bouts of sneezing are frequently observed in individuals with atopic sensitization to airborne allergens. When the nasal mucosa encounters an allergen to which the individual is sensitized, inflammatory mediators are released from mast cells and basophils, and these may cause sneezing.

Michael Gleeson

SNORING

Snoring is the noise produced in sleep by the vibration of the soft palate and the tongue base. A differentiation is made between simple snorers and patients with obstructive sleep apnoea (OSA) (see also SLEEP, DISORDERS OF, p. 655). Whilst in simple snorers the blood oxygen saturation does not fall significantly, in patients with OSA the upper airway collapse results in recurrent periods of apnoea, blood oxygen desaturation and subsequent arousal reactions. This disorder may lead to fatigue, loss of energy during the day, changes in personality and, in severe cases, to pulmonary hypertension and right ventricular strain.

It is now considered that a continuous spectrum exists between uncomplicated simple snoring and the obstructive sleep apnoea syndrome. Simple snorers may develop OSA after the ingestion of alcohol. Snoring is more common in obese people, and in many patients a change in lifestyle (loss of weight, reduction of alcohol consumption) may improve their symptoms. In selected cases, appropriate surgical treatment aiming at the portion of the airways that is responsible for the vibration or collapse may be beneficial. In children, snoring is most often due to adenoid or tonsillar hypertrophy, and may be cured by adenotonsillectomy. Patients with nasal obstruction may benefit from septoplasty or sinus surgery.

If redundancy of the soft palate and lateral pharyngeal walls are the source of the problem, surgical resection may be effective, a procedure known as uvulopharyngopalatoplasty (UPPP). Cases of tongue base collapse are more difficult to treat surgically, but may be improved by use of a mandibular advancement device.

Michael Gleeson

SPEECH, ABNORMALITIES OF

Speech and language are complex functions that are critical for normal human social interaction. Language disorders involve the abnormal production or comprehension of written or spoken language; those due to acquired brain disease (usually focal) are termed dysphasia or aphasia. Although speech production is often disrupted in disorders of language, this entry is limited to speech disorders in which language function is preserved. The disorders to be considered here are dysarthria and dysphonia.

Dysarthria is a motor disorder of speech production due to dysfunction of the muscles of articulation. *Dysphonia* is a motor disorder of voice production. *Apraxia of speech* is a rare disorder of speech motor function unaccounted for by disease of the muscles of articulation or their innervation, and is considered elsewhere (see APRAXIA, p. 39).

A classification of developmental speech and language delay is provided in Table S.10.

Table S.10 Classification of developmental speech and language delay

Cerebral palsy
Hearing disorders
Acquired lesions causing aphasia (e.g. Landau–Kleffner syndrome)
Congenital deafness
Congenital word deafness
Congenital inarticulation
Stuttering and stammering
Cluttered speech
Other articulatory defects
Developmental dyslexia
Developmental dysgraphia
Developmental dyscalculia

Dysarthria

Speech production requires a complex integration of motor actions, and consists of respiration, phonation, articulation, resonance and prosody. The respiratory muscles are important so that expiration occurs with appropriate duration, force and flexibility. Intact anatomy and function of the respiratory muscles, larynx, palate, nasal passages, tongue and lips are required for normal speech. The respiratory muscles (intercostal muscles and diaphragm) are supplied by the phrenic nerve, which arises from cervical segments 3, 4 and 5. The larynx, pharynx, tongue and lips receive lower motor neurone innervation from the trigeminal, facial, vagus and hypoglossal cranial nerve nuclei. The nuclei of these nerves are in turn controlled by upper motor neurone descending pathways from the speech motor cortex (the corticobulbar tracts). Pure dysarthria does not involve a dysfunction of cortical language functions, so that comprehension, reading and writing are intact. It is convenient to subdivide dysarthria into lower motor neurone, upper motor neurone (pseudobulbar), cerebellar (ataxic), hyperkinetic and hypokinetic. The dysarthria that commonly results from a unilateral cortical or subcortical stroke does not fall into any of the above categories.

Lower motor neurone dysarthria

Involvement of the lower motor neurone innervation of the bulbar muscles (cranial nerve nuclei or below) produces this type of speech, which is characterized by weak, imprecise articulation and poor breathing support. Air escaping through the nose due to palatal weakness causes hypernasality. The tongue may be weak and fasciculating, palatal movements may be reduced, and the ability to cough explosively may be lost due to vocal cord paralysis. This pattern may also be termed a *bulbar palsy*. The lesion can be in the cranial nerve nuclei, the cranial nerves themselves, or the muscles of the pharynx and tongue. Causes include the motor neurone diseases, though in the commonest form – amyotrophic lateral sclerosis – upper motor neurone features will also be present. Pure lower motor neurone diseases include X-linked bulbospinal neuronopathy (Kennedy syndrome, with gynaecomastia and diabetes), multifocal motor neuropathy and the post-polio syndrome. Other causes of bulbar palsy include cranial polyneuropathies due to meningeal disease, myasthenia gravis, lower brainstem stroke, or muscle diseases involving the bulbar muscles such as polymyositis, dermatomyositis or oculopharyngeal muscular dystrophy.

Upper motor neurone dysarthria

Involvement of the upper motor neurone pathway to the bulbar cranial nerves produces a pseudobulbar palsy. The type of speech that results is termed *spastic dysarthria*; the tongue is immobile and spastic, so that speech has a strangled, effortful quality, sometimes with associated spastic dysphonia, and it is often slow. Bilateral involvement of either the cortex or descending pathways is necessary to produce pseudobulbar palsy, though in the case of multiple strokes there may be old pre-existing lesions followed by a strategically placed acute infarct causing a sudden presentation with dysarthria or anarthria (inability to produce any intelligible speech). Other causes of pseudobulbar palsy include motor neurone disease with upper motor neurone involvement, multiple sclerosis, large frontal tumours and cerebral palsy. Associated features of a classical pseudobulbar palsy (reflecting damage to frontal cortex descending projections) are emotional lability with inability to suppress laughter or crying, and a 'frontal' gait disturbance with small stuttering steps, termed *marche à petit pas*.

Cerebellar dysarthria

Cerebellar dysarthria may present with slurred speech, superficially resembling alcohol intoxication. However, there are often additional problems of 'scanning' or explosive speech, due to an inability to modulate accurately the rhythm, rate and force of speech. Cerebellar dysarthria may result from focal damage to the vermis or to more widespread damage to the whole cerebellum (or its connections). Any disease affecting the cerebellum can cause this pattern of dysarthria; causes include multiple sclerosis, cerebellar degeneration (e.g. paraneoplastic cerebellar degeneration, spinocerebellar degenerations, alcohol), stroke, vitamin E deficiency, hypothyroidism and coeliac disease.

Extrapyramidal dysarthria

Extrapyramidal diseases result from pathology of the basal ganglia, are attributed to neurotransmitter abnormalities (e.g. dopaminergic neurone loss in Parkinson's disease), and cause abnormal control of volitional movement. Some extrapyramidal diseases (e.g. Parkinson's disease) cause slowness of movement and rigidity (hence the term 'akinetic–rigid syndrome'), which may impact on speech as well as limb motor control. In other extrapyramidal disorders (e.g. Huntington's disease), basal ganglia pathology causes an excess of involuntary movements that interfere with normal volitional movement. It follows from the above that two types of speech disorder may be seen in extrapyramidal diseases: hypokinetic and hyperkinetic.

In Parkinson's disease, the speech is hypokinetic. The range of articulation is reduced, breathing support is poor, and the volume is low. The speech may be either slow and monotonous, or produced in short, rapid phrases. In the early stages the only abnormality might be a slight loss of prosody (emphasis and inflections), whereas in the late stages of Parkinson's disease the speech may be virtually inaudible and unintelligible. Palilalia may be seen, in which there is repetition of a phrase, which the patient reiterates with increasing rapidity.

Hyperkinetic dysarthria results from chorea, orofacial dyskinesia and athetosis (see CHOREA, p. 109). Articulation is interrupted by involuntary movements, producing jerky and irregular speech with reduced intelligibility.

Dysphonia

Spastic dysphonia

Spastic dysphonia, also termed spasmodic dysphonia or laryngeal dystonia, is a form of focal dystonia (i.e. a disorder of involuntary muscle movement and postures), thought to be due to abnormal functioning in the basal ganglia. It may be primary or secondary to another neurological disorder. The muscles of the larynx contract so that, in the adductor type, the vocal cords are brought together and speech is effortful, strained and strangled. Symptoms may improve or disappear temporarily either spontaneously or when yawning, laughing, singing or relaxing. In the abductor type, there is an excessive action of the muscles that open up the vocal cords, resulting in a disjointed, breathy, whispering voice pattern. Adductor and abductor spasms may co-exist, causing an irregular voice tremor. Upper motor neurone disorders affecting the vagus – and hence the recurrent laryngeal innervated muscles – may produce a spastic dysphonia, which can be associated with spastic dysarthria.

Flaccid dysphonia

Lower motor neurone damage to either the vagus nerve, the recurrent laryngeal nerve or the vocal cord muscles, may cause the more common flaccid dysphonia. Patients may also have a 'bovine cough'. This type of dysphonia most commonly results from isolated damage to one of the recurrent laryngeal nerves. It may also be seen in poliomyelitis, motor neurone disease, cranial polyneuropathies, myasthenia gravis and some rare forms of muscle disease.

David Werring

SPINE, DEFORMITY OF

Definitions of terms

Unfortunately, these are confusing since the same terms, kyphosis and lordosis, are used to describe both normal and abnormal curves:

- Kyphosis: this is a smooth flexion curve.
  - *Normal thoracic kyphosis* describes the normal gentle forward curve of the thoracic spine.
  - *Postural kyphosis* describes a poor posture with 'drooping shoulders', which is voluntarily correctable.
  - *Compensatory kyphosis* means an increased curve of the thoracic spine secondary to some other fixed deformity such as increased lumbar lordosis.
  - *Structural kyphosis* is fixed and is associated with changes in the shape of several vertebrae with increased wedging anteriorly. Causes include Scheurmann's disease (adolescent kyphosis), osteoporosis and ankylosing spondylitis.
- Kyphos: this is also referred to as a 'gibbus'. In contradistinction to a kyphosis, a kyphos is a sharp, acute-angle deformity due to localized collapse or wedging of one or more vertebrae. A kyphos due to the collapse of just one vertebra is surprisingly easy to overlook. The best way to detect it is to run a finger down the spine with the patient lying prone. A progressive kyphos has a high risk of being complicated by paraplegia. Therefore this deformity is an important sign to be able to detect. The changes on a lateral X-ray are always more dramatic than the physical signs.
- Lordosis: this is a smooth extension curve.
  - *Normal cervical or lumbar lordosis* describes the standing posture of these two areas of the spine.

◆ *Compensatory lordosis* indicates an increased curve secondary to a structural kyphosis of the thoracic spine.

◆ *An increased structural lordosis* does not fully correct on forward flexion and is associated with underlying bony abnormality, for example a spondylolisthesis.

■ Scoliosis: this is a lateral curve. It is designated left or right according to the direction of the convexity of the curve. In reality it is not a simple lateral curve as it is always associated with a rotational deformity of the spine. The bodies rotate towards the convexity and the spines and neural arches rotate into the concavity.

■ Spondylolisthesis: this is a forward slip of a vertebral body on the vertebra immediately below.

Kyphosis

Congenital kyphosis occurs when there is a failure of vertebral segmentation involving several vertebrae and the anterior bone block acts as a tether.

Adolescent kyphosis (Scheuermann's disease) is, as the name implies, a condition that starts at puberty. The patient becomes progressively more round-shouldered, and there is a smooth thoracic kyphosis with a compensatory lumbar lordosis. Boys are affected twice as commonly as girls. Approximately 50 per cent of children will have some pain over the apex of the curve, but this is usually mild. Neurological complications can occur, but are rare. Very occasionally, if the deformity is severe, it may interfere with normal lung function.

Inflammatory kyphosis (also termed 'ankylosing spondylitis; see BACK, PAIN IN, p. 58) is a condition that usually progresses from the sacroiliac joints to involve the lumbar spine, thoracic spine and finally the cervical spine. It is usually associated with a kyphotic deformity, a straightening out of the lumbar lordosis and increased thoracic kyphosis. These deformities are often associated with fixed flexion deformities of the hips which greatly exaggerate the bent posture (see Figs B.3 and B.4).

Metabolic causes of kyphosis

Osteoporosis is the most common cause of an increased thoracic kyphosis in which anterior wedging of the bodies of the vertebrae produces a structural deformity. The kyphosis can be so severe as to result in impingement of the costal margin onto the iliac crest. If the deformity is of relatively sudden onset it is important to exclude other serious underlying diseases such as multiple myeloma. It is also easy to assume that

the cause is osteoporosis and to miss the diagnosis of osteomalacia.

Kyphos

Due to the sharp, acute-angle deformity there is a much greater risk of neurological involvement, particularly when it affects the thoracic spine. The cord is at greater risk of compression than the cauda equina, which commences at the level of the L1 vertebra.

Congenital kyphos: this results from a defect of the formation of one or more vertebral bodies. In mild cases there may be a failure of just part of a single vertebra, while in severe types there may be a total absence of the vertebral body. The deformity increases markedly during growth, and may lead to paraplegia.

Traumatic kyphos results from a wedge crush fracture. The most common cause is osteoporosis, but the differential diagnosis includes metastatic disease and multiple myeloma. A sharp, angulated kyphos can also occur after a major fracture dislocation, the thoracolumbar region being the most commonly affected site.

Infective kyphos due to pyogenic infection is increasing in frequency due to the longevity of the population in general and the rising incidence of specific illnesses, for example diabetes, HIV and drug addiction. It is an easily missed cause of pyrexia in intensive care units, where it is usually secondary to blood-borne infection from intravenous cannulae. Classically, X-rays show destruction of the intervertebral disc and adjacent end plates – 'two bodies and the intervening disc' (see SPINE, TENDERNESS OF, p. 664, and Figs S.49–S.53).

Chronic infection: tuberculosis

Classically, this is a paradiskal infection affecting the anterior distal aspect of the 'body above' and the anterior superior aspect of the 'body below'. While cervical spinal tuberculosis is the most common site in children, thoracic disease classically affects adolescents and young adults. As with pyogenic infection, the lateral X-ray shows the involvement of two bodies and the intervening disc. With progression of the disease the adjacent vertebral bodies become involved and the predominantly anterior destruction of the bodies leads to a sharp angular kyphos (Fig. S.39). Large abscesses may develop and migrate considerable distances; for example, a psoas abscess presenting in the groin (Fig. S.40). Spinal cord compression (Pott's paraplegia) may supervene, either with the active disease due to a compression by caseous pus, inflammatory oedema and angulation, or late in the healed disease due to stretching of the cord over the bony ridge of the apex of the deformity. In the former situation, where the compression is 'soft', there is usually a good response to conservative therapy, antibiotics and, if necessary, drainage (now possible by aspiration under CT guidance). In the latter situation, surgery is essential to relieve the mechanical compression from the hard bony ridge.

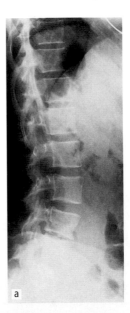

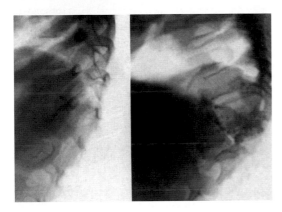

Figure S.39 Tuberculosis of the spine. The thoracic spine is particularly at risk from progressive deformity and neurological complications as the vertebral bodies subsequently collapse. The natural lordotic posture of the lumbar spine provides some protection against vertebral collapse, while the cauda equina is less susceptible to compression than the cord.

Lordosis

An increased lumbar lordosis is most commonly compensatory, secondary to fixed flexion deformities of the hips, and is therefore found in nearly all hip disease. An increased lumbar lordosis is one of the classical signs of untreated congenital dislocation of the hips and also infantile coxa vara.

Scoliosis

There are two fundamental types of scoliosis: postural and structural (Table S.11).

Postural scoliosis

This is secondary to some other condition. For example, a short lower limb will produce compensatory

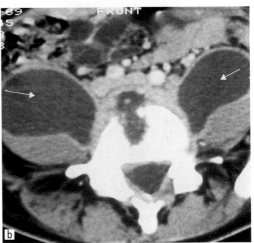

Figure S.40 Note loss of the lumbar lordosis but absence of vertebral body collapse (a), despite the extent of vertebral body infection and the presence of large psoas abscesses (arrowed) shown by the MRI scan.

scoliosis convex to the side of the short leg. The scoliosis therefore disappears and the spine reverts to its straight position when the patient is examined sitting. If it is secondary to a poor stance, then scoliosis disappears on forward flexion to touch the toes. This type of scoliosis is of little importance.

Structural scoliosis

This type does not disappear on sitting or on forward flexion. It is always associated with rotation, which produces the characteristic rib hump and is most noticeable on forward flexion. On the concave side, the scapula is usually elevated and the hip is prominent (Figs S.41–S.43).

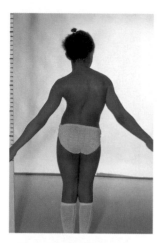

Figure S.41 Adolescent kyphoscoliosis. Thoracic curve convex to the right.

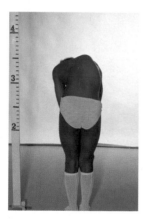

Figure S.42 The rib hump, indicative of the rotational component, becomes evident on forward flexion.

Idiopathic adolescent scoliosis accounts for 80 per cent of patients presenting with a structural scoliosis. It is important to exclude the other causes and to monitor the rate of progression of the deformity. This type of scoliosis is familial. Pain is an uncommon feature in childhood, although it may occur later in life secondary to degenerative change occurring in the curve segment. The classical cause of a painful scoliosis in a teenager or young adult is an osteoid osteoma

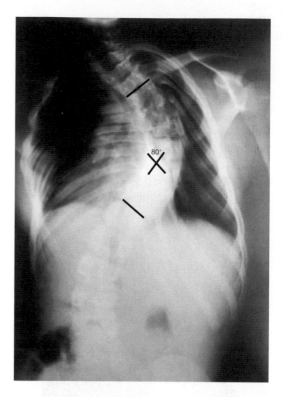

Figure S.43 Same patient as Fig. S.41. Standing X-ray taken postero-anteriorly. The deformity (the Cobb angle) is 80°. Note the clinical deformity seen in Fig. S.41 underestimates the true deformity as the spinous processes rotate inwards to the concavity (i.e. they remain more central) (see Fig. C.3).

Table S.11 Classification of structural scoliosis

Idiopathic
  Early onset (infantile)
  Adolescent

Congenital
  Failure of formation
  Failure of segmentation

Trauma
  Vertebral injuries
  Spondylolisthesis

Infection
  Pyogenic infection
  Tuberculosis

Neuromuscular (paralytic)
  Myelodysplasia
    (spinal dysraphism)
  Diastematomyelia
  Syringomyelia

  Muscular dystrophies
  Cerebral palsy
  Friedreich's ataxia
  Poliomyelitis

Syndromal (dystrophic)
  Neurofibromatosis
  Osteogenesis imperfecta
  Ehlers–Danlos syndrome
  Marfan's syndrome
  Osteochondrodystrophies
  Mucopolysaccharidoses

Tumours and 'tumour-like' conditions
  Intradural
  Extradural
  Osteoid osteoma (N.B. this
    causes painful scoliosis)

(Figs S.44–S.46) (see also LOWER LIMB, PAIN IN, p. 404, Figs L.54–56; and BACK, PAIN IN, Spinal tumours, p. 61).

Infantile scoliosis develops before the age of 3 years but, unlike the congenital variety (Fig. S.47), there are no vertebral bony abnormalities. The curve improves, or even resolves spontaneously. There is an association with plagiocephaly, and sometimes a postural adduction contracture of one hip.

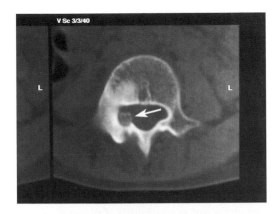

Figure S.46 Same patient as Fig. S.44. CT scan showing the lesion (arrowed) and the reactive sclerosis.

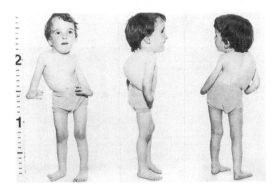

Figure S.47 Congenital kyphoscoliosis. Note the radial club hands due to absence of the radii.

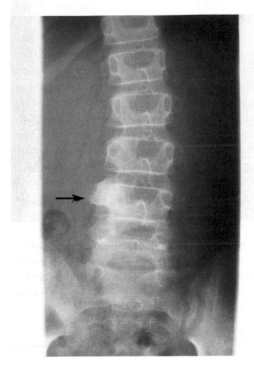

Figure S.44 Osteoid osteoma is a rare but classical cause of a painful scoliosis, though in this example the spinal deformity is minimal. Analgesics, especially aspirin, give excellent pain relief. Anteroposterior X-ray showing dense sclerosis of the pedicle of L4 (arrowed).

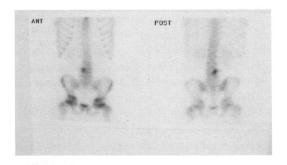

Figure S.45 Same patient as Fig. S.44. Technetium scan with a localized 'hot-spot'.

Torticollis (wry neck)

The congenital variety is due to a unilateral contracture of the sternocleidomastoid muscle, and produces a deformity in which the head is tilted to the ipsilateral side whilst the chin is rotated to the contralateral side. A rare cause of a torticollis is the Klippel–Feil syndrome, which is a congenital fusion of two or more vertebrae in the cervical region. There may be other associated abnormalities such as a congenital high scapula, or Sprengel's deformity (see UPPER LIMB, PAIN IN, p. 741, Fig. U.2).

Spondylolisthesis

This is a forward shift of one vertebral body on another. The levels are nearly always L4 on L5, or L5 on the sacrum. The whole lumbar spine therefore slips forward in relation to the sacrum and the pelvis. As a consequence, the lumbar spine appears shortened, transverse skin creases are present, and the sacrum seems to extend upwards towards the waist. A 'step' may be present; this is best felt by running a finger down the lumbar spine. There is often associated hamstring tightness.

Spondylolisthesis is subdivided into: 'dysplastic', in which the slip is secondary to congenital changes in the upper part of the sacrum and vertebral arch of L5; 'isthmic', which accounts for the majority of the cases and is caused by a stress fracture through, or elongation of, the pars interarticularis of the vertebral arch (Fig. S.48); 'traumatic', due to an acute fracture; and 'degenerative', which occurs as a result of disc degeneration and facet joint osteoarthritis. The term 'spondylolysis' refers to a defect of the pars

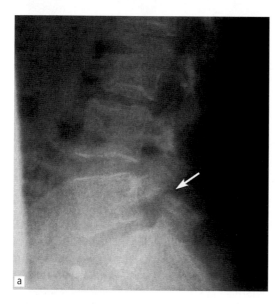

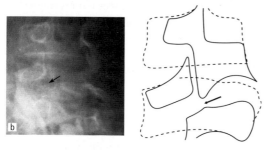

Figure S.48 Spondylolysis. A stress fracture (arrowed) through the pars interarticularis in an athlete presenting with backache. (a) Lateral X-ray; (b) oblique view: 'the collar on the Scottie dog'.

interarticularis but the vertebral bodies remain aligned (i.e. there is no forward slip).

Fred Heatley

SPINE, TENDERNESS OF

See also BACK, PAIN IN (p. 51) and SPINE, DEFORMITY OF (p. 659).

Tenderness of the spine is usually due to local disease of, or injury to, the tissues at the site of tenderness. Such tenderness is always deep, but may also be associated with cutaneous hyperalgesia. In a second and less important group, the tenderness is partly or entirely cutaneous, and is a referred phenomenon found in visceral disease. In testing for spinal tenderness it is therefore desirable to differentiate between cutaneous and deep tenderness and, in the case of the latter, between tenderness elicited by pressing upon the spinous processes and tenderness in the adjacent muscles. This is because spinal disease is usually accompanied by local muscular spasm and the muscles thus affected become tender, although they are not themselves the site of the disease. Failure to allow for this fact is the usual explanation of the mistakes – sometimes serious – which are often made in attributing muscle tenderness to a strain or to a rheumatic condition when in reality it is due to local spasm in response to disease of the vertebrae, the intervertebral discs, or to the spinal cord and its membranes.

The chief conditions in which spinal tenderness occurs are summarized in Table S.12.

The investigation of spinal tenderness requires an exhaustive case history, a careful examination and certain special investigations.

The *history* is of particular importance, because not only will it disclose the duration, site and severity of the spinal symptoms, but it will also indicate whether the spinal cord or nerve roots are involved (root pain, girdle sensations, paraesthesiae in the limb, muscular weakness or stiffness, sphincter disturbances). A systematic interrogation as to general health, previous diseases, and symptoms referable to the other systems of the body may bring out facts relevant to the spinal condition. There is no laboratory procedure which can provide this information, and a further advantage of the historical approach is that it provides a guide to the

Table S.12 The main conditions in which spinal tenderness occurs

Diseases of the overlying skin and subcutaneous tissue
These are rare and clinically obvious

Diseases of the vertebral column
Traumatic
Fracture
Dislocation
Disc herniation
Spondylolisthesis
Infective
Pyogenic
Staphylococcus
A wide variety of organisms may be present in spinal
infection in immunocompromised/AIDS/drug-addicted patients
Chronic
Tubercular: Pott's disease
Salmonella typhi: typhoid spine
Brucellosis
Actinomycosis
Hydatid disease
Inflammatory
Ankylosing spondylitis
Degenerative (mechanical)
Herniation of nucleus pulposus (prolapsed disc)
Spondylosis
Osteochondritis (rarely causes tenderness)
Spondylolisthesis
Neoplastic
Metastases
Myeloma (see NECK, PAIN IN; Fig. N.16, p. 475)

Leukaemic deposits
Benign and malignant bone tumours (see LOWER LIMB PAIN, in
and around the knee; tumours, p. 400)
Erosion by aortic aneurysm

Diseases of the spinal cord and meninges
Metastatic epidural abscess or tumour
Meningioma
Neurofibroma
Herpes zoster
Meningitis serosa circumscripta
Tumour of the spinal cord
Syringomyelia

Metabolic disorders
Osteoporosis
Osteomalacia
Hyperparathyroidism
Paget's disease

Referred causes
N.B. Tenderness over the spine corresponds to segmental
innervation of the viscus

Hysteria and malingering
Compensation neurosis (see BACKACHE, p. 62)

---

patient's mental and emotional conditions, which is invaluable in assessing the reality and severity of the spinal symptoms.

The second step, a *physical examination*, must cover the whole body in a search for factors which may throw light on the spinal tenderness. Reference has already been made to the need for care in determining that the tenderness is really in the spine itself, and not in the adjacent muscles or the overlying skin. (A useful method for examining the vertebrae is to gently 'spring' each spinous process, starting proximally and moving distally. To do this, lie the patient down prone, and using the hypothenar eminence of one's hand apply a sudden but relatively gentle pressure to each spinous process in turn.) Acute tenderness of organic origin is always associated with limitation of movement in one or more directions. Beware of the spine that has loss of movement in all directions. Assume that such a spine has an infective, inflammatory or neoplastic problem until proven otherwise. The characteristic of

mechanical derangement in the spine is that movement in at least one direction remains almost full. For example, a patient presenting with an acute lumbar disc associated with a lumbar tilt/scoliosis will retain a good range of movement on lateral flexion towards the side of the tilt. The examination of sensation, power and reflexes below the level of tenderness is important for significant neurological abnormalities may be found in the absence of any subjective symptoms. Attention must be paid to the chest, cardiovascular system, abdomen and prostate. The long bones should receive attention, and the skull must not be forgotten, because in carcinomatosis painless secondary deposits may be found in the latter.

Of the special investigations, X-ray examination of the spine takes the first place. The earliest X-ray changes of pyogenic infection are often fluffiness along the lower border of the body (i.e. at the inferior end plate). The characteristic of established infection is involvement of two bodies and the intervening disc (Figs S.49–S.51).

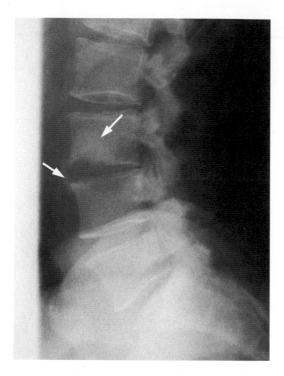

Figure S.49 *Staphylococcus aureus* infection. This began either as a discitis (left arrow) or an osteomyelitis (right arrow) of the distal aspect of the body of L3.

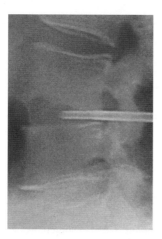

Figure S.50 Same patient as Fig. S.49. Aspiration under radiological guidance to establish the bacterial diagnosis. Note: a wide variety of organisms can be found in immunocompromised/AIDS patients and drug addicts.

Anatomically, the infection is reflecting the original segmentation which is half a vertebral body, the disc and half a vertebral body. Metastatic deposits classically show as loss of a pedicle on the anteroposterior film of

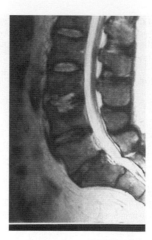

Figure S.51 Same patient as Fig. S.49. MRI reveals that the disease is more extensive than was suggested on the plain X-rays. Both bodies, L3 and L4, are involved – 'two bodies and the intervening disc' – which is the classical pattern of spinal infection.

the spine, and this is easy to miss in a poor-quality X-ray. Lesions in the sacrum are notoriously difficult to appreciate on plain films. Evidence of local disease may be long delayed, and it is dangerous to assume that a negative finding is conclusive. CT scanning provides very accurate delineation of the spinal anatomy, especially the bony anatomy. In general, the soft tissue anatomy is best shown on an MRI scan.

Check the ESR as well as the haemoglobin, WBC and electrolytes. A raised ESR requires further thought before attributing backache to a mechanical cause. A rise in the serum acid phosphatase or serum or prostate-specific antigen will suggest the presence of a secondary growth from the prostate, whilst a high alkaline phosphatase is found in Paget's disease. A raised serum calcium level may suggest hyperparathyroidism.

Tenderness in the spine due to disease in other parts of the body

Superficial tenderness over the spine is a common association of visceral disease, and the tenderness is situated over the portion of the spine corresponding to the segmental innervation of the affected viscus. The tenderness is not associated with local rigidity, and there is invariably well-marked evidence of the visceral disease, so that such tenderness should not be mistaken for a manifestation of spinal disease (Figs S.52 and S.53). However, it is easy to be confused.

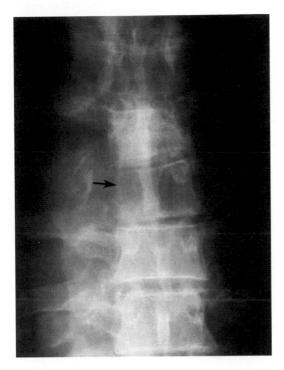

Figure S.52 Spinal metastasis. This patient presented with persistent backache and weight loss. Tenderness was localized over the spinous process of T8. There was a loss of the right pedicle on anteroposterior X-ray (arrowed).

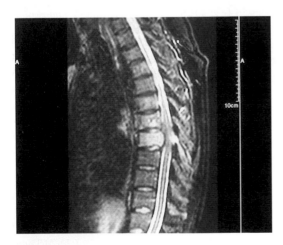

Figure S.53 Same patient as Fig. S.52. MRI scan showing involvement of the body with early collapse posteriorly onto the cord.

This is particularly the case in the elderly, the majority of whom will of course have abnormal findings on plain spinal X-rays. Thus, for example, attributing chest pain to a mechanical problem in the thoracic spine in a 70-year-old is a diagnosis that should only be made by *exclusion*!

Suspected intercostal nerve root entrapments can be confirmed by use of local anaesthetic. In the abdomen, these nerve roots are classically 'trapped' at the edge of the lateral border of the rectus abdominis. A useful physical sign is that the tenderness, which is often diffuse, will localize to this site if the abdominal muscles are contracted by asking the patient simply to raise the head and torso slightly off the bed whilst lying supine. In right iliac fossa tenderness these nerve root entrapments are a differential diagnosis for appendicitis, especially in patients in middle age.

Hysteria, malingering, compensation neurosis

Psychogenic factors are important to assess, especially in patients with chronic backache (see BACK, PAIN IN, p. 51). Excessive spinal tenderness is one of the 'inappropriate signs'. Characteristically, even the lightest touch to the skin of the back causes 'severe pain'. Frequently patients 'wobble' and may even lose their balance. By contrast, it is uncommon to find marked tenderness in most cases with serious underlying disease. For example, in spinal infection or ankylosing spondylitis one may need to 'spring the spine' to elicit any tenderness (see above).

Fred Heatley

SPLENOMEGALY

The causes of splenomegaly are numerous, and the most likely diagnosis varies considerably with the age, geographical location and social habits of the patient (Table S.13).

Patients with splenomegaly may present with the symptoms and signs of pancytopenia due to hypersplenism which may occur with only a modest enlargement of the organ. There is usually an approximately parallel reduction in erythrocytes, leucocytes and platelets, although on occasions there may be a more marked reduction of only one cell line. In the presence of such haematological abnormalities it is important to demonstrate normal or hyperplastic bone marrow morphology. In addition to the cellular elements being pooled and preferentially destroyed in the spleen, the cytopenias are often exacerbated by a consistent increase in plasma volume.

Table S.13 Causes of splenomegaly

Infections
Viruses
  Glandular fever
Bacterial
  Typhus
  Typhoid
  Septicaemia ('septic spleen')
Protozoal
  Malaria
  Kala-azar
  Egyptian splenomegaly (schistosomiasis)
Parasitic
  Hydatid

Congestion (portal hypertension)
Hepatic cirrhosis
Portal vein obstruction
Splenic vein obstruction
Budd–Chiari syndrome
Cardiac failure

Haemolytic anaemias
Haemolytic anaemia
Hereditary spherocytosis
Thalassaemias
Red-cell enzyme defects
Immune-mediated haemolysis

Haematological malignancies
Chronic myeloid leukaemia
Acute leukaemias
Chronic lymphatic leukaemia
Macroglobulinaemia
Polycythaemia rubra vera
Myelofibrosis
Essential thrombocythaemia
Lymphomas
  Hodgkin's disease
  Non-Hodgkin's disease
Hairy-cell leukaemia

Connective-tissue disorders
Systemic lupus erythematosus
Felty's syndrome

Storage disorders
Gaucher's disease
Niemann–Pick disease
Histiocytosis X

Space-occupying lesions
Abscess
Metastatic tumour
Cysts
  Hydatid
  Haemangioma
  Dermoid

Many diseases may result in enlargement of the spleen by several different mechanisms. For example, in schistosomiasis the spleen may be enlarged because of chronic infection as well as portal hypertension secondary to portal fibrosis. A grossly enlarged spleen has a vastly increased blood supply, and portal hypertension may result from the high blood flow. In myelofibrosis with gross splenomegaly, for example, such a high flow of its own accord may cause portal hypertension such that ascites develops. When this is observed the prognosis is usually poor and splenectomy should be considered.

A careful history and examination along with a full blood count and liver function tests will often provide a short differential diagnosis. If an infection is suspected, appropriate microbiological tests will need to be carried out. When difficulty is encountered it is usually necessary to undertake fairly wide-ranging investigations. These should start by confirming that the mass palpated is spleen and not another pathology. A trans-abdominal ultrasound examination will confirm the presence of a mass and also provide accurate dimensions; it is usually possible to distinguish between spleen and the other causes of a left upper quadrant mass (e.g. enlarged kidney). Furthermore, it may be valuable both for detecting space-occupying lesions (e.g. cysts or abscesses) and cases of portal hypertension or segmental portal hypertension (e.g. due to chronic pancreatitis). Endoscopic ultrasound does not seem to have any particular role. An abdominal CT scan with intravenous contrast delineates the size and consistency of the spleen, and is the investigation of choice if a lymphoma is suspected as it is useful for delineating retroperitoneal and mesenteric lymph nodes. Direct splenic puncture appears to be generally safe, and permits tissue sampling for infective causes of splenomegaly. It also enables a contrast splenic-portogram to be performed. Almost all causes of lymphadenopathy may be associated with splenomegaly and, failing positive findings in other investigations, a biopsy of an enlarged lymph node often renders a diagnosis.

John Meenan

SPUTUM

Normally about 100 ml of bronchial secretion is removed daily by ciliary action from the airways of the lung through the larynx and disposed of into the alimentary tract by unconscious acts of swallowing. Sputum consists of: (i) bronchial secretions in excess of the amount that can be disposed of in this way; (ii) pathological secretions, exudates and pus from abnormal bronchi, bronchioles and alveoli, or from abscesses, cavities or cysts in the lung; or (iii) material derived from morbid processes in pleura, lymph nodes, mediastinum, oesophagus, subphrenic space and liver which have ulcerated into the lung. It may be mixed with saliva and secretions from the upper respiratory tract, but should be distinguished from these.

The patient's account of its mode of production, quantity and quality of the sputum, and the physician's observations – especially the naked-eye appearances – often provide information at least as important as that derived from laboratory procedures.

Although the production of sputum is usually associated with cough, some chronic bronchitic patients deny cough, regarding the expectoration of mucus or even mucopus in the mornings as so 'normal' that they refer to it as 'clearing the throat'. Other patients, who evidently raise excess secretions from their lower respiratory tracts by cough, deny producing sputum because they habitually swallow the material expectorated.

Sputum arising from the bronchi may be mucoid, mucopurulent or frankly purulent. It is important to remember that in asthmatic patients a yellow sputum does not necessarily indicate the presence of pus (i.e. neutrophil polymorphs); instead, it may be due to eosinophil polymorphs, associated with allergic reactions rather than infection.

In acute pulmonary oedema the material expectorated is derived largely from the oedema fluid transuded into the alveoli; it is thin, frothy, and may be pink from uniform blood-staining.

When sputum is profuse and purulent, it is likely that it arises from a localized abnormality, such as bronchiectasis, lung abscess or empyema with pleura bronchial fistula. Inquiry should be made about the effect of posture upon sputum production; the patient may have noticed that certain postures lead to cough and expectoration; the posture that they adopt for sleeping may be significant since it may have been chosen because it does not lead to cough. The sudden production of a large volume of sputum suggests the evacuation of a localized collection of liquid into a bronchus from a pleural empyema, a cyst (infected or otherwise), a lung abscess or a mediastinal, subphrenic

or intrahepatic abscess. An episode of this sort may be followed by persistent expectoration, or may cease temporarily when the bronchial communication becomes occluded, and recur later. Rupture of a hydatid cyst in the lung may result in the sudden expectoration of a large amount of thin watery material, which may be accompanied or followed by an anaphylactic reaction.

The uniformly purulent sputum of a patient with a localized source of suppuration in the lungs or pleura is generally distinguishable from that of a patient with a diffuse mucopurulent bronchitis with or without bronchiectasis; it is often evidently thinner with little or no viscid mucoid secretion mixed with it, and flows easily.

Sputum may be odourless, and this provides no indication of the likely pathogens. However, if it has a sickeningly offensive smell it is virtually certain that there is an infection with anaerobic organisms, as may occur in some types of lung abscess, empyema with pleurobronchial fistula and severely infected bronchiectasis. The pus in acute specific lung abscesses due to Staphylococcus aureus or Klebsiella pneumoniae, and in empyemas due to these organisms, to pneumococcus or to Streptococcus pyogenes, is not malodorous.

In addition to the yellow of pus or eosinophil pseudopus, other colours may be observed in the sputum. A uniformly purulent sputum may be green rather than yellow, either because of degeneration of leucocytes in specimens that have been left standing, or because of infection by Pseudomonas aeruginosa. The ulceration of an amoebic liver abscess into the lung gives rise to the expectoration of reddish-brown, so-called 'anchovy-sauce' pus. Sputum may be stained with fresh or altered blood, or mixed with larger quantities of blood; this is considered under HAEMOPTYSIS (see p. 257). The sputum of those patients exposed to dust will contain the dust that has settled on the bronchi, often aggregated by ciliary streaming to give a mottled appearance. The sputum of coal-miners contains coal-dust. In coalminers with complicated pneumoconiosis, the confluent collagenous masses incorporating coal-dust that constitute progressive massive fibrosis sometimes liquefy centrally; when this occurs, the liquid black contents are expectorated, resulting in an episode of expectoration of inky black material, or 'melanoptysis'.

Formed elements may be visible in sputum. In patients with asthma or with diffuse bronchitis, a careful search by floating the sputum in water may reveal fragments which are evidently casts of small parts of the peripheral bronchial tree, but large casts with multiple branching are rarely seen. They occur in the very rare plastic or fibrinous bronchitis; the patient, often an asthmatic, suffers recurrent febrile illnesses with collapse-consolidation of a lobe or lobes of the lung, re-expanding after expectoration of the cast. Much more frequently identified is allergic bronchopulmonary aspergillosis, in which the sputum may contain 'plugs', generally about 4–5 mm in diameter and 15–20 mm in length. Usually, these are roughly spindle-shaped, without the multiple branching of bronchial casts, though occasionally there is a single bifurcation at one end. They consist mainly of tough mucus, containing many eosinophils, and with a little *Aspergillus mycelium* in the centre, usually demonstrable only by special staining. This disease occurs in extrinsic atopic asthmatics, and the sputum may also have the microscopic features seen in asthma (see below). A careful search in the sputum of asthmatic patients suspected of allergic aspergillosis may be required to demonstrate the 'plugs', but patients on inquiry will often be found to have noticed the presence from time to time of a tough fragment in the sputum. Very rarely, a patient with a bronchial carcinoma coughs out a gross fragment of the tumour. Another rare event is the expectoration of a fragment of calcified caseous material from an old tuberculous focus, either in lung or in a bronchopulmonary lymph node. If a previous chest radiograph is available, it is sometimes possible to see that one of the calcified foci evident in it has disappeared in a subsequent film.

The principal laboratory examinations to which sputum should be submitted are microscopy and bacteriological culture.

The presence of pus can be confirmed microscopically by the finding of large numbers of neutrophil polymorphs. As already noted, it is important to distinguish the eosinophil pseudopus which appears in the sputum of some asthmatics from true pus. Additionally, in the mucoid sputum of asthmatics, many eosinophils may be present. This finding is of especial importance in the differential diagnosis between late-onset intrinsic asthma and chronic bronchitis. The sputum of asthmatic patients may also contain Curschmann's spirals and Charcot–Leyden crystals. Curschmann's spirals consist of whitish, twisted threads of mucus, often including eosinophils; Charcot–Leyden crystals are colourless, elongated octahedrons which appear to be associated with eosinophils. Occasionally, small clumps

of desquamated bronchiolar epithelial cells – the so-called 'Creola bodies' – may be seen in the sputum of asthmatic patients, especially after a severe attack or during a prolonged attack.

Examination of the sputum for cancer cells is an important investigation in the diagnosis of bronchial carcinoma. This is a specialized procedure, its reliability depending very much upon the skill and experience of the cytologist. Clinicians should be aware of some possibly confusing factors. In asthmatic patients, a report that clumps of adenocarcinoma cells have been seen should be interpreted in the knowledge that the 'Creola bodies' (see above) may mimic such cells very closely; likewise, in patients with chronic tuberculous or other cavities in the lung, which may be lined with metaplastic squamous cells, these cells may be desquamated and prove difficult to distinguish with certainty from squamous carcinoma cells.

After haemoptysis from any cause, and in the presence of pulmonary congestion associated with heart disease, iron-containing macrophages or siderocytes may be seen in the sputum. They also appear in the sputum in idiopathic pulmonary haemosiderosis, but are not of specific significance in this disease.

Persons who have been exposed to asbestos dust produce 'asbestos bodies' in their sputum. These consist of very thin, needle-like fibres of asbestos surrounded by a clear brownish coating of proteinaceous material containing iron, often arranged in an irregular beaded distribution or with a terminal bead or beads that cause the whole to resemble a drumstick or dumbbell. The presence of these bodies indicates only exposure to asbestos – it is not necessarily associated with pulmonary *asbestosis*. Apart from this, microscopy of the sputum provides no specific information on pneumoconioses. Similarly, although orf-containing macrophages may be found in the sputum of patients with *exogenous oil inhalation pneumonia*, they may also be found in users of oily nasal drops – but without pathological consequences in the lungs.

In pulmonary *alveolar proteinosis*, microscopy of the sputum shows amorphous eosinophilic periodic acid–Schiff (PAS)-positive material, while electron microscopy shows the presence of lamellar bodies, presumably derived from type II pneumocytes, which may be diagnostic.

Microscopy of suitably stained sputum-smears is an essential part of the examination of the sputum for *mycobacteria*. It has been estimated that sputum specimens must contain as many as 100 000 bacilli per ml if acid-fast bacilli can be reliably demonstrated in them by microscopy after Ziehl–Neelsen staining. Examination by fluorescence microscopy (after suitable staining) has a somewhat higher sensitivity. Appropriate methods of culture demonstrate *mycobacteria* in specimens containing far fewer organisms, but there is a delay of several weeks before the results are available. For this reason, persistent attempts should be made to identify acid-fast bacilli by microscopy in any patient who is acutely ill with an inflammatory process in the lung that might be tuberculous. In this interpretation of negative findings it is important to remember that failure to find acid-fast bacilli in a scanty mucoid sputum in a patient with acute pneumonic changes without cavitation militates very little against a diagnosis of tuberculosis. In contrast, in a patient with a cavitated inflammatory process and frankly purulent sputum, repeated negative findings are much more significant.

Microscopy of Gram-stained smears of sputum is of value in acute pneumonias; for example, a preponderance of Gram-positive diplococci suggests a *pneumococcal infection*, while clumps of Gram-positive cocci indicate a *staphylococcal infection*. However, in bacterial infections culture is generally required both to identify organisms and to provide information about their sensitivity to antibiotics. Sputum is usually cultured only aerobically. The culture of expectorated sputum anaerobically is useless because the sputum is inevitably contaminated by oropharyngeal organisms which include many anaerobic species. If infection with anaerobic organisms is suspected, then specimens must be obtained from the lower respiratory tract, either by transtracheal aspiration or at fibre-optic bronchoscopy using a sheathed brush to obtain the specimens.

In patients suspected of *Pneumocystis pneumonia*, specimens of alveolar secretion may be obtained by alveolar lavage and examined by immunofluorescence staining techniques for *Pneumocystis carinii*. It should be remembered that in the sputum of patients receiving broad-spectrum antibiotics, organisms other than the original pathogens often become predominant. These may be organisms that rarely become pathogenic, such as *Proteus* and coliform organisms, as well as some that can assume independent pathogenicity, such as *Pseudomonas pyocyanea* and *Candida*. Even with the latter organism, it is often difficult to be certain whether or not they are truly pathogenic in an individual case of chronic mucopurulent bronchitis.

Spore-producing organisms such as *Aspergillus* species, the spores of which are frequently present in the air, appear as contaminants in a proportion of all sputum cultures. For this reason, the finding of *Aspergillus* in the sputum is of no significance unless supported by clinical and immunological evidence. When infection with other pathogenic fungi is suspected, special culture media are required. It must be noted, however, that these cultures, if positive, can be highly infectious and may represent a major laboratory hazard.

Boris Lams

SQUINT (STRABISMUS)

Squints may be classified according to their direction, into convergent (Fig. S.54), divergent or vertical; and according to their cause, into paralytic and non-paralytic (concomitant). The differential diagnosis between a paralytic and a non-paralytic squint is, as a rule, straightforward. In a paralytic squint, the degree of deviation of the two eyes varies, as the farther the eyes are moved in the direction of the action of the paralysed muscle, the greater will be the angle of squint. In a concomitant squint, the eyes always bear the same relative position to each other in whichever direction they are turned. Concomitant squint is characteristically a disorder of childhood, while paralytic squint more frequently occurs later in life.

The diagnosis of the cause of a paralytic squint is discussed under DIPLOPIA (p. 153).

Concomitant squints are usually the sequel to disharmony of the accommodation–convergence synkinesis (as with high hypermetropia, poor development in the power of fusion or anatomical fascio-muscular abnormalities) of the eyes – all of which may have a congenital basis. They may be aggravated

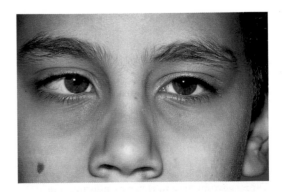

Figure S.54 Convergent squint. [Moorfields Eye Hospital.]

by any sensory or central impediment to the acquisition of the binocular fixation reflex, for example poor vision from a congenital cataract, or poor coordination from mental deficiency.

Reginald Daniel

STATURE, SHORT

Patients can be described as suffering from 'short stature' when they are shown to be below the 3rd centile of a normal population of their sex and age. Charts have been devised by Tanner and Whitehouse for a normal British population, but these are not necessarily applicable to people of a different ethnic origin. Most short British children are so because they have small parents, are socially deprived or are suffering from delayed puberty, whereas in developing countries of the world common causes of short stature are malnutrition and chronic debilitating disease in childhood. Rarer causes include skeletal deformities and hormonal deficiencies. The causes of short stature are listed in Table S.14.

Normal genetic short stature (normal variant short stature, NVSS)

Most children who present with short stature are short because they have small parents. This can be readily ascertained by plotting the child's height on a growth chart for the relevant population and comparing it with the parents' heights.

The short child whose centile falls within his or her parents' normal range should be seen in 6 months' time, to make sure that the growth velocity is normal.

Growth delay (normal variant constitutional delay NVCD)

Growth delay, which is often associated with delayed puberty, is a common cause of short stature. There is often a family history of both. The bone age, assessed from a radiograph of the wrist and hand, will usually be delayed by 3 years or more. Ultimately, normal growth and sexual development is the rule.

Chromosomal abnormalities

The most common chromosomal abnormalities are Turner's syndrome and Down's syndrome.

Turner's syndrome

Turner's syndrome occurs in girls and is characterized by gonadal dysgenesis, a lack of sexual development, and short stature. It occurs with a prevalence of 1 per 3000 female births. The karyotype is 45,XO and the buccal smear will show no Barr bodies. The average height reached is 140 cm, and rarely is a height above 152 cm achieved. However, about one-quarter of all patients with Turner's syndrome have mosaicism, such as XO,XX or XO,XXX, and they may grow to a greater height. These patients may show one, or in the latter case, even two Barr bodies on buccal smear. It is wise in such circumstances to perform a full chromosome analysis.

Because the ovaries are represented only by a fibrous streak, no estrogens are secreted and so both the internal and external genitalia remain infantile. No breast development occurs, and there is primary amenorrhoea. In addition, there are various physical abnormalities that are not hormonally mediated. The short stature is in contrast to most other types of primary hypogonadism, in which tall stature due to a lack of epiphysial fusion is a feature. There may be webbing of the neck and a low hairline at the back of the neck. There is an increased carrying angle at the elbows (cubitus valgus), shortened fourth and/or fifth metatarsals and metacarpals, Madelung's deformity of the wrist (abnormal carpal angle), a shield-like chest and abnormal fingerprints (dermatoglyphics). Pigmented naevi are often present on the skin, and intestinal telangiectasia sometimes occurs. Congenital cardiovascular anomalies exist in about one-fifth of cases; these consist of coarction of the aorta, aortic stenosis and both atrial and ventricular septal defects. Renal abnormalities such as horseshoe kidney or double ureter may occur. Hypertension is not uncommon. Subcutaneous oedema may be present in infancy. Minor abnormalities of the facies frequently draw attention to the diagnosis. The features include a flattened bridge to the nose, wide separation of the eyes (hypertelorism) and epicanthic folds. Osteoporosis may develop late in life due to the lack of oestrogens. Autoimmune thyroid disease is more common in patients with Turner's syndrome than it is amongst the general female population.

Noonan's syndrome

This syndrome may occur in boys as well as girls, and is somewhat like Turner's syndrome. The prevalence is

Table S.14 Causes of short stature

1. Normal genetic short stature
2. Growth delay
3. Chromosomal abnormalities
   - Gonadal dysgenesis
     - Turner's syndrome
     - Noonan's syndrome
   - Autosomal anomalies
     - Trisomy 21 (Down's syndrome)
     - Trisomy 18 (Edward's syndrome)
     - Trisomy 13 (Patau's syndrome)
4. Disease in childhood
   - Calorie deficiency (marasmus)
   - Protein malnutrition (kwashiorkor)
   - Vitamin D deficiency (rickets)
   - Tuberculosis
   - Bronchiectasis
   - Cystic fibrosis
   - Chronic asthma (particularly when treated with steroids)
   - Gluten enteropathy (coeliac disease)
   - Other malabsorption syndromes
   - Hookworm infection
   - Malaria
   - Cyanotic congenital heart disease
   - Chronic renal disease
   - Congenital syphilis
   - Glycogen storage disease
   - Thalassaemia major
5. Psychological causes
6. Skeletal abnormalities
   - Congenital
     - Achondroplasia, hypochondroplasia
     - Morquio's disease (chondro-osteodystrophy)
     - Dysostosis multiplex (gargoylism or Hurler's syndrome)
     - Chondrodystrophia calcificans congenita (Conradi's syndrome)
     - Epiphysial dysplasia multiplex
     - Chondro-ectodermal dysplasia (Ellis–van Creveld syndrome)
     - Osteogenesis imperfecta (fragilitas ossium)
     - Approximately 50 others
   - Acquired
     - Rickets (see below)
     - Tuberculosis and other infections of the spine
     - Deformities secondary to neurological and joint diseases (e.g. poliomyelitis, Still's disease)
7. Endocrine abnormalities
   - Growth hormone deficiency (GHD)
     - Familial
       - Type IA (complete, autosomal recessive)
       - Type IB (incomplete, autosomal recessive)
       - Type II (autosomal dominant)
       - Type III (X-linked GHD)
       - Deficiency of pituitary transcription factor *Prop1* (panhypopituitarism)
       - Deficiency of pituitary transcription factor *Pit 1* (hypopituitarism)
   - Hypothalamic/pituitary dysfunction
     - Destructive lesions
       - Craniopharyngioma
       - Pituitary tumour
       - Tuberculosis
       - Meningitis
       - Sarcoidosis
       - Toxoplasmosis
       - Histiocytosis X
       - Trauma
       - Intracranial irradiation
       - Chemotherapy
     - Pituitary agenesis
     - Biologically inactive GH
     - Neurosecretory dysfunction
     - Growth hormone resistance
       - Genetic: Laron syndrome
       - Acquired: liver disease
     - Frohlich's syndrome
     - Laurence–Moon–Biedl syndrome
   - Laron-type short stature
   - Somatomedin resistance (Pygmies)
   - Hypothyroidism
     - Thyroid agenesis
     - Solitary TSH deficiency
     - Dyshormonogenesis
     - Autoimmune thyroiditis
     - Ectopic thyroid tissue
   - Poorly controlled Type I diabetes mellitus
   - Sexual precocity
     - True precocity
       - Physiological precocious puberty
       - Space-occupying lesions of the central nervous system
       - Congenital and acquired hypothalamic lesions
     - False precocity
       - Congenital and adrenal hyperplasia
       - Cushing's syndrome
       - Adrenocortical tumour
       - Interstitial cell tumour of testis
       - Granulosa cell tumour of ovary
   - Pseudohypoparathyroidism and pseudo-pseudohypoparathyroidism
   - Rickets
     - Vitamin D deficiency
     - Renal impairment
     - Vitamin D resistance
8. Intra-uterine maldevelopment
   - Small-for-date babies
   - Fetal alcohol syndrome
   - Russell–Silver syndrome
   - Progeria (Hutchinson–Gilford syndrome)
   - Cornelia de Lange syndrome ('Amsterdam dwarfism')
   - Cockayne syndrome
   - Prader–Willi syndrome
9. Drugs
   - Glucocorticoids
   - Androgens
   - Anabolic steroids
   - Oestrogens
   - Thyroid hormones
   - Anti-thyroid drugs
   - Vitamin D

1 in 8000 births. In both boys and girls the karyotype is normal. Short stature is perhaps not so marked as in Turner's syndrome, but there may be webbing of the neck with a low hairline and a shield-like chest with widely spaced nipples. Pectus excavatum is present in 50 per cent of cases. The face shows some typical features: a slant of the eyes, which are widely spaced, may have epicanthic folds and show ptosis; the face may be triangular in shape, the ears low-set and the brow prominent. A high-arched palate is not infrequently present. The cardiovascular abnormalities differ in frequency from those of Turner's syndrome. Although coarctation of the aorta and aortic stenosis have been described, the characteristic cardiac diseases have been pulmonary stenosis (in approximately 50% of cases) and atrial septal defect. Sometimes, both conditions occur together. Ventricular septal defect and persistent ductus arteriosus have also been associated with Noonan's syndrome. Cubitus valgus is common, and mental retardation may be a feature. In males, undescended testes are common and androgen deficiency may manifest itself at puberty. Girls usually show delayed puberty, but eventually normal ovarian function develops.

Down's syndrome (Trisomy 21)

This is the most common autosomal abnormality leading to short stature. There is disordered growth of the skull and long bones. The mouth and ears are small, the tongue is large and tends to protrude, and there are epicanthic folds on the eyes. There is invariably mental retardation. Autoimmune thyroiditis is much more common than in the general population.

Trisomy 18

Trisomy 18, also known as Edward's syndrome, is the second most common autosomal condition, and is characterized by a small face and cardiac malformations that nearly always lead to an early death. It occurs with a prevalence of 1 per 8000 births.

Trisomy 13

Trisomy 13, also known as Patau's syndrome, is much more rare, and occurs only once in 20 000 live births. Death tends to occur in the first year of life.

Malnutrition and chronic debilitating disease in childhood

General calorie deficiency (marasmus) or protein deficiency (kwashiorkor) are common causes of short stature in under-developed parts of the world. Rickets, which is now unusual among the indigenous population of Britain, but relatively frequent among Asian children resident in this country, leads to retarded bone age and short stature. Self-inflicted malnutrition due to anorexia nervosa and bulimia are also common in the developed world. Growth failure in these circumstances is characterized by a normal or elevated growth hormone with decreased somatomedin levels.

The existence of chronic debilitating disease is readily apparent on taking the patient's history or performing the physical examination. Tuberculosis and bronchiectasis are not nearly as common as they used to be in the developed countries. Cystic fibrosis occurs in approximately 1 in 1700 live births among Caucasians, but is much rarer in other ethnic groups. Recurrent pulmonary infections are usually the predominant feature. Chronic asthma, particularly when treated with steroids, leads to stunting, probably because excess glucocorticoids block the action of growth factors at the cellular level.

Malabsorption of food may lead to short stature. Gluten enteropathy (coeliac disease) is the most common such condition, occurring in approximately 1 in 2000 children. Although characteristic symptoms of chronic diarrhoea, pale bulky stools, anorexia and cramping abdominal pain may be present, they are by no means invariable. Sometimes, the only clue in a short child is a rather protuberant abdomen and scanty subcutaneous fat. If other causes of short stature have been excluded, a small-bowel biopsy to show flattened villi is a useful investigation, for once the diagnosis has been confirmed and a gluten-free diet instituted, normal growth should occur. Less common causes of malabsorption include cystic fibrosis (see above), lactose intolerance, Crohn's disease and infection with Giardia lamblia.

Children who either live in the tropics or have recently returned from there may have hookworm infestation or malaria. Thalassaemia major may be associated with short stature and delayed puberty. Cyanotic congenital heart disease and chronic renal failure are usually obvious clinically as causes of growth failure. Less commonly seen are congenital syphilis and glycogen storage disease.

Psychological causes

An adverse psychological environment, with emotional deprivation and child abuse, is a very important cause of failure of growth. This has been shown to be due to suppression of growth hormone secretion by the pituitary, but nutritional factors undoubtedly play a role. It is reversible when the child is removed to happier and more secure surroundings.

Skeletal disorders

Congenital skeletal disorders

These are rare, and many of them are inherited. The most common is *achondroplasia* (*chondrodystrophy*). The condition, which is autosomal dominantly inherited, is caused by a disturbance of endochondral ossification in which the growth cartilages are invaded by connective tissue. The trunk is of normal length, but the limbs are shortened. The fingers are short and are of equal length. The head is large, the forehead being particularly prominent, but the nose is small and the bridge is flattened. There is often a marked lumbar lordosis and the buttocks are prominent. Delayed puberty is not a feature.

Hypochondroplasia is similar to achondroplasia, but the face is usually normal. Again, the inheritance is autosomal dominant.

Morquio's disease (*chondro-osteo-dystrophy*) is a rare type of skeletal deformity affecting both the limbs and the spine, and which is often familial. The epiphyses are deformed or fragmented, and a variety of deformities of the long bones have been described. The glenoid fossae and acetabulae are poorly formed. The intervertebral spaces are widened and, owing to the irregularity, flattening or wedge-shaped deformity of the vertebral bodies occurs and there is a dorso-lumbar kyphosis and shortening of the neck, the head appearing to be pushed down onto the shoulders. Many cases show a gross pigeon-breast deformity, and the short stature is further accentuated by a limitation of extension of the hips and knees. Characteristic changes are seen on X-ray examination.

Dysostosis multiplex (*gargoylism* or *Hurler's syndrome*) shows similar bony deformities to the above, though a peculiar sabot-shaped deformity of the second and third lumbar vertebral bodies appears more constantly, giving rise to angular kyphosis. The skull commonly is conical (oxycephalic) or hydrocephalic, and there may be enlargement of the pituitary fossa. The face shows widely spaced eyes (hypertelorism), a prominent forehead and a large tongue and lips. The liver and spleen may be enlarged. Mental retardation, corneal opacities and deafness are the rule. Distortion

of the heart valves and thickening of coronary arteries are frequent findings. The condition is inherited as an autosomal recessive trait, and is due to the deposition of the mucopolysaccharides heparan sulphate and dermatan sulphate. Infantilism may be associated with the short stature, but this is not always the case. However, most children do not survive longer than about the age of 14 years.

Chondrodystrophia calcificans congenita (*Conradi's syndrome*) is a rare autosomal recessive condition in which the epiphysial centres of the long and small bones ossify and fuse during early childhood.

Epiphysial dysplasia multiplex can be transmitted as an autosomal dominant or as a recessive type of inheritance. It manifests itself in older children (usually under the age of 10 years) as a disorder of gait and short stature. The pathology lies in the epiphyses, which are fragmented.

Chondro-ectodermal dysplasia (*Ellis–van Creveld syndrome*) causes short stature because of a reduction in length of the extremities. The fingers are also short and there may be polydactyly. Hypoplasia of the teeth, nails and hair occurs, and there may be both cardiac and renal abnormalities.

Osteogenesis imperfecta (*fragilitas ossium*) is characterized by extreme brittleness of the bones. The multiple fractures which occur during intra-uterine life or in childhood, coupled with the fragility of the spine, result in gross deformity and short stature. The disease is inherited as an autosomal dominant trait, and there may be a family history of otosclerosis. The patient may have slaty-blue sclerae. Radiographically, the long bones are seen to be both shorter and more slender than normal, poorly calcified, with extreme thinning of the cortex. The appearances are quite distinct from those of rickets.

Acquired skeletal disorders

Any disorder leading to damage of the long bones or spine will lead to stunted growth. *Rickets* (see p. 350) is not uncommon amongst Asian immigrant communities in Britain, particularly those who are vegetarians. *Tuberculosis of the spine* (*Pott's disease, spinal caries*) is much less common than it used to be. It is recognized by pain and tenderness localized to one or more of the vertebrae, associated with angular kyphosis. Radiographs show destruction and collapse of the affected vertebral bodies, and there may be evidence of a 'cold abscess'. These features serve to distinguish spinal tuberculosis from congenital abnormality of the vertebrae and kyphosis or scoliosis from other causes (e.g. poliomyelitis), in which weakness of the muscles of the back, perhaps unrecognized, is liable to result in a severe degree of postural deformity.

Still's disease (*chronic juvenile arthritis*; see p. 352) may lead to a stunting of growth because of premature fusion of epiphyses in affected joints.

Endocrine disorders

Endocrine abnormalities account for approximately 10 per cent of cases of short stature. It is important to make the diagnosis promptly in children as appropriate therapy can normalize growth. The most common endocrine causes of short stature are growth hormone deficiency (GHD), which may be partial rather than total, and hypothyroidism. Less common are adrenal disorders, for example glucocorticoid excess either iatrogenic or secondary to Cushing's disease, and primary adrenal hypercortisolism. The remaining causes listed in Table S.11 are much more rare.

Growth hormone deficiency is a mixture of genetic abnormalities. GHD is recognized early in life, because the children tend to be fat with small genitalia, short stature and hypoglycaemia. They have delayed bone age and delayed puberty, but enter puberty when their bone age is appropriate. There are two variants of Type 1 GHD, depending on the degree of genetic mutation. Type 1A GHD is due to gene deletion or point mutations, and there is complete GHD. These patients develop growth hormone (GH) antibodies when treated. Type 1B GHD is associated with splice-site mutations in the GH gene. Patients retain the ability to produce small amounts of GH, and they do not develop antibodies when treated with GH. Destructive lesions involving the pituitary and hypothalamus may cause pan-hypopituitarism. These include tumours, of which the most common in childhood is a craniopharyngioma, but other causes are meningitis (e.g. tuberculous), sarcoidosis, xanthomas (e.g. Hand–Schüller–Christian syndrome, histiocytosis X), trauma (especially basal skull fractures) and following intracranial irradiation and/or chemotherapy. A subset of children with normal GH responses to stimulatory testing may still respond to GH treatment. These children are thought to be suffering from a *neurosecretary dysfunction of GH secretion*. A more comprehensive system of interpreting GHD may therefore come from

the combination of short stature, decreased growth velocity, delayed bone age and low serum *insulin-like growth factor* (IGF)-I in addition to low levels of *IGF binding protein* (IGFBP-3) and another binding protein called the *acid-labile subunit* (ALS). Collectively, the IGFs have been known as the somatomedins, and play a role in somatic growth on binding of GH to its receptor.

Frohlich's syndrome is mentioned if only to be dismissed. Frohlich originally described a patient with obesity, somnolence, retarded skeletal and sexual development and optic atrophy. The pathology in this case was a suprasellar tumour pressing on the hypothalamus, and clearly pituitary hormone deficiencies secondary to hypothalamic damage were likely to have been present. Unfortunately, the term 'Frohlich's syndrome' tends to be attached to any short, fat boy with delayed sexual development and small genitalia. It is best forgotten.

Laurence–Moon–Biedl syndrome may sometimes be associated with short stature. The condition is autosomal recessive. Clinical features include obesity, retarded sexual development, mental retardation, retinitis pigmentosa and either polydactylism or syndactylism.

The rare *Laron type* of short stature is caused by mutations or deletions of the GH receptor gene, and is associated with increased GH levels and decreased levels of IGFs and IGFBP-3. It can now be diagnosed by measuring levels of GH-binding protein and can be treated with IGF-I.

The pygmies of Africa have normal GH and somatomedin levels; an absence of somatomedin receptors has been postulated.

Hypothyroidism is a common cause of short stature. Somatomedin levels are below normal. Among babies born in Britain, 1 in 3300 is hypothyroid, usually due to thyroid agenesis. The diagnosis is now made early by neonatal thyroid-stimulating hormone (TSH) screening. However, it must be noted that neonatal hypothyroidism may be secondary to isolated TSH deficiency. This will be missed on TSH screening, but will be diagnosed if serum thyroxine is measured. In addition, hypothyroidism may co-exist with GH deficiency and may render false-negative stimulatory tests of GH production. It is important therefore to rule out hypothyroidism in the first instance. Dyshormonogenesis, which may be due to one of six defects in the synthesis of thyroid hormones, tends to lead to goitre and hypothyroidism in early life, though those with partial defects may present later. After the age of round about 6 years, autoimmune thyroiditis begins to become an increasingly important cause of hypothyroidism. A goitre is usually palpable and thyroid antibodies are present in blood. Sometimes at the time of puberty an ectopic, often sublingual, thyroid may be the cause of hypothyroidism.

Uncontrolled Type 1 diabetes mellitus is associated with decreased somatomedin levels and poor growth. Restoration of the growth rate occurs with improved nutrition and diabetes control.

When *precocious sexual development* occurs, the production of sex hormones causes initially an acceleration of growth, but bone maturation is more rapid than normal, fusion of the epiphyses takes place, and the final stature is shorter than would be expected from parental height (Fig. S.55). Precocious sexual development is five times more common in girls than in boys, and in the majority of girls the cause is some unknown triggering mechanism in the hypothalamus which initiates a normal, albeit early, physiological puberty. In boys, on the other hand, a pathological cause is found in about half the cases.

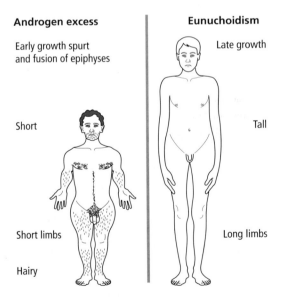

Androgen excess

Early growth spurt
and fusion of epiphyses

Short

Short limbs

Hairy

Eunuchoidism

Late growth

Tall

Long limbs

Figure S.55 Comparison of short stature due to early closure of epiphyses and tall stature due to late closure of epiphyses because of hypogonadism, but with normal growth hormone secretion. [Courtesy of the Departments of Medical Illustration, Guy's and Westminster Hospitals.]

It is important to separate true precocity from false precocity. In true precocity, puberty is 'physiological'

and thus follows the pattern of normal development. While the majority are constitutional, it is important to look for space-occupying lesions of the central nervous system. These include craniopharyngioma, pineal tumour, hamartoma, neurofibroma, astrocytoma and cysts of the third ventricle. Hypothyroidism may cause the premature release of follicle-stimulating hormone (FSH) from the pituitary. Tuberose sclerosis, McCune–Albright syndrome (polyostotic fibrous dysplasia with cutaneous pigmentation), encephalitis and hydrocephalus may all lead to true precocity. On the other hand, 'false' precocity is due to the action of sex hormones produced by the gonad or by the adrenals. The common causes are congenital adrenal hyperplasia due to a 21-hydroxylase defect and Cushing's syndrome. Testicular and ovarian tumours are very rare. For further details, see PUBERTY, PRECOCIOUS (p. 563).

Pseudohypoparathyroidism is a disorder in which the renal tubules are resistant to the action of parathyroid hormone. As a result, the production of 1,25-dihydroxyvitamin D by the kidneys is reduced and, as a consequence, the absorption of calcium from the gut is diminished. The patient is usually short and mentally retarded, has short fourth and fifth metacarpals, and may have cataracts and ectopic subcutaneous calcification with ulceration. Serum calcium levels are low and parathyroid hormone levels are increased. Some patients have the short stature and skeletal abnormalities, but with a normal calcium level. This is called 'pseudo-pseudohypoparathyroidism'.

Rickets may lead to stunting of growth and bowing of the legs. The commonest cause is vitamin D deficiency due to lack of ultraviolet light, so that the precursor of the vitamin, 7-dehydrocholesterol, is not converted into vitamin D. The normal British diet contains very little vitamin D. Groups particularly at risk are Indian and Pakistani immigrants, especially if they are vegetarian (Fig. S.56). Small-bowel and biliary diseases also cause malabsorption of vitamin D.

Other rarer causes of rickets are congenital renal tubular defects and 25-hydroxyvitamin D-1-α-hydroxylase deficiency (vitamin D-resistant rickets).

Intra-uterine maldevelopment

Most small-for-date babies subsequently grow at a normal rate, though they may not achieve a final stature appropriate for their parents' centiles. Some, however, fail to grow normally and may be examples

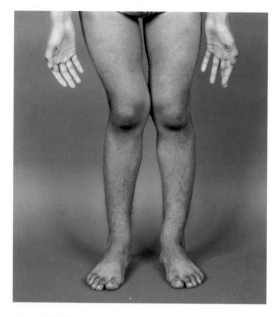

Figure S.56 Rickets in a vegetarian Indian boy. Note the genu valgum.

of specific syndromes, of which the most common is the Russell–Silver syndrome. This is characterized by a lack of subcutaneous fat, a triangular face with a large forehead, small jaw, low-set ears and a turned-down mouth. There is incurving and shortening of the fifth fingers.

The *fetal alcohol syndrome* is being increasingly recognized; this is probably related to the rising consumption of alcohol. In addition to growth retardation, there is mental subnormality and a characteristic facial appearance. This consists of a small jaw, short nose, under-developed upper lip and a reduction in length of the palpebral fissures. More serious conditions are congenital heart defects and flexion contractures.

Progeria (Hutchinson–Giford syndrome) is characterized by premature ageing, and death usually occurs before the age of 20 years. Appearances are normal at birth, but growth ceases – owing to epiphysial closure – within a period ranging from a few months to 3 years. There is no subcutaneous fat, the nose is beaky and the ears prominent. There may be premature baldness, some mental retardation, periarticular fibrosis and arteriosclerosis.

Cornelia de Lange syndrome (Amsterdam dwarfism) is characterized by poor growth, mental deficiency, a small head with a flattened occiput, abnormal lips and mouth, bushy eyebrows that meet in the middle, short nose with anteverted nostrils and abnormalities

of the extremities, particularly of the upper limbs. Hirsutism may be a feature.

Patients with *Cockayne syndrome* have a somewhat similar appearance to that of progeria, except that mental retardation is more marked, and there is retinal degeneration, photosensitive dermatitis, deafness, unsteady gait and tremor.

The *Prader–Willi syndrome* is characterized by poor growth, obesity, hypogonadism, cryptorchidism, hypotonia and mental retardation. The hands and feet are small in relation to the rest of the body.

Drugs

The administration of various drugs, particularly in high doses, may lead to stunting of growth in a child. *Glucocorticoids*, used particularly in asthma and Still's disease, may cause short stature due to interference with growth at the cellular level. The dosage should therefore be kept to the minimum possible and should preferably be given on alternate days.

Anabolic steroids have sometimes been used to try to increase the height of a short child. The danger is that they accelerate bone age, cause epiphysial fusion, and may thus actually decrease potential height. The same may happen when androgens or oestrogens are used in boys and girls, respectively, to bring about sexual maturation. Specialist advice should be sought before using any of these drugs in children.

A lack of thyroid hormone (hypothyroidism) causes delayed bone maturation and short stature, but it must be remembered that the condition may be iatrogenic, when too much anti-thyroid drug is given, and that iodides may lead to goitre formation and hypothyroidism in some individuals who are predisposed to autoimmune thyroid disease. Conversely, over-treatment of hypothyroidism in childhood with thyroxine will lead initially to a growth spurt due to stimulation of somatomedin production by the liver but, by accelerating bone maturation, may reduce potential stature in the long term.

Vitamin D preparations, given to children for conditions such as hypoparathyroidism, pseudohypoparathyroidism and rickets, may give rise to hypercalcaemia which, if chronic, will cause renal failure. If the renal failure is severe enough, then stunting of growth will result. Vitamin D treatment should always be monitored with regular measurement of the serum calcium.

Sharon O'Byrne

STATURE, TALL

A patient is usually defined as exhibiting tall stature if the height is above the 97th centile for the normal population. In most cases, tallness is inherited from tall parents; pathological causes are much less common. However, a child may be below the 97th centile, but still be inappropriately tall compared with the parents. If a period of observation shows that the growth velocity is greater than normal, the appropriate investigations should be carried out. The classification of tall stature is listed in Table S.15.

Table S.15 Causes of tall stature

1. Constitutional
2. Overnutrition
3. Endocrine abnormalities
   ■ Sexual precocity and virilizing syndromes
   ■ Hypogonadism
   ■ Thyrotoxicosis
   ■ Pituitary acidophil over-activity ('gigantism')
4. Chromosomal abnormalities
   ■ Klinefelter's syndrome (47,XXY)
   ■ 'Supermale' (47,XYY)
   ■ 'Superfemale' (47,XXX)
5. Miscellaneous
   ■ Marfan's syndrome
   ■ Homocystinuria
   ■ Cerebral 'gigantism' (Sotos' syndrome)
   ■ Brain damage
   ■ Lipodystrophy
   ■ Beckwith–Wiedemann syndrome

Constitutional

Constitutional tall stature can be identified by plotting the patient's height relative to age on a growth-development chart relevant to the child population and ethnicity. Some children who enter puberty relatively early may initially become taller than their contemporaries because of an early growth spurt, but their epiphyses will also fuse earlier and so the ultimate adult height attained will be appropriate for their family. Enhanced growth hormone (GH) secretion and a greater efficiency of GH-mediated insulin-like growth factor (IGF-I) production may be potential causes of familial tall stature.

Over-nutrition

Over-nutrition leading to obesity in early childhood may lead to accelerated linear growth, but fusion of the epiphyses at an earlier age than usual normalizes the final height. The GH levels may be low, but GH binding protein (GHBP) and IGF-I levels are normal to high.

Endocrine abnormalities

The commonest endocrine causes of tall stature in childhood are true precocious puberty and false precocious puberty (see p. 563). True precocious puberty is either physiological (which is the commonest), or is due to space-occupying or other lesions affecting the hypothalamus. False precocious puberty can be caused by either adrenal disease (congenital adrenal hyperplasia, e.g. 21-hydroxylase defect, and adrenocortical tumour) or by very rare hormone-secreting testicular or ovarian tumours. The increased amounts of sex hormones produced in these various conditions lead to an increased maturation of bone, with an acceleration of growth so that the child is inappropriately tall compared with peers of the same age-group. Unfortunately, epiphyses fuse early and a normal adult height is not achieved. A similar growth acceleration is seen in *thyrotoxicosis* and in hypothyroid patients who are over-treated with thyroxine. Somatomedin levels are high. Thyrotoxic children are usually round about the 75th centile for height. However, tall stature is rarely a presenting feature in these children, and ultimate stature is not usually abnormal because the epiphyses fuse early.

Hypogonadism will cause increased stature with long arms and legs (eunuchoidism), because of delayed fusion of the epiphyses, as long as normal amounts of GH and thyroid hormone are present. Disease of the hypothalamus, pituitary or gonad may cause hypogonadism, leading to tall stature. *Solitary deficiency of the hypothalamic gonadotrophin releasing hormone* is well recognized. When it is associated with anosmia due to agenesis of the olfactory bulbs it is called *Kallmann's syndrome*. *Pituitary deficiency of luteinizing hormone* has been described in males. There is little or no testosterone production by the testes and the seminiferous tubules are immature. However, full maturation of both secondary sexual characteristics and of the seminiferous tubules can be achieved by means of human chorionic gonadotrophin injections, hence accounting for the alternative title of the *fertile eunuch syndrome*.

In primary gonadal disorders leading to hypogonadism the characteristic biochemical feature is high serum gonadotrophins. *Anorchia* is a rare congenital cause in males. More usual causes are *trauma, tuberculous orchitis* or *oophoritis* and *radiation damage to the gonads*. Rarely, there may be *autoimmune ovarian failure*; this is usually associated with other autoimmune disease such as Addison's disease. Boys with *Klinefelter's syndrome* (XXY) are usually tall and have abnormally long limbs before puberty, but if testosterone levels are low in the middle to late teens an element of hypogonadism is added (see below).

Either *adenoma* or *hyperplasia of the pituitary acidophil cells* can lead to the excessive secretion of GH and the rare condition of *'gigantism' analagous to acromegaly in the adult*. Sometimes, the adenoma may be of chromophobe cells or of mixed cell type. GH-secreting tumours also occur in multiple endocrine neoplasia (MEN), neurofibromatosis and tuberous sclerosis. If the condition arises before puberty, then the main feature is excessive growth of the long bones, resulting in a wide span and an increased lower segment to upper segment ratio. Heights of over 2.4 metres (8 feet) have been recorded. If hypogonadism does not supervene, then the epiphyses may fuse and acromegalic features may begin to develop. Acromegaly means enlargement of the extremities; the bones of the hands and feet become broadened and the soft tissues become thicker, so that it is difficult for the patient to get shoes and gloves to fit. The facial appearance gradually changes, the skin and subcutaneous tissues becoming thicker, so that the skin folds are more prominent, the nose enlarged, and the general impression is one of coarsened features. The frontal air sinuses enlarge and so the supraorbital ridges are more prominent. The lower jaw elongates and causes prognathism; dental malocclusion may become a problem. Radiographs may show enlargement of the pituitary fossa, but by no means always. Characteristic tufting of the terminal phalanges and widening of the joint spaces may be seen on hand radiographs. Increased heel pad thickness is usually demonstrated on radiographs. If it is above 23 mm acromegaly is possibly present; if above 27 mm, acromegaly is certain.

Enlargement of the tongue, lips and ears occurs. Thickening of the vocal cords leads to deepening of the voice. Overgrowth of soft tissues at the wrist causes carpal tunnel syndrome in 35 per cent of cases. Evidence of a proximal myopathy is found in one-third of patients. Persistent sweating is a common problem, and girls may be troubled by hirsutism. Persistent headaches caused by stretching of the diaphragma sellae by the enlarging adenoma are a feature in one-third of the patients. Other local pressure effects include visual field loss due to the tumour encroaching upon the optic chiasm. A very early feature may be loss of central vision for red objects; subsequently, the classic bitemporal hemianopia develops and this may lead on to optic atrophy and total blindness.

All organs enlarge, particularly the heart and liver. A cardiomyopathy may be present and hypertension is a common feature. Frank diabetes mellitus is present in 10 per cent of cases, and a further 33 per cent have impaired tolerance to oral glucose. Goitre may be present and thyrotoxicosis occurs in 3 per cent of patients. Galactorrhoea due to excessive prolactin secretion may be a feature. In long-standing cases, hypopituitarism develops in about 50 per cent of patients.

A resting GH in the fasting state of more than 10 mU/l (5 ng/ml) which does not suppress to less than 2 mU/l (1 ng/ml) after 75 g of oral glucose is diagnostic of acromegaly or 'gigantism'. Most patients have much higher fasting levels than this, and they may even show a rise in GH levels following glucose. Serum IGF-I levels are also elevated.

Chromosomal abnormalities

The most commonly recognized chromosomal anomaly leading to tall stature is *Klinefelter's syndrome*. This syndrome, occurring once in every 500 live male births, is caused by an extra X chromosome, giving a karyotype of 47,XXY. The patient is tall and has eunuchoid proportions (Fig. S.57). The tallness may not be particularly apparent in childhood, but becomes noticeable during the teens because the hypogonadism delays epiphysial fusion. The testes are small and firm, and histology shows tubular sclerosis and hyalinization. Variable numbers of Leydig cells may be present, and this accounts for the fact that the serum testosterone may be frankly low or be in the low normal range, FSH is elevated and LH usually so, but not if the testosterone is normal. There is a female escutcheon of pubic hair, and facial and body hair is usually diminished. Gynaecomastia is a usual finding. Infertility is the rule, but occasional exceptions have been described.

Another syndrome – the *supermale*, with a karyotype of 47,XYY – also occurs, with a frequency of 1 per 1000 live male births. These individuals are usually very tall. The testes may be normal or small; in the latter case, the testosterone level is low and FSH and LH are elevated.

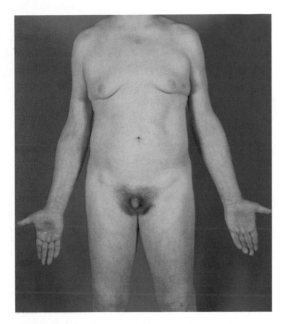

Figure S.57 Klinefelter's syndrome. The arms and legs are long in proportion to the trunk, and there is gynaecomastia.

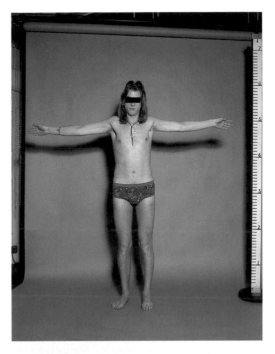

Figure S.58 A young male with Marfan's syndrome.

In some cases mental retardation and a tendency to aggressive behaviour are noted.

The *superfemale* (47,XXX) tends to have long legs and long fingers, but with a relatively normal span. The face is long and narrow, there is sometimes amenorrhoea and the secondary sexual characteristics may be poorly developed. Mild mental subnormality is a feature.

Miscellaneous causes

There is a group of miscellaneous causes of tall stature in children of which *Marfan's syndrome* is the most commonly recognized (Fig. S.58). This is an autosomal dominant disorder of collagen metabolism. The child is usually within the normal height range for his/her age-group, but may be inappropriately tall for their family. The extremities are long and thin, and the fingers and toes are spider-like (*arachnodactly*). The joints are hyperextensible. There may be dilatation of the aorta, aortic regurgitation, dislocation of the lenses of the eye, a high arched palate and long patellar ligaments. Although the skeletal proportions appear 'eunuchoidal', bone maturation, in fact, proceeds at a normal rate. From a radiograph of the hands the metacarpal index can be calculated by dividing the mean of the lengths by the mean of the widths. An index of more than 8.4 indicates arachnodactyly.

Patients with *homocystinuria* are rather similar in appearance to those with Marfan's syndrome. The condition is an autosomal recessive disease. Additional features are mental retardation, a tendency to spontaneous thromboses in arteries and veins, and the presence of homocystine in the urine.

Cerebral gigantism (*Sotos' syndrome*) is characterized by accelerated growth in the first few years of life, though puberty is usually early and causes premature closure of the epiphyses such that a normal adult stature is achieved. The hands and feet are large, and the appearance is somewhat acromegalic, though GH and IGF levels are normal. Mental subnormality is common. No cause has been identified.

Some children who may have suffered *brain damage* and mental retardation from birth trauma become excessively tall. The cause is unknown.

Lipodystrophy is a rare condition with absent fatty tissue, hyperlipidaemia and diabetes; there may be increased GH levels, and tall stature is a feature.

The *Beckwith–Wiedemann syndrome* is rare, and consists of accelerated fetal growth, enlarged tongue, omphalocele, renal medullary hyperplasia and neonatal hypoglycaemia secondary to islet cell hyperplasia and raised insulin levels. Early epiphyseal fusion occurs, and therefore there is no increase in adult height. This syndrome may be associated with disordered regulation of the *IGF-II* gene transcription.

Failure to enter puberty and complete sexual maturation may result in sustained growth during adult life. The result is a tall stature with eunuchoid appearances. This has been described in conditions where mutation of the oestrogen receptor has taken place, or in cases of aromatase deficiency (enzymatic conversion of androstenedione to oestrogen in extraglandular sites). These abnormalities emphasize the role of oestrogen in epiphyseal closure and termination of skeletal growth.

Sharon O'Byrne

STOMACH, DILATATION OF

See also ABDOMINAL SWELLINGS (p. 11).

Dilatation of the stomach presents itself clinically under two totally different aspects: (i) acute; and (ii) chronic.

Acute dilatation of the stomach

This is generally a serious, but fortunately rare, complication or even a fatal catastrophe arising in the course of some other condition, especially after operations (notably laparotomy), or after abdominal injury.

The diagnosis is generally easy. The abdomen is distended and tympanitic; there is constant effort to bring up wind, sometimes in vain, sometimes with copious and recurrent eructations, often with intractable hiccoughs. Sometimes, immense quantities of blackish-brown or greenish-brown fluid flow effortlessly from the mouth and nostrils. The dilatation itself is of the nature of an acute paralysis of the stomach. Diagnosis is confirmed, and indeed treatment initiated, by the passage of a stomach tube which deflates the gastric dilatation.

Chronic dilatation of the stomach

This is due to conditions which cause stenosis at, or more commonly on either side of, the pylorus.

Causes of stenosis

These include the following:

- Peptic ulcer, particularly of the duodenum, although much less commonly a benign gastric ulcer at the pylorus or in the antrum may be responsible.
- Carcinoma of the pylorus or antrum.
- Other tumours in this region; these include leiomyoma, leiomyosarcoma, infiltration with Hodgkin's disease or lymphosarcoma or invasion from an adjacent carcinoma of the pancreas or gall bladder.
- Congenital pyloric septum.
- Adult hypertrophy of the pylorus.
- Heterotopic pancreatic tissue.
- Adhesions of the duodenum to the liver bed following cholecystectomy.

The history in an established case of pyloric stenosis may be absolutely typical. In the case of a peptic ulcer, there may be a long preceding story of ulcer pain. Vomiting is an important symptom, and it occurs in at least nine out of every ten patients. Typically, copious amounts of vomitus are produced in a projectile manner, and the patient will recall (but often only on direct questioning) that he or she has noticed fragments of food, particularly vegetable or fruit debris, which had been ingested one day and vomited up the next, or even 2–3 days later. There is really no condition other than obstruction to the gastric outlet in which this state of affairs obtains. Obstruction due to carcinoma, in contrast, often has a shorter history, perhaps of only a few months, and pain is completely absent in about one-third of patients.

Examination of the patient often reveals features of importance. There may be evidence of dehydration and loss of weight; indeed the classic 'ulcer facies' applies only rarely to uncomplicated examples of peptic ulcer, but is perfectly mirrored in the usual appearance of the victim of long-standing stenosis. A gastric splash which is present 3–4 hours after a meal or drink is elicited in two-thirds of patients with benign stenosis. Often, the patient – when asked directly – will agree that they have noticed a splashing sound when walking or moving about. Visible gastric peristalsis, passing from left to right, is present much less frequently, and still less often the loaded and hypertrophied stomach may actually be palpable as well as audible and visible (see PERISTALSIS, VISIBLE, p. 540). About half of the patients with malignant obstruction will reveal a palpable tumour at the pylorus. Such a mass may, it is true, be felt rarely in the benign case, when a large inflammatory mass is present around the first part of the duodenum. Because of the more rapid progression in the malignant case, gross dilatation of the stomach is much less often seen than in benign obstruction, so that gastric splash and visible peristalsis may not be elicited.

Radiological investigation in these cases is mandatory. The findings can be divided into two groups: the first group confirms the presence of an obstruction at the gastric outlet; and the second indicates its pathology. A plain radiograph of the abdomen may itself be at least suggestive of pyloric stenosis by demonstrating a large gastric gas bubble with considerable quantities of retained food particles, as indicated by patchy, translucent areas. A sign of obstruction at the gastric outlet on the barium meal is the large residue of food within the stomach shown after taking a few mouthfuls of barium. Instead of the normal appearance of the barium running down the lesser curvature, the particles of barium can be seen to sink through a layer of fluid and then to rest at the bottom of the greater curve, like a saucer. In the erect position, three layers can be seen: the air bubble above; then the layer of gastric juice; and finally the lowermost layer of barium (Fig. S.59). In the early phase of pyloric stenosis giant peristaltic waves may be seen passing along the gastric wall, but in late decompensated obstruction the stomach is a large atonic bag. Obstruction of the gastric outlet is confirmed by taking further films at 4–6 hours, when it will be seen that a large residue of barium remains in the stomach (Fig. S.60). Under normal circumstances the stomach is all but empty at the end of 2 hours. It is not always easy to tell the exact cause of the pyloric obstruction. Radiological evidence that a duodenal ulcer is responsible is given by the presence of an active ulcer crater or severe scarring in the duodenal cap. If the obstruction is situated in the antrum of the stomach, it is most probable that the diagnosis is cancer (Fig. S.61), but occasionally a similar appearance

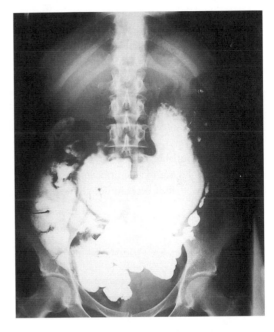

Figure S.60 Pyloric stenosis due to a chronic duodenal ulcer. X-ray taken 24 hours after a barium meal. Note the considerable residue of barium.

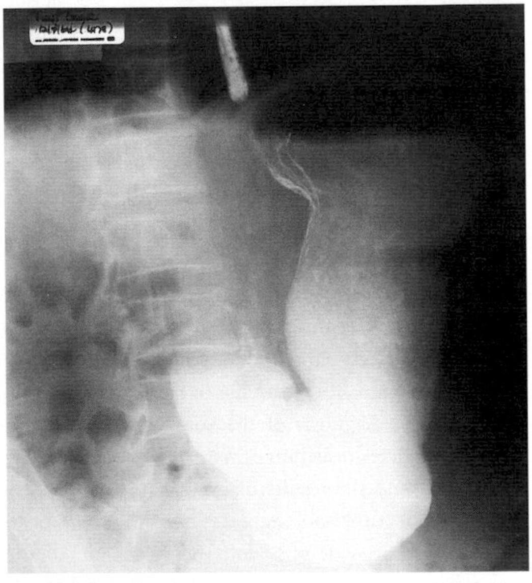

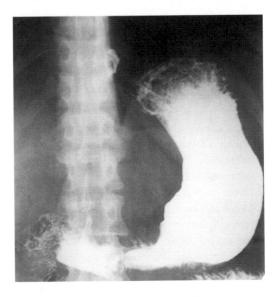

Figure S.59 Pyloric stenosis due to a chronic duodenal ulcer; barium meal examination. Note the three layers: air, gastric juice, and barium.

Figure S.61 Barium meal of pyloric obstruction due to an extensive antral carcinoma.

is given by a penetrating benign gastric ulcer. A further sign of duodenal bulb obstruction that has been found useful is abnormal dilatability of the pyloric canal, which may be seen on screening to dilate up to 2.5 cm or more in width, and then to contract down again to its usual size proximal to the point of stenosis.

Gastroscopy by means of a fibre-optic endoscope may visualize the obstructing ulcer and allow a biopsy to be performed, but often adherent gastric contents obscure the view. This can be obviated by careful pre-examination gastric lavage.

The less common causes of pyloric obstruction mentioned above which may be associated with chronic dilatation of the stomach are rarely diagnosed before laparotomy. However, since obstruction of the gastric outlet almost invariably requires surgical intervention, elucidation of the exact cause preceding operation is a luxury rather than a necessity for the experienced surgeon.

Harold Ellis

STOOLS, MUCUS IN

Mucus in the stools is not pathognomonic. It occurs in malignant disease of the colon as a clear glairy substance, often blood-stained, and it has the same character in intussusception. The obstruction in both of these conditions accounts for the absence of faecal colouring. Large amounts of mucus may be secreted by extensive benign papillomatous tumours of the colon and rectum. Since this material is rich in potassium, profound potassium depletion may occur in this condition, leading to weakness, paraesthesiae and even paralysis and vascular collapse. The volume of fluid passed may amount to 2–3-litres daily. ·

Mucus is often seen with constipated motions, the hard faeces having led to irritation of the large bowel with consequent increased secretion of mucus as a defensive mechanism against misguided therapy, especially colonic lavage. In severe cases, a motion may consist almost entirely of coagulated shreds, with little faecal matter. In other cases, complete casts of the bowel formed from coagulated mucus are passed; these may be 30 cm or more in length. They may have become broken into fragments which the patient describes as 'skins', which look not unlike segments of tapeworm for

which indeed they are, on inadequate examination, easily mistaken.

Patients passing this variety of mucus are said to have membranous or spastic colitis; this is an incorrect term, as no inflammatory process occurs. The term 'irritable colon syndrome' is also used for this disorder, which is characterized by colonic abdominal pain, abnormal stools and alteration in bowel habits. It is more common in females aged 15 to 45 years, but it may occur in either sex under conditions of emotional tension. The patients on examination often appear anxious and tense, and perspire excessively. Curiously enough, this hypersecretion of mucus has almost disappeared during the past 40 years, although the general symptomatology is still recognized. It may be added that the popular treatment of lavage to remove the mucus will be responsible for its continued secretion as a protest against irritation of the mucosa. In the more acute varieties of inflammation of the bowel the mucus passed is jelly-like and semi-liquid, of varying colour according to the amount of faecal staining. In polyposis coli and severe cases of ulcerative colitis, Crohn's colitis, enteritis and dysentery, the motions consist of nothing but mucus and blood. Differentiation between the numerous varieties of enteritis and colitis cannot be made upon the basis of the mucus in the stools alone.

Harold Ellis

STOOLS, PUS IN

Pus in the stools in sufficient amounts to be recognizable by the naked eye indicates the rupture of an abscess into the intestinal tract. Such recognition is, however, unusual, for even when a large appendicular abscess perforates into the caecum the pus becomes indistinguishable either from admixture with the faeces (the patient believing they simply have diarrhoea), or on account of its digestion and decomposition. The less the pus is mixed with other intestinal contents, the nearer to the anus must the site of rupture have been. However, the diagnosis of the source of the abscess needs to be determined on other grounds, particularly the history and the results of examination, including that of the rectum and vagina. Abscesses most apt to cause a discharge of pus with the stools are of the appendicular, pericolic, pelvic or other local peritoneal types; of prostatic or perirectal origin; or a pyosalpinx.

Microscopical quantities of pus in the stools may be due to any of the causes already mentioned and, in addition, to affections of the mucous membrane itself. These comprise acute or chronic ulcerative colitis, Crohn's colitis, dysentery, cholera, dengue, malignant, tuberculous, typhoidal, carcinomatous or venereal ulceration of the bowel. The pus cells may be recognizable as such under the microscope. Examination with the sigmoidoscope, followed by a barium enema X-ray and/or colonoscopy, is invaluable in deciding the diagnosis.

Harold Ellis

STRANGURY

Strangury differs somewhat from mere pain on micturition in that, in addition to severe pain before, during or after the act, the patient is troubled constantly by urgent and repeated necessity to pass urine, sometimes as often as every few minutes, yet without satisfactory relief to their discomfort. The condition is also spoken of as 'vesical tenesmus'. Very little urine is passed each time; sometimes, the desire and the necessity are urgent when there is no urine in the bladder at all. The most common cause of strangury worldwide is a vesicle calculus abutting against the bladder outlet, but other aetiologies are legion. The causes resolve themselves into five groups, as follows:

1   Nervous conditions, especially:
 ■ Hysteria
 ■ Anxiety state
 ■ Tabes dorsalis (vesical crises)

2   Obstruction to the urine outflow
 ■ Urethral stricture
 ■ Benign enlargement of the prostate
 ■ Carcinoma of the prostate
 ■ Retroverted gravid uterus
 ■ Uterine fibroid ⎫
 ■ Ovarian cyst ⎬ impacted in the pelvis
 ■ Ovarian carcinoma ⎭
 ■ Extreme prolapse of the uterus and bladder
 ■ Calculus impacted in the urethra
 ■ Inflamed urethral caruncle
 ■ Gonorrhoea
 ■ Urethritis other than gonococcal
 ■ Periprostatic abscess
 ■ Ischiorectal abscess

3   Local affections of the bladder wall
 ■ Calculus irritating the trigone
 ■ Injury
 ■ Acute cystitis
 ■ Chronic cystitis
 ■ Interstitial cystitis (Hunner's ulcer)
 ■ Tuberculous cystitis
 ■ Carcinoma
 ■ Bilharziasis
 ■ Infiltration by:
  ◆ Carcinoma of the uterus
  ◆ Carcinoma of the rectum

4   Reflex conditions
 ■ Inflamed haemorrhoids
 ■ Tuberculous kidney, before the bladder is involved
 ■ *E. coli* bacilluria ⎫ even before there is infection of
 ■ Pyelitis ⎭ the bladder wall

5   The effects of certain drugs, especially:
 ■ Cantharides
 ■ Oxalic acid
 ■ Turpentine
 ■ Hexamine and its derivatives

Most of the conditions mentioned above, and the methods of distinguishing between them, are discussed in the section on MICTURITION, FREQUENCY OF (see p. 439).

Interstitial cystitis (Hunner's ulcer) is probably not an infectious disease. Histologically, there is inflammatory infiltration of the bladder wall, unifocal or multifocal with mucosal ulceration and scarring, leading to contraction of smooth muscle, diminished capacity and frequent painful micturition with haematuria. The patients are usually middle-aged women.

Another point that merits attention is the strangury produced by certain drugs. *Cantharides* is familiar in this respect, but more from its prominence in textbooks upon forensic medicine than from its occurrence in actual practice. The same applies to *oxalic acid* and to *turpentine*. Hexamine and similar drugs derived from it are important. These have in the past been employed in the treatment of pyuria, as well as other conditions, but have now been largely replaced by sulpha drugs and antibiotics. If given for pyuria, when there may have been frequent and painful micturition already, the increased frequency and pain that sometimes ensue when any of the above drugs are administered are apt to be attributed to an increase in the cystitis or other genitourinary lesion, and the dose of the drug may be increased instead of diminished. The important point is that hexamine and other drugs of like nature may be responsible for such strangury as may simulate local disease of the bladder, and unless this is borne in mind an erroneous diagnosis is liable to be made.

Harold Ellis

STRIAE ATROPHICAE

Striae or 'stretch marks' are unsightly linear marks due to disruption of the dermal support tissue (e.g. collagen and elastic fibres). Although initially reddish-purple, they later fade to an opalescent whitish colour. They commonly occur following rapid distension, for example during the growth phase of adolescence (lumbosacral region in boys (Fig. S.62) and thighs, buttocks and breasts in girls) and during pregnancy (breasts and abdomen). They are also caused by corticosteroids, which reduce the bulk of dermal support tissue (e.g. Cushing's syndrome; flexures), and after steroid therapy, both systemic and topical.

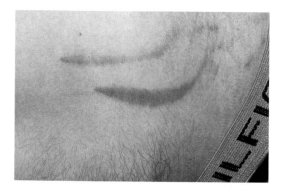

Figure S.62 Striae.

Striae are usually only a cosmetic problem but can, if extensive, ulcerate, particularly following trauma.

Barry Monk

STRIDOR

Stridor is a harsh noise produced during breathing, typically heard as a high-pitched inspiratory wheeze audible at a distance. It is commonly caused by obstruction affecting the larynx or extrathoracic trachea. The intensity of sound is accentuated by inspiratory negative pressure tending to collapse the extrathoracic airways. Stridor may not be evident on quiet breathing, and is best heard after exercise or during hyperventilation through the open mouth. On auscultation, a fixed inspiratory wheeze is heard over the trachea, becoming fainter over the lungs. When narrowing affects the portion of the trachea within the thorax, the carina or main bronchi, stridor tends to be louder on expiration because the intrathoracic airways partially collapse due to the expiratory rise in intrathoracic pressure. In this situation it may be difficult to differentiate stridor from abnormal noisy breath sounds commonly present on quiet breathing in widespread airflow obstruction. These differences, and also the distinction between main airway narrowing and diffuse distal airway narrowing, as in asthma or chronic obstructive pulmonary disease, may be demonstrated by flow–volume loops (Fig. S.63).

Stridor is generated by vibration of the walls of critically narrowed airways, and the pitch is dependent upon the speed of airflow and the density of the inspired air. A low-density gas mixture (helium and oxygen) produces much less turbulence and stridor than conventional nitrogen and oxygen mixtures, and therefore may provide useful temporary relief of symptoms in critically breathless patients. With extreme degrees of tracheal narrowing, violent ineffectual respiratory effort, cyanosis and sudden death may result when a relatively minor additional insult, such as a mucous plug, occludes the narrowed trachea.

In children, the onset of stridor is usually alarmingly sudden and due to acute infective conditions (Table S.16), whereas in adults the onset tends to be insidious and may be confused with late-onset bronchial asthma, chronic bronchitis, or other chronic pulmonary disorders (Table S.17).

In many patients the cause of stridor is obvious, for example when it is caused by secretions lodging in the larynx or trachea in seriously ill patients, or in patients in coma from any cause. In others, local examination of the upper respiratory tract and larynx will provide the diagnosis without much difficulty.

Fibre-optic laryngoscopy and bronchoscopy will often be diagnostic. The greatest difficulty is likely to be encountered in children in whom the possibility of stridor of acute onset being due to diphtheria should never be forgotten, and in less acute cases retropharyngeal abscess must be borne in mind. Foreign bodies

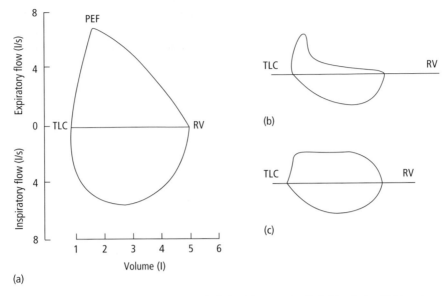

Figure S.63 Maximum flow–volume curves represented diagrammatically for: (a) a normal subject; (b) patients with intrapulmonary airflow obstruction (chronic obstructive pulmonary disease); or (c) obstruction of the upper (extrathoracic) trachea (fixed upper airway). In extrathoracic tracheal obstruction the reduction in inspiratory flow is equal to or greater than the reduction in expiratory flow, whereas in intrapulmonary airways obstruction maximum expiratory flow is reduced more than maximum inspiratory flow. TLC, total lung capacity; RV, residual lung volume; PEF, peak expiratory flow.

Table S.16 Causes of acute inspiratory stridor in infants and young children

Congenital
- Choanal atresia in newborn
- Congenital laryngeal paralysis in newborn

Inhaled foreign body
- Small plastic toys in crawling children
- Peanuts in older children

Croup syndrome
- Diphtheria – any age
- Acute laryngotracheobronchitis – usually in 2-year-olds
- Acute epiglottitis – usually in 2- to 7-year-olds
- Acute pseudo-membranous croup
- Upper airway burns
- Angioneurotic oedema
- Infectious mononucleosis

in the larynx or the main air passages are also a possible source of difficulty in children who are often too young to provide a clear history.

Inspiratory stridor is common in early childhood. The most frequent cause is acute viral laryngotracheobronchitis (croup), but it is essential to consider the full differential diagnosis if tragic and preventable death from acute airway obstruction is to be avoided (see Table S.17).

Acute laryngotracheobronchitis is the common cause of croup in the second year of life. Males are affected most frequently. The main pathogens are parainfluenza virus (50%), respiratory syncytial virus, influenza A and B, rhinovirus, adenovirus and measles. It is usually preceded for 1–2 days by an upper respiratory tract infection before developing a harsh, barking cough and hoarse voice due to inflammatory swelling of the subglottic region. With more severe airway obstruction chest wall recession occurs and stridor may be inspiratory and expiratory. Fever, restlessness, hypoxia, tachypnoea, tachycardia and eventually cyanosis herald the risk of sudden collapse and death.

Acute epiglottitis is often mistaken for acute laryngotracheobronchitis, but its pathology and clinical course are quite different. The onset is usually rapid and the patient pyrexial and lethargic, complaining of a sore throat. Within a short time, upper airway obstruction becomes obvious with a soft inspiratory stridor and expiratory sound resembling a snore. The child prefers

Table S.17 Causes of stridor in adults

Causes above the larynx ■ Retropharyngeal abscess ■ New growths of the pharynx ■ Lingual angio-oedema	**Compression of larynx or trachea from without** ■ Goitre, especially haemorrhage into an adenomatous goitre. Hashimoto's disease, intrathoracic goitre ■ Riedel's thyroiditis ■ Carcinoma of the thyroid ■ Aneurysm of the arch of the aorta ■ Malformations of the aorta – double aortic arch ■ Mediastinal new growths, including metastatic involvement of mediastinal lymph nodes ■ Mediastinal Hodgkin's disease and other reticuloses ■ Carcinoma of oesophagus invading the trachea ■ Malignant disease of lower cervical lymph nodes ■ Cellulitis of neck ■ Ludwig's angina ■ Tuberculous nodes in mediastinum ■ Fungal infections ■ Histoplasmosis ■ Coccidicidomycosis ■ Blastomycosis

Causes above the larynx

- Retropharyngeal abscess
- New growths of the pharynx
- Lingual angio-oedema

Causes inside the larynx or trachea

- Mucus or mucopus in patients enfeebled by illness or in whom a defect of the cough mechanism (laryngeal or respiratory muscle paralysis) leads to inability to expel these secretions

Affections of the wall of the larynx or trachea

- Inflammatory
  - Acute diphtheria, acute laryngitis, due to exposure to irritant gases.
  - Chronic tuberculous or syphilitic laryngitis with stenosis
  - Wegener's granulomatosis
  - Sarcoidosis
- Traumatic or post-traumatic
  - Injuries of larynx or trachea
  - Post-traumatic stenosis of larynx or trachea (e.g. after tracheostomy, after attempted suicidal 'cut-throat' and after prolonged use of a cuffed endotracheal tube with or without tracheostomy)
- Neoplastic
  - Carcinoma of larynx
  - Carcinoma of trachea
  - Benign tumours of larynx or trachea
- Oedema of the glottis
  - Burn injuries
  - Angio-oedema
  - Inhalation of toxic gas
- Ankylosis of crico-arytenoid joint in rheumatoid arthritis
- Tracheopathia osteoplastica

Compression of larynx or trachea from without

- Goitre, especially haemorrhage into an adenomatous goitre. Hashimoto's disease, intrathoracic goitre
- Riedel's thyroiditis
- Carcinoma of the thyroid
- Aneurysm of the arch of the aorta
- Malformations of the aorta – double aortic arch
- Mediastinal new growths, including metastatic involvement of mediastinal lymph nodes
- Mediastinal Hodgkin's disease and other reticuloses
- Carcinoma of oesophagus invading the trachea
- Malignant disease of lower cervical lymph nodes
- Cellulitis of neck
- Ludwig's angina
- Tuberculous nodes in mediastinum
- Fungal infections
- Histoplasmosis
- Coccidicidomycosis
- Blastomycosis

Laryngeal nerve palsies

- Bulbar or pseudobulbar palsy
- Bilateral lesions of recurrent laryngeal nerves (postoperative or inflammatory)

Narrowing of both main bronchi

- Bronchial carcinoma arising in main bronchus or metastasizing to subcarinal lymph nodes
- Mediastinal tumours
- Tuberculous strictures of main bronchi
- Strictures of main bronchi in sarcoidosis
- Amyloidosis
- Bronchopathia osteoplastica
- Tracheomalacia

to sit upright, mouth-breathe, and often drools saliva. Acute epiglottitis is an acute life-threatening form of laryngeal obstruction due to oedema and hyperaemia of the epiglottis, aryepiglottic folds and hypopharynx which results in considerable oedema around the laryngeal inlet obstructing respiration and swallowing. The changes do not extend below the vocal cords. Septicaemia is invariably present, the usual organism being *Haemophilus influenzae* type B. The clinical features are similar to those of acute obstructive laryngo-tracheobronchitis, except that there is rapid onset of dysphagia and drooling saliva as well as respiratory distress with stridor and a thick muffled voice.

The child is toxic, and complete respiratory obstruction may supervene very quickly. No attempt should be made to examine the pharynx with a tongue depressor as this may precipitate complete obstruction. Because of the risk of laryngeal obstruction, immediate transfer of the child to a hospital with appropriate facilities should be arranged for full assessment with a view to nasal or oral intubation and appropriate antibiotic treatment (see also WHEEZE, p. 799).

Boris Lams

SUCCUSSION SOUNDS

Succussion sounds may be heard when a viscus or cavity that contains both liquid and air or gas is shaken whilst the ear or the stethoscope is applied over it. The sounds may be loud enough to be audible at a distance from the patient. A good example of succussion is often afforded by the normal stomach after a quantity of liquid has been swallowed. Gastric succussion sounds are not necessarily evidence of abnormality, they merely indicate that the viscus contains liquid and gas. Succussion sound may be heard in the chest in cases of *hydropneumothorax* when the patient oscillates their trunk to and fro. Less often, succussion sounds may be produced by a pyopneumothorax or a haemopneumothorax, the difference between these being decided by a pleural tap. Other succussion sounds are uncommon.

A list of all possible causes of succussion sounds is provided in Table S.18.

Table S.18 Causes of succussion sounds

In the thorax
- Hydropneumothorax
- Pyopneumothorax
- Haemopneumothorax
- Diaphragmatic hernia
- Subdiaphragmatic abscess communicating with the stomach or duodenum, or infected with *E. coli*: in either case, gas and pus are present
- Hydropheumopericardium
- Pyopneumopericardium

In the abdomen
- The normal stomach
- Dilatation of the stomach
- Gross dilatation of the caecum
- Gross dilatation of the colon
- Pneumoperitoneum due to:
  - Perforated gastric ulcer
  - Perforated duodenal ulcer
  - Perforated typhoid ulcer of the intestine
  - Perforated carcinoma of the colon
  - Production of gas by *E. coli*, either in a local abscess (e.g. appendicular or subdiaphragmatic) or in the general peritoneum
- Subdiaphragmatic abscess communicating with the interior of the stomach
- Air and urine in the bladder (see PNEUMATURIA, p. 547)
- Gas production by *E. coli* in a large pyonephrosis infection by a gas-producing micro-organism of an ovarian cyst or other collection of fluid

Succussion sounds in the chest

It is almost unknown for a *tuberculous cavity* to give succussion sounds. Should it do so, the situation would be subapical rather than basal, and thus distinguishable from most cases of hydro- or pyopneumothorax. *Hydro-* and *pyopneumopericardium* are also rare: they are identified by the churning sounds made by the heart beating within the mixture of air and liquid. The cause is generally a tumour of the oesophagus or bronchus opening the pericardium from behind, a foreign body such as dental plate ulcerating through from the oesophagus, the opening of an air-containing subdiaphragmatic abscess through the diaphragm into the pericardium, or infection of the pericardial sac by a gas-producing micro-organism.

A *subdiaphragmatic abscess* containing air due to communication with a hole in a gastric or duodenal ulcer may elevate the diaphragm so high that the condition may be mistaken for hydro- or pyopneumothorax. A decision may be impossible until the position of the diaphragm is ascertained by X-rays and ultrasonography. When the pathology is subdiaphragmatic, the tendency is to displace the heart upwards rather than towards the opposite side of the chest; the contrary is usual in the case of pneumothorax.

Diaphragmatic hernias, if large and if the stomach is herniated into the thorax, will show the effect of eating and drinking upon the physical signs and may point to the diagnosis. X-rays will demonstrate the condition on barium meal.

Most cases of *hydropneumothorax* present little difficulty in diagnosis, although it may not be easy to ascertain the cause of the condition. If the onset has been sudden, with acute pain in the affected side of the chest, cyanosis and dyspnoea, the most likely cause is *tuberculosis*. In some instances, an injury or a ruptured emphysematous bulla may have been responsible, but injury seldom produces hydropneumothorax unless a tuberculous or other lesion in the lung was present at the time of the accident. Hydropneumothorax may result from *paracentesis thoracis*; if bleeding occurs during the puncture, *haemopneumothorax* will be produced. This is also common after bullet wounds of the chest. Either a hydro- or a haemopneumothorax may become infected with pyogenic organisms and converted into a *pyopneumothorax*. This may develop in cases of gangrene of the lung, obstruction of a bronchus by a foreign body or a tumour, the breaking down of an infective bronchopneumonia or pulmonary infarct, or the conversion of a pleural haematoma into a mixture of pus and gas as the result of infection by gas-gangrene organisms after gunshot or other wounds of the chest.

Fluid often collects in the pleural cavity when an artificial (therapeutic) pneumothorax has been induced, giving succussion sounds.

Succussion sounds in the abdomen

The first point in the differential diagnosis of succussion sounds in the abdomen is to decide whether the sounds are, or are not, of gastric origin. This is usually obvious, but any doubt can be at once resolved by a barium meal. Dilatation of the stomach has three causes, namely atony, non-malignant pyloric, or duodenal obstruction, especially by a healed simple ulcer, and malignant pyloric obstruction by primary gastric carcinoma (see PERISTALSIS, VISIBLE, p. 540). The presence of visible peristaltic waves or the occurrence of vomiting will indicate some degree of pyloric obstruction. Such obstruction will usually result in periodic vomiting, when the particles of food eaten a day or more previously can be recognized. Visible peristaltic waves corresponding to the stomach are another confirmatory feature. The most certain method of detecting gastric outflow obstruction is by means of a barium meal examination.

If there are well-marked abdominal succussion sounds that can be definitely shown to be of non-gastric origin, there are generally other signs and symptoms to assist the diagnosis. Succussion sounds in the peritoneal cavity are exceedingly rare, for even though this cavity should contain both gas and liquid – for example, after perforation of a typhoid ulcer – the coils of bowel prevent the sounds from being readily produced. The most common cause is iatrogenic, occurring when air is introduced into the peritoneum, when ascites is tapped or when carbon dioxide is introduced at laparoscopy in the presence of ascites. It would clearly be next to impossible to diagnose most of the conditions listed above unless the previous state of the patient was known, or without a laparotomy. *Escherichia coli* produces gas so that intra-abdominal abscesses – appendicular and otherwise – are occasionally resonant; the occurrence, however, of marked non-gastric succussion sounds in the abdomen of a patient who is not acutely ill will support the conclusion that there is distension with gas and liquid of some part of the large bowel, especially the caecum or the sigmoid colon. This distension is generally the result of either chronic constipation or intestinal stenosis. In cases of idiopathic dilatation of the colon, volvulus of the sigmoid colon or

Hirschsprung's disease, the sigmoid dilatation may be so extreme that this part of the intestine bulges up as far as the diaphragm.

John Meenan

SWEATING, ABNORMALITIES OF

Hyperhidrosis, or excess of sweating, may be either generalized or local (see Table S.19).

Table S.19 Hyperhidrosis

Generalized	Local
Exercise	Organic nerve lesions, brain
Raised ambient temperature	tumours, spinal cord injuries
Anxiety	Palms/soles
Infections/pyrogens	Pachydermoperiostosis
Drugs: alcohol, pilocarpines,	Granulosis rubra nasi
tricyclic antidepressants	
Hypoglycaemia	
Dumping syndrome	
Alcohol/drug withdrawal	
Shock/syncope	
Intense pain	
Rickets	
Infantile scurvy	
Pink disease	
Hyperthyroidism	
Hyperpituitarism	
Acromegaly	
Phaeochromocytoma	
Carcinoid	
Gout	

Generalized hyperhidrosis

The sweat glands are controlled via the sympathetic nerves by thermoregulatory centres in the hypothalamus. Sweating is the normal response to exercise or excessive heat, though there is marked physiological variation between individuals. Fever and sweating accompany infections, and drenching sweats usually occur with a fall of temperature. Sweat regulation can be unbalanced by pyrogens, and sweating may occur out of phase with the fever, for example in some cases of tuberculosis, brucellosis, HIV and lymphoma. These conditions are often associated with night sweats. Generalized hyperhidrosis may also be produced by drugs (e.g. alcohol, pilocarpines and tricyclic anti-depressants). Hyperhydrosis may cause maceration of the skin, increasing the risk of fungal or pyogenic skin infection.

A 'cold and clammy skin', where sweating is associated with cutaneous vasoconstriction, occurs in hypoglycaemia, the dumping syndrome, alcohol and drug withdrawal, shock and syncopal states, and also in intense pain. Increased sweating is seen in many endocrinological disturbances – hyperthyroidism, hyperpituitarism and acromegaly. It has also been described with phaeochromocytoma, the carcinoid syndrome and gout. Sweating is a feature of rickets, pink disease and infantile scurvy (Barlow's disease).

Local hyperhidrosis

Local increase in sweat production is seen with organic neurological lesions (e.g. brain tumours and spinal cord injuries), and can help to localize the neurological defect. Local hyperhidrosis of the palms, soles and/or axillae is not uncommon, and this occurs in patients who are otherwise perfectly normal; the sweating increases with embarrassment, anxiety and during the summer months. Sweat can literally drip from the hands, making paperwork extremely difficult. The keratin of the soles becomes macerated, and secondary infection causes an offensive odour (osmidrosis). In pachydermoperiostosis, local hyperhidrosis occurs over the skin folds of forehead and extremities.

Granulosis rubra nasi is a rare, genetically determined disease where profuse sweating of the tip of the nose is associated with a diffuse erythema and the formation of minute, dark-red papules. The disorder usually begins in early childhood and subsides at puberty. It must be distinguished from rosacea, lupus erythematosus and lupus vulgaris.

Miliaria

Miliaria are lesions caused by blockage and rupture of sweat ducts; they are most often seen in tropical conditions of heat and high humidity, which are simulated in the UK by polythene occlusion of the skin, or in neonatal nurseries. There are three forms depending on the depth of duct obstruction:

1 *Miliaria crystallina* (sudamina). Superficial blockage causes 'crystal'-clear vesicles just below the epidermal surface with little inflammatory reaction and few symptoms. These are often seen on the trunk during febrile illnesses.

2 *Miliaria rubra* (prickly heat). The rupture occurs in mid-epidermis, resulting in tiny, intensely pricking red papules. These may erupt widely in persons recently arrived in tropical conditions, or they may be confined to friction areas and flexures.

3 *Miliaria profunda* (mamillaria). The blockage occurs within the dermis. Lesions are easily overlooked as they are neither red nor uncomfortable but appear as firm papules (1–3 mm) on the body or limbs. They may follow repeated attacks of miliaria rubra. The natural history of miliaria depends on environmental factors; if sweating continues the lesions continue to erupt, but if sweating is arrested (e.g. by entering an air-conditioned or cool area), then healing can commence.

Anhidrosis

Anhidrosis is much less common than hyperhidrosis; sweating may be either diminished or totally suppressed, and either the whole skin or only some particular area is affected. A lack of sweat glands may occur with skin dystrophies (e.g. congenital ectodermal dysplasia) or atrophy (e.g. scleroderma). The sweat gland population may also be diminished in ichthyosis and Anderson–Tabry's disease. In these situations heat regulation may be impaired. Suppression of sweating is characteristic of heat-stroke, though the mechanism of heat stress and acclimatization is still poorly understood. Organic brain damage at any level, especially of the hypothalamus, can result in complete anhidrosis. Localized anhidrosis can follow spinal cord lesions, for example syringomyelia or neuropathy of diabetes or leprosy. It can thus help in localizing neurological lesions. Sympathectomy abolishes sweating.

Generalized decreased sweating and dry skin is a well-known sign in myxoedema. Blockage of sweat ducts can occur in atopic eczema, psoriasis and lichen planus and be associated with crises of itching, as in miliaria rubra.

Osmidrosis

Osmidrosis is foul-smelling sweat. Sweat is usually odourless, but various substances may be excreted in sweat, including garlic, drugs (e.g. dimethyl sulphoxide) and arsenic. In the past, physicians have remarked on the particular odour of sweat: in diabetes, gout, scurvy, typhoid, uraemia (see also SMELL, ABNOR-MALITIES OF, p. 655). Hyperhidrosis, especially of the soles, is commonly accompanied by a foul odour due to bacterial overgrowth. Imaginary osmidrosis is a well-recognized paranoid delusional symptom. Personal body odour is largely determined by apocrine gland secretion.

Chromhidrosis

Chromhidrosis is usually due to coloured sweat. Perhaps 10 per cent of normal people have coloured apocrine sweat (blue, yellow or green), and rarely areas of ectopic apocrine glands can give rise to areas of discolored skin, where it is possible to see tiny beads of coloured sweat. The pigments are lipofuscins. In pseudochromhidrosis, colourless sweat becomes coloured on the surface of the skin, due usually to chromogenic bacteria. Occasionally, workers in the chemical industry can develop coloured eccrine sweat which can be shown to contain dyes. Certain drugs may give rise to coloured sweat (e.g. rifampicin).

Urhidrosis

The urea content of sweat increases with serum urea concentration. Uraemic sweat has a particular odour, and after evaporation leaves a visible deposit of urea crystals on the skin; this is known as 'uraemic frost'.

Danielle Harari

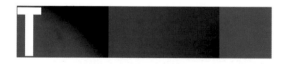

TACHYPNOEA

Tachypnoea signifies an increase in the rate of breathing, as may occur normally during exercise or abnormally with a number of clinical disturbances, especially those associated with hypoxia. In most clinical situations, tachypnoea is associated with symptoms of breathlessness (see DYSPNOEA, p. 159).

In health, both the rate and depth of respiration are controlled by brainstem respiratory centres to maintain a constant arterial blood oxygen level. The relationship between ventilatory rate and depth, demands for oxygen uptake and requirements for CO_2 elimination is controlled by complex interaction between: (i) mechanoreceptors in the airways and lung parenchyma; (ii) peripheral chemoreceptors in the carotid and aortic bodies; and (iii) central chemoreceptors mostly located on or beneath the ventral surface of the medulla. The automatic control system situated in the brainstem is concerned primarily with oxygen, CO_2 and acid–base homeostasis. When metabolic requirements are modest, this automatic system can be overridden by the voluntary control system which arises in the cerebral cortex to allow other activities such as talking, coughing and singing to occur. A low arterial PO_2, high arterial PCO_2 or acid pH all stimulate ventilation.

There are many causes for tachypnoea. The increased metabolic demands of fever or circulatory shock from myocardial infarction, haemorrhage, trauma or pulmonary embolism often manifest clinically with rapid breathing. Stimulation of the central chemoreceptors by metabolic acidosis in uncontrolled diabetes mellitus, renal or hepatic failure or acute circulatory collapse as well as salicylate overdose may all cause tachypnoea. Stimulation of lung stretch receptors with reflex increase in ventilatory drive may follow acute pulmonary emboli, acute pneumonias, asthma, aspiration of gastrointestinal contents, pulmonary fibrosis or buflous lung disease and provoke tachypnoea out of proportion to the hypoxia so commonly associated with these conditions. Neurological causes of tachypnoea include cerebral haemorrhage, meningitis, encephalitis, head injury or primary abnormalities in the brainstem.

Breathing is under voluntary control, and deep inspiration in excess of ventilatory requirements can be taken to anticipate exercise or facilitate talking or singing. Inappropriate hyperventilation is common and may present with complaints of breathlessness, associated with lightheadedness, dizziness, peripheral paraesthesiae, headache or anxiety. Even tetany may occur if a significant respiratory alkalosis results from over-breathing.

Clinical features suggesting a diagnosis of the hyperventilation syndrome (HVS) include complaints of breathlessness at rest for no apparent reason, paradoxical absence of significant breathlessness on exercise, and marked variability of symptoms. Clinical examination with routine respiratory investigations (including a chest radiograph) may reveal no abnormality, although the occasional patient does exhibit a sighing, irregular pattern of breathing. The most common cause of this condition is anxiety.

Boris Lams

TASTE, ABNORMAL PERCEPTION OF

Taste perception comprises the basic elements of sweet, salty, bitter and sour. Disorders of taste are much less common than those of smell. In fact, the complaint of abnormal taste is usually found to be due to olfactory dysfunction with preserved taste. This is because in the overall perception of 'taste', smell and taste proper are inextricably linked; a patient with anosmia will complain that food is 'tasteless' because the normal tongue can only distinguish the basic tastes of sweet, salt, sour and bitter. Patients with altered or lost taste should therefore be asked about symptoms of head injury or recent upper respiratory illness (which could disturb smell) as well as Bell's palsy (which may disturb taste). Both taste and smell may be lost in acute upper respiratory infection due to a coated tongue and inflamed nose. Smell and taste must be tested separately in every case. Taste can be tested with solutions of sugar, sodium chloride or quinine applied to each quadrant with a cotton applicator. Cards are used for the patient to point to their impression of taste, and water is used to rinse the mouth between applications.

True loss of taste is found in disease of the tongue itself, the facial nerve (chorda tympani branch), the glossopharyngeal nerve, and the glossopharyngeal nucleus in the medulla. Loss of smell by itself occurs in inflammatory conditions of the nose, in tumours of the anterior fossa (which compress the olfactory nerves), and frequently as a result of fractures of the cribriform plate (see SMELL, ABNORMALITIES OF, p. 655). The appreciation of taste is a function of the tongue; fibres from the anterior two-thirds pass via the chorda tympani to the geniculate ganglion, passing from there to the pons by the nervus intermedius. Fibres from the posterior third travel in the glossopharyngeal nerve. In the pons, taste fibres pass into the tractus solitarius and

from the nucleus of this tract a gustatory lemniscus is formed which, after decussating, passes upwards near the midline to the thalamus and from there to the gustatory cortex at the bottom of the postcentral gyrus. Disorders of taste can be classified as absence of taste (ageusia), diminished taste (hypogeusia), increased sensitivity to some or all taste qualities (hypergeusia), distortion of taste (parageusia or dysgeusia), or gustatory hallucinations. Persistent foul taste can be considered as a specific form of dysgeusia and termed cacogeusia. Common causes of taste disturbance are listed in Table T.1.

Table T.1 Disorders of taste

Ageusia (impairment or loss)
- Local mouth disorders
  - Coated or geographic tongue
  - Epithelioma
  - Glossitis
  - Xerostomia (dry mouth): Sjögren's syndrome, radiation therapy, pandysautonomia
- Neurological causes
  - Glossopharyngeal nerve damage (e.g. meningeal infiltration, skull base tumour, carotid dissection)
  - Facial nerve chorda tympani damage (e.g. Bell's palsy)
  - Thalamic damage (e.g. stroke, tumour)
  - Pontine damage (e.g. stroke, demyelination)
- Drugs (e.g. penicillamine, ACE inhibitors, calcium-channel blockers, nasal sumatriptan)
- Other causes
  - Diabetes
  - Hypogonadism

Parageusia/dysgeusia (altered taste)
- Pregnancy or menstrual cycle changes
- Glossitis
- Hysteria
- Drugs (e.g. metronidazole, corticosteroids, lamotrigine)
- Cortical damage (e.g. stroke, rare)

Gustatory hallucinations
- Uncinate pathology (e.g. tumour, demyelination)
- Psychiatric disease

Cacogeusia (foul taste)
- Local oral disease: caries, stomatitis, gingivitis, glossitis
- Gastrointestinal disease: carcinoma, gastritis, pyloric stenosis
- Lung disease: abscess, tuberculosis, bronchiectasis

From the diagnostic point of view, impairment of taste sensation is important only when it is persistent or recurrent, and even then it is usually due to a primary condition of the mouth, nose, lung or gastrointestinal tract. In the absence of one of these explanations, diagnosis becomes difficult, and a neurological cause should be considered. The most common neurological cause of loss of taste is Bell's palsy, in which it often occurs as an early and transient feature, the loss being confined to the anterior two-thirds of the tongue on the same side as the facial paralysis. This may be asymptomatic or symptomatic. Recovery of taste within 14 days usually indicates that a full recovery will occur.

A persistent facial palsy and loss of taste may be due to the spread of inflammatory disease from the middle ear. Taste may be impaired due to disease process affecting lower cranial nerves (e.g. carcinomatous meningitis or skull base tumours), but will usually be accompanied by more obvious symptoms and signs. Organic lesions of the temporal lobe uncus (glioma, demyelination, stroke, arteriovenous malformation, cortical dysplasia) can cause *uncinate* fits in which there is a hallucination of smell or taste, usually unpleasant, followed by salivation, chewing or sucking movements of the mouth and jaws, and disturbance of consciousness which may be mild or progress to loss of consciousness and a generalized convulsion. The distortions of taste that occur during pregnancy are neither delusional nor hallucinatory, but their origin is not understood. Disturbances of smell or taste are uncommon manifestations of hysteria. Loss of taste and smell occasionally occurs as part of a migraine aura.

David Werring

TESTICULAR ATROPHY

Apart from the physiological atrophy of the testes which occurs with advancing age, and may begin as early as the age of 50 years, the causes of testicular atrophy can be classified under the headings hypothalamic/pituitary conditions, testicular conditions, adrenal disorders, general disease and drugs (Table T.2).

Hypothalamic/pituitary conditions

The testes contain two main components: the seminiferous tubules, which are responsible for the production of spermatozoa; and the interstitial tissue which contains Leydig cells that secrete testosterone. Spermatogenesis is under the control of one gonadotrophin, follicle-stimulating hormone (FSH), and testosterone secretion is stimulated by the other

gonadotrophin, luteinizing hormone (LH), both of which are produced by the pituitary gland in response to the secretion of the hypothalamic hormone gonadotrophin-releasing hormone (GnRH). It follows from this that any hypothalamic or pituitary condition that reduces GnRH or gonadotrophin secretion is likely to lead to testicular atrophy. Probably the most common hypothalamic condition is a congenital lack of GnRH which, when associated with anosmia, is called *Kallmann's syndrome* (see PUBERTY, DELAYED p. 560). In this condition there is a midline defect with agenesis of the olfactory bulbs and other midline anomalies such as cleft palate and hare lip. The patients are sexually immature and are tall, with eunuchoidal skeletal proportions, having long arms and legs relative to the trunk. Kallmann's syndrome is an autosomal dominant condition with variable penetrance, and it occurs in 1 in 10 000 male births and 1 in 50 000 female births.

Isolated LH deficiency is a rare condition causing the 'fertile eunuch syndrome'. There is little or no testosterone production by the Leydig cells, and the seminiferous tubules are immature because an adequate concentration of intracellular testosterone is necessary for this development and for the production of spermatozoa. The patients are sexually immature and have eunuchoidal skeletal proportions. They can be made sexually mature by treatment with human chorionic gonadotrophin (HCG), which has LH-like activity, and this also fully develops the seminiferous tubules.

The Laurence–Moon–Biedl syndrome is an uncommon condition which is an hereditary autosomal recessive disorder with variable penetrance. There are low levels of gonadotrophins with consequent retarded sexual development, obesity, mental retardation, retinitis pigmentosa and either polydactylism or syndactylism.

Raised prolactin levels produced in men by macroprolactinomas of the pituitary or as a consequence of drug therapy (phenothiazines, metoclopramide, haloperidol, pimozide, methyldopa, reserpine, cimetidine) lead to reduced gonadotrophin secretion by the pituitary and consequently to impotence, infertility and testicular atrophy.

Testicular conditions

Conditions affecting the testes directly are a much more common cause of atrophy than are those secondarily

Table T.2 Causes of testicular atrophy

Physiological
■ Old age
 	
Hypothalamic/pituitary conditions
■ GnRH deficiency (e.g. Kallmann's syndrome)
■ Hypopituitarism
■ Isolated LH deficiency
■ Hyperprolactinaemia
■ Haemochromatosis
■ Laurence–Moon–Biedl syndrome
 	
Testicular conditions
■ Trauma*
■ Disturbances of blood supply
  ◆ Bilateral torsion of testes
  ◆ Inguinal hernia
  ◆ Ill-fitting truss
  ◆ Hydrocele
  ◆ Haematocele
  ◆ Varicocele
  ◆ Postoperative
  ◆ Elephantiasis
■ Destructive lesions
  ◆ Orchitis or epididymitis
	■ Mumps*
	■ Lymphocytic choriomeningitis virus
	■ Echovirus
	■ Arbovirus
	■ Chickenpox
	■ Tuberculosis
	■ Syphilis
	■ Gonorrhoea
	■ Typhoid fever
	■ Brucellosis
	■ Leptospirosis
	■ Lepromatosis leprosy
	■ Autoimmune orchitis
	■ Congenital lesions
	  ◆ Cryptorchidism
	  ◆ Klinefelter's syndrome*
	  ◆ XX male
	  ◆ Reifenstein's syndrome
	  ◆ Noonan's syndrome
	  ◆ Dystrophia myotonica
	  ◆ Sertoli-cell only syndrome
	  ◆ Haemochromatosis
		■ Tumour
		  ◆ Feminizing tumour
		
		Suprarenal disorders
		■ Cushing's syndrome
		■ Congenital adrenal hyperplasia
		■ Feminizing (oestrogen secreting) tumour
		
		General disease
		■ Alcoholism*
		■ Cirrhosis of liver*
		■ Renal failure
		■ Sickle-cell anaemia
		■ AIDS
		
		Drugs
		■ GnRH analogues
		■ Oestrogen therapy
		■ Spironolactone
		■ Marijuana
		■ Cyclophosphamide
		■ Chlorambucil

*Most common causes.

related to hypothalamic or pituitary disorders. Trauma, such as being struck in the testes by a cricket ball or falling astride a fence, may lead to an intratesticular haematoma which causes pressure necrosis of the seminiferous tubules and eventual atrophy of the testis. Any disturbance of the blood supply to the testes, particularly torsion, can lead to testicular atrophy.

Mumps occurring in males after the age of 13 years is an important cause of testicular atrophy. Permanent atrophy may occur in 36 per cent of cases. A wide range of other infections mentioned in Table T.2 may have the same effect.

Testes which have been situated in the inguinal canal (cryptorchidism) or ectopically in the superficial inguinal pouch, perineum or upper thigh may fail to develop properly and remain small. Cryptorchidism which is unilateral in 84 per cent of cases occurs in 3 per 1000 of the adult male population. Cryptorchidism may be associated with Kallmann's syndrome (see above) but, more importantly, also with *Klinefelter's syndrome* (see Fig. S.57). This condition is relatively common, occurring in 1 per 500 male births. It is due to the presence of an extra X chromosome giving a

karyotype of 47,XXY, though sometimes mosaicism occurs with a karyotype of 46,XY/47,XXY. The patients are tall with eunuchoidal proportions, and they have small, firm testes which, if biopsied, show tubular sclerosis and hyalinization. Variable numbers of Leydig cells are present. There is invariably gynaecomastia, and there is a tendency to low intelligence. The gonadotrophins LH and FSH are increased.

Patients with partial androgen resistance (*Reifenstein's syndrome*) may present with small testes, though there is usually also hypospadias and a small penis. The condition is an X-linked recessive with a 46,XY karyotype.

Noonan's syndrome may present with atrophic testes, though more commonly the testes are undescended.

Dystrophia myotonica (Fig. T.1) is an autosomal dominant condition with a considerable degree of penetrance. Although it commonly appears to present in early middle age, careful studies have shown that evidence of it is usually present in adolescence. Testicular atrophy, cataract and baldness are usual features accompanying the muscular features, which consist of atrophy of the sternomastoids, facial muscles and distal muscles of the limbs, and the

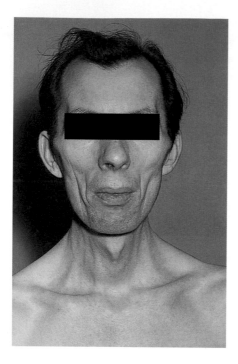

Figure T.1 A patient with dystrophia myotonica, showing wasting of facial muscles and sternomastoids and also frontal balding.

characteristic delay in the ability to relax the muscles, exemplified in the prolonged handshake. In addition, the patient usually displays progressive intellectual and psychological impairment.

Haemochromatosis leads to iron deposition in many tissues, including the pituitary and testes. The patient usually has testicular atrophy secondary to low levels of gonadotrophins. The patient has slate-grey skin and may have an enlarged liver and spleen. Feminizing tumours of the ovary or suprarenal are extremely rare, but may cause atrophy of non-tumorous testicular tissue because of oestrogen secretion. The patient usually also displays gynaecomastia.

Suprarenal disorders

Cushing's syndrome may lead to some degree of testicular atrophy because the high levels of plasma cortisol reduce LH secretion. Similarly, children with congenital suprarenal hyperplasia have small testes, despite development of the penis and secondary sexual hair, because the raised concentrations of androgens suppress the gonadotrophins.

General disease

Alcohol abuse and cirrhosis of the liver are important causes of testicular atrophy. Alcohol impairs gonadotrophin release from the pituitary, but also has a direct effect on the testes, lowering testosterone synthesis. Spermatogenesis is also impaired. Testicular atrophy is found in 10–50 per cent of alcoholics without liver disease. Cirrhosis of the liver causes decreased testosterone secretion and an increased conversion of testosterone to oestrogen. This leads to an increase in the carrier protein, sex hormone-binding globulin (SHBG), which binds more avidly with what testosterone there is so that the level of free testosterone falls even further. Between 30 and 75 per cent of alcoholics with cirrhosis have testicular atrophy.

Approximately one-third of males with sickle-cell anaemia have testicular atrophy, presumably secondary to impairment of blood supply or infarction of testicular tissue.

Testicular atrophy is frequently found in men with the acquired immune deficiency syndrome (AIDS). The hormonal changes present in AIDS suggest a non-specific response to systemic illness – low testosterone without an appropriate increase in LH. The disease may involve the testes directly, as virus has been found in lymphocytes in the seminiferous tubules, in the interstitial cells of the testes and within spermatogonia. Opportunistic infections (e.g. cytomegalovirus infection of the testes) have been noted in approximately 30 per cent of cases at post-mortem examination. These patients suffer from hypogonadism.

Drugs

Drugs used in the treatment of carcinoma of the prostate lead to testicular atrophy. Oestrogen therapy was commonly used in the past, but recently long-acting analogues of GnRH have been used. These act by exhausting the pituitary gonadotroph cells and lowering the levels of gonadotrophins so that a medical 'orchidectomy' occurs.

Chemotherapy, particularly with cyclophosphamide and chlorambucil, leads to testicular damage. Pubertal, but not prepubertal, boys seem most vulnerable. Marijuana has a direct effect on the hypothalamus, pituitary and testis, and spironolactone not only impairs testosterone synthesis but also antagonizes the action of testosterone.

Sharon O'Byrne

TESTICULAR PAIN

See also TESTICULAR SWELLING (p. 702).

Pain in the testicle of varying degree may be present in many conditions, which may be discussed under separate headings as follows:

- Diseases of the body of the testis or epididymis.
- Affections of the coverings of the testicle.
- Affections of the spermatic cord.
- A retained or misplaced testicle.
- Pain from lesions remote from the testis.

Diseases of the body of the testis or epididymis

Inflammatory lesions

Inflammatory lesions may attack the testis proper or, as is more common, may begin in the epididymis. The investing tunica vaginalis distends with inflammatory exudate to form a secondary hydrocele. This tender mass may be mistaken for a swelling of the testis proper, and the condition is frequently labelled an 'acute epididymo-orchitis'. However, surgical exploration and histological study reveal that the testis proper is rarely implicated, and it is accurate therefore to speak of 'acute epididymitis'. An inflammatory affection of the testicle may be acute, subacute or chronic, the last state often being the terminal result of the others.

An acute epididymitis arises most commonly by spread of infection to the organ from the urethra via the vas deferens, or by the lymphatics accompanying the vas. When any inflammation has reached the prostatic portion of the urethra the orifices of the vasa deferentia may become infected, and inflammation spreads along the duct to the epididymis.

Causes of testicular or epididymal conditions are listed in Table T.3.

Acute epididymitis begins as a painful thickening of the epididymis associated with febrile symptoms. Before any actual pain is noticed in the testis, there is

Table T.3 Causes of testicular or epididymal conditions

Acute epididymitis
- Causes of urethral origin
  - ◆ Urethritis due to *Neisseria gonorrhoeae*
  - ◆ Urethritis due to *Chlamydia trachomatis*
  - ◆ Septic urethritis
  - ◆ Passage of catheters
  - ◆ Urethral instrumentation
  - ◆ Infection behind a stricture
  - ◆ Ulceration around an impacted calculus
  - ◆ Injections into the posterior urethra
  - ◆ After operations on the prostate
  - ◆ Urinary infections
  - ◆ Non-specific epididymitis

Acute orchitis
- Parotitis (mumps)
- Injury

Chronic epididymitis
- Tuberculosis
- Resolving acute epididymitis

Syphilitic disease of the testis
- Diffuse interstitial orchitis
- Gummatous orchitis

Other diseases
- Malignant tumours of the testis
- Torsion of the testis
- Cysts of the epididymis

often a sense of discomfort and weight over the external abdominal ring and inguinal canal due to the inflammatory process extending along the vas deferens. The swelling of the epididymis increases, and with it there is a secondary effusion of exudate into the tunica vaginalis (secondary hydrocele), causing swelling of its body and increase of pain. The whole organ thus becomes enlarged, and it is often exquisitely tender, with the touch of the clothes or the gentlest examination causing pain. The swollen gland is often flattened on the outer and posterior aspect from pressure against the adductor muscles of the thigh; the vas deferens and tissues of the spermatic cord are thickened.

By far the most common cause of an acute epididymitis was formerly an *acute gonorrhoeal urethritis*; however, under the more effective modern antibiotic treatment of gonorrhoea it occurs much less often. During the disease the prostatic portion of the channel frequently becomes infected, when the orifices of the ejaculatory ducts may share in the inflammation, and infection be conveyed by the vas deferens to the testicle. Infection may also arise following an attack of non-specific urethritis, acquired as a result of sexual intercourse with a partner suffering from a non-specific genital infection. Non-specific urethritis today is the most common sexually transmitted disease in the Western world, and at least 1 per cent of all male cases develop epididymitis. *Chlamydia trachomatis* is commonly found, and this organism appears to be the cause in around 50 per cent of cases. The gonorrhoeal form of acute epididymitis usually resolves slowly, and shows little liability to suppurate, whereas the inflammation resulting from a staphylococcal or streptococcal infection may break down into a testicular abscess.

Acute epididymitis may also arise from septic processes in the urethra following the *passage of catheters*, of *instruments* for vesical operations, transurethral prostatic resection or lithotrity for example, from infection behind a *urethral stricture* or about a calculus in the prostatic urethra, occasionally after the *instillation of strong solutions* into the posterior urethra in the treatment of a chronic urethritis, or after operations on the prostate (especially prostatectomy), or as a complication of a urinary infection by *E. coli* or other micro-organisms. It may follow prostatic massage. In any case, the onset of pyrexia with pain and rapid swelling of the testis should lead to suspicion of a urinary tract infection. Bacteriological examination of any urethral discharge and of the urine is essential (see URETHRAL DISCHARGE, p. 762).

In *non-specific epididymitis* there may be no evidence of urethral infection and the bacteriological studies are entirely negative. The condition sometimes arises after unaccustomed exercise, and has been attributed to a reflux of urine down the vas deferens. The testicle becomes painful, and enlarges rapidly in the same manner as in acute inflammation from urethral infection and, under appropriate conservative treatment by means of a scrotal support, gradually resolves. Less frequently, testicular inflammation may occur after a direct injury to the organ, such as a blow or squeeze.

Initially, the pain in an acute inflammation is generally of an aching character, felt not only in the testis but also at the external abdominal ring, and often as a heavy dragging pain in the inguinal or iliac areas of the affected side. As the testis enlarges, the local pain becomes more severe, so that the swollen gland is exquisitely tender to pressure or to the touch. After a few days the pain subsides to a large extent, but remains as a dull ache until the swelling is greatly reduced, and it usually does not disappear entirely until the organ returns to the normal size. In a few cases in which a fibrous scar remains in the epididymis, pain may remain and cause some difficulty in the diagnosis from an incipient tuberculous lesion, but the earlier history of acute inflammation will help in forming an opinion. In other cases the persistence of the pain and swelling may indicate the formation of an abscess in the testicle when, after decreasing at first, the swelling increases, the skin covering it becomes reddened and oedematous, and a soft area becomes evident in one aspect of the organ.

Acute orchitis

Acute orchitis may complicate *acute specific parotitis* (mumps), especially when this occurs in adolescents or adults. The testicular pain and swelling occurs usually within a week of the parotid swelling. Both testes may be affected, and the result may be bilateral testicular atrophy with resultant infertility. Much less often the testis may be affected in *typhoid, scarlet fever* or *influenza*.

Tuberculosis of the testicle

Tuberculosis of the testicle is still common today in many parts of the world, including India and the Far East, but is comparatively rare in the UK. It arises with extreme rarity as a primary disease, but more commonly as secondary to tuberculous disease of the kidney, bladder, prostate or seminal vesicles. It is most frequently seen in young adults. It begins as a localized deposit in almost all cases, causing a rounded, firm nodule in the epididymis, usually in the lower pole. This nodule may remain unaltered for many months, or may enlarge, soften, become adherent to the skin and coverings of the testicle, or actually ulcerate through them to form a discharging sinus in the scrotum. The small nodule in the epididymis is usually painless at first and may be found by accident, but later, as it gradually enlarges, it causes an aching pain in the organ. There may be an associated hydrocele of the tunica vaginalis. Other nodules may be formed in the epididymis, or the body of the testis may become involved, while commonly small shot-like thickenings may be felt in the course of the vas deferens, or a progressively increasing thickening as it is traced down to the epididymis. In the more advanced stages nodules may be felt upon rectal examination in the seminal vesicles or prostate, or there may be some in the epididymis of the other side.

Tuberculous disease of the testicle usually presents some difficulty in its diagnosis from non-specific epididymitis, particularly when it has an acute onset, as sometimes happens. In an early case the occurrence of one or more nodules in the epididymis, which are painful on pressure and which have not resulted from a preceding acute epididymitis, should always suggest a tuberculous focus, and a careful search should be made for other tuberculous lesions in the body. The urine is cultured for *Mycobacterium tuberculosum*, and intravenous pyelography performed. If no evidence of tuberculosis is found, the gradual subsidence of the lesion under careful observation will indicate that it was a non-specific epididymitis. At later stages the diagnosis is less difficult; the gradual enlargement of the nodules, their craggy or bossy feel, the infection of the vas deferens or other genitourinary organs with tuberculosis – and above all the tendency of the focus in the epididymis to soften and to become adherent to the scrotal coverings and to produce an indolent sinus – arc points to be looked for.

Syphilitic disease of the testis

Syphilitic disease of the testis, once common, but now a rarity, causes very little pain in the organ, but there is often a sense of dragging or heaviness. Syphilis may attack the testicle in several different ways, producing:

- In acquired syphilis:
  - ◆ Diffuse interstitial orchitis
  - ◆ Localized gummatous orchitis
- In congenital syphilis:
  - ◆ Interstitial orchitis
  - ◆ Localized gummatous orchitis

The outstanding feature of syphilitic disease of the testicle is that it affects the body of the testis rather than the epididymis, thus differing in a marked degree from tuberculous disease. In the interstitial form there is thickening of the intertubular connective tissue, with an infiltration of spindle cells which, in forming young connective tissue, yield fibrous tissue. The subsequent contraction of this fibrous tissue may cause atrophy of the testis. The testis may, on section, show small gummas in addition to the diffuse orchitis. Alternatively, if the inflammation is more localized, gummas may be the main feature, these varying in size from that of a pea to that of a walnut, or larger. The epididymis is affected rarely, though cases are on record of a nodular swelling in the epididymis during the secondary stage of syphilis which disappears rapidly under anti-syphilitic treatment.

In *congenital syphilis*, both the interstitial and gummatous forms exist; they usually occur in childhood or in young adult life, and in many cases the affection is bilateral. Syphilitic inflammation of the testicle may be accompanied in either the acquired or the congenital form by a vaginal hydrocele. A gummatous testis may ulcerate through the scrotum, usually in front, producing a circular 'punched-out' ulcer with a slough in the base.

There is a sense of weight in the scrotum rather than pain, and often an aching or dragging feeling in the inguinal or lumbar region. On palpation, the body of the testis feels enlarged and nodular with the gummatous deposits, but the epididymis can usually be distinguished from the testis and found to be unaffected. Testicular sensation is lost. The tissues of the cord remain unthickened. Tertiary syphilitic lesions of the testicle give rise to very little tenderness on palpation.

The diagnosis of syphilitic disease of the testis is usually simple. There may or may not be a history of syphilis, but other signs of the disease should be looked for: in the acquired form, any scar of previous ulceration or periosteal thickening, or, in the congenital variety, signs in the teeth, eyes or ears. Syphilitic disease is distinguished from *tuberculous disease* of the testis by the fact that the epididymis is usually free; that the cord, prostate and vesicles remain normal; and that pressure applied directly to the testicle gives little or no pain. Tuberculous deposits tend to soften and to involve the scrotal coverings in spite of treatment. The condition is differentiated from haematocele by the history of injury or by an absence of the history or signs of syphilis. It is distinguished from *malignant tumours of the testis* by the history of syphilis, the tendency of syphilitic disease to be bilateral, the slow enlargement, and positive serological tests. In malignant disease, the increase in the size of the testicle is more rapid, while the tumour often shows areas of varying consistence; the cord is often thickened in malignant or in tuberculous cases, but seldom in syphilitic cases.

It should be pointed out that gumma of the testis is so rare in the UK today, compared with its former frequency, that it is safer to regard any solid swelling in the testicle itself as the much more common and more likely malignant tumour of the testis, and treat it as such by orchidectomy. In the unlikely event that a gumma is thus removed, the surgeon can comfort him/herself with the fact that a functionally useless organ has been excised.

Malignant tumours of the testis

Malignant tumours of the testis may give rise to pain in the organ, but as a rule pain is experienced only in the later stages of the disease. For a fuller consideration of this topic, see TESTICULAR SWELLINGS (p. 704).

Torsion of the testis

Torsion of the testis on its vascular pedicle may occur in a testis which has a mesorchium, or in one which is ectopic. It occurs most commonly in infants or in youths soon after puberty; the exciting cause may be some mild exertion or movement such as crossing the legs or turning over in bed. There may be a history of repeated minor attacks before complete torsion takes place, and the other testis may have suffered similar incomplete attacks or be found to be unduly mobile or horizontally placed. At the moment of torsion there is severe sickening pain which may be felt at first in the abdomen, but is quickly localized to the testis; the boy may even say that his testicle has 'twisted'. There is usually nausea and sometimes vomiting. The testis forms a tense tender swelling in the upper part of the scrotum or at the external abdominal ring, and the scrotum below is empty. This sign serves to distinguish the condition from a strangulated hernia or an inflamed lymph node. In acute epididymitis the testis is in its normal position, and there may be evidence of urethral discharge or of a urinary tract infection. Because of the initial abdominal pain and vomiting, the condition has been mistaken for acute appendicitis, but adherence to the rule of examining the scrotal contents in all abdominal cases should prevent this error.

Cysts of the epididymis

Cysts occur most frequently in connection with the epididymis. These cysts are quite different from hydrocele of the tunica vaginalis, and are often spoken of as a spermatocele, although all do not contain spermatozoa and the term is thus better avoided. They cause a swelling of varying degree in the scrotum, and usually an aching in the testicle, groin or lumbar region. These cysts are usually placed above and to the outer side of the testis, but occasionally behind it. They move with the organ, and can usually be distinguished from the latter by the test of translucency. They may be multiple and are frequently bilateral. Their increase in size is very slow, but they may cause aching pain in the testicle by pressure upon, or stretching of, the tissues of the epididymis. They can be distinguished from hydrocele of the tunica vaginalis by the position of the swelling relative to the testicle, and by the fact that the fluid contained in them is colourless or slightly opalescent from the contained spermatozoa, in distinction from the straw-coloured clear fluid of a vaginal hydrocele.

A small cyst on the upper pole of the testis, a few millimetres in diameter (*appendix testis*) or at the upper end of the epididymis (*appendix epididymis*), are not uncommon findings at autopsy, and are symptomless. Occasionally, one or other may undergo acute torsion and result in sudden and sever testicular pain which mimics testicular torsion.

Affections of the coverings of the testis causing pain in the organ

The only common lesions of the coverings of the testis are *hydrocele* and *haematocele*: new growths of the testicular tunics are so rare as to render them surgical curiosities and they rarely cause pain.

Hydrocele

Hydrocele may occur occasionally as an acute affection accompanying an acute epididymitis, injury to the scrotum, or in the course of acute specific fevers such as mumps. Acute hydrocele has been described in conjunction with acute lesions of other serous membranes (e.g. polyserositis). The more usual form of hydrocele is the chronic variety, which may be due to some disease of the testicle, but for which, in the majority of cases, no ascertainable cause can be found (primary or idiopathic hydrocele).

A hydrocele is usually painless, but may cause some aching in the testicle, or a dragging sensation in the inguinal or iliac areas from the mechanical effect of its weight. It forms an oval swelling on one side of the scrotum with a smooth uniform surface; it gives a distinct sense of fluctuation. The swelling is limited above from the cord or external abdominal ring, and gives no sense of impulse on coughing. With a good light it can be found in most cases to be translucent, the testicle occupying a posterior and low position in the swelling. The diagnosis of hydrocele is usually easy, but difficulty may be experienced in long-standing cases in which the walls are much thickened. A hydrocele must be distinguished from: (i) a scrotal hernia; (ii) haematocele; (iii) new growth; and (iv) a cyst of the epididymis.

Usually, an *inguino-scrotal hernia* gives an impulse on coughing, can be reduced into the abdomen with a sudden slip or gurgle, and varies in size with the position of the patient. A hernia comes from above and descends into the scrotum. In a large irreducible hernia, some part of it is usually resonant from the contained intestine, the swelling is not limited above, and the testis can be distinguished at the bottom of the scrotum. A hydrocele is distinctly limited above so that the examining fingers can meet above it, gives no impulse on coughing, is translucent, and the spermatic cord can be distinguished easily (see Fig. T.3). The testis in a hydrocele cannot usually be distinguished in the scrotum as in a hernia. Difficulty may arise between the two conditions when the hydrocele extends along the funicular process in the inguinal canal and thus gives an impulse on coughing, or if the translucency is lost owing to the thickness of the walls of the sac. A scrotal hernia in an infant may be translucent.

Haematocele is distinguished from hydrocele by the absence of translucency and the rapidity of the onset, usually after an injury or puncture (see also below).

A hydrocele is of much slower rate of increase in size than a *new growth*. It has a smooth surface and uniform consistence, and is translucent.

In cases of doubt, ultrasonography of the swelling usually enables accurate anatomical delineation of the mass to be made, and distinguishes between a *cystic* and a solid swelling.

Haematocele

Haematocele may occur from puncture of a vein in the sac or of the testicle as the result of tapping a hydrocele, or by the occurrence of bleeding into a hydrocele. It may occur quite independently of a hydrocele, usually after direct injury. As a rule there is a rapid onset of swelling in the scrotum following the injury, with ecchymosis of the scrotal skin; the resulting tumour resembles a hydrocele in its clinical symptoms, save that it is not translucent. In other cases, the swelling arises more slowly, when a pyriform or oval swelling is present in one side of the scrotum covered by normal skin; the surface of the swelling is smooth, and gives a sense of fluctuation and elasticity. There is no translucency, and on tapping, dark blood-stained fluid is withdrawn.

The diagnosis in the less acute cases often presents a difficulty, especially with regard to *malignant disease of the testicle* (see above); this is particularly so when the haematoma is organized. Haematocele is distinguished from *hydrocele* by the absence of translucency, and from *hernia* by the same points, except for translucency, as mentioned above in the differential diagnosis between hydrocele and hernia.

Affections of the spermatic cord causing testicular pain

An inflammatory affection of the cord secondary to urethral infection is not uncommon. Tuberculous infection of the cord is practically never present without corresponding infection of the epididymis. New growths of the cord, lipomas, sarcomas (extremely rare) and hydroceles of the cord cause no pain in the testis. A *varicocele*, especially if large, and in a pendulous scrotum, is a frequent cause of a dull, aching pain in the testicle; it is nearly always left-sided, though the reason for this is obscure. The characteristic feel of the enlarged veins in the erect position (like a 'bag of worms'), and the slight impulse and thrill on coughing, will readily point to the correct diagnosis.

Retained or misplaced testis

This, in its various situations, may give rise to pain. A testis may be arrested in its descent at the external abdominal ring, in the inguinal canal, it may remain inside the abdomen, or it may pass upwards and outwards from the external abdominal ring into the superficial inguinal pouch where it can be felt readily. It is doubtful if a testis retained within the inguinal canal is ever palpable. Occasionally, it passes into the perineum after traversing the inguinal canal, to the upper part of the thigh via the crural ring, or to the root of the penis in front of the pubis. In one-fifth of all cases, the undescended testes are bilateral.

In the various situations in which an undescended or ectopic testicle is placed, it may be attacked by several diseases which affect the normally placed organ, and thus give rise to pain. However, in addition, owing to the effect of recurrent muscular strains and the comparative immobility of the organ, it is particularly liable to attacks of inflammation, especially when the testis is retained in the inguinal canal. In the intra-abdominal position it remains protected from muscular injury, while an ectopic testicle has a greater range of mobility than does one that is retained in the inguinal canal and is thus especially prone to torsion. The inflammation of an undescended testicle may be so acute as to lead to gangrene of the organ, with or without torsion of the cord. The pain may be complained of first when the testes begin to enlarge at puberty, at which time an undescended right testicle may produce symptoms which can be easily mistaken for appendicitis.

The diagnosis of undescended testicle rests upon the following points: the fact that one side of the scrotum is empty; the outline and situation of the swelling in the superficial inguinal region or elsewhere; the testicular sensation upon pressure; and the recurrent attacks of pain. An undescended testicle may give rise to acute pain from inflammatory lesions or from acute torsion of the organ and may, if it is in the inguinal canal, give rise to symptoms suggesting a strangulated hernia. A partially descended testicle is often accompanied by an inguinal hernia. The misplaced testis is especially liable to become the seat of malignant disease.

It should be remembered that an imperfectly descended testis is a small and poorly developed organ, and the spermatogenesis from the gland may be absent or only last for a short time after puberty.

Testicular pain from lesions other than in the testicle

Complaint may be made of testicular pain when, on clinical examination, the testis is found to be normal. After an acute inflammation of the organ, even when no palpable nodule remains, the resulting cicatrization may cause aching in the organ, especially after *sexual excitement* or prolonged desire. Apart from former testicular disease, referred pain may be felt in the organ if a *calculus* is present in the *pelvis of the kidney* or *upper ureter*, or from stimulation of the peripheral nerves by *secondary deposits in the bodies of the lumbar vertebrae*, pressure from an *extramedullary intraspinal tumour* such as a neurofibroma, meningioma or ependymoma, or the pressure of an *aneurysm* in this situation. Pain in the testicle is occasionally present in *appendiceal inflammation* when the appendix turns down into the pelvis. Finally, when no organic cause of any sort is present, the condition is usually called *neuralgia testis*; this is pain of an aching character which may occur in patients of a neurotic tendency.

Harold Ellis

TESTICULAR SWELLING

See also TESTICULAR PAIN (p. 697).

It is first essential to prove that the swelling is really testicular and not an inguino-scrotal hernia. This is done by grasping the root of the scrotum between the thumb and index fingers to determine whether any of the swelling extends along the cord into the inguinal region. True scrotal swellings may arise in: (i) skin; (ii) the various connective tissue coverings of the testicle; (iii) tunica vaginalis; (iv) testicle; (v) epididymis; and (vi) the lower end of the spermatic cord.

Swellings affecting the skin

The nature of these is usually obvious. The only common ones are sebaceous cysts. Much less common are soft sores, chancre, warts and epithelioma. The last-named soon ulcerates, and was once commonly seen in chimney-sweeps or in those who work with tar, tar products or petroleum. It is now relatively rare.

Swellings of the various connective tissue coverings

These are rare, but occasionally a fibrosarcoma may occur. These swellings are movable upon the testicle. The symmetrical enlargement called elephantiasis scroti (Fig. T.2), due to *Wuchereria bancrofti*, is limited to filiarial infection in the tropics, though sometimes a similar state of scrotal distension and over-growth results in the UK from lymphatic obstruction due to pelvic cellulitis or to congenital abnormality. The enlarged scrotum resulting from acute generalized oedema in acute or chronic renal disease

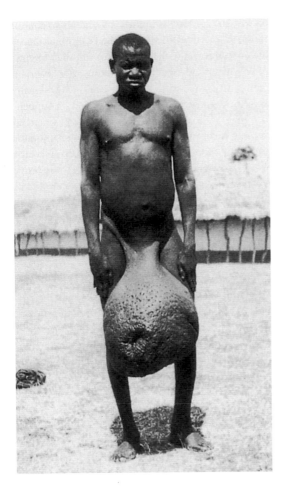

Figure T.2 Elephantiasis of the scrotum due to filariasis. [Dr C. J. Hackett, Wellcome Museum of Medical Science.]

is seldom difficult to recognize. The penis and prepuce are generally distended by oedema at the same time as are the legs, loins, eyelids and other parts. The diagnosis is confirmed by the albumin and tube-casts in the urine.

Gross oedematous scrotal swelling also occurs with ascites or inferior vena caval thrombosis, and may accompany the abdominal swelling of pellagra and infantile kwashiorkor.

The tunica vaginalis

The tunica vaginalis may become distended with serous fluid, blood or pus: distension with fluid may be primary, the idiopathic vaginal hydrocele, or secondary to disease of the testis or epididymis. *Vaginal*

hydrocele usually arises slowly, though some follow injury and give a short history. The patient is well, with no pain or urinary complaint, and merely complains of the lump, or of the drag that it causes. The swelling is large, heavy, ovoid, tense and elastic rather than fluctuating, though fluctuation can be proved if the swelling is fixed by an assistant or the patient; neither testis nor epididymis can be felt apart from the swelling. A hydrocele can be transilluminated, but it needs a dark room and a strong light (Fig. T.3); when transilluminated, the testicular shadow will be noticed at one edge of the swelling, usually behind. Tapping withdraws a golden fluid of soapy feel, with a specific gravity of about 1.030, that coagulates solid on boiling.

Secondary hydrocele follows disease of the testis or epididymis: the amount of fluid is usually small, and the swelling lax, so that the finger can be passed through it to touch the testis. The complaint is of the causative disease rather than of the hydrocele, which is usually discovered on examination. Transillumination will confirm the presence of fluid. A *haematocele* has the physical characters of a hydrocele except that it is not translucent. Vaginal hydroceles vary very much in this respect, for their wall becomes thicker from fibrosis or deposition of fibrin, particularly after repeated tapping, and the fluid becomes stained with blood-pigment and hazy with cholesterol crystals, so that the strongest light may only just be perceptible across them. Tapping may be required to establish the presence of blood. Haematocele is due to injury, torsion or growth of the testis, and its discovery is therefore the indication for exploration, unless the history of trauma is recent and definite – for example, as the result of tapping a hydrocele. A *pyocele* is merely part of a suppurative process arising in the testis or the epididymis. The differential diagnosis of hydrocele is from translucent swellings in the epididymis and cord-cyst of the epididymis and encysted hydrocele.

Ultrasonography has proved to be invaluable in the investigation of a testicular mass, in particular in determining whether or not there is underlying testicular disease in a patient with hydrocele.

Swellings of the testicle

These usually affect either the body of the testis or the epididymis, rarely the two together. The first group includes torsion, mumps, gumma and new growth;

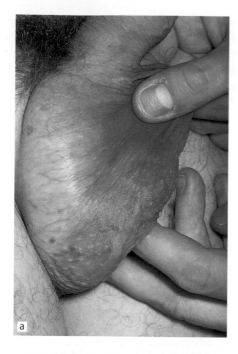

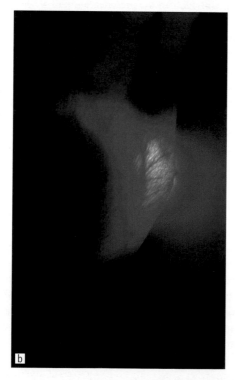

Figure T.3 (a) Left vaginal hydrocele; the fingers reach above it, thus excluding inguinoscrotal hernia. (b) The hydrocele transilluminates brilliantly.

the second group comprises tuberculosis, gonorrhoea, *E. coli* infection and cysts. Determination of the anatomical site of the swelling will therefore go some way towards settling its pathological nature.

Swelling of the body of the testicle

Torsion is met with as an acute condition accompanied by abdominal pain and vomiting, and it often occurs in the undescended testis (see INGUINAL SWELLING, p. 245). Torsion of a fully descended testis, giving rise to a scrotal swelling, is seldom seen after adolescence. The local signs, in addition to the abdominal pain and vomiting, are moderate enlargement of the testicle, tenderness, the presence of a small haematocele and the appearance after a few hours of oedema of the scrotal wall on the affected side. Recurring subacute torsion of the testicle is not uncommon, and in these cases the signs and symptoms are less pronounced than in the acute variety into which they eventually pass. The main points of distinction between the less acute enlargements of the corpus testis are listed in Table T.4.

Mumps orchitis usually occurs within a week of the parotid swelling, and results in an acutely tender enlargement of the testis. It especially complicates the acute parotitis of adolescents or adults. The affected testis often undergoes atrophy. If the condition is bilateral, the result may be infertility.

It is often difficult to distinguish syphilitic *enlargement of the testicles* from that due to growth; however, a course of anti-syphilitic therapy and the serological reactions may settle the matter. Gumma of the testis, once common, is now a clinical rarity in Western communities (see also TESTICULAR PAIN, p. 697), so that today a solid mass in the testis is highly suspicious of a neoplasm.

Tumours of the testis

Nearly all tumours of the testis are highly malignant. They fall into two main pathological varieties, *seminoma* and *teratoma*, the latter including the subgroups of *chorionepithelioma*, *dermoid* and *fibrocystic disease*. The *seminoma* (Fig. T.4) is a soft vascular solid growth composed of large spheroidal cells derived from the germinal epithelium of the seminiferous tubules. It occurs at about the age of 40 years, and is less malignant – but more radiosensitive – than

Table T.4 Swellings of the body of the testicle

	Mumps	*Syphilis*	*Tumour*
Age	Puberty or adolescence	Any age, but usually 18 to 30 years	Any age, more common after 20 years
History and other symptoms	Short history with pyrexia Previous contact with mumps Parotids enlarged	Previous history of exposure to venereal disease; usually has had chancre and rash Gumma or tertiary rashes may be found elsewhere	Onset insidious History of months
Scrotum	Normal or red and hot	Normal or adherent in front Later, ulcer with sharp edges and slough at base, or hernia testis	Normal or merely stretched until growth is size of tennis ball, when it may be invaded
Testis Size and shape	Moderately enlarged, shape normal	Enlarged; up to two or three times normal May be nodular	Increases steadily and may reach diameter of 10–13 cm Initially smooth, later nodular
Sensation	Tender and painful Testicular sensation present	Not tender or painful Testicular sensation lost	Painful, but not tender
Tunica vaginalis	Slight hydrocele in most	Hydrocele in 60%	Hydrocele in early stages: later haematocele
Epididymis	Unaltered	Usually unaltered	Flattened
Cord	May be tender	Normal	Usually normal, but may have nodules of growth in lymphatics
Lymph nodes	Not characteristically enlarged	Not characteristically enlarged	Drainage to para-aortic nodes at kidney level. These may form very large mass Eventually left supraclavicular nodes involved. Inguinal nodes not enlarged unless scrotal skin is invaded

teratoma. It tends to retain the shape of the testis as it enlarges.

The *teratoma* (Fig. T.5) or mixed tumour is a solid or multilocular cystic growth in which one or other of the germinal layers may preponderate. Dermoids, containing hair or teeth, are less common than in the ovary but sometimes occur in childhood and are relatively benign.

Fibrocystic disease pursues an even more benign course, and may be present for 10 or more years before exhibiting its malignant characteristics by sudden rapid growth and the formation of metastases. Most cases of teratoma occur at the age of 25–30 years; they give a short history, are more resistant to X-ray treatment, and show early metastases. There may be enlargement of the breasts and chorionic hormone may be present in the urine; in seminoma, the pituitary gonadotrophic hormone is sometimes found in the urine. Either type may follow injury in a significant proportion of cases, although it is likely that trauma merely draws attention to the testicular mass.

The undescended testis is more prone to develop malignant disease than is the normally placed one. The testis which has been initially undescended and subsequently brought down into the scrotum maintains this higher tendency to malignant change, estimated at about ten times that of the normal organ.

A testicle that is the seat of a malignant growth enlarges slowly or rapidly, but as pain is at first absent there may be nothing to arouse the patient's suspicions. As long as the tunica albuginea remains intact, the swelling retains the shape of the testis, but when perforation of the fibrous covering takes place nodular projections appear and render the tumour irregular. A rapidly growing malignant tumour of the testis may be so soft as to appear to be a fluid collection in the tunica vaginalis. Generally, however, although a growth may be accompanied by a small amount of fluid in the tunica vaginalis, the more solid mass can be felt through the fluid on careful examination; this fluid is often blood-stained. The epididymis may become incorporated in the growth so that it cannot

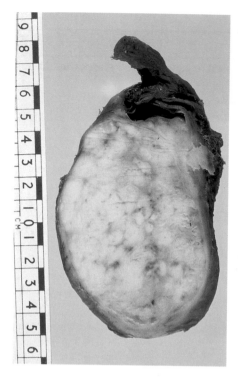

Figure T.4 Seminoma of the testis.

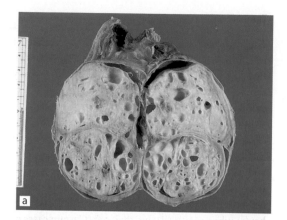

be distinguished, and the tissues of the cord become thickened. The coverings of the testis become stretched over the tumour; the mass does not become adherent to the scrotal skin until late in the disease.

Clinically, it is impossible to distinguish between a teratoma and a seminoma. In both types the para-aortic lymph nodes become enlarged, and may be felt in a thin subject to one or other side of the epigastric area, and pain due to the pressure of these nodes upon nerve structures may become marked (see Fig. T.5b). The inguinal nodes are usually not enlarged unless the scrotal skin is affected; retrograde spread may then occur to the iliac nodes, which may be felt at the brim of the pelvis. In advanced cases, the left supraclavicular lymph nodes are involved and become palpably enlarged. Mediastinal or pulmonary metastases are frequent, the latter giving the characteristic radiological appearance of 'cannon-ball' secondaries. The diagnosis of malignant disease of the testis may be quite easy in the case of rapidly growing tumours, but in others – and especially in the early stages – it may present great difficulty. Rarely, an interstitial cell tumour occurs in a child and produces sexual precocity.

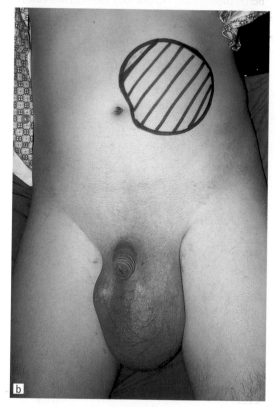

Figure T.5 (a) Teratoma of the testis; operative specimen. (b) Teratoma of the left testis with a large mass of para-aortic nodes.

Ultrasonography of the testis can be very useful in localizing the exact site of the mass and in differentiating between a solid and a cystic mass. If any doubt exists, it is advisable to excise the testis, first dividing the cord at the internal ring. Incision into a testis which is the seat of a growth is almost invariably followed by rapid recurrence.

The epididymis

The epididymis may become enlarged as the result of inflammation, new growth or cystic degeneration. Primary new growth of the epididymis is excessively rare and need not give rise to much concern in differential diagnosis.

Inflammatory swellings are characterized by being elongated in a vertical direction; by their relation to the testicle, which they overlap at its posterior border and its upper and lower poles; and by being flattened from side to side. There may be an associated small, lax secondary hydrocele. Inflammatory swellings may be: (i) tuberculous; (ii) due to E. coli (Certain cases of epididymitis, indistinguishable clinically from E. coli infection, are of very obscure aetiology. Some say that they are due to irritation by urine passing by reflux up the vas deferens, others that a virus is responsible. They are grouped as 'non-specific' epididymitis, and they tend to settle spontaneously in about 3–4 weeks.); (iii) *Chlamydia trachomatis*; (iv) gonorrhoeal; and (v) septic, secondary to some infection of the urethra. The main points of the distinction are shown in Table T.5.

It will be seen that *E. coli* epididymitis may bear a close resemblance to a tuberculous lesion, particularly when the acute infection has been partially aborted by antibiotic therapy, but lacks any distant or constitutional evidence of the disease. Support of the testicle in a suspensory bandage and the administration of suitable antibiotic therapy will cause marked improvement in a few days, and thus settle the diagnosis. Apart from the history and an increased liability to suppuration in septic epididymitis, there is little to distinguish the latter from the gonococcal variety.

Cysts of the epididymis may be either solitary or multiple, and may be bilateral. A cyst of the epididymis is placed above and behind the testicle, from which it is distinct; though attached to the epididymis, it is rounded, but being thin-walled it does not feel as tense as a hydrocele. It tends to have several rounded projections rather than a simple surface, and the fluid withdrawn by tapping is milky or opalescent, of low specific gravity, containing little albumin but showing numerous cells under the microscope, some of which may be spermatozoa. *Multiple cysts* occur in men past middle age, are painless, and

Table T.5 Inflammatory swellings of the epididymis

	Tuberculosis	E. coli and 'non- septic specific'	Gonorrhoeal	Septic
History	Previous tuberculous infection, especially urinary	Usually none	Recent infection, with gleet, and pain on micturition	Recent catheterization or operation on bladder or prostate
Other signs and symptoms	? Cough, wasting. ? Evidence of phthisis in lungs ? Tubercle bacilli in urine	Usually none Urine may smell fishy and contain E. coli	Urethral discharge Gram-negative diplococci: other manifestations such as joints	Pus in alkaline urine
Scrotum	May be adherent behind May have sinus discharging thin pus	Normal	Red, hot, swollen and tender	Red, hot, swollen and tender May suppurate
Testes	Usually normal	Normal	Normal, but outline obscured by surroundings	Normal, but outline obscured by surroundings
Tunica vaginalis	Hydrocele in 30%	Normal	Small hydrocele usually present	Hydrocele or pyocele
Epididymis	Nodular enlargement Nodules, hard and very tender Later break down to abscess, with sinus	No local nodules or much enlargement, but affected part hard and tender Does not break down	Whole epididymis large, hard and broad; hot and tender	Globus minor or whole epididymis enlarged and broad; hot and tender
Cord	Oedema of cord Vas may be thickened	Normal	Whole cord tender and swollen	Whole cord tender and swollen
Prostate and seminal vesicles	Vesicle on affected side may be hard and tender	Normal	Prostate may be hot and tender Tenderness along vesicles	Swollen and tender Vesicles may be felt

increase in size very slowly. These swellings are strikingly translucent.

Swellings of the lower end of the cord

The most important swelling of the lower part of the spermatic cord is *varicocele*. It is apt to be mistaken for an inguinal hernia, but this mistake should never be made because of the characteristic feel of the varicocele (like a 'bag of worms'), and the reappearance of the swelling after it has been completely reduced by elevation of the scrotum and the finger firmly pressed on the external abdominal ring. Varicocele is far more common on the left than the right testis.

Harold Ellis

TETANY

See also CRAMPS (p. 130), TIC (p. 719), VERTIGO (p. 773).

Tetany is a condition where abnormal muscle cramps are caused by increased neuromuscular excitability induced by a fall in the concentration of ionized calcium. Important precipitating factors include a low-calcium diet, pregnancy and lactation. Early symptoms of acute tetany include paraesthesiae and numbness of the extremities and around the mouth. Then muscle cramps may occur, particularly in the extremities. The wrist and elbow may become flexed, the fingers flexed at the metacarpophalangeal joint, but extended at the terminal interphalangeal joint, and the fingers all pressed together, with the thumb adducted into the palm of the hand so that the whole hand forms the 'main d'accoucheur' (obstetrician's hand). When the legs are affected the knees and ankles are extended, the foot is arched and inverted, and the toes flexed and pressed together. The cramps may be painful and last from several minutes to a couple of hours. In severe cases the face and neck muscles may be involved, and laryngospasm may cause respiratory obstruction and lead to loss of consciousness and death. Generalized epileptic convulsions may occur, especially in children. Hypocalcaemia may also lead to prolongation of the QT interval on the ECG and predispose to ventricular tachyarrhythmias.

Latent tetany may be revealed by special signs:

- *Chvostek's sign.* Twitching of the muscles of the upper lip may be elicited by tapping on the facial nerve in front

of the ear. However, note that this sign can be present in some people with normal calcium levels.
- *Trousseau's sign.* Spasm of the fingers and hand to form the 'main d'accoucheur' is induced by obstruction of the brachial artery for up to 3 minutes by a sphygmomanometer cuff.

Additional features, which may be present in patients with chronic tetany, include:

- Ectodermal changes (particularly in idiopathic hypoparathyroidism). The skin is dry and scaly, the tongue atrophic, the hair sparse and brittle, and the nails ridged; cataracts may be present.
- Central nervous system changes: general fatigue, irritability, anxiety, depression, paranoia and epilepsy. Papilloedema is sometimes found.

Causes of tetany

The causes of reduced serum calcium (hypocalcaemia) are listed in Table T.6.

Table T.6 Causes of hypocalcaemia

Most common
- Chronic renal failure
- Postoperative (thyroidectomy, parathyroidectomy)
- Osteomalacia/rickets

Less common
- Acute pancreatitis
- Alkalosis
- Magnesium deficiency
- Massive blood transfusion
- Drug therapy: bisphosphonates, calcitonin, phosphates

Rare
- Vitamin D resistance
- Pseudohypoparathyroidism
- Idiopathic hypoparathyroidism: autoimmune/congenital (DiGeorge syndrome)

- *Renal failure.* In acute renal failure, hypocalcaemia may occur secondary to phosphate retention and the formation of insoluble calcium compounds. In chronic renal failure, calcium levels may fall due to a fall in the renal hydroxylation of vitamin D.
- *Vitamin D deficiency.* Skin irradiation is the most important source of vitamin D, blood levels of which rises in the summer and fall in the winter. Elderly people and certain ethnic groups who do not venture outside very much are most at risk for vitamin D deficiency. It is difficult to

provide enough vitamin D from even a normal diet. Vitamin D is found in wheatgerm, eggs and fish. Margarine and milk is fortified with vitamin D in some countries. Malabsorption syndrome of all types may cause vitamin D deficiency. Since vitamin D must be hydroxylated in the liver and kidney in order to create its most potent form, diseases of these organs may lead to hypocalcaemia. The problem of vitamin D deficiency is always exacerbated by prolonged lactation.

■ *Acute pancreatitis.* Hypocalcaemia may occur early on in acute pancreatitis. The mechanism is not clearly understood, but part of it may be due to the formation of calcium soaps.

■ *Magnesium deficiency.* This leads to reduced secretion of parathyroid hormone (PTH) and to peripheral resistance to the actions of PTH. It occurs in: (i) patients on prolonged intravenous therapy who are not receiving magnesium supplements; (ii) severe diarrhoea; (iii) malabsorption syndrome; (iv) small-bowel resection or bypass; (v) chronic alcoholism; (vi) diuretic phase after recovery from renal tubular necrosis; and (vii) hyperaldosteronism.

■ *Alkalosis.* This condition, from any cause, may be associated with hypokalaemia and can lead to a decrease in the ionized fraction of calcium and cause tetany. The causes of alkalosis are: (i) the excessive ingestion of alkali; (ii) frequent vomiting; (iii) hyperventilation, especially hysterical; and (iv) hyperaldosteronism, where magnesium deficiency also plays an accessory role.

■ *Pseudohypoparathyroidism.* This is a rare disorder in which the hypocalcaemia is due to end-organ resistance to the actions of PTH, the concentration of which is raised. The patients have certain phenotypic characteristics (see also STATURE, SHORT, p. 672).

Melvin Lobo

THINKING, DISORDERS OF

Disorders of thinking are commonly considered under two separate headings:

1 Disorders of the content of thinking. These include adherence to delusional beliefs as found in psychotic individuals, and the presence of unwelcome, intrusive obsessional thoughts found in patients with obsessional neurosis. These are discussed in other sections (see DELUSIONS, p. 145; OBSESSIONS, p. 494).

2 Disorders of the thinking process including abnormalities of the flow and the *form* of thoughts.

A person's thought processes can only be inferred from their words and actions. We may consider that a person's thoughts are racing when they have pressure of speech or flight of ideas, as in *mania*. Here, there are logical connections between the ideas expressed, but the subject's thinking is so speeded up that it tends to jump from topic to topic, often in response to environmental distractions. The speaker is difficult to interrupt, loud, emphatic, and may use clang associations when the choice of words is governed by their sound rather than by a logical relationship. Sentences may be linked by rhyming and punning, often with amusing consequences. The above description is typical of mania, but lesser degrees of increased flow of thinking may be found in acute reactions to stress, major depressive illness with marked features of anxiety and, occasionally, in schizophrenia and organic mental disorders. A reduced flow of speech may reflect *poverty of thought* when the subject makes no spontaneous conversation and responds to questions with only brief unelaborated replies in a flat, monotonous tone. In its most severe form it may lead to muteness, and this occurs frequently in major depressive episodes, schizophrenia and the dementias. However, when assessing a mute patient, *hysterical aphonia* should always be considered as a possible cause.

Disorders in the form of thinking (formal thought disorder) are of enormous importance in the diagnosis of schizophrenia, but similar features may also occur in normal subjects who are tense or fatigued, and in patients with organic brain diseases. An important symptom in schizophrenia – and one which can often be observed in patients with longstanding chronic disability – is *loosening* of association of thoughts leading to *incoherence* of speech. These characteristic changes may be accompanied by other so-called *negative symptoms* of schizophrenia, including a degree of apathy with diminished drive and volition which may be the principal feature of the disease after the more florid symptoms of delusions and hallucinations have resolved in response to antipsychotic medication. *Loosening* of association describes a thought disorder characterized by speech in which ideas shift from one subject to another, completely unrelated, topic without the speaker being aware that the topics are disconnected. Unlike flight of ideas, the flow of talk may be normal or even reduced. *Derailment* is a description sometimes used for such idiosyncratic moves from one frame of reference to another and, if severe, speech becomes *word salad* and totally incoherent. In very severe schizophrenic thought disorder, the speech has some of the characteristics of a fluent aphasia (schizophasia), becoming a series of totally incomprehensible sentences often admixed with *neologisms. Thought blocking* is expressed as an interruption in the normal flow of speech, usually in a patient with schizophrenia. The subject, moreover, is aware and will spontaneously describe how their train of thought was suddenly stopped and they had no control over it. The symptom is quite different from mere absentmindedness, and sometimes the patient may elaborate the paranoid delusion that an external force is responsible for taking their thoughts away. *Concrete thinking* is another term which is frequently applies to schizophrenic patients, but is also observed in patients with a low IQ, who are brain damaged, and also in autistic individuals. It describes a difficulty in handling abstract and symbolic language, leading for example to very literal interpretations of proverbs. When mild, this feature has no diagnostic value as it reflects cultural, educational and personality factors. In *perseveration*, which is found in organic brain disorders and in schizophrenia, the patient continues to hold ideas after they have ceased to be appropriate, so that the same word or idea will crop up in the patient's speech many times in a few sentences. It may be quite marked, for example, 'I think I'll put on my hat, hat, hat, hat', when the term *logoclonus* or syllable repetition would apply.

Obsessional and anxious people may betray aspects of their thinking by *circumstantiality*. Here, speech may be produced in a slow stream but with a great excess of unnecessary detail that can entirely obscure the main answer to the question. Circumstantiality, however, is commonly found in those with no mental illness.

Andrew Hodgkiss

THORACIC WALL VEINS

Venous blood from the posterior chest wall muscles, skin and vertebral venous plexuses drains into 11 posterior intercostal veins. On the right side, the second, third and often fourth posterior intercostal veins unite to form the right superior intercostal vein, which then drains directly into the azygos vein. The lower posterior intercostal veins individually drain into the azygos vein. On the left side, the second, third and sometimes fourth posterior intercostal veins unite to form the left superior intercostal vein to open directly into the left brachiocephalic (innominate) vein. The lower left posterior intercostal veins drain individually into the hemiazygos vein to then cross the midline behind the mediastinal structures to the azygos vein and on to the superior vena cava just above the pericardium. The superior vena cava arises from the brachiocephalic (innominate), jugular and azygos veins.

The thoracic wall veins may become distended in a number of conditions, usually associated with partial or complete obstruction of blood flow in the innominate or vena cava to cause a rise in pressure in the azygos, hemiazygos or jugular venous systems.

Superior vena caval syndrome

This may be caused by either partial or complete obstruction of the superior vena cava (SVC). The condition was first described by William Hunter in 1757 in a patient in whom the SVC was obstructed by a syphilitic aortic aneurysm. The signs and symptoms can be subtle and may evolve slowly over a few weeks. Characteristic signs include cyanosis, oedema, venous engorgement of the head, neck and arms, chest and upper abdomen, brawny non-pitting oedema of the neck and dysphonia due to laryngeal oedema. The symptoms – which frequently worsen when the patient lies down or leans forward – include facial congestion and swelling, breathlessness, cough, dysphagia, headache, stupor, seizures and syncope. Malignant disease accounts for most cases, especially from small cell carcinoma involving the right upper lobe and causing paratracheal gland enlargement and mediastinal infiltration. Lymphomas, malignant thymomas, germ cell tumours and, to a lesser extent, metastatic carcinomas may also give rise to SVC obstruction. Benign lesions account for about 5 per cent of cases. Aneurysms of the ascending aorta and innominate artery are now rare.

Large retrosternal goitres or chronic fibrous mediastinitis account for some cases, the latter being secondary to tuberculosis, histoplasmosis, coccidioidomycosis, blastomycosis or filarial mediastinal lymphadenitis.

In a proportion of patients the cause of mediastinal fibrosis remains obscure. *Iatrogenic causes* of SVC obstruction include thrombosis following the introduction of subclavian lines for venous access, or the insertion of temporary pacemaking wires. Superior venal caval obstruction is seldom a medical emergency, but does warrant prompt investigation and treatment. Whenever possible, a histological diagnosis should be obtained, by either bronchoscopy, mediastinoscopy or thoracotomy, to facilitate effective treatment for lymphoma, small-cell carcinoma, other tumours or non-malignant conditions.

Lesser degrees of localized chest wall venous distention may occur secondary to axillary vein thrombosis. This is not an uncommon condition and may occur after vigorous use of the arm, allowing the vein to be compressed and damaged between the clavicle and first rib. Painful congestion and oedema of the affected arm follow with collateral vein distension on the upper chest. The condition usually settles over 3 months.

Thrombophlebitis of the superficial veins of the breast and anterior chest wall (Mondor's disease) are also encountered. This condition may also affect the arm. The essential characteristic physical sign is an indurated subcutaneous thrombophlebitic cord about 3 mm in diameter. The cause is uncertain, and the condition gradually subsides over a few months.

Boris Lams

THRILLS

See also HEART, MURMURS IN (p. 291).

A thrill is a palpable vibration of vascular origin. It indicates vascular turbulence close to the site where it is felt. Thrills can be divided into: (i) those of cardiac origin, which can be regarded virtually as palpable heart murmurs; and (ii) those which arise in the extracardiac vessels. Cardiac thrills are discussed, along with heart murmurs, on page 291. Extracardiac thrills are usually accompanied by an audible component, termed a 'bruit'.

Carotid thrills usually arise from turbulence generated at the aortic valve rather than from a local carotid stenosis. This is perhaps because turbulence in the relatively small carotid vessel generates a high-frequency sound which is more easily heard than felt.

A slow-rising carotid pulse with a thrill is virtually pathognomonic of aortic stenosis, and this is confirmed by hearing an aortic ejection systolic murmur and demonstrating aortic valve disease by electrocardiography. It must be remembered that intracardiac and carotid lesions may co-exist.

Subclavian thrills may be generated locally or arise from the aortic valve. A difference in timing of the pulse at the two wrists, and unequal blood pressures in the arms, should be sought. A subclavian aneurysm may cause a thrill, but these are rare.

Peri-scapular thrills are a feature of aortic coarctartion, and are due to dilatation and increased flow in the peri-scapular vessels, as these form part of an anastomotic circulation around the aortic obstruction. There is often an associated bruit, together with upper segment hypertension and delayed or absent femoral pulses.

Cimino–Brescia arteriovenous fistulae created surgically in the vessels of the forearm (less commonly the leg), to allow easy venous access for haemodialysis in patients with renal failure, are probably the most common cause of peripheral vascular thrills in modern practice. The presence of a thrill indicates that the anastomosis remains functional. Sometimes these fistulae enlarge excessively, and have adverse haemodynamic effects.

Congenital arteriovenous fistulae are much less common. In children, they may cause excessive lengthening of a limb. There is usually conspicuous dilatation of superficial vessels.

Abdominal thrills are uncommon. An arteriovenous malformation in the liver, or a very vascular tumour such as an angiosarcoma, may cause a palpable thrill usually accompanied by a bruit.

Femoral artery thrills are usually the result of iliac atheroma, and are accompanied by a bruit and evidence of peripheral vascular disease elsewhere. Very occasionally, they may be due to a femoral arteriovenous fistula, which is a rare complication of cardiac catheterization by the femoral route.

Melvin Lobo

THROAT, SORE

Sore throats affect everyone from time to time. Most are part of a viral upper respiratory infection. Others do not progress in that way, and the infection remains restricted to the pharynx. While a large number of these infections have a viral cause, other sore throats are caused by bacterial infection, and an increasing number are fungal. The development of a persistent sore throat in a middle-aged or elderly smoker should raise concern, as it might be the first symptom produced by an upper aerodigestive tract neoplasm. A past history of excessive spirit consumption should heighten this concern and prompt a thorough clinical examination of the oral cavity, oropharynx, hypopharynx, larynx and neck. The pain experienced on swallowing in this group of patients often radiates to the ear.

The causes of sore throat are listed in Table T.7. Influenza, herpes simplex, adenovirus, rhinovirus, Coxsackie and the Epstein–Barr viruses cause *viral pharyngitis*. Patients usually complain of severe pain with, perversely, very little to find on clinical examination. There will probably be redness and oedema of the pharynx, especially along the pillars of fauces, the tonsils and the posterior pharyngeal wall. Lymphoid aggregates in the pharyngeal mucosa swell to produce a nodular or granular appearance on the posterior pharyngeal wall. Symptomatic relief with analgesics and mouthwashes is all that can be offered, other than sympathy. The condition resolves spontaneously in about 2–3 days.

Table T.7 Causes of sore throat

Tonsillitis
- Bacterial: streptococcal
- Viral: infectious mononucleosis

Pharyngitis
- Viral: rhinovirus, Coxsackie, Epstein–Barr virus, adenovirus, herpes, HIV
- Fungal: *Candida*, phycomycetes, blastomycetes

Mucocutaneous disorders
- Aphthae, lichen planus, pemphigus, pemphigoid, Behçets.

Neuralgias
- Glossopharyngeal
- Eagle's syndrome
- First bite pain

Neoplasia
- Carcinoma of the tongue, palate, pharynx and hypopharynx

Miscellaneous
- Thyroiditis
- Gastro-oesophageal reflux disease (GORD)
- Angina

Apart from *pharyngitis, acute tonsillitis* is probably the most common cause of a sore throat. This condition mainly affects the young, with peak incidences between 4 and 6 years of age and again later in adolescence. Acute tonsillitis in patients presents with malaise, pain and dysphagia. They are pyrexial and have enlarged tonsils with pus exuding from the crypts together with a jugulo-digastric adenopathy. There is usually a good response to antibiotics, and penicillin should be used in the first instance. Complete recovery takes 5–7 days, considerably longer than recovery from a viral pharyngitis. However, some do not respond to treatment or present late when the infection has spread beyond the tonsillar capsule and pus has collected in the peri-tonsillar space – a *quinsy*. These patients are extremely toxic, have marked trismus and a very 'plummy-sounding' voice. Only a limited view of the oropharynx is possible in these unfortunate patients, but it is usually sufficient to appreciate the swelling and faucial oedema of one tonsil together with displacement of the uvula to the other side (Fig. T.6). Apart from being very unpleasant, this can develop into an extremely serious condition if the infection continues to spread and involve the parapharyngeal space; this is termed *parapharyngeal space abscess*.

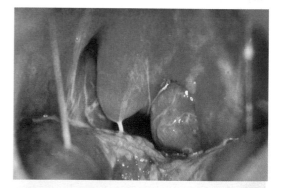

Figure T.6 A left-sided quinsy. The anterior pillar of fauces is swollen and the tonsil has displaced the uvula to the right side.

Infectious mononucleosis (*glandular fever*) is caused by infection with the Epstein–Barr virus. In this condition, which normally affects adolescents, there is malaise, pyrexia, tonsillitis and a marked cervical lymphadenopathy. The tonsils are covered with a thick, white plaque and there may be petaechial haemorrhages at the junction of the hard and soft palate

(Fig. T.7). In some, the tonsillar enlargement can be so severe that the airway becomes compromised and the patient has stertor. Some patients will also have hepatosplenomegaly.

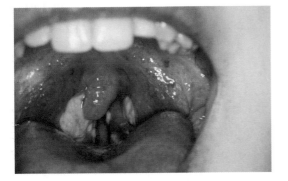

Figure T.7 The typical appearance of the tonsils in infectious mononucleosis. There is a thick, confluent plaque developing on the surface and two small petaechial haemorrhages on the left anterior pillar of fauces. Similar haemorrhages can often be seen at the junction of the hard and soft palate.

Fungal pharyngitis caused by *Candida albicans* is increasingly being seen. It is associated with the use of inhaled steroids and, in an otherwise fit young man, may be one of the presenting features of HIV infection (Fig. T.8). Other immunocompromised patients are also susceptible to this form of infection. Less common is infection with the phycomycetes and blastomyces fungi, and these are usually confined to selected geographical areas.

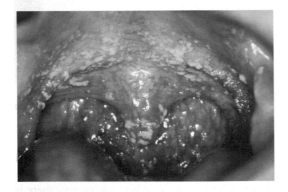

Figure T.8 Pharyngeal candidiasis caused by inhaled steroids.

Aphthous ulceration, Behçet's syndrome, pemphigus, pemphigoid and *erosive lichen planus* can all affect the mucosa of the pharynx. These conditions give rise to painful superficial ulceration that often also involves the mucosa of the oral cavity. In the case of pemphigus and pemphigoid, ulceration is preceded by a bullous lesion. The recurrent nature of these lesions and other cutaneous lesions suggests the diagnosis in most cases. Patients with major aphthae always have relatively few ulcers, and in some cases they may be solitary. Healing can take a number of weeks in these patients, and this may cause concern that the diagnosis might be incorrect. If in doubt, a biopsy is prudent (Fig. T.9).

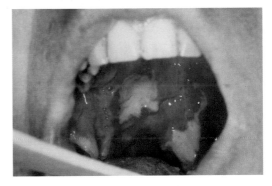

Figure T.9 Major aphthae affecting the soft palate. If there had been just one ulcer in this patient it would have been difficult to differentiate it from a carcinoma, other than by biopsy.

A number of conditions can give rise to neuralgic pain in the throat that is either spontaneous or precipitated by swallowing. *Glossopharyngeal neuralgia* is the immediate counterpart of trigeminal neuralgia. Patients with this condition experience paroxysms of excruciating pain, sometimes spontaneous but at other times triggered by eating or swallowing. In *Eagle's syndrome*, a similar type of pain is also experienced when swallowing. It is caused by friction between the glossopharyngeal nerve and an elongated styloid process. *First bite pain* is again similar in character and affects those patients who have undergone surgery on carotid body tumours or the cervical sympathetic chain. Their pain is triggered by chewing food or swallowing. Characteristically, it only affects these patients during the first meal of the day, but in some it is more prolonged.

Acute or subacute thyroiditis can cause pain in the neck or throat. In the acute phase of the disorder, the patient has no difficulty in localizing the problem to the neck. Patients with subacute thyroiditis, however, frequently complain of a persistent soreness in the throat. Discomfort is constant and aggravated by swallowing; it is associated with the sensation of a lump in the throat. Patients are intolerant of constriction of the neck, for example by shirt collars.

Reflux oesophagitis usually causes vague symptoms of soreness in the throat or a sensation of a lump in the throat caused by cricopharyngeal spasm. The patient may have chronic hoarseness or a constant feeling of wanting to clear their throat. The pain may be aggravated after meals or at night, when the patient is recumbent and subject to free reflux.

Without doubt, the most important issue in middle-aged and elderly patients with a sore throat is to exclude a *carcinoma*. This almost always affects those who have smoked heavily for a prolonged period, many of whom will also have consumed large amounts of spirits. Most of these tumours can only be seen on mirror examination of pharynx or with endoscopes (Fig. T.10). The pain is progressive, often radiates to the ear, and may become or be associated with a husky voice, haemoptysis, cervical adenopathy and weight loss.

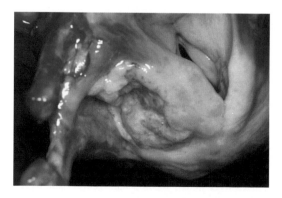

Figure T.10 Squamous cell carcinoma of the left piriform sinus that developed in a patient who had smoked 60 cigarettes per day for his entire life.

When the diagnosis of sore throat is not immediately obvious on physical examination, cultures for bacteria and viruses, haematological studies, lateral X-rays of the neck, barium studies of the pharynx, oesophagus and stomach and CT scanning of the neck and examination under anaesthetic may be required. If pain in the throat is initiated or accentuated

by exertion, then a thorough cardiac assessment is also wise, as angina can be experienced in this way. As stated previously, frequent recurrent infections of the pharynx may be an expression of immunodeficiency, as seen in the diGeorge syndrome or AIDS. It is also seen in subclass deficiencies of immunoglobulins.

Michael Gleeson

THYROID ENLARGEMENT

See also NECK, THYROID, PAIN IN (p. 473).

An enlarged thyroid gland gives rise to a swelling in the front of the neck, medial and deep to the sternocleidomastoid muscles and medial to the carotid vessels which, if the swelling is large enough, are displaced laterally and backwards. The gland is connected intimately with the larynx so that it rises and falls with the larynx and trachea during deglutition. This sign alone is generally sufficient to establish the diagnosis of an enlarged thryroid gland. The only other lump in the neck which moves on swallowing is a thyroglossal cyst, which characteristically, and in addition, moves upwards when the patient protrudes the tongue. This is because of the attachment of the cyst by a fibrous strand extending to the foramen caecum of the tongue.

Inspection with the patient at rest and on swallowing may alone be enough to render a diagnosis of thyroid swelling extremely likely. Palpation will confirm this, and is usually best performed while standing behind the patient with the neck flexed and relaxed. The lateral lobes are palpated with the appropriate sternocleidomastoid muscle relaxed. If the enlargement is only slight, help may be obtained by displacing the trachea towards the side being examined, when it is possible to introduce the fingers under the relaxed sternocleidomastoid to feel the posterior border of the lobe. The trachea and larynx may of course already be the subject of pathological displacement by pressure of the enlarged gland, and this should be determined at the time of palpation. The larynx should also be examined with a mirror for paralysis or asymmetry of the vocal cords. Vocal cord paresis will usually be accompanied by alteration in the voice and, if both cords are affected, possibly with dyspnoea and stridor as well.

The possibility of pressure effects always requires investigation, and these may be enumerated as follows:

- Pressure on the trachea causing deviation or compression or both, with varying degrees of dyspnoea and stridor.
- Pressure on the oesophagus causing dysphagia.
- Pressure on nerves, usually the recurrent laryngeal nerves, producing various forms of vocal cord palsy with or without alteration in the voice, dyspnoea, stridor and 'brassy' cough. The cervical sympathetic is occasionally involved, as shown by contracted pupil and ptosis (Horner's syndrome). Such nerve palsies are almost invariably associated with invasive tumours of the thyroid gland.
- Pressure on veins giving rise to engorgement and setting up of anastomotic channels, as a result of superior mediastinal obstruction from a large retrosternal extension of the gland.
- Acute pressure symptoms may arise, or those already present may become acutely aggravated, by haemorrhage into a thyroid cyst.

Retrosternal prolongation of the thyroid should not be forgotten, and may be recognized by a dullness on percussion over the manubrium, but this sign is unreliable. When the patient is asked to swallow or cough, it is sometimes possible to feel the lower limit of the gland as it rises; at the end of deglutition it slips back behind the sternum ('plunging goitre'). The thyroid in the neck may occasionally appear of normal size in the presence of a retrosternal enlargement, and in a few rare cases the whole gland lies behind the sternum. Pressure symptoms are liable to be great when part or the whole of the gland is in this position, and sometimes the result of pressure on the great veins is seen in the presence of dilated anastomotic skin veins over the upper anterior part of the thorax.

Radiographic examination is a most useful adjunct in the diagnosis of thyroid enlargement, showing both the presence of retrosternal prolongation and tracheal displacement and compression. Other aids may be useful with individual cases.

Varieties of enlargement and their differential diagnosis

It should be noted that the term 'goitre' is in common use; this simply means an enlargement of the thyroid, from whatever cause.

- Physiological enlargement: this occurs at puberty and during menstruation and pregnancy, and is usually symptomless.
- Inflammatory enlargement:
  - *Acute*: In acute thyroiditis, symptoms include the usual signs of acute inflammation; this condition is rare.
  - *Chronic*: Tuberculosis, syphilis, Riedel's disease; all of these conditions are rare.
- Simple goitre (endemic and sporadic). Parenchymatous goitre, colloid goitre, nodular goitre, solitary (fetal) adenoma.
- Hyperthyroid (thyrotoxic) goitre:
  - Primary hyperthyroidism (Fig. T.11)
  - Secondary hyperthyroidism
- Goitre of thyroid deficiency:
  - Cretinism
  - Hypothyroidism (myxoedema)
  - Lymphadenoid goitre (Hashimoto's disease)
  - Drugs (e.g. resorcinol, phenylbutazone)
- Malignant enlargement:
  - Carcinoma
  - Sarcoma (rare).

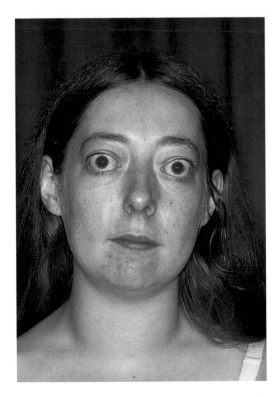

Figure T.11 Primary hyperthyroidism. Note the diffuse thyroid swelling and the exophthalmos.

These conditions can be regrouped for diagnostic purposes as follows:

- Thyroid enlargement with hyperthyroidism
  - ◆ Primary hyperthyroidism (enlargement general)
  - ◆ Secondary hyperthyroidism:
    - Localized enlargement: toxic adenoma (rare)
    - Generalized enlargement: nodular goitre in which one nodule may be so large as to suggest a solitary adenoma, occasionally parenchymatous or even malignant goitre
- Thyroid enlargement with signs of deficient secretion:
  - ◆ Congenital
    - Cretinism
  - ◆ Acquired
    - Hypothyroidism (myxoedema: mild deficiency may be exhibited by calloid or malignant goitre)
    - Hashimoto's disease
- Thyroid enlargement: uncomplicated
  - ◆ Localized enlargement: one large nodule in a small nodular goitre, cyst, adenoma, Riedel's disease (early stages), malignant disease (early stages)
  - ◆ Generalized enlargement: nodular calloid goitre, lymphadenoid goitre, Riedel's disease (late stages), malignant goitre (late stages).

Thyroid enlargement with hyperthyroidism

Hyperthyroidism is characterized by the presence of symptoms of hyperthyroidism from the onset of the disease. In secondary thyrotoxicosis, these symptoms develop after a simple goitre has been present for a variable period, often many years. The diagnostic points of each condition are listed in Table T.8.

Various eye signs are described in connection with exophthalmos, of which the following are the best known:

- von Graefe's sign: lagging behind of the upper lid as the patient looks downward.
- Dalrymple's sign: retracted lids causing a wide palpebral opening.
- Stellwag's sign: diminished frequency of blinking.
- Moebius' sign: inability to maintain convergence for close vision.

Dalrymple's sign is fairly constantly present, but may be found in other conditions, while the other signs are neither constantly present nor confined to exophthalmic goitre. Indeed, lid retraction alone may be found without true exophthalmos.

Cretinism

Usually, the thyroid is atrophic in this condition, but a goitre is occasionally present, especially in a long-standing case. An untreated patient is easily recognizable, but one is seldom seen nowadays. Slow development, either physical or mental, should rouse a suspicion of thyroid deficiency, remembering other possible causes of backward development such as rickets, renal rickets and achondroplasia. The diagnosis of cretinism will not be detailed further as it is barely relevant.

Table T.8 Diagnostic points of hyperthyroidism

	Primary hyperthyroidism	*Secondary hyperthyroidism*
Age of onset	Young	Middle-aged
Onset	Acute	Insidious
Thyroid swelling	Not present before onset. Generalized soft elastic and vascular swelling, enlargement not gross. May harden if iodine has been given	Present before onset. Enlargement may be considerable; frequently nodular
Exophthalmos	Generally present, often gross	Rare and, if present, slight
Heart	Tachycardia, but fibrillation and heart failure not common except in late or severe cases	Tachycardia. Cardiovascular failure most prominent symptom. Atrial fibrillation fairly common
Tremor and general excitability	Marked	Slight
Loss of weight	Marked	Present, not so marked
Increased perspiration	Marked	Present, not so marked
Results of iodine medication	Often striking improvement	Improvement, but of a lesser degree
Thyroid function tests	Raised	Raised
Radio-iodine uptake	Raised	Raised

Hypothyroidism

As in cretinism, the thyroid is only occasionally enlarged, and here again a detailed account will not be given. The characteristic symptoms of hypothyroidism include slowed mentality, coarse features, dry skin, brittle nails and sparse coarse hair, and a gain in weight, often gross.

Certain drugs (e.g. resorcinol as an external application and phenylbutazone by mouth) may occasionally be associated with thyroid enlargement, with signs of hypothyroidism reversible on stopping drug administration. Occasionally, a moderately enlarged gland may increase in size during treatment with an antithyroid agent (e.g. neomercazole).

Lymphadenoid goitre (Hashimoto's disease)

In this disorder the thyroid gland becomes infiltrated with lymphoid tissue as a result of an autoimmune reaction. Interestingly, it was the first autoimmune disease to be described. It is a disease occurring in women in middle life, and usually produces a uniform, firm enlargement of the thyroid with evidence of hypothyroidism. Laboratory tests for thyroid function show low levels. There is an increased serum cholesterol, a raised erythrocyte sedimentation rate, and autoimmune antibodies are present in the blood. Occasionally, lymphadenomatous goitre will occur with normal thyroid function and, very exceptionally, with hyperthyroidism. In the past, diagnosis has often been made after operation as a result of histological section of the tissue removed, but with careful investigation this should not be necessary in a typical case.

Carcinoma of the thyroid may cause confusion, but this condition is practically never associated with hypothyroidism in an untreated case.

Riedel's disease

This is an interesting and rare condition where an intense sclerosing fibrosis starts in one area of the gland and spreads first to the whole gland and then to surrounding structures. Its aetiology is unknown, but it may represent an end stage of Hashimoto's disease. The progress is slow as a rule, but gradually the trachea, the oesophagus and the great vessels all suffer from constriction, while the recurrent laryngeal nerves are affected early. The differential diagnosis from malignant disease is very difficult, but the condition should be suspected when an intensely hard goitre with pressure symptoms out of all proportion to its size is found in a young adult. Diagnosis is confirmed by histological examination of biopsy material.

Uncomplicated thyroid enlargement

A true *adenoma* is an uncommon condition, but a particularly large nodule in an otherwise small nodular goitre forming an asymmetrical swelling in the thyroid tissue is common (Fig. T.12). The lesion may be either cystic or solid, but palpation is not always reliable in determining this. *Nodular goitre* may give rise to a uniform enlargement, as also may *colloid goitre*. This last condition may present a smooth surface, as is usually the case in *parenchymatous* enlargement. A *simple cyst* is quite common, but may suddenly enlarge from haemorrhage into it.

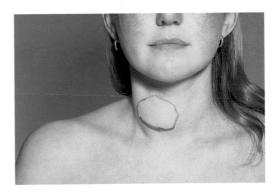

Figure T.12 A large colloid mass in the right lobe of the thyroid gland has been outlined with a skin pencil.

Malignant disease starts in one area and spreads to involve the whole gland, finally breaking through the capsule to invade the surrounding structures. Movement on deglutition may be lost, the recurrent laryngeal nerve is involved early, and the growth tends to surround the carotid sheath rather than push it back, as is the case with large simple goitres, so that pulsation of this vessel may be impalpable in the middle of the neck. The sympathetic chain is often involved late in the disease, with a resultant Horner's syndrome. The swelling is usually hard, as in Riedel's disease, but tends to be much greater in size and more rapid in growth. Pressure symptoms are early, and pain is often a marked feature, particularly on swallowing. Bone and lung metastases are not uncommon.

One type of thyroid carcinoma – namely the papillary carcinoma – deserves special mention. This lesion typically occurs in the fourth and fifth decades of life, when it metastasizes to the lymph nodes. The secondary deposits may be much larger than the primary, which cannot be detected, so that these cases often present with soft lumps in the side of the neck that used to be called (erroneously) 'lateral aberrant thyroids'. Thyroid tissue so situated is always a secondary deposit from a small primary in the thyroid.

Laboratory investigations

These include the following:

- *Serum free thyroxine (T4) and free tri-iodothyronine (T3)*. Measurement of the biologically active unbound fraction is more accurate than measurement of total T3 and T4; elevation suggests hyperthyroidism.
- *Thyroid-stimulating hormone (TSH) level* is raised in myxoedema, but suppressed in hyperthyroidism, where the gland secretes T4 autonomously.
- *Thyroid scintogram*. Radioiodine studies of the thyroid gland provide very useful information. A small tracer dose of γ-ray emitting iodine-131 is injected intravenously, and the gland scanned with a γ-ray detector to map areas of high uptake reflecting high activity. A nodule in the thyroid gland that is hyperactive can be pinpointed by this method, a so-called '*hot nodule*'. Similarly, a nodule that is not producing T4 will not take up the radioiodine, for example a cyst or tumour ('*cold nodule*').
- *Thyroid antibodies*, against thyroglobulin or the 'microsomal' antigen (now identified as thyroid peroxidase), indicate an autoimmune pathology (Hashimoto's thyroiditis); other autoantibodies are often present.
- *Thyroid ultrasound* provides valuable information as to whether a mass is solid or cystic.
- *Fine needle aspiration* and *biopsy* allows material to be obtained for cytological and histological examination. It is now the principal investigation for all solitary nodules, often under ultrasound guidance.
- *Serum cholesterol* is usually raised in myxoedema and may be normal or a little low in hyperthyroidism.
- *Electrocardiogram* in hyperthyroid cardiac involvement will show low electrical activity with small complexes. Atrial fibrillation complicating hyperthyroidism will be confirmed.

Harold Ellis

THYROID, PAIN IN

A painful thyroid swelling is not a common clinical situation. The two most likely causes to be encountered are either haemorrhage into a pre-existing thyroid cyst or inflammation of a thyroglossal cyst. The following conditions may give rise to this pain symptom:

- Inflammatory:
  - ◆ Acute (suppurative) thyroiditis
  - ◆ Subacute thyroiditis (De Quervain's disease)
  - ◆ Inflammation of a thyroglossal cyst or fistula
- Haemorrhage into a cyst of the thyroid
- Hashimoto's disease (rarely)
- Carcinoma of the thyroid in its late stages.

Acute (suppurative) thyroiditis

This is a rare condition which is nearly always bacterial in origin. Fungal and parasitic causes can be regarded as medical oddities. The usual organisms producing this condition are *Staphylococcus aureus*, haemolytic *Streptococcus*, *Pneumococcus*, and occasionally *Salmonella* and *E. coli*. In two-thirds of cases, there is pre-existing thyroid disease. The sexes are equally affected.

The source of the bacterial invasion is either extension from an adjacent infection or bacteraemia secondary to a distant focus. Commencing as an acute inflammation, the condition usually progresses to suppuration.

The clinical features are a sudden onset with severe pain in the neck which may be referred to the ear, the lower jaw or the occiput and which is aggravated by swallowing and movement of the neck. There is associated malaise and fever.

Examination reveals a febrile patient (the temperature in the range of 38–40°C), and tachycardia. Swelling, tenderness and redness in the region of the thyroid generally appears later and, more characteristically, only one lobe of the thyroid is involved. Regional lymphadenopathy is variable. The neck is held flexed and neck movement is painful. Fluctuation is not usually elicited because of induration of the surrounding tissues. There is leucocytosis and, if untreated, the mass progresses to the formation of an obvious abscess.

Subacute (non-suppurative) thyroiditis

This condition, also known as De Quervain's thyroiditis, is viral in origin. Any age may be affected, ranging from 3 to 76 years, although it occurs most commonly in the fifth decade of life. Females are far more often affected than males. Usually, the condition involves a previously normal gland.

The illness is preceded frequently by an upper respiratory infection, and the thyroid symptoms are often anteceded by muscular aches and malaise with fever (in the region of 39°C) and weight loss. Pain then develops in the thyroid gland, and possibly radiates to the ears. Pain is aggravated by movement of the neck and swallowing. Usually, both lobes are enlarged, although in one-third of cases one lobe is involved first and the inflammation then spreads to the opposite side. Examination of the neck reveals a tender, firm or hard enlargement of the thyroid gland. Quite often there are accompanying symptoms and signs of hyperthyroidism.

Laboratory tests reveal a raised white cell count and ESR. Usually, the T4 is raised, the elevation persisting for 1–3 months.

The condition runs a variable course of weeks or months, and even if untreated it usually subsides without sequelae. Rarely it is followed by clinical hypothyroidism. As its name implies, it does not proceed to frank suppuration.

Inflammation of a thyroglossal cyst or fistula

The typical thyroglossal cyst lies in the midline of the neck, usually at the cricothyroid space, less commonly at a higher or lower level, although it may deviate somewhat to one or other side of the midline. It usually presents in children or young adults, and characteristically moves upwards on protrusion of the tongue, as well as on swallowing (see NECK, SWELLING OF, p. 478). Infection of the cyst is not uncommon, when it presents as an obvious inflammatory mass above the anatomical region of the thyroid gland. A thyroglossal fistula is occasionally congenital, but it may follow infection or inadequate removal of a thyroglossal cyst. The fistula discharges mucus and is frequently the site of recurrent attacks of inflammation.

Thyroid cyst

Haemorrhage into a pre-existing thyroid cyst produces a sudden, painful enlargement of a lump in the

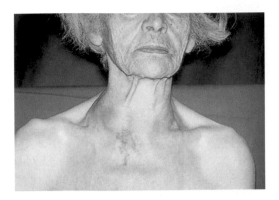

Figure T.13 An advanced carcinoma of the thyroid. The sternocleidomastoid muscle is involved, and the cervical lymph nodes are enlarged and hard.

thyroid gland which may or may not have already been noted by the patient. The danger is that it may also produce a sudden and dangerous compression of the trachea, with respiratory obstruction. The symptoms may require urgent surgical treatment but, if less severe than this, the swelling gradually subsides over the succeeding few days.

The cystic nature of the swelling can be confirmed by ultrasound examination of the mass.

Hashimoto's disease

This condition (see p. 717) is usually painless, but from time to time the thyroid enlargement may be painful and tender.

Carcinoma of the thyroid

Poorly differentiated (anaplastic) carcinomas of the thyroid usually occur in elderly patients. In their advanced stages, the lesions produce a tender and painful infiltrating mass in the neck, usually with local lymphadenopathy (Fig. T.13). Clinical diagnosis is not usually in doubt, but it can be confirmed by needle biopsy.

Harold Ellis

TIC

See also TETANY (p. 708); VERTIGO (p. 773).

'Tics' or 'habit spasms' are the terms which cover a variety of twitching or jerking movements that occur irregularly and tend particularly to involve the muscles around the eyes, the face and the shoulders. These are voluntary movements, and patients usually obtain relief from tension by their repetitive performance. In many instances, the condition is exaggerated by anxiety or neurosis. Often, with the passage of time, the movements become so habitual as to be almost involuntary.

In most instances the movement is the same and repeated in an identical fashion. Multiple tics may occur in the syndrome of Gilles de la Tourette. In this syndrome, the multiple tics may be accompanied by involuntary utterances and grunts. Although tics in isolation are thought to be functional in nature, there is some evidence to suggest that this particular syndrome has an organic neural basis. Multiple tics need to be differentiated from involuntary movement disorders such as chorea.

Mark Kinirons

TINNITUS

Tinnitus is a symptom that can be defined as any sound perceived by the patient when no external source of the sound exists. In the past, tinnitus was subclassified as either objective or subjective, depending on whether it was audible to the physician, or not. However, objective tinnitus is extremely rare – albeit fascinating for the physician and alarming for the patient. A more appropriate and clinically useful classification is provided in Table T.9.

From a clinical perspective, there are two types of tinnitus that demand careful investigation:

- Pulsatile tinnitus, which may indicate the presence of a vascular abnormality or tumour.
- Unilateral tinnitus, in which a space-occupying lesion within the cerebello-pontine angle or petrous apex must be excluded.

In all other respects, the quality of the tinnitus – no matter how disturbing for the patient – has little diagnostic relevance.

Tinnitus is a very common symptom which most people experience from time to time. Most normal people perceive some tinnitus if placed in a completely silent environment. The majority of people manage to suppress the tinnitus from conscious awareness; this is compensated tinnitus. A few are

Table T.9 Causes of tinnitus

Otological causes
- External ear
  - ◆ Otitis externa
  - ◆ Foreign bodies
  - ◆ Wax
- Middle ear
  - ◆ Otosclerosis
  - ◆ Chronic suppurative otitis media
  - ◆ Acute otitis media
  - ◆ Tympanosclerosis
  - ◆ Middle-ear tumours
- Inner ear
  - ◆ Presbyacusis
  - ◆ Noise-induced hearing loss
  - ◆ Idiopathic sensorineural hearing loss
  - ◆ Labyrinthitis
  - ◆ Menière's disease
  - ◆ Ototoxicity
  - ◆ Skull base fracture

Neurological causes
- ◆ Myoclonus of middle-ear muscles
- ◆ VIIIth nerve tumours
- ◆ Temporal lobe epilepsy
- ◆ Palatal myoclonus
- ◆ Multiple sclerosis

Vascular causes
- ◆ Glomus jugulare
- ◆ Glomus tympanicum
- ◆ Arteriovenous malformations
- ◆ Carotid artery stenosis
- ◆ Jugular bulb turbulence (venous bands)

unable to suppress their tinnitus and, regardless of its intensity, find that it interferes with every second and activity of their life; this is uncompensated tinnitus.

All patients with tinnitus should undergo a careful general and otologic/clinical examination in order to exclude any pre-existing conditions that may suggest the underlying cause. Most important, a thorough inspection of the ears, nervous system and neck, together with pure tone audiometry should be undertaken. Only when all underlying conditions have been excluded can the patient be considered to have idiopathic tinnitus.

Unilateral tinnitus always demands further investigation. It is a common and early presenting feature of VIIIth nerve tumours, and is not necessarily accompanied by hearing loss or vertigo. Patients with unilateral tinnitus should always have an MR scan of their cerebello-pontine angles.

Pulsatile tinnitus usually infers vascular abnormality. Light pressure on the neck over the internal jugular vein may abolish tinnitus in those patients with venous turbulence. An audible murmur on auscultation over the carotid artery or mastoid, or a palpable thrill, may suggest an arteriovenous malformation or carotid stenosis that can be confirmed by arteriography. Pulsatile tinnitus is the most common presenting symptom of patients with glomus tumours of the middle ear or skull base. These paraganglia are not always visible or palpable on clinical examination, and again, an MR scan is necessary for diagnosis.

If there is an obvious cause in the external or middle ear (foreign bodies, wax impaction, otitis externa, otitis media), treatment of this cause may eradicate or reduce the intensity of the tinnitus. In those patients where the tinnitus is an accompanying feature of a significant hearing loss, it may be improved by fitting an appropriate hearing aid.

Rarer and treatable causes of tinnitus include palatal myoclonus and spasms of the middle ear muscles. Clenching the teeth often intensifies or changes the quality of the tinnitus in this group of patients. Botulinum toxin injection or section of the tensor tympani or stapedius tendons can prove effective.

In the majority of patients, the precise cause of their tinnitus is not immediately obvious. The cause is then usually attributed to minor degrees of age-related hearing loss. It must be remembered that tinnitus is an extremely disturbing symptom for the patient. Many become convinced that they have a brain tumour, or even something worse. An explanation of their symptoms, together with sensitive reassurance, allows many to live happily with their tinnitus. Tinnitus maskers have limited benefit for a minority, and trials of various medications have met with only minor success.

Michael Gleeson

TOES, DEFORMITIES OF

See LOWER LIMB, PAIN IN (p. 419).

TONGUE, DISCOLORATION OF

The mucous membrane of the tongue is covered mainly by filiform papillae which cover the major portion of the tongue, and vary in length from 1 to 3 mm. Fungiform papillae are found at the apex and along the lateral aspect of the tongue. They are barely visible by eye, but on occasion even in the normal patient they may be red, large, smooth and round.

Today, discoloration of the tongue has much less of a diagnostic role in gastrointestinal disease than in the past. Changes that are thought to take place with constipation, appendicitis and other gastrointestinal diseases are insignificant and unreliable. On the other hand, there are more important changes which are associated with infectious diseases, deficiency states and metabolic disorders.

The tongue surface may be dry, brown and slightly furred in patients who are *mouth breathers* or who are *dehydrated*. A brown, dry tongue is common in *tobacco smokers*. Furring of the tongue is due to heaping up of the squamous epithelium on the filiform papillae, probably from inadequate cleansing of the tongue which ordinarily occurs during chewing. The term 'geographic tongue' is used when an area of filiform papillae is lost from the dorsum of the tongue. Smooth, pink mucosa is seen that contrasts sharply against that mucosa which is covered with normal papillae. A feature of the condition is that the appearance of the tongue will change from day to day, creating a 'wandering rash' across the surface of the tongue. This condition can be regarded as a variant of normal.

Very marked overgrowth of the filiform papillae produces a black, hairy tongue. This rare condition is encountered in patients on antibiotic therapy and some smokers. Hypertrophy of the fungiform papillae in *scarlet fever* produces the classic 'strawberry' or 'raspberry' tongue.

Leucoplakia describes white patches on the surface or lateral aspect of the tongue. These, on histology, show hyperkeratosis, acanthosis and dyskeratosis. The white areas may be seen as a patch or a raised plaque, and are usually painless. Leucoplakia is regarded as a precancerous lesion, as is the asymptomatic red, velvety lesion which may sometimes be seen on the ventrolateral aspect of the tongue. 'Hairy' leucoplakia is unique to *HIV infection*, and is found particularly along the side of the tongue, although it may occur anywhere in the mouth. The lesions are slightly raised, poorly demarcated, and show a corrugated white 'hairy' surface which does not rub off; they are asymptomatic. The histology is distinctive, showing keratin projections, parakeratosis, acanthosis, and a characteristic ballooning change in the pickle-cell layer.

Mucosal infection with the yeast *Candida albicans* produces the clinical picture of *moniliasis*, or candidosis or thrush. Creamy white, curd-like patches occur on the tongue and other areas of the buccal mucosa. When scraped, they reveal a raw bleeding area. The lesion can be quite painful and is found particularly in sick infants, debilitated patients, or those receiving broad-spectrum antibiotics or high doses of corticosteroids. Candidiasis is a common manifestation of *immunodeficiency*, particularly HIV infection. In infants, thrush is distinguished from milk curds by the difficulty with which the former are removed, leaving an underlying patch of inflamed mucosa.

The tongue will appear blue in patients who are centrally *cyanosed*, and pale in *anaemic* patients. Many anaemic patients however have a red, painful, bald tongue. This is the consequence of complete atrophy of the papillae which may occur in *pernicious anaemia*, severe *iron-deficiency anaemia* and/or *deficiency states involving other B vitamins*. The red, painful tongue may be associated with other evidence of mucosal atrophy in the mouth and fissuring at the corner of the lips known as 'angular stomatitis'. The mucosal lesions of folic acid deficiency are often more marked than those encountered in vitamin B_{12} deficiency. Other terms which have been used to describe the colour changes taking place in vitamin B deficiencies are the 'beefy red' tongue of *pellagra* and the 'magenta' tongue of *riboflavin deficiency*. The *Plummer–Vinson* (or *Patterson–Kelly*) syndrome describes the iron-deficiency state in which the tongue is painful, reddened and smooth. There is cheilitis, postcricoid webs and koflonychia.

Pigmentation of the tongue may be found in *Addison's disease* and *acanthosis nigricans*, in which the tongue undergoes hypertrophy of the filiform papillae to produce a shaggy, papillomatous dorsum. *Acrodermatitis enteropathica* is a rare autosomal recessive disorder related to zinc deficiency. Intra-oral features include a white coating to the tongue and buccal mucosa, with marked halitosis. There is chronic diarrhoea, hair loss, severe dermatitis and failure to thrive. The condition may also occur in patients on maintained hyperalimentation who become deficient in zinc.

In *hereditary haemorrhagic telangiectasia* (Osler–Weber–Rendu syndrome), telangiectasia occur throughout the gastrointestinal tract. They most commonly occur in areas of the oral cavity including the lips, gingiva, buccal mucosa and tongue. The lesions are dilated capillary vessels and small arterioles. The pigmentary changes involving *Peutz–Jegher's syndrome* and *pseudoxanthoma elasticum* do not normally involve the tongue. Granulomatous involvement of the tongue and buccal mucosa in *Crohn's disease* produces raised, smooth, red nodules and hyperplastic ridges on the tongue. These may appear erythematous. A number of dermatological diseases may affect the mouth, including *erythema multiforme*, *lichen planus*, *pemphigus* and *pemphigoid*, but involvement of the tongue in these conditions is rare.

John Meenan

TONGUE, PAIN IN

Pain in the tongue may be attributable to an obvious lesion, usually with breach of the surface such as a carcinoma. These conditions are discussed elsewhere (see TONGUE, ULCERATION OF, p. 727). On the other hand, pain in the tongue or soreness of the tongue may be an insistent complaint when there is no superficial evidence of abnormality. The conditions that must be considered include the following:

1 When the pain complained of is not on the dorsum, tip or sides of the tongue but underneath or deeper:
   - Injury to the frenulum linguae
   - Ranula
   - Calculus in the duct of a submandibular salivary gland
   - Foreign body in the tongue
   - Myositis
   - Trichinosis

2 When the pain complained of appears to be upon the surface of the tongue, even if it also affects the tongue as a whole:
   - Bitten tongue
   - After an anaesthetic (mouth-gag)
   - Injury by tooth or dental plate
   - Antibiotic glossitis, associated with lichen planus, Behçet's disease or pemphigus vulgaris
   - Congenital fissured tongue
   - Geographical tongue
   - Median rhomboid glossitis
   - Moeller's glossitis

- Glossitis of deficiency disease
- Smoking
- The effects of over-hot beverages or foodstuffs
- The effects of pungent condiments such as cayenne pepper
- Minor viral diseases
- Carcinoma.

The differential diagnosis depends upon the following considerations.

Pain underneath the tongue, or deeper

Injury to the frenulum linguae may cause visible abrasion or a definite ulcer. The most injured spot is tender as well as painful, the diagnosis depending on careful attention to the appearance and to the site of greatest tenderness. The cause may be injury by a fish bone or other sharp or puncturing objects. In violent coughing bouts, as in whooping cough, the protruded tongue may be forced against the lower incisor teeth with such violence that the frenulum becomes abraded, inflamed or ulcerated.

Ranula is not painful unless it becomes inflamed. It is an asymmetrical red smooth cystic swelling in the floor of the mouth under the tongue on one or other side of the fraenum. It may result from obstruction of the duct of one of the sublingual salivary glands, but more often it is a retention cyst arising in one of the many mucous glands in the floor of the mouth.

Calculus in the duct of a submandibular salivary gland is not necessarily painful. It may produce discomfort or more or less severe pain recurrent or constant according to the degree of inflammation. The stone may be very small and difficult to detect either with a probe or by X-rays. However, its existence may be suspected by the situation of discomfort, or by the corresponding salivary gland swelling when the patient begins to eat, when the stone interferes with the free passage of increased saliva flow. The calculus can frequently be palpated bimanually in the floor of the mouth, and is occasionally seen to protrude through the duct orifice. An X-ray will confirm the diagnosis.

A foreign body in the tongue is uncommon, though a fish-bone may become impacted in it. More often, the foreign body injures the tongue, itself escaping but leaving the pain behind. The diagnosis depends on the accuracy of the story obtained, or the discovery of the foreign body by palpation or by radiography.

Myositis of the tongue is seldom (if ever) a localized condition. It may, however, be a prominent feature in *polymyositis* or in *trichinosis*, in which the embryo trichinellae have a special predilection for the muscles at the base of the tongue, which become stiff, painful and tender. The diagnosis of trichinosis is difficult, especially as it will hardly be thought of unless there is an epidemic at the time. The blood exhibits eosinophilia, but the only way of clinching the diagnosis is by demonstrating the trichinellae embryos microscopically in portions of the muscles excised.

Pain on the surface of the tongue

A *bitten tongue* will usually present an obvious lesion, but the pain may persist after a tongue-bite, even when no obvious bruising or breach of surface can be detected. The patient may be unaware of having accidentally inflicted the bite, notably if the accident occurred during sleep or during an epileptic seizure. Indeed, the occurrence of a local painful area in the tongue suggesting the effect of tongue-bite may be the first indication that the patient is an epileptic. In tetanus, traumatic glossitis is common and may cause airway obstruction.

After *general anaesthetics*, patients may complain of soreness of the tongue resulting from the use of tongue forceps or of a mouth-gag.

Injury by a tooth or dental plate may cause a local painful place on one side of the tongue, often fairly far back, the pain being increased by movements of the tongue in speaking, eating or swallowing. Fear of cancer is usual until the cause is found in the jagged edge of the adjacent tooth, or of the dental plate at the corresponding site. The condition needs to be watched carefully to be certain that the lesion disappears after the offending irritant is smoothed down or removed, and to allay any anxiety that the jagged tooth or plate may have initiated an epithelioma. Tuberculosis of the tongue, presenting as a painful deep persistent ulcer, is now rarely seen.

Antibiotic glossitis is a common cause of diffuse soreness of the tongue from the taking of antibiotics by mouth. The pain is sometimes due to infection with *Monilia albicans*, which can be grown from the surface. Its preponderance is favoured by the wide-spectrum antibiotics. In other cases of antibiotic glossitis no such cause can be found, and the change is attributed to vitamin deficiencies arising from the suppression of normal gut flora. The tongue is clean, red and very sensitive to heat (Fig. T.14). Glossitis occurs in deficiencies of vitamin B_{12} and folic acid, in pellagra, malabsorption syndrome and the Plummer–Vinson syndrome, but seldom causes acute pain in these conditions.

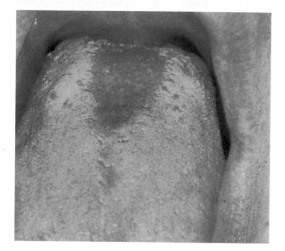

Figure T.14 Glossitis due to oral antibiotic. [Prof. Martin Rushton.]

Lichen planus affecting the tongue may be confused with monilia glossitis because both conditions produce small whitish patches on the surface. The lichen tends to produce lines or a mesh of pearly dots, and to favour the cheeks near the occlusal line of the molars.

The tongue may also become inflamed and painful in Behçet's disease, erythema multiforme or pemphigus vulgaris.

Congenital fissured tongue (Fig. T.15) or 'scrotal tongue' is thick, deeply fissured and usually symptomless. If food particles lodge in the fissures infection may arise and thus cause pain.

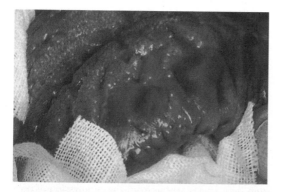

Figure T.15 Congenital fissuring of the tongue. [Prof. Martin Rushton.]

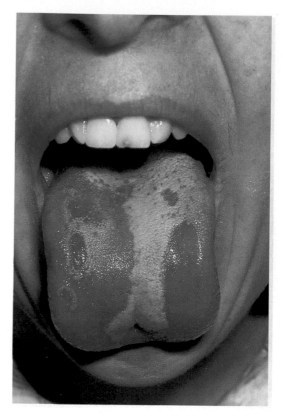

Figure T.16 Geographical tongue.

Geographical tongue (Fig. T.16) shows red denuded patches of irregular outline which often change their position. It causes anxiety rather than pain.

Median rhomboid glossitis (Fig. T.17) is a rare congenital abnormality caused by persistence of the tuberculum impar between the two halves of the tongue. It occupies the middle third of the dorsum and is smooth, shiny and red. It carries no filiform papillae. Opalescent nodules may be scattered over the surface. The area may become inflamed and thus cause soreness and often an unfounded fear of cancer.

Moeller's glossitis, often confused with the glossitis of pernicious anaemia, presents atrophic sharply defined red patches on the dorsum and sides: the atrophy in pernicious anaemia is evenly spread and the mucosa is pale and dry. Spiced food causes pain. The condition may be met in allergic states, nutritional deficiencies and with certain drug eruptions (e.g. reserpine).

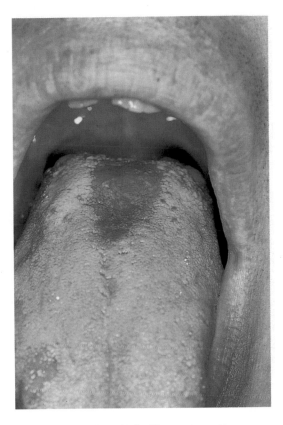

Figure T.17 Median rhomboid glossitis.

Glossitis of deficiency disease occurs with avitaminosis, particularly of the B group, as in pellagra, but also with iron-deficiency and pernicious anaemia.

Smoking and the effects of tea or other *hot liquid* or *food* may cause acute pain in the tongue lasting for days after the cause has ceased to act. *Pungent condiments* such as capsicum, cayenne pepper, ginger and the like may similarly be responsible.

Foot-and-mouth disease may rarely be contracted by humans from infected farm animals or consumed milk or milk products from infected herds. Vesicles appear in the mouth and on the tongue. In the so-called 'hand-foot-and-mouth disease', which is probably due to Coxsackie A viruses, children are affected. Vesicular stomatitis contracted from horses, cattle and pigs occurs in North and South America.

Carcinoma of the tongue (Fig. T.18) starts as a nodule, fissure or ulcer, usually on the lateral border of the organ. At first painless, it becomes painful as it invades and becomes grossly septic. The pain often radiates to the ear, being referred from the lingual branch of the trigeminal nerve supplying the tongue along its auriculotemporal branch. Ulceration is accompanied by bleeding; hence the typical picture of late disease is an old man spitting blood into his handkerchief with a plug of cotton-wool in his ear.

Harold Ellis

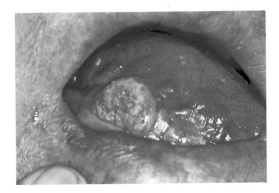

Figure T.18 Carcinoma of the tongue.

TONGUE, SWELLING OF

Swelling of the tongue is a condition the nature of which is generally obvious on inspection and palpation, if the history is taken into account at the same time. Causes of tongue swelling are listed in Table T.10, though many require little detailed discussion.

If the nature of the tongue enlargement is not obvious from the history and simple inspection and palpation – as will probably be the case when it is due to a *bite, sting, injury, corrosive* or *irritant* application, after the use of *serum, mercury, aspirin* or other drugs, *variola, pemphigus* or *erythema multiforme* – it may be so from the concomitant symptoms, as in the case of *cretinism, acromegaly, mongolism* or *myxoedema*.

Simple *macroglossia* is rare; when it does occur the history is that it dates from youth or childhood and the patient may otherwise be perfectly normal, unless he or she also has some other congenital peculiarity, such as macrocheilia (blubber-lips).

The chronic local lesions associated with swelling are in many cases accompanied by superficial ulceration, and the difficulties that may arise in distinguishing *simple, syphilitic* and *carcinomatous* ulcers are

Table T.10 Causes of swelling in the tongue

Acute swelling
- A bite or sting
- Injury (e.g. by a fish-bone, or by biting during an epileptic fit)
- Corrosives or acute irritant applications
- Acute oedema, secondary to:
  - Inflammatory conditions within the mouth: stomatitis
  - The effects of certain drugs (e.g. mercury, rarely aspirin)
  - Erythema bullosum or pemphigus
  - Variola
  - Serum injections and other conditions liable to cause giant urticaria
  - Angioneurotic oedema (angio-oedema)
- Haemorrhage into the substance of the tongue (e.g. in scurvy, leukaemia and other haemorrhagic states)

Chronic or persistent swelling
General swelling
- Macroglossia
- Cretinism
- Myxoedema
- Mongolism
- Acromegaly
- Primary amyloidosis

Local or asymmetrical swelling
- Irritation of a dental plate or decayed tooth
- Carcinoma
- Gumma
- Leucoplakia (chronic superficial glossitis)
- Tuberculous infiltration
- Actinomycosis
- Ranula
- Calculus in a sublingual salivary gland
- Suprahyoid cyst
- Haemangioma or lymphangioma
- Sarcoma
- Lipoma

discussed under TONGUE, ULCERATION OF (p. 727). *Tuberculous* and *actinomycotic glossitis* are both rare, and may be mistaken for malignant or syphilitic disease. Tuberculous lesions are usually painful, and this cause should always be thought of when considering the possible causes of a painful swollen tongue, particularly as the manifestations of tuberculosis of the tongue may assume unusual and bizarre forms. *Ranula* and *sublingual salivary gland calculus* or *cyst* both cause swellings that are beneath the front part of the tongue rather than in its substance, generally bulging up one side of the floor of the mouth near the frenulum linguae. A ranula is a distended mucous gland, and after growing to perhaps the size of a chestnut it often ceases to enlarge further; it does not

fluctuate in its dimensions in relationship to meals, as a salivary gland swelling often does.

A *suprahyoid cyst* is situated in the root of the tongue posteriorly, when it arises from remains of the embryological thyroglossal duct. It is seldom large; its nature is suggested by its situation.

An *angioma* of the tongue is rare (Fig. T.19). Sometimes, however, after remaining latent for years, it grows with rapidity and necessitates an operation. The diagnosis may be suggested by the colour of the tumour, but histological examination subsequent to removal may be required before one can be sure whether the tumour is a simple angioma, an angiosarcoma or a *sarcoma*.

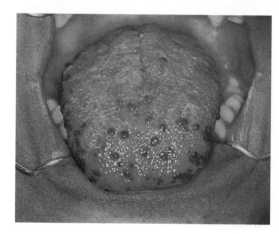

Figure T.19 Angioma of the tongue.

A *lipoma* occurs infrequently in the tongue, and its lobulated form generally breaks surface and presents like a cluster of soft white cherries.

Haemorrhage into the substance of the tongue, with swelling and inability to speak or eat, may result from certain blood disorders, such as acute leukaemia or primary or secondary thrombocytopenic purpura (see PURPURA, p. 583).

Acute oedema of the tongue may be due to *severe stomatitis*, *angioneurotic oedema of the tongue* or *Ludwig's angina*. This is an acute inflammatory condition, often streptococcal in origin, affecting the floor of the mouth and tongue, and spreading rapidly through the deeper structures of the mouth, throat and neck, causing extreme swelling of the adjacent tissues.

Angioneurotic oedema of the tongue is rare, but it is important because it may, rarely, prove fatal. As a rule there is a history of previous similar attacks in other parts of the body, and other members of the family may have had similar episodes. Tracheostomy may, though very rarely, be necessary as a life-saving measure, the diagnosis becoming clear only when the oedema of the tongue and adjacent parts subsides almost as rapidly as it came on, and the patient develops similar episodes (angio-oedema), probably in other parts, on subsequent occasions.

Harold Ellis

TONGUE, ULCERATION OF

To enable a good view to be obtained of the affected part, the patient should be seated in a good light and the protruded tongue gently dried with a piece of gauze. The presence of an ulcer being ascertained, its nature may be considered under the following heads:

- Carcinomatous
- Syphilitic
- Dental
- Tuberculous
- Ulcer in connection with stomatitis

Carcinomatous ulcer

Carcinomatous ulcer (see Fig. T.18) is much more common in men than in women. It is very unusual before the age of 30, and rarely starts before 45. The foul smell of the breath and the ill and wearied expression of the patient may awaken suspicion before the tongue is seen, for the sloughing ulcer is usually heavily infected, and the toxic absorption combined with pain and loss of sleep have a rapid and marked effect upon health. The tongue in a normal individual can be protruded 3–4 cm beyond the teeth; if the protrusion is limited, or if the tongue is not protruded straight, it can generally be inferred – except in cases of paralysis – that there is some tumour binding it down (ankyloglossia). The position of the ulcer is to be studied, and its relation to any sharp and carious tooth. A carcinoma is usually on the side of the tongue, but it may be anywhere on the upper, lateral or under-surface or on the floor of the mouth, but is hardly ever exactly in the midline.

As regards the ulcer itself, the typical appearance when fairly developed may be described as irregular, deep, foul, sloughy, with raised nodular everted edges and a surrounding area of induration. Other types associated with minimal ulceration of the mucous membrane are: the *scirrhous*, where there is an excessive fibroblastic reaction, and the affected part of the tongue is shrivelled up as in the similar atrophic scirrhous cancer of the breast; and the *nodular*, where the lesion is mostly buried within the substance of the tongue and, like an iceberg, broaches the surface over a deceptively small area. In addition, the papilliferous type and multiple ulcerations are not uncommon.

Lastly, there is the fissure carcinoma associated with *leucoplakia* (Fig. T.20) with thickened white patches of mucosa. This may have been predisposed to by smoking, syphilis, sepsis, spices, sore tooth or spirits, but often no cause can be found.

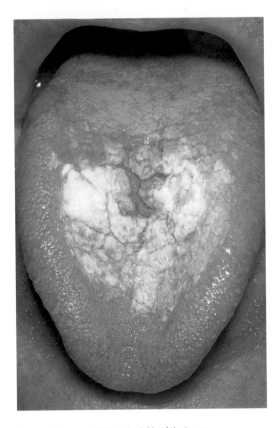

Figure T.20 Non-syphilitic leukoplakia of the tongue.

Except in early cases, some of the lymph nodes are enlarged and hard, and they may be fixed. The submandibular group is generally the first affected, but the disease sometimes misses these and invades the jugular and even the supraclavicular nodes. Examination, therefore, should not be concluded before the whole of the neck has been palpated. The diagnosis should have been made, however, before the disease has developed thus far. In its earliest stages a carcinoma may be represented by a superficial ulcer no more than 1.5 cm (one-sixteenth of an inch) in diameter, by a crack or a small lump, without any enlargement of the nodes. In all of these conditions, however, the ulcer is already hard and very resistant to any form of simple topical treatment. Any ulcer of the tongue occurring in a middle-aged man, and lasting for more than 2–3 weeks, should always awaken suspicion (Figs T.21 and T.22).

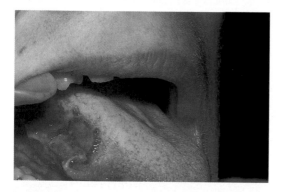

Figure T.21 Carcinomatous ulcer of the tongue. Surprisingly, the patient was an otherwise completely normal girl aged 17 years.

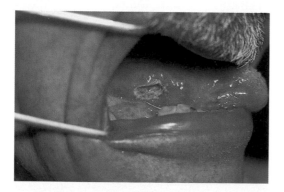

Figure T.22 Ulceration from epithelioma (carcinoma) of tongue.

Differential diagnosis

From syphilitic ulcer

This may be a very real difficulty, owing to the fact that the two conditions may exist side by side, and that the syphilitic leucoplakia may be the actual precursor of a cancer. Positive serological reactions, therefore, are not proof that a carcinoma is not present. If a well-formed gumma is present, anti-syphilitic remedies soon make a great change in its appearance. Although a biopsy is necessary for a definite diagnosis, certain clinical criteria are characteristic, and a putative diagnosis of gumma may be made when the ulcer is centrally situated, painless, serpiginous in outline, and has the steep-cut edges and wash-leather slough base typical of syphilitic ulcers elsewhere.

From dental ulcer

The ulcer in this case is caused by a carious or otherwise jagged tooth, and therefore is in a corresponding position on the tongue. Further, the ulcer is soft to the touch and heals rapidly when the offending tooth is stopped or extracted. There is seldom difficulty in differentiation, except when the ulcer is of very long standing.

Syphilitic ulcer

This may be primary, secondary or tertiary.

Primary syphilis or chancre is certainly rare on the tongue and, owing partly to its rarity and partly to the fact that it is unexpected, it is frequently missed. It is more common in men than in women, but it may occur even in children. It starts as a small pimple which ulcerates and becomes indurated, though the induration is not so marked as when it is situated on the glans penis. The appearance of a secondary rash with general enlargement of the lymph nodes would indicate the true diagnosis. Further proof is supplied by positive serological tests, and the detection of spirochaetes in serum from the sore. Furthermore, the sore heals rapidly under the influence of treatment.

Secondary syphilis manifests itself by the formation of mucous patches and superficial ulcers. The latter are almost always multiple, and situated along the edges and tip of the tongue, and with them are also found similar sores on the mucous membrane of the cheek, lips, palate and tonsil, and at the edges of the mouth. The ulcers are small, round, painful, with sharply cut edges and a greyish floor. Other secondary symptoms will be present to make the diagnosis clear.

Tertiary syphilis or *gummatous ulcerations* are now extremely rare and are divided into superficial and deep. *Superficial gummas* begin as small, round-celled infiltrations in the mucous and submucous tissue.

The ulcers are usually shallow, often irregular, and associated with chronic glossitis, fissures and leucoplakia. Though rare today, they are extremely important as they may be followed by carcinomatous change. The ulcers themselves are not at first indurated, but if surrounded by interstitial fibrosis they may appear hard; a histological examination is essential if there is the least doubt. A *deep gumma* starts as a hard swelling in the substance of the tongue. It is usually situated in the midline, and in the posterior half. Later it softens, breaks down and shows itself as a deep cavity with irregular soft, steep-cut walls, and a wash-leather-like slough at its base. It is not painful, and does not increase progressively in size. The important thing is to distinguish it from carcinoma and tuberculous disease. Unlike carcinoma, it does not infiltrate widely or fix the tongue, its history is short, and it causes no pain. Furthermore, it yields rapidly to anti-syphilitic treatment.

Dental ulcer

Dental ulcer is due to repeated small injuries from the sharp edge of a decayed tooth or damaged denture, and is situated opposite the tooth, generally on the side of the tongue. The ulcer is small, superficial and not indurated, unless it is of long standing. It is therefore not easily mistaken for any other kind of ulcer, but if doubt arises it is allayed by the healing of the ulcer on appropriate dental treatment. Failure to heal within a fortnight suggests that it is a carcinoma.

There is a form of dental ulcer which is found on the fraenum of the tongue in children suffering from whooping cough. During the violent expiratory spasms peculiar to the illness, the under-surface of the tongue may suffer from rubbing over the lower incisor teeth.

Tuberculous ulcer

This is rare in the Western world, but it occurs at that period of life during which tuberculous disease of the lung is common, between the ages of 15 and 35 years. It is due to infection with tubercle bacilli brought up into the mouth. The ulcer itself is usually on the tip of the tongue or the side in its anterior half and is generally painful, although sometimes it is entirely painless. The outline is irregular. The edges are usually thin and undermined, and the base is covered by pale granulations, or excavated clearly down to the underlying muscle fibres. Less commonly the edges are raised, though never everted or hard, and the base is nodular,

sloughy or caseous. It has often been mistaken for a carcinoma or gumma. The fact that it is not hard, that it is usually painful, and that pulmonary tuberculosis is present should point to the true diagnosis. Negative serological tests exclude a syphilitic gumma, though histological proof may be necessary by biopsy, and cultures carried out for bacteriological confirmation.

A further example of tuberculous ulceration is the so-called 'truncated tongue'. In this type there is an oedematous infiltration of the parenchyma of the tongue, causing it to become swollen and almost 'woody'. There is also a shallow ulceration of the tip, giving an appearance as if part of the tongue had been amputated. In fact, the clinical manifestations of tuberculosis of the tongue are so protean that this disease should always be suspected in unusual lesions, especially if associated with pain.

Ulcers in connection with stomatitis (ulcerative stomatitis)

Septic infection of the mouth due to a variety of causes, such as irritation from decayed teeth, alkalis, acids or mercury, may be accompanied by the formation of small vesicles which, on bursting, give rise to superficial ulcers (Fig. T.23). They are not limited to the tongue, but also appear on the mucous membrane of the cheeks and gums. Aphthous stomatitis commonly occurs in conjunction with the febrile diseases of childhood. It is characterized by the formation of whitish spots on the buccal mucous membrane, and small superficial ulcers may be formed by shedding of the epithelium. The ulcers of the tongue here occur during the course of a general inflammation of the mouth. One type that may be resistant to treatment is

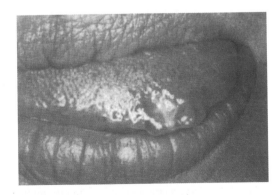

Figure T.23 Aphthous ulcer. [Prof. Martin Rushton.]

produced by Vincent's angina organisms; bacteriological tests provide the diagnosis, but it may be suggested by the extreme foetor of the breath.

When ulceration of the tongue – and at the same time, very probably of the inside of the mouth in general – occurs in such conditions as chickenpox, pemphigus and other conditions that may affect the buccal mucosa as well as the skin, the diagnosis depends, not upon the appearances of the ulcers or the tongue, but upon the concomitant skin eruption.

Harold Ellis

TONSILS, ENLARGEMENT OF

The tonsils are situated between the anterior and posterior faucial pillars of the oropharynx. They consist of lymphoid tissue and play an important role in the development of the immune system during childhood. There is a physiological increase in size of the tonsils between the ages of 4 and 6 years, and subsequently the tonsils involute. During childhood, tonsillar enlargement is usually accompanied by a synchronous enlargement of the adenoids. Extreme hyperplasia of the tonsils at this age ('kissing tonsils') can lead to respiratory obstruction and obstructive sleep apnoea. These patients improve dramatically with adenotonsillectomy.

In adult life, enlargement of the tonsils is most commonly caused by infectious diseases. Symmetrical enlargement may be caused by bacterial infection, glandular fever or toxoplasmosis, and is then accompanied by severe malaise and lymphadenopathy.

A peritonsillar abscess ('quinsy') develops when infection spreads through the capsule of the tonsil (see Fig. T.6). Pus and oedema displaces the tonsil medially and causes trismus, drooling, dysphagia, and change in quality of the voice ('hot potato voice'). Dramatic relief of many of these symptoms is experienced when the pus is evacuated.

The head and neck is the commonest region for the development of lymphoma, and many of these present as unilateral enlargement of the tonsil. This may, or may not, be accompanied by enlargement of the cervical lymph nodes.

In adults, deep lobe or parapharyngeal parotid tumours can cause displacement of the tonsil that can

be mistaken for tonsillar enlargement. Other lesions in the parapharyngeal space, such as chemodectoma, glomus vagale or schwannoma, can cause the same tonsillar displacement and apparent enlargement of the tonsil.

Michael Gleeson

TRACHEAL DEVIATION

The trachea extends downwards from the lower border of the cricoid cartilage to the bifurcation into the two main bronchi at the level of the fifth thoracic vertebra. In normal individuals the upper half of the trachea lies in the midline of the neck, while the lower intrathoracic portion inclines slightly to the right of the midline. Palpation of the trachea in the neck may provide information about the position of the mediastinum, provided that the thoracic spine is straight and the thyroid gland not enlarged.

Displacement of the trachea from the mid-sternal line will usually signify disease of the pleura, lung or occasionally the mediastinum. In conjunction with conventional physical examination of the chest to assess chest wall movement, air entry, percussion note, vocal fremitus and breath sounds, the position of the trachea should be carefully palpated. Deviation

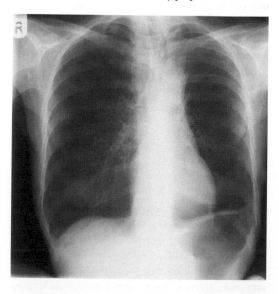

Figure T.24 Tracheal deviation due to left upper lobectomy for lung tumour.

of the trachea away from the abnormal side will suggest volume displacement, perhaps due to a large pleural effusion, pneumothorax under tension, bullous emphysema, or rarely, a massive lung or mediastinal tumour (Fig. T.24). Deviation towards the abnormal side will suggest collapse of the underlying upper lobe or lung. In adults, deviation of the trachea towards the affected side in conjunction with flattening of the upper anterior chest raises the possibility of long-standing fibrotic contracture of the lobe or lung, possibly with associated pleural thickening, secondary to healed pulmonary tuberculosis.

The trachea is not displaced by consolidation without collapse of the underlying lung. It may remain centrally positioned when carcinoma has caused a combination of lung collapse with pleural effusion.

A confirmatory chest radiograph should be taken if the physical signs suggest underlying lung or pleural disease.

Boris Lams

TREMOR

Tremor may be defined as a regular, rhythmic oscillation of one part of the body from a fixed point usually in one plane. It results from alternating or synchronous contractions of reciprocally innervated antagonistic muscles. Any body part including the limbs, neck, tongue, chin or vocal cords may be affected. There are three basic types of tremor: (i) a resting tremor is present with the relevant body part completely reposed; (ii) a postural tremor is elicited by extending a limb against gravity (this term is often used interchangeably with action tremor); and (iii) an intention tremor is elicited by moving a limb to and from a target. The differential diagnosis for each type is listed in Table T.11.

Resting tremor

The most important causes of resting tremor are Parkinson's disease and other parkinsonian syndromes (e.g. multiple system atrophy). The cardinal features of Parkinson's disease are slowness of voluntary movements (bradykinesia), rigidity and tremor. Typically these symptoms are initially manifest as asymmetrical or unilateral limb clumsiness, often in

Table T.11 Types of tremor

Resting tremor
- Idiopathic Parkinson's disease
- Other Parkinsonian syndromes (e.g. MSA-P)
- Essential tremor (resting tremor usually much less prominent than postural/intention tremor)
- Wilson's disease

Postural tremor
- Physiological
- Exaggerated physiological tremor
- Stress/anxiety
- Thyrotoxicosis, phaeochromocytoma, hypoglycaemia
- Drugs (beta-receptor agonists, amphetamine, lithium, theophylline, caffeine, alcohol withdrawal)
- Essential tremor
- Orthostatic tremor
- Task-specific tremors (e.g. primary writing tremor)
- Parkinson's disease
- Corticobasal ganglionic degeneration
- Dystonias

Peripheral neuropathies
- Charcot–Marie–Tooth syndrome
- Paraproteinaemic neuropathies

Intention tremor
- Disease affecting cerebellum and its connections (e.g. dentate nuclei, superior cerebellar peduncles)
- Multiple sclerosis
- Stroke
- Tumour
- Drugs
- Cerebellar degenerations (e.g. paraneoplastic, spinocerebellar ataxias)
- Rubral tremor

Hysterical tremor

Mixed tremors not classifiable in any of the above

one hand. Additional problems may develop, including postural instability, hypophonia (soft voice), dysarthria and facial hypomimia (poverty of expression). The tremor usually involves the hands, but may also involve the arms, legs, lower jaw or tongue. The tremor is coarse and regular, with a frequency of approximately 3–4 per second. The classical description is of pronation–supination of the forearm with flexion–extension of the fingers and adduction–abduction of the thumb, though this 'pill-rolling' is actually seen in only a minority of patients. The tremor can be exaggerated by distraction, for example by asking the patient to close their eyes and recite the days of the week. It may also be worsened by excitement or walking, where there may be reduced arm swing. Usually, the tremor itself causes little disability in daily tasks as it is markedly suppressed during volitional movements. The associated bradykinesia and rigidity, if present, do interfere with motor tasks. Rest tremor may be a feature of the parkinsonian variant of multiple system atrophy (MSA-P). Tremor is not characteristic of progressive supranuclear palsy, and is uncommon in drug-induced or post-encephalitis parkinsonism compared to idiopathic Parkinson's disease.

Postural tremor

The most important causes of a postural tremor are physiological tremor and essential tremor. Physiological tremor is a normal, small-amplitude oscillation that is usually asymptomatic, with a frequency of 8–13 per second. It most often affects the hands, and is best elicited by asking the patient to hold their arms outstretched with the fingers wide apart. The tremor is not present when completely at rest. Many factors can exaggerate physiological tremor, including metabolic disturbances (hyperthyroidism, hypoglycaemia) and intense anxiety or fright. Drugs including beta-receptor agonists, theophylline, caffeine and corticosteroids may increase physiological tremor.

Essential tremor is the most common type of postural (or action) tremor. It is slower than physiological tremor, being of frequency 4–8 Hz, and usually affects the upper limbs. There may be an associated 'No-No' or 'Yes-Yes' head tremor that disappears when the head is supported. The jaw, lips, tongue and larynx can also be involved, causing voice disturbance, but isolated jaw or head tremor is reported not to be a feature of essential tremor. The disorder may be inherited in an autosomal dominant manner, with complete penetrance. Though it is often termed 'benign essential tremor', it may cause marked disability by preventing normal activities such as carrying objects accurately. It can be brought out during examination by asking the patient to maintain the arms outstretched. It is worsened by emotion, stress and fatigue, and may show a striking response to small doses of alcohol. Unlike Parkinson's disease, the tremor is usually symmetrical, and asymmetric onset (particularly in the legs) should call the diagnosis into question.

Orthostatic tremor may be considered a special form of postural tremor. Unlike essential tremor, it affects mainly the legs, and is most prominent during standing. It diminishes with walking and disappears on sitting or lying flat. A buzzing noise may be heard on listening over the thigh or calf muscles with a stethoscope.

Intention tremor

The most important cause of intention tremor is cerebellar (and cerebellar outflow tract) disease, which may be due to many underlying disorders including demyelination, stroke, tumour or degenerative conditions. This tremor is perhaps inappropriately named as it occurs not on intention but on actual movement. Intention tremor can also be accurately termed ataxic, as it is always associated with cerebellar ataxia. Performing a precise guided movement, such as reaching with a finger to touch the examiner's finger, brings it out. It is absent at rest or during the early part of a reaching movement, but is manifest as the body part approaches its target requiring fine adjustments of position. It is irregular, of frequency 2–4 Hz, and continues for several cycles after the target has been reached. It may be disabling for fine motor task performance.

Rubral (Holmes) tremor

This tremor is a mixture of resting, postural and intention tremor. Lifting the arm slightly, or maintaining an outstretched posture, causes a large-amplitude 2–5 Hz tremor that can be dramatic and cause the patient to lose balance. The lesion, as postulated by Gordon Holmes, an eminent British neurologist, was stated to be in the red nucleus of the midbrain (hence rubral). Experimental data now indicate that the tremor may be due to dentatothalamic cerebellar outflow fibres traversing the red nucleus. The commonest causes of a rubral tremor are stroke, demyelination and Wilson's disease.

Hysterical tremor

Tremor is quite a rare manifestation of hysterical conversion. When it occurs, it is often confined to one limb, is of large amplitude and diminished by distraction – for example, performing a complex motor task with another body part. It is usually present equally at rest and during movement, unlike most organic tremors.

It should be remembered that tremors cannot always be fitted into the above groups, and that they may have features of more than one type. For example, in Parkinson's disease a resting tremor may be combined with an intention tremor, whilst in a cerebellar lesion the tremor may (rarely) resemble a parkinsonian resting tremor.

David Werring

TRISMUS (LOCKJAW)

See also FACE, ABNORMALITIES OF APPEARANCE AND MOVEMENT (p. 190).

Trismus, or lockjaw, signifies a maintained muscular spasm tending to closure of the jaws so that the mouth cannot be opened. The term does not include mechanical inability to open the jaws owing to such affections as mumps, alveolar abscess with surrounding inflammatory oedema, injury, Ludwig's angina, quinsy or severe tonsillitis, an odontoma, epithelioma of the mouth, myositis ossificans or cervicofacial actinomycosis. There are two conditions which may not at first sight be obvious, but may lock the jaws together and simulate true trismus. These are *impaction of a wisdom tooth* and *arthritic changes in the temporomandibular joint*. Diagnosis is by careful local examination of the teeth and of the joint respectively; in the latter case there may be arthritic changes in other joints also. X-ray examination may be required to detect the joint changes or the impacted wisdom teeth.

Circumstantial evidence will generally serve to distinguish trismus due to *hysteria* or to *facial neuralgia*; any doubt at first experienced is dispelled if the patient is watched for a while. Convulsive seizures in a hysterical patient with trismus can generally be distinguished from those due to tetanus or to strychnine poisoning by their polymorphous character, and by the fact that touching the patient, and other similar stimulation, does not bring them on so certainly as would be the case with strychnine or tetanus.

In fits, for example epilepsy, the trismus is of short duration and offers no difficulty in diagnosis. Malingering may sometimes take the form of lockjaw, and it may be a little while before the fraud can be detected. In sleep the malingerer's muscles relax completely.

Trichiniasis is rare, but if infected pork is eaten raw, or insufficiently cooked, the larvae of the parasites find their way to many different muscles, but they show a predilection for those of the tongue, mouth and jaws. The resultant irritation, pain and stiffness can cause trismus, the origin of which may be difficult to determine unless the history points to pork. The patient is very ill in the earlier stages, with high fever, and the condition may be fatal. The malady may be epidemic. The blood exhibits eosinophilia. The final criterion of the diagnosis is the discovery of the typical parasites coiled up in small oval cysts among the affected muscle fibres.

Hydrophobia (*rabies*) and *tetany* seldom exhibit trismus as a prominent symptom. The former, though now almost unknown in the UK, would suggest itself if a convulsive illness developed after a bite by a dog, fox or other similar animal, particularly if the spasmodic muscular difficulty is markedly increased by efforts at swallowing. The symptoms may not develop for weeks or months after the bite, so that the patient may fall ill when he or she has come from a country overseas where rabies is endemic. *Tetany*, also rare, is at once distinguished by its typical carpopedal contractions; trismus, which is almost constant in tetanus, is nearly always absent in tetany.

Strychnine poisoning gives rise to generalized twitchings and convulsions long before trismus, the lateness of the development of the latter serving to distinguish it from tetanus. Furthermore, there is complete muscular relaxation between spasms. There may be evidence of strychnine having been taken or administered, either by mouth or hypodermically; the symptoms develop very acutely, and are often rapidly fatal.

Tetanus is the cause par excellence of trismus, which develops in days, following introduction of infection (e.g. from small penetrating wound, burns, surgery, intravenous drug abuse, post-partum). Muscle stiffness starts usually in the neck muscles, spreading to those of the face and jaw, and thence to the rest of the trunk and limbs. Patients may have extremely painful generalized muscle spasms from the slightest stimulation (e.g. feather stroke or banging of a door). Muscle stiffness results in dysphagia, risus sardonicus and opisthotonos, and muscular relaxation is not possible unless an anaesthetic is given. It may be possible to demonstrate the presence of the drumstick bacilli in films prepared from the deeper parts of the wound. Diagnostic difficulty may arise when there is no clear history, or when the wound has been so small that it has healed or cannot be found; even then, most cases are typical, particularly the combination of normal conscious level and normal cerebrospinal fluid despite recurrent generalized convulsions. Unnecessary anxiety in a non-immunized individual may arise in cases of an impacted wisdom tooth, or of hysteria, where tetanus may be suspected at first; the subsequent course of the malady soon serves to exclude this. Involvement of the temporomandibular joint in a *serum reaction*, especially if prophylactic tetanus antitoxin has been given, may lead to the belief that tetanus has in fact set in.

Trismus may be simulated by *scleroderma* of the face, but here the condition is rather one of fixation of the skin than of the muscles. The skin becomes like parchment so that one cannot pick it up between the fingers, it feels firm or almost hard, and the patient becomes unable to open the mouth properly. The disease is of slow onset and gradual progress, so that there is seldom difficulty in diagnosis.

Danielle Harari

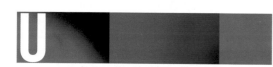

UNDER-ACTIVITY

The causes of under-activity are listed in Table U.1. Under-activity will most commonly be a normal response to fatigue and insomnia. The complaint of under-activity may also come from someone suffering an adjustment reaction from recent severe stress, such as marital or business problems or chronic illness. The response to stress may include anxious and depressed mood, physical complaints, disturbance of conduct including antisocial behaviour, or it may take the form of withdrawal from normal activities, without any clear evidence of mood change. Timely intervention with counselling may help the situation to resolve. Feelings of tiredness, fatigue and lack of drive accompany almost every form of debilitating illness and a complaint of under-activity may be due, for example, to anaemia, endocrine disorders such as hypothyroidism or Addison's disease; cardiac, renal or hepatic impairment; chronic infections; post-viral states.

Table U.1 Causes of under-activity

Common causes
- Insomnia and physical fatigue
- Physical illness
    - Hypothyroidism
    - Addison's disease
    - Chronic infections
    - Cardiac, renal, hepatic failure
    - Anaemias
    - Under-nourishment
- Adjustment reaction
- Uncomplicated bereavement
- Depressive illness
- Organic brain disease
- Frontal lobe syndrome
- Causes of confusion
- Schizophrenia
- Drug abuse
    - Opioid
    - Barbiturate
    - Cannabis
- Inhalent intoxication
- Post head injury

Less common causes`
- Obsessive–compulsive disorder
- Psychogenic stupor

Malnutrition caused by malabsorption will similarly cause symptoms related to debility. However, in people who are malnourished and also living in conditions of poverty and extreme deprivation, there can develop a profound state of apathy and under-activity as a result of a combination of adverse physical and social factors.

Many drugs of abuse are taken because they generate euphoria and under-activity. These include opioids, cannabis, hallucinogens (LSD, mescaline, magic mushrooms), barbiturates, benzodiazepines and other hypnotics and sedatives. More innocent drugs include codeine.

In depression, patients may show a slowing of all motor activity including speech, gestures and facial movements. There is usually retardation of thinking and complaint of difficulty in initiating and executing all voluntary acts. Severe depression with retardation may pose diagnostic problems in an elderly person when a gradual onset may lead the clinician erroneously to diagnose dementia in a patient whose apparent memory loss and cognitive impairment is due to their slowness in performing the tasks rather than to real cognitive change. Pseudodementia due to depression often responds well to antidepressant treatments, and it is important to bear in mind that during the early stages of treatment retardation may improve more quickly than the mood state, and there is a high risk of a patient making a suicide attempt. Depression is undoubtedly the most common cause of retardation, and even when retardation develops in a patient with another condition such as schizophrenia or obsessional illness, depression may be an important contributing factor. In obsessive–compulsive disorder (see OBSESSIONS, p. 494), some patients are so preoccupied by obsessional thoughts and inner rituals that they appear uncommunicative and slow in all their activities. In schizophrenia, under-activity may be the result of several different processes. Catatonic schizophrenia describes a relatively uncommon presentation of the psychosis, in which motor disorders dominate the picture. Patients may become mute or stuperose, and in rare cases adopt strange postures, exhibiting a disturbance of muscle tone by which their limbs will remain in any new position – however uncomfortable – for minutes at a time (waxy flexibility). They may show automatic obedience, responding to all requests without question; negativism, responding in exactly the opposite way to that requested; or sometimes they will remain mute and unresponsive, unwilling to engage at all with the interviewer. A detailed history and follow-up assessment is the only way that the diagnosis can be confirmed.

A rather more common type of under-activity affecting many patients with schizophrenia occurs with so-called 'negative' symptoms. These patients lose their sense of drive and volition, and become apathetic and careless about their appearance. They have a paucity of speech and emotional blunting which limits their full enjoyment of anything. They are poor time-keepers at work, and will be described as lazy, egotistical and inconsiderate by family and friends who are not made aware of the true nature of the condition. Depressive symptoms are common in chronic schizophrenia, and may exacerbate the underlying slowness and apathy. The side effects of anti-psychotic medication is a further cause of slowness in these patients, since higher doses of most anti-psychotic drugs cause a combination of motor and psychological slowing which adds to the negative symptoms.

Stupor describes a state in which a subject is fully conscious but makes no spontaneous movements and does not respond to stimuli. Occasionally, this may be psychogenic in origin, in which case the onset is sudden and stress-related and the patient may sit motionless for long periods without moving or talking, although their muscle tone, posture and eye movements indicate that they are neither asleep nor unconscious.

Patients with damage to their frontal lobes show changes in behaviour, mood and volition, typically with loss of initiative and spontaneity and a marked reduction in motor behaviour. Such people have particular difficulties in starting any new initiatives. Despite their mood – which can be euphoric – they perform tasks slowly and incompetently. A frontal lobe syndrome may follow head injury, be due to vascular or space-occupying lesions, or other pathologies such as demyelination involving the frontal lobes.

Mark Kinirons

UPPER LIMB, PAIN IN

Principles of diagnosis

The presenting features of disease and injury of the upper limb are pain, deformity, stiffness, weakness and paraesthesiae, swelling, instability and loss of function. Pain is by far the most common symptom. This may be localized (e.g. the pain of DeQuervain's tenosynovitis localizes to the radial styloid) or, more often, presents as a pattern. Dual pathology is common, for example cervical spondylosis and carpal tunnel syndrome. Routine examination therefore involves examination of the whole arm including the cervical spine, the neurology and the vascular system. In comparison to the lower limb, nerve entrapments and tendonitis/tenosynovitis are more common, while vascular disease is less frequent (Table U.2).

Pain referred into the arm

This falls into two main categories. Sharp, well-localized neuralgia often associated with paraesthesia is usually caused by nerve root or trunk compression. Diffuse discomfort in the upper limb, which is often difficult for the patient to describe and which may be accompanied by changes in skin temperature, vascularity and sweating, suggests involvement of the autonomic pathways. With this type of 'cylindrical' limb pain, an origin within the thorax, the thoracic spine or the involvement of T1 nerve root/stellate ganglion should be sought.

Table U.2 Causes of radicular/referred pain to the arm

Fractures/dislocation	Major trauma
	Complication of rheumatoid
	arthritis/ankylosing spondylitis
Cervical spondylosis	
Cervical disc prolapse	
Radiculitis	Viral (e.g. herpes zoster)
	Paralytic brachial (neuralgic
	amyotrophy)
Spinal abscess	Pyogenic
	Tuberculosis/brucellosis
	Fungal (in immunocompromised/
	AIDS patients)
Epidural abscess	
Pachymeningitis cervicalis	
Tumours	Spinal cord
	Meninges
	Nerve roots
	Vertebrae
	■ Primary
	■ Secondary

Many musculoskeletal pains are also transmitted via the autonomic system. For example, the pain from a frozen shoulder can temporarily be relieved by blocking the stellate ganglion with local anaesthetic.

Lesions in the cervical spine

Note. X-ray changes of cervical spondylosis are a normal finding after the age of 40 years. Over the age of 60, neurological symptoms and signs referred from the cervical roots are common. Therefore, great care must be taken before ascribing patients' symptoms solely to spondylosis, as there is often dual pathology.

Cervical spondylosis can produce three clinical syndromes which may occur alone or in combination: (i) pain and stiffness of the neck, which is often recurrent and may be aggravated by tension, anxiety and posture; (ii) radicular pain radiating down one or both arms and which may or may not be associated with muscle wasting, weakness and reflex changes (this is often referred to as brachial neuralgia); (iii) compression of the cervical cord, which may produce three sets of symptoms and signs:

■ Weakness, wasting and fibrillation in the upper limbs with reduction or loss of the tendon reflexes at the level of the compression.
■ Paraesthesiae in the arm and legs with or without impaired sensation in the hands and feet.
■ Pyramidal tract involvement with weakness, spasticity, hyperreflexia and extensor plantar responses in the feet.

The combination of weakness and wasting in the arms and spastic weakness in the legs resembles amyotrophic lateral sclerosis; spondylosis may usually be distinguished from this by the history of paraesthesiae, evidence of sensory impairment and radiographic or MRI evidence of cord compression. L'Hermitte's sign may be demonstrable – electric shock sensation on neck flexion.

Disc herniation at the C5/6 and C6/7 intervertebral spaces is a common cause of pain in the upper limb. Onset may be acute, with well-localized pain radiating from the back of the neck, across the back of the shoulder, down the arm and forearm to the wrist or fingers. More commonly the onset is less dramatic, often after a period of recurrent aching and stiffness in the neck. Pain may be aggravated by movements of the neck, by downward pressure on the head (the compression test) and by changing the position of the arm. Pain relief by applying traction implies entrapment at an exit foramen – with the patient sitting, place one hand under the mandible the other under the occiput and lift. Pain may radiate downwards into the scapular region and to the upper chest. Sensory disturbances are common and they may be detected in a dermatomal distribution (Fig. U.1). Muscle weakness may be detected in the appropriate muscles. The clinical signs

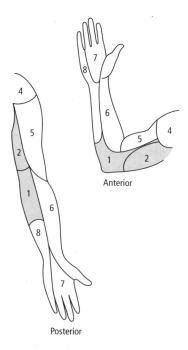

Figure U.1 Dermatomes of the arm from C4–8 and T1–2.

Table U.3 Signs and symptoms associated with common nerve root lesions affecting the arms

Root	Paraesthesiae/ numbness	Muscle weakness	Reflex change
C5	Radial aspect of forearm	Shoulder abduction Elbow flexion	Biceps jerk diminished
C6	Thumb and index finger	Wrist extension and pronation	Brachioradialis jerk diminished
C7	Middle finger, back of hand	Elbow extension and finger extension	Triceps jerk diminished
C8	Little finger, ulnar border of hand	Finger and wrist flexion	–
T1	Ulnar border of forearm and elbow	Intrinsic muscles of hand	–

N.B. 1. The biceps jerk is predominantly C5 but also has a component from C6.
2. The brachioradialis jerk, C6, is often though erroneously called the supinator jerk.

associated with the most common root lesions are indicated in Table U.3. Depression of the biceps jerk indicates a lesion of the C5 root; paraesthesiae in the thumb and index finger with depression of the brachioradialis jerk indicates a lesion of the C6 root; and paraesthesiae in the index and middle fingers with loss of the triceps jerk are associated with a lesion of the C7 root. Note, there are no specific reflexes for the C8 or T1 roots. For C8, test the power of finger flexion and check sensation in the little finger and the ulnar border of the hand. For T1, evaluate the intrinsic muscles of the hand, in particular the power of finger abduction. Ask the patient to 'spread out' the fingers; the examiner then squeezes them together. Compare both hands, and test sensation of the ulnar border of the elbow and the upper arm. Check for paraesthesiae in the feet, spasticity in the legs and examine the plantar response in case there is associated cord compression.

X-rays of the cervical spine may show disc space narrowing especially at the C5/6 or C6/7 levels with lipping of the adjacent margins of the vertebral bodies. In the acute stage, X-rays may not reveal a relevant abnormality, as disc space narrowing in the lower cervical spine is an extremely common appearance in normal individuals over the age of 40. CT or MRI is the investigation of choice in demonstrating a disc herniation, including herniation into the lateral recess. Spinal fluid examination is not a routine investigation for disc

prolapse as it is usually normal; however, it is worth recalling that the protein content may be raised in a large herniation, especially in the presence of cord compression.

Other causes of brachial neuralgia are uncommon but viral, bacterial and fungal infections not only occur but can also be diagnostically deceptive in their early stages. *Herpes zoster* is a good example. Later, the presence of a vesicular rash and residual pigmented scars in a dermatomal distribution provide an obvious explanation for the persistent pain. Weakness of one or more muscles in the limb with cutaneous hyperalgesia or hypoaesthesia may occasionally be present. *Acute viral radiculitis* (paralytic brachial radiculitis, neuralgic amyotrophy) produces severe pain in the shoulder and upper arm, often with rapid onset of muscle wasting and weakness. Symptoms usually subside after a few days, though there may be some persisting weakness and ache, for example winging of the scapula after involvement of the long thoracic nerve (see Fig. U.5).

Vertebral and paravertebral abscesses may result from tuberculosis or brucellosis, or be caused by more common pyogenic organisms such as *Staphylococcus aureus*. The incidence of spinal infection is increasing due to the rise in drug addiction and AIDS. Fungal or parasitic lesions are occasionally encountered in both these groups. Such lesions may or may not be accompanied by fever, and initial symptoms may closely resemble a cervical disc prolapse. Occasionally, there are no other pointers to a septic lesion so that severe root symptoms in the arms in the absence of clear radiographic abnormalities should prompt CT or MRI examination of the neck. Neurological signs will be present in about 15 per cent of cases of spinal infection, while quadriplegia can be a presenting feature. *Epidural abscesses* are fortunately rare, as there is a tendency for them to spread throughout the epidural space, causing a rapid onset of neurological deterioration with quadriplegia or paraplegia. *Pachymeningitis cervicalis hypertrophica* is a rare condition, sometimes syphilitic in origin, which causes diffuse pain in both arms together with paraesthesiae, widespread atrophy, loss of reflexes and variable sensory loss; more than one root is implicated. Positive syphilitic serology alone should not be taken to indicate this rare condition in the absence of other diagnostic features.

Primary (rare) or *secondary neoplasms* of the vertebral bodies may give rise to root pain with our without motor, sensory and reflex changes. X-rays are usually abnormal – collapse of a body, loss of a pedicle, cystic or sclerotic lesions are the common features, though only approximately 50 per cent of metastases will show on plain films. In multiple myeloma, X-rays may show nothing more than diffuse osteoporosis until the body collapses. Technetium bone scanning can be helpful, though spurious 'hot spots' may be seen in the presence of marked degenerative disease of the spine, and it is important to bear in mind that plasmacytomas and myeloma deposits may (as with plain X-rays) not be detected by this technique. CT and MRI scanning are particularly helpful in early lesions and also in determining the extent of any extra–osseous extension. In 60 per cent of cases of multiple myeloma, Bence–Jones protein (which precipitates at 60°C) is present in the urine. Electrophoresis of the serum shows a distinctive spike close to the gamma position. *Tumours of the meninges and roots* usually cause symptoms in the legs from compression of the pyramidal and sensory tracts, as well as pain in the arm. Scalloping of the pedicles is the classical picture on plain X-rays. Root lesions in the presence of multiple cutaneous neurofibromata (von Recklinghausen's disease) should raise the possibility of transformation to a malignant neurofibrosarcoma. *Syringomyelia* occasionally causes pain in the arm, but only as a late feature. By this stage the classical features of dissociated sensory loss, muscle wasting and hyporeflexia in the arms with pyramidal signs below the level of the lesion are likely to be apparent.

Traumatic injuries to an otherwise intact cervical spine are remarkably easy to miss. There are two reasons for this. First, these injuries are not all due to high-velocity forces; for example, 'hangman's fracture' – fractures through the pedicles of C2 – can occur with a blow to the forehead in a relatively straightforward fall while skiing. The second reason for misdiagnosis is that X-rays, particularly of the cervical thoracic junction, are difficult to interpret due to the overlying shadows of the shoulders on the lateral views. Any patient presenting with stiffness and spasm in the cervical spine, especially if there is a radiating pain into an arm, should be presumed to have major cervical spine injury until proven otherwise, and not assumed to merely have a whiplash injury. *Fracture dislocations* of the cervical spine are especially likely in the presence of *rheumatoid arthritis* or *ankylosing spondylitis*. In the former condition, atlanto-axial and/or subaxial subluxation of the spine may lead to upper and lower limb symptoms

(see NECK, PAIN AND/OR STIFFNESS, p. 476; see Figs N.17, N.18 and N.19), while the fused segments of a spondylitic spine are particularly at risk of fracture with or without displacement. Fractures of cervical vertebrae due to osteoporosis are unusual.

Lesions of the brachial plexus and subclavian/brachial arteries

The causes of these lesions are as follows:

- Thoracic outlet syndrome:
  - Cervical rib/fibrous band
  - Scalenus anterior syndrome
  - Subclavian aneurysm
  - 'Drooping shoulder' syndrome
- Malignant infiltration:
  - Axillary lymph nodes (e.g. lymphoma, metastatic carcinoma)
  - Posterior triangle disease (e.g. metastatic carcinoma)
  - Apical bronchial carcinoma (Pancoast's tumour)

The *thoracic outlet syndrome* is due to compression of the neurovascular bundle. Causes include an abnormal insertion of the scalenus anterior muscle, the presence of a cervical rib or a vestigial fibrous band and poor posture from drooping of the shoulder with consequent stretching of the plexus over a normal first rib (most commonly seen in middle-aged overweight women). Typically, pain is felt behind the clavicle and down the inner aspect of the arm. Paraesthesiae and hypoaesthesia in the C8 and T1 dermatomes with associated vasospastic features are common findings (i.e. in the little finger and ulnar border of the hand and forearm). Symptoms may be aggravated by carrying heavy weights, although this is not diagnostic. There may be atrophy of the hypothenar eminence and interossei muscles. The diagnosis is usually based on induction of paraesthesiae and numbness by abduction of the arm to 90° with external rotation; detection of an arterial bruit in the supraclavicular fossa during this manoeuvre; and disappearance of symptoms and bruit with return of the arm to the neutral position. Finding a position of the arm in which the radial pulse is obliterated has been considered a key diagnostic finding. However, this may be demonstrated in normal subjects and symptoms can be due to compression of the brachial plexus without involvement of the subclavian artery. The diagnosis is not, therefore, dependent on demonstration of arterial compression. When chronic or recurrent subclavian artery compression is present, this may (occasionally) lead to the development of aneurysmal dilatation of the subclavian artery and consequently to emboli causing infarcts in the fingers. In a few patients the accessory rib may be palpable and also visible on X-ray; not infrequently the rib is vestigial, being replaced by a fibrous band which cannot be detected. There is a tendency to over-diagnose thoracic outlet syndrome as a cause of pain in the arm. The alternative diagnoses of cervical spondylosis, cervical disc lesion or a peripheral nerve lesion are much more common.

Pain in the arm is occasionally due to pressure on, or infiltration of, the brachial plexus by *malignant tumours*. Lymphadenopathy associated with lymphomas or metastatic carcinoma will usually be detectable by palpation of the axilla and of the posterior triangle of the neck. However, infiltration of the plexus by metastatic carcinoma, especially from the breast, may take time to become evident. Involvement of the plexus by upward spread of an apical bronchial carcinoma (Pancoast tumour) or more rarely by apical inflammatory lung disease can produce unilateral Horner's syndrome in addition to arm pain. Such lesions can usually be detected on a chest X-ray. In all of these conditions severe pain may be present without any accompanying signs in the early stages. Further infiltration usually leads to paralysis with relative sparing of sensation.

Lesions in the thorax, thoracic spine and abdomen

The causes of these lesions are as follows:

- Cardiac ischaemia
- Syphilitic aortitis
- Thoracic disc
- Oesophagitis
- Diaphragmatic irritation
  - ◆ Subphrenic abscess
  - ◆ Ruptured abdominal viscus
  - ◆ Lesions of the spleen and pancreas

In contrast to the characteristically searing localized pain of nerve root involvement, pain in the arm originating in the chest has a dull, poorly localized quality, sometimes described as cylindrical. Autonomic controlled functions, including temperature of the arm and sweating, are often altered.

Pain associated with *myocardial infarction* and the exercise or stress-related pain of angina pectoris is usually readily recognized and confirmed by ECG or exercise testing. *Syphilitic aortitis* may induce similar referred pain. *Oesophagitis* can produce cylindrical arm pain with or without more classical 'heart-burn'. Such pain may also be accompanied by ECG abnormalities, so that accurate distinction from myocardial ischaemia may rest upon exercise testing, trial of glyceryl trinitrate and visualization of the upper gastrointestinal tract. Referral from the thoracic spine is a major but little recognized cause of aching in the arm or 'fibrositis'. *Thoracic disc prolapse* usually presents with an insidious onset of thoracic back pain which is occasionally referred into the arm. There is local thoracic spine tenderness, best elicited by sequentially pressing on the thoracic vertebrae with the patient prone. Pain is exacerbated by thoracic rotation. Other causes of stiffness of the thoracic spine, including spondylosis, may lead to similar symptoms.

In a minority of instances myocardial infarction leads to the development of pain and stiffness at one shoulder with varying degrees of pain, swelling, osteoporosis, vasomotor disturbance and trophic skin changes more distally in the limb. This 'shoulder–hand syndrome' is an example of a reflex sympathetic dystrophy or algodystrophy. This can also occur following nerve injuries, fractures such as a Colles fracture or a sprained wrist. The pain is usually described as 'burning'. The fingers, wrist and shoulder stiffen, but the elbow is often less affected. The condition can last for many months. Local anaesthetic blockade of the stellate ganglion is often effective in relieving the pain, thereby confirming the diagnosis and shortening the period of disability. However, when severe, full finger mobility in particular is not usually recovered.

Since the C5 nerve root supplies the diaphragm and the shoulder, several upper abdominal conditions can present with shoulder pain – subphrenic abscess, lesions of the spleen and pancreas, subdiaphragmatic irritation from a perforated viscus, etc.

Pain, stiffness and weakness of the shoulder girdle

This includes the clavicle, acromioclavicular joint, scapula and glenohumeral joint. A good knowledge of the anatomy is essential to making a diagnosis (Table U.4).

Pain may be referred, may arise locally or be a combination of both – for example, cervical spondylosis

latter injuries being due to high-velocity force. The minor sprains result in tenderness around the joint; with disruption of the capsule there is subluxation and more pronounced pain and swelling; while rupture of the conoid/trapezoid ligament complex will permit dislocation of the clavicle from the acromion causing an obvious deformity; this is best visualized from behind with the patient sitting and the arm hanging down by the side. These injuries are frequently missed or minimized on routine shoulder X-rays. The correct view is an anteroposterior (AP) film taken with a 15° superior tilt and the arm unsupported.

Rheumatoid arthritis of the acromioclavicular and sternoclavicular joints may affect up to 60 per cent of patients with rheumatoid disease. This is frequently overlooked, but it is a potent cause of unnecessary loss of shoulder function as it is easily treated. Pain is usually felt anteriorly and radiates across the point of the shoulder. To demonstrate the degree of destruction requires a 15° tilted AP X-ray. Patients often present late with fixed internal rotation and very little other movement remaining in the shoulder. *Osteoarthritis* is an important entity since osteophytes on the underside of the joint are a major cause of subacromial impingement and tears of the rotator cuff. The pain is usually well localized to the joint and is exacerbated by using the arm above the head. The joint is swollen, tender and abduction produces a high painful arc (i.e. above 120°). The diagnosis may be confirmed by injecting local anaesthetic, which abolishes the painful arc.

Osteonecrosis of the medial clavicular epiphysis (*Friedreich's disease*) is a rare condition that is usually only diagnosed in retrospect by the late development of osteoarthritis of the joint. *Condenscens osteitis* also affects the medial end of the clavicle but the joint space is preserved. It is usually seen in women in the middle years. They present with pain at the medial end of the clavicle, and X-rays confirm the diagnosis.

Winging of the scapula usually results from trauma to the long thoracic nerve (C5, 6 and 7) which supplies serratus anterior – 'backpackers shoulder' (Fig. U.5). A spontaneous onset is attributed to a post-viral neuritis. *Paralysis of the trapezius muscle* is due to injury to the spinal accessory nerve which is easily damaged by operations, including 'minor' operations, to remove a lump in the neck. Loss of trapezius results in drooping of the shoulder and inability to control scapulothoracic movement, thus causing a major loss of shoulder function.

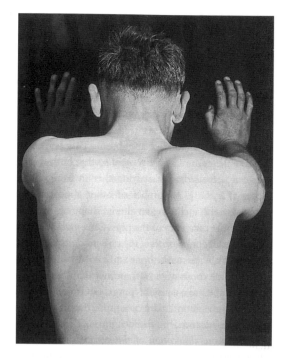

Figure U.5 Winging of right scapula secondary to paralysis of serratus anterior. The scapula becomes prominent when the patient pushes against a wall with his hands.

Injuries and diseases of the glenohumeral joint

Testing the shoulder muscles should follow the procedure in Table U.5.

Table U.5
Put the muscle under test in the optimal position and test against resistance

Muscle	Position
Deltoid	Test all three components (i.e. flexion, abduction and extension)
Supraspinatus	In plane of scapula (i.e. slight flexion and 15° of abduction)
Subscapularis	Internal rotation against resistance with the elbow flexed to 90° and held behind the back (get the patient to lift the hand away from the back/buttocks)
Infraspinatus	External rotation against resistance with the elbow flexed to 90° teres minor and held by the side
Trapezius	Shrug shoulders upwards
Serratus anterior	Press with both hands against a wall. Weakness causes 'winging' of the scapula (see Fig. U.5)

See Table U.6 on page 746 for a summary of the diagnostic categories for pain arising from the glenohumeral joint and humerus.

Lesions of the rotator cuff

The rotator cuff is a common source of symptoms as it is liable to: (i) compression between the humeral head and the acromion/coraco-acromial ligament; and (ii) degenerative tears due to its relatively poor blood supply. Osteophytic lipping on the inferior aspect of the acromioclavicular joint or the anterior lip of the acromion may further reduce the space for the supraspinatus component of the cuff, and consequently this is the most common site for *impingement*. The classical presentation is the 'painful arc' which typically occurs between 70–120° of active abduction. The pain is usually localized to the anterolateral aspect of the shoulder, with radiation down to the deltoid insertion. It is a common condition, particularly in older athletes and in those whose work puts repetitive demands on the shoulder, for example carpenters. The syndrome is relatively uncommon under the age of 40.

In addition to the standard examination of the shoulder and the demonstration of a painful arch in abduction, there are two useful special tests: (i) the impingement test – press down on the shoulder with one hand and forcibly fully flex the arm with the other hand; (ii) place the arm in forward flexion at 90° with the elbow at 90° and then passively internally rotate the humerus. An injection of local anaesthetic into the subacromial space should abolish the pain of impingement.

The subacromial space is best visualized by a lateral X-ray taken along the line of the scapula with a 5–10° caudal tilt. This will reveal any calcification in the tendon or abnormalities of the acromion. An AP view with a 15° superior tilt will show the acromioclavicular joint. MRI imaging is excellent for showing the rotator cuff (Fig. U.6), as is ultrasound examination by an experienced doctor.

Acute calcification most commonly affects the supraspinatus tendon, followed by infraspinatus and teres minor. Subscapularis calcification is uncommon. It is a disease of middle age, usually between 40–50 years, and is rarely seen over 70 years. While the majority are asymptomatic, the calcification showing as an incidental finding on plain X-rays, a

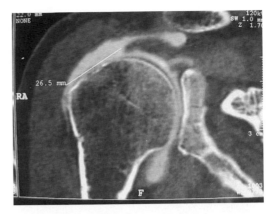

Figure U.6 Rupture of the supraspinatus tendon. A MRI scan reveals that the rotator cuff has retracted by over 2.5 cm. Synovial fluid, displayed as a white zone, fills the resulting gap. The subacromial bursa and the glenohumeral joint are in continuity.

few present with severe pain and inability to move the arm (Fig. U.7a). As the calcification disperses (Fig. U.7b) the pain settles, usually over 5–7 days and the shoulder returns to normal, though a painful arc may persist.

Ruptures of the rotator cuff (see Fig. U.4) begin on the under-surface of supraspinatus tendon near its insertion, progressing to a full-thickness tear and then spreading posteriorly to involve the infraspinatus. The rotator cuff retracts posteriorly and inferiorly, allowing the humeral head to migrate through the gap, so that it wears against the acromion. Onset can be acute or gradual, and is often precipitated by relatively minor trauma, for example, grabbing something to prevent a fall. In addition to the features of impingement, which are commonly present, there is evidence of weakness.

The *frozen shoulder* is a painful, stiff shoulder secondary to global loss of glenohumeral movement. It is more common in women than men, with an average age on presentation of 55 years (range 40–70 years). It is of slow onset and has three clinical stages, each of which last between 3 to 9 months – the painful stage, the painful stiff stage, and the resolving stage. It rarely recurs in the same shoulder, but it can affect the opposite shoulder. In the vast majority of cases, the shoulder returns to near normality. Characteristically there is slow onset of painful restriction of movement, especially external rotation and abduction, with the pain being most prominent at night. Biopsies show

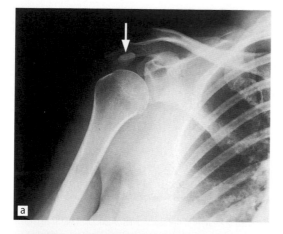

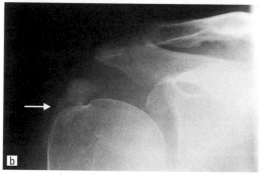

Figure U.7 (a) Supraspinitus tendon calcification (arrowed). The patient presented with a severe 'painful arc' of acute onset. (b) Calcification dispersing (arrowed).

an active fibroblast proliferation and transformation to myofibroblasts in the capsule and the coraco-humeral ligament. There is an increased incidence in patients with diabetes, hyperthyroidism and Dupuytren's contracture. Radiologically, the joint is normal apart from some osteopenia. This, together with the history, will distinguish a frozen shoulder from other causes of a stiff painful shoulder such as osteoarthritis or an undiagnosed posterior disloca-tion of the shoulder.

Instability

Anterior dislocation is a common sports injury. The anterior capsule and labrum are torn off the glenoid rim and the humeral head is held anteromedially deep to the glenoid. It may reduce spontaneously, in which case the diagnosis can be difficult, or remain dislocated due to the pain and consequent muscle spasm. The

diagnosis is then obvious, for not only is the shoulder held immobile but the absence of the head from the socket also unmasks the lateral prominence of the acromion. If, following reduction, the capsular tear does not heal, then recurrent subluxation/dislocation is likely to occur. *Posterior dislocation* is fortunately rare, since it is difficult to diagnose as there is no gross deformity as the humeral head moves posteriorly to lie directly under the acromion. Close inspection from above the shoulder is the best way to observe the altered outline. The smooth, rounded prominence of the anterior aspect of the head is missing, and instead there is a fullness posteriorly. The deception is increased by: (i) there may be no history of injury, since posterior dislocation can occur in an epileptic fit – these patients may not present for a few weeks and as the hallmark is a gross restriction of movement, especially internal rotation and abduction, an erroneous diagnosis of frozen shoulder can easily be made; and (ii) AP X-rays appear to show the head in correct alignment with the glenoid (Fig. U.8). An axillary view will confirm that the head is lying posteriorly.

The integrity of the axillary nerve should be established prior to reducing any dislocation. Failure to do so may result in medicolegal litigation. Since the deltoid will be inhibited by the pain of the dislo-cation, carefully examine the sensory distribution of the nerve which is in the small area of the lateral aspect of the shoulder over the distal part of the deltoid.

In many instances the dislocation, whether it be anterior or posterior, reduces spontaneously, but the patient may be left with instability and recurrent weak-ness in performing certain movements. While this diag-nosis is easy to suspect, it can be difficult to prove. Furthermore, instability must be differentiated from normal laxity. It is therefore essential to examine and compare both shoulders. The classical test for anterior dislocation is the apprehension test (Fig. U.9). Place the arm at 90° of abduction and maximum external rota-tion, with the elbow flexed to 90°. The examiner then stabilizes the scapula with one hand, while increasing the external rotation abduction force with the other hand. If the shoulder is unstable, the patient will resist the movement and also recognize that this is the pos-ition in which the shoulder 'pops out'. To distinguish between instability and impingement, the shoulder is placed in a similar position to the apprehension test (i.e. abduction and external rotation), but this time

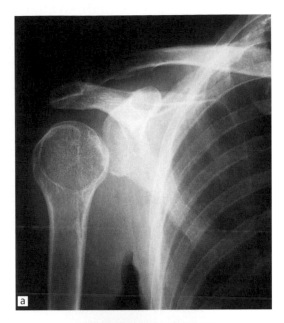

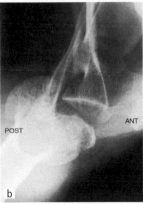

Figure U.8 Posterior dislocation of the shoulder. (a) Anteroposterior X-ray showing 'false congruity'. In fact, the humerus is lying directly posterior to the glenoid. The proximal humerus shows the 'light-bulb appearance' due to the altered rotation. (b) This posterior dislocation occurred during an epileptic fit and was initially treated as a frozen shoulder. The axillary view confirms that there is an impaction fracture of the humeral head on the posterior rim of the glenoid.

with the patient lying supine, place one hand over the head of the humerus to prevent its anterior displacement. With instability there is now no apprehension and no muscle contracture on further externally rotating with the examiner's other hand; however, if there is impingement the pain will still be reproduced.

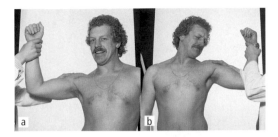

Figure U.9 (a) Full external rotation in abduction is present in the right shoulder. (b) In the unstable left shoulder, this movement is resisted – the 'apprehension' test for anterior subluxation. The patient's facial expression changes from a confident smile with the right arm to an apprehensive grimace on the left.

Multi-directional instability is due to a combination of anterior inferior plus posterior instability, and is often associated with general ligamentous laxity. The sulcus sign is a useful test. This is done by distracting the humerus out of the glenoid by applying longitudinal traction – that is, with the patient upright or supine, pull on the arm. As the humeral head moves inferiorly, so a dent or a sulcus appears below the acromion. A gap of over 1 cm is abnormal.

Arthritis

Rheumatoid arthritis of the glenohumeral joint is variable both in its severity and in the pattern of presentation. Three clinical pictures are recognized; the 'dry form' which presents as stiffness and bony crepitus secondary to loss of the joint space; the 'wet form' with marked synovial reaction; and the 'resorptive form' in which there is marked bone erosion of both the glenoid and the humeral head. *Primary osteoarthritis* was, until recently, uncommon in the shoulder but is now increasing in frequency due to the longevity of the population – most cases present over the age of 75 (Fig. U.10). Osteoarthritis below this age is nearly always secondary to previous injury (e.g. dislocation and fractures involving the humeral head) or to massive unrepairable tears of the rotator cuff which allow the humeral head to migrate proximally and eventually articulate against the underside of the acromion.

The shoulder is the second most common site after the hip to be affected by *osteonecrosis* (Fig. U.11). This reflects the fragile vascular supply to the large humeral

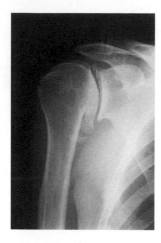

Figure U.10 Osteoarthritis of the shoulder in a man aged 85 years.

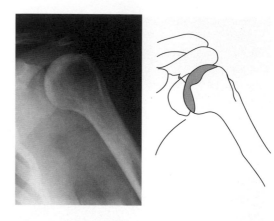

Figure U.11 Marked subchondral sclerosis of the humeral head secondary to avascular change in sickle cell disease.

head. In contrast to the hip, most cases have a well-defined precipitating cause. High-dose steroid treatment, for example as used in the treatment of head injuries, appears to have a particular affinity for precipitating osteonecrosis in the shoulder. It is also the most commonly affected joint in Caisson disease (the 'bends'

in deep sea divers and tunnel workers). MRI is the investigation of choice, especially in the early stages when plain X-rays are normal.

Infection

Both the glenohumeral joint and the humerus are uncommon sites for *acute pyogenic infection*. As a

Table U.6 Diagnostic categories for pain arising from the glenohumeral joint and humerus

Lesions of the rotator cuff	Impingement syndromes	
	Cuff rupture	
	Acute calcification	
	Frozen shoulder	
Instability	Anterior subluxation/dislocation	
	Posterior subluxation/dislocation	
	Multidirectional instability	
Arthritis	Rheumatoid arthritis	
	Osteoarthritis	Primary
		Post-traumatic
		Post-rotator cuff disintegration
	Osteonecrosis	Post-traumatic
		Steroids, alcohol, etc.
		Haemoglobinopathies (e.g. sickle cell disease)
		Caisson disease (the 'bends')
Infection	Acute pyogenic	Septic arthritis
		Osteomyelitis
	Chronic	Tuberculosis
		Infected implant surgery
Tumours/tumour like conditions See Pain in and around the knee (p. 389); Tumours and tumour-like conditions (p. 400)	Metastatic disease	
	Primary malignant bone tumours	
	Benign bone tumours	
	Tumour-like conditions	
	Benign	
Miscellaneous	Rupture of biceps	Long head
		Distal insertion

consequence, there may be a delay in making the diagnosis, which is often falsely attributed to trauma – in particular, fracture separation of the proximal humeral epiphysis due to a misinterpretation of the normal X-ray. (An AP film taken in slight rotation produces an appearance of a slight offset step between the metaphysis and the epiphysis at the level of the epiphyseal plate.) *Tuberculous infection* of the shoulder is also uncommon. It is easily mistaken for a frozen shoulder from which it remains an important but little known differential diagnosis. The historic name 'Caries Sicca' (dry tuberculosis) is a testament to diagnostic confusion in an earlier generation, with most cases probably being a frozen shoulder rather than tuberculosis!

Tumours and tumour-like conditions

These are discussed under PAIN IN AND AROUND THE KNEE; Tumours and tumour-like conditions (see p. 400).

Miscellaneous

Rupture of the tendon of the long head of the biceps affects elderly men, and usually occurs after lifting (Fig. U.12). Something is felt to snap in the shoulder. There is usually some bruising in the upper arm, but the most dramatic sign is that the belly of the muscle rolls up into a ball when the biceps is tensed. Patients often think they have developed a tumour. Occasionally, the biceps can avulse from its distal attachment to the radial neck. *Bicipital tendinitis* presents in two ways: either in association with a rotator cuff impingement; or as an isolated condition in young adults. In the latter, tenderness is localized to the bicipital groove and aggravated by resisted active use of the biceps and resisted supination of the forearm with the elbow flexed to 90°.

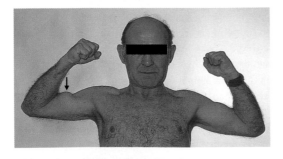

Figure U.12 Rupture of the biceps (arrowed). The outline of the biceps is exaggerated, and there is a deep sulcus proximally.

Pain in the elbow

Pain in the elbow is often well-localized and characteristic, for instance a tennis elbow. However, there is frequently dual pathology – for example, cervical spondylosis with referred pain plus stiffness in the wrist causing abnormal use and stresses to the elbow, etc. A full history and examination of the upper limb plus the cervical spine including the peripheral neurology should be routine. On examination, check for any deformity (in particular the carrying angle) by comparing both elbows fully extended, or in comparable positions if extension is limited. Swellings of the olecranon bursa and subcutaneous nodules from rheumatoid arthritis or gout are usually obvious, but synovial thickening and an effusion can be easily overlooked. This is best checked by inspecting and feeling the soft tissues on each side of the olecranon. The joint line can be easily found on the lateral side. Feel just distal to the lateral epicondyle while pronating and supinating the forearm to 'outline' the radial head. On the medial side, the joint space is obscured by the muscle mass of the forearm flexors arising from the medial epicondyle. The ulnar nerve is easily palpated behind the medial epicondyle. Check the alignment of the three bony points – with the elbow flexed to 90° the olecranon lies distally at the apex of a triangle formed with the two epicondyles; compare flexion and extension in both elbows. Since the elbow joint works in mid range for most activities, many patients do not actually notice that they have lost 20–30° of extension. Full extension is useful for carrying heavy objects such as a bucket, but only seems essential for bowling at cricket! Check pronation and supination, which is often markedly reduced by relatively minor incongruity between the head of the radius and the capitulum.

Epicondylitis is considered first as it is an extremely common symptom (Table U.7). The name itself is a misnomer, for not only is there no inflammation but the problem is also situated slightly more distally in origins of the extensor or flexor muscles. *Tennis elbow* affects 1–3 per cent of the total population in the 40- to 50-year age bracket, and if one considers all ages the incidence rises to 20 per cent of men and 10 per cent of women. At least 50 per cent of patients 'put up' with their symptoms and do not trouble their doctor. It is caused by overuse of the extensors, particularly extensor carpi radialis brevis – classically the backhand stroke at tennis. The pain comes on gradually,

Table U.7 Diagnostic categories of elbow pain

Epicondylitis	Lateral elbow pain	Tennis elbow
		Posterior interosseus nerve entrapment
		Lesions of the radiocapitellar joint
	Medial elbow pain	Golfer's elbow
		Medial collateral ligament sprain
		Ulnar neuritis
Arthritis	Rheumatoid arthritis	
	Osteoarthritis	Primary
		Post-traumatic
		Haemophilia
Infection	Acute pyogenic	Septic arthritis
		Osteomyelitis
	Chronic	Tuberculosis
Loose bodies/locked elbow	Osteochondritis dissecans	
	Osteoarthritis	
Instability	Synovial chondromatosis	
	Neuropathic joint	
	Tabes dorsalis	
	Congenital indifference to pain	
Nerve entrapments	Ulnar nerve	
	Median nerve	
	Posterior interosseous nerve	
Swellings	Olecranon bursitis	Non-infective, mechanically induced
		Inflammatory
		Infective
	Nodules	Rheumatoid
		Gout

often after a period of unaccustomed excessive exercise. It usually localizes to the lateral epicondyle, but when severe it can radiate widely. It is aggravated by simple activities which use the forearm in pronation, for example, pouring tea from a teapot. As with other tendonitides there is a triad of signs; tenderness just below the lateral epicondyle; pain on resisted active extension of the wrist; and pain on passive stretch (i.e. combined pronation and palmar flexion of the wrist with the elbow at 90°). X-rays are usually normal, but occasionally there is calcification seen at the extensor origin. Rarely this calcification may precipitate an *acute calcification syndrome* which is extremely painful and is accompanied by marked inflammation with warmth and swelling over the lateral side of the elbow to the extent that it can be easily mistaken for an acute severe infection. Other causes of lateral elbow pain are *entrapment of the posterior interosseous nerve* between the two heads of the supinator muscle at the level of the radial neck (see Nerve entrapments, below) and osteoarthritis affecting the radiocapitular joint. With the latter, pronation/supination is restricted. *Golfer's elbow* is similar to tennis elbow but involves

the flexor origin from the medial epicondyle. The diagnosis is often less clear-cut, and it can be difficult to distinguish from an ulnar neuritis, or sprains of the medial ligament. The triad of signs are: local tenderness just distal to the epicondyle; pain on resisted palmar flexion of the wrist; and pain on combined supination and extension of the wrist.

Arthritis

Rheumatoid arthritis commonly affects the elbow; approximately 75 per cent of patients complain of some pain, and in 20 per cent the joint is severely involved. X-ray features vary from osteoporosis and soft tissue swelling in the early stages, to gross bone loss of the distal humerus with erosion into the olecranon in later stages, when a fracture secondary to a fall can easily result in a flail elbow. The ulnar nerve is at risk both from the early synovitis or the deformity secondary to the destructive arthropathy. The surprising feature about *osteoarthritis* is that, while it frequently involves the elbow, many patients are unaware that they have a problem since they are not inconvenienced by loss of 20–30° of flexion provided they can get their hand up to eat, wash and comb their hair. Loss of supination is more troublesome than an equivalent loss of pronation as the latter can be compensated for by abduction of the shoulder. The elbow is the second most common joint (after the knee) which is affected by *haemophiliac arthropathy*; this eventually may lead to severe ankylosis. The most common cause of a very stiff and painful elbow is *traumatic osteoarthritis* secondary to severe intra-articular fractures.

Infection

Symptoms and signs of an *acute septic arthritis* are similar to those described for the knee – fever, synovial thickening, warmth, tenderness and immobility. The X-rays are normal, and the diagnosis is made on aspirating the joint (see PAIN IN AND AROUND THE KNEE, p. 399). *Osteomyelitis* can affect the metaphyseal area of any of the three bones, but it is much less common than in the lower limb. There is frequently a delay in diagnosing both *tuberculous osteitis* or *synovitis*. Furthermore, a discharging sinus is easily mistaken for a discharging olecranon bursa if it points at the back of the elbow.

Loose bodies/locked elbow

The elbow is the second most common joint, after the knee, for loose bodies. The convex surface of the capitulum is one of the classic sites for *osteochondritis dissecans*. This can present with lateral elbow pain, or if the fragments separate as a loose body can cause locking. It occurs in adolescents, but it may remain asymptomatic until later in life when the elbow locks. An X-ray usually reveals two or three significantly sized loose bodies. The reason for the time delay is that the loose bodies, by deriving their nutrition from the synovial fluid, can continue to grow in size, eventually becoming large enough to limit movement. Multiple loose bodies are due to *synovial chondromatosis* (Fig. U.13), which is now regarded as a benign synovial neoplasm (see PAIN IN AND AROUND THE KNEE, p. 390).

Instability

The elbow is particularly prone to trauma; it is the second most common joint, after the shoulder, to suffer dislocation. Dislocations, fracture dislocations (especially fractures of the coronoid or the radial

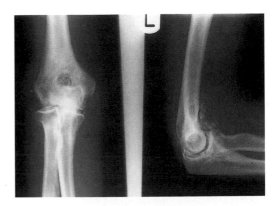

Figure U.13 Synovial chondromatosis of the elbow with multiple loose bodies.

head), and fractures (the radial head in combination with the medial ligament injury) can result in major instability. Elbow injuries are deceptive; in particular, dislocation can spontaneously reduce and small bony avulsions are easily missed on X-rays. Always be suspicious of a bruised swollen elbow, and check for any neurovascular complications. A good example is entrapment of the medial epicondyle together with the ulnar nerve within the joint in a child (see Nerve entrapments, below). The main causes of *neuropathic arthropathy* are tabes dorsalis, syringomyelia, diabetes and congenital indifference to pain. Tabes dorsalis predominantly affects the lower limb, while syringomyelia involves the upper limbs. Diabetes particularly affects the foot. Charcot joints can be painful in their early stages before the joint disintegrates. Excessive osteophyte formation in the presence of gross instability is the hallmark of a Charcot joint.

Sprains of the medial collateral ligament are an occupational hazard of baseball players, in particular 'pitchers'.

Nerve entrapments

The ulnar nerve can be compromised at several anatomical sites around the elbow: (i) in the intermuscular septum as the nerve passes from the anterior to the posterior compartment of the arm; (ii) in the cubital tunnel behind the medial epicondyle where it is vulnerable from direct injury, pressure from synovitis of the elbow in rheumatoid or osteophytes in osteoarthritis; and (iii) where it passes between the two heads of flexor carpi ulnaris, just distal to the elbow. In addition there are two specific childhood fractures.

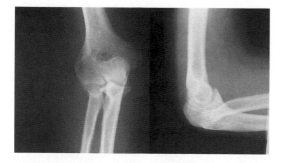

Figure U.14 This patient presented with an ulnar nerve palsy secondary to a childhood injury at the age of 8 years. Left: there was a marked valgus deformity of the elbow. Right: the lateral X-ray reveals that the radial head had been dislocated and never reduced.

The childhood lateral condylar fracture of the distal humerus, if poorly treated, can leave a valgus deformity (increase in the carrying angle) which may eventually cause an ulnar nerve paresis many years later (Fig. U.14). The other injury causes acute ulnar nerve symptoms. In a dislocation of the elbow with an avulsion of the medial epicondyle, the joint often spontaneously relocates, but the medial epicondyle – together with the flexor origin and the ulnar nerve – may become trapped within the elbow joint. Since the small bony fragment is obscured by the overlying bone, this injury and its complication can be easily missed by the unwary. A comparative X-ray of the opposite elbow will confirm that the epicondyle is missing.

In the early stages of *ulnar neuritis*, symptoms predominate over signs. The patient presents with a history of paraesthesia and numbness which on close questioning affect the ring and little fingers. The first sign is a loss of sweating (e.g. dryness of the little finger and ulnar half of the ring finger). Continuing compression or irritation leads to weakness in using the hand. Look for wasting of the hypothenar eminence, weakness of abduction and adduction of the fingers and loss of power of pinch. Muscle wasting is best seen and felt in the web space between the thumb and index metacarpals (adductor pollicis and the first dorsal interosseus muscles). Due to the loss of this muscle the pinch grip is affected and the thumb collapses into hyperextension at the metacarpophalangeal joint with flexion at the interphalangeal joint (Froment's sign).

The *median nerve* is particularly at risk with major elbow injuries, for example the supracondylar fracture of the humerus in children or a posterior dislocation of the elbow, since the nerve has a relative fixed point where it passes between the two heads of pronator teres. A chronic entrapment can also occur at this site. In addition to the altered sensation in the median nerve distribution in the hand, look for local tenderness by compressing the nerve as it passes under pronator teres whilst simultaneously resisting the patient pronating the forearm. Entrapment of the *posterior interosseous branch of the radial nerve* where it passes through the supinator muscle is difficult to distinguish from tennis elbow. The tenderness is situated more anteriorly over the radial neck and becomes localized to this site during resisted supination of the forearm. The patient may complain of weakness of grip due to the failure of the extensor muscles to stabilize the wrist. Electromyography is useful in confirming the clinical diagnosis of a nerve entrapment, especially if there is symptomatic cervical spondylosis with nerve root irritation – the 'double-hit' phenomenon in which a nerve is irritated at two sites.

Swellings

Anatomically there are a considerable number of bursae around the elbow joint. The majority are deep, for example, the bursa between the biceps tendon and the radial tuberosity. Only the *olecranon bursa* is of clinical relevance, the common cause of bursitis being recurrent minor trauma. Often referred to as 'students elbow', it is most frequently seen in office workers – leaning on the elbow whilst using a telephone is a common culprit. It presents as a fluctuant, non-tender, clearly defined swelling without tenderness or other signs of inflammation and with full elbow mobility (Fig. U.15). If there are any signs of inflammation, look for an underlying diagnosis. The common inflammatory causes are rheumatoid arthritis, gout or infection; typically, 20–30 per cent of all olecranon bursitis will be infected. If there is any suspicion of infection, aspirate and culture the fluid. In the presence of chronic infection – particularly if there is a discharging sinus – an X-ray is required to check that there is no pathology such as tuberculosis within the joint or the bones.

The posterior subcutaneous border of the ulna is a common site for *inflammatory subcutaneous nodules*. Rheumatoid arthritis or gout are the common cause.

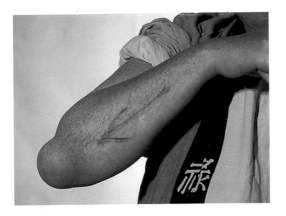

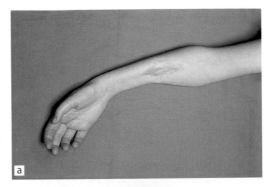

Figure U.15 A large olecranon bursa.

Pain in the forearm

Tendinitis and tenosynovitis are considered in the next section (see Pain in and around the wrist). The forearm is the second most common anatomical site after the lower leg, for a *compartment syndrome*. In both situations there are two bones, a tough interosseous membrane and well-defined compartments bounded by a strong overlying deep fascia. If undiagnosed, it leads to *Volkmann's ischaemic contracture* (Fig. U.16) in which loss of the forearm flexors to the fingers and thumb, together with loss of median and sometimes the radial nerve, results in a useless hand. Muscles supplying the wrist usually survive, but the fingers show a fixed length phenomenon – that is, palmar flexion of the wrist automatically causes extension of the finger at the interphalangeal and metacarpal phalangeal joints, while on dorsiflexion the fingers become clawed. Classically, the condition is due to a displaced supracondylar fracture of the distal humerus in a child, the brachial artery being occluded and damaged against the sharp distal end of the proximal fragment (i.e. across the metaphysis of the humerus). Other causes are crush injuries to the forearm; postoperatively after both vascular and orthopaedic surgery (there is a particular risk following plating of the radius); and bleeding disorders. The signs and symptoms are similar to those described for the lower limb. The cardinal symptom is pain, and the cardinal sign is pain on passive extension of the fingers. Other features include paraesthesiae progressing to numbness and paralysis and a solid woody feel to the forearm on palpation. The pulse can be highly misleading as it may be transmitted down

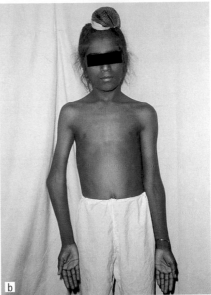

Figure U.16 (a) Complications of a supracondylar fracture of the distal humerus. Volkmann's ischaemic contracture of the forearm and the hand. Surgical decompression of the forearm muscles was carried out too late to prevent ischaemic necrosis. In addition, there was loss of both the median and ulnar nerves. (b) Varus deformity of the right elbow (the gun-stock deformity) due to a malunion.

an artery that is not passing through the involved compartment.

The wrist: pain and deformity

Causes of pain and deformity in the wrist are shown in Table U.8.

Deformity

Congenital deformities are rare and complex. In general, they are due either to failure of formation of part

Table U.8 Diagnostic categories of wrist pain and deformity

Deformity	Congenital	Radial club hand
		Ulnar club hand
		Distal ulnar dysplasia
	Acquired	Post-traumatic
		malunion
		growth plate injuries
		Rheumatoid arthritis
		Nerve injuries (e.g. wrist drop)
Nerve entrapments	Carpal tunnel syndrome	
	Ulnar nerve – distal entrapment	
Conditions of tendons	Tenosynovitis	Infective
		Inflammatory
		Mechanical
	Tendon ruptures	
Arthritis	Rheumatoid arthritis	
	Osteoarthritis	Wrist joint
		Distal radio-ulnar joint
	Osteonecrosis of lunate	
	(Keinboch's disease)	
Infection	Acute – pyogenic	
	Chronic – tuberculous	
Tumours/tumour-like conditions		
Miscellaneous	Ganglion	
	Chronic wrist pain/carpal instability	

of the skeleton or occur as part of a generalized disease. Radial and ulnar club hands are examples of 'arrest of development' in which a ray may be partially or completely absent (see Fig. S.47). For example, in a radial club hand the thumb, first metacarpal, scaphoid and trapezium will be absent and the radius only partially developed. Without an adequate wrist joint the hand falls off the ulna and collapses into radial deviation. Failure of development on the ulnar side produces the opposite deformity. *Distal ulnar dysplasia* is an example of a generalized disease and is associated with multiple exostosis. Secondary to the ulnar defect the radius is bowed and the radial head dislocated at the elbow.

Acquired deformities around the wrist are common. Displaced *Colles' fractures* invariably heal with some deformity despite an initial satisfactory reduction. *Premature fusion of the distal radial epiphysis* occasionally occurs following a fracture separation in childhood. This can produce a marked deformity with a radial tilt and relative overgrowth of the ulna. Severe destruction of the wrist and carpal joints is a hallmark of *rheumatoid arthritis*. A 'wrist drop' is of course not a true deformity but results from an injury to the radial nerve and paralysis of the extensor muscles – in order to grip it is essential to be able to extend the wrist.

Nerve entrapments/injuries

The *carpal tunnel syndrome*, in which median nerve function is impaired beneath the carpal ligament, is the most common of all entrapment syndromes. Although in most cases it is idiopathic, it should not be considered a primary diagnosis since it may be secondary to systemic disease such as diabetes and thyroid dysfunction, or local disease such as rheumatoid arthritis, which causes mechanical impingement into the carpal tunnel. It commonly occurs in pregnancy, but the symptoms are usually mild and transient, disappearing once the baby is born. The features are paraesthesiae and numbness, most noticeable at night, affecting the median nerve distribution. The symptoms are relieved by shaking the hand or holding it over the side of the bed (Fig. U.17a). Prolonged and severe compression will eventually cause motor weakness – weakness of thumb opposition (Fig. U.17b). Frequently, no abnormal physical signs can be detected in the clinic. Occasionally, there is a positive Tinel sign over the carpal tunnel and sometimes paraesthesiae can be precipitated by keeping the wrist in full palmar flexion for a minute. Wasting of the thenar eminence is a late feature. Electromyography (EMG) is particularly useful when the diagnosis is either not clear-cut, or when there are associated radicular problems in the arm secondary to cervical

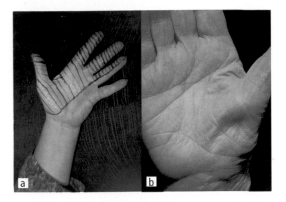

Figure U.17 Carpal tunnel syndrome. (a) The patient, who initially stated that her whole hand tingled when she woke at night, has marked the precise area involved. The outline shows the median nerve distribution. (b) Thenar wasting is uncommon, but can occur in a long-standing carpal tunnel syndrome.

spondylosis. *Compression of the ulnar nerve* in the palm of the hand in the ulnar tunnel is a well-described (although uncommon) condition. Diagnostically it can be confusing since, depending on the precise location of the compression in relation to the division of the nerve into a superficial sensory branch and a deep motor branch, the signs may be purely sensory, purely motor, or a mixture of both. Isolated motor loss with gradual onset of clumsiness in the hand is easy to miss. Ulnar clawing of the ring and little fingers is much more obvious in distal ulnar nerve injuries than in proximal injuries around the elbow, as the clawing will be less marked when the medial ulnar half of the flexor digitorum profundus and the distal small muscles to the ring and little finger are both paralysed.

Tendons

Acute pyogenic infection of the flexor tendon sheaths is considered later (see Conditions affecting the hands and fingers). An important anatomical point is that the synovial sheath of flexor pollicis longus extends from the tendon insertion on the distal phalanx proximally through the carpal tunnel into the distal forearm. The common sheath of the digital flexors also passes under the carpal ligament into the palm, and then continues down into the flexor sheath of the little finger. The extensor tendon sheaths extend distal and proximal to the extensor retinaculum, but do not extend down into the fingers. Acute infection of

the extensor sheaths is usually due to a penetrating injury. There is often an associated overlying cellulitis, which can obscure infection in the underlying sheath.

Inflammatory tenosynovitis is common in *rheumatoid disease* and affects both the flexor and the extensor tendons. The thickened swollen synovium is more obvious around the dorsal extensor tendons than the palmar flexor tendons (Fig. U.18), where the swelling is confined to the proximal palm and the distal forearm by the constriction of the tight carpal ligament. Pain on flexion of the fingers in the presence of good individual finger function is the main feature of the rheumatoid flexor tenosynovitis at the wrist. *Extensor tendon ruptures in rheumatoid* are not only common but easily overlooked by both the patient and the doctor in a severely affected rheumatoid hand. They present with a 'dropped finger'; this is an inability actively to extend the metacarpophalangeal joint. Due to the action of the interossei muscles extension at the proximal interphalangeal joint is retained, hence the deception. Rupture is due to two factors, rheumatoid synovium from the

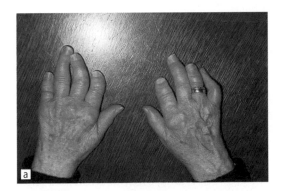

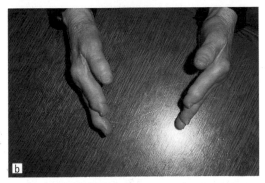

Figure U.18 (a) Hands in rheumatoid arthritis. (b) Note the swan-neck deformities of the fingers on the lateral views.

tendon sheath invading into the tendon, and abrasion over the ulnar head. Failure to make the diagnosis early will lead to sequential dropping of the fingers and an unnecessary additional loss of function in the hand.

Some ruptures are mechanical, for example, *rupture of the extensor pollicis longus* approximately 6 weeks after a minimally displaced Colles' fracture, which results in loss of extension of the distal phalanx of the thumb. Mechanical or stress-induced tenosynovitis around the wrist is common, usually following a period of repetitive unaccustomed activity, for example an office worker using a pick-axe and causing de Quervain's syndrome (tenosynovitis of the tendon sheath of extensor pollicis brevis and abductor pollicis longus where they pass through a tunnel over the radial styloid). The triad of signs are local tenderness over the radial styloid, pain on resisted ulnar deviation with the thumb abducted, and pain on passive stretch into radial deviation with the thumb first placed fully opposed across the palm. Differential diagnosis is from a fractured scaphoid and carpometacarpal osteoarthritis between the trapezium and the thumb metacarpal.

Arthritis

The wrist joints are the second most commonly involved joints in rheumatoid arthritis, after the metacarpophalangeal joints. Initial involvement is often on the ulnar side, especially the distal radioulnar joint. As the disease progresses into the radial carpal and intercarpal joints, so the wrist develops the classical deformity with radial deviation and palmar subluxation. As mentioned above, the synovial sheaths of the tendons are frequently involved. Without a well-aligned balanced wrist, it is impossible to have a good finger grip. In contradistinction to rheumatoid, *osteoarthritis* of the wrist is uncommon unless there has been a previous intra-articular fracture or dislocation. *Osteonecrosis* affects the proximal convex surface of the lunate. There is usually an associated relative shortening of the ulna. The condition presents in early adult life with discomfort following exercise. Grip strength is usually diminished. In the early stages, the X-rays are normal, followed in time by sclerosis, then collapse of the articular surface and finally osteoarthritic change in the wrist joint (Fig. U.19). The proximal pole of the scaphoid is at risk following fractures across the proximal part of the wrist. The long-term result is osteoarthritis of the wrist (Fig. U.20).

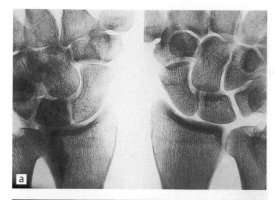

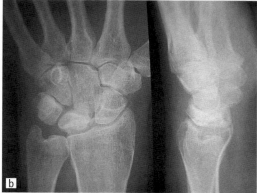

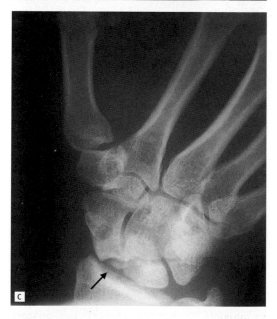

Figure U.19 Osteonecrosis of the lunate (Keinboch's disease). (a) Note the increased sclerosis in the left lunate. (b) Collapse of the proximal convex surface. (c) Osteonecrosis of the proximal pole of the scaphoid (arrow) following a transverse fracture across the proximal part of the waist of the scaphoid.

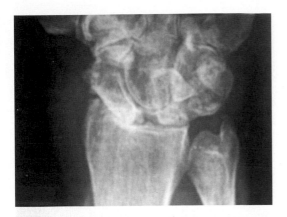

Figure U.20 Osteoarthritis of the wrist is the long-term result of osteonecrosis of the lunate.

Infection

Acute pyogenic infection of the wrist joint is uncommon unless there has been a penetrating injury. However, the wrist is a common site for *tuberculous infection*, which often presents relatively late as there is a gradual onset of pain and stiffness. With progressive destruction there is palmar subluxation and it is easy to mistake for monoarticular rheumatoid. There is usually marked wasting of the forearm muscles. Involvement of the flexor sheath leads to large fluctuant swellings in the palm and distal anterior forearm, the two being connected under, but constricted by, the carpal ligament (a *compound palmar ganglion*). In the early stage, tuberculous arthritis shows local osteoporosis with pencilling of the cortical margins. With progression there is bone erosion, leading eventually to destruction of the carpus and the wrist.

Tumours and tumour-like conditions

For discussion on benign tumours, cysts of bone, tumour-like conditions and primary malignant bone tumours, see LOWER LIMB, PAIN IN (p. 400).

The distal radius is the third most common site for an *osteoclastoma* (*giant-cell tumour*). This presents with aching discomfort and bony swelling of the distal radius. On plain X-rays these tumours have a characteristic appearance as the cystic lesion extends up to the joint margin. It affects patients in the 20- to 40-year age group.

Miscellaneous

The most common site for a *ganglion* is the dorsum of the wrist, where they arise as a result of mucoid degeneration of the joint capsule. The patient is usually a young adult but may be middle-aged. Ganglia are rarely (if ever) seen in the elderly – that is, they eventually resolve. Many simply present with a painless lump. Symptoms are usually caused by pressure on adjacent structures; for example, a ganglion on the palmar aspect of the wrist may be associated with a carpal tunnel syndrome or ulnar nerve compression. On examination there is a non-tender, well-defined smooth lump that is usually slightly fluctuant but may appear hard if it is small and beneath the deep fascia.

Chronic wrist pain is a complex subject. In brief, recent advances in MRI imaging and arthroscopy have revealed that the carpus is the site of complex ligamentous injuries and tears, the latter triangular fibrocartilage, which binds the radius and ulna together but separates the inferior radioulnar joint from the wrist joint, can be torn rather like a meniscus in the knee. The most common type of carpal instability is *scapholunate disassociation* secondary to disruption of the ligaments connecting the scaphoid to the lunate. This injury can occur following relatively

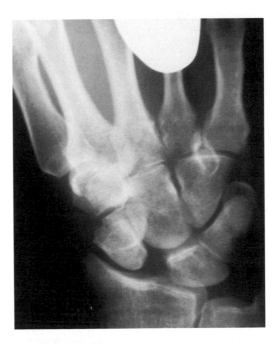

Figure U.21 Scapholunate disassociation. Note the gap between the scaphoid and the lunate.

minor 'sprains' of the wrists. Plain X-rays show widening of the gap between the scaphoid and the lunate (Fig. U.21) on the AP film and collapse of the normal alignment on the lateral film – the longitudinal axis of the radius, the capitate and third metacarpal should form a straight line. Patients present with pain, or weakness of the wrist and diminished grip, while certain movements may cause a click or a snap. These injuries are the cause of osteoarthritis later in life.

Conditions affecting the hands and fingers

The hands and the fingers are affected by many systemic diseases (see JOINTS, AFFECTIONS OF, p. 343, which deals with the generality of joint diseases). This section is concerned either with conditions local to the hands or fingers, or else the local manifestation of generalized disease (Table U.9).

Deformity

This is a complex group of conditions which may be local to the hand, or occur as part of a generalized skeletal abnormality. *Syndactyly* is the most common congenital hand deformity. The fingers and thumb may be joined by complete or partial webs of skin. *Duplication* affects any digit. There are a number of different types which have different incidences in different populations. For example, in the black American population replication of the little finger is very common. *Macrodactyly* can affect any of the fingers or the thumbs and is secondary to a local hamartomatous enlargement. *Microdactyly* is the reverse.

Table U.9 Diagnostic categories affecting the hand and fingers

Deformity	Congenital	Localized defects are generalized (i.e. due to skeletal dysplasia)
	Acquired	Neurological (e.g. cerebral palsy, nerve injuries)
		Arthritis (see below)
		Contracture of palmar fascia (Dupuytren's disease)
Conditions of tendons	'Locking'	Trigger finger
		Trigger thumb
		– children (congenital)
		– adults
	'Ruptures'	Mallet finger
		'Dropped' finger
		Boutonnière deformity
		Swan-neck deformity
		Tenosynovitis (non-infective)
Infections	Acute pyogenic	Cellulitis/lymphangitis
		Paronychia (nail-fold)
		Finger pulp infection
		Infective tenosynovitis
		Septic arthritis
		Osteomyelitis
		Necrotizing fasciitis
		Deep palmar space infections
	Chronic	Tuberculous
		Leprosy
		Fungal
		Infection from bites
Arthritis	Inflammatory	Rheumatoid arthritis
		Gout
		Psoriatic arthropathy
	Osteoarthritis	Heberden's nodes
		Carpometacarpal osteoarthritis of thumb
Tumours and tumour-like conditions	Enchrondroma	
	Epidermoid cyst	
	Pigmented villonodular synovitis (giant cell tumour of tendon sheath)	
	Soft tissue sarcoma	
Miscellaneous	Ganglion/mucous cyst	
	Ligament injuries – ulnar collateral ligament of thumb	

Acquired deformities are common, with most being due to local trauma. For example, failure to regain movement in a digit following a laceration of a tendon; rotational malalignment of the finger secondary to a fracture, etc. An important group is contracture secondary to neurological disease, for example cerebral palsy or an ulnar clawed hand secondary to a laceration of the ulnar nerve (see earlier discussion on high and low ulnar nerve injuries). *Dupuytren's disease*, which is due to contracture of the palmar fascia (Fig. U.22), is common in Northern Europe and rare in Asia.

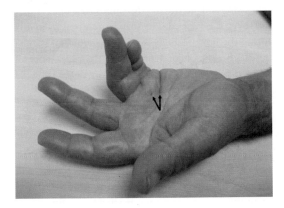

Figure U.22 Dupuytren's contracture of the palmar fascia involving the ring and little fingers. Note the flexion deformity at the metacarpal, phalangeal and proximal interphalangeal joints, and a thickening and pitting of the palmar skin.

It is probably an autosomal dominant condition, but other risk factors are involved such as smoking, alcohol, diabetes and (possibly) epilepsy. The ring and little fingers are the most commonly affected. In the early stages, there is a thickening in the palm, which manifests itself as firm nodules with puckering and pitting of the overlying skin. With time this develops into inextensible thickened bands, which usually run up into the fingers causing loss of extension of the metacarpophalangeal joint and contractures of the interphalangeal joints. In severe cases of Dupuytren's disease the fingernails will be held impacted down into the palm. Knuckle pads may be present over the dorsum of the proximal interphalangeal joints. The condition can also affect the feet (the plantar fascia) and may occasionally be associated with fibrosis of the corpus cavernosum (Peyronie's disease). In early cases the differential diagnosis is from an implantation dermoid cyst,

which causes a more superficial nodule in the skin and a contracture of a flexor tendon in which, contrary to Dupuytren's, the tight band moves on passively flexing the finger.

Tendons

'*Triggering*' can affect any finger including the thumb, but is most frequently seen in the middle and ring fingers. Flexion (often accompanied by a click) is full, but on trying to extend the finger remains stuck until the patient applies an extra active extension effort or unlocks the finger passively with the other hand. Most cases arise spontaneously due to thickening in the flexor tendon accompanied by thickening and stenosis at the entrance to the fibrous flexor profundus tunnel in the palm. However, it is important to exclude associated underlying disease such as rheumatoid arthritis, gout or amyloid. There is a well-recognized association with diabetes. *Congenital trigger thumb* is a well-recognized entity in children, although there is a dispute as to whether it is really congenital as it is rarely (if ever) seen under the age of 6 months.

Mallet finger results from a loss of active extension at the distal interphalangeal joint secondary to a traumatic avulsion of the extensor tendon at its insertion into the base of the distal phalanx. It is a common injury in cricketers and baseball players, where the hard ball can catch the tip of the finger, forcing it into sudden flexion. While passive extension is present there is a loss of active extension. A lateral X-ray will distinguish between a pure tendon rupture and an avulsion fracture. The most common cause of a dropped terminal phalanx of the thumb is a traumatic rupture of extensor pollicis longus at the wrist (see The wrist: pain and deformity, p. 751). *Boutonnière (button-hole) deformity* is due to a rupture or attenuation of the central slip of the extensor hood at its insertion onto the base of the proximal phalanx. As the name implies, the proximal interphalangeal joint button-holes through the resulting defect, the adjacent extensor slips being pushed aside. This allows an excessive extensor pull at the distal interphalangeal joint so that in the final deformity the finger is fixed flexed at the proximal interphalangeal joint and in hyperextension at the distal joint. The reverse deformity to a boutonnière is the *swan-neck finger*, in which there is extensor over-activity at the proximal interphalangeal joint and a simultaneous flexion deformity at the distal joint. There are a number of causes, including contracture of the intrinsic muscles acting at the proximal interphalangeal joint: mallet finger deformity at the distal phalangeal joint and paralysis or division of flexor digitorum superficialis, which causes weakening of the flexor action at the proximal interphalangeal joint. As with the boutonnière, the swan-neck is commonly seen in a rheumatoid hand (see Fig. U.18). *Non-infective tenosynovitis* occurs with inflammatory disorders such as rheumatoid arthritis, or occasionally from unaccustomed repetitive over-use of a finger. It is only seen with flexor tendons since the extensor tendons do not have synovial sheaths in the fingers.

Infections

Infections in the hand and fingers are common, important, but often poorly diagnosed and managed. It is all too easy to confuse the common superficial infections with the destructive, though fortunately less frequent, deep infections. Furthermore, due to the tough compact nature of skin and subcutaneous tissues of the palm and palmar surface of the fingers, the swelling of inflammatory oedema appears on the back of the hand, thereby masking the anatomical site of origin of many deep infections. The serious complication of lymphangitis and septicaemia can rapidly supervene. Therefore, as well as assessing the hand, always take the temperature and feel the regional lymph nodes.

In examining the hand, look not only for signs of inflammation but also think anatomically. For example, a deep infection involving the little finger will spread along the tendon sheath – that is, through the palm, under the carpal tunnel and up into the forearm. A full medical history and examination is required to exclude diseases such as diabetes, steroids, HIV and other immunocompromising conditions. Check the tetanus status. A full blood count should be performed, and cultures obtained prior to starting antibiotic treatment. The ESR can be useful in monitoring the response, especially to deep infections and osteomyelitis. X-rays will show the presence of osteomyelitis, gas in the tissues or fractures which are sometimes difficult to distinguish from infection. Ultrasound is useful in localizing deep abscesses and displaying fluid in flexor tendon sheaths. Technetium bone scans and MRI are helpful in localizing or excluding osteomyelitis, particularly in the early stages when the X-rays are normal.

Cellulitis is an infection of the skin and subcutaneous tissues. It is very important to distinguish a true cellulitis from the local signs of infection in the skin overlying an abscess. *Necrotizing fasciitis*, in its early stages, often presents as a widespread, very painful cellulitis with marked systemic symptoms. Fortunately it is rare, but it carries a high mortality. Drug addicts, immunocompromised patients and diabetics are most at risk from this form of severe cellulitis.

Paronychia (a *nailfold infection*) is the most common of all hand infections. When acute, there is erythema, swelling and tenderness around the nailfold and extending across the dorsum of the distal phalanx over the nailbed. Pus may be released by gently lifting the nail. *Chronic paronychia* requires a bacterial diagnosis as it may be due to the persistence of pyogenic infection, a fungal infection, or occasionally be tuberculous. An X-ray should be taken to rule out chronic osteomyelitis. A *felon* or *whitlow* is a finger pulp infection, and presents with a swollen, red and acutely tender fingertip. *Infective tenosynovitis* is usually secondary to a puncture wound, and involves the fibrous flexor sheath of a finger. The ring, middle and index fingers are the most commonly affected, and in these fingers the infection is limited to the finger and palm distal to the distal palmar skin crease (i.e. distal to the metacarpophalangeal joint). The finger will be painful, swollen, held rigidly semi-flexed, very tender, and any movement will be firmly resisted. Infections involving the tendon sheaths of the thumb and little finger will extend through the palm under the carpal ligament and into the distal forearm.

Web space infections often start as abrasions, blisters or callosities on the distal part of the palm, with infection spreading into the subfascial space. Due to the tough overlying palmar skin, signs of inflammation and swelling are most obvious on the dorsal aspect of the hand in the interval between the adjacent metacarpals. An abscess in this region may be of the collar stud variety – that is, the pus pointing on the dorsum but the main abscess lies much more anteriorly, deep to the palmar skin. *Deep palmar space infections* are fortunately uncommon. They form in the space between the palmar aponeurosis and the third, fourth and fifth metacarpals, which is traversed by the flexor tendons to the little, ring and middle fingers, the appropriate digital nerves and vessels and the superficial palmar arch. The hand is markedly swollen, and in particular the concavity of the palm is lost. If this sign is present, do not be deceived by the excessive swelling on the dorsum.

Deep thenar space infection occurs in the potential space between the palmar aponeurosis and the fascia overlying adductor pollicis, which contains not only flexor pollicis longus tendon plus the neurovascular bundles to the thumb but also the neurovascular bundle on the radial side of the index plus the flexor tendons of the index. Therefore, a deep thenar space infection can involve both the thumb and the index finger.

Acute pyogenic septic arthritis may result from a penetrating wound or as a complication in rheumatoid arthritis – an acute onset of inflammation in a single joint in a multiply involved rheumatoid hand should alert the physician to this complication. Differential diagnosis in an otherwise normal hand is from gout. *Osteomyelitis* is easy to miss in the hand as it is mistaken for an overlying soft tissue infection. It can also occur as a result of poorly treated soft tissue or joint infections. The usual error is to omit to take an X-ray.

Tuberculosis presents with a variety of pathologies – most commonly as a chronic tenosynovitis – but it can cause osteomyelitis or a joint synovitis. A biopsy is usually required for diagnosis. Other mycobacteria may be encountered, for example *M. marinum* from seawater. *Leprosy* (*M. lepraum*) usually presents with trophic changes in the hands and feet.

Fungal infections

There are a wide variety of fungal infections, which can involve any of the tissues or anatomical spaces discussed under pyogenic infections. Therefore, these must be included in any differential diagnosis for a sub-acute or chronic infection. Diabetic and immunocompromised patients are particularly at risk. Unfortunately, the diagnosis is often delayed as fungal infections tend to be overlooked. They are particularly common in chronic paronychia, chronic infection of the nailplate (onychomycosis) and granulomas, especially if the original wound was from a thorn. When fungi cause deep infections (fortunately uncommon), the organism can be difficult to isolate. *Mycetomas* (*Madura ulcer*) are due to subcutaneous implantation of fungal spores or actinomycosis. These can affect the fingers and present with pseudo-tumours and discharging sinuses.

Bites

One of the common wounds to a hand is a bite, the most frequent culprit being a dog. Fortunately most wounds do not become infected, but when they do a wide variety of organisms can be involved. Cat bites, while less frequent, have a greater tendency to infection. Cat-scratch fever can be a further complication. Bites from animals are also an entry point for rabies. Human bites are unpleasant and have a particular propensity to infection, usually by several species of organisms. Most are caused by fighting between children, but when they result from adult domestic violence they can be deceptive as the recipient often fails to give a full history. Venomous bites and stings from snakes, bees, spiders and other insects may, in addition to systemic affects, often cause widespread local or regional inflammation, which can progress to local necrosis and which in turn may become secondarily infected. As the onset is so acute there is usually a clear history, but occasionally bee or mosquito stings can be confused with a cellulitis.

Arthritis

The hand is involved in many inflammatory arthropathies. The peculiar feature of *rheumatoid arthritis* is the sparing of the distal inter-phalangeal joints, whereas the other small joints of the hand and the carpus are almost invariably involved. The disease often presents with early morning stiffness affecting, in particular, the metacarpophalangeal joints and the proximal interphalangeal joints. In the early stages there is a synovitis with swelling, warmth, tenderness, stiffness and painful movement of some or all of these joints. In long-standing disease, the classical deformities of ulnar drift at the metacarpophalangeal joints with progressive palmar subluxation and eventual dislocation of the fingers become evident. Swan-neck and boutonnière deformities are particularly destructive of finger function.

It is easy to overlook 'dropped fingers'; the initial finger affected is usually the little finger. The cause is extensor tendon rupture in the region of the inferior radioulnar joint due to a combination of synovitis and bony impingement. If the diagnosis is missed there can be a sequential 'dropping' of all the other fingers. Involvement of the thumb causes a loss of pinch grip as the thumb assumes a swan-neck or boutonnière type of deformity – there is either fixed flexion of the carpometacarpal joint with hyperextension at the interphalangeal joint or vice versa. The extent of bone and joint destruction on X-rays is usually greater than one would expect from the clinical examination. Early features are soft tissue swelling, periarticular erosions and osteoporosis, followed later by loss of joint space, bony destruction and joint disintegration, subluxation and then dislocation. *Psoriatic arthropathy* (see Fig. J.22) is often extremely destructive, and in addition involves the distal interphalangeal joints. Small joint polyarthritis is also a complication of many medical diseases (see JOINT, AFFECTIONS OF, p. 353). *Gout* (Fig. U.23) can be deceptive if the initial presentation is in the hand rather than the foot.

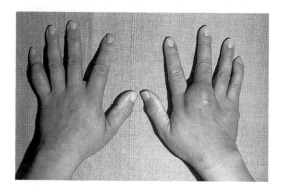

Figure U.23 Acute gouty arthritis of the metacarpal-phalangeal joint of the right third finger and the interphalangeal joint of the left little finger.

Osteoarthritis commonly affects the joints of the hand – in decreasing frequency the distal interphalangeal joint, the proximal interphalangeal joint, the carpometacarpal joint of the thumb, the other carpometacarpal joints, and finally the intercarpal joints. The presenting symptoms are a gradual onset of stiffness, discomfort and weakness. Similarly, the physical signs slowly become more evident. Heberden's nodes are smooth, bony hard swellings situated dorsally on the radial and ulnar sides over the distal interphalangeal joint. They are due to osteophytes with overlying soft tissue thickening. Occasionally, destruction of the joint may be more rapid. This is particularly seen in the proximal interphalangeal joint, and presents as a 'spindle finger'. This must be differentiated from an acute ligamentous injury or early rheumatoid arthritis, which can produce similar physical signs. With very advanced finger osteoarthritis there can be marked deformities with lateral or medial subluxation

secondary to erosion of the articular surface. Bony crepitus can then be elicited on passive movement. All joints of the thumb can be involved. The classical deformity is fixed flexion of the trapezium–metacarpal joint with hyperextension at the metacarpophalangeal joint and flexion at the interphalangeal joint (Fig. U.24). Isolated painful trapezium–metacarpal osteoarthritis is most commonly seen in middle-aged women, and is accompanied by weakness; for example, knitting, writing and unscrewing jars can be difficult.

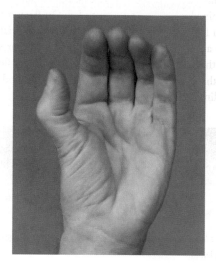

Figure U.24 Osteoarthritis of the carpometacarpal joint of the left thumb producing a 'z-thumb' deformity (swan-necking of the thumb). Note also the fixed adduction deformity of the thumb, the metacarpal having moved across into the palm.

Tumours and tumour-like conditions

See Pain in and around the knee; tumours (p. 400). Almost all varieties of this complex pathological group can affect the hand. Fortunately, the most common bone lesions are benign. The *enchondroma* classically presents with a swelling of a phalanx, and on X-rays has a well-defined lytic lesion with a good margin and punctate areas of calcification. Unless complicated by a pathological fracture, they are usually asymptomatic. Lytic lesions in the terminal phalanx are most likely to be due to an *epidermoid inclusion cyst* which is filled with keratin debris. The flexor tendon sheaths are a classical site for pigmented villonodular synovitis (giant-cell tumour of tendon sheath). It presents either with a soft tissue swelling on the palmar aspect of the finger along the tendon sheath or as a trigger finger. It can be locally aggressive. Beware of soft tissue masses within the palm as these are most likely to be a malignant soft tissue sarcoma. A biopsy is required to establish precise diagnosis.

Miscellaneous

Ganglia/mucous cysts are common in the hand, usually on the extensor surface overlying a joint (Fig. U.25). In the fingers they are usually small, smooth, and have a hint of mobility and compressibility when examined with the finger extended. On flexion they often feel bony hard. They may occur in association with an underlying osteophyte. On the palmar surface they arise in conjunction with the fibrous flexor sheaths of tendons forming small, smooth, nodular swellings.

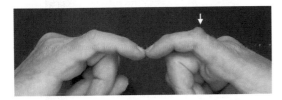

Figure U.25 Mucous cyst overlying the proximal interphalangeal joint of the left little finger (arrow).

Dislocations and *sprains* are common in the fingers. Dislocation of the terminal joint can easily be overlooked if the finger is examined a few hours after the injury due to the surrounding soft tissue swelling. Sprains (partial tears) of the collateral ligaments of the proximal interphalangeal joints are a cause of a 'spindle finger' with a tapered cylindrical swelling around the joint, which is often stiff and painful for several weeks. The X-ray is normal, in contradistinction to the spindle finger caused by osteoarthritis or rheumatoid. *Gamekeeper's thumb* is due to a rupture of the ulnar collateral ligament of the metacarpophalangeal joint of the thumb. As with other complete ligamentous disruptions, this can be relatively painless and is easily missed unless the finger is correctly examined for instability; the thumb will collapse into abduction on making a pinch grip between the thumb and index finger. It is a common skiing injury.

Fred Heatley

URETHRA, FAECES PASSED THROUGH

Faeces or faecal fluid are passed per urethram only when the bladder is in fistulous communication with some part of the bowel, or with an abscess infected with *Escherichia coli* (see PNEUMATURIA, p. 548). The chief causes are as follows:

- Diverticular disease of the sigmoid colon with a fistula into the bladder (the commonest cause).
- Carcinoma of the bladder opening into the rectum or into some loop of bowel which has become adherent to the bladder.
- Carcinoma of the:
  - ◆ rectum
  - ◆ sigmoid colon
  - ◆ caecum

  opening into the bladder either directly or through the medium of an intervening abscess.
- Carcinoma of the uterus opening both into the bladder and into the rectum.
- Crohn's disease of large or small bowel with vesical fistula.
- Prostatis or prostatic abscess opening into the rectum.
- Rectovesical fistula from injury and sloughing, particularly after childbirth.
- Appendicular abscess opening into the bladder.
- Pelvic actinomycosis.

The passage of faeces into the urine may be simulated by some cases of very foetid cystitis due to infection by *E. coli*, especially in diabetic subjects.

If the symptom is due to carcinoma, it matters little which viscus is the primary site by the time the growth has involved both bladder and bowel. The differentiation resolves itself, therefore, between malignant and non-malignant conditions. If malignant disease is not obvious, it will nearly always be advisable to resort to surgical measures in the hope of discovering some curable primary condition – rectal, appendicular, prostatic or otherwise. This diagnosis will be suggested by the history and confirmed by local examination. Special investigations may include cystoscopy, barium enema and colonoscopy.

Harold Ellis

URETHRAL DISCHARGE

Discharge of secretions or fluid from the urethra is usually only recognized in the male. Urethral discharge (Fig. U.25) is most commonly an accompaniment of sexually acquired urethral infection from gonorrhoea, *Chlamydia* or, less often, *Mycoplasma genitalium*, *Trichomonas vaginalis*, *Ureaplasma urealyticum* and herpes simplex. In this setting, urethral discharge is commonly associated with dysuria, and may also be complicated by epididymitis, orchitis or prostatitis. The diagnosis may be made by microbiological examination of appropriate samples of discharge fluid and urine.

Post-micturition dribble (PMD), which is the passage of a few drops of urine after micturition is completed, is a normal finding in most males, but becomes a problem for a few. Reassurance is all that is usually necessary. A urethral diverticulum, which is rare in males, may be a cause of urethral discharge, if infected, or leakage of urine after micturition (PMD). After patch urethroplasty, the urethra may become baggy and dilated and be associated also with PMD. Infection within the Cowper's glands in the proximal urethra may give rise to urethral discharge.

Females may develop urethral discharge, which usually comes from a urethral diverticulum. The discharge in females is usually purulent in nature as it is infected.

Julian Shah

URINE, ABNORMAL COLOUR OF

The normal amber colour of urine is due mainly to urobilinogen; the depth of colour naturally varies with the concentration, and very dilute urine is nearly colourless. In very concentrated urine the depth of colour may raise suspicions of biliuria. Several substances can alter the colour of the urine. This is usually of no pathological significance, although a patient may seek an explanation. In a few conditions the colour is characteristic and of diagnostic significance.

Bile pigment imparts a deep *orange colour* to the urine; in high concentration, the appearance resembles beer. This occurs mainly when there is bile outflow obstruction. Senna and rhubarb ingestion can produce a similar colour.

A *red colour* in the urine can be due to a number of substances. Haemoglobin is the most important, either in intact red cells when the urine has a turbid or 'smoky' appearance or as free pigment when the urine is clear. This may be confirmed by urine dipstick. If large amounts are present – and particularly if some of the haemoglobin has been oxidized to methaemoglobin – the colour may be brownish-black. In porphyrinuria, the colour is typically that of 'port wine', but it may be pink or red. Myoglobinuria may give a red or brown colour in the urine. Other substances causing red urine include beetroot, blackberries, phenolphthalein in purgatives (if the urine is alkaline) and certain aniline dyes in sweets.

Apart from methaemoglobin, a *dark brown* or *black* urine may be due to phenol (carboluria), melanin, homogentisic acid or *p*-hydroxyphenyl-pyruvic acid. In carboluria, due to phenol poisoning, the urine may be greenish-brown. Melanin is found in the urine in some cases of disseminated malignant melanoma; the urine may be of normal colour when passed, but turns black on standing, from above downwards. A similar colour change on standing occurs in the urine in alkaptonuria, in which homogentisic acid is excreted. This substance also accumulates in the cartilage of the ear and in the sclera, which may become black, and in joint cartilage causing severe arthritis; this syndrome is known as ochronosis. The urine may also darken in air in the very rare tyrosinosis in which *p*-hydroxyphenyl-pyruvic acid is excreted. The antimicrobial drug metronidazole also causes the urine to become dark brown. Rifampicin causes urine to go orange, which may be used as a measure of compliance with therapy.

Due to the presence in normal urine of urobilinogen, any blue compound in low concentration may produce a green colour. *Green* and *blue* urines are most commonly due to biliverdin in long-standing obstructive jaundice, or to methylene blue in pills or sweets. Indigo-carmine and indigo-blue can also colour the urine. The former may rarely be present after exposure to industrial dyes, while the latter is the consequence of oxidation of indican. Indicanuria is due to intestinal malabsorption of tryptophan, which is metabolized to indole by intestinal bacteria in such conditions as coeliac disease and Hartnup disease.

Mark Kinirons

URINE, INCONTINENCE OF

Incontinence is the involuntary loss of urine from the bladder at times and in places which are inappropriate and inconvenient. Preservation of continence depends on the integrity of the lower urinary tract, both anatomically and physiologically. Incontinence secondary to an anatomical abnormality occurs congenitally, as in ectopic ureter, or is acquired, as in vesico-vaginal fistula; physiological disturbance occurs because of imbalance between the tone of the detrusor muscle and that of the external urethral sphincter.

Sphincter weakness results in genuine stress incontinence, sometimes called simply stress incontinence; detrusor incontinence occurs when detrusor activity is sufficiently enhanced to overcome the resistance offered by a normal sphincter mechanism. Overflow incontinence occurs when the detrusor is flaccid so that urine trickles out when the fully distended bladder can hold no more, in much the same way that water trickles over the lip of a dam.

The common causes of incontinence of urine can be divided into: (i) sphincter damage; and (ii) neurological lesions.

Sphincter damage

Mechanical damage to the sphincter is the most common cause of genuine stress incontinence. Broadly speaking, the sphincter apparatus in both sexes consists of three components: the bladder neck, which is a muscle group derived from the detrusor muscle of the bladder wall; the intrinsic urethral apparatus, which consists of muscle components from both bladder neck and external sphincter together with fibrous and vascular components; and the external sphincter, which consists of the striated muscle of the pelvic floor.

In women, all three components can be affected by stretch or direct damage during the passage of the fetal head during labour, giving rise to stress incontinence.

In men, prostatectomy is a common cause of stress incontinence; the bladder neck has been ablated inevitably during prostatectomy itself, but there is additional damage to the intrinsic apparatus and even occasionally to the external sphincter. Prostatectomy inevitably implies internal sphincter ablation and considerable resection of the intrinsic apparatus, but provided that this procedure is limited to the zone proximal to the verumontanum in the urethra, the remaining intrinsic urethral mechanism and the external sphincter together will allow preservation of continence. Incontinence is common following radical prostatectomy carried out for carcinoma of the prostate. Sphincter involvement by malignant extension from prostatic carcinoma is rarely enough in itself to give rise to stress incontinence as the simultaneous obstruction produced by the enlarged malignant gland will compensate for loss of sphincter tone.

The pelvic floor can be injured by trauma, such as gunshot wounds, and is particularly vulnerable to injury when the pelvis is fractured. A dual mechanism is often responsible for incontinence in the latter as direct damage to the pelvic floor is compounded by damage to its nerve supply, particularly the pudendal nerves.

Stress incontinence

Genuine stress incontinence in women is related to urethral sphincter damage during childbirth, and to the weakening of the supporting pelvic floor muscles. The sphincter apparatus falls below the level at which it can be protected by transmitted pressure during coughing and other activity, so that the intra-abdominal pressure acts in an unopposed manner on the bladder dome. Increases in abdominal pressure produce a simultaneous leak of urine. The condition is usually associated with anterior and posterior vaginal wall prolapses, manifested as cystocele and rectocele respectively, but this is by no means invariable. Supporting the bladder neck by inserting the index and middle finger against the anterior vaginal wall and pushing upwards will control the leaking. This test mimics the effect of a successful surgical procedure. Genuine stress incontinence also occurs in some congenital abnormalities, such as the short urethra, the wide urethra and epispadias.

Some degree of stress incontinence in men is usual after prostatectomy, but this clears up as the prostatic cavity heals and infection is eradicated. If there has been sphincter damage as a result of the procedure, the resulting incontinence improves slowly with time. A period of some 12 months must elapse before the degree of remaining incontinence can be judged permanent.

Urge incontinence

Incontinence after prostatectomy also usually relates to the irritability of the bladder base through the oedema of the healing zone. This incontinence is called urge incontinence, where the desire to micturate is so strong that it overrides all attempts of the sphincters to retain urine. Urge incontinence is frequent in both sexes, and is the major differential diagnosis from genuine stress incontinence. The detrusor contracts in an abnormal manner and, as it does so, it opens the bladder neck and thus decreases the outflow resistance. This kind of incontinence is sometimes called 'unstable bladder' incontinence. It is not related to any neurological factor, but is seen in association with acute cystitis, chronic cystitis, post-radiotherapy, in tuberculous cystitis, interstitial cystitis, in the presence of a foreign body in the bladder, when a stone is impacted at the ureterovesical junction, in outflow tract obstruction secondary to prostatic hypertrophy and bladder neck stenosis. In most cases, no specific aetiological feature can be discovered. It is difficult to distinguish from genuine stress incontinence on clinical grounds as, during the circumstances of examination, the first cough may not precipitate incontinence but subsequent coughing on request may initiate a detrusor contraction which is strong enough to open the sphincter.

Neurological lesions

Incontinence related to neurological causes may be due to upper or lower motor neurone lesions. In upper motor neurone lesions, the central inhibitory impulses to the micturition centre in the sacral segments are lost. Sudden contractions of the detrusor muscle occur, resulting in unheralded precipitate micturition. The volume of urine lost in upper motor neurone lesions is almost always greater than that lost in simple detrusor instability. The condition is associated with spinal cord injuries, disseminated sclerosis, and cerebrovascular accidents. It is seen in some cases of Parkinson's disease, syringomyelia and is a feature of normal-pressure hydrocephalus (Fig. U.26). The reflex centre in the cord is intact so that the stretching of the bladder wall causes reflex detrusor spasm and micturition. The difficulty arises because the sphincter mechanism is also subject to a similar degree of spasm. The result is bladder wall hypertrophy with trabeculation, formation of saccules and diverticula and the

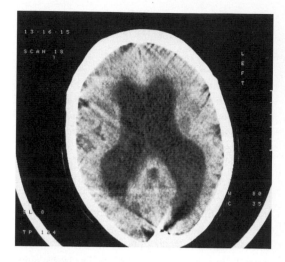

Figure U.26 Computed tomogram showing normal-pressure hydrocephalus.

presence of a urine residue. If the patient is paraplegic, management becomes extremely difficult as sepsis, excoriation of the genitalia and perineum, and areas of pressure necrosis occur.

In lower motor neurone lesions which affect the afferent and efferent portions of the sacral reflex arc as well as the reflex centre itself, the bladder is cut off from this spinal regulatory centre. As the pathognomonic feature of an upper motor neurone lesion is spasticity, so is flaccidity the feature of a lower motor neurone lesion. The detrusor muscle becomes flaccid, often insensitive to stretch, and the bladder distends enormously. The concomitant weakness of the sphincter mechanism eventually leads to overflow incontinence where urine trickles through the urethra. The bladder is readily palpable, is asymmetrical, often enormous, not tender and relatively soft; from the side the huge bulge above the symphysis pubic is readily apparent and unchanging during respiration while the upper abdomen adopts a scaphoid shape. Pressure on the bladder dome often results in the expression of urine, a diagnostic test which, in itself, can sometimes be adapted as a therapeutic technique to promote bladder emptying.

Lower motor neurone lesions are also associated with peripheral neuritis, as in diabetes. In diabetes, a selective peripheral neuropathy can affect bladder behaviour, and the mechanism of erection in the male, without any peripheral signs of such a neuropathy. Damage to the autonomic supply to the bladder also follows pelvic surgery, especially abdominoperineal excision of the rectum, Wertheim hysterectomy and radical cystectomy. Operations which spare the autonomic supply to the pelvis and genitalia have been developed.

A similar picture of incontinence with overflow is also seen in chronic outflow obstruction, almost always secondary to prostatic enlargement or bladder neck stenosis. Enuresis is a pathognomonic clinical feature of this condition.

All of the conditions described so far present as incontinence of an intermittent variety. Continuous incontinence, day and night, is found in some congenital abnormalities. The most severe of these is ectopia vesicae (bladder extrophy) where there is failure of development of the abdominal wall and anterior wall of the bladder so that the mucosa of the bladder is exposed and the two ureteric orifices can be seen with urine dripping from them. There is wide separation of the two pubic rami (pubic diastasis).

An ectopic ureter occasionally opens into the vagina in the female or into the urethra beyond the sphincter apparatus in either sex. Urine leaks continually. The ectopic ureter usually drains a duplex kidney, and when a pyelogram shows a duplex system in a case of incontinence an ectopic ureter should be sought. The opening is often extremely difficult to find, but the intravenous injection of indigocarmine or methylene blue will facilitate its location. The rule in duplex kidneys is that the ureter of the lower moiety opens normally into the bladder, the ureter of the upper moiety is always heterotopic and opening inferior to the orthotopic ureter. The upper moiety ureter will always be the ectopic ureter and the affected moiety is usually hydronephrotic; it may drain only one calicine system.

Incontinence from a fistula is usually continuous, but if the abnormal opening is between the ureter and vagina, the leakage may appear to be intermittent. Fistulae from the urinary tract may communicate with the uterus (in which case urine can be seen escaping from the cervical os), or with the vagina (when the fistula can usually be seen on speculum examination of the anterior vaginal wall). Ureterovaginal fistula may arise in the female from erosion of a calculus into one of the vaginal fornices, and also after gynaecological surgery. Vesico-vaginal fistulae are secondary to malignant processes within the upper vagina or in the posterior bladder wall, invading anteriorly or posteriorly respectively. They may follow surgery.

The investigation and diagnosis of incontinence, when there is no overt cause such as fistula or congenital abnormality, depends on urodynamic assessment of the patient. The study consists of:

1 *Sphincterometry*, where the pressure exerted by the sphincter apparatus is measured and the configuration of the sphincter complex observed. When there is sphincter incompetence the pressure is low, and when the sphincter is in spasm, as in an upper motor neurone lesion, the pressure is high.

2 *Cystometry*, where bladder pressure is monitored during filling. Two parameters are measured – the intra-abdominal pressure through a vaginal or rectal transducer, and the total bladder pressure through a bladder transducer. Electronic subtraction of the former from the latter gives a reading of true or intrinsic bladder pressure.

The bladder is a perfectly compliant organ in that intrinsic bladder pressure does not rise as the bladder fills. The normal curve is observed in genuine stress incontinence. In enuresis and in minor degrees of bladder disturbance secondary to upper motor neurone lesions, a 'delayed voiding contraction' is seen, the bladder contracting vigorously near capacity. When the bladder is extremely irritable, as in acute cystitis, or when there is an upper motor neurone lesion affecting the bladder to a considerable degree, an uninhibited pattern of behaviour is seen. The 'unstable detrusor' is manifest as waves of contraction of a pressure which exceeds $10\,cmH_2O$. In lower motor neurone lesions, or in bladders affected by chronic retention, filling goes on and on with little alteration in intrinsic bladder pressure.

3 *Voiding pressure and flow rate*. During the void phase, the bladder voiding pressure and the flow rate are measured. When there is sphincter incompetence, the voided pressure is low while the flow rate is often abnormally high; in obstruction, the voiding pressure will be high and the flow rate low.

Harold Ellis

URINE, RETENTION OF

Retention of urine is the inability to empty the bladder completely; the end result is the acute or gradual accumulation of urine within the bladder. In *acute retention* there is a sudden inability to pass urine. The condition is painful and presents as a surgical emergency. In chronic retention there is a gradual increase in bladder size; it can often reach enormous proportions, occasionally reaching as high as the xiphisternum (Fig. U.27). Pressure effects on the upper tract are not uncommon, and an elevation of the blood urea, in association with bilateral hydronephrosis and hydroureters, is observed. The condition is a medical emergency in that stabilization of the biochemical changes is a prerequisite to surgical correction of the cause. Retention of the urine must be distinguished from anuria, when the kidneys fail to secrete urine. In retention – whether acute or chronic – the kidneys still function and urine continues to collect in the distended bladder.

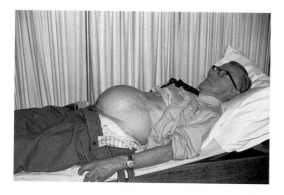

Figure U.27 Distension of the bladder to the umbilicus in chronic retention of urine due to benign prostatic hypertrophy.

Acute retention

Acute retention produces severe pain. The bladder is palpable some two fingers' breadths above the symphysis pubis, and it is central, tense, tender and dull to percussion. The most common cause is outflow tract obstruction in the male, secondary to *prostatic enlargement* or *bladder neck stenosis*. It should be noted that the severity of outflow tract obstruction bears no relation to the size of the prostate, a tiny prostate often being responsible for an acute retentive episode, whilst the largest prostate may remain asymptomatic.

Acute retention from urethral stricture alone is uncommon, but secondary spasm and congestion proximal to the stricture, especially involving the sphincter apparatus, may result in retention.

Acute retention may be precipitated by exposure to cold, over-indulgence in *alcohol*, the administration of *anticholinergic agents* in order to relieve the urinary frequency which the patient almost invariably has, and *bronchodilating agents*, thus explaining the increased frequency of acute retention in elderly men with chronic bronchitis in winter when their chests need treatment. Under some circumstances, particularly delay in the act of micturition beyond reasonable limits – a feat often accomplished while the patient is 'anaesthetized' with alcohol – the prostate becomes acutely congested and retention follows. The retention is relieved by catheterization, the congestion subsides, and normal micturition can be re-established, to recur with the next bout of excess.

Acute retention in women is sometimes associated with *pregnancy*, especially when the *gravid uterus is retroverted*, while large *uterine fibroids* may produce the same effect. In young women, *herpes genitalis*, acquired as a sexually transmitted disease, may also precipitate acute retention, not only because of the urethral oedema associated with the herpetic lesions, but also by neurological involvement of the sacral reflex arc in such a way that detrusor activity is lost. *Herpes zoster* may give rise to acute retention in both sexes; in this case, the pathognomonic herpetic eruptions will be seen over the buttock area or the sacrum.

Chronic retention

Chronic retention is insidious in its onset, and symptoms develop so slowly that the patient may deny urinary difficulty. It is only in retrospect and after surgical correction that the patient admits that there were significant lower urinary track symptoms preoperatively. Enuresis (bed-wetting) is a frequent presenting feature.

Retention secondary to *urethral stricture* can be related to previous episodes of sexually transmitted diseases, *Chlamydia trachomatis* being a potent cause of extensive stricture formation. Primary infection with gonorrhoea is now almost exclusive to the male homosexual population in the UK, but the heterosexual male may acquire gonorrhoea as a result of sexual contact overseas.

The history in stricture is of a gradual increasing difficulty with micturition, slowing of the stream, and dribbling after micturition; this last symptom occurs because of the column of urine which is trapped between the sphincter apparatus and the stricture. An important distinction between stricture and prostatic obstruction is that straining assists urine flow in the former and reduces flow in the latter. The investigation of choice is urethrography, but if instrumentation is undertaken as a primary investigation direct vision urethroscopy is obligatory. The stricture may then be visualized before it has been traumatized and divided appropriately by direct vision urethrotomy. *Prostatic enlargement* is unusual below the age of 50, but bladder neck stenosis can occur much earlier.

On rectal examination, prostatic enlargement may be found. The gland may be smooth, uniform in consistency, elastic and movable within the pelvis when the enlargement is benign. A nodular, hard, irregular prostate may indicate *carcinoma*, while fixation to either side of the pelvic walls implies malignant extension well beyond the confines of the capsule. With bladder neck stenosis the prostate is of normal size.

When retention of urine follows *acute prostatitis* or a prostatic *abscess,* a history of recent urethral discharge will be obtained. The patient will be obviously ill, with a fever, rigors, frequency of micturition, pain on micturition, and perineal and pelvic discomfort.

Acute retention of urine secondary to urethral intra-luminal causes is most commonly caused by the *impaction of a calculus* in the urethra. A calculus may impact at the site of a stricture, when it can often be felt on examination of the penis, or at the external urethral meatus, in which case it can usually be seen. The history in such a case is dramatic in that a normal flow of micturition is quite suddenly interrupted, causing a sudden pain along the urethra, a feeling similar to receiving a blow in the bladder area, and the dribbling of a few drops of blood.

Blood clot may impact in the urethra ('clot retention') as a complication of bleeding from any cause along the urinary tract, for example, a renal carcinoma, or following any operation on the urinary system. Thus, clot retention is not an uncommon complication following prostatectomy.

As transurethral resection is now the favoured procedure for correction of prostatic enlargement, and the removal of all the resulting chips is often difficult, especially if there are bladder diverticula, 'chip retention' is a relatively new but not uncommon phenomenon, having the same symptoms as retention secondary to impaction of a stone.

Blockage of the bladder neck by the free-floating area of a *pedunculated bladder tumour* is rare; the growth is forced into the orifice during micturition, causing obstruction.

Complete *traumatic rupture of the urethra* leads to acute retention of urine. It almost always follows rupture of the pelvis, but may follow a blow to the perineum, for example from a boot or from falling astride a bar. There will be history of injury, and blood will appear at the external urethral meatus; perineal haematoma may not be too evident in pelvic fracture, but will certainly indicate local urethral trauma. If urethral rupture is incomplete, the patient should be encouraged not to pass urine as extravasation may occur and cause a haemato-urinoma in the perineum.

Prolapse of an intervertebral disc or a *spinal tumour* will occasionally cause acute neurological urinary retention from direct pressure on the nerve roots. Retention may occasionally be the presenting feature of the condition which, from the spinal point of view, remains asymptomatic. Acute, but painless, retention of urine will invariably occur after traumatic transection of the spinal cord.

Acute retention is a fairly common complication of *surgery on the rectum* and neighbouring organs. It may also follow operations on the hip (in both sexes) and hernia repairs. The mechanism in these cases must be reflex spasm of the sphincter apparatus. When there is dual pathology – for example, hernia or haemorrhoids in the presence of benign prostatic enlargement – it may be as well to combine the two surgical procedures to avoid the acute retention that the hernia or haemorrhoid operation may cause.

Acute retention of urine may be a manifestation of *hysteria*, but in common with all other diagnoses, medical and surgical, an organic cause should be sought and excluded before any psychogenic element is ascribed to the diagnosis. Hysterical retention usually occurs in children and in young women. Retention due to psychiatric illness is more usually a complication of therapy, as tricyclic antidepressants are powerful anticholinergic agents which suppress detrusor activity to the extent that retention – either acute or chronic – may occur.

Acute retention in female children is unusual, but it not infrequently occurs in males. While the male infant is still wearing nappies, *ammoniacal ulceration of the foreskin* (or of the meatus if circumcised) can give rise to acute retention because micturition is so painful that the child refuses to allow the act to continue. Retention in the presence of a tight phimosis is unusual, but the pathognomonic feature will be ballooning of the foreskin during micturition. Meatal stenosis following ulceration secondary to circumcision can occasionally lead to acute retention in young males. When micturition is attempted, the urethra can often be felt as a distended and rigid band on the ventrum of the penis. Retention may also follow the inadvertent insertion of a *foreign body*, such as a bean or screw, into the anterior urethra.

Harold Ellis

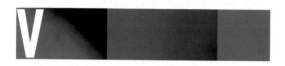

VAGINA AND UTERUS, PROLAPSE OF

A prolapse is the protrusion of an organ or structure beyond its normal anatomical position. The pelvic organs are supported by the pelvic floor, which in turn is comprised of muscle, fascia and ligamentous support. The pelvic floor is made up from the levator ani, internal obturator and piriformis muscles as well and the superficial and deep perineal muscles. The vagina is normally held in place by the transverse cervical ligaments (of Mackenrodt), the pubo-cervical ligament (pubo-cervical fascia) and the utero-sacral ligaments.

If the patient is examined in the left lateral or Sims' position, with a Sims' speculum holding back first the posterior and then the anterior vaginal wall, it is possible to determine which part of the vagina is prolapsing:

- Prolapse of the anterior vaginal wall if close to the introitus is classed as a urethrocele.
- The deeper part of the anterior vaginal wall would constitute a cystocele. Very often, these two may be combined in a cystourethrocele.
- Uterine prolapse is classed in three degrees (Fig. V.1):
  - First degree: the cervix descends to the vulva but no protrusion through the introitus.
  - Second degree: the cervix protrudes through the vulva.
  - Third degree (procidentia): the whole of the uterus is outside the vulva.
- Vault prolapse can occur after hysterectomy when the vaginal vault descends.
- Enterocele is prolapse of the posterior fornix, which is related to the pouch of Douglas and may contain loops of small bowel.
- Rectocele is a prolapse of the lower part of the vagina posterior, which is the rectum.

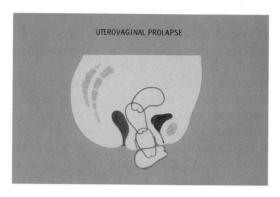

Figure V.1 Uterovaginal prolapse. Diagram of the position of the normal uterus and the three degrees of prolapse.

Predisposing factors for the development of prolapse include weakening of the support mechanisms. The most common of these is injury as a consequence of childbirth and pregnancy, but atrophy of the supporting tissues may also be implicated. Prolapse does occur in nulliparous women, but it is an unusual occurrence and this suggests congenital or developmental weakness of the support structures.

There are several activating factors which will increase the chances of prolapse development. These include obesity, increase in intra-abdominal pressure in the form of chronic cough, constipation requiring continued straining, increased weight of the uterus, and if any undue traction has been put on the cervix at any time.

Symptomatology is related to the anatomical aspect of the prolapse, and many women complain of 'something coming down' or sitting on an egg. Though not painful as such, the patient may complain of backache. The woman may have urinary symptoms in the form of urgency and difficulty in emptying the bowel; indeed, the patient may be required to empty the bowel digitally. There may be some discharge, and even bleeding and ulceration with a complete procidentia.

The differential diagnosis includes tumours of the vulva, vagina and cervix, which are not common tumours in England and Wales, hypertrophy of the cervix, a urethral diverticulum and true uterine inversion, which again is a very uncommon event. Fibroid polyp, chronic inversion of the uterus, vaginal cyst and endometrial polyp completes the list.

Management of these weaknesses can be either conservative or surgical, with the ring pessary being used in a number of patients while they await surgery. Surgery would address the problem, using either a suprapubic approach (particularly if there is any element of genuine stress incontinence) or a vaginal approach. The mainstay is vaginal hysterectomy and repair. A complete procidentia would need to be reduced to prevent ulceration. Prior to surgery, the condition can be kept reduced by packing the vagina and using local oestrogen cream. This would be the preferred option unless there is a contraindication to surgery.

Antony Hollingworth

VAGINA, DISCHARGE FROM

Discharge from the vagina can be classified in the following manner:

- Physiological, which varies with age and the time of the menstrual cycle.
- Pathological:
  ◆ Prepubertal
  ◆ During the reproductive life
  ◆ Postmenopausal

Physiological discharge

The normal discharge from the vagina is a mixture of secretions from the uterine body, cervix, and vaginal wall, the bulk of which originates from the cervix (Fig. V.2), as there are more glands there than in any other part of the genital tract. There are no glands in the vagina, and as such is not a mucosa but a skin. The secretions vary during the menstrual cycle, being abundant, clear, and almost free from leucocytes at the time of ovulation. At this time its elasticity is greatest (Spinnbarkeit), and this allows easier

penetration by the spermatozoa. At other times of the month the cervical mucus is scanty, opaque and tenacious. The secretion from Bartholin's gland, which is thin and mucoid, may be copious under sexual excitement, but under normal conditions it is scanty, and so does not contribute to a vaginal discharge. The vaginal mixed secretion is acid in reaction, owing to the presence of lactic acid produced by Doderlein's bacillus from the glycogen in the basal cells of the vaginal epithelium. This bacillus is normally found in the vagina from puberty to the menopause. The pH of the vagina is 4.5, the vaginal acidity being a bar to vaginal infection; unmixed uterine secretion is alkaline.

Normally, the amount of mixed vaginal discharge should do no more than just moisten the vaginal orifice; it may be increased with the presence of an ectropion (Fig. V.3), where there is eversion of the

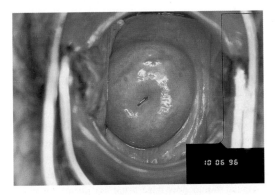

Figure V.2 Normal cervix.

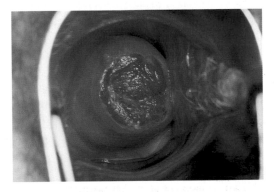

Figure V.3 Normal cervical ectropion, normal physiological appearance. The area appears reddened as the columnar epithelium is one cell thick, and translucent.

columnar epithelium towards the vagina. If excessive, the ectropion may require cautery or cryotherapy. Girls before puberty and women after the menopause do not have the protection of an acid secretion in the vagina.

Pathological discharge

Prepubertal

The main causes of discharge in a prepubertal girl include:

- Poor hygiene
- Foreign body
- Threadworms
- Sexual abuse
- Sarcoma botyroides

In young girls presenting with vaginal discharge the most common diagnosis is due to a foreign body; this may necessitate ultrasound scanning or an examination under anaesthetic (EUA). At the time of EUA, a small hysteroscope can be inserted into the vagina, whereupon the irrigating fluid used may flush the foreign body out and so treat the problem. Poor hygiene again is not uncommon, and appropriate advice can be given to the mother. Threadworms may produce intense itching, especially at night. One needs to be cautious if sexual abuse is considered, and the paediatric leader for child protection should be consulted. Each hospital should now have a named doctor for child abuse following the recent Klimbie report. Sarcoma botyroides is a rare tumour that may present with discharge or bleeding in young girls, and this would need referral to a cancer centre for further management.

Reproductive age

These are mostly infective causes, and include *Candida*, trichomoniasis, gonorrhoea, streptococci, anaerobes, *Chlamydia*, pelvic inflammatory disease, bacterial vaginosis and retained tampon.

Candida

This is a common infection in women, and gives rise to white patches of thrush on the vagina walls and cervix (Fig. V.4). It causes itching, discomfort and redness. It may also complicate diabetes and pregnancy,

as well as the use of antibiotics or the combined oral contraceptive pill. A swab may be taken for recognition of the mycelium and spores of *Candida albicans* in stained smears and for culture. Treatment may be either topical or systemic.

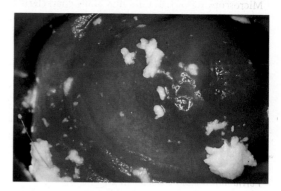

Figure V.4 *Candida* on the cervix.

Trichomonas vaginalis

This flagellate parasite produces a frothy, purulent discharge that causes local pain and soreness, in addition to extreme irritation of the external genitalia. The discharge is green or greenish-yellow, contains small bubbles of gas, and has a characteristic odour. The protozoon can be identified on microscopy. *Trichomonas* lives in the vagina in symbiosis with the micrococcus *Aerogenes alcaligenes*, which forms the froth or bubbles so characteristic of the discharge. *A. alcaligenes* is a Gram-negative organism, and causes the vaginal walls to have a typical red stippled ('strawberry') appearance. Treatment is with metronidazole.

Neisseria gonorrhoeae

Gonorrhoea causes the cervix to be red, swollen and oedematous, being bathed in pus. There is nothing characteristic of gonorrhoeal discharge that is visible to the naked eye. The detection of the gonococcus can alone decide the question. This is often a matter of difficulty, because it is only in the few days immediately after infection that the organism can be found in the discharge. In chronic cases, the gonococcus must be sought in one of three locations: in the interior of the cervical canal; in the urethra; or in discharge squeezed from the orifices of Bartholin's glands. Gram's method stains the discharge, and the organisms are Gram-negative intracellular diplococci.

Bacterial vaginosis

This is characterized by a copious whitish discharge, which may be offensive or have a fishy smell. It is caused by *Gardnerella*, *Mycoplasma* and anaerobes. The vaginal pH is >5 and the vagina is not inflamed. Microscopy of vaginal fluid may show characteristic 'clue' cells. Treatment is with either metronidazole or local clindamycin cream.

Chlamydia trachomatis

This is an obligate intracellular parasite, which lives in the columnar cells of the endocervical canal. It may cause discharge, or may not give any symptoms at all. An endocervical swab is needed for culture. Treatment is usually with doxycycline or azithromycin.

Pelvic inflammatory disease (PID)

This condition presents with bilateral lower abdominal pain, discharge, low-grade pyrexia, tachycardia, bilateral adnexal tenderness and cervical excitation. The organisms involved include *C. trachomatis*, *N. gonorrhoeae*, *Mycoplasma hominis* and anaerobes. It is treated with antibiotics, and it is important to treat properly on the first occasion as successive bouts of PID may lead to infertility, tubal pregnancy, chronic lower abdominal pain and menstrual problems.

Retained tampons

These are sometimes found, and removal will allow the discharge to settle quite quickly.

Contact tracing of a partner should ideally be undertaken for *Chlamydia*, gonorrhoea and PID.

Post-menopausal women

There are essentially two diagnoses, namely *atrophic changes* and *malignancy*.

In post-menopausal women, the amount of vaginal discharge produced is reduced unless they are taking hormone replacement therapy (HRT). If the woman develops vaginal discharge that is especially offensive in nature, then a malignancy should be excluded. She will not have the infections that occur during reproductive age, except for *Candida*. It would be necessary to exclude either an endometrial or cervical lesion. In elderly women, a foul discharge may come from the interior of the uterus, a *pyometra*. In this case pus can be made to flow from the os uteri by squeezing the uterus or passing a sound. The condition is due to senile endometritis, or it may be associated with carcinoma of the uterine body or cervix.

Fistulae may develop as a late manifestation of malignant disease, though this is not common, and it can also occur in bowel tumours and Crohn's disease. The remainder of the women will have atrophic changes, and may present with post-menopausal bleeding rather than discharge. If the woman requires a ring pessary to be inserted, this should be regularly changed or discharge may develop.

Antony Hollingworth

VAGINA, SWELLING IN

Generalized swelling within the vagina may occur secondary to infection. Condyloma (warts) may occur with a frond-like surface. Biopsy may be useful before instituting treatment. Otherwise, there are few structures that present as swellings within the vagina. Patients may present with a lump in the vagina, and the vast majority of these will be due to some form of prolapse (see VAGINA AND UTERUS, PROLAPSE OF, p. 768).

Benign swellings

These include the following:

- *Simple mesonephric (Gartner's)* or *paramesonephric cysts* may be seen high up in the vagina in the fornices. They are embryological remnants, which have failed to be obliterated. They may be small, asymptomatic and found incidentally on vaginal examination. Occasionally, they can grow and give some degree of dyspareunia. The characteristic position and cystic feel serve to differentiate them from the various types of vaginal prolapse. They can be treated by marsupialization if necessary.

- *Small implantation cysts* may be seen at the vaginal orifice posteriorly; they are small, and may follow operations on the perineum, or lacerations at childbirth. They may cause dyspareunia, and occasionally the scarring from removal means that there is no improvement of the symptoms.

- Occasionally an *endometrioma* may burrow through into the posterior vaginal fornix from the floor of the pouch of Douglas into the rectovaginal septum, forming nodular growths, which tend to bleed at the time of menstruation. This condition may be confused with a primary carcinoma of the vagina, but it is not friable. Microscopic section will settle its nature. It can also cause dyspareunia and may require elaborate surgery to resolve it.

- *Benign tumours.* Sessile and pedunculated swellings arise in the vaginal wall which, on histology, are found to be papilloma, fibroma or lipoma. They are uncommon, and excision may be necessary if they interfere with intercourse.

Malignant swellings

As in any type of malignancy, there is the possibility of primary or secondary tumours. Primary tumours of the vagina are rare and management needs to be undertaken at a gynaecological cancer centre. By and large, the prognosis from these tumours is poor despite radical surgery, radiotherapy and chemotherapy. The types of tumour are as follows:

- Squamous lesions: the vast majority usually occurs in the upper vagina.
- Clear cell carcinomas: these were thought at one time to be related to in-utero exposure to diethylstilboestrol, but with more information this may not be the case.
- Malignant melanomas: these have a poor prognosis, and may present as bleeding rather than swelling.
- Endodermal sinus tumour: this is a very rare type of adenocarcinoma.
- Rhabdomyosarcoma (sarcoma botryoides): this is a rare tumour found in girls aged less than 5 years. It usually presents as vaginal bleeding. It has a characteristic appearance, like a bunch of grapes, and microscopic section proves its nature.
- Secondary tumours: these usually originate from the local organs, namely the cervix and uterus, though there have been reports of secondaries from primary tumours in the ovary, colon and hypernephroma.

Antony Hollingworth

VEINS, VARICOSE ABDOMINAL

The point at which distension of veins becomes varicosity is arbitrary; most conditions that produce undoubted varicosity of the veins of the abdominal wall in some cases merely dilate them in others. When this dilatation is considerable it nearly always has much diagnostic significance, particularly if the direction of blood flow is reversed.

Veins, when dilated, may be clearly seen as such, but they are unduly visible owing to wasting of the subcutaneous fat. Alternatively, in rare cases they may be simply varicose, like veins in the leg, owing to idiosyncrasy or hereditary predisposition. In neither of these cases, however, is the blood flow in them reversed. To test the direction of blood flow, part of a vein should be chosen where there are no side branches, and the blood expressed from it by means of two fingers pressed gently down on the vein close together and then drawn apart while pressure over the vein is maintained by each. When a length of the distended vein has been emptied in this way, one of the two fingers is lifted, and the time taken by the vein in refilling is noted. The procedure is repeated, the other finger being lifted off this time. It is then generally easy to decide whether the vein fills from below upwards, or from above downwards. Normally, blood flows from above downwards in the veins of the lower two-thirds of the abdominal wall. When the blood flow is from below upwards, there is almost certainly an obstruction to the inferior vena cava, the blood which is unable to return finding a collateral circulation via the abdominal wall to the superior vena cava.

Obstruction to the inferior vena cava is due to one or other of three main groups of conditions, namely:

- *Great general increase in the intra-abdominal tension*, owing to such conditions as ascites, ovarian cyst, great splenic or hepatic enlargement.
- *Thrombosis* without external obstruction.
- *Obstruction by local compression*, especially by secondary deposits in the retroperitoneal lymph nodes.

When the obstruction of the inferior vena cava is due not to the vein itself being thrombosed or invaded by new growth, but to the *general intra-abdominal pressure* becoming so great that the vein is, so to speak, flattened out, the varicosity of the veins upon the abdominal wall is but a late symptom. At this point the diagnosis of the cause of the great abdominal distension, generally ascites or a large tumour, will already have been made. If there is a marked varicosity of the superficial veins early in a case of ascites the probability is that both are due to malignant disease.

When the inferior vena cava is obstructed by *thrombosis* without evidence of external compression, the clotting will probably have started, not in the inferior vena cava itself, but below it, either in the deep veins of the legs or in the pelvis. Oedema of the legs will be pronounced. The higher the thrombosis extends, the higher up the back will the oedema spread. Moreover, when the renal veins have been reached, albuminuria, haematuria and ascites may ensue, and acute nephritis may be simulated. Distension or varicosity of the veins of the abdominal wall assists in distinguishing such a case from one of acute or subacute nephritis, besides which there will be no oedema of the eyelids or face.

If there is no very tense distension of the abdomen; if the way the case began does not suggest thrombosis in one leg, or in the pelvis, extending upwards; and if, nevertheless, there is marked varicosity of the veins of the lower part of the abdominal wall, with the blood flow in them reversed, so as to be from below upwards (the history being a relatively short one), the probability is that the inferior vena cava is being obstructed by something that is in immediate contact with it. There will very likely be symmetrical oedema of the legs, and possibly albuminuria and haematuria. It is remarkable how seldom an aortic aneurysm or other non-malignant mass obstructs a large vein sufficiently to produce this collateral varicosity; hence, the presumption is that such varicosity indicates *malignant disease*. It is worthy of note that carcinoma of the kidney is prone to extend into the renal veins and thus into the inferior vena cava by direct extension. Sometimes, the tumour mass reaches as far as the right atrium, and may produce therein a pedunculated polyp. In such cases there has generally been haematuria or other renal symptoms before evidence of inferior vena caval obstruction arises. In thus situation, cases of growth in the kidney invading the inferior vena cava may be distinguished from cases of secondary growth in the retroperitoneal nodes which, if they produced haematuria at all, would do so by first obstructing the inferior vena cava, and thence involving the renal veins. In such cases there are often other symptoms pointing to primary growth in some organ from which the lymphatics drain into the retroperitoneal nodes; the testes and ovaries should not be overlooked in this respect.

It is said that *cirrhosis of the liver* leads to varicosity of the veins around the umbilicus – the *caput medusae*.

Most cases of cirrhosis of the liver cause no distension of the superficial abdominal veins until the general intra-abdominal tension has been greatly increased by the tenseness of the ascites, which occurs late. Not even the telangiectases that occur so commonly in men past middle age around the lower part of the chest, in a line with the attachment of the diaphragm, indicate cirrhosis; these are quite as common in cases of emphysema without cirrhosis.

In summary, varicosity of the superficial abdominal veins generally indicates either thrombosis of the inferior vena cava, secondary to direct spread of thrombosis up to it from veins in the pelvis or in the leg, or else obstruction of the vena cava by secondary malignant disease.

Harold Ellis

VERTIGO

Vertigo is a symptom for which there is a multitude of causes (Table V.1). Misdiagnosis must be avoided at all cost, and every effort should be made to establish the correct diagnosis by careful documentation of the patient's history, a thorough clinical examination, followed by the selection and interpretation of specific investigations. While the patient may find accurate description of their symptoms difficult or beyond their capability to express, the physician should be absolutely clear that vertigo arising from the vestibular system is a subjective sensation of movement which is usually rotatory. Patients may say that they feel either themselves or their environment moving. General sensations of light-headedness, dizziness or instability are rarely the result of labyrinthine or vestibular nerve disorders, and in these cases alternative causes should be sought.

Associated auditory symptoms, hearing loss and tinnitus are important features to establish and to define, as they are strongly indicative of an otological lesion. Assessment of this deficit is pivotal in subsequent management decisions. Almost all otological conditions that cause vertigo do so by involvement of the inner ear structures. A *labyrinthine fistula* should be seriously considered in patients with otorrhoea and those who have previously undergone surgery for chronic infection or otosclerosis. Hennebert's sign

Table V.1 Causes of vertigo and dizziness

General systemic	Haematological	Anaemia
		Hyperviscosity
	Cardiovascular	Postural hypotension
		Carotid sinus syndrome
		Dysrrhythmias
		Shock
	Metabolic	Hypoglycaemia
		Hyperventilation
Neurological	Supra-tentorial	Epilepsy
		Syncope
		Psychogenic
	Infra-tentorial	Multiple sclerosis
		Vertebrobasilar ischaemia
		Infections (e.g. syphilis, TB, herpes zoster)
		CPA tumours
		Foramen magnum abnormalities
Otological		Menière's disease
		Post-traumatic syndrome
		Positional vertigo
		Vestibular neuronitis
		Perilymph fistula
		Labyrinthitis
		Otosclerosis/Paget's disease
		Vascular accidents
		Tumours
		Autoimmune disorders
		Drug intoxication
Miscellaneous		Ocular disorders
		Odontogenic
		Orthopaedic (e.g. cervical spine disease)

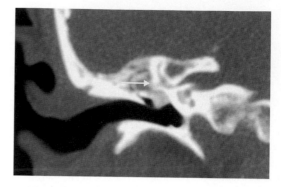

Figure V.5 Computed tomogram of the labyrinth, showing a defect in the lateral semicircular canal caused by an osteoma that had developed in the mastoid antrum.

(the fistula sign) should be sought in these patients by applying pressure to the external meatus and, if present, horizontal nystagmus will be observed. Careful otoscopy together with micro-suction will most likely reveal a cholesteatoma or attic defect. Failing that, a defect in the otic capsule will be seen on a CT scan (Fig. V.5).

Menière's disease is caused by fluctuation in endolymph production or resorption that results in distension of the membranous labyrinth, endolymphatic hydrops. The condition is characterized by episodes of vertigo that last for more than a few minutes and often several hours. They are often accompanied by pallor, prostration and vomiting and preceded by a feeling of fullness in the affected ear, together with tinnitus that steadily increases in intensity. Marked nystagmus develops during the attack.

As the vertigo subsides, the patient becomes aware of deafness in the affected ear, which over the course of several hours or days slowly resolves.

Positional vertigo is diagnosed when the history indicates that changes in head position precipitate vertigo, or that it can be demonstrated clinically. It can be caused by either a peripheral or central lesion. If peripheral, the condition is commonly attributed to disease of the otolith organ, *cupulolithiasis*, and severe vertigo is experienced, usually accompanied by rotatory nystagmus, when the head is lowered so that the affected otolith organ is undermost. The vertigo and nystagmus fades quickly while the head is maintained in this position. Usually, if the manoeuvre is repeated, the response is diminished or absent. This condition may develop after head injury, after a viral infection, or for no apparent reason. In these circumstances this condition is referred to as *benign paroxysmal positional vertigo*.

Positional vertigo may also develop in association with central lesions such as multiple sclerosis or cerebellar tumours, often metastatases. In such cases there is no adaptation or fatigue of the response. Instead, the vertigo is present and persists for as long as the head is held in the critical position.

In *cervical vertigo* (which should not be confused with positional vertigo), the vertigo is induced by turning the head in a particular way. It can develop in patients suffering from atheromatous stenosis of the internal carotid artery or a similar narrowing of the vertebral arteries. It is thought that movement of the head causes obstruction to the cerebral blood flow, and there is some evidence that the vertebral artery may also be compressed within its bony canal by osteophytes in those with severe cervical spondylosis. Unlike positional vertigo, it is a movement of the neck, and not the position of the head, that determines the symptoms and, in some, it is not vertigo that they perceive but light headedness; a few suffer syncope.

Vestibular neuronitis is thought to be a viral affection of the vestibular nerve. It is associated with intense vertigo with which a patient may waken and which may be accompanied by vomiting unless they lie absolutely still. There is no associated deafness or tinnitus. The intense vertigo usually passes off within a few days, but there remains a liability to brief vertigo on head movement which may persist for weeks or even months. Bithermal caloric tests of vestibular function show absent or severely reduced responses on one side.

Less common than any of the above are tumours of the VIIIth nerve or space-occupying lesions of the cerebello-pontine angle or petrous apex, for example *vestibular schwannoma, meningioma, petrous apex cysts* and *cholesteatoma*. The most common of these is *vestibular schwannoma* (acoustic neuroma). Most patients with vestibular schwannoma present with a progressive unilateral hearing loss associated with tinnitus and episodic vertigo or instability of gait. As the tumour enlarges, other cranial nerve deficits develop that include facial paraesthesia and anaesthesia, trigeminal neuralgia caused by distortion of the Vth cranial nerve, dysarthria, dysphagia and voice disturbance secondary to IXth, Xth and XIIth cranial nerve palsies. Eventually, the brainstem becomes so severely moulded and compressed that hydrocephalus ensues with increasing headache and visual disturbance (Fig. V.6).

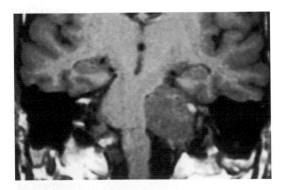

Figure V.6 A large left-sided vestibular schwannoma that presented with hearing loss, ataxia, headaches and facial anaesthesia.

More central lesions in the *medulla* and *lower pons* also cause vertigo. The vertigo in these conditions may be paroxysmal or continuous, but generally speaking the diagnosis depends less upon the quality of the giddiness than on other symptoms and signs arising from simultaneous involvement of structures adjacent to the vestibular nuclei. There is seldom tinnitus or deafness in any of these conditions, but long tracts may be involved and nystagmus is present even when the patient is not actually feeling vertiginous. Moreover, the nystagmus is different in that in labyrinthine and vestibular nerve lesions the quick component is always towards the affected side, whereas in central lesions it is towards the left when the patient looks to the left and to the right when he or she looks to the right. The diseases that produce vertigo in this situation include *multiple sclerosis, thrombosis of the posterior inferior cerebellar artery, stenosis of the basilar artery, brainstem tumours* and *syringobulbia*. Cerebellar disease can give rise to vertigo, more especially if the lesion is acute, as in penetrating injuries and infarction, but generally speaking chronic lesions cause a sense of disequilibrium rather than a sense of movement.

Systemic disorders also cause vertigo. *Hypertension* is common, *dysrrhythmias* less so, while vertigo as the side effect of *drug therapy* is not infrequent. *Demyelination* and even *syphilis* should also be considered, if only to be excluded. Light headedness often confused with vertigo accompanies *anaemia* and *hypotensive states*.

It is the authors' practice to undertake a neuro-otological examination for all patients with vertigo. This initial examination includes otoscopy, audiometry, evaluation of the central nervous system, and measurement of blood pressure and pulse rate, together with auscultation of the carotid arteries.

Audiometric and vestibular tests are tailored to each individual patient's needs. A pure tone audiogram alone may be adequate for some with absolutely normal, symmetrical hearing who give a classic history of a non-otological condition, for example vertebrobasilar ischaemia. The addition of a caloric test might be sufficient investigation for a patient with symptoms and signs of a benign otological condition, for example post-traumatic vertigo. More sophisticated tests are indicated and essential in other patients, for example those with asymmetrical or fluctuating sensorineural hearing loss, and absolutely mandatory for those in whom surgery is considered. They should also have a battery of basic blood tests to include a full blood picture, indices, biochemical screen and syphilis serology. An MR scan is almost always arranged to exclude an intra-canalicular tumour, and a CT scan performed if surgical intervention is deemed necessary.

Containment of expense in the investigation of patients with vertigo has always been a problem for the otologist. Healthcare resources are becoming increasingly limited each year, and attempts to force economies on clinicians are more frequent. The surgeon should continually remember the potential consequences for the patient of missing the diagnosis of an acoustic neuroma or other cerebello-pontine angle lesion at an early stage. For some, this could mean a permanently paralysed face and a lifetime's misery. We should not be shy or slow to remind our institutions that the consequence for them could be a very substantial claim for negligence that would be difficult to defend.

In the UK, incapacitating vertigo precludes driving and also many other activities that might place either the patient or others at risk of bodily harm. While surgical treatment is often successful, the patient should not resume driving until they have been free from spontaneous attacks of vertigo for a period of at least 3 months. Standards of medical fitness to hold Heavy Goods Vehicles and Public Service Vehicles licences are much more stringent. In this respect, a history of recurrent vertigo or significant unilateral deafness is more than sufficient to disbar the patient from obtaining or renewing their licence.

Michael Gleeson

VESICLES

See BULLAE AND VESICLES (p. 85).

VISION, DEFECTS OF

See also EYE, BLINDNESS OF (p. 186).

In diagnosing the cause of visual loss it is helpful to consider the speed of onset and permanence of loss, and whether one or both eyes are involved (see Table V.2).

Table V.2 Differential diagnosis of visual loss

Transient monocular loss
- Carotid territory thromboembolism
- Retinal migraine
- Anterior visual pathway hypoperfusion (hypotension, hyperviscosity)
- Ophthalmological disease (e.g. intermittent angle-closure glaucoma)
- Vasculitis
- Demyelination (Uhtoff's phenomenon)
- Visual obscuration

Transient binocular visual loss
- Migraine
- Cerebral hypoperfusion (thromboembolism, large-vessel stenosis, hypotension, hyperviscosity)
- Occipital seizures
- Visual obscurations (papilloedema)

Sudden monocular non-progressive visual loss
- Central retinal arterial or venous occlusion/Branch retinal arterial or venous occlusion
- Traumatic optic neuropathy
- Retinal detachment
- Vitreous haemorrhage
- Anterior ischaemic optic neuropathy
- Hysteria

Sudden binocular non-progressive visual loss
- Bilateral occipital infarction
- Pituitary apoplexy
- Leber's hereditary optic neuropathy

Progressive visual loss (monocular or binocular)
- Optic neuritis (demyelinating, infectious, granulomatous)
- Toxic amblyopia, drug-induced optic neuropathy
- Anterior visual pathway tumour (e.g. parasellar meningioma)
- Anterior visual pathway aneurysm (e.g. giant aneurysm of the supraclinoid carotid artery)
- Radionecrosis
- Drusen
- Chronic papilloedema (e.g. idiopathic intracranial hypertension or tumour)
- Cataract
- Macular degeneration
- Cancer-associated retinopathy

In addition, the pattern of visual field loss is helpful in localizing the lesion to a particular part of the visual pathway, and sometimes may be characteristic of particular disorders (Table V.3). Lesions anterior to the optic chiasm (e.g. retina, optic nerve) cause monocular field loss. Chiasmal lesions (e.g. pituitary tumours) cause binocular, non-homonymous field defects (classically bitemporal hemianopia). Retrochiasmal lesions (optic tract, optic radiation, occipital cortex) cause

Table V.3 Anatomical localizing value of visual field defects with possible causes

Visual field defect	Anatomical localization of lesion	Possible causes
Total monocular loss	Anterior to optic chiasm (optic nerve, retina, ocular)	Central retinal artery or vein occlusion
Central scotoma	Optic nerve, central retina	Optic neuritis
Centrocaecal scotoma (between and blind spot)	Optic nerve, central retina	Leber's optic neuropathy
		Toxic amblyopia
Arcuate scotoma	Optic nerve	Glaucoma
Altitudinal defect	Optic nerve	Anterior ischaemic optic neuropathy
Binocular, non-homonymous field loss (e.g. bitemporal hemianopia)	Optic chiasm	Pituitary tumour, inflammatory or granulomatous disease
Binocular, homonymous hemianopia	Retrochiasmal disease (e.g. optic tract)	Pituitary region tumours (adenoma/craniopharyngioma)
Binocular homonymous upper quadrantanopia	Optic radiation (temporal lobe fibres)	Tumour (glioma, metastasis), demyelination, stroke, degenerative diseases, vasculitis
Binocular homonymous lower quadrantanopia	Optic radiation (parietal lobe fibres)	
Macular-sparing hemianopia	Optic radiation (posterior occipital lobe)	
Peripheral constriction	Retina or optic nerve head	Chronic papilloedema, retinitis pigmentosa, hysteria

homonymous field defects with varying congruity. A focal defect in the visual field is called a 'scotoma'. A central scotoma is rapidly noticed and reported, and is due to disease of the central retina or optic nerve. A centrocaecal scotoma (between the fixation point and the physiological blind spot) also localize the lesion to retina or optic nerve, and may be seen with Leber's hereditary optic neuropathy or toxic amblyopia. An arcuate scotoma is characteristic of glaucoma, but may also be seen in optic disc drusen, optic neuritis and ischaemic optic neuropathy. An altitudinal scotoma (respecting the horizontal meridian) is typical of anterior ischaemic optic neuropathy. Peripheral constriction of the visual field occurs in open-angle glaucoma, retinitis pigmentosa and hysterical visual loss. In glaucoma, there is also cupping of the optic disc. Central vision may remain good, even though the field of vision is extremely limited. In retinitis pigmentosa, there may be associated night-blindness. Retinitis pigmentosa may occur in isolation or in the context of a more widespread neurodegenerative condition, for example abetalipoproteinaemia, Refsum disease or adrenoleucodystrophy (typical bone spicule retinopathy), or mitochondrial cytopathy ('salt and pepper' retinopathy). The mode of transmission is variable, and there may be a range of associated neurological features depending on the underlying cause.

Constriction of the field of vision may also occur in *hysterical blindness*, but is often variable or manipulable. A distinct psychological trigger can sometimes be identified, that is presumed to be somehow converted into a physical symptom (hence conversion disorder). Before making this diagnosis, all evidence of visual pathway disease must be carefully excluded.

Other localizing symptoms include metamorphopsia (distortion of straight edges), which is characteristic of retinal disease, and acquired loss of colour vision, which is characteristic of an optic nerve lesion.

Transient monocular visual loss

The possible causes are listed in Table V.2. Of these, the most common manifestation is with classical amaurosis fugax, where the patient reports a black curtain coming from above or below to extinguish vision, either completely or in one hemifield. The visual loss typically lasts for a few minutes, with recovery over 15–20 minutes (in the reverse direction to the onset). This presentation suggests an embolus passing across the retinal circulation, resulting in temporary occlusion of the central retinal artery) (or a proximal branch) before dissolving and moving to the periphery. This implies an embolic source, which in a patient aged under 40 years is likely to be cardiac (e.g. due to mitral valve prolapse, endocarditis or atrial myxoma), and in those aged over 40 from the ipsilateral carotid or aorta (due to atheromatous disease). Amaurosis fugax may be a premonitory symptom of central retinal artery occlusion, which causes permanent monocular blindness. Amaurosis fugax requires prompt investigation, and if a patient presents very acutely during an attack, it can be treated with ocular massage and intravenous acetazolamide.

Transient binocular visual loss

Visual obscurations are fleeting, usually fading visual loss on performing a Valsalva manoeuvre, coughing or changing posture. This is an important symptom of raised intracranial pressure with papilloedema. Migrainous aura can usually be recognized by the time course (up to 30 minutes), with an evolving pattern of visual disturbance often with typical positive phenomena (teichopsia) as well as visual loss in the form of hemianopic or scotomatous loss. Cerebral hypoperfusion in presyncope is characteristically a fading of vision over seconds, always on standing, and usually associated with a dulling of hearing, feeling of faintness and sometimes a 'coat-hanger' ache of the neck and shoulders before the patient collapses. Recurrent episodes in particular circumstances may suggest a vasovagal mechanism (e.g. precipitation by emotional or unpleasant stimuli). Particularly in older patients, extracranial large vessel arterial stenosis can also cause posture-induced cerebral hypoperfusion with similar visual fading and other focal neurological deficits.

Sudden monocular non-progressive visual loss

The important causes of sudden monocular blindness include acute central retinal artery or vein occlusion, anterior ischaemic optic neuropathy (which may be secondary to giant cell arteritis), vitreous haemorrhage and retinal detachment. In embolic central retinal arterial occlusion there may be warning episodes of amaurosis fugax. Other causes of central retinal artery occlusion include in-situ occlusion due to extensive atheroma (often in older patients in the context of diabetes and/or hypertension), and vasculitis (giant-cell arteritis, polyarteritis nodosa, Raynaud's disease). A waxing and waning or stuttering onset is particularly characteristic of anterior ischaemic optic neuropathy, which may be either arteritic (due to giant-cell arteritis) or non-arteritic (due to in-situ atheroma). Papilloedema is usually seen due to optic disc infarction. It is important to recognize anterior ischaemic optic neuropathy due to giant-cell arteritis, since urgent treatment with

high-dose corticosteroids may save vision. Associated features include systemic malaise, fatigue, headache (with scalp tenderness), myalgia, jaw claudication and on examination the temporal arteries may be pulseless and thickened. The ESR may be markedly elevated, sometimes above 100 mm/hour. Giant-cell arteritis is nearly always limited to patients aged over 60 years. Posterior ischaemic optic neuropathy is less common, and may result from prolonged or severe perioperative hypotension.

The features of vitreous haemorrhage or retinal detachment can be detected on detailed ocular examination, including fundoscopy.

Sudden binocular non-progressive visual loss

This is usually caused by vascular pathology, either pituitary apoplexy or bilateral occipito-parietal infarction. Pituitary apoplexy is haemorrhagic infarction, and necrosis of the pituitary gland, usually in the context of a pituitary adenoma. The associated features of this dramatic condition may include sudden collapse, headache, meningism and ophthalmoplegia. Pituitary apoplexy can occur post-partum with no adenoma present (*Sheehan's syndrome*). Bilateral occipital infarction may be due to thrombotic or embolic occlusion of the posterior cerebral arteries (or the distal basilar artery from which they arise). It can also occur with border zone (watershed) ischaemia and infarction due to prolonged reduced cerebral perfusion pressure, usually in the context of persistent systemic hypotension (e.g. after cardiac arrest). The pupillary light reflexes are preserved. *Anton's syndrome* – the combination of cortical blindness, denial of the visual defect and confabulation – may result from bilateral posterior cerebral infarction.

Leber's hereditary optic neuropathy is a mitochondrial disorder (maternal inheritance) that usually affects males in the second or third decade of life, and causes sudden central visual loss. Typically, one eye is affected, followed by the second eye after an interval of weeks to months, but simultaneous loss can occur.

Progressive visual loss

Optic neuritis

The most important cause of monocular progressive visual loss in patients aged under 50 years is optic neuritis, which may be either 'idiopathic' or in association with multiple sclerosis. Visual loss progresses over hours to a few days, and reaches its nadir within a week. The severity of loss ranges from impaired colour saturation or contrast sensitivity with normal acuity to no perception of light. Pain is usually present on eye movement at onset or shortly afterwards; the pain does not usually persist beyond a few days. Recovery begins within a month, stabilizes by about 6 weeks and, in the vast majority, is good (better than 6/9 acuity). Partial recovery occurs, but no recovery is rare. Papilloedema may be present if the anterior portion of the nerve is affected. If the optic neuritis affects the more posterior retrobulbar portion of the optic nerve, initial fundoscopy is normal. Optic atrophy subsequently develops, but does not correlate with the extent of visual recovery. Atypical features such as age greater than 50 years, lack of pain or prolonged pain, and an absence of the typical natural history of recovery, should alert the clinician to other causes, for example ischaemic optic neuropathy, 'atypical' optic neuritis (e.g. post-infectious, infectious, post-viral, granulomatous, vasculitic) or compression by tumour. Bilateral simultaneous or sequential optic neuritis may occur, particularly in childhood. Treatment with corticosteroids may speed up visual recovery (though not improve final outcome), and may be offered to patients with bilateral involvement, pre-existing poor vision in the fellow eye, or those with severe visual loss and severe pain.

Optic neuritis may be associated with multiple sclerosis (MS); about 50 per cent of patients with isolated optic neuritis will subsequently develop multiple sclerosis, though the interval is very variable. The presence of typical lesions on MRI scanning increases the likelihood of developing MS, and the extent of MRI disease is predictive of future disability. Follow-up studies indicate that MS presenting with optic neuritis has a relatively benign prognosis. The association of optic neuritis (usually bilateral) and subsequent or preceding spinal cord inflammation is termed *Devic's neuromyelitis optica*; there are usually few cerebral lesions, and no oligoclonal bands are found in the cerebrospinal fluid (in contrast to multiple sclerosis in which lesions and oligoclonal bands are almost invariably detected).

Toxic amblyopia (nutritional optic neuropathy)

The patient reports dimness or blurring of near or distant vision progressing over days to weeks. There is typically a central loss of vision for colours, green

only in the earlier stages, subsequently green and red. On examination, there may be a central or centrocaecal scotoma, larger for coloured than for white objects. The fundus may be normal, but pallor of the temporal portion of the optic disc may be seen in some cases. Although it is often termed 'tobacco-alcohol amblyopia', there is strong evidence that it is due to nutritional deficiency, rather than to toxicity from alcohol and tobacco use, though the precise deficiency is not known. B vitamins have been suggested; a B_{12} deficiency can cause an optic neuropathy, but does not fully explain the majority of cases.

Drug-induced optic neuropathy

Treatment with drugs including ethambutol, isoniazid, streptomycin, chloramphenicol, or quinine can cause an optic neuropathy. In the case of ethambutol and isoniazid, the optic nerve damage is dose-dependent. A careful history of the duration and timing of exposure to drugs in relation to visual symptoms is needed to make an accurate diagnosis.

Compressive lesions of anterior visual pathways

The hallmark of visual loss due to a compressive lesion is a slowly progressive onset without recovery (in contrast to typical optic neuritis). Other features that raise the possibility of a mass lesion include complete absence of pain on eye movement, persistent pain over more than a week or two, proptosis, or spread to involve the other eye. The most common compressive lesions are pituitary region tumours (adenoma, craniopharyngioma), meningiomas, gliomas, or aneurysms. In any case of visual loss without a history of typical optic neuritis, urgent imaging of the anterior visual pathways with CT or MRI (if available) is mandatory. The other main causes of progressive visual loss are listed in Table V.2.

Chronic papilloedema

Progressive visual loss may result from very long-standing chronic papilloedema due to raised intracranial pressure. This may be due to a mass lesion and hydrocephalus, meningeal disease or, if no underlying cause is identified, to idiopathic intracranial hypertension. Visual acuity is usually well preserved despite marked papilloedema, as the pathology does not directly damage the optic nerve fibres until late on in the illness.

Cancer-associated retinopathy

This rare retinal degeneration is a paraneoplastic manifestation of a remote systemic carcinoma. The typical presenting complaint is of shimmering visual disturbance. Specialist retinal electrodiagnostics are required for an accurate diagnosis.

Developmental amblyopia

Binocular fusion of images from both eyes is normally achieved by 6 months of age. If one eye receives a defective image – for example from an uncorrected high refractive error – the less-clear image is suppressed. If uncorrected, the eye becomes amblyopic and cannot be corrected by refraction. Alternatively, an imbalance of extraocular muscles that would cause diplopia in adults leads to a failure of development of visual pathways in the affected eye (strabismic amblyopia). Severe amblyopia may result from obstruction of the light pathway to the retina from birth, for example congenital cataract or ptosis (stimulus-deprivation amblyopia).

David Werring

VISION, SUBJECTIVE DISTURBANCES OF

The main categories of visual loss have been described under VISION, DEFECTS OF (p. 776). There are other visual disturbances that do not fit easily into the above-described scheme, and some of these are now briefly considered. They can be divided into positive symptoms (an abnormal 'excess' of an aspect of visual perception) or negative symptoms (an abnormal loss of an aspect of visual perception), or distortions of normal visual perception. Some of the main causes are listed in Table V.4.

Positive disturbances

Subjective visual disturbances, positive more than negative, are common in migraine. There are a wide

Table V.4 Subjective disturbances of vision

Positive disturbances
- Migranous visual aura (including teichopsia)
- Floaters
- Phosphenes
- Palinopsia (visual perseveration)
- Visual hallucinations including Charles Bonnet syndrome
- Polyopia

Negative disturbances
- Disturbance of colour vision (achromatopsia)
- Visual agnosia
- Prosopagnosia
- Alexia without agraphia
- Disturbance of motion perception (akinetopsia)
- Balint syndrome (visual disorientation, optic ataxia, optic apraxia)

Distortions
- Micropsia or macropsia

Metamorphopsia

variety of reported visual symptoms, including flashing lights (photopsia), shimmering, and transient spots before the eyes (scotomata). Fortification spectra (teichopsia), comprised of zig-zag lines, are particularly frequent and are pathognomonic of migraine. The time course and evolution of migrainous visual aura is characteristic, with evolution of symptoms over minutes (with movement or spreading across the visual field, classically one hemi-field) and a total duration of less than 30 minutes. The pathophysiological basis is thought to be spreading cortical depression (excitation followed by inhibition) moving anteriorly across the visual cortex. Other brief flashing visual phenomena (phosphenes) elicited by eye movements have been described in normal individuals and in myopic patients with vitreous opacities. Eye movement-induced phosphenes are found in patients with optic neuritis and multiple sclerosis and may be related to abnormal excitability of optic nerve fibres. *Floaters* (moving spots before the eyes) are very commonly seen against a bright background; they often appear suddenly, and then very gradually fade. They are probably due to condensations in the vitreous gel, which either break up and disappear, or sink. They are very common in high myopia. If there is associated eye pain, uveitis should be considered; in this case the floating particles are composed of an inflammatory exudate.

Palinopsia is a symptom of continuing to perceive an object that is no longer in view; it may be confined to a hemi-anopic field, and is due to a lesion in the occipitoparietal region. Polyopia is where more than one image is perceived with one eye despite no intra-ocular structural damage or extra-ocular movement abnormality, and is probably related to occipital cortex damage. Visual hallucinations are images seen in the absence of an objective external visual stimulus. They are rarely seen in psychiatric disease, unlike auditory hallucinations, and may be due to a state of delirium due to systemic disease. The Charles Bonnet syndrome is seen usually in elderly patients, who report vivid scenes of detailed patterns, often in tessellating patterns; figures in ornate period costume are also typical. The hallucinations typically last minutes only, and are often seen at twilight. They are benign and non-threatening. The mental state is normal, and the rest of the visual world is normally perceived. This syndrome is probably due to cortical mechanisms resulting from defective visual input of any ocular or neurological cause (e.g. cataract or macular degeneration).

Negative disturbances

Disturbances of colour vision are a hallmark of optic nerve disease, but they can also be caused by cortical lesions (e.g. stroke, demyelination, tumour, degenerative disorders) of the ventral occipito-temporal region (area V4), in which case visual acuity will be preserved. An inability to recognize familiar faces (or to learn new ones) despite normal objective tests of visual acuity is termed 'prosopagnosia', and may be caused by lesions in the nearby fusiform gyrus. *Visual agnosia* refers to an inability to identify objects despite normal visual acuity, and is due to a lesion in the dorsolateral visual association pathway (superior occipito-parietal region). *Balint's syndrome* is classically due to a lesion in the occipitoparietal region, and comprises an inability to reach for objects accurately (optic ataxia), an inability to fixate on a target (psychic paralysis of gaze) and an inability to perceive a scene as a whole despite perceiving its individual elements (simultanagnosia). *Alexia* is an inability to read despite normal visual acuity, and when not associated with a more general language (aphasic disorder), is termed 'alexia without agraphia'. The syndrome is due to stroke in the posterior cerebral artery territory (occipitotemporal cortex).

Disturbance of motion perception (akinetopsia) has also been rarely reported with lateral occipitotemporal cortical lesions.

Distortions

Metamorphopsia (distortion of straight lines) is usually due to retinal disease. Distortions of the sizes of objects (*micropsia* or *macropsia*) may be a manifestation of occipital lobe seizures or migraine aura. Micropsia and macropsia may accompany distortions of body image; this phenomenon has been termed '*Alice in Wonderland syndrome*', in reference to the illusions described in the book by Lewis Carrol (Charles Dodgson), himself a migraine sufferer.

David Werring

VOICE, DISORDERS OF

Voice is created by the modulation of sound produced by vocal fold vibration as air is forced or injected through the larynx from the lungs. *Pitch* is determined by the length and tension or stiffness of the vibrating vocal fold. *Loudness of voice* is a character largely determined by the pressure of air presented to, or allowed to develop in, the larynx. The subtlety and complexity of vocal fold vibration has only been appreciated in recent years with the development and widespread use of optical rods and stroboscopic light in clinical practice. With these tools it is possible to see that the vocal folds vibrate in both planes of space, vertical and horizontal. A mucosal wave is generated during the production of voice as the epithelium covering the fold is able to slip on the underlying muscle and cord. Modulation of the sound produced in the larynx takes place in the upper airway, the vocal tract, and the quality or character of voice produced is largely determined by the shape and competence of these structures.

Even from this relatively simplistic outline of voice production it can be appreciated that there are a multitude of causes of abnormal voice that range from structural lesions of the airway to disorders that affect laryngeal biomechanics. There is no entirely satisfactory classification of these disorders but, from a clinical standpoint, the broad division into 'structural'

Table V.5 Causes of voice disorders

Structural causes
- Inflammation
  - Acute laryngitis: bacterial, viral, fungal, chemical and allergic
  - Chronic laryngitis: non-specific or specific
- Trauma
  - Acute: haematoma, fracture
  - Chronic: vocal cord nodules, Reinke's oedema, inter-arytenoid pachydermia
- Neoplasia
  - Benign: papilloma, dysplasia
  - Malignant: carcinoma
- Miscellaneous
  - Myxoedema
  - Amyloid
  - Relapsing polychondritis
  - Systemic lupus erythematosus

Functional causes
- Neurological
  - Vocal cord palsy
    - Vagal nerve palsy
    - Recurrent laryngeal nerve palsy
    - Superior laryngeal nerve palsy
  - Laryngeal dystonia
  - Parkinson's disease
  - Myaesthenia gravis
  - Multiple sclerosis
- Muscle tension dysphonia
  - Dysphonia plicae ventricularis
  - Laryngeal myasthenia: prebylarynges
- Degenerative
  - Fixation of the crico-arytenoid joint
- Psychological

and 'functional' conditions has much to commend it (Table V.5). The major weakness of this system lies in the fact that the larynx can compensate for disability, and that some voice abnormalities caused by covert structural lesions may present and be misdiagnosed at the outset as functional disorders.

While structural lesions cause hoarseness, functional disorders may produce a variety of more subtle voice changes, some of which are characteristic of their cause. The trained ear can detect these, and phoniatrists refer to them in terms of 'jitter', 'shimmer', 'breathiness' etc. – descriptors that indicate the stability of a particular sound or smoothness of transition from one frequency to another. These abnormalities can be documented by waveform and spectral analysis of vocal fold vibration and voice frequency.

Structural lesions

Acute laryngitis

The most common cause in adults is a viral infection that accompanies a common cold or upper respiratory tract infection. Rhinovirus, parainfluenza virus, respiratory syncytial virus and adenovirus are most frequently implicated. Secondary bacterial infection often takes place. Patients present with generalized malaise, complete or intermittent loss of voice and cough. Spontaneous recovery takes place in a few days aided by steam inhalations, cough suppressants and voice rest. Some require antibiotics, and it goes without saying that those who smoke should not.

Laryngitis in children is known as *croup*, and is a more serious condition than its adult counterpart. The oedema associated with the infection in childhood may cause significant narrowing of the airway and critical obstruction. In addition to loss or alteration of voice, the child may develop stridor with intercostal and supraclavicular recession as he or she struggles to breathe. In severe cases infection can spread down the airway, as *laryngotracheitis* and *laryngotracheobronchitis*. These children can be extremely unwell, and both of these conditions can reach life-threatening proportions.

Bacterial infection of the supraglottis, known as *supraglottitis* in adults and *epiglottitis* in children, is fortunately becoming less common as a result of immunization programmes against *Haemophilus influenzae* infection. While *H. influenzae* is the most common organism, *Streptococcus pneumoniae*, *Staphylococcus aureus* and haemolytic streptococci may also cause the condition. Supraglottitis, and particularly epiglottitis, presents as a rapidly progressive illness with fever, sore throat, hoarseness or muffled voice and dyspnoea. The diagnosis should be made on the basis of the clinical history and the speed of progression of the illness, which can be frighteningly fast. Inspection of the larynx in the awake child in order to see the swollen epiglottis is dangerous as it may incite acute laryngeal spasm and respiratory arrest. Delay in management to obtain a lateral neck X-ray that will show the epiglottic swelling can also be critical. It is better to examine the child under anaesthesia with the ability to secure the airway by tube or tracheostomy. In adults, the infection is rarely as severe, but suppuration is more common with the development of an epiglottic abscess. Nevertheless, the condition demands close observation, humidification of inspired air, antibiotics and occasionally steroids.

Angio-oedema or *allergic laryngitis* of the larynx can be life-threatening, and precipitated by a number of substances that include food colorants and common medications such as ACE inhibitors and NSAIDs. In some, the condition is inherited through an autosomal dominant gene that causes C1 esterase inhibitor deficiency. In an attack, patients lose their voice, experience difficulty swallowing their saliva, and also develop swelling of lips, tongue and periorbital tissues.

Diphtheria of the larynx is very uncommon nowadays, but is still seen in the developing world and in those travelling from it. Caused by *Corynebacterium diphtheriae*, it usually affects young persons, and presents with a fever, progressively severe sore throat, loss of voice and increasing airway obstruction. An exudative inflammatory response can be seen in the throat as a thick, grey-green, plaque-like membrane over the fauces, pharynx and larynx that, if removed, cause bleeding of the underlying tissues. The diagnosis is made by bacteriological examination of swabs, smears and cultures. Administration of diphtheria antitoxin and the establishment of a secure airway by tracheostomy are life-saving measures, as mortality is largely due to cardiac arrhythmias and neuropathic effects of toxins and airway obstruction. The organism is still sensitive to penicillin.

Chronic laryngitis

Regardless of the cause, chronic inflammation of the larynx can result in the development of erythema and/or oedema over the vocal folds (Reinke's oedema), discrete polyps or more widespread *polypoid degeneration* of the laryngeal mucosa and granuloma formation. Smoking, vocal abuse such as excessive shouting, intubation injury, radiation, chronic bronchitis, emphysema and laryngopharyngeal reflux are most often implicated; these are sometimes loosely grouped together as non-specific causes of chronic laryngitis. Chronic candidal infection may be associated with inhaled steroid preparations. All of these patients have a persistent and long-standing voice disturbance, with no associated swallowing problem or pain. Dyspnoea is extremely unusual. The mainstay of treatment in this condition is correction or avoidance of the precipitating cause, vocal hygiene (voice rest, steam inhalations and avoidance of dehydration), anti-reflux measures and speech therapy. In some, the inflammatory reaction will subside, the larynx and voice returning to normal. Unfortunately, in others it does not, and microsurgical procedures become necessary, for example, stripping excessive redundant mucosa from the cords or removing polyps.

A number of specific causes of chronic laryngitis are still seen, especially in developing countries and in immunocompromised patients. These include *tuberculosis*, *syphilis*, *scleroma*, *leprosy*, *blastomycosis*, *histoplasmosis*, *sarcoidosis* and *Wegener's granulomatosis*. It is important to exclude these conditions in patients who fail to respond to conventional therapy or who have an unusual history, with progressive dyspnoea and malaise being prominent. Diagnosis is made by biopsy, smears and cultures from swabs in infective disorders. In Wegener's, the laryngeal condition may be part of a multi-system disorder affecting all parts of the respiratory system and the kidneys. Raised serum anti-neutrophil cytoplasmic antibodies (ANCA) levels and biopsies confirm the diagnosis.

Trauma

In its simplest form, constant *vocal abuse* through shouting inflicts various degrees of hoarseness that can be reversible as *nodules* (*singer's nodes*), *Reinke's oedema*, and submucosal haemorrhages subside. In contrast, blunt injury to the neck may result in a *fracture of the larynx*. The voice abnormality in this situation is associated with subcutaneous emphysema that is palpable and visible on X-rays, painful dysphagia and, in severe cases, dyspnoea.

Neoplasia

Papillomata are the most common benign laryngeal neoplasm, and tend to affect children rather than adults. Multiple lesions develop within the larynx and cause hoarseness and progressive dyspnoea. In some, complete remission takes place at puberty. In a few patients the papillomata spread into the trachea and bronchi. Diagnosis is made by biopsy. Malignant transformation is most unusual, but is occasionally seen in adults who smoke.

Dysplasia of the laryngeal epithelium may also cause a change in voice quality. Degrees of dysplasia from mild to severe and *in-situ carcinoma* are recognized on the basis of histological criteria. On laryngoscopy, they appear as white plaques, sometimes with adjacent erythematous areas. Some – though not all – progress to frank malignancy.

The majority of *laryngeal cancers* are squamous cell carcinomas. Three distinct sites within the larynx are recognized, and tumours developing in them tend to present and behave in slightly different ways. At the outset, supraglottic tumours cause a sensation of a persistent lump in the throat that may be painful when swallowing, the pain often radiating to the ear. As the tumour grows and spreads onto the vocal cords, hoarseness develops followed by progressive dyspnoea. Some patients experience minor haemoptyses. In contrast, tumours that develop on the vocal cord present with huskiness and progressive dyspnoea, only developing problems with swallowing at a late stage. Subglottic tumours are most uncommon and present with dyspnoea. Nodal metastases in the neck are found at presentation in up to 25 per cent of patients with supraglottic tumours and 5 per cent with glottic carcinomas. Laryngeal cancer develops in heavy smokers. Any middle-aged smoker who develops hoarseness must have the diagnosis of laryngeal cancer excluded without delay by laryngoscopy, and biopsy of any suspicious lesion. Squamous cancers respond well to radiotherapy when small, but more advanced tumours require surgical treatment. As this is a smoking-related disease, 15–20 per cent of patients will develop second primary neoplasms in the upper aerodigestive tract, either synchronously or metachronously.

Miscellaneous

Early *myxoedema* can present as a subtle voice change, huskiness or restriction of vocal range. With increasing oedema deposited in the vocal folds, dyspnoea and critical airway obstruction can develop alongside more classical signs of hypothyroidism.

Amyloid infiltration of the larynx may be seen in both the primary and secondary forms of the disease. Abnormalities of voice develop when the infiltrate involves the vocal cord, and in severe cases dyspnoea from airway obstruction may develop. The diagnosis is made on the basis of biopsies and plasma immunophoresis.

Functional lesions

Neurological

Vocal cord palsy may be either unilateral or bilateral, and caused by lesions of the vagus or recurrent laryngeal nerves. Paralysis of the left vocal cord is more common than the right cord. The longer course of the left recurrent nerve accounts for this difference. Palsies are not uncommon in clinical practice, and present with sudden voice change that may be relatively subtle or very obvious. The degree of abnormality depends on the size of the glottic chink that develops as a result of loss of vocal cord adduction. High lesions that affect both superior and recurrent laryngeal nerve function tend to be worse, and the voice change is associated with aspiration of fluids and a bovine cough. Over time, the larynx often compensates for unilateral paresis and the voice quality can return to normal without recovery of vocal cord movement.

Iatrogenic trauma acquired during thyroid, oesophageal, carotid, cardiac and skull base surgery accounts for about 40 per cent of palsies. Malignant infiltration of the nerves at the skull base by glomus tumours, in the neck from thyroid or oesophageal carcinomas and in the mediastinum from bronchial carcinoma, metastases or lymphomas are responsible for about 25 per cent of cases. No cause is apparent in 25 per cent, while knife and bullet wounds produce 25 per cent; the remainder are due to various neuropathies.

Muscle tension dysphonia

This is caused by disproportionate, ineffective or uncoordinated contraction of the intrinsic and extrinsic laryngeal musculature. In some patients, endoscopy will show incomplete closure of the vocal folds on phonation with excessive contraction of the vocalis muscle causing adduction of the false cords – dysphonia plicae ventricularis. In contrast, others show ineffective glottic closure with bowing of the vocal folds, as if the folds were intrinsically weak or subject to fatigue – laryngeal myaesthenia or presbylarynges. This is particularly common in the elderly. Various surgical procedures have been suggested for both of these conditions, but speech therapy and vocal rehabilitation is helpful (if not curative) in most.

Psychological

Hysterical dysphonia or aphonia is not common, and can be extremely difficult to treat. It may result from emotional trauma or reflect emotional instability. The important issue in this condition is to recognize it, together with the fact that the patient may have a serious underlying psychiatric illness that requires treatment in its own right.

Michael Gleeson

VOMITING

Vomiting is the forceful ejection of material from the upper gastrointestinal tract. Obstruction or partial obstruction of the gut lumen immediately comes to mind on considering possible causes. Intra-abdominal pathologies, however, as well as metabolic, systemic, psychogenic disorders and physiological causes such as pregnancy must be considered.

Vomiting is a significant feature of mechanical obstruction secondary to lumen narrowing caused by inflammation (peptic ulcer disease, Crohn's disease, ischaemia), fibrosis (healing of inflammation, surgery), neoplasia (adenocarcinoma, lymphoma, polyps) or foreign bodies (bezoar, worm infestation, gallstone).

It is important to bear in mind that obstruction of the gastrointestinal tract at any level may result in vomiting. It may be, consequently, a feature of obstruction of both the small and large bowel. Certain conditions are common to both areas (Crohn's disease, anastamotic stricture, adenomatous polyps, adenocarcinoma, lipomata, stromal cell tumours, ischaemic strictures, endometriosis). Some conditions, however, are limited or more likely to occur in the small bowel, or be more problematic should they occur in this area (adhesions, herniae, lymphoma, hamartomatous polyps, Henoch–Schönlein purpura, mesenteric adenitis, serosal secondary deposits, ulcerative jejunitis, neuroendocrine tumours, bezoar, foreign body or gallstone impaction). Colonic causes of obstruction include diverticular disease, faecal impaction, invasive cancer (prostate, ovary, uterus), rectal carcinoid, mega-rectum, Hirschsprung's disease, anal canal stenosis (Crohn's disease, surgery, squamous cell cancer) and pelvic radiation therapy.

Mechanical causes for vomiting include *volvulus*. Volvulus of the stomach is an uncommon surgical emergency, and presents with upper abdominal pain and 'fruitless' vomiting. Volvulus of the rectosigmoid colon is not uncommon in the elderly, and tends to recur if not addressed by surgical or endoscopic fixation. Zenker's and oesophageal diverticula may cause vomiting, but are more usually associated with non-forceful regurgitation of food. Muscle hypertrophy of the pylorus is well-described in infants, and presents with projectile vomiting.

Vomiting is a feature of acute appendicitis, where it is preceded by pain localizing to the right lower quadrant. It is, additionally, a common feature of both biliary and renal colic.

Paresis of the stomach (pancreatitis, diabetic, viral, post-surgical, or due to retroperitoneal cancer such as pancreatic adenocarcinoma, lymphoma) or of the small bowel (post-surgical ileus) may lead to recurrent, chronic vomiting.

Infective causes of vomiting include food poisoning (*Staphylococcus aureus*, *Bacillus cereus*), epidemic viruses (Norwalk virus), viral and bacterial meningitis and syphilis (tabes dorsalis).

The 'morning sickness' associated with the first trimester of pregnancy is normally self-limiting and mild. Persistent vomiting associated with weight loss, dehydration and acidosis is termed 'hyperemesis gravidarum', and is part of a wider spectrum of conditions, including fatty liver or pancreas. The presence of haemorrhagic retinitis is a poor sign.

Iatrogenic causes of vomiting, in addition to adhesions and anastomotic strictures, include tight fundoplication, post-vagotomy/oesophagectomy pyloric obstruction, medication (opiates, NSAIDs, steroids, azathioprine, cisplatin/chemotherapy, allergic reactions) and ileus which may occur following any surgical operation, and is not limited to intra-abdominal procedures alone.

Vomiting is a well recognized feature of intracranial pathology (space-occupying lesions, meningitis, cerebrovascular accident, hydrocephalus, middle-ear disease). The presence of the vomiting centre and chemoreceptor trigger zone in the medulla oblongata and fourth ventricle, respectively, give rise to vomiting being a feature of systemic disease such as sepsis, malaria, pyrexia and diabetic ketoacidosis. Psychiatric and behavioural disorders are commonly associated with recurrent vomiting.

The complications of vomiting include Mallory–Weiss tear of the oesophagus, suggested by vomiting followed by haematemesis; rupture of the oesophagus (Boerhave's syndrome), suggested by vomiting with severe, acute retrosternal chest pain and vomiting during childbirth leading to the aspiration of gastric acid (Mendelson's syndrome). Persistent vomiting leads to the development of a hypokalaemic alkalosis secondary to renal correction of volume disturbance. In cases of bulimia, the dental enamel becomes eroded.

The cause of a patient's vomiting is often indicated by the clinical setting and other organ-specific symptoms or signs. In cases of mechanical obstruction, the interval between eating and vomiting gives some indication as to the level of a mechanical obstruction. The contents of the vomitus rarely gives an indication as to cause. In particular, the presence of a small volume of fresh or altered ('coffee-grounds') blood is as likely to be due to a secondary gastritis as indicating peptic ulcer disease to be present. Similarly, the presence of bile implies little. *Projectile vomiting* is classically associated with pyloric channel obstruction and raised intracranial pressure; it occurs also in those with large antral gastric ulcers with no physical obstruction. The demonstration of a succussion splash is more likely to be due to some degree of gastroparesis than outlet obstruction, to which it is traditionally ascribed.

Investigations

The investigation of vomiting aims to determine both the underlying cause and its consequences (metabolic disturbance, aspiration pneumonia). General blood tests (full blood count, urea/electrolytes, serum calcium/phosphate, amylase, liver blood tests and serum glucose) can be very useful in both of these respects. Likely upper gastrointestinal pathology is most easily accessed by endoscopy, though care must be taken to prevent aspiration. Colonoscopy can be attempted and may prove useful, but an oral bowel preparation will not be possible. X-ray studies (contrast meal and enema) can be used to identify obstruction and paresis, but are best performed using water-soluble contrast rather than barium on account of the risks of aspiration or worsening lower-bowel obstruction. They are, however, less sensitive than their barium counterparts. In the absence of any other positive findings, nuclear gastric emptying studies can quantify gastroparesis. The main role of oesophageal motility studies is to identify conditions such as achalasia or oesophageal scleroderma. If no gastrointestinal or systemic cause

can be elicited, it is important to exclude intracranial pathology through a CT, or preferably MRI of the head. Lumbar puncture will be necessary in cases of syphilis.

John Meenan

VULVA, SWELLINGS OF

The differential diagnosis of vulval swellings includes not only tumours of the vulva itself, but also swellings that appear at the vulva as a result of the displacement of other structures, as in cases of uterine prolapse and cystocele (see VAGINA AND UTERUS PROLAPSE, p. 768). Hernias into this region can occur, and no further discussion is included in this section. Inflammatory lesions and ulceration of the vulva may be accompanied by swelling of the vulva due to oedema; for details, see VULVA, ULCERATION OF (p. 789). Conditions presenting with itching of the vulva as the main complaint are described under PRURITUS VULVAE (p. 557).

Vulval swellings may be classified as either infective or cystic.

Infective swellings

Warts (condyloma acuminatum)

Warts on the vulva are usually multiple (Fig. V.7). They are caused by the human papillomavirus types 6 and 11, and are almost invariably transmitted sexually. They may spread throughout the lower genital tract and anal region, and have also been associated with premalignant disease of the cervix. Vulval warts may proliferate and coalesce, in which case they are referred to as *condyloma acuminata*. This situation can be problematic in pregnancy and in patients who are immunocompromised (e.g. HIV, SLE patients on long-term steroids).

Bartholin's abscess

This presents as an extremely painful swelling in the region of Bartholin's gland, which occurs at the entrance to the vagina. Pressure on the gland causes much pain, and the area appears reddened. The duct of the gland has become blocked and the secretions within the gland infected. The abscess may discharge by itself, but surgical treatment in the form of of the labium majus; this projects medially so as to encroach on the vaginal entrance, causing dyspareunia. It is not particularly tender unless it becomes infected and forms an abscess (see above). The cyst tends gradually to increase in size, causing local discomfort until marsupialization is performed.

Sebaceous cysts are fairly common affecting the labia majora as a rule. They may occur in groups. Mucous, inclusion (Fig. V.9) and implantation cysts also occur, as do vestigial cysts of mesonephric origin (Gartner's duct cysts). The true nature of these cysts is not usually known without histological examination.

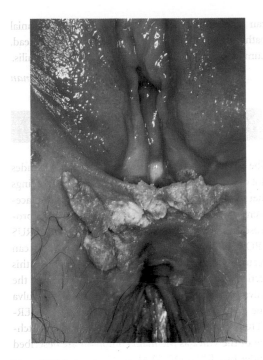

Figure V.7 Vulval warts.

marsupialization to create a new duct is likely. The abscess my recur.

Cystic swellings

These include Bartholin's cyst, sebaceous cyst, mucous cyst, implantation cyst, dermoid cyst and hydrocele of the canal of Nuck Vestigial (mesonephric) cyst.

The most common is a *Bartholin's cyst* (Fig. V.8). This is usually a swelling in the duct of the Bartholin's gland, and produces a swelling in the posterior third

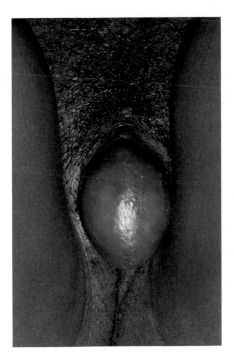

Figure V.9 Inclusion cyst following female circumcision.

Blood cysts

These include varicocele, traumatic haematoma and endometrioma.

Varicocele of the vulva occurs mainly in pregnancy, and can become worse with successive pregnancies. These cysts give a typical varicose appearance in the labia majora, and the patient can become conscious of an uncomfortable swelling on standing. The veins seldom rupture during delivery. Varicocele must be differentiated from an inguinal hernia extending into

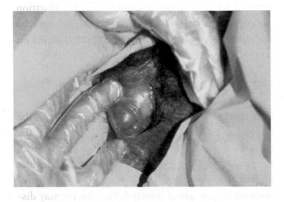

Figure V.8 Bartholin's cyst.

the labium majus, and from a cyst of the canal of Nuck (the processus vaginalis which has failed to become completely obliterated). Both of the latter tend to involve only the anterior parts of the labium majus, but all of these conditions extend to the groin. Whereas a hernia is reducible as a rule, a cyst of the canal of Nuck is not. Inguinal hernias usually disappear as pregnancy progresses, but varicoceles become worse. If a hernia contains bowel, it is resonant to percussion. A strangulated hernia will not be reducible, but the accompanying acute symptoms and the history should make the diagnosis clear.

A *haematoma of the vulva* may follow delivery or occur as the result of direct trauma. It is recognized as a bluish swelling, which is painful and tender and spreads up into the pelvis by the side of the vagina. The appearance is characteristic and the diagnosis is made on the history. An endometrioma is a rare cause of a blood-containing cyst on the vulva.

Benign new growths

These include caruncle, fibroma, fibromyoma, lipoma, hidradenoma, papilloma, lymphangioma, myxoma, angioma, melanoma and neuroma.

Benign new growths

As the vulva is comprised of skin, any swelling that can occur in a skin appendage can be found in the vulval region. Both *fibroma* and *lipoma* are seen in the vulva, and may become pedunculated. They may occur at any age, are soft, oval or rounded, and covered by vulval skin. They may grow slowly to reach the size of a fist. A lipoma is usually broader based than a fibroma. Several other benign swellings are found on the vulva; these are usually solitary and small (about 1 cm or so in diameter), and their nature is arrived at on histology. A *papilloma* is a sessile benign tumour of the skin of the labia in women of middle or old age. A *hidradenoma* is a tumour of sweat gland origin which may be solid or cystic, and which may ulcerate to allow a red papillomatous growth to be extruded. When ulcerated, it may suggest (clinically) the diagnosis of carcinoma, but the problem is solved by biopsy. Less commonly are found *fibromyoma, myxoma, angioma, lymphangioma, benign melanoma* and *neuroma*, with each being distinguished by microscopic examination.

Tumours at the urethral meatus

Urethral caruncles are frequent, especially in older women. A caruncle appears as a small, reddish sessile growth arising from the posterior wall of the urethral meatus, and causing bleeding and painful micturition. It is often very tender, but it may be symptomless. It is usually granulomatous, but may be polypoidal and papillomatous. This condition must be distinguished from prolapse of the urethral mucosa, in which there is a ring of protruding red tissue all round the urethral opening.

Malignant new growths

These include squamous cell carcinoma, rodent ulcer, adenocarcinoma, sarcoma, melanoma and chorioncarcinoma.

In malignant new growth (Fig. V.10) it must be emphasized that cancer within the vulva is a very uncommon condition, and that any tumour occurring in the skin can also occur in the vulval region. The most common type is *squamous cell carcinoma*, which may have been preceded by pruritus but might be completely asymptomatic. This lesion occurs mainly in post-menopausal women, usually as a

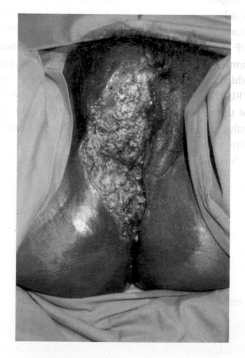

Figure V.10 Vulval carcinoma.

single tumour, although on occasion it may present as 'kissing ulcers'. The most common site is on the labia, where it first extends locally before spreading to the inguinal lymph nodes. Squamous lesions account for 85 per cent of vulval cancers; the remainder comprise tumours of the skin and vulval appendages. Other malignant tumours found in the vulva include:

- Rodent ulcer (basal cell carcinoma), which forms a flat plaque with a characteristic rolled edge
- Malignant melanoma (pigmented and non-pigmented)
- Adenocarcinoma arising in Bartholin's gland or in the urethra
- Sarcoma
- Undifferentiated tumours
- Metastatic tumours from primaries in the cervix, uterine body and ovary, but these occur only rarely
- Choriocarcinoma, which has occasionally been described.

Antony Hollingworth

VULVA, ULCERATION OF

Malignancy of the vulva produces a localized swelling that becomes ulcerated. The various types of malignancy are summarized under VULVA, SWELLINGS OF (p. 786). Vulval dystrophies are chronic conditions that cause intense itching of the vulva, and which may lead to breaching of the epithelium (see PRURITUS VULVAE, p. 557). Pre-malignant lesions of the vulva do not usually cause ulceration of the vulva unless there has been scratching from pruritic symptoms.

Vulval ulceration can therefore be classified thus:

- Infective
  - ◆ Sexually transmitted
  - ◆ Non-sexually transmitted
- Systemic-type disease association
- Vulval dystrophies
- Malignancy

Infective: sexually transmitted

Herpes

Primary infection occurs from 2–7 days after inoculation with herpes simplex virus (HSV). Prodromal symptoms of tingling or itching are followed by vesicular eruptions, which rapidly erode resulting in painful, shallow ulcers all over the vulva (Fig. V.11). These give rise to dysuria and, if secondarily infected, may lead to retention of urine, bilateral inguinal lymphadenopathy, fever and malaise. Herpes virus can be obtained from the vesicular fluid in the early stages, with 85 per cent of cases being due to the HSV type 2. The lesions, which are very painful, persist for 2–6 weeks before healing occurs and antibody appears in the blood. The ulcers tend to recur at intervals of weeks or months, and the virus may be recovered from them. Coitus with a non-immune partner will pass on the infection. The disease is self-limiting in time, and the lesions eventually heal spontaneously. During pregnancy the fetus is at risk if the episode is a primary infection.

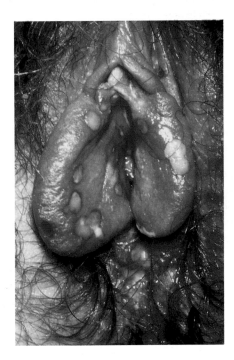

Figure V.11 Vulval herpes.

Syphilis

Primary syphilis gives rise to an indurated ulcer that characteristically is painless unless it becomes secondarily infected. The incubation period is between 10 and 90 days following contact. Genital lesions in women often escape notice because they are hidden inside the vagina or are on the cervix. The lesion must be differentiated from an epithelioma. The serum from a chancre contains the spirochete *Treponema pallidum*, which can be seen microscopically with the aid of dark-ground illumination. If an epithelioma is suspected, the ulcer and swelling should be excised and examined microscopically. The chancre persists for 1–5 weeks, but serological tests for syphilis do not become positive for about 4–6 weeks after appearance of the chancre. The serological tests most commonly performed are the VDRL slide test and the FTA-ABS (fluorescent treponemal antibody absorption) test, which have replaced the Wassermann, Kahn and TPI (treponemal immobilization) tests. To exclude primary syphilis, serological tests must be conducted weekly for 6 weeks after the appearance of the chancre. Between 2 weeks and 6 months after the chancre has healed, the generalized cutaneous eruption of secondary syphilis appears. Numerous moist flat-topped papules occur on the vulva and round the anus. These are known as 'condyloma latum'. In only one-third of untreated cases does tertiary syphilis occur, but not until some years after the primary lesion.

Lymphogranuloma venereum

This is a sexually transmitted disease which is found in the tropical and subtropical regions of Africa, Asia and south-eastern USA. It is due to a subtype of *Chlamydia trachomatis*, and begins with a vesicopustular eruption on the vulva. This soon disappears, but there follows a painful suppuration in the inguinal glands with hypertrophy and ulceration of the groins, vulva and perineum. Later scarring may cause anal stricture or severe dyspareunia. The diagnosis may be made by isolating the organism, by the intradermal injection of virus antigen when a cutaneous reaction develops (Frei test), or by a complement-fixation test.

Granuloma inguinale

This is a chronic venereal infective condition with a tendency to ulceration and massive granulation tissue affecting the vulva and groins. It is almost non-existent in the UK, but is seen in India, Brazil and the West Indies, islands of the South Pacific, Australia, China and Africa. It starts as a raised papilloma, which soon ulcerates, the ulcer having a typical serpiginous outline. The granuloma in the groin rarely suppurates, but much scarring develops. Scrapings from the ulcers reveal the causative organism, the Donovan body, a small bacterium encapsulated in mononuclear leucocytes with a curved rod-like nucleus.

Chancroid

This is a very common cause of genital ulceration in tropical parts of the world, and occurs at 3–5 days after coitus. It begins as a vesicopustule, which becomes a punched-out ulcer with a red base, or as a saucer-shaped, ragged ulcer. The lesion, which is contagious, is extremely tender and produces a heavy, foul discharge. The lesion contains the causative organism, Ducrey's bacillus (*Haemophilus ducreyi*), a Gram-negative rod. The lesion may be solitary, or there may be several ulcers and associated painful inguinal adenitis, which may break down and discharge.

Yaws

This occurs in tropical countries, and produces lesions similar in appearance to the condyloma latum of secondary syphilis.

Infective: non-sexually transmitted

- Aphthous ulcers: these are analogous to the painful small ulcers which can be found in the mouth.
- Tuberculous: this is a rare cause of vulval ulceration, but it may be associated with inguinal lymphadenopathy. They are very indolent and can only be diagnosed with certainty on microscopic section.
- Furunculosis: these are boils caused by staphylococcal infection of the hair follicles. They are common, and affect the labia majora in particular; shaving the area may predispose to this problem.
- Diphtheria: this condition produces ulceration with a characteristic membranous exudate.
- Candidal: mycotic and diabetic vulvitis due to *Candida* can cause soreness and pruritus of the vulva, with redness, excoriation and oedema of the skin and a characteristic white curd-like discharge containing the mycelium of *Candida albicans*.

Systemic disease

- Behçet's syndrome: this is a rare disorder of unknown cause characterized by oral and vulval ulceration. Iridocyclitis, arthritis and nervous system involvement are complications of severe cases.

- Crohn's disease: here, the vulva and perineum may be affected in up to 30 per cent of cases, and may pre-date gastrointestinal symptoms. The lesions resemble knife-cuts in the skin; however, discharging sinuses and irregular ulcers are more common.
- Lipschutz ulcers: these mainly occur on the labia minora, and are of acute onset with an associated fever and lymphadenopathy. The cause is not known, but it may be due to Epstein–Barr virus.

Malignancy

This subject has been discussed previously, but in summary the types of tumours arising in this area are:

- Squamous carcinomas
- Melanomas
- Sarcomas
- Basal cell carcinomas
- Bartholin's glands adenocarcinomas
- Undifferentiated
- Possible secondary tumours

Antony Hollingworth

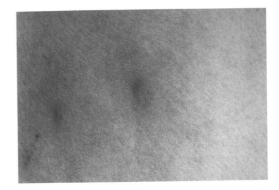

Figure W.1 Urticaria.

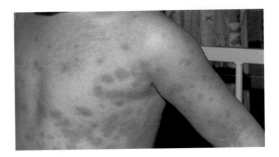

Figure W.2 Giant urticaria.

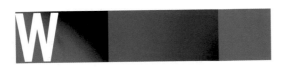

WEALS

A weal is a transient erythematous lesion arising from the release of inflammatory mediators in the skin. It is a component of the Lewis triple response, and may thus arise as a normal physiological response to firming stroking of the skin. In some susceptible individuals, there is an exaggeration of the normal wealing process, producing *symptomatic dermographism*, with wealing occurring from such innocent phenomena as the pressure of clothing on the skin. The investigation of such patients is invariably unrewarding, but antihistamines may provide some symptomatic relief.

Urticaria (Figs W.1 and W.2) is a common condition where weals arise in the skin spontaneously, presenting

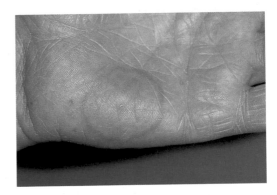

Figure W.3 Angio-oedema.

as randomly scattered evanescent erythematous lesions, sometimes with a rim of pallor at their margins, and sometimes associated with subcutaneous or mucosal swelling (*angio-oedema*) (Fig. W.3) which, if it affects the respiratory passages, may be life-threatening. Individual lesions may last for a matter of minutes or hours (normally not more than 24 hours), vanishing without trace, though new neighbouring weals may continue cropping. Weals can be produced experimentally by intradermal injection of histamine, and are largely blocked by antihistamines. The release of histamine from dermal mast cells is the suggested mechanism in most cases, though other inflammatory mediators may be involved (e.g. acetylcholine, kinins, prostaglandins and platelet activating factor).

Urticaria is very common (probably 10% of the population will experience an attack at some stage), and despite the clamour of sufferers for 'allergy tests' a careful history is the most important part of investigation. In acute urticaria, the onset is abrupt, and the condition may last from a day or two to several weeks. In most cases there is a history of reaction to a food (strawberries, shell-fish, etc.) or a drug. Peanut sensitivity can provoke especially violent episodes, often associated with angio-oedema or bronchospasm, and in susceptible individuals, even a minute quantity may provoke an attack. There is a specific IgE radioallergosorbent test (RAST) test for peanuts.

Chronic urticaria is usually idiopathic, and may have an autoimmune basis. It may continue for years, but prophylactic antihistamines may help. Aspirin may trigger flares, without itself being the primary cause. If angio-oedema is a prominent feature, and there is a family history, the possibility of hereditary C1 esterase inhibitor deficiency should be entertained. The diagnosis may be confirmed by a blood test; it is an important diagnosis, because attacks may be associated with abdominal pain and, if the true cause is known, a laparotomy may be avoided.

In some cases of urticaria, the triggering factor is a physical rather than an allergic one, and this is termed a *physical urticaria* (Fig. W.4). The condition is chronic and of unknown cause, and often relatively resistant to treatment. An important example is *cold-induced urticaria*. Attacks may be triggered off by for example eating an ice-cream; jumping into a cold swimming pool (or the sea) may be especially hazardous. The diagnosis may be confirmed by performing a provocation test with an ice cube. In *delayed pressure urticaria*, the attacks occur several hours after the event, and lesions arise in areas of the skin that have been subject to pressure (e.g. carrying a heavy shopping bag or walking on cobblestones). The episodes may last for some days, and are associated with mild systemic upset. Other recognized triggers of physical urticaria include ultraviolet light, vibration and water; indeed, *aquagenic urticaria* is surprisingly common.

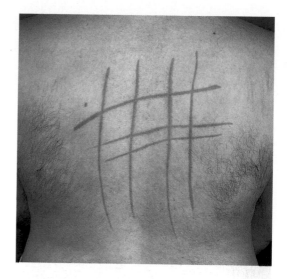

Figure W.4 Dermographism.

Cholinergic urticaria is a distinctive condition where numerous intensely itchy pinhead papules develop some 10 minutes after sweating. Some patients can be induced to exhibit their symptoms by asking them to do mental arithmetic in the outpatient clinic. Susceptible individuals show an exaggerated reaction to the introduction of acetylcholine derivatives into the skin. Severe attacks are followed by a refractory period of 24–48 hours.

A very important form of urticaria, only relatively recently recognized, is that of *contact urticaria* to *latex*. Rubber is produced from the sap of the tree *Hevea braziliensis*, and prolonged exposure to rubber – especially in rubber gloves used by nurses or doctors – results in a type I sensitivity. Itching and swelling start within minutes of contact, and can be associated with severe systemic reactions. A specific IgE RAST test to latex will be positive. Latex-sensitive individuals must also avoid certain fruits (e.g. avocado, strawberry, kiwi fruit, and banana) which contain cross-reactants.

Serum sickness

Type III hypersensitivity causes weals of longer duration. Wealing is a rare feature of several general medical conditions and infections. In thyrotoxicosis and lymphoma, other signs and symptoms can be found, but in the early stages of systemic lupus erythematosus urticaria may be the only clinical abnormality, the weals often persist for an unusually long time

(2–4 days), and they may cause bruising. Viral hepatitis can begin with urticaria, the fever and icterus following 2–3 days later. A particular urticarial eruption appearing dramatically each evening often accompanies adult *Still's disease.*

Weals can be the presenting feature of other dermatoses (e.g. pemphigoid, dermatitis herpetiformis or vasculitis). In a few atopic individuals a contact urticaria occurs soon after the skin is touched by, for example, certain grasses, animal hair or saliva, or foods such as fish or fruits.

Barry Monk

WEIGHT GAIN

The hypothalamus is central to the control of energy homeostasis in the body. This involves the control of hunger (via the lateral hypothalamic nucleus, LHA), which stimulates food intake, and satiety (via the ventromedial hypothalamic nucleus, VMH), which inhibits food intake. Body weight is influenced by the rate of energy expenditure, which is regulated by the secretion of hormones involved in the build-up of energy stores. Short-term signals for food intake affect the size and timing of individual meals. These involve internal sites in the gut and external stimuli such as food cues in the environment and higher brain centres associated with the cognitive and emotional aspects of food intake. Long-term signals are mediated through the fat-derived hormone, leptin, which gives a peripheral signal to the brain of adipose stores; leptin levels decrease in states of starvation. Neuropeptide Y (NPY) is present in the peripheral and central nervous system, and promotes anabolism by stimulating the secretion of insulin (independent of increased food intake) and also stimulates adipose tissue lipoprotein lipase activity. Corticotrophin-releasing hormone has the opposite effect to NPY by having a catabolic effect.

The major causes of weight gain are highlighted in Table W.1.

Although it is usually simple to differentiate the major causes – especially where pregnancy or oedema are apparent – a scientific assessment of fat and muscle mass can be made by using skinfold-thickness measurements or by measuring electrical impedance.

Table W.1 Causes of weight gain

Pregnancy
Excess fluid retention
- Cardiac failure
- Liver failure
- Renal failure
- Nephrotic syndrome
- Periodic oedema
- Hypoproteinaemic states

Lymphatic obstruction
- Milroy's syndrome
- Elephantiasis
- Metastatic carcinoma

Excess muscle
- Precocious puberty
- Androgenic steroids
- Growth hormone
- Athletes, especially weightlifters

Fat excess
- Obesity

Organ enlargement
- Ovarian cyst

Overweight and obesity refer to conditions where body fat is in excess. The term 'overweight' is used when body weight is 110–119 per cent of the upper limit of an acceptable range (which is itself defined as 100%), while the term 'obesity' refers to a body weight of 120 per cent or above. The acceptable range is based on life assurance figures of mortality, drawn up for height and body weight. The degree of obesity is often expressed as the *body mass index* (BMI), which is calculated from the equation:

$$\frac{\text{bodyweight (in kg)}}{\text{height}^2 \text{ (in metres)}}$$

A BMI of 25 to 29.9 is graded as overweight (Garrow Obesity Scale 1), 30–40 as Grade II obesity, and greater than 40 as morbidly obese (Grade III).

Recent surveys have indicated the enormity of the problem in Western society. Both sexes show a rapid increase in weight in their mid-20s. Males tend to become progressively heavier until they reach their 50s, whereas in women, weight remains fairly static until the menopause, when there is a substantial weight gain. By the age of 25 years about 30 per cent of males and females are overweight, whereas at 60 years of age about half have a weight problem considered to be a risk to health. In the 1990 census in the UK, 8 per cent of males and 12 per cent of females had a BMI of 30 or above. Although the risk to health increases with the degree of obesity, the configuration of adipose tissue may be an independent risk factor associated with an increased risk of hyperinsulinaemia, hyperlipidaemia, hypertension, ischaemic heart disease, cardiovascular events and death. A comparison of the circumference of waist and hip indicates that a ratio of over 0.8 in females and 0.95 in males is hazardous to health.

The cause of obesity in everyone is an energy intake in excess of energy expenditure. The scientific arguments arise over whether some individuals with a predisposition for obesity have a lower energy expenditure at the outset. Recent reports suggest a degree of variability in energy expenditure in any obese population, and if this is matched by a similar variability in appetite, this possibly explains in a simple manner the aetiology of obesity. Studies of twins indicate a degree of genetic involvement in the development of obesity, but there is no doubt that the cause is multifactorial, with environmental influences playing a major role. Much emphasis has been made for an aetiological role for brown fat, which is a potent thermogenic tissue in rodents. Certainly, in adults brown fat is present, but is thought to contribute little to daily energy expenditure and could not by itself account for the variations in energy expenditure reported.

Although the vast majority of obese individuals could be said to have 'idiopathic' or 'simple' obesity, it is always worthwhile considering the other rare causes of obesity (Table W.2).

Any *hypothalamic lesion* which destroys the ventromedial nucleus (classical 'satiety' area) may result in obesity. Often other hypothalamic manifestations may be present in such patients. These include panhypopituitarism, diabetes insipidus, and also lethargy and somnolence. If the condition arises in childhood, then the genitalia are usually poorly developed. In Frohlich's original case, a craniopharyngioma was pressing upon the hypothalamus, and hence such obesity associated with a hypogonadal state and poor growth are often referred to as Frohlich's syndrome. Most boys in whom the diagnosis of Frohlich's syndrome is entertained are in fact suffering from 'simple' obesity in which the pre-pubertal genitalia are buried in a pubic pad of fat.

Hypothyroidism leads to weight gain due to both a reduction in the metabolic rate and to the deposition of hydrophilic mucopolysaccharides all over the body, which causes fluid retention. Most cases are due to thyroid gland dysfunction, and in such patients the serum thyroid-stimulating hormone (TSH) level is elevated. Hypothalamic pituitary lesions can result in a similar dysfunction (known as *secondary hypothyroidism*) with a low serum TSH and an absent or delayed TSH response to thyroid-releasing hormone (TRH). Weight loss can be rapid following the introduction of replacement thyroxine therapy in severely hypothyroid patients. Nevertheless, in those whose obesity precedes the development of mild hypothyroidism, weight loss can be slight with thyroid replacement. This is a source of disappointment to many, but indicative of an underlying 'simple' obese problem. In most cases of thyrotoxicosis, weight decreases due to an increase in energy expenditure. In some rare cases of thyrotoxicosis the increase in appetite produces an energy intake in excess of the rise in energy expenditure, hence resulting in an increase in weight.

Pseudohypoparathyroidism is associated with some degree of obesity. These patients are short, with stubby hands and feet due to the shortening of one or more (which can include all five) metacarpals and metatarsals. Ectopic calcification, including basal ganglia calcification, and cataracts have been reported. The cause appears to be due to a peripheral resistance to the metabolic effects of parathyroid hormone, producing serum hypocalcaemia. This is most likely as a consequence of a deficiency in the membrane regulatory or coupling proteins (known as N or G). This membrane protein dysfunction can extend to other hormone receptors, hence explaining the abnormalities in secretion and in the effects of thyrotrophin, prolactin, gonadotrophin, vasopressin, glucagon and insulin sometimes encountered in this syndrome. There is also a variant disorder of similar phenotype, but normal biochemistry, termed *pseudo-pseudohypoparathyroidism*, which can occur independently or in relatives of patients with pseudohypoparathyroidism.

Cushing's syndrome is rare, but can be differentiated from 'simple' obesity by its four cardinal signs, namely: thin skin, conjunctival oedema (chemosis), frontal balding (most notably in women) and proximal myopathy. In a florid case obesity is central, with thin arms and legs due to muscle wasting and a moon plethoric face (see Fig. F.7). Oedema, hypertension,

Table W.2 Causes of obesity

Idiopathic or simple
- Energy intake in excess of energy expenditure; multifactorial causes

Genetic
- Prader–Willi syndrome
- Laurence–Moon–Biedl syndrome
- Alstrom syndrome
- Morel syndrome
- Morgagni syndrome
- Morgagni–Stewart–Morel syndrome
- Carpenter's syndrome
- Cohen's syndrome
- DIDMOAD

Hypothalamic
- Trauma
- Tumours
  - Craniopharygioma
  - Astrocytoma
- Inflammation
  - Meningitis
  - Encephalitis
  - Tuberculosis
  - Syphilis
- Infiltration
  - Sarcoidosis
  - Histiocytosis X

Endocrine
- Hypothalamus
  - Hypogonadotrophic hypogonadism
  - Growth hormone failure
- Pituitary
  - Laron dwarf
  - Hyperprolactinaemia
  - Cushing's disease
  - Nelson's syndrome
  - Hypopituitarism (Fröhlich)

Thyroid
- Cretin
- Primary and secondary hypothyroidism
- Rare cases of thyrotoxicosis

Parathyroid
- Pseudohypoparathyroidism
- Pseudo-pseudohypoparathyroidism

Adrenal
- Cushing's syndrome (ectopic source, adenoma, carcinoma)

Pancreas
- Nesidioblastoma
- Insulinoma
- Beckwith–Wiedemann syndrome

Ovaries
- Polycystic ovarian syndrome
- Post-menopausal

Testes
- Primary hypogonadism

Inactivity
- Mental retardation (e.g. Down's)
- Physical disability (e.g. spina bifida)

Drugs
- Insulin
- Cessation of smoking
- Sulphonylurea agents
- Corticosteroids
- Oestrogen
- Alcohol excess (pseudo-Cushing's)
- Cyproheptadine

Abnormal fat distribution
- Multiple lipomatosis
- Partial lipodystrophy

Painful fat
- Dercum's disease

diabetes mellitus and severe osteoporosis are usually present. The latter often results in spontaneous rib and spine fractures, and in turn a loss of height and kyphosis. The latter condition must also be distinguished from the buffalo hump associated with fat over the upper thoracic spine. Acne, virilism, hirsutism and spontaneous bruising are often present. In children, this disease slows growth – unlike simple obesity, where growth is accelerated in the early years. Striae can be found in Cushing's syndrome, but the absence does not exclude the condition. Striae are not pathognomic of Cushing's syndrome, for they are often found in healthy individuals who have had a rapid weight change.

In mild cases of Cushing's syndrome, the differential diagnosis from simple obesity is not easy. If suspected, then 24-hour urine samples should be measured for free cortisol, as this is elevated in Cushing's syndrome. Some use an overnight 1 mg dexamethasone suppression test, the drug being taken at midnight and a blood cortisol value measured at 9:00 a.m. the next morning; a value of less than 100 nmol/l is considered normal. Although the simple overnight dexamethasone test is helpful, no test is ever totally reliable, and if clinical suspicion persists then further investigations should be carried out on an inpatient basis. Alcohol can mimic Cushing's syndrome both in clinical features and by increasing urine free cortisol output; this situation is termed *pseudo-Cushing's*. Admission to hospital with a total ban on alcohol will eventually result in normal cortisol values.

Patients with *insulinoma* are said to be mildly obese as insulin stimulates appetite. Hyperinsulinaemia due to islet cell hyperplasia can occur in the rare abnormality of *Weidmann–Beckman syndrome*. These children grow more rapidly, have an enlarged tongue, omphalocele and tend to be mildly obese.

In the *polycystic ovarian syndrome* over half the patients are obese. The reason for this is not known, but obesity tends to perpetuate the syndrome because of the conversion in adipose tissue of ovarian androstenedione to oestrone. The other features of the syndrome are oligomenorrhoea or menorrhoea, infertility, hirsutism and enlarged, polycystic ovaries. Biochemically, serum luteinizing hormone (LH) is elevated in comparison to follicle-stimulating hormone (FSH), associated with a raised serum testosterone and androstenedione. Many have wondered whether *hyperprolactinaemia* induces weight gain, for the clinical impression is that many such woman are obese. One survey disputed whether obesity was more prevalent in hyperprolactinaemia, but the impression still remains.

Males with *hypogonadism* of whatever cause tend to be slightly obese. The distribution of fat is of a female distribution over the lower abdomen, hips and thighs. *Growth hormone failure* in children is associated with mild obesity, as is the rare *Laron dwarf* who has decreased levels of IGFs and IGFBP-3 (see STATURE, SHORT, p. 676).

There are various other congenital syndromes associated with obesity. The *Prader–Willi* syndrome is characterized by muscular hypotonia, short stature, small body and feet, mental retardation, hypogonadism and gross obesity. Hyperappetite appears to be the principal cause of their obesity, although a hypothalamic thermic abnormality has been reported. Recently, deletions of chromosome 15 have been implicated as the cause of this condition. In *Laurence–Moon–Biedl* syndrome, obesity is associated with short stature (in some), retarded sexual development, mental retardation, retinitis pigmentosa, and either polydactylism or syndactylism.

In *Alstrom's syndrome* there is obesity, diabetes mellitus, nerve deafness, retinal degeneration and cataracts producing childhood blindness and late-onset nephropathy. Many patients with *Down's syndrome* are obese, as are many children with mental or physical retardation, possibly due to inactivity associated with too high an energy intake.

Morgagni–Stewart–Morel syndrome is a combination of the syndromes described by Morel and Morgagni. In *Morel's syndrome* there is obesity, hyperostosis of the frontal bone and headache. In *Morgagni syndrome*, the obesity is associated with internal frontal hyperostosis and virilism.

Carpenter's syndrome is associated with acrocephaly, polydactyly and syndactyly, mental retardation, male hypogonadism and mild obesity. In *Cohen's syndrome*, obesity is associated with severe mental retardation, microcephaly and short stature and facial abnormalities.

DIDMOAD is an acronym for the major features of the syndrome consisting of diabetes insipidus, diabetes mellitus, optic atrophy and deafness. Most such patients are associated with mild obesity as well as bladder and ureter atonia.

Effects of drug intake on obesity

Some drugs may cause obesity or a worsening of a pre-existing weight problem. Insulin given to diabetics tends to lead to weight gain, as do the sulphonylurea drugs, but usually this is not seen with the biguanide metformin. Weight gain noted when glycaemic control is improved with insulin is partly due to a reduction in both energy expenditure and urine glucose losses. Glucocorticoids in excess rapidly cause weight gain and produce iatrogenic Cushing's syndrome. Oestrogen can also induce weight gain. Although water retention has been implicated, a reduction in energy expenditure in the second half of the menstrual cycle due to a lack of ovulation also plays a role. A frequent finding is of weight gain on cessation of smoking. Recent studies have shown that a smoked cigarette increases sympathetic drive, and on average one cigarette increases energy expenditure by about 9 kcal. Hence, if smoking is ceased then energy intake must be appropriately reduced to prevent weight gain. Nevertheless, many people tend to over-eat on cessation of smoking, which exacerbates the problem.

Body fat distribution

An abnormal distribution of fat occurs in *lipodystrophies*; these comprise a group of disorders ranging from generalized lipo-atrophy to partial forms. *Partial lipoatrophy* (lipodystrophia progressiva) is characterized by a symmetrical loss of subcutaneous fat over dermatome areas of the face and upper body, with a normal or even excessive amount of adipose tissue below the waist. Occasionally, the atrophy is confined below the waist without upper body involvement. This condition, which mainly affects females, is associated with hyperglycaemia, hyperinsulinaemia, marked insulin resistance, hyperlipaemia and hepatosplenomegaly. In *Dercum's* disease, obesity is generalized but there is pain and tenderness in the more prominent fatty deposits, for reasons as yet unknown.

Abnormal body fat distribution may occur in patients with AIDS. Dorso-cervical fat pad enlargement (buffalo hump), benign symmetrical lipomatosis, abdominal girth enlargement and breast hypertrophy (see WEIGHT LOSS, HIV INFECTION, p. 799) have all been documented in patients with AIDS. It remains unclear whether this change in body fat distribution is related to or aggravated by drug therapy (e.g. with the protease inhibitors), as some aspects of the change in body fat distribution have been documented in patients not receiving therapy. The redistribution of body fat occurs in association with peripheral and gluteal wasting, and although this is a very similar clinical picture to that seen in Cushing's syndrome, the cortisol biochemistry is not abnormal.

Sharon O'Byrne

WEIGHT LOSS

Loss of weight may be the result of inadequate food intake, absorption or retention. It may also be due to increased utilization. It is important to distinguish between those patients who lose weight in spite of normal food intake and those whose calorie intake is diminished. In children, the most common causes are malnutrition from injudicious feeding, gastrointestinal disease and infections (see MARASMUS, p. 428). In adults, when loss of weight is considerable, one thinks first of *malignant disease*, infection such as HIV, *tuberculosis*, or endocrine abnormalities such as *hyperthyroidism* and *diabetes mellitus*. Without any evidence of organic disease, other conditions to consider include *depression* or an eating disorder.

Research indicates that in 35 per cent of patients losing weight, no specific cause is usually found. In the remainder, a serious underlying cause is discovered, with 10 per cent having a psychiatric aetiology, the others having a physical disorder, the most common being cancer, gastrointestinal disease, heart failure, alcohol abuse, obstructive airways disease, poorly controlled diabetes mellitus, thyrotoxicosis and HIV. Taking a good history and performing a thorough physical examination will provide direction as to the area for investigation. The single most helpful investigation is a chest radiograph, which often reveals masses, infiltrates (e.g. opportunistic infection), heart failure or lymph node enlargement.

Weight loss with adequate food intake

1　Increased utilization
- Hyperthyroidism
- Chronic infections (e.g. pulmonary tuberculosis)
- Anxiety states, food phobias
- Drugs: L-thyroxine, amphetamine

2　Diminished absorption
- Intestinal hypermotility states
- Chronic pancreatitis
- Carcinoid
- Gluten enteropathy
- Short-circuit operations
- Post-colectomy and post-gastrectomy states
- Chronic hepatic disease
- Dysphagia, e.g. scleroderma
- Whipple's disease
- Lymphatic obstruction
- Drugs: serotonin re-uptake inhibitors (paroxetine, fluoxetine, citalopram); sibutramine and orlistat both used in the treatment of obesity

3　Abnormal calorie loss
- Diabetes mellitus
- Fistulas
- Intestinal parasites

Weight loss with diminished food intake

1 Psychogenic
   - Depression
   - Anorexia nervosa
   - Psychoses

2 Gastrointestinal
   - Gastric ulcer
   - Malignancy
   - Chronic colitis
   - Hepatobiliary disease

3 Malignant conditions
   - Lymphoma
   - Leukaemia
   - Carcinoma: adenocarcinoma/squamous cell carcinoma
   - Sarcoma

4 Uraemia

5 Chronic infections

6 Chronic non-infective inflammatory conditions
   - Rheumatoid arthritis
   - Systemic lupus erythematosus
   - Dermatomyositis
   - Polyarteritis nodosa
   - Giant-cell arthritis
   - Systemic sclerosis

7 Chronic intoxications
   - Alcohol
   - Additive drugs
   - Heavy smoking
   - Lead

8 Endocrine disease
   - Addison's disease and some cases of hypopituitarism (Simmond's disease)
   - Phaeochromocytoma
   - Gut hormone tumours (e.g. vipoma)

9 Food intolerance

10 Chronic cardiac conditions

11 Chronic lung conditions (e.g. obstructive airways disease)

12 HIV infection

Any condition of the gastrointestinal tract that interferes with intake, digestion and absorption of food may produce loss of weight; for example, gastrointestinal neoplasia anywhere from the oral cavity to the anal canal; gastritis or gastric ulcer, inflammatory bowel disease and bowel surgery; and partial or total gastrectomy, small bowel surgery or colectomy.

Chronic infections may produce loss of weight by interfering with general nutrition. This is seen in many who have returned from the tropics after infection by dysentery, yellow fever, malaria, dengue or hepatitis. The chronic infection of a joint, the skin, or the renal tract may produce loss of weight in a similar way.

Liver disorders may affect general nutrition, and loss of weight may occur in some sufferers from cirrhosis; loss of body weight may be masked by the weight gain due to ascites. Malignant change in cirrhotic livers is not uncommon. Hepatocellular carcinoma may develop in patients with haemochromatosis and hepatitis C virus infection. In drug addiction and HIV (see below), weight loss is often considerable.

The effect of *alcohol* upon body weight is variable, with some persons becoming stout, others thin, and others changing little. This depends greatly on food (calorie) intake, but beer-drinkers tend to become obese and pot-bellied. Broadly speaking, it is heavy spirit drinkers who lose weight, and in some cases serious doubts may arise whether the weight loss in such a patient is due to alcoholic habits alone or whether there is underlying neoplasia or tuberculous infection. When alcoholism leads to peripheral neuropathy there is often a rapid and extreme loss of weight. In *chronic debilitating disorders* such as rheumatoid arthritis, multiple sclerosis or hemiplegia, a marked loss of weight may occur, as it may in chronic congestive heart failure, where oedema may mask the wasting.

The loss of weight in *old age*, due to diminished intake of and lessened interest in food, is usually gradual and slow: if otherwise, neoplasia or chronic infection, such as tuberculosis, depression, giant-cell arteritis or some other cause should be suspected.

Diabetes mellitus, especially in the young, may have loss of weight as its earliest symptom.

In *Addison's disease*, the loss of weight may be marked. There may or may not have been attacks of syncope or of diarrhoea. The diagnosis is suggested by brown pigmentation of the skin, particularly in the flexures and groins (Fig. W.5), and also beneath the mucous membranes – particularly of the mouth, inside the lips or within the cheeks – where it is a grey colour. The blood pressure is usually low, and shows a marked postural fall.

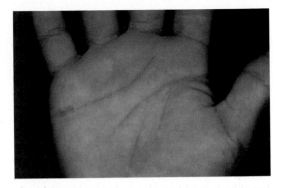

Figure W.5 Crease pigmentation indicated Addison's disease in this patient, who had noted progressive and rapid weight loss associated with diarrhoea and lassitude.

Loss of weight is a prominent feature in cases of *hyperthyroidism*; indeed, it may be the first symptom to attract attention, preceding those of tachycardia, nervousness, excessive perspiration, fine tremor of the outstretched fingers, exophthalmos and symmetrical enlargement of the thyroid gland.

Anorexia nervosa is a condition in which wasting is the prominent symptom, but amenorrhoea often occurs very early in the disease.

HIV infection

Between 11 and 18 per cent of AIDS patients suffer from the wasting syndrome, which is an involuntary loss of ≥10 per cent of their body weight. The wasting that occurs in AIDS results from a combination of abnormalities, including hypermetabolism, infection, malabsorption and anorexia. It remains unclear whether the testosterone deficiency found in patients with AIDS contributes to the weight loss and muscle wasting. The wasting syndrome is associated with progressive HIV infection, and contributes directly to mortality. During the evaluation of weight loss in patients with AIDS, mucosal, gastrointestinal and systemic infection, as well as malignancy and hypogonadism, must be searched for. A rapid loss of weight is usually associated with active secondary infection. The compensatory decrease in resting energy expenditure (REE), that usually occurs during decreased caloric intake, does not take place in AIDS patients, who appear to maintain a high REE in the presence of a decreased caloric intake. A syndrome of lipodystrophy characterized by

subcutaneous fat loss in the face and extremities has been observed in people with HIV treated with antiretroviral drugs, particularly the nucleoside analogue, stavudine.

Sharon O'Byrne

WHEEZE

Wheezes are continuous, musical sounds with a definite pitch, typically loudest during expiration, which may be heard at the mouth or with the aid of a stethoscope. These sounds are generated by vibration of an airway, not only narrowed, but almost closed to allow the walls to touch lightly. Air accelerating through the narrowed airway generates pressure fluctuations, causing the airway walls to oscillate rapidly and produce a musical wheeze. The pitch of the wheeze depends upon the speed of vibration rather than the length or calibre of the airway. Four clinical types of wheeze may be identified.

Expiratory polyphonic wheeze

This is a complex musical sound that is commonly associated with widespread airflow obstruction due to chronic obstructive pulmonary disease or bronchial asthma. The wheeze, together with a background of loud noisy breathing, is audible at the mouth. When listened to on the chest wall, the higher frequencies of the breath sounds are filtered out and the wheezes dominate. Polyphonic wheeze present during tidal breathing is a reliable sign of severe airways obstruction. Normal subjects can generate polyphonic wheezes, but only on forced expiratory effort.

Fixed monophonic wheeze

When a bronchus is narrowed by stenosis of an intrabronchial tumour, a low-pitched monophonic wheeze may be heard, often on inspiration in association with noisy breathing. The low note of the wheeze is related to the tumour mass, which is set in slow oscillation by high-velocity gas flow. The pitch can be varied within a narrow range by altering the velocity of gas flow. Stridor is a special example of this sound.

Random monophonic wheeze

A particular variety of wheeze distinct from the polyphonic expiratory sounds may be heard in widespread airflow obstruction, overlapping throughout inspiration and expiration with varying duration, timing and pitch.

Sequential inspiratory wheeze

In patients with lung restriction due to pulmonary fibrosis, oedema or infiltration, a brief high-pitched wheeze can frequently be heard late in inspiration in association with inspiratory crackles. The musical note may repeat from breath to breath, or disappear and reappear at different times. These sounds occur in deflated areas of lung, and are therefore heard in various forms of pulmonary fibrosis, especially extrinsic allergic alveolitis.

The paradoxical absence of wheezing may be of great clinical importance, indicating severe and widespread airflow obstruction. The production of a wheeze requires an airway on the point of closure and an optimum velocity of gas flow at the site of stenosis to set the bronchial walls in oscillation. In patients with severe ventilatory failure, wheezing may be absent because the velocity of flow is too slow to oscillate the airways on the point of closure. For the same reasons, deteriorating asthmatic patients may become less wheezy and eventually develop a silent chest, indicating an ominous airways obstruction (see also STRIDOR, p. 686).

Boris Lams

WRIST, DEFORMITIES OF

See UPPER LIMB, PAIN IN (p. 751).

WRIST, PAIN IN

See UPPER LIMB, PAIN IN (p. 751).

Index

Page numbers in *italics* refer to figures and tables, those in **bold** indicate main discussion.